Optical Coherence Tomography of Ocular Diseases

Second Edition

Optical Coherence Tomography of Ocular Diseases

Second Edition

Joel S. Schuman, MD

Eye and Ear Foundation Professor and Chairman
UPMC Eye Center, Department of Ophthalmology
Professor of Bioengineering
University of Pittsburgh School of Medicine
Pittsburgh, Pennsylvania

Carmen A. Puliafito, MD

Professor and Chairman
Kathleen and Stanley Glaser Chair
Bascom Palmer Eye Institute
Department of Ophthalmology
University of Miami School of Medicine
Miami, Florida

James G. Fujimoto, PhD

Professor of Electrical Engineering and Computer Science
Research Laboratory of Electronics and Department of Electrical Engineering and Computer Science
Massachusetts Institute of Technology
Cambridge, Massachusetts

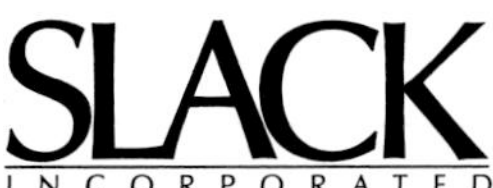

An innovative information, education, and management company
6900 Grove Road • Thorofare, NJ 08086

The procedures and practices described in this book should be implemented in a manner consistent with the professional standards set for the circumstances that apply in each specific situation. Every effort has been made to confirm the accuracy of the information presented and to correctly relate generally accepted practices. The authors, editor, and publisher cannot accept responsibility for errors or exclusions or for the outcome of the application of the material presented herein. There is no expressed or implied warranty of this book or information imparted by it.

The work SLACK Incorporated publishes is peer reviewed. Prior to publication, recognized leaders in the field, educators, and clinicians provide important feedback on the concept and content that we publish. We welcome feedback on this work.

Printed in the United States of America.

Library of Congress Cataloging-in-Publication Data

Optical coherence tomography of ocular diseases / [edited by] Joel S. Schuman, Carmen A. Puliafito, James G. Fujimoto.-- 2nd ed.

p. ; cm.

Includes bibliographical references and index.

ISBN 1-55642-609-7 (alk. paper)

1. Retina--Tomography. 2. Eye--Tomography.

[DNLM: 1. Retinal Diseases--diagnosis. 2. Glaucoma--diagnosis. 3. Tomography, Optical Coherence--methods. WW 270 O21 2004] I. Schuman, Joel S. II. Puliafito, Carmen A., 1951- III. Fujimoto, James G.

RE551.O28 2004

617.7'350757--dc22

2004002675

Published by: SLACK Incorporated
6900 Grove Road
Thorofare, NJ 08086 USA
Telephone: 856-848-1000
Fax: 856-853-5991
www.slackbooks.com

Contact SLACK Incorporated for more information about other books in this field or about the availability of our books from distributors outside the United States.

Last digit is print number: 10 9 8 7 6 5 4 3

Dedication

To our families for their dedication and support, and to our students and trainees—past and present—

for their commitment to advancing scientific knowledge and clinical care

Contents

Dedication . . . . *v*
Contributors . . . . *xi*
Preface . . . . *xiii*

Section I — Principles of Operation and Interpretation

Chapter 1 — **Principles of Optical Coherence Tomography** 3
James G. Fujimoto, PhD; Michael R. Hee, MD, PhD; David Huang, MD, PhD; Joel S. Schuman, MD; Carmen A. Puliafito, MD; and Eric Swanson, MS
Introduction
How Optical Coherence Tomography Works
Optical Coherence Tomography Instrumentation
Summary

Chapter 2 — **Interpretation of the Optical Coherence Tomography Image** 21
Michael R. Hee, MD, PhD; James G. Fujimoto, PhD; Tony Ko, MS; Ji Eun Lee, MD; Joel S. Schuman, MD; Jay Duker, MD; and Carmen A. Puliafito, MD
Introduction
Optical Coherence Tomography Image Generation and Optical Properties of Tissue
Interpreting Optical Coherence Tomography Images of the Normal Retina
Interpreting Optical Coherence Tomography Images of the Normal Anterior Eye
Optical Coherence Tomography Scanning and Imaging Protocols
Quantitative Measurements of Retinal Morphology
Interpreting Optical Coherence Tomography Images of Retinal Pathologies
Quality, Artifacts, and Errors in Optical Coherence Tomography Images
Summary

Section II — Optical Coherence Tomography in Retinal Diseases

Chapter 3 — **Vitreoretinal Interface Disorders** 57
Elias C. Mavrofrides, MD; Adam H. Rogers, MD; Steven Truong, MD; Carmen A. Puliafito, MD; and James G. Fujimoto, PhD
Idiopathic Epiretinal Membrane
Vitreomacular Traction Syndrome
Idiopathic Macular Hole
Full-Thickness Macular Hole
Lamellar Macular Hole

Chapter 4 — **Retinal Vascular Diseases** 103
Vanessa Cruz-Villegas, MD; Carmen A. Puliafito, MD; and James G. Fujimoto, PhD
Branch Retinal Artery Occlusion
Central Retinal Artery Occlusion
Branch Retinal Vein Occlusion
Central Retinal Vein Occlusion
Bilateral Idiopathic Juxtafoveal Retinal Telangiectasis
Retinal Arterial Macroaneurysm

Chapter 5 — **Diabetic Retinopathy** 157
Vanessa Cruz-Villegas, MD and Harry W. Flynn Jr, MD
Nonproliferative Diabetic Retinopathy
Diabetic Macular Edema
Proliferative Diabetic Retinopathy

Chapter 6 **Central Serous Chorioretinopathy** 215
Elias C. Mavrofrides, MD; Carmen A. Puliafito, MD; and James G. Fujimoto, PhD
Typical Central Serous Chorioretinopathy
Chronic Central Serous Chorioretinopathy
Bullous Central Serous Chorioretinopathy
Laser Treatment for Central Serous Chorioretinopathy
Photodynamic Therapy Treatment for Central Serous Chorioretinopathy

Chapter 7 **Age-Related Macular Degeneration** 243
Elias C. Mavrofrides, MD; Natalia Villate, MD; Philip J. Rosenfeld, MD; and Carmen A. Puliafito, MD
Drusen
Vitelliform Macular Degeneration
Geographic Atrophy
Choroidal Neovascularization
Retinal Angiomatous Proliferation
Retinal Pigment Epithelial Tear
Subretinal Hemorrhage
Disciform Scarring

Chapter 8 **Miscellaneous Macular Degenerations** 345
Elias C. Mavrofrides, MD and Carmen A. Puliafito, MD
Pathologic Myopia
Angioid Streaks
Idiopathic Choroidal Neovascularization
Central Serous Chorioretinopathy With Choroidal Neovascularization
Juxtafoveal Telangiectasis With Choroidal Neovascularization
Presumed Ocular Histoplasmosis

Chapter 9 **Chorioretinal Inflammatory Diseases** 371
Natalia Villate, MD; Elias C. Mavrofrides, MD; and Janet Davis, MD
Intermediate Uveitis
Idiopathic Retina Vasculitis and Neuroretinitis
Multifocal Choroiditis
Sarcoidosis
Vogt-Koyanagi-Harada Disease
Sympathetic Ophthalmia
Birdshot Chorioretinopathy
Toxoplasmosis
Syphilitic Uveitis
Cytomegalovirus Retinitis With Immune Recovery Uveitis

Chapter 10 **Retinal Dystrophies** 413
Vanessa Cruz-Villegas, MD; Philip J. Rosenfeld, MD; and Carmen A. Puliafito, MD
Retinitis Pigmentosa
Cone-Rod Dystrophy
Stargardt's Disease
Best's Disease
Pattern Dystrophy
X-Linked Juvenile Retinoschisis

Chapter 11 **Miscellaneous Retinal Diseases** 457
Elias C. Mavrofrides, MD; Vanessa Cruz-Villegas, MD; and Carmen A. Puliafito, MD
Pseudophakic Cystoid Macular Edema
Cystoid Macular Edema Associated With Glaucoma Therapy
Rhegmatogenous Retinal Detachment
Posterior Segment Trauma
Congenital Pit of the Optic Disc
Myelinated Nerve Fiber Layer
Cancer-Associated Retinopathy

Section III Optical Coherence Tomography in Glaucoma, Neuro-Ophthalmology, and the Anterior Segment

Chapter 12 **Optical Coherence Tomography in Glaucoma** 483
Gadi Wollstein, MD; Siobahn Beaton; Adelina Paunescu, PhD; Hiroshi Ishikawa, MD; James G. Fujimoto, PhD; and Joel S. Schuman, MD
Normal Eyes
Structure-Function Correspondence
The Utility of Imaging in Early Glaucoma
Glaucoma is Global
Imaging Supports Early, Questionable Visual Field Findings
Imaging Discloses Functional Artifact
Imaging Suggests Actual Glaucoma Damage Exceeds Visual Fields
Beware Artifact
Nerve Fiber Layer is Superior to Optic Nerve Head and Macula in Sensitivity to Glaucomatous Damage
Abnormal Structure With Normal Function May Suggest Future Functional Loss
Longitudinal Analysis

Chapter 13 **Optical Coherence Tomography in Neuro-Ophthalmology** 611
Thomas R. Hedges III, MD
Optic Atrophy
Optic Disc Swelling
Anomalies

Chapter 14 **Corneal and Anterior Segment Optical Coherence Tomography** 663
David Huang, MD, PhD; Yan Li, MS; Sunita Radhakrishnan, MD; and Maria Regina Chalita, MD, PhD

Section IV Appendices

Appendix A **Physical Principles of Optical Coherence Tomography** 677
James G. Fujimoto, PhD; David Huang, MD, PhD; Michael R. Hee, MD, PhD; Tony Ko, MS; Eric Swanson, MS; Carmen A. Puliafito, MD; and Joel S. Schuman, MD
Introduction
Optical Interferometry
Low-Coherence Interferometry Measurement of Light Echoes
Sensitivity
Spatial Resolution
Pixel Density and Image Acquisition Time
Advances in Optical Coherence Tomography Technology
Summary

Appendix B **Optical Coherence Tomography Scanning and Image-Processing Protocols 691**
Ji Eun Lee, MD; Joel S. Schuman, MD; James G. Fujimoto, PhD; and Carmen A. Puliafito, MD
Line Scan Protocols
Circle Scan Protocols
Time-Efficient or Fast Scans
Image-Processing Protocols
Retinal Thickness and Retinal Thickness Map
Nerve Fiber Layer
Optic Disc

***Index*. 701**

Contributors

Siobahn Beaton
UPMC Eye Center
University of Pittsburgh School of Medicine
Pittsburgh, Pennsylvania

Maria Regina Chalita, MD, PhD
Medical Director
Vision Institute-Ipepo Department of Ophthalmology
Federal University of Sao Paulo
Sao Paulo, Brazil

Vanessa Cruz-Villegas, MD
Formerly Instructor in Ophthalmology
Bascom Palmer Eye Institute
University of Miami School of Medicine
Miami, Florida

Janet Davis, MD
Professor of Ophthalmology
Bascom Palmer Eye Institute
University of Miami School of Medicine
Miami, Florida

Jay S. Duker, MD
Professor and Chair
New England Eye Center
Tufts-New England Medical Center
Tufts University School of Medicine
Boston, Massachusetts

Harry W. Flynn Jr, MD
Professor of Ophthalmology
J. Donald M. Gass, MD Distinguished Chair
Bascom Palmer Eye Institute
University of Miami School of Medicine
Miami, Florida

James G. Fujimoto, PhD
Professor of Electrical Engineering and Computer Science
Research Laboratory of Electronics and Department of Electrical Engineering and Computer Science
Massachusetts Institute of Technology
Cambridge, Massachusetts

Thomas R. Hedges III, MD
New England Eye Center
Professor of Ophthalmology and Neurology
Tufts University School of Medicine
Boston, Massachusetts

Michael R. Hee, MD, PhD
Pacific Eye Specialists at Seton Medical Center
Daly City, California
Clinical Faculty, Department of Ophthalmology
University of California, San Francisco
San Francisco, California

David Huang, MD, PhD
Associate Staff
Cole Eye Institute
Cleveland Clinic Foundation
Cleveland, Ohio
Assistant Professor of Biomedical Engineering
Case Western Reserve University
Cleveland, Ohio

Hiroshi Ishikawa, MD
Assistant Professor
UPMC Eye Center
Department of Ophthalmology
University of Pittsburgh School of Medicine
Pittsburgh, Pennsylvania

Tony Ko, MS
Research Laboratory of Electronics and Department of Electrical Engineering and Computer Science
Massachusetts Institute of Technology
Cambridge, Massachusetts

Ji Eun Lee, MD
Bascom Palmer Eye Institute
Miami, Florida
Pusan National University
Busan, Korea

Yan Li, MS
Case Western Reserve University
Cleveland Clinic Foundation
Cleveland, Ohio

Elias C. Mavrofrides, MD
Lecturer on Ophthalmology
Bascom Palmer Eye Institute
University of Miami School of Medicine
Miami, Florida

Adelina Paunescu, PhD
Postdoctoral Fellow
New England Eye Center
Department of Ophthalmology
Tufts University School of Medicine
Boston, Massachusetts

Carmen A. Puliafito, MD
Professor and Chairman
Kathleen and Stanley Glaser Chair
Bascom Palmer Eye Institute
Department of Ophthalmology
University of Miami School of Medicine
Miami, Florida

Sunita Radhakrishnan, MD
Cleveland Clinic Foundation
Cleveland, Ohio

Adam H. Rogers, MD
Assistant Professor of Ophthalmology
New England Eye Center
Tufts University School of Medicine
Boston, Massachusetts

Philip J. Rosenfeld, MD
Associate Professor of Ophthalmology
Bascom Palmer Eye Institute
University of Miami School of Medicine
Miami, Florida

Joel S. Schuman, MD
Eye and Ear Foundation Professor and Chairman
UPMC Eye Center, Department of Ophthalmology
Professor of Bioengineering
University of Pittsburgh School of Medicine
Pittsburgh, Pennsylvania

Eric Swanson, MS
Entrepreneur and Consultant
Carlisle, Massachusetts

Steven Truong, MD
Clinical Fellow in Ophthalmology
New England Eye Center
Tufts University School of Medicine
Boston, Massachusetts

Natalia Villate, MD
Formerly Clinical Fellow in Ophthalmology
Bascom Palmer Eye Institute
University of Miami School of Medicine
Miami, Florida

Gadi Wollstein, MD
Assistant Professor
UPMC Eye Center
Department of Ophthalmology
University of Pittsburgh Medical Center Eye Center
Pittsburgh, Pennsylvania

Preface

The history of ophthalmology as a medical specialty began with a collaboration between a physicist and an ophthalmic surgeon when Herrmann von Helmholtz invented the ophthalmoscope in 1851 and Albrecht von Graefe used it to revolutionize ophthalmic diagnosis and therapy. And so it was with optical coherence tomography (OCT), which was born of a collaboration between physical scientists and ophthalmologists (James Fujimoto, David Huang, Charles Lin, Carmen Puliafito, Joel Schuman, and Eric Swanson).

Since the invention of OCT by our groups in the early 1990s and its first scientific description by Huang et al in *Science* (1991;254(5035):1178-1181), this technology has emerged to become a widely used tool that has already revolutionized the diagnosis and therapy of eye disease. OCT also marks the beginning of a new field that might be called structural imaging of the eye. We believe that these and other technologic developments in ophthalmic structural imaging will produce widespread changes in the way the eye is examined and eye disease is treated.

Several individuals played a special role in the development of OCT. David Huang, MD, PhD, a student in the Harvard-Massachusetts Institute of Technology (MIT) MD PhD program, conceived the idea of cross-sectional imaging while working on his PhD in Dr. Fujimoto's laboratory at MIT. Eric Swanson, MS ,working at Lincoln Laboratory of MIT, built the first OCT system. Mr. Swanson was also a cofounder, along with Drs. Puliafito and Fujimoto, of the startup company Advanced Ophthalmic Diagnostics, which was acquired by Humphrey Instruments/Carl Zeiss Meditec and transferred OCT ophthalmic imaging technology to industry. Michael Hee, MD, PhD wrote all the original OCT imaging processing algorithms and analysis protocols, which are now in standard clinical use, as well as coauthored the first edition of this book. Charles P. Lin, PhD and Joseph A. Izatt, PhD also played important roles in the initial laboratory and clinical investigations. Tony Ko, a student in the Medical Engineering and Medical Physics Program at MIT, made critical contributions to advanced OCT development.

OCT was first implemented as a practical clinical tool at the New England Eye Center of the Tufts University School of Medicine in Boston, where both Drs. Puliafito and Dr. Schuman were founding faculty members. Our valued clinical collaborators at the New England Eye Center have included Jay S. Duker, MD, Cynthia Mattox, MD, Elias Reichel, MD, and Caroline Baumal, MD. Christine Kiernan, Director of Photography at the New England Eye Center from its inception, and her photography staff played a vital role.

Dr. Schuman's group established the value of OCT as a valuable tool in eyes with glaucoma. Tamar Pedut-Kloizman, MD, Helena Pakter, MD, Viviane Guedes, MD, and Gadi Wollstein, MD participated in OCT's development as research fellows. Hiroshi Ishikawa, MD, in Dr. Schuman's laboratory, has advanced the analysis algorithms of this device.

The authors are grateful to the retina faculty at the Bascom Palmer Eye Institute for their support in this undertaking. We recognize the invaluable help of Ms. Ditte Hesse, Director of Photography at the Bascom Palmer Eye Institute, and Carl Denis, head OCT technician.

The transition of OCT into a clinical technology would not have been possible without the commitment of industry. The team at Carl Zeiss Meditec played a critical role in engineering the technology and making it available to the general clinical community.

We believe that OCT opens a new window to the eye that promises not only to enable earlier and more sensitive diagnosis of disease, but also to contribute to a better understanding of the mechanisms of disease itself. We hope that this book will prove valuable to both clinicians and researchers who wish to learn more about optical coherence tomography.

Joel S. Schuman, MD
Carmen A. Puliafito, MD
James G. Fujimoto, PhD

Section I

Principles of Operation and Interpretation

Chapter 1

Principles of Optical Coherence Tomography

James G. Fujimoto, PhD; Michael R. Hee, MD, PhD; David Huang, MD, PhD; Joel S. Schuman, MD; Carmen A. Puliafito, MD; and Eric Swanson, MS

- Introduction
- How Optical Coherence Tomography Works
- Optical Coherence Tomography Instrumentation
- Summary

Introduction

Optical coherence tomography (OCT) is a fundamentally new type of medical diagnostic imaging modality. OCT performs high-resolution, micron-scale, cross-sectional, or tomographic imaging of the internal microstructure in biological tissues by measuring the echo time delay and intensity of backscattered or backreflected light.[1-5] OCT is a powerful imaging technology because it enables real-time in situ imaging of tissue structure or pathology with resolutions of 1 to 15 microns (μm), which is one to two orders of magnitude higher than conventional clinical imaging technologies such as ultrasound, magnetic resonance (MR), or computer tomography (CT). Since its development in 1991, OCT has been investigated in a wide range of clinical applications.[4-6]

Figure 1-1 shows the first demonstration of OCT imaging as reported by Huang et al.[1] The first OCT images were demonstrated in the human retina and coronary artery in vitro. Figure 1-1 shows an OCT image of the human retina in the region of the optic disc and corresponding histology. The OCT image shown has an axial image resolution of 15 μm, which is almost one order of magnitude finer than ultrasound. Imaging was performed with infrared light at ~800 nanometer (nm) wavelength. The image is displayed using a false color map that corresponds to detected backscattered light levels ranging between 4×10^{-10} to 10^{-6} of the incident light. The OCT image clearly shows the contour of the optic disc, as well as retinal vasculature near the disc region. The retinal nerve fiber layer can also be visualized. This image was performed in vitro, so postmortem retinal detachment with subretinal fluid accumulation is evident.

Figure 1-2 shows one of the first examples of in vivo imaging of the normal human retina as reported by Hee et al.[3] The axial image resolution was 10 μm in tissue, and imaging was performed at ~800 nm wavelength. A prototype OCT instrument was developed based upon a modified slit-lamp biomicroscope, which enabled a simultaneous view of the fundus and the OCT imaging beam as it scanned across the retina. This early device and measurement protocol formed the basis for current OCT ophthalmic imaging instrumentation. The OCT image shows the normal contour of the foveal pit and the optic nerve head. The retinal nerve fiber layer is evident as a highly backscattering layer that decreases in thickness away from the optic disc. The retinal pigment epithelium and choroid are evident as a thin, highly backscattering layer posterior to the retina. These early results demonstrated that OCT can image retinal structure and pathology with unprecedented resolution.[3,7]

Figure 1-3 shows the first demonstration of OCT imaging of the anterior eye as reported by Izatt et al.[2] The axial image resolution was 10 μm in tissue and was performed at ~800 nm wavelength. The image spanned a transverse dimension of 21 mm, thus allowing cross-sectional imaging of the entire anterior chamber. The OCT image clearly shows the corneal thickness and the depth of the anterior chamber. The curvature of the anterior and posterior surfaces of the cornea can be measured. The sclera and iris are visible as highly optically scattering structures that produce shadowing of posterior features.

To date, OCT has had its largest clinical impact in ophthalmology for retinal imaging. However, OCT can be applied to image pathology in a wide range of tissues other than the eye.[4-6] Figure 1-4 shows an example of an OCT image of arterial plaque and corresponding histology reproduced from Brezinski et al.[8] This figure shows an example

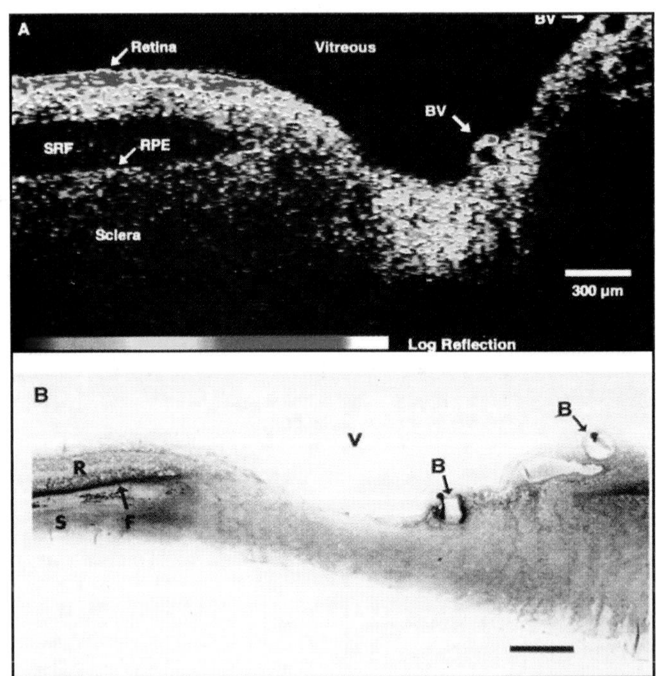

Figure 1-1. The first demonstration of OCT imaging. OCT imaging is analogous to ultrasound B-mode imaging, except light is used instead of sound. A cross-sectional image is generated by scanning a light beam across the tissue and measuring the echo time delay and intensity of backscattered or backreflected light. This figure depicts an OCT image of the human retina in vitro and the corresponding histology. The axial image resolution was 10 µm, and imaging was performed using infrared light at ~800 nm wavelength. The scale bar is 300 µm. (Reproduced from Huang D, Swanson EA, Lin CP, et al. Optical coherence tomography. *Science.* 1991;254(5035):1178-1181.)

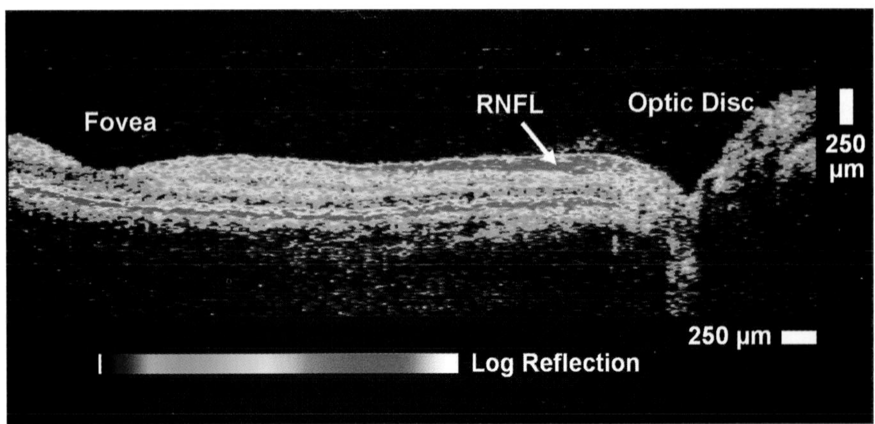

Figure 1-2. Early OCT image of the human retina in vivo. The axial image resolution is 10 µm, and imaging was performed with light at ~800 nm wavelength. The image is displayed using a logarithmic false-color scale, which maps the log of the backscattered or backreflected light intensity to a rainbow color scale. As in other medical imaging modalities, the use of false color does not necessarily correspond to microstructural features, but it can aid in differentiating different structures in an image. The maximum signal is approximately -50 dB of the incident signal, while the minimum detectable signal is approximately -95 dB. The image shows the normal retinal contour in the fovea and the optic disc region. The retinal nerve fiber layer is evident as a highly backscattering layer that emanates from the optic disc and decreases in thickness as it approaches the fovea. (Reproduced from Hee MR, Izatt JA, Swanson EA, et al. Optical coherence tomography of the human retina. *Arch Ophthalmol.* 1995;113(3): 325-332.)

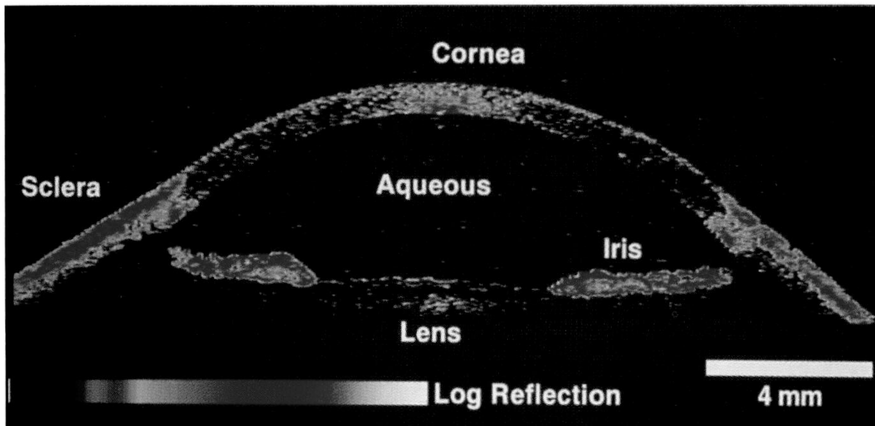

Figure 1-3. OCT image of the anterior chamber in vivo. This image is the first demonstration of anterior eye imaging. The axial image resolution is 10 μm, and imaging was performed with light at ~800 nm wavelength. The image shows the curvature of the anterior and posterior surfaces of the cornea, as well as the depth of the anterior chamber. The iris is visible, but it scatters light strongly, so deeper structures are shadowed. (Reproduced from Izatt JA, Hee MR, Swanson EA, et al. Micrometer-scale resolution imaging of the anterior eye in vivo with optical coherence tomography. *Arch Ophthalmol.* 1994;112(12):1584-1589. Copyright © 1994, American Medical Association. All rights reserved.)

of unstable plaque, characterized by a thin intimal cap layer adjacent to calcified plaque with low lipid content. Although these tissues are optically scattering, OCT image penetration depths of 2 to 3 mm may be achieved by using longer wavelength infrared light at ~1300 nm. The axial image resolution was ~15 μm in tissue.

OCT is a powerful medical imaging technology because it enables real-time in situ visualization of tissue microstructure without the need to excise and process a specimen as in conventional biopsy and histopathology. The nonexcisional "optical biopsy" performed by OCT and the ability to visualize tissue morphology in real-time under operator guidance can be used both for diagnostic imaging as well as to guide intervention.[4-6] OCT promises to have applications in three general types of clinical situations:

1. Where conventional excisional biopsy is hazardous or impossible, such as imaging the eye, coronary arteries, or nervous tissues
2. Where excisional biopsy suffers from sampling errors. Biopsy followed by histopathology is the standard for cancer diagnosis; however, if the biopsy misses the lesion, then a false-negative result is obtained. OCT might be used to guide biopsy in order to reduce sampling error. In selected applications in which sufficient sensitivity and specificity can be achieved, it may ultimately provide direct, real-time diagnostic information
3. To guide interventional procedures. The ability to see beneath the surface of tissue enables the assessment and guidance of microsurgical procedures, such as vessel and nerve anastomosis, or the guidance of stent placement and atherectomy in interventional cardiology

Coupled with catheter, endoscopic, or laparoscopic delivery, OCT promises to have a powerful impact on many medical applications, from improving the screening and diagnosis of neoplasia, to enabling new microsurgical and minimally invasive surgical procedures.

OCT is especially powerful in ophthalmology because it provides real-time, noncontact cross-sectional imaging of the retina or the anterior eye with unprecedented resolution. Since OCT generates a cross-sectional image of retinal morphology, it can provide vital diagnostic information that is complementary to conventional fundus photography and fluorescein angiography. OCT enables visualization of structural features of the retina, including the fovea and optic disc, as well as the internal architectural morphology of the retina, such as the nerve fiber layer, ganglion cell layer, or photoreceptors.[3] OCT imaging of the anterior eye enables visualization of the cornea, iris, lens, and angle.[2] OCT was demonstrated for the detection and monitoring of a variety of macular diseases, including macular edema, macular holes, central serous chorioretinopathy, age-related macular degeneration and choroidal neovascularization, and epiretinal membranes.[7,9-15] OCT imaging can also be used to perform quantitative measurements or morphometry of the retina. OCT is especially powerful for the diagnosis and monitoring of diseases such as glaucoma or macular edema associated with diabetic retinopathy because it can provide quantitative information, which is a measure of disease progression. Images can be analyzed quantitatively and processed using image processing algorithms to automatically extract features such as retinal thickness or retinal nerve fiber layer thickness.[16-18] The retinal nerve fiber layer thickness, a diagnostic indicator for early glaucoma and disease progression, can be quantified and correlated with measurements of optic nerve head structure or visual function.[19-23] Mapping and display techniques have been developed to represent OCT image data in alternate forms, such as topographic thickness maps, in order to better facilitate interpretation and comparison to fundus images.[15] Finally, since structural image information can be assessed quantitatively, OCT imaging can be used as a diagnostic tool to predict the probability of disease and to monitor the effectiveness of treatment.

This chapter presents an overview of the principles of operation of OCT imaging. This will provide the interested reader with a foundation on how OCT functions and how OCT imaging compares to other diagnostic imaging technologies such as ultrasound. In addition, we will briefly describe OCT technology and OCT instruments. A more detailed description of the physical principles of OCT is included in Appendix A. This information is useful for the researcher who wishes to understand the factors that govern OCT imaging resolution and performance. A detailed discussion of OCT imaging of the retina and baselines for interpreting OCT images of the normal retina and retinal pathology are presented in Chapter 2.

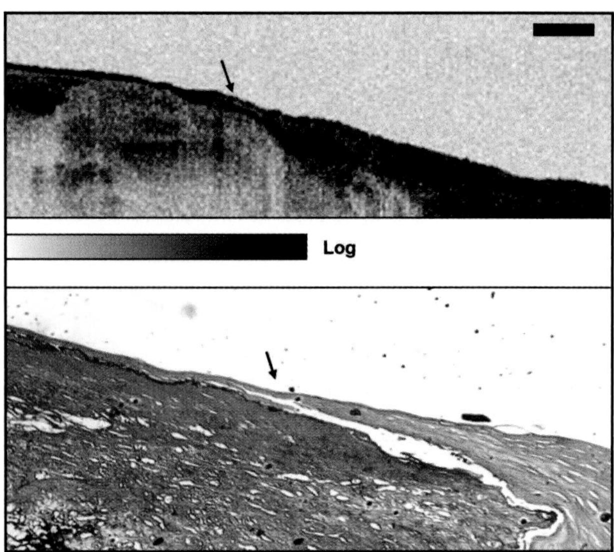

Figure 1-4. OCT image of arterial plaque in vitro and the corresponding histology. OCT imaging can be used in a wide range of applications other than ophthalmology. This example shows an OCT image of calcified plaque with a thin intimal cap layer and corresponding histology. The axial image resolution is 15 μm, and imaging was performed with light at 1300 nm wavelength. The high resolution of OCT, when compared to ultrasound, enables important architectural features to be visualized. This image exhibits strong attenuation of the signal with depth as well as speckle noise, features that are common in many scattering tissues. For this reason, OCT images in scattering tissues are usually displayed using a gray scale rather than a false-color scale. The scale bar is 500 μm. (Reproduced from Brezinski ME, Tearney GJ, Bouma BE, et al. Optical coherence tomography for optical biopsy. Properties and demonstration of vascular pathology. *Circulation.* 1996;93(6):1206-1213.)

How Optical Coherence Tomography Works

Optical Versus Ultrasound Imaging

OCT imaging is analogous to ultrasound B-mode imaging, except that it uses light instead of sound. There are several different embodiments of OCT, but essentially OCT performs cross-sectional imaging by measuring the echo time delay and intensity of backscattered or backreflected light from microstructure inside tissues. OCT images are two-dimensional or three-dimensional data sets representing variations in optical backscattering or backreflection in a cross-sectional plane or volume of tissue.

Because of the analogy between OCT and ultrasound, it is helpful to begin by considering the factors that govern OCT imaging as compared to ultrasound imaging. Ultrasound is widely used clinically for quantitative measurements of intraocular distances as well as for imaging the anterior eye and globe.[24-28] Since ultrasound imaging depends on the reflection of sound waves from intraocular structures, it requires direct contact of the ultrasound probe to the cornea, or immersion of the eye in a liquid that enables the transmission of sound waves into the globe. The resolution of ultrasound measurement depends on the frequency or wavelength of the sound waves that are used. For typical ultrasound systems, sound wave frequencies are in the 10-megahertz (10 mHz) regime, which yield spatial resolutions of approximately 150 μm. Ultrasound imaging also has the advantage that sound waves are readily transmitted into most biological tissues; therefore, it is possible to obtain images of structures deep within the body. High-resolution ultrasound imaging systems have been developed that use higher frequency sound waves and that have resolutions on the 20-μm scale.[26,27]

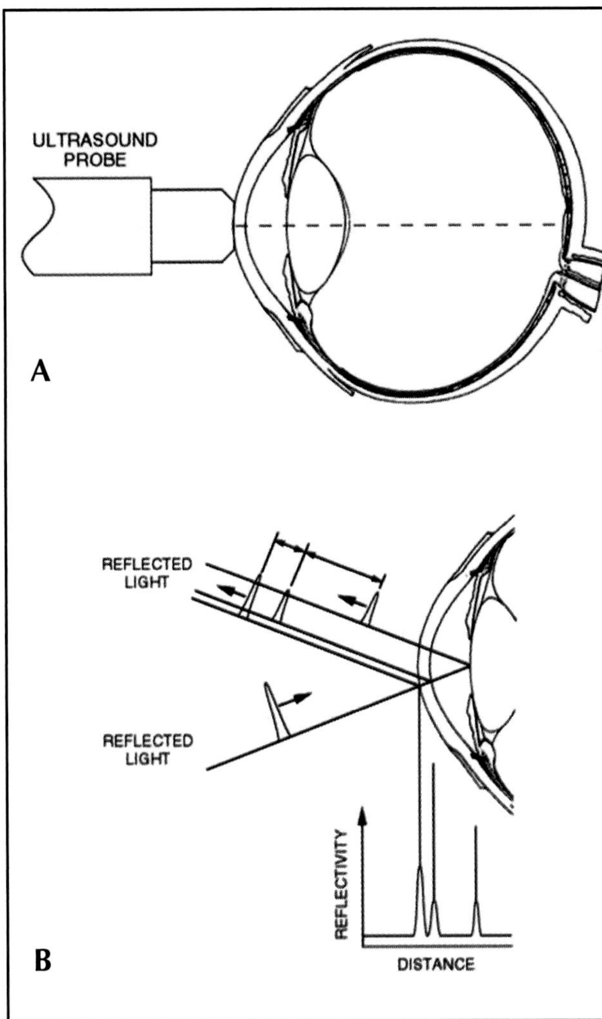

Figure 1-5. Reflection of light and sound from the eye. (A) Ultrasonic axial measurement (A-mode) and imaging (B-mode) function by measuring the time delay for sound to be reflected from different intraocular structures. Ultrasound measurement requires direct contact with the eye in order to transmit and receive the sound waves. (B) Optical axial ranging and imaging works by measuring the time delay when light is reflected from different structures. Optical techniques have higher spatial resolution than ultrasound and do not require direct contact with the eye.

However, high-frequency ultrasound is strongly attenuated in biological tissues. High-frequency ultrasound imaging can be performed to depths of only 4 to 5 mm, thus limiting its application to the anterior eye.

In contrast, OCT is an optical measurement and imaging technique that uses light rather than sound waves. The principal disadvantage of optical techniques is that light is highly scattered or absorbed in most biological tissues; therefore, optical imaging is constrained to tissues that are optically accessible either directly or by devices such as endoscopes or catheters. OCT is ideally suited for ophthalmology because of the ease of optical access to the eye. In addition, OCT can be performed without physical contact to the eye, thereby minimizing patient discomfort during examination. Imaging using light rather than sound provides a significantly higher spatial resolution than what is possible with ultrasound. Standard-resolution ophthalmic OCT images have axial resolutions of ~10 µm, which is approximately 10 to 20 times finer than standard ultrasound B-mode imaging.[3] Research OCT systems for ultrahigh-resolution ophthalmic imaging can achieve even finer resolutions of ~3 µm.[29] The inherently high resolution of OCT imaging permits visualization of the morphology of individual retinal layers, thus facilitating the diagnosis of a wide range of retinal pathologies.

In order to perform cross-sectional or tomographic optical imaging in biological systems, it is first necessary to measure the internal structure of biological tissues. In OCT, the first step in obtaining a tomographic image is the measurement of axial distance or range information within the tissue, which is similar to ultrasound A-mode scanning. Figure 1-5 shows a schematic that contrasts the use of sound waves versus light waves for the measurement of distances in the eye. In ultrasound, a high-frequency, pulsed sound wave is launched into the eye from an ultrasonic probe. The sound wave travels into the eye and is reflected from boundaries or different microstructural features in the eye. These sound wave echoes are reflected back to the ultrasonic probe and their time delay and intensity are measured. Distances in the eye are determined from the echo time delay of the sound pulse. The principle of operation is similar to radar detection of aircraft, where distance or range is determined by measuring the echo delay of a radio wave pulse. In OCT, measurements of distance and microstructure are performed by directing light into the eye and measuring the echo time delay and intensity of backreflection or backscattering from different structures in the eye. For the purpose of illustration, it is possible to understand OCT imaging by thinking of the light beam as being composed of short pulses of light. However, it is important to note that OCT systems operate using a continuous beam of low-coherence light rather than short pulses of light. The operation of OCT is based on an optical measurement technique known as *low-coherence interferometry*. A detailed description of the physical principles of low-coherence interferometry is presented in Appendix A.

When a beam of light is directed onto the eye, it is backreflected from boundaries between different tissues and backscattered differently from tissues that have different optical properties. The distances and dimensions of different tissue structures can be determined by measuring the echo time delay of light that is backreflected or

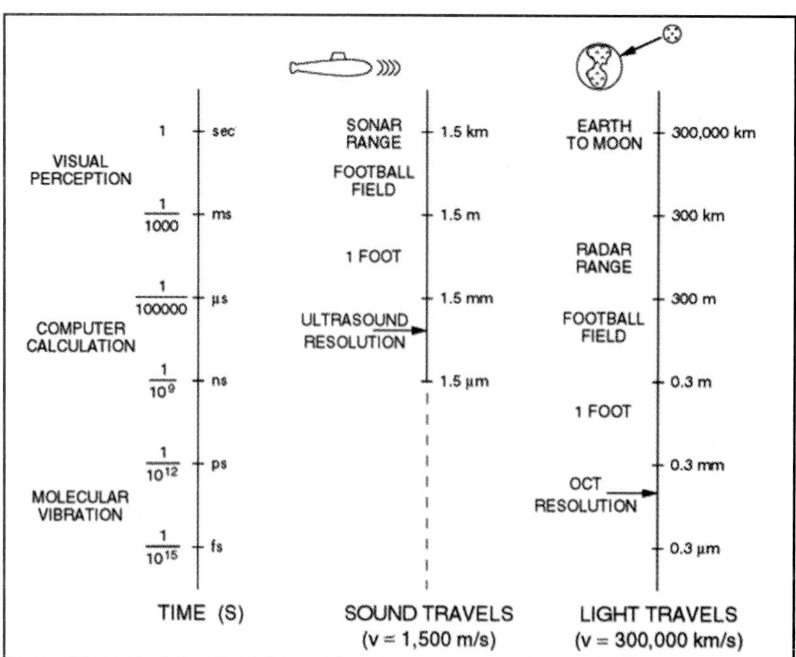

Figure 1-6. Distance and time scales for light and sound. The velocity of sound is approximately 1500 meters/s, while the velocity of light is 3 x 10^8 m/s. Standard ultrasound has a resolution limit of 150 µm, which corresponds to a time measurement of 100 nanoseconds (100 x 10^{-9} s). In contrast, standard OCT imaging has a resolution of 10 µm, corresponding to a time measurement of 30 femtoseconds (30 x 10^{-15} s). In order to measure echoes of light from small structures, extremely fine time resolution is required. The above scales are logarithmic; each vertical division represents a factor of 1000. Notice that light from the moon takes approximately 1.3 s to reach the earth.

backscattered from the different structures at varying axial (longitudinal) distances.[30,31] The principal difference between ultrasound and optical imaging is that the velocity of light is almost a million times faster than the velocity of sound. Since distances within the biological tissue are measured using the echo time delay of reflected sound waves or light waves, distance measurement involving light requires faster time resolution compared to distance measurements using sound.

Figure 1-6 describes distance and time scales for light and sound. The velocity of sound in water is approximately 1500 meters per second, while the velocity of light is approximately 3 x 10^8 meters per second. Distance or range information may be determined from the time delay of echoes according to the formula $\Delta T = \Delta z/v$, where ΔT is the echo delay, Δz is the distance that the echo travels, and v is the velocity of the sound wave or light wave. Thus, the measurement of distances or structures with a resolution of ~100 µm, which would be typical for ultrasound, requires a time resolution of approximately 100 nanoseconds (100 x 10^{-9} s). In contrast, the measurement of structures with a resolution of ~10 µm, which is achieved by OCT, requires a time resolution of approximately 30 femtoseconds (30 x 10^{-15} s). Fortunately, it is possible to perform ultrahigh-resolution time and distance measurements using low-coherence interferometry.

Measuring Echoes of Light Using Low-Coherence Interferometry

OCT uses low-coherence interferometry to perform ultrahigh-resolution time and distance measurements for imaging. The technique of "low-coherence" or white-light interferometry is well established and was first described by Sir Isaac Newton.[32] During the last several years, low-coherence interferometry was developed as a technique for performing high-resolution optical measurements in fiberoptic and optoelectronic components.[33-35] In order to perform distance measurements with tens-of-micron resolution (corresponding to echo delay times of tens of femtoseconds), it is necessary to use an optical instrument that compares or correlates one optical beam or light wave with another reference optical beam or light

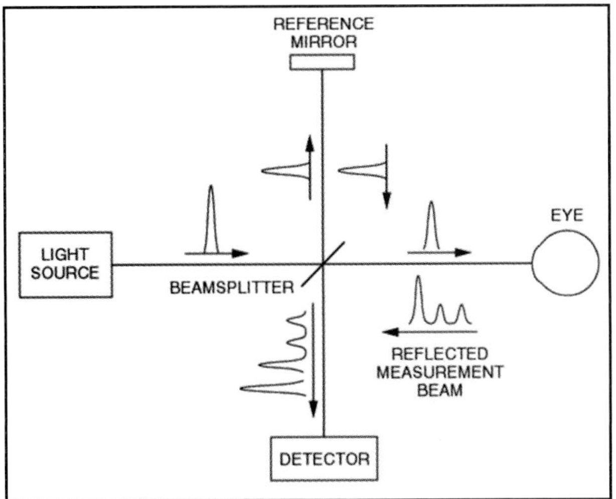

Figure 1-7. Low-coherence interferometry for high-resolution time and distance measurement. The echo delay time of light can be measured with high resolution by comparing or correlating one light beam with another. Light from a source is directed onto a partially reflecting mirror (ie, beamsplitter) and is split into measurement and reference beams. The measurement beam is backreflected or backscattered from the tissue with different echo time delays, depending upon its internal microstructure. The light in the reference beam is reflected from a reference mirror at a known distance, which produces a known time delay. The light signal from the tissue, consisting of multiple echoes, and the light from the reference mirror, consisting of a single echo at a known delay, are combined by the interferometer and detected. The echo structure of the backreflected or backscattered light signal may be measured by scanning the position of the reference mirror in order to produce different time delays for the reference light while electronically processing the detector output. This generates echo versus distance and is analogous to ultrasound A-mode ranging. A more detailed discussion of how low-coherence interferometry works is provided in Appendix A.

wave. This type of measurement may be performed by an optical device known as an *interferometer*.

Figure 1-7 shows a schematic of an optical interferometer. The light source is a laser or other device that emits either short pulses of light or short coherence-length light. The optical beam from the light source is directed onto a partially reflecting mirror (ie, beamsplitter). The partially reflecting mirror splits the light into two parts; one beam is reflected and the other is transmitted. One light beam is directed onto the patient's eye and is reflected from intraocular structures at different distances. The reflected light beam from the eye consists of multiple echoes that give information about the distance and thickness of different intraocular structures. The second beam is reflected from a reference mirror at a known spatial position. This backreflected reference optical beam travels back to the partial mirror (beamsplitter) where it combines with the optical beam reflected from the eye.

The operation of the system can be understood qualitatively if one thinks of the light beam as being composed of short pulses of light. The light pulse reflected from the reference mirror will coincide with the light pulse reflected from a given structure in the eye only if both pulses arrive at the same time. This will occur only if the distance that light travels to and from the reference mirror precisely matches the distance that light travels when it is reflected from a given structure in the eye. When the two light pulses coincide, they produce a phenomenon known as *interference*, which is measured by a light-sensitive detector (ie, photodetector).

In order to measure the time delays of light echoes from different structures within the eye, the position of the reference mirror is varied so that the time delay of the reference light pulse is adjusted accordingly. The signal from the detector will then be related to the echo structure of the light backreflected from the eye. If there are multiple reflections, then there will be a peak observed each time the reference pulse is delayed, so that it coincides with an echo pulse from a particular structure in the eye. Thus, the interferometer can precisely measure the echo structure of reflected light and perform high-resolution measurements of the distance and thickness of different tissue structures.[36-39] While the explanation presented here assumes that the light is composed of short optical pulses, the measurement is usually performed using continuous wavelight having a short or low coherence length. A more detailed description of how the interferometer operates is presented in Appendix A. For the purposes of this current discussion, the important feature of the interferometer is that it measures the time delays of optical echoes by comparing or correlating the light with reference light that travels a reference path.

Technological advances in fiber optics and photonics communications technology have made it possible to engineer an extremely compact, robust, and low-cost measurement system using optical fibers and diode light sources.[39] Figure 1-8 shows a schematic representation of a fiberoptic version of the interferometer. The light source for the interferometer is a compact superluminescent diode that is coupled directly into an optical fiber. This light source in OCT is similar to laser diodes used in compact disc players, except that the diode source is designed to emit light that has a short coherence length. The interferometer is constructed using a fiberoptic coupler that functions analogously to a beamsplitter. The optical fiber in one path of the interferometer is connected to the

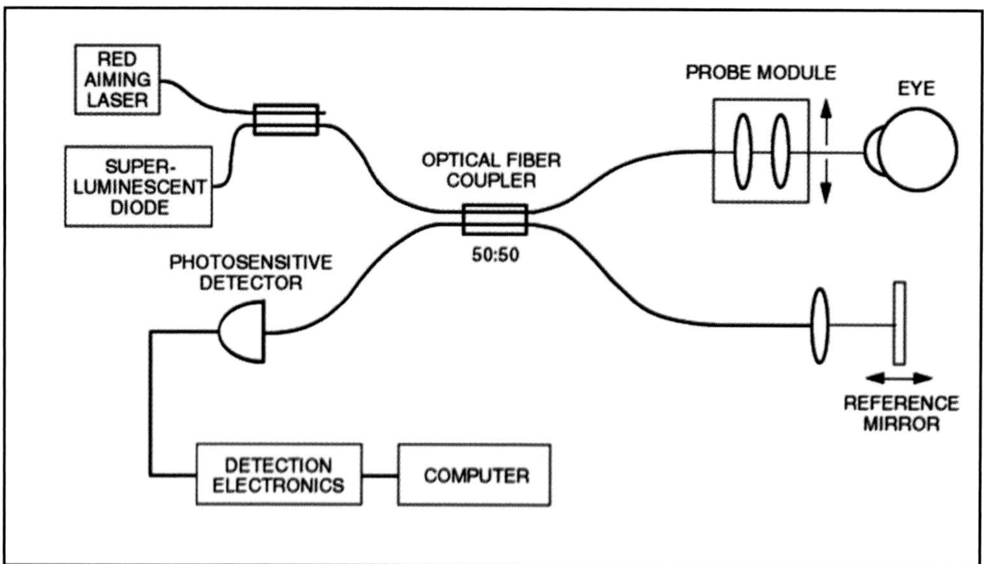

Figure 1-8. A fiberoptic interferometer forms the heart of the OCT imaging system. The interferometer shown in the previous figure can be built using fiberoptic components, thus yielding a compact and modular system. The light source used in most OCT systems is a compact, low-coherence, superluminescent diode that is directly coupled into an optical fiber. The interferometer is built using an optical fiber coupler (beamsplitter), where one fiber forms the measurement path of the interferometer and the other fiber forms the reference path. The fiber in the measurement path is connected to a clinical imaging device, such as the fundus camera and a slit-lamp biomicroscope.

OCT ophthalmic instrument, which resembles a fundus camera. The reference path of the interferometer consists of a reference mirror located within the instrument. In other applications, the OCT system can be fiberoptically coupled to endoscopes or catheters imaging luminal structures inside the body.[40] OCT technology draws upon well-developed fiberoptic and device technologies that are used in the fiberoptic and photonic industries. Thus, OCT systems are inherently reliable and robust.

Axial Scans and Optical Coherence Tomography Image Generation

The simplest type of measurement that can be performed by OCT is analogous to the ultrasound A-mode scanning measurement of axial range or distance. Information on tissue distances or thicknesses is determined by detecting the output signal from the interferometer, then processing the signal electronically and displaying it on a computer. Figure 1-9 shows an example of axial distance measurements or axial scans performed on the anterior chamber.[37] The plot shows the intensity of the backreflected or backscattered light from different structures within the anterior eye as a function of echo time delay or axial (longitudinal) distance. Echoes are observed from the anterior and posterior surfaces of the cornea as well as from the anterior capsule of the lens. The intensity of the backreflected light is a measure of the discontinuity of the index of refraction between different tissues. The reflection of the light beam from the anterior surface of the cornea is relatively large. However, reflections from internal boundaries between different tissue types, such as between the cornea and aqueous, or different layers of the retina, are relatively small. In addition, different tissues, such as the cornea, lens, and sclera of the anterior eye or the different layers of the retina, will produce varying amounts of optical backscattering. This variation or differential in backscattering is also observed in the OCT axial scan measurement.

The axial (longitudinal) distance measurement shown in Figure 1-9 permits a direct measurement of the corneal thickness as well as anterior chamber depth. The thickness of the tissue is calculated by measuring the optical echo delay and multiplying it by the speed of light in the tissue. The speed of light in the tissue is given by the speed of light in vacuum multiplied by the index of refraction of the tissue. Therefore, the measurement of physical thickness in OCT relies upon knowing or assuming a value for the index of refraction of the tissue. The strength or intensity of the backreflected or backscattered light is extremely small; approximately 10^{-5} to 10^{-9} (-50 decibels [dB] to -90 dB) of the incident light intensity. Thus, very high detection sensitivity to extremely weak reflected light echoes is required for the measurement of structures within the eye.

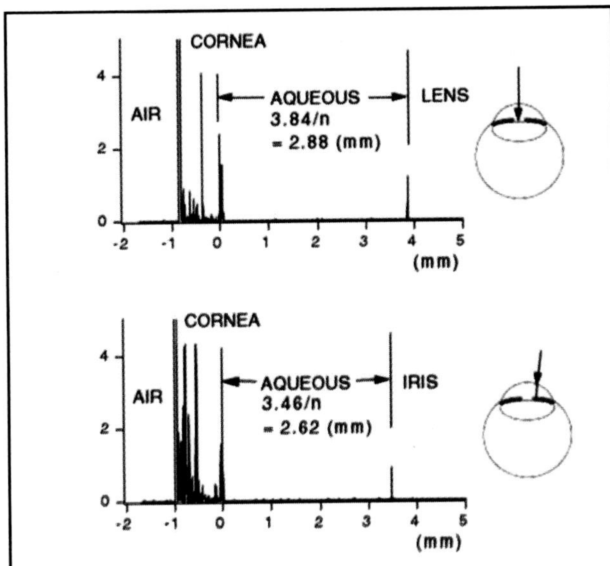

Figure 1-9. Measurement of anterior chamber depth using optical low-coherence interferometry. The graphs display the magnitude of the backreflected or backscattered optical intensity as a function of echo delay or distance. This measurement is analogous to ultrasound A-mode ranging, except that light is used rather than sound. A large reflection is observed from the anterior surface of the cornea, while smaller reflections originate from the posterior corneal surface (cornea-aqueous boundary), and the lens or iris. Note the presence of scattered light that originates from within the cornea. The graphs show the structural features that occur along the axis of the optical beam. If the transverse position of the optical beam is changed, then different features are measured (the depth of the anterior chamber versus the depth to the iris). (Reproduced from Huang D, Wang J, Lin CP, Puliafito CA, Fujimoto JG. Micron-resolution ranging of cornea and anterior chamber by optical reflectometry. *Lasers Surg Med.* 1991;11:419-425. Copyright © 1991. Reprinted by permission of Wiley-Liss, Inc, a subsidiary of John Wiley & Sons, Inc.)

Once an axial measurement or A-mode scan has been made, the relative positions of different structures may be measured by scanning the transverse position of the optical beam within the eye. Figure 1-9 shows a second axial measurement, with the optical beam aimed at the iris rather than at the anterior capsule of the lens. Because the light beam can be focused to a small spot size, the transverse position of the beam can be known with high precision. Thus, information on both the axial (or longitudinal) and the transverse microstructure of tissue can be measured. This is how OCT performs cross-sectional imaging.

OCT cross-sectional imaging of tissue is achieved by performing successive axial (longitudinal) measurements or A-mode scans of the tissue at different transverse positions, which is analogous to ultrasound B-mode imaging.[1-3,41] Figure 1-10 illustrates how an OCT image is acquired. Successive, rapid axial measurements or A-mode scans are performed while scanning the optical beam in the transverse direction. The result is a set of many axial scans similar to that shown in Figure 1-9, where each scan represents the backreflection or backscattering of the light as a function of depth in the tissue. Different scans describe the axial (or longitudinal) information at a different transverse position. For purposes of visualization, this two-dimensional data set is processed by computer and displayed as a gray-scale or false-color image.

Gray-Scale Versus False-Color Optical Coherence Tomography Images

OCT images can be displayed by mapping the backreflected or backscattered signal intensity into either a gray-scale or false-color scale. Figure 1-11 shows examples of an OCT image of the foveal region of the retina in which the logarithm of the optical backscatter signal is displayed in gray scale and false color. These images are examples of typical images generated by commercial OCT instruments (StratusOCT, Carl Zeiss Meditec, Dublin, Calif) and have an axial image resolution of 10 µm. This image was generated from 512 axial scans and consists of 512 transverse pixels spanning a 6-mm transverse dimension. The scale of the image is expanded in the axial direction in order to permit better visualization of the thin retinal features over the large transverse dimension. The backscattered signal level typically ranges approximately from -50 dB, the maximum signal, to -95 dB, the detection sensitivity limit. Because the backreflected or backscattered signal varies over approximately five orders of magnitude, or ~50 dB, it is convenient to use the logarithm of the signal to display the image. This expands the dynamic range of the image display so that both strong and weak signals can be visualized on the same image, but it results in compression of relative variations in signal.

Gray-scale image display is extensively used in ultrasound imaging and has the advantage that it gives a good intuitive interpretation of the image. White and black correspond to the strongest and weakest backreflected or backscattered optical signal intensities, respectively. The background noise is typically "threshold segmented," so that noise signals below a certain threshold level are set to display as black in order to remove the background noise. Images can also be displayed in reversed gray scale, where the roles of black and white are reversed, and black rather than white corresponds to the highest signal. The disadvantage of gray-scale display is that the ability to differen-

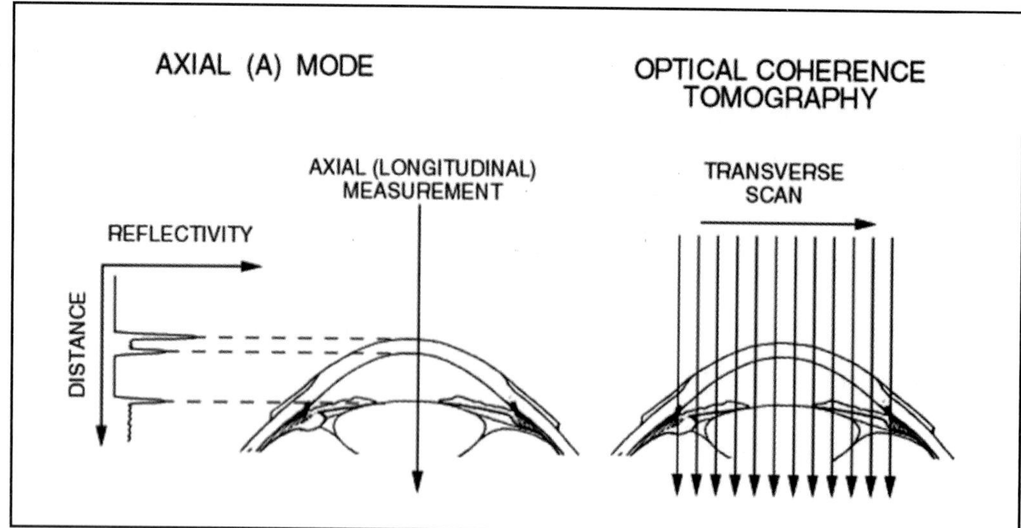

Figure 1-10. Image generation using OCT. OCT imaging is analogous to ultrasound B-mode imaging. OCT images are constructed by performing rapid, successive axial (longitudinal) measurements at different transverse points. Each axial measurement represents the echo delay of backreflection and backscatter from microstructures inside tissue and gives a measurement of tissue dimensions and properties along the optical beam. By scanning the optical beam transversely while performing successive axial measurements, a two-dimensional data set can be acquired. These data are a cross-sectional map of the backreflection and backscatter within the tissue and can be displayed as a cross-sectional image.

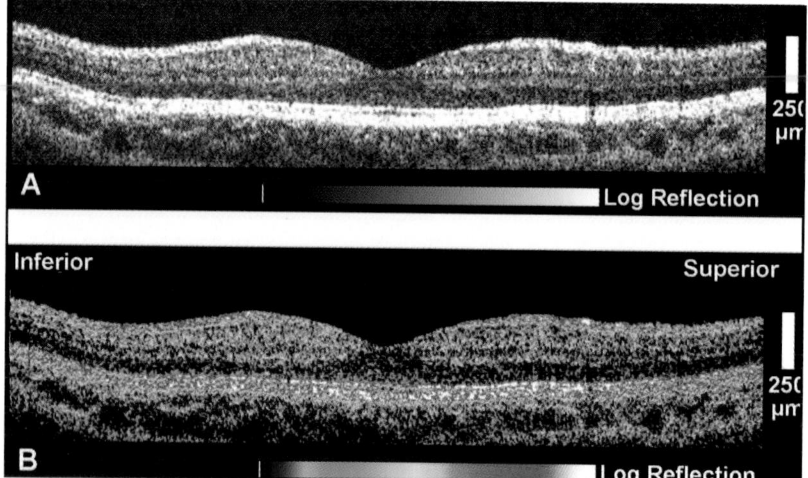

Figure 1-11. Gray-scale and false-color display of OCT images. (A) Gray-scale OCT retinal image. The image is displayed using a logarithmic mapping of the signal intensity onto a gray scale ranging from white to black. The maximum signal is approximately -50 dB, while the minimum detectable signal, or noise level, is approximately -95 dB. The disadvantage of gray-scale image display is that the dynamic range is poor, and it is difficult to visualize differences in the gray level. (B) False-color OCT retinal image. The image is displayed using a logarithmic mapping of the signal intensity to color. The maximum signal is represented by a red-white color, while the minimum detectable signal is represented by a blue-black color. The colors do not necessarily correspond to microstructural features in the tissue, but they enhance the ability to differentiate small differences in the signal level.

tiate variations in intensities is very limited. Computer monitors provide only 8-bit gray resolution, or 256 gray levels. In addition, the eye has a limited ability to distinguish different gray levels, so that gray-scale images cannot correctly represent the full dynamic range available in OCT images.

In contrast to gray levels, computer monitors typically have 24-bit or more color levels, and the human eye can differentiate between millions of distinct colors. In order to enhance the ability to differentiate between subtle structures within the image, false-color representations are often used in OCT images, as shown in Figure 1-11B. In false-color images, the logarithm of the optical backreflection or backscattering signal is mapped into different colors. Although many different false-color maps are possible, the optical signal intensity is usually mapped into a "rainbow" of colors for ophthalmic imaging. The highest intensity signal is represented by white and red colors, and typically corresponds to -50 dB of the incident intensity, while the lowest intensity signal is represented by black and blue colors, and typically corresponds to -95 dB of the intensity. This lowest detectable intensity is set by the sensitivity of the instrument. The retinal images in Figure 1-11 demonstrate that false-color mapping can improve the ability to differentiate tissue structures. However, one disadvantage of false-color display is that it can produce artifacts in the image. If the signal intensity is changed, this can produce a change in color of structures in the image. Careful calibration of signal levels is required.

Tissue structures that have different optical reflection or scattering properties will be displayed as different colors in a false-color image. However, it is important to note that although the OCT image represents true dimensions (correcting for index of refraction and beam refraction effects), the coloring of different structures in a false-color image represents different optical properties and is not necessarily different tissue morphology. Care must be taken to avoid interpreting images like histopathology. In histopathology, tissue sections are stained in order to produce color differences or a contrast between different tissue structures, and the staining is specific to certain structures, such as nuclei. However, OCT imaging is similar to ultrasound in which different degrees of ultrasound backscattering produce image contrast. In OCT images, tissue structures are visualized because they have different optical backreflection or backscattering properties. False-color display enhances this visualization, but the colors are associated with different signal intensities and are not analogous to histological staining. A detailed discussion of the interpretation of OCT retinal images and retinal architectural morphology will be presented in Chapter 2.

Finally, it is interesting to note that in highly scattering tissues, such as in the coronary artery image shown in Figure 1-4, light is rapidly attenuated with depth, resulting in a strong gradation in the image. There can also be significant amounts of speckle or other noise arising from the microstructural features in the tissue. This can produce artifacts if the image is displayed using a false-color scale. Therefore, it is more common to display OCT images of scattering tissues using a gray scale.[6]

Image Resolution

The resolution of OCT images in the axial (longitudinal) and transverse directions is determined by different mechanisms. A more detailed description of the image resolution is presented in Appendix A. The quantitative information presented here is intended only as an approximate guide to understanding image resolution, since different OCT systems may have significantly different performance, depending upon their design and intended application.

The resolution of the OCT image in the axial (longitudinal) direction is determined by the resolution of the optical distance measurement. This is determined by the physical properties of the light source that is used in the interferometer. If a short pulse laser is used, the axial resolution is determined by the pulse duration. If a continuous-wave low-coherence light source is used, the axial resolution is determined by the coherence length of the light source. For standard OCT systems used clinically, the axial resolution is approximately 10 μm in tissue.[3] However, state-of-the-art systems used in the research laboratory can achieve ultrahigh resolutions of 3 μm for retinal imaging and as fine as 1 to 2 μm for other applications.[29,42] The axial resolution is the full-width at half-maximum (FWHM) on a linear scale of an isolated backreflection, or the so-called "point spread function." The axial resolution is a measure of the smallest feature that can be seen in an image. It is important to note that the measurement of distance or tissue thickness can often be performed with higher resolution than the actual axial resolution.

The resolution of the image in the transverse direction is determined by the focused spot size of the optical beam. This is analogous to optical microscopy. The spot size is a function of the optics used to project the beam into the eye and is determined by factors such as whether or not imaging is performed over a large depth, such as in the anterior eye, or whether or not the focusing angle is restricted, as in imaging the retina. The typical transverse resolution for OCT retinal imaging is 20 to 25 μm. Although the pupil limits the available aperture for focusing on the retina, the absolute minimum spot size is limited by the aberrations in the optics of the eye. In other imaging applications, much finer transverse resolutions can be achieved by using high numerical aperture focusing.

The resolution of an OCT image also depends on the number of pixels in the image, as well as the fundamental resolution of the instrument. Even if the instrument has a high resolution, images will still appear grainy if there is an insufficient number of pixels. This concept is analogous to pixel resolution in digital photography. Larger images with finer features require more pixels. The pixel number is especially important for the transverse dimension of an OCT image. Since the OCT image is generated by taking multiple axial (longitudinal) data sets or axial scans at different transverse points, the number of pixels in the transverse direction is determined by the number of these axial scans. The image acquisition time increases in proportion to the number of axial scans (number of transverse pixels), so higher transverse pixel density images require longer acquisition times. However, the number of pixels in the axial (longitudinal) direction is independent of the transverse direction and is determined by the speed of the detection electronics and computer. Since computers and electronics are relatively fast, large numbers of axial pixels can be acquired. Fortunately, for most ophthalmic applications, much finer resolution is required in the axial direction than in the transverse direction because the retina has a thin-layered structure and retinal pathology is characterized by changes in the layers of the retina. A more detailed discussion of image acquisition speed and pixel densities is presented in Chapter 2, as well as in Appendix A.

Computer Image Processing and the Correction of Eye Motion

Since OCT has extremely high resolution, it is essential to compensate for eye motion during the image acquisition because it can cause image blurring. Movements of the eye can be caused by a variety of processes, including fluctuations in intraocular pressure produced by the pulse, microsaccades and tremor, and changes in the patient's fixation point. The axial (longitudinal) resolution of OCT is finer than the transverse resolution, and retinal architecture has fine features in the axial direction because of the layered structure of the retina. Therefore, axial (longitudinal) eye motion has the most severe effect in blurring OCT images. Fortunately, since OCT measures the distance or absolution range of the tissue, it is possible to correct images for axial eye motion. Powerful, yet simple computer image processing techniques can be used to dramatically enhance imaging performance by virtually eliminating image blurring in the axial direction from involuntary patient eye motion.[41]

Figure 1-12 is an example of OCT of the fovea showing the raw image data without image processing and the image achieved after processing to correct for axial eye motion. These changes in the axial position of the eye may be corrected because the optical distance measurement itself determines the distance of the retina. The OCT image is constructed by performing sequential axial measurements at different transverse positions within the eye. However, if the eye moves on a micron scale in the axial direction between the times that successive axial data sets are acquired, then the positions of different features will be observed at different axial (longitudinal) ranges. Thus, the position of the patient's eye in the axial (longitudinal) direction may be measured by correlating adjacent axial data sets. Once the axial position of the patient's eye is known, the axial scans in the OCT image may be displaced in the axial direction so that the microstructural features will be realigned.

Changes in transverse eye position are not eliminated using this simple image-processing technique. However, small changes in transverse position do not produce significant degradation in image quality because the typical retinal features in the transverse dimension are larger than in the axial (longitudinal) direction. Larger drifts in patient fixation are not compensated, so it is important to acquire OCT images at high speed in order to minimize possible eye motion. It is also important to examine OCT images for errors due to patient fixation changes, which may produce artifacts in the image. A discussion of these artifacts is presented in Chapter 2.

Optical Coherence Tomography Instrumentation

OCT imaging can be performed in the retina or the anterior eye. In this section, we describe OCT instrumentation and imaging techniques that are used in these two generic cases. The instruments used for retinal and anterior segment imaging operate analogously to the fundus camera and slit-lamp biomicroscope, respectively. The OCT instrument permits the operator to view the retinal fundus or anterior segment using a video camera. The wavelength of the OCT beam is typically in the near-infrared 800 nm wavelength; thus it is minimally visible to the patient. This reduces patient discomfort during the examination. From the instrument operator's viewpoint, the acquisition of OCT images is straightforward. The optical beam from the OCT device is scanned and aimed at the structure that is to be cross-sectionally imaged. The patient's fixation point can be adjusted using an operator-controlled fixation target visible to the eye that is being scanned or with an external fixation target used for the other eye.

The scanning OCT beam is visible on the video image and defines the location on the retinal fundus or anterior eye where the cross-sectional OCT image is being

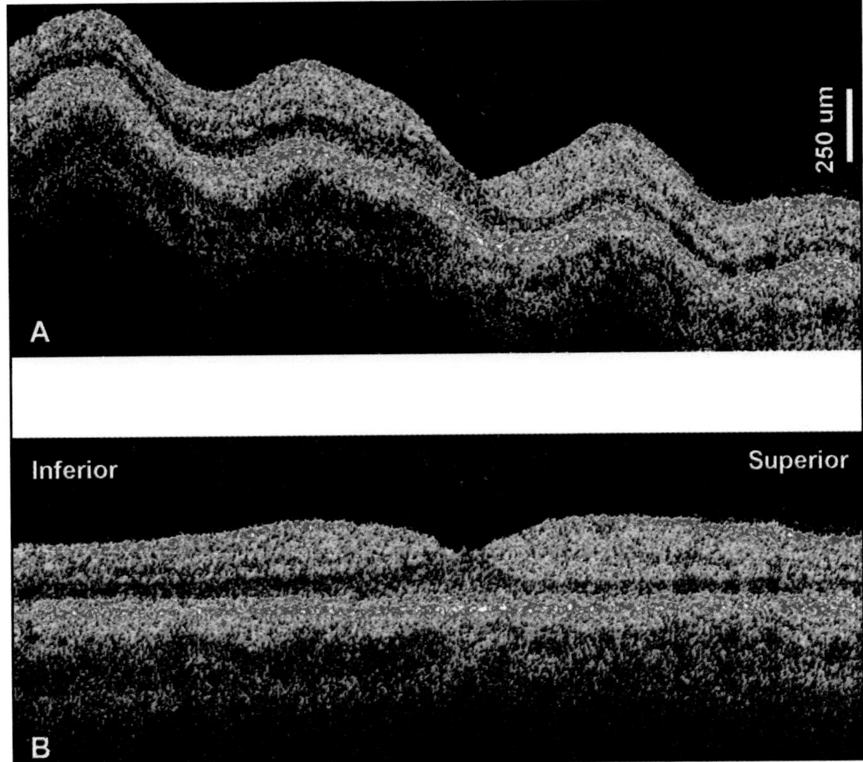

Figure 1-12. OCT images of the macula showing computer image-processing to correct for patient eye motion. (A) Original, unprocessed image with motion artifacts because of instability in the patient's axial eye position. (B) Processed image with axial motion correction. Since OCT can measure absolution distance or range, it is possible to measure the eye motion in the axial direction and correct the image by realigning the axial scans in the image. Because OCT images have high resolution, motion correction is used as a standard feature on all ophthalmic OCT imaging systems.

acquired. In retinal imaging, the scanning pattern of the OCT beam is also visible to the patient and appears as a low-intensity, fine red line. The OCT instrument records axial (longitudinal) scan information at different transverse positions and generates an OCT image continuously as it is being acquired. When the OCT image is recorded for the patient record, the instrument can store both the OCT image as well as a fundus photograph showing the registration of the OCT image on the retina. Acquiring the fundus image requires illumination of the fundus with a brief flash of visible light. The scan pattern of the OCT beam is controlled by software, and cross-sectional images along arbitrary cross-sectional planes or curves can be acquired. Software options also allow post-processing of the image in order to perform quantitative measurements or to construct topographic maps. Multiple software scanning and image-processing protocols, which are designed for various applications such as assessing macular edema or retinal nerve fiber layer thickness in glaucoma, can be performed. A more detailed description of scanning and image-processing protocols is presented in Appendix B.

Retinal Imaging

The most common application of OCT in ophthalmology is retinal imaging. The instrument design for OCT retinal imaging is similar to a fundus camera. Figure 1-13 shows a schematic diagram of the optical design used for OCT retinal imaging. A high-power objective lens, similar to a handheld 78 diopter lens, is used so that the retina is relay imaged onto an image plane inside the instrument. The instrument then relays the retinal image onto a video camera that enables real-time operator viewing of the fundus. The magnification and field of view of the retinal image are determined by the refractive power of the objective lens and other optics. Standard instruments have a ~30 degree field of view. The OCT imaging beam is coupled into the optical path of the instrument

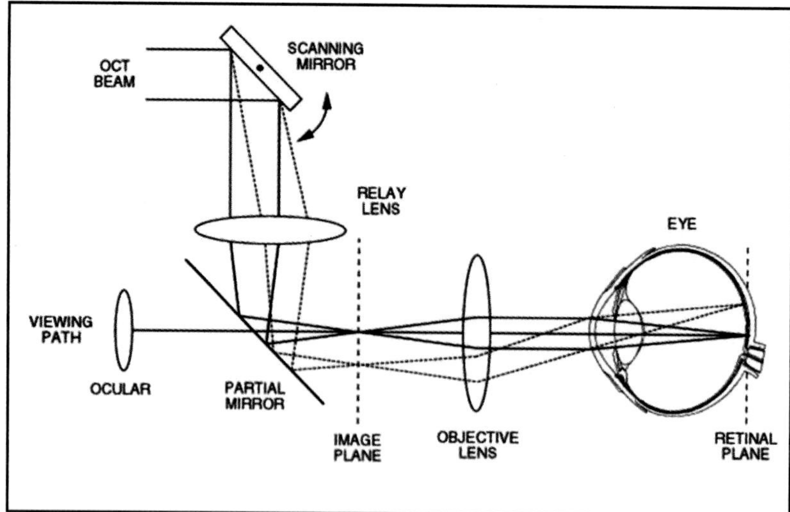

Figure 1-13. Schematic of the optical system for OCT imaging of the retina. The instrument for retinal imaging is similar to a fundus camera. An objective lens produces an image of the retina on a plane inside the OCT instrument. Operator viewing of the fundus is performed by imaging with a video camera. A computer-controlled, two-axis scanning mirror positions and scans the OCT measurement beam. A relay lens focuses the OCT beam onto the image plane, and the objective lens directs the OCT beam through the pupil onto the retina. The OCT beam is focused on the retina by adjusting the objective lens. During imaging, the beam pivots about the pupil of the eye when the OCT beam is scanned in order to minimize vignetting.

using a partially reflective mirror (beamsplitter). The OCT beam is focused onto the retinal image plane using a relay lens. The focused OCT beam is then relay imaged onto the retina by the ocular objective lens and the patient's eye. The transverse spot size of the OCT beam on the retina is typically ~20 µm. Prior to OCT image acquisition, the instrument must be focused by adjusting the ocular objective lens position so that the OCT beam is focused on the retina. This also focuses the video fundus image. The instrument also emits a beam that illuminates the fundus to enable video viewing.

The transverse position of the OCT beam is scanned by two perpendicularly oriented x-y scanning mirrors that are inside the instrument. The optical system is designed so that the beam pivots about the pupil of the eye when the angle of the mirrors are scanned to control the transverse position of the OCT beam on the retina, as shown in Figure 1-13. This prevents the OCT beam from being vignetted by the pupil and it enables access to a wide field of view on the retina. In order to ensure that the OCT pivots about the pupil of the eye, the patient's eye must be located at a given distance from the ocular objective lens. If the patient's eye is too close or too far from this position, the OCT beam will change position instead of pivoting about the pupil, and vignetting will occur.

OCT imaging can be performed at different locations on the fundus, controlling the scanning of the OCT beam under computer control. The location of the OCT image can also be controlled by changing the patient's point of fixation. The instrument has an internal fixation target, visible to the patient's eye that is being imaged, which can be adjusted under computer control. The operator can view the fundus image in real-time by video, which is displayed in a window on the computer monitor. This enables precise aiming of the OCT imaging beam. When the OCT beam is scanned, it produces a scan pattern on the retina that is visible to the operator. The OCT beam is also visible to the patient as a thin, red line whose position in the patient's visual field corresponds to the points on the retina that are being scanned.

The OCT instrument can be aligned and focused by scanning the OCT beam at high speed and simultaneously viewing the fundus image and the OCT image as it is acquired. Once OCT image data are acquired, the OCT beam is scanned slower in order to acquire a higher pixel resolution image. The position of the OCT image on the fundus can be recorded immediately after OCT image

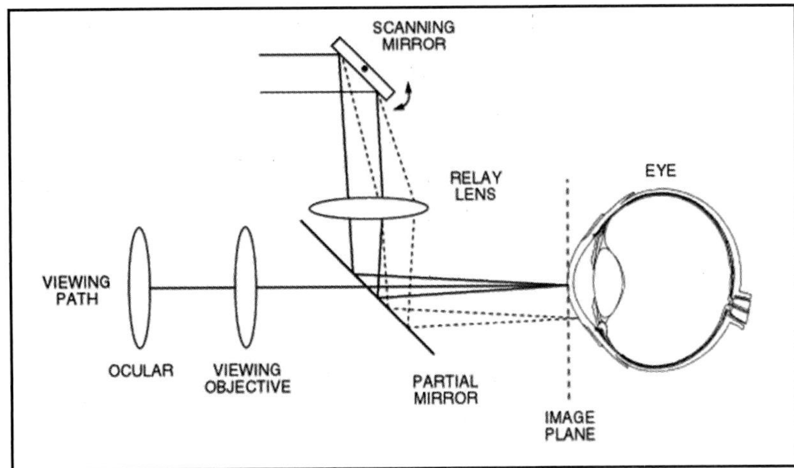

Figure 1-14. Schematic of the optical system for OCT imaging the anterior eye. The instrument for anterior eye imaging is similar to a slit-lamp biomicroscope. A viewing objective and ocular lens function as a microscope to produce an image of the anterior eye that can be viewed directly or with a video camera. A computer-controlled, two-axis scanning mirror positions and scans the OCT measurement beam. The OCT beam is focused with a relay lens so that it is coincident with the image plane. The OCT beam can be positioned and scanned under operator control so that it generates real-time cross-sectional images of selected structures in the anterior eye.

acquisition by capturing the video fundus image. Thus, the OCT image can be exactly registered with respect to landmarks or pathology on the fundus.

Since the scanning pattern of the OCT beam on the retina can be controlled by computer, different scan patterns can be designed and adopted as part of the diagnostic protocol for different retinal diseases. The use of different scan patterns to image different retinal features is described in more detail in Chapter 2. Scanning and imaging-processing protocols are also described in more detail in Appendix B.

Finally, retinal imaging is performed using infrared light at 800 nm wavelengths. The allowable limits for safe retinal exposure have been thoroughly investigated and are governed by international standards such as the American National Standards Institute (ANSI) standard. The maximum safe, permissible exposure depends upon the wavelength, the spot size, the duration of exposure, as well as repeated exposures. Because OCT instruments have extremely high detection sensitivities, instruments require low power levels of <1 milliwatt (mW), which are well within safe exposure limits.

Anterior Segment Imaging

OCT imaging of the anterior segment is somewhat simpler than retinal imaging. The instrument design for OCT anterior eye imaging is similar to a slit-lamp biomicroscope. Figure 1-14 shows a schematic diagram of the optical system design used to image the anterior segment. A viewing objective in combination with an ocular lens forms a microscope that provides a direct or video view of the anterior eye and is similar to a slit-lamp biomicroscope. The operator's view of the anterior segment is determined by the magnification of the viewing objective and ocular lens.

The OCT beam is focused using a relay lens and is coupled into the viewing path of the instrument using a partially reflecting mirror (beamsplitter). The focal position of the OCT beam is coincident with the image plane of the viewing optics. The transverse position of the OCT beam is scanned by two perpendicularly oriented x-y scanning mirrors that are inside the instrument. The OCT beam's focused spot size and depth of field or range over which the beam is in focus are determined by the relay lens optics. For imaging the anterior segment, a large depth of field is required, thus the focused spot size of the OCT beam must be large. As a result, the OCT image resolution in the transverse direction is usually coarse. In contrast to retinal imaging, which is performed with light at 800 nm wavelengths, imaging of the anterior eye is typically performed using 1300-nm wavelengths.[2,43] Longer wavelengths are scattered less and they enable deeper image penetration depths into the anterior angle. Since the allowable, safe ocular light exposure levels are higher for these longer wavelengths, higher incident powers can be used than those used for retinal imaging. This enables high-speed, real-time imaging at several frames per second. The 1300 nm wavelengths are not visible to the patient. However, since these wavelengths are also not visible to the operator using conventional video cameras, a visible aiming beam is used to guide the positioning of the OCT beam. The OCT beam can be positioned under operator control to generate real-time cross-sectional images of selected structures in the anterior eye.

Summary

OCT can generate cross-sectional images of the retina or anterior eye with unprecedented resolution; greater than any previously available ophthalmic clinical imaging technology. Because OCT images can be acquired rapidly without contacting the eye, and the OCT measurement beam is in the infrared, imaging is well-tolerated by patients. The rapid acquisition time of OCT permits multiple images to be acquired with different cross-sectional image planes, thus enabling a comprehensive assessment of the macula and optic disc. OCT can provide diagnostically important information that complements standard fundus photography or fluorescein angiography. OCT images allow a direct visualization of retinal pathology and enable the visualization of internal retinal structure on the level of architectural morphology. Furthermore, OCT can provide quantitative information of retinal architecture or other intraocular structures. These morphometric measurements can be used to diagnose disease or to assess disease progression and response to therapy. For these reasons, OCT imaging is rapidly becoming the standard of care in clinical ophthalmology.

References

1. Huang D, Swanson EA, Lin CP, et al. Optical coherence tomography. *Science*. 1991;254(5035):1178-1181.
2. Izatt JA, Hee MR, Swanson EA, et al. Micrometer-scale resolution imaging of the anterior eye in vivo with optical coherence tomography. *Arch Ophthalmol*. 1994;112(12):1584-1589.
3. Hee MR, Izatt JA, Swanson EA, et al. Optical coherence tomography of the human retina. *Arch Ophthalmol*. 1995;113(3):325-332.
4. Fujimoto JG, Pitris C, Boppart SA, Brezinski ME. Optical coherence tomography: an emerging technology for biomedical imaging and optical biopsy. *Neoplasia*. 2000;2(1-2):9-25.
5. Fujimoto JG. Optical coherence tomography for ultrahigh resolution in vivo imaging. *Nat Biotechnol*. 2003;21(11):1361-1367.
6. Fujimoto JG, Brezinski ME, Tearney GJ, et al. Optical biopsy and imaging using optical coherence tomography. *Nat Med*. 1995;1(9):970-972.
7. Puliafito CA, Hee MR, Lin CP, et al. Imaging of macular diseases with optical coherence tomography. *Ophthalmology*. 1995;102(2):217-229.
8. Brezinski ME, Tearney GJ, Bouma BE, et al. Optical coherence tomography for optical biopsy. Properties and demonstration of vascular pathology. *Circulation*. 1996;93(6):1206-1213.
9. Puliafito CA, Hee MR, Schuman JS, Fujimoto JG. *Optical Coherence Tomography of Ocular Diseases*. Thorofare, NJ: SLACK Incorporated; 1996.
10. Hee MR, Puliafito CA, Wong C, et al. Quantitative assessment of macular edema with optical coherence tomography. *Arch Ophthalmol*. 1995;113(8):1019-1029.
11. Hee MR, Puliafito CA, Wong C, et al. Optical coherence tomography of macular holes. *Ophthalmology*. 1995;102(5):748-756.
12. Hee MR, Puliafito CA, Wong C, et al. Optical coherence tomography of central serous chorioretinopathy. *Am J Ophthalmol*. 1995;120(1):65-74.
13. Hee MR, Baumal CR, Puliafito CA, et al. Optical coherence tomography of age-related macular degeneration and choroidal neovascularization. *Ophthalmology*. 1996;103(8):1260-1270.
14. Wilkins JR, Puliafito CA, Hee MR, et al. Characterization of epiretinal membranes using optical coherence tomography. *Ophthalmology*. 1996;103(12):2142-2151.
15. Hee MR, Puliafito CA, Duker JS, et al. Topography of diabetic macular edema with optical coherence tomography. *Ophthalmology*. 1998;105(2):360-370.
16. Schuman JS, Hee MR, Arya AV, et al. Optical coherence tomography: a new tool for glaucoma diagnosis. *Curr Opin Ophthalmol*. 1995;6(2):89-95.
17. Schuman JS, Hee MR, Puliafito CA, et al. Quantification of nerve fiber layer thickness in normal and glaucomatous eyes using optical coherence tomography. *Arch Ophthalmol*. 1995;113(5):586-596.
18. Schuman JS, Pedut-Kloizman T, Hertzmark E, et al. Reproducibility of nerve fiber layer thickness measurements using optical coherence tomography. *Ophthalmology*. 1996;103(11):1889-1898.
19. Bowd C, Weinreb RN, Williams JM, Zangwill LM. The retinal nerve fiber layer thickness in ocular hypertensive, normal, and glaucomatous eyes with optical coherence tomography. *Arch Ophthalmol*. 2000;118(1):22-26.
20. Zangwill LM, Williams J, Berry CC, Knauer S, Weinreb RN. A comparison of optical coherence tomography and retinal nerve fiber layer photography for detection of nerve fiber layer damage in glaucoma. *Ophthalmology*. 2000;107(7):1309-1315.

21. Bowd C, Zangwill LM, Berry CC, et al. Detecting early glaucoma by assessment of retinal nerve fiber layer thickness and visual function. *Invest Ophthalmol Vis Sci*. 2001;42(9):1993-2003.
22. Schuman JS, Wollstein G, Farra T, et al. Comparison of optic nerve head measurements obtained by optical coherence tomography and confocal scanning laser ophthalmoscopy. *Am J Ophthalmol*. 2003;135(4):504-512.
23. Guedes V, Schuman JS, Hertzmark E, et al. Optical coherence tomography measurement of macular and nerve fiber layer thickness in normal and glaucomatous human eyes. *Ophthalmology*. 2003;110(1):177-189.
24. Olsen T. Calculating axial length in the aphakic and the pseudophakic eye. *J Cataract Refract Surg*. 1988;14(4):413-416.
25. Olsen T. The accuracy of ultrasonic determination of axial length in pseudophakic eyes. *Acta Ophthalmologica*. 1989; 67(2):141-144.
26. Pavlin CJ, Sherar MD, Foster FS. Subsurface ultrasound microscopic imaging of the intact eye. *Ophthalmology*. 1990;97(2):244-250.
27. Pavlin CJ, Harasiewicz K, Sherar MD, Foster FS. Clinical use of ultrasound biomicroscopy. *Ophthalmology*. 1991; 98(3):287-295.
28. Pavlin CJ, Foster FS. Ultrasound biomicroscopy. High-frequency ultrasound imaging of the eye at microscopic resolution. *Radiol Clin North Am*. 1998;36(6):1047-1058.
29. Drexler W, Morgner U, Ghanta RK, Kärtner FX, Schuman JS, Fujimoto JG. Ultrahigh-resolution ophthalmic optical coherence tomography. *Nat Med*. 2001;7(4):502-507.
30. Fujimoto JG, De Silvestri S, Ippen EP, Puliafito CA, Margolis R, Oseroff A. Femtosecond optical ranging in biological systems. *Optics Letters*. 1986;11(3):150-153.
31. Stern D, Lin WZ, Puliafito CA, Fujimoto JG. Femtosecond optical ranging of corneal incision depth. *Invest Ophthalmol Vis Sci*. 1989;30(1):99-104.
32. Born M, Wolf E, Bhatia AB. *Principles of Optics: Electromagnetic Theory of Propagation, Interference and Diffraction of Light*. 7th (expanded) ed. Cambridge, England: Cambridge University Press; 1999.
33. Youngquist R, Carr S, Davies D. Optical coherence-domain reflectometry: a new optical evaluation technique. *Optics Letters*. 1987;12(3):158.
34. Takada K, Yokohama I, Chida K, Noda J. New measurement system for fault location in optical waveguide devices based on an interferometric technique. *Appl Opt*. 1987;26:1603-1608.
35. Gilgen HH, Novak RP, Salathe RP, Hodel W, Beaud P. Submillimeter optical reflectometry. *IEEE Journal of Lightwave Technology*. 1989;7:1225-1233.
36. Fercher AF, Mengedoht K, Werner W. Eye-length measurement by interferometry with partially coherent light. *Optics Letters*. 1988;13:1867-1869.
37. Huang D, Wang J, Lin CP, Puliafito CA, Fujimoto JG. Micron-resolution ranging of cornea and anterior chamber by optical reflectometry. *Lasers Surg Med*. 1991;11:419-425.
38. Hitzenberger CK. Measurement of corneal thickness by low-coherence interferometry. *Appl Opt*. 1992;31(31): 6637-6642.
39. Swanson EA, Huang D, Hee MR, Fujimoto JG, Lin CP, Puliafito CA. High-speed optical coherence domain reflectometry. *Optics Letters*. 1992;17:151-153.
40. Tearney GJ, Brezinski ME, Bouma BE, et al. In vivo endoscopic optical biopsy with optical coherence tomography. *Science*. 1997;276(5321):2037-2039.
41. Swanson EA, Izatt JA, Hee MR, et al. In vivo retinal imaging by optical coherence tomography. *Optics Letters*. 1993;18(21):1864-1866.
42. Drexler W, Morgner U, Kartner FX, et al. In vivo ultrahigh-resolution optical coherence tomography. *Optics Letters*. 1999;24(17):1221-1223.
43. Radhakrishnan S, Rollins AM, Roth JE, et al. Real-time optical coherence tomography of the anterior segment at 1310 nm. *Arch Ophthalmol*. 2001;119(8):1179-1185.

Chapter 2

Interpretation of the Optical Coherence Tomography Image

Michael R. Hee, MD, PhD; James G. Fujimoto, PhD; Tony Ko, MS; Ji Eun Lee, MD; Joel S. Schuman, MD; Jay Duker, MD; and Carmen A. Puliafito, MD

- Introduction
- Optical Coherence Tomography Image Generation and Optical Properties of Tissue
- Interpreting Optical Coherence Tomography Images of the Normal Retina
- Interpreting Optical Coherence Tomography Images of the Normal Anterior Eye
- Optical Coherence Tomography Scanning and Imaging Protocols
- Quantitative Measurements of Retinal Morphology
- Interpreting Optical Coherence Tomography Images of Retinal Pathologies
- Quality, Artifacts, and Errors in Optical Coherence Tomography Images
- Summary

Introduction

Optical coherence tomography (OCT) generates cross-sectional images of the internal structure in tissues by measuring the echo time delay and intensity of backscattered or backreflected light.[1-5] OCT is a powerful adjunct to the standard clinical techniques of slit-lamp biomicroscopy, indirect ophthalmoscopy, fluorescein angiography, and visual field testing. OCT provides non-contact, real-time, high-resolution, cross-sectional imaging of the eye, which cannot be obtained by any other method.

The interpretation of OCT images is intuitive and provides diagnostically important information on a wide range of pathologies, including macular edema, retinal detachment, alterations in the vitreoretinal interface, macular hole, age-related macular degeneration, diabetic retinopathy, and glaucoma. In addition to providing direct visualization of a cross-sectional slice of retina, thus enabling the identification of alterations in retinal morphology, OCT imaging may also be used to quantitatively measure structures such as retinal thickness or retinal nerve fiber layer thickness. A wide range of OCT scanning protocols may be used to obtain optimum diagnostic information on specific structures such as the macula or optic disc. Computer image-processing may be applied to identify and measure layers of the retina automatically. Quantitative measurements may be displayed with *en face* topographic maps, such as retinal thickness maps, which facilitate direct comparison and registration with fundus images or fluorescein angiography. The ability of OCT to provide direct visualization as well as quantitative information makes it useful to longitudinally track small alterations in tissue structure associated with the progression or resolution of disease.

This chapter provides a brief explanation of how light propagates through tissue, guidelines on how to interpret OCT images of the normal anterior eye and retina as well as key retinal pathologies, and an overview of OCT image-processing for quantitative structural measurement. A more detailed description of scanning protocols is provided in Appendix B.

Optical Coherence Tomography Image Generation and Optical Properties of Tissue

OCT is analogous to conventional ultrasound imaging, except that light, rather than sound, is used so that optical properties rather than acoustic properties of tissues are imaged. OCT generates cross-sectional images of tissue, which depend upon the backreflection or backscattering of light from structures at different depths. OCT image contrast depends upon differences in optical backreflection or backscattering between different types of tissue. Since light that reaches deeper tissue layers must pass through more superficial layers, shadowing effects, similar to those in ultrasound, can sometimes occur. Before discussing the detailed interpretation of OCT images of the retina and anterior eye, it is helpful to consider the general concepts of light propagation through tissue as a basis for interpreting OCT images.

Light incident onto tissue—an optically scattering or turbid medium—is either transmitted, absorbed, or scattered.[6-9] Transmitted light remains unaffected and is free to interact with deeper tissue layers. Absorbed light is essentially removed from the incident beam. Absorption occurs because tissue chromophores, such as hemoglobin or melanin, have absorption spectra that match the energy of the incident light. At the near-infrared wavelengths used in OCT imaging, most of the light absorbed produces only thermal effects, in contrast to visible wavelengths that produce photochemical effects. The average incident optical power used in OCT imaging is extremely low, so the local temperature changes are negligible and well within safe exposure limits. Optical scattering is a property of a heterogeneous medium and occurs because of microscopic spatial variations in the refractive index within tissue. These index variations can be caused by subcellular structures, such as nuclei, cytoplasm, or cell membranes, or bundles of smaller structures, such as nerve fibers or axons. Optical scattering causes incident light to be redirected in multiple directions. Light that completely reverses direction when scattered is called *backscattered* light. Backreflection of light can also occur when light is incident on a boundary between two homogenous materials that have different indices of refraction.

In tissues that are strongly absorbing or scattering, the intensity of the incident beam decreases exponentially with depth at a rate characterized by an absorption or scattering coefficient. In tissues other than the eye, attenuation of the optical beam from scattering limits the image penetration depth for OCT imaging, although the high sensitivity of OCT enables the detection of light from depths up to 2 mm in most scattering tissues.[10,11] In ophthalmic imaging, the retina backscatters weakly, generating low optical signal levels. In this case, the high sensitivity of OCT allows these weak optical signals to be detected so that retinal tissues can be imaged, although they are virtually transparent.

OCT imaging is performed by detecting the echo time delay and intensity of backscattered and backreflected light. When a beam of light is incident onto tissue, it is first attenuated by absorption and scattering as it propagates into the tissue. Then, the light is backscattered by structures at different depths. Finally, the returning light is attenuated by absorption and scattering as it propagates out of the tissue before being detected by the OCT instrument. OCT imaging depends upon the ability to resolve the time-of-flight of the detected light in order to distinguish the echo reflections from tissue structures at different depths. In addition, OCT also uses the spatial properties of the focused light beam to eliminate unwanted scattered light. As a result, the OCT image may be considered to be comprised of "single backscattered" light (ie, light that has propagated into tissue, has been backscattered once from the structure being imaged, and has then propagated out of the tissue). The strength of the OCT signal from a particular tissue structure at a given depth is defined by the amount of incident light that is transmitted without absorption or scattering to that depth layer, by the proportion of this light that is directly backscattered, and by the fraction of the directly backscattered light that returns to the detector. Specular reflections can also occur at the boundary of two media that have different indices of refraction, such as between the tear film and cornea in the anterior eye. When there is strong absorption or scattering, such as from hemorrhage, light is strongly attenuated and shadowing of deeper structures can occur.

It is important to note that although OCT images display the true dimensions of the structures being imaged (after correcting for index of refraction and refraction effects), the contrast in the OCT images arises from different mechanisms than in histopathology. Thus, care must be taken in interpreting OCT images because they are not analogous to conventional histology. In histology, selective stains are used to identify specific cellular or subcelluar features. In OCT, image contrast arises from differences in tissue optical properties. In the next sections, we describe examples of OCT imaging of the normal retina and anterior eye, as well as selected retinal pathologies, in order to provide a baseline for OCT image interpretation.

Interpreting Optical Coherence Tomography Images of the Normal Retina

Papillomacular Axis

OCT can visualize the cross-sectional structure of the retina and posterior eye.[2] Figure 2-1A shows a large field-of-view OCT tomogram of the normal retina, including both the macular and peripapillary region. The image was performed with 10 micron (µm) axial resolution at 800-nanometer (nm) wavelength. The image spans a transverse width of 10 mm and is shown in the fundus photograph of Figure 2-1B. Because the retina is very thin but

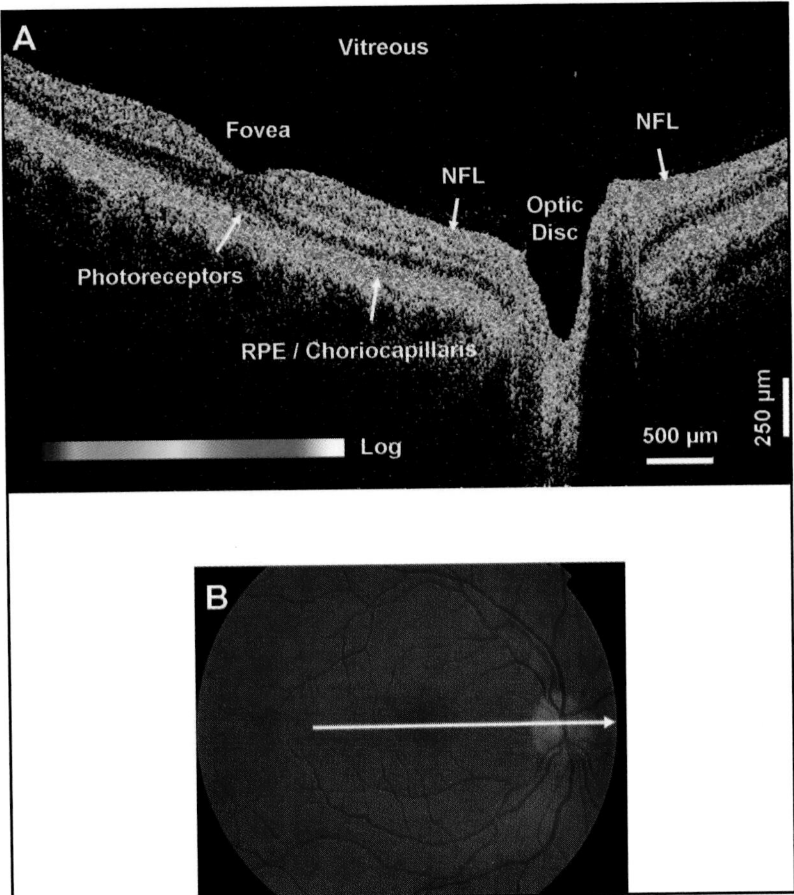

Figure 2-1. OCT tomogram (A) of a normal fovea and optic disc taken along the papillomacular axis. The OCT scan is 10 mm long and its location is shown on a corresponding fundus photograph (B). The fovea and optic disc are identifiable by their characteristic morphology, and the layered structure of the retina is apparent. The retinal NFL is highly reflective and increases in thickness toward the disc.

the transverse field of view is large, the OCT image is expanded in the axial direction in order to better visualize the microstructure of the retina. Large-scale anatomic features of the retina, such as the fovea, optic disc, retinal profile, and curvature, are evident, and they can be identified by their characteristic morphology.

The vitreoretinal interface is identified by the increase in backscattering between the transparent vitreous and the surface of the inner retina. The fovea appears as a characteristic thinning of the retina with the absence of inner retinal layers and an increase in thickness of the photoreceptor layer. The optic disc appears with the characteristic contour of the optic nerve. A highly scattering layer, which is visible as red in the false-color image, delineates the posterior boundary of the retina in the tomogram and corresponds to the retinal pigment epithelium (RPE) and choriocapillaris. A second, closely spaced, highly scattering layer, which is immediately anterior, arises from a reflection between the inner and outer segments of the photoreceptors. These posterior layers terminate at the margin of the optic disc and are consistent with the termination of choroidal circulation at the lamina cribrosa. Posterior to the choriocapillaris, relatively weak signals are visible from the deep choroid and sclera due to attenuation of the optical beam after passing through the retina, RPE, and choriocapillaris. A variable thickness, highly scattering layer at the inner margin of the retina, which is visible as red in the false-color image, corresponds to the nerve fiber layer (NFL). The NFL is thicker in the region of the optic disc and becomes thinner toward the macula. The other inner retinal layers also become thinner approaching the fovea, with only the outer nuclear layer and photoreceptors present in the fovea, in agreement with well-established retinal morphology.

Retinal Microstructure

OCT images can also visualize the microscopic anatomy of the retina. Figure 2-2A shows an OCT image of the normal macula. The image is 6 mm in transverse width, consists of 512 transverse pixels, and is oriented in the temporal-nasal direction. Figure 2-2B shows a higher magnification OCT image of the normal fovea. The OCT image is 3 mm in transverse width and consists of 512 transverse pixels. The microstructure of the various retinal layers can be differentiated in the OCT image and correlates with the well-known morphology of the retina in the foveal and parafoveal region.[12-15] For comparison, Figure 2-2B (bottom) shows a schematic of the different retinal cell types. Histologically, the retina can be seen as divided into 10 distinct layers, including four cell layers and two layers of neuronal interconnections. Several of these layers can be resolved in ophthalmic OCT images. The interpretation of OCT imaging is supported by studies that compare OCT to histology, as well as ultrahigh-resolution OCT imaging studies.[16-20] The interpretation of features in OCT images is also confirmed by imaging pathologies that produce known alterations of retinal architecture.

The NFL and plexiform layers consist of axonal structures that are highly optically backscattering and appear as red in the false-color OCT images. In contrast, nuclear layers are weakly backscattering and appear as blue-black. The first highly backscattering layer, visible nasal to the fovea, is the NFL. This layer is thin in the macular region. The three, weakly backscattering layers are the ganglion cell layer (GCL), inner nuclear layer (INL), and outer nuclear layer (ONL). The GCL increases in thickness in the parafoveal region. The moderately backscattering inner plexiform layer (IPL) is adjacent to the GCL and INL. The obliquely running photoreceptor axons, sometimes considered as a separate layer in the outer plexiform layer (OPL) known as *Henle's fiber layer*, are highly backscattering.

The boundary between the photoreceptor inner segments (IS) and outer segments (OS) is visible as a thin, highly backscattering band immediately anterior to the RPE and choroid. The reflection arising from this structure may be the result of a refractive index difference between the photoreceptor IS and the highly organized structure of the OS, which contain stacks of membranous discs, rich in the visual pigment rhodopsin.[14,15,21] The thickness of the photoreceptor IS and OS increases in the foveal region, which corresponds to the well-known increase in the length of the OS of the cones in this region. The external limiting membrane (ELM) can sometimes be visualized a thin backscattering layer posterior to the ONL and anterior to the boundary between the photoreceptor IS and OS. The ELM is not a physical membrane but is an alignment of structures between the photoreceptors and the Müller cells.

The RPE, which contains melanin, is a very strongly backscattering layer. Bruch's membrane, which is only 1 to 4 µm thick, cannot be visualized as an independent structure. Finally, the choriocapillaris is vascular and strongly backscattering. Since the RPE is in close contact with the choriocapillaris, it is often not distinguishable as a separate layer in the OCT images. The vascular structures of the choriocapillaris and choroid are highly optically scattering, and they produce shadowing effects that limit the OCT imaging depth for deeper structures. In some cases, retinal blood vessels can be identified by their increased backscatter and by their shadowing of the deeper structures.

Optic Nerve Head

OCT images can directly visualize the contour of the optic disc. Figure 2-3 shows an OCT image of the normal optic disc. The contour of the optic disc is demarcated by the boundary between the low backscattering vitreous and the highly backscattering NFL. The normal cupping of the disc is evident. The OCT image shows an increase in NFL thickness approaching the neuroretinal rim where the NFL is nearly the entire thickness of the retina. The retinal nerve fibers exhibit a directional reflectance. The reflected signal intensity from the nerve fibers decreases at the disc rim where the nerve fibers are no longer perpendicular to the incident OCT optical beam, but bend into the optic nerve head.

The RPE and choriocapillaris are visible as a highly backscattering layer that terminates at the lamina cribrosa. The boundary between the photoreceptor IS and OS is also visible as a thin, highly backscattering feature immediately anterior to the RPE and choroid. The photoreceptor layer and RPE terminate in the region approaching the disc and can be used as a landmark to define the disc margin. The IPL and OPL are moderately reflective, while the INL and ONL are weakly reflective.

OCT imaging of the optic nerve and neuroretinal rim is valuable in assessing glaucoma or neuro-ophthalmic diseases. In evaluating the contour of the disc, it is important to note that OCT images are often displayed with an expanded scale in the axial direction in order to allow better visualization of the thin retinal layers while still encompassing a several-millimeter transverse scan. Quantitative morphometry of the images using the correct axial and transverse scales are, therefore, important. The

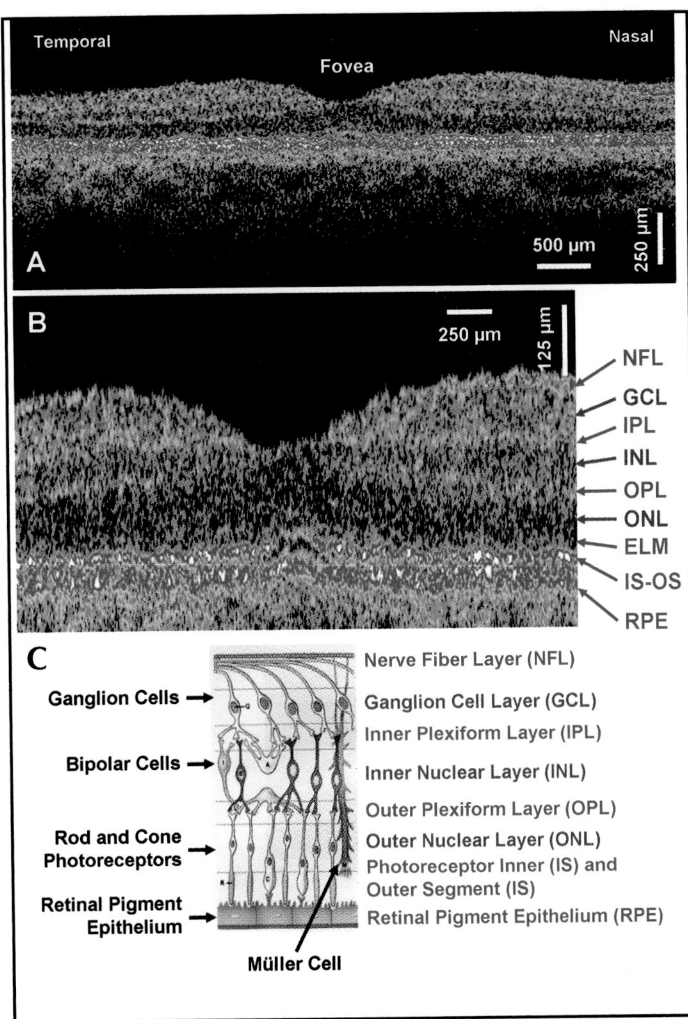

Figure 2-2. OCT images (A and B) of the macular region. (A) OCT image with 6 mm transverse width and 512 transverse pixels. (B) High magnification OCT image with 3 mm transverse width and 512 transverse pixels. The images are shown expanded in the vertical direction for better visibility. The NFL is highly backscattering. The IPL and OPL are more highly scattering than the INL and ONL. There is an isolated reflection from the boundary between the IS and OS of the photoreceptors. A small reflection from the ELM can sometimes be seen immediately anterior to this feature. The RPE and choriocapillaris are visible as a highly backscattering boundary at the posterior retina. (C) Morphology of the retina. The retina can be divided into 10 distinct layers, including four cell layers and two layers of neuronal interconnections. Proceeding from inner retina to the outer retina, these layers are the inner limiting membrane (not shown), the nerve fiber layer, ganglion cell layer, inner plexiform layer, inner nuclear layer, outer plexiform layer, outer nuclear layer, the external limiting membrane (not shown), the inner and outer segments of the photoreceptor layer, and the retinal pigment epithelium. The choriocapillaris and choroid are immediately posterior to the RPE.

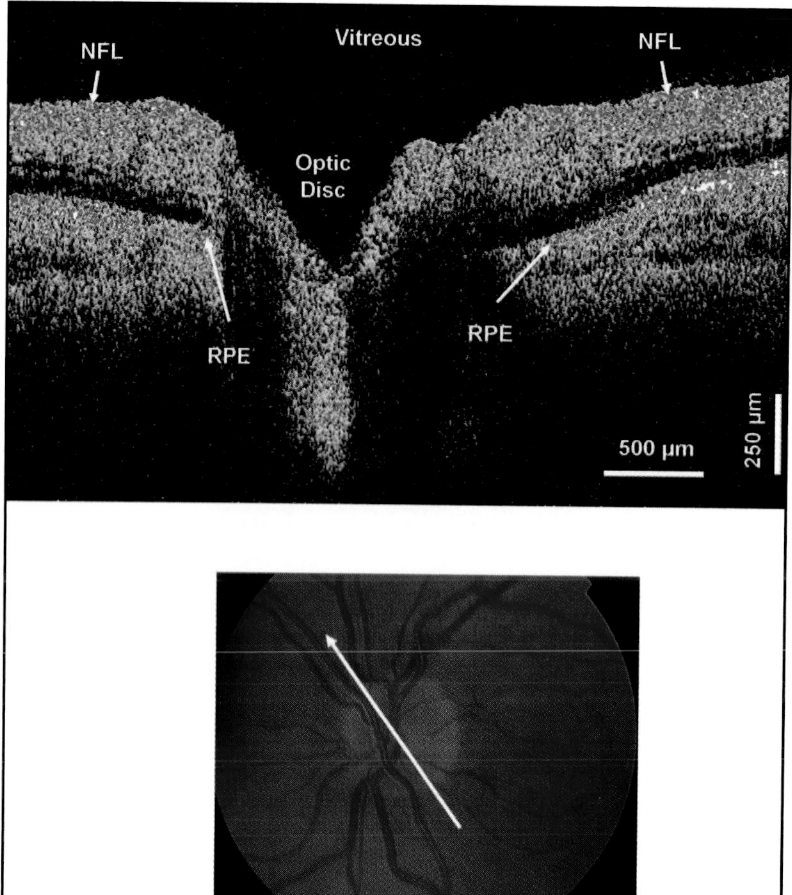

Figure 2-3. OCT showing the cross-section of the optic nerve head. The NFL is visible and increases in thickness approaching the disc rim. The termination of the RPE/choriocapillaris and photoreceptors near the lamina cribrosa can be clearly visualized. Disc parameters such as cup and disc diameter, neuroretinal rim area, and cup-to-disc ratio may be measured using this feature as a landmark.

use of intelligent algorithms to assess the morphology of the optic disc will be discussed in a later section.

Circular Tomograms in the Peripapillary Region

Documentation of NFL thickness and degeneration in the peripapillary region is important in the diagnosis and treatment of glaucoma. A protocol used to assess the NFL was developed by Schuman and Hee and was introduced in 1995.[22-24] Circumpapillary OCT scans are performed, creating cylindrical sections of the retina centered around the optic disc so that all nerves emanating from the nerve head cross the OCT image plane. Figure 2-4 shows circumpapillary OCT scans with diameters of 2.3 mm and 3.4 mm centered on the nerve head. The region scanned is shown in the corresponding fundus photograph. The OCT image is displayed "unwrapped," and the superior, inferior, temporal, and nasal quadrants around the optic nerve head are labeled.

The NFL is visible as a well-demarcated, highly backscattering layer in the OCT image. The thickness of the NFL varies with position around the optic nerve head, with the thickest NFL corresponding to the superotemporal and inferotemporal nerve fiber bundles. The RPE and choriocapillaris, as well as the junction between the inner and outer segments of the photoreceptors, are evident as thin, highly backscattering layers at the posterior surface of the retina. Retinal vessels originating from the optic disc can be visualized in cross section and are evident by

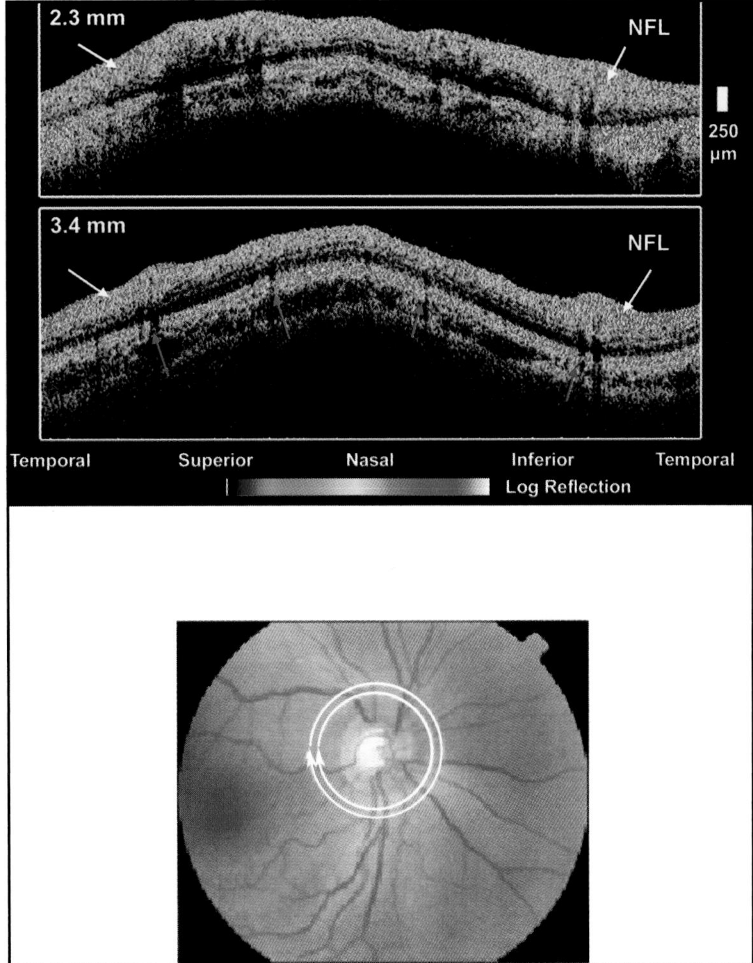

Figure 2-4. Circumpapillary OCT image used to assess the NFL. Circular OCT tomograms acquired around the optic disc at diameters of 2.3 and 3.4 mm. The cylindrical sections correspond to a clockwise scan around the disc and are displayed unwrapped. The superotemporal and inferotemporal bundling of the NFL is evident (white arrows). Retinal blood vessels are evident by their shadowing of the RPE and choriocapillaris (red arrows). The location of the scan is shown on the corresponding fundus photograph.

their increased backscatter and by their shadowing of deeper structures. The retinal NFL can be detected automatically using segmentation or boundary detection algorithms and its thickness quantitatively measured. These image-processing and analysis techniques will be discussed in a later section.

Interpreting Optical Coherence Tomography Images of the Normal Anterior Eye

Anterior Chamber

In addition to retinal imaging, OCT can also be used to image the anterior eye.[3,25] Figure 2-5 shows OCT imaging of the anterior chamber of a normal human eye. The image has 15 to 20 µm axial resolution, using a wavelength of 1300 nm. In comparison to the 800 nm light source typically used for retinal imaging, the longer wavelength used for imaging the anterior eye reduces the attenuation from optical scattering and enables increased image penetration depth and better visualization of the angle.[10,11,26] In addition, since the safe ocular exposure limit is higher for longer wavelength light, higher incident powers than those used in retinal imaging can be used to image the anterior eye, allowing high-speed image acquisition at several frames per second.

Figure 2-5A shows clearly identifiable structures, including the cornea, sclera, iris, and lens anterior capsule. The strongest signals arise from the epithelial surface of the cornea and the highly scattering sclera and iris. Smaller amounts of backscatter are visible from within the nominally transparent cornea and lens. The backscatter intensity gradually decreases from central to peripheral cornea. This signal fading may be related to highly angle-dependent backscattering from the stromal collagen lamellae, which runs parallel to the corneal surface. The limbus appears as the angled interface between the cornea and the sclera. The normal "watch glass" insertion of the cornea into the sclera is clearly visible. Structures in the angle are also visible. Because light is refracted or bent when it is incident at an angle between two media with different indices of refraction, such as the air and the cornea, the OCT image of the anterior chamber must be corrected for this refraction in order to correctly show the geometry of the anterior chamber. This correction can be performed with computer image-processing techniques.[25] Clinically relevant parameters may be quantitatively extracted from the image, including corneal thickness and curvature, anterior chamber depth, and anterior chamber angle.

Cornea and Angle

By narrowing the field of view, higher transverse magnification images of the anterior eye can be obtained. A close-up view of the angle region (see Figure 2-5B) shows the iris contour and epithelium, the corneoscleral limbus, and the anterior chamber angle. Structures in the angle region, such as the trabecular meshwork, ciliary body, and Schlemm's canal, aren't visualized as well, since light is attenuated after penetrating the overlying scleral tissue. Figure 2-5C shows a higher magnification view of the cornea, again highlighting the demarcation between the epithelium and stroma.

Optical Coherence Tomography Scanning and Imaging Protocols

Image Pixel Density and Acquisition Speed

OCT images are generated by performing a sequence of rapid axial measurements of backreflected or backscattered light at successive transverse positions. Therefore, the transverse image resolution, or pixel density, is directly related to the acquisition time. Fast image acquisition time implies low pixel density, while higher pixel density requires a longer image acquisition time.

Current OCT instruments scan at a rate of approximately 400 axial scans per second. Figure 2-6 demonstrates the tradeoff between transverse resolution and acquisition speed. The image in Figure 2-6A has a high (512) transverse pixel density, but it requires T = 512/400 = 1.28 seconds to acquire. In contrast, the image in Figure 2-6B can be acquired in T = 128/400 = 0.32 seconds, but has low (128) transverse pixel density. Higher transverse pixel density (512 and higher transverse pixels) images are typically used to image macular pathology because they display more retinal detail, but they take longer to acquire and are increasingly subject to eye motion artifacts. Lower transverse pixel density images can be acquired very rapidly and are less sensitive to eye motion. These images are typically used when mapping the optic nerve head contour or retinal thickness in order to minimize eye motion artifacts.

The fundamental resolution of the OCT instrument can be different from the pixel density in an image. In the transverse direction, the resolution of the OCT instrument is determined by the spot size of the OCT light beam on the retina. Typical ophthalmic OCT instruments employ a spot size of approximately 20 µm. A typical OCT scan across the macula is 6 mm in length, so an image containing 128 transverse pixels has a transverse pixel size of 6 mm/128 = 48 µm. In contrast, a 512 pixel image has a transverse pixel size of 6 mm/512 = 11.7 µm. Thus, the pixel size in the transverse direction for a low-density, fast-acquisition image is much coarser than the actual transverse resolution of the instrument.

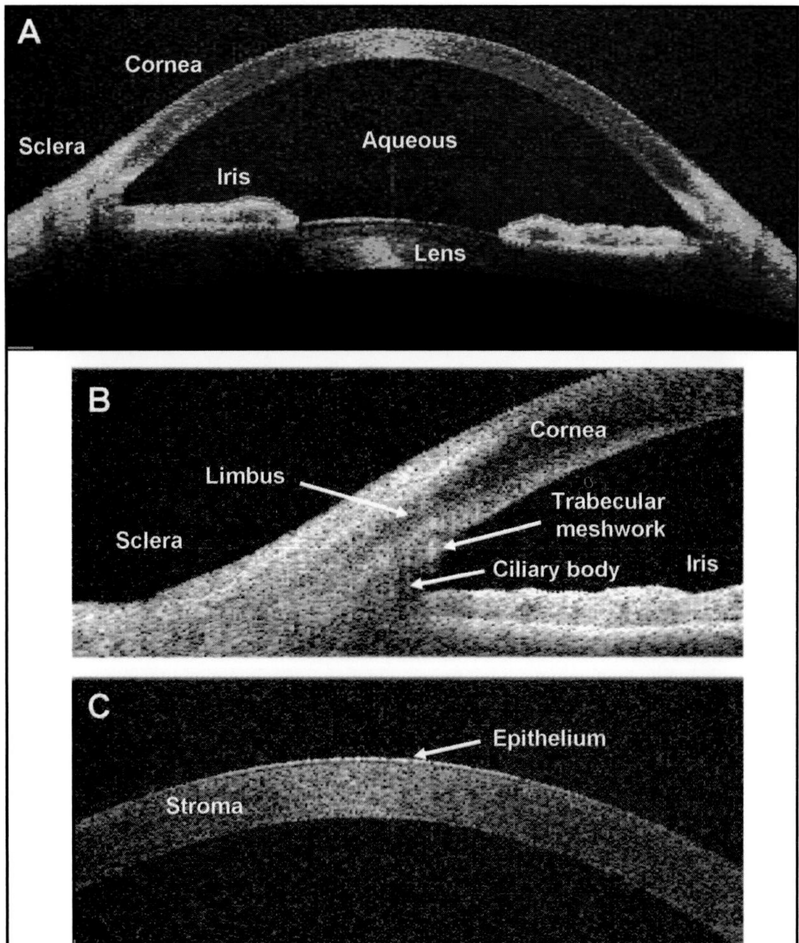

Figure 2-5. OCT imaging of the anterior eye. Imaging was performed at a wavelength of 1300 nm in order to reduce scattering and to improve image penetration. (A) OCT image of a normal anterior eye chamber. The anterior and posterior surfaces of the cornea are evident as well as the angle. The iris produces shadowing of the lens, and the lens is visible through the pupil of the iris. The anterior lens capsule and scattering from within the lens are also evident. (B) Higher magnification, narrower field of view, OCT image of the normal anterior chamber angle. OCT imaging can measure the angle. Features such as the trabecular meshwork and ciliary body can be visualized but are shadowed by the sclera. (C) Higher magnification OCT image of the normal cornea showing the contrast in optical reflectivity between the corneal epithelium and stroma. (Courtesy of Carl Zeiss Meditec.)

In the axial or longitudinal direction, a typical retinal OCT image is 2 mm deep in tissue and consists of 1024 pixels, leading to a longitudinal pixel size of 2 mm/1024 = 1.9 µm. The number of axial pixels is determined by the analog-to-digital (A/D) sampling rate of the instrument, which can be made as fast as necessary and usually does not limit the image acquisition time. In contrast, the fundamental axial or longitudinal resolution of the instrument is approximately 10 µm and is determined by the coherence length of the light source. Therefore, the pixel size in the axial direction is much finer that the axial resolution of the instrument, thus providing good visualization of fine features. A more detailed discussion of the imaging parameters governing resolution and pixel density is presented in Appendix A.

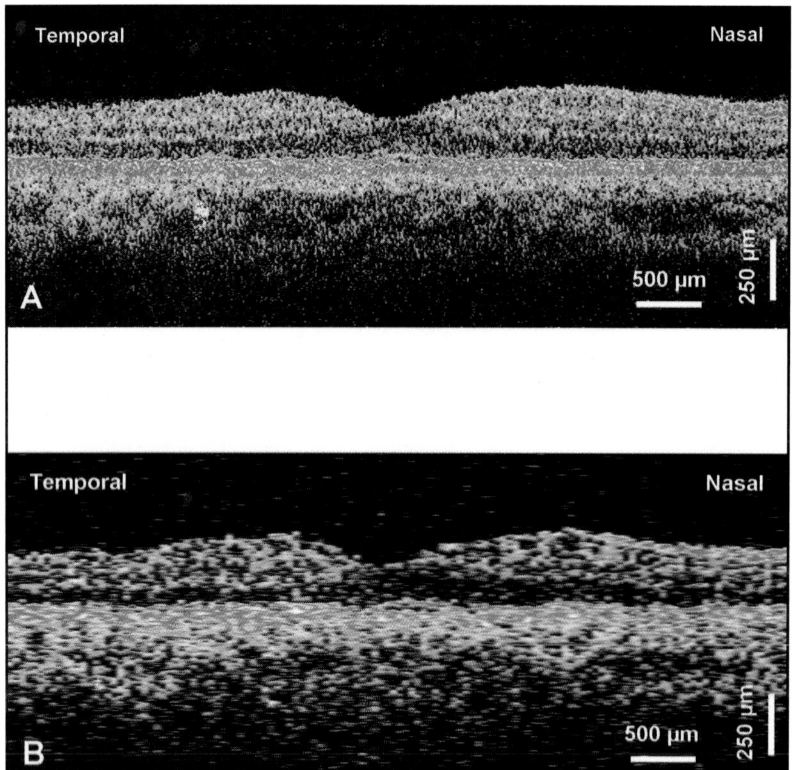

Figure 2-6. Pixel density versus image acquisition speed. (A) High transverse pixel density, slow acquisition image. The image consists of 512 transverse pixels and is acquired in 1.3 seconds. High pixel density images provide more detail of retinal architecture. (B) Low transverse pixel density, fast acquisition image. The image consists of 128 transverse pixels and is acquired in 0.3 seconds. High-speed images have less motion artifacts and are useful in more complex three-dimensional scanning protocols.

Serial Raster Scans Through the Macula

In analogy to other imaging modalities, such as X-ray, computed tomography (CT), or magnetic resonance imaging (MRI), information on three-dimensional structure may be obtained by using the optical sectioning capability of OCT to acquire serial images of consecutive slices through the retina. As an example, Figure 2-7 shows six horizontal OCT images obtained consecutively from the macula of a human subject with a lateral displacement of 200 μm between each image. The locations of each OCT scan on the retina are labeled on a corresponding fundus photograph in Figure 2-7.

Characteristic features of the retina appear consistently in the serial sections. The anterior and posterior surfaces of the neural retina are demarcated by backscattering at the NFL and the highly backscattering red layer that represents the RPE and choriocapillaris. The sequence of images shows cross sections of the foveal depression, which reaches its maximal depth at the fovea centralis. As expected, the ONL is thickest and most pronounced in the image through the fovea centralis. Serial scans of this type are often helpful in visualizing the three-dimensional extent of structural alterations of the macula, such as macular holes or edema.[2]

Serial Radial Tomograms Through the Optic Disc

OCT imaging can be performed with an arbitrary orientation of the cross-sectional imaging plane. Figure 2-8 displays OCT images taken through radial planes with different angular orientations, each passing through the center of the optic nerve head. The orientation of each image is labeled on a corresponding fundus photograph and corresponds to planes oriented along different clock hours as shown in Figure 2-8. In the 90 degree tomogram (perpendicular to the papillomacular axis), high backscattering (red) is visible from the NFL and from a band defining the posterior boundary of the sensory retina, which corresponds to the RPE and choriocapillaris. The OCT image shows the NFL increasing in thickness

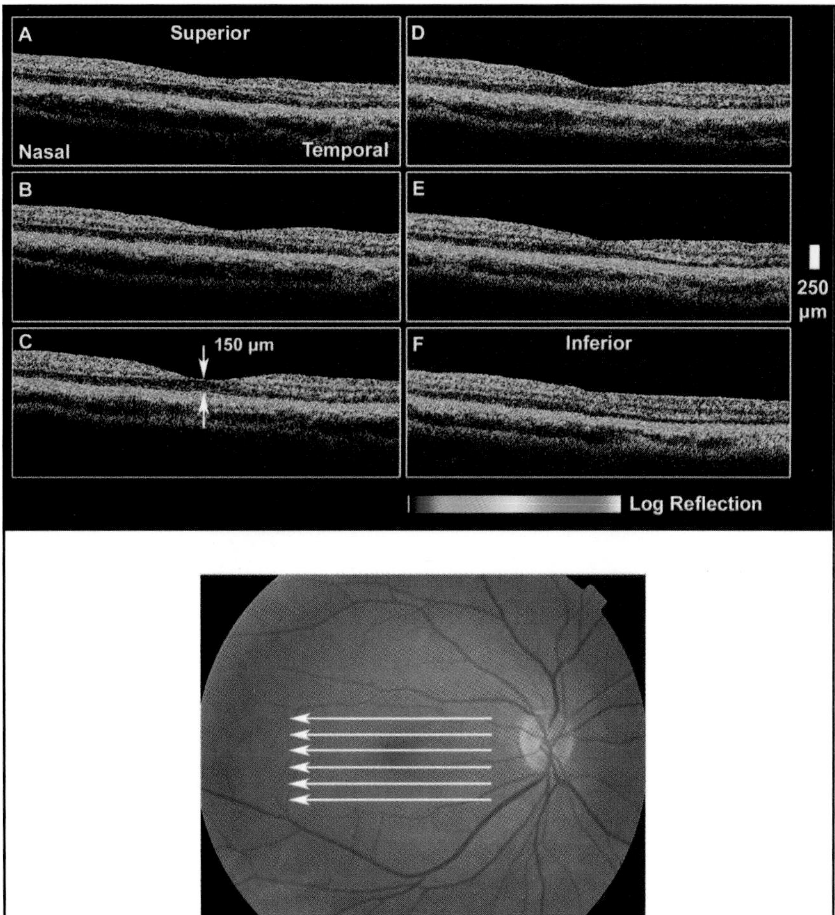

Figure 2-7. (A to F) Serial horizontal tomograms through the normal macula showing the three-dimensional structure of the fovea. The location of the scans is shown on the corresponding fundus photograph (bottom). Serial OCT images show the normal foveal contour with the increase in the GCL thickness and an absence of layers other than the photoreceptor layer in the foveola. This scanning pattern provides comprehensive coverage of the macula.

toward the optic disc to occupy nearly the entire retinal thickness, which is commensurate with the presence of the inferior and superior arcuate nerve fiber bundles. In comparison, the 0 degree tomogram (taken parallel to the papillomacular axis) exhibits a thinner NFL, which is consistent with fewer nerve fibers in this area. The surface contour and normal cupping of the disc are visualized in all of the tomograms. The termination of the RPE and choroid as well as the photoreceptors at the lamina cribrosa are also visible.

This scanning protocol is useful for assessing the profile of the optic disc and for comparing nerve fiber thickness through different planes. Intelligent algorithms can be applied to measure features of the optic disc such as the disc, cup, and rim diameter, as well as two-dimensional features such as the disc, cup, and rim areas, and cup-to-disc ratios. These will be discussed in more detail in a later section.

A similar radial scanning protocol can be used to assess the macula. Six OCT images can be taken through radial planes with different angular orientations, each passing through the fovea. This set of images provides a means of imaging the entire macula, including extrafoveal pathologies, while still allowing each individual image to intercept the fovea. In combination with segmentation or boundary detection algorithms, this scanning protocol enables macular thickness to be topographically mapped.[27]

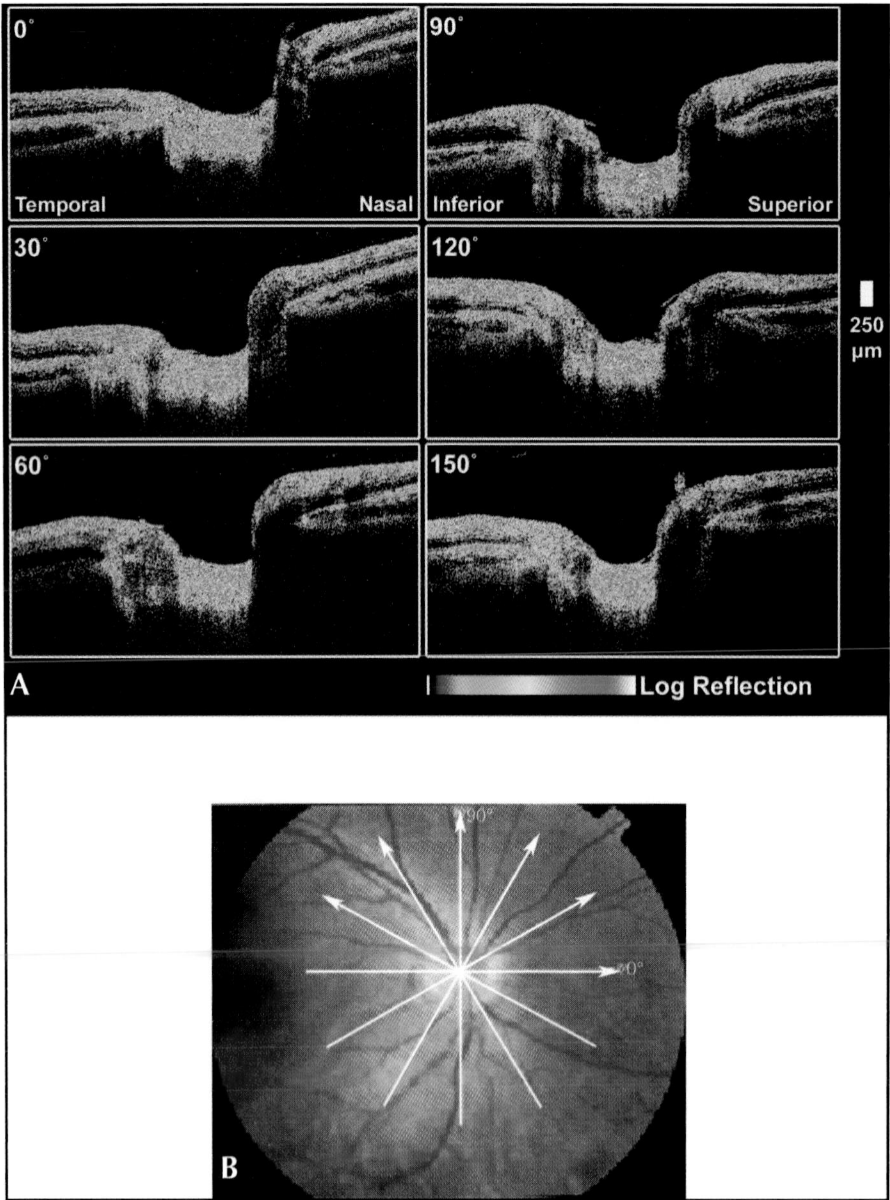

Figure 2-8. Radial OCT sections (A) through the optic disc and peripapillary region taken at equally spaced angular orientations showing the three-dimensional structure of the disc. The contour of the disc, including cupping, is well visualized. The location of the scans is shown on the corresponding fundus photograph (B). This scan pattern is useful for mapping the optic disc. A similar scan pattern can be used to map the macula.

Quantitative Measurements of Retinal Morphology

Detection of Retinal Layers by Segmentation

OCT is especially powerful for diagnosing and monitoring conditions such as retinal NFL atrophy in glaucoma or macular edema associated with diabetic retinopathy because it can provide quantitative information on retinal morphology. OCT images can be analyzed quantitatively and processed using intelligent algorithms to extract features such as retinal or retinal NFL thickness.[22-24,27] Mapping and display techniques have been developed to represent the image data in alternate forms, such as topographic thickness maps, in order to better facilitate interpretation.

Retinal Thickness Measurement

Computer image-processing algorithms have been developed to automatically identify the superficial and deep neurosensory retinal boundaries to measure retinal thickness. The measurement of retinal thickness is important in quantifying macular edema or abnormal fluid accumulation within the neurosensory retina, which often leads to retinal thickening. Macular edema is a potential consequence of many ocular conditions such as diabetic retinopathy, epiretinal membrane formation, ocular inflammation, retinal vascular occlusion, and cataract extraction. It is important to measure macular thickness in order to track the progression and treatment of macular edema. Macular thickness measurement might also be a potentially useful screening method for the development of macular edema, especially in patients with diabetes.

The challenge is to identify the retinal boundaries, despite varying intraretinal morphology and signal-to-noise conditions in the images. Retinal morphology may be disrupted in many diseases. Diabetic retinopathy, in particular, often leads to the presence of hard exudate and cyst formation, which manifest as abnormally high or low intraretinal backscattering, respectively. Signal-to-noise conditions can vary with instrument alignment, cataracts, and other media opacity. In high signal-to-noise conditions and in ocular inflammation, intravitreal reflections might be confused with retinal reflections. In low signal-to-noise conditions, retinal reflections are minimally visible, particularly in the fovea. The signal-to-noise ratio can vary within a given OCT image (eg, if the pupil obstructs part of the scanning beam). Although automated image-processing algorithms are reasonably robust, if the OCT image quality is sufficiently degraded, it is possible to have incorrect measurements or artifacts. Therefore, it is important to assess the quality of OCT images and the results of automated image-processing. The impact of image quality on the performance of image-processing algorithms will be discussed in more detail in a later section.

The first step in quantitatively measuring retinal thickness is boundary detection, which is also known as *segmentation.* Boundary detection algorithms have been developed that consist of the following steps: smoothing, edge detection, and error correction. Special consideration is required to achieve good performance in low signal-to-noise conditions. Figure 2-9A shows an example of a processed image of the macula that has been segmented to detect retinal thickness. The lines in the image are produced automatically by the image-processing algorithm. The anterior boundary of the retina is assumed to lie at the vitreoretinal interface and is detected from the increase in backscattering signal that occurs at this interface. The boundary between the IS and OS of the photoreceptor layer is identified by detecting the thin, high backscattering boundary at the posterior retina.

After the anterior and posterior boundaries of the retina have been detected on the OCT image, the retinal thickness at any transverse position can be measured, as shown in Figure 2-9B. In addition, average measurements may be performed over a range of transverse positions. As noted previously, both the junction between the photoreceptor IS and OS and the RPE/choriocapillaris complex produce a high backscattering signal. These two features are not always resolved separately in all OCT images. Current retinal thickness image-processing techniques detect the most anterior feature. Although this measurement does not always include the photoreceptor's OS in the retinal thickness measurement, the approach has the advantage of being very robust, and it can be used on a wide range of images with varying signal-to-noise quality and different pathologies. Absolute anatomic measurement of the retinal thickness is not as critical for diagnostic purposes as is the ability to perform measurements in a robust and consistent manner.

Retinal Topographic Mapping and Analysis

The utility of OCT in clinical practice depends on the ability of the physician to accurately and quickly interpret the OCT results in the context of conventional clinical examination. In standard ophthalmoscopic examination, retinal features are assessed on the appearance of the fundus. Therefore, topographic methods of displaying retinal and NFL thickness, which could be directly and intuitively compared with fundus examination, were developed for OCT. In these methods, multiple OCT cross-sectional images are acquired in a variety of scan patterns on the retina in order to create a three-dimensional data set. Then, retinal or NFL thickness can be extracted to form a two-dimensional topographic data set that can also be displayed in false color.

Measurement of retinal thickness in the macula is particularly important in patients with diabetic macular edema, where it is necessary to determine whether macular thickening involves the fovea. Thus, a scanning pattern is used that concentrates measurements in the central fovea, where accurate information is most important, and enables the distance to the central fovea of any macular thickening to be measured accurately. A protocol for scanning and topographically displaying macular thickness with OCT was developed by Hee et al.[27] Six consecutive OCT scans are obtained at equally spaced angular orientations in a radial spoke pattern centered on the fovea. The retinal thickness data are displayed in two complementary manners, as shown in Figure 2-9C. For quantitative interpretation, the macula is divided into

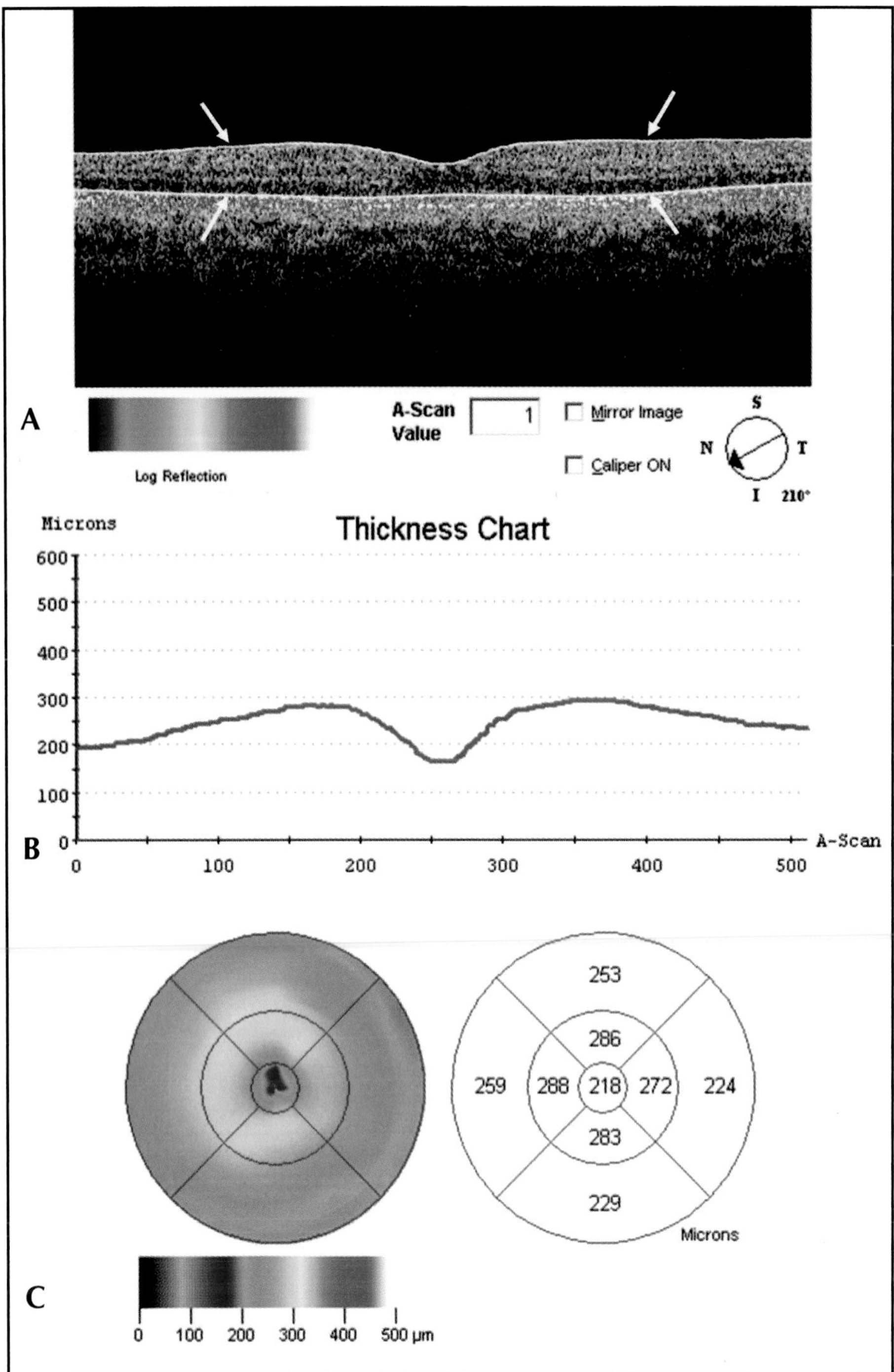

Figure 2-9. Computer image-processing to quantitatively measure retinal features. Measurement of retinal thickness. (A) Image of the macula that has been computer processed to perform boundary detection or segmentation in order to measure retinal thickness. The anterior and posterior retinal surfaces are automatically identified. (B) Quantitative measurement of retinal thickness based on the segmented OCT image. (C) Topographic map of retinal thickness in the macula. The topographic map is constructed by processing multiple OCT scans in the macula, measuring the retinal thickness profile of these scans, and estimating or interpolating the retinal thickness in the regions between the scans. The retinal thickness is represented by a color table. This display has the advantage that it can be directly compared with the fundus image.

nine regions, including a central circle of 500 μm radius (the foveal region), and an inner and outer ring, each divided into four quadrants, with outer diameters of one and two disc diameters, respectively. An average retinal thickness is reported for each of the nine regions. Retinal thickness for every point within two disc diameters from the center can also be converted to a false-color topographic thickness map. Bilinear interpolation in polar coordinates is performed to estimate thicknesses in the wedged regions between the radial OCT scans. Retinal thickness values between 0 and 500 mm are displayed by colors ranging from blue to red.

The ability to reduce image information to numerical information is important because it allows a normative database to be developed and statistics to be calculated. The topographic thickness mapping protocol demonstrates how OCT images can be processed to yield different levels of diagnostic information and detail. On the coarsest level, the foveal thickness—a single number—can provide a diagnostic indicator of central macular edema in a patient. This type of information might be useful in a screening context in which a high-risk patient population (eg, patients with insulin-dependent diabetes) is screened for macular edema in a nonspecialist setting. On the next, more detailed level, regional retinal thickness values can be used to more specifically localize the presence of macular edema and to improve the statistical accuracy of the assessment. The topographic false-color map provides more graphic information that can be compared directly to the fundus image of the retina. Finally, the original OCT images contain the most specific information on retinal pathology and can be interpreted to diagnose the presence of other retinal pathologies, in addition to macular edema.

Retinal Nerve Fiber Layer Thickness Measurement

Precise measurement of retinal NFL thickness is useful for evaluating patients with glaucoma, for distinguishing between patients with papilledema and crowded optic nerves, and for evaluating other neurodegenerative diseases. Computer image-processing algorithms have been developed to estimate NFL thickness from circumpapillary OCT images acquired in cylindrical sections surrounding the optic disc. A circumpapillary scan pattern, which is typically 3.4 mm diameter, is used because this effectively intercepts all of the nerve fibers that emanate from the optic disc while avoiding inaccurate measurements resulting from peripapillary atrophy.[22-24] This pattern also enables quantitative measurement of the circumferential variation in NFL thickness around the optic disc and visualization of the nerve fiber bundles.

In OCT, the NFL appears as a highly backscattering "red" layer at the vitreoretinal interface. Again, the challenge is to develop image-processing methods that are relatively insensitive to varying morphology or signal-to-noise conditions in the images. As in the measurement of retinal thickness, the first step in image-processing is boundary detection or segmentation. Figure 2-10A shows an example of a processed circumpapillary OCT image that has been segmented to detect NFL thickness. The lines in the image are produced automatically by the image-processing algorithm. The anterior boundary of the NFL is assumed to lie at the vitreoretinal interface. The posterior boundary of the NFL must occur between the vitreoretinal interface and boundary of the posterior retina. The most commonly used method to detect the posterior boundary of the NFL is to detect the edge of the NFL, based upon changes in the optical backscattering signal intensity. After image smoothing, each A-mode scan, which corresponds to a vertical line of pixels in the image, is evaluated in order to detect where the signal crosses a threshold level representing the posterior boundary of the NFL. Information from adjacent A-mode scans is also incorporated to assist boundary detection and to correct errors. The NFL boundary detection algorithms are more sensitive to OCT image quality variations than the simpler retinal thickness measurement algorithms. Therefore, special care is required to ensure that the initial OCT images are of sufficient quality before accepting the results of automated NFL measurements.

Nerve Fiber Layer Thickness Analysis

NFL thickness can be analyzed and displayed in several complementary ways. Figure 2-10B shows an example of an NFL analysis from a standard 3.4 mm diameter circumpapillary OCT scan of a normal subject. The measurement can be displayed as a graph of the NFL thickness versus the position around the optic nerve head. Average values of NFL thickness can be calculated in the four quadrants around the optic disc (ie, superior, inferior, nasal, temporal) or the 12 o'clock position sectors around the optic disc. Finally, the average NFL thickness around the entire disc can also be calculated. These display conventions enable the graph of NFL thickness versus position to be simplified and reduced to numerical values.

In order to be used for screening or diagnosis, measured values of the NFL thickness may be compared to a normative database. A normative database accounts for the variation in NFL thickness among normal subjects in the population and may be used to assess the probability that a given NFL thickness measurement is abnormal. Since normal subjects lose retinal nerve fibers as a function of age, this normative database must be age adjusted. Figure 2-10C shows an example of a circumpapillary NFL thick-

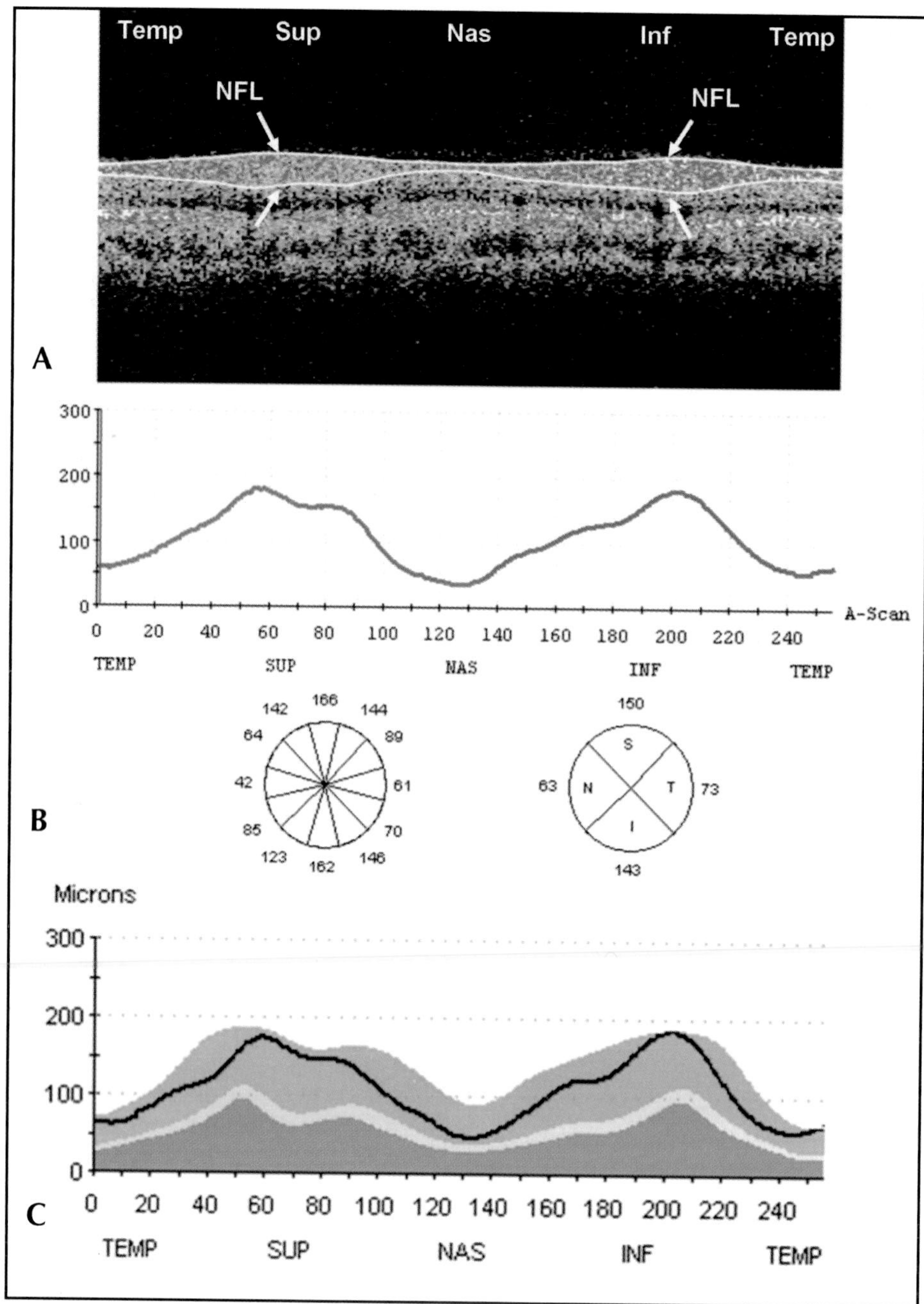

Figure 2-10. Measurement of NFL thickness. (A) Circumpapillary OCT image representing a cylindrical section around the optic disc at a diameter of 3.4 mm. The lines indicate the computer-generated profiles of the anterior retinal boundary and the posterior margin of the retinal NFL. (B) NFL analysis. Graphs and quantitative measures of NFL. Thicknesses also can be averaged over quadrant and clock hour. (C) Measurement of NFL thickness compared to a normative population. The colored areas represent variations in the normal population. The normative curves are age adjusted.

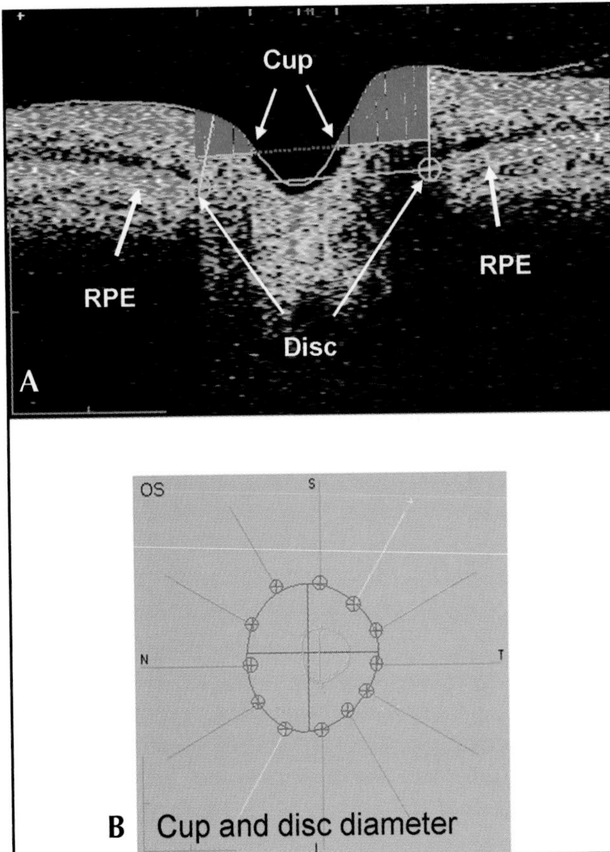

Figure 2-11. Optic nerve head analysis with image-processing. (A) OCT of optic nerve head that has been image processed to identify features of the disc. The points where the RPE/choriocapillaris and photoreceptors terminate serve as landmarks for the disc diameter. The image-processing algorithm measures the cup diameter by using an offset parallel line. (B) Analysis of the optic nerve head generated from six radial OCT scans. The disc and cup margins are shown. Other parameters such as cup-to-disc ratio can be calculated.

ness measurement with normative data. Superotemporal and inferotemporal variations in NFL thickness can be seen. The normative values of NFL thickness are represented by the different color-coded graphs. Extensive cross-sectional studies have been performed to develop criteria for diagnosing glaucoma based upon OCT measurements on NFL thickness.[23,24,28-36] A detailed discussion of NFL thickness and glaucoma is presented in Chapter 12.

Expert Algorithms and Optic Nerve Head Analysis

Changes in the optic nerve head are a well-established marker for glaucoma. Expert algorithms can also be used to perform OCT image analysis in order to assess the optic nerve head and measure cup and disc parameters. Optic disc topography measured by OCT has shown to be in agreement with other disc measuring instruments.[31,37]

The optic nerve head is typically imaged using six radial OCT scans at varying angular orientations, as shown previously in Figure 2-8. The boundary of the disc can be determined from each OCT image by the point at which the photoreceptor layer, RPE, and choriocapillaris terminate at the lamina cribrosa. This point can be located automatically by expert image-processing algorithms and then viewed by the operator for inspection and confirmation. The disc diameter can be determined by measuring the distance between the disc boundaries on opposite sides of the disc. As shown in Figure 2-11A, the cup diameter can be measured by constructing a line parallel to and offset anteriorly by a standard amount to the line that defines the disc diameter. Measurements from the multiple radial OCT images can be used to construct a two-dimensional map of the optic nerve head, as shown in Figure 2-11B. The disc area, cup area, neuroretinal rim area, as well as various cup-to-disc ratios, can also be calculated.

Interpreting Optical Coherence Tomography Images of Retinal Pathologies

OCT enables cross-sectional imaging of the retina with unprecedented resolution and provides a direct visualization of retinal pathology. On OCT images, pathologies such as macular hole, vitreomacular traction, or accumulation of subretinal fluid (retinal detachment) can be manifest as a major structural alteration. Macular disease can also produce abnormalities that change the optical properties of the retina, such as edema, hemorrhage, or drusen. Disease can also result in retinal atrophy, such as loss of the NFL in glaucoma, or atrophy of internal retinal layers in macular dystrophies. Many diseases may involve combinations of these alterations.

As discussed previously, OCT imaging can be used in conjunction with image-processing algorithms to perform quantitative measurements of retinal architecture. This approach, called *morphometry*, provides an objective measure for diagnosing disease, tracking disease progression, and evaluating response to therapy. The unprecedented resolution and high speed of OCT imaging enables excellent reproducibility of morphometric measurements and sensitivity to small changes in retinal architecture. In this section, we present an overview of how to interpret OCT images of retinal pathologies.

General Features Associated With Pathology

Many retinal diseases are manifest as a major structural disruption of the normal retinal architecture. For example, changes in the morphology of the fovea in macular hole, vitreomacular traction, and retinal detachment are often indicative of disease. Steepening of the foveal contour is commonly associated with epiretinal membranes and macular pseudoholes or lamellar holes. Loss or flattening of the foveal contour may occur with impending macular holes, foveal edema, or foveal retinal detachments. OCT can distinguish between various stages of macular holes, pseudoholes, and lamellar holes.[38,39] OCT is also able to image the various stages of macular hole formation. Impending macular holes, for example, can be identified by thickening of the fovea with the formation of cystic spaces and disruption between the inner retina and photoreceptor layer. Vitreomacular traction can be assessed by visualizing the vitreal detachment and its disruption of retinal architecture in the fovea. Surgically repaired macular holes often have varying morphologies on OCT images.[39-42]

Retinal thickness is an important consideration in the assessment of many macular diseases. Retinal thickness may be increased with edema, vitreomacular traction, retinal detachment, retinoschisis, and retinal vascular occlusion. The accumulation of intraretinal fluid leads both to increased retinal thickness as well as change in the scattering properties of the tissue. It is especially important to characterize retinal thickening in the fovea, where edema can have a profound effect on visual acuity. The high axial image resolution of OCT, combined with its ability to clearly identify the anterior and posterior boundaries of the retina, make OCT well suited for the quantitative measurement of retinal thicknesses. OCT can directly image changes in retinal architecture as well as provide objective and reproducible measurements of retinal thickness.[27,43-45] Retinal edema may be further characterized by direct visualization of intraretinal cystic spaces or traction from the posterior hyaloid or an epiretinal membrane.

Retinal abnormalities can also be associated with changes in optical properties that can be detected in OCT images. Backscattering may increase with inflammation, or infiltrate into layers of the retina or choroid; fibrosis (such as in a disciform or other scar); hard exudate; and hemorrhage. Both hard exudate and hemorrhage are highly backscattering while producing pronounced shadowing of deeper retinal structures. Blood vessels, for example, are most readily identified by their shadowing effects upon deeper structures. The distinction between blood, serous fluid, and exudate may also be made based on backscattering. Serous fluid, which contains few cells, is optically transparent, so it is clearly recognizable on OCT images as a region devoid of backscattering, in contrast to blood, which exhibits enhanced reflectivity and increased attenuation of the incident light. Cloudy subretinal exudate typically has an intermediate appearance between blood and serous fluid on OCT images. Decreased backscattering may be caused by retinal edema, in which fluid accumulation leads to a decreased density of tissue and cyst formation, with a corresponding reduction in the backscattering. Alterations in cellular structure, such as hypopigmentation of the RPE, may also result in reduced backscattering.

The intensity of the OCT image is determined by both the feature being imaged and the scattering and absorption characteristics of the overlying tissue. Thus, care is required in interpreting OCT images because the brightness of various features may be affected by abnormalities in the cornea, aqueous, lens, vitreous, as well as anterior retinal layers, which can produce shadowing. Morphological causes of reduced backscattering must be distinguished from alterations in the incident light caused by dense cataracts, cloudy media, astigmatism, poorly centered intraocular lens implants, or poor alignment of the OCT instrument while imaging. Abnormalities in the intervening structures typically cause a diffuse decrease in intensity throughout the OCT image in all retinal layers. Focal decreases in backscattering may be caused by shadowing from hyperreflective tissues, such as hemorrhage, hard exudate, or a detached RPE.

Macular Holes

OCT imaging can provide important diagnostic information on pathologies such as macular hole and is a powerful adjunct to fundus examination or fluorescein angiography for the staging of macular holes.[38,39] OCT can differentiate macular holes from partial thickness lamellar holes or pseudoholes. Figure 2-12A shows an OCT image of a full thickness macular hole. The full-thickness macular hole is characterized by a loss of the normal foveal contour and disruption of the normal retinal organization extending throughout the full thickness of the retina. Intraretinal edema and cystic changes are seen adjacent to the hole. The RPE is intact in the base of the hole, and the adjacent retina has the appearance of being lifted

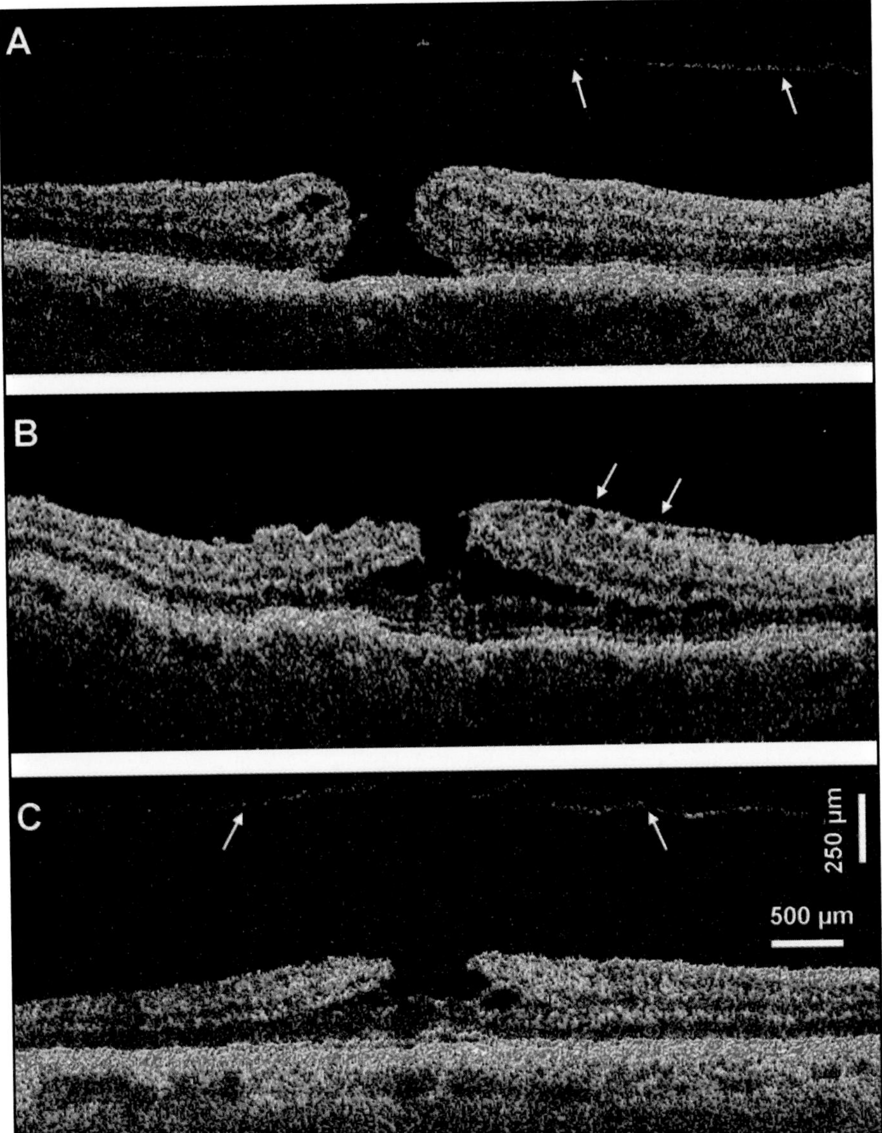

Figure 2-12. Macular holes exhibit disruption of normal retinal structure. (A) An idiopathic full thickness macular hole. The retina appears lifted away from the RPE at the edges of the hole. Edema with cystic changes are evident adjacent to the hole. The vitreous is detached and visible as a thin backscattering line above the retina (arrows). (B) Macular pseudohole due to an epiretinal membrane. The pseudohole is characterized by a steepened foveal pit contour due to traction by the epiretinal membrane. The epiretinal membrane is sometimes visible when it is separated from the sensory retina (arrows). The photoreceptor layer is intact with a separation between the ONL and OPL. (C) Lamellar or partial-thickness hole. There is a separation between the ONL and OPL. The vitreous is detached and is visible as a thin backscattering line above the retina (arrows).

away from the RPE. Cystic changes are present and appear in the inner and outer nuclear layers. The vitreous is detached and visible as a thin line above the retina.

Figure 2-12B shows a macular pseudohole with an epiretinal membrane. There is a disruption of the inner retina in the area of the hole with adjacent separation of the retina between the OPL and ONL. However, the ONL and IS and OS of the photoreceptors are intact. Strands, which may be Müller cells, are seen spanning the separation in retinal layers. The epiretinal membrane is visible as a thin, highly backscattering line between the vitreous and retinal NFL. The epiretinal membrane is producing traction on the inner retina with a wavy appearance of the inner retina and the formation of small cystic spaces in the NFL.

Figure 2-12C shows a lamellar or partial-thickness macular hole. A partial-thickness hole is visible centrally, with the photoreceptor layer appearing largely intact in the region of the hole. There is a separation between the OPL and the ONL. The retina adjacent to the hole appears normal, with all major retinal layers intact. The vitreous is detached and visible as a thin line above the retina.

OCT can be used to stage macular holes based upon their characteristic cross-sectional appearance and it has provided information on the pathogenesis of macular hole development.[38,39] OCT imaging can also provide objective, quantitative information about a macular hole, including the diameter of the hole, the extent of intraretinal cystic edema, and the extent of surrounding subretinal fluid accumulation. OCT imaging performed pre- and postoperatively can be used to assess the effectiveness of surgical treatment.[41,43,46-48]

Vitreous and Vitreoretinal Interface Abnormalities

OCT can provide structural information on the vitreous and vitreoretinal interface.[38,49-52] The normal vitreous gel is highly optically transparent and, therefore, not visible in OCT imaging. However, the vitreoretinal interface can be seen in OCT images as a high-contrast boundary between the vitreous and retina. Pathologies where the vitreous has inflammatory infiltrate, vitreous condensations, or hemorrhage result in increased optical scattering and are visible in the OCT image.

The posterior hyaloid is nominally indistinguishable from the superficial retina on the OCT image, but it becomes visible when the posterior vitreous is detached. Figure 2-13A shows an example of a posterior vitreous detachment, with the hyaloid visible as a thin, weakly reflecting surface located a few hundred microns above the retina. The reflection from the hyaloid is typically weak and appears patchy because the vitreous gel and the intervening fluid have similar indices of refraction. OCT can often detect the initial, partial detachment of posterior vitreous more accurately than biomicroscopy. When present, an operculum or pseudo-operculum can be visualized as a focal, thin area of backscatter anterior to the retinal surface. A complete posterior vitreous detachment often may not appear on an OCT image if it is more than 1 or 2 mm from the retina.

Figure 2-13B shows an example of vitreomacular traction syndrome. The vitreous is detached peripheral to the fovea and is exerting foveal traction, causing a separation between the ONL and the OPL. Strands, which may be Müller cells, are seen spanning the separation in retinal layers.

As seen in Figure 2-13C, OCT can also be used to visualize epiretinal membranes.[49,51] An epiretinal membrane that is separated from the retina can be distinguished from the posterior hyaloid based on the epiretinal membrane's higher reflectivity, greater thickness, and differences in contour. An epiretinal membrane in contact with the retina usually has a flatter contour than a detached posterior hyaloid, indicating greater tension. Structural deformation of the retina and alteration of the normal foveal contour can also be present. OCT can be used also to assess the outcome of epiretinal membrane surgical treatment.[49,51,53]

Subretinal Fluid, Hemorrhage, and Fibrovascular Proliferation

OCT is extremely useful for evaluating detachments of the neurosensory retina and retinal pigment epithelium.[54] Figure 2-14A shows an example of an OCT image of central serous chorioretinopathy. The OCT image shows a neurosensory retinal detachment with a shallow elevation of the retina. Subretinal fluid is present as an optically clear space between the retina and RPE. The normal retinal architectural morphology is preserved in the area of the detachment with all retinal layers present and intact. The photoreceptor layer is thicker than normal with increased backscattering, possibly indicative of a disruption in normal photoreceptor metabolism. The OCT image shows a well defined boundary between the retina and subretinal fluid. The RPE and choriocapillaris are visible as a highly scattering layer and the RPE is in contact with the choriocapillaris. OCT imaging is sensitive to small collections of subretinal fluid, which may be difficult to visualize with ophthalmoscopy or biomicroscopy, and can also longitudinally track the resolution of subretinal fluid upon treatment.

Figure 2-14B shows an example of a retinal pigment epithelial detachment (RPED), which has distinctive features on OCT. The RPE is visible as a thin, highly scattering band attached posteriorly to the outer retina. Although there is distortion of the normal retinal contour, the retinal architectural morphology is preserved

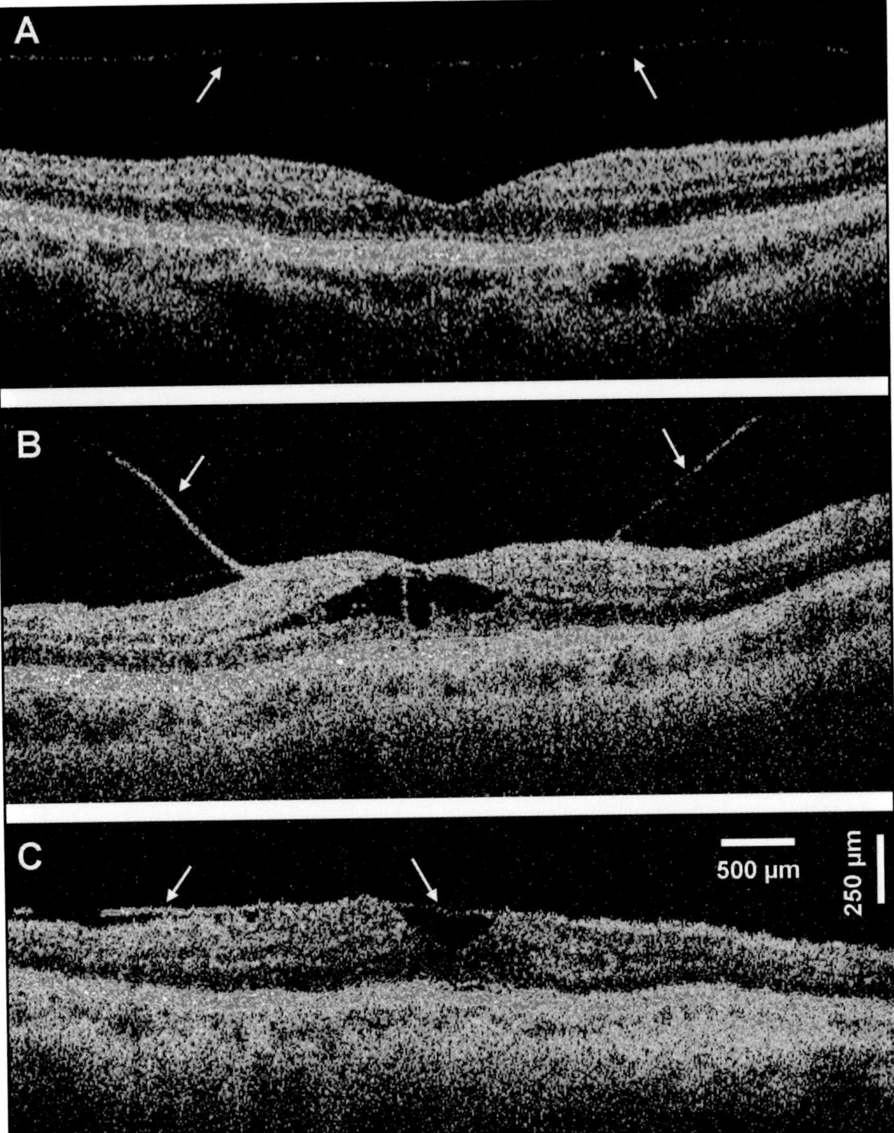

Figure 2-13. Vitreoretinal interface. (A) Vitreous detachment. The posterior hyaloid is visible as a thin line above the retina (arrows). (B) Vitreomacular traction. There is an incomplete posterior vitreous detachment with vitreoretinal adhesion at the fovea. This produces a characteristic mechanical deformation of the retina. There is a separation between the ONL and OPL with formation of cystic spaces. (C) Epiretinal membrane. Epiretinal membranes can be directly visualized when they are separated from the retina or indirectly manifest by a deformation of the retina. In this case, the epiretinal membrane spans the fovea and produces deformation of the normal foveal contour.

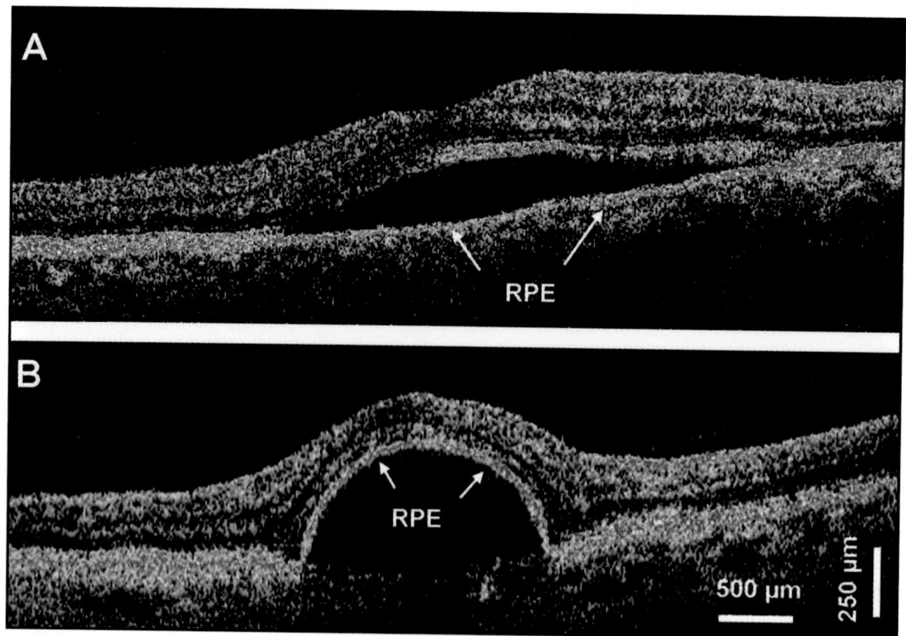

Figure 2-14. Subretinal fluid. (A) Central serous chorioretinopathy. The detachment is manifest as an optically clear space beneath the retina. The RPE is attached to the choroid and is visible as a thin, flat, highly backscattering layer. The retinal layers in the detached area are intact, but the photoreceptor OS appear thicker than normal and have increased backscattering. (B) RPED. The pigment epithelium detachment is evident by the thin, curved, highly backscattering layer that is continuous with the sensory retina. The detached RPE produces shadowing of the choroid below.

and all retinal layers are present and intact. The detached RPE exhibits increased backscattering, perhaps due to the refractive index difference between serous fluid and the choriocapillaris, or due to morphological changes in the RPE itself. The increased backscattering from the RPE produces shadowing of the choroid below the detachment. The angle of the detachment is often more acute in a pigment epithelial detachment (PED) compared to a neurosensory detachment because of the tight adherence of RPE cells to the basement membrane, which supports an increased fluid pressure. If an RPE tear is present, focal interruptions of the RPE can be detected.[55] The PED tends to have a pleated or tent profile, rather than the dome-shaped profile associated with neurosensory retinal detachment, and the retracted RPE exhibits increased backscattering. The bare choroid also exhibits increased backscattering from choroidal vessels and appears brighter than normal as a result of reduced shadowing because the RPE is absent.

The increased reflectivity from the photoreceptors in a neurosensory detachment may mimic the high reflectivity from the pigment epithelium, but usually it does not produce significant shadowing of the RPE and choroid. Thus, the differentiation between neurosensory retinal detachment and PEDs often relies upon assessing the strength of the backscattering below the serous fluid collection and evaluating the angle of the detachment. OCT images of neurosensory detachments may occasionally be confused with severe retinal edema, since, in many cases, the fluid accumulation and reduced backscattering that occur with edema are preferentially seen in the outer retinal layers. In these cases, it is important to identify a smooth and continuous fluid-retina boundary to establish the diagnosis of a sensory retinal detachment. OCT imaging can also distinguish retinoschisis from retinal detachment as a splitting between the layers of the neuroretina.[56-58]

Figure 2-15A shows an example of a hemorrhagic detachment of the RPE. OCT images of hemorrhagic detachments of the RPE have characteristics similar to a serous RPE detachment, but they can be differentiated by the presence of optical backscattering arising from blood directly beneath the detached RPE. In this case, the blood usually appears moderately, rather than highly, backscattering because of the attenuation of the incident light through the detached RPE. The image penetration

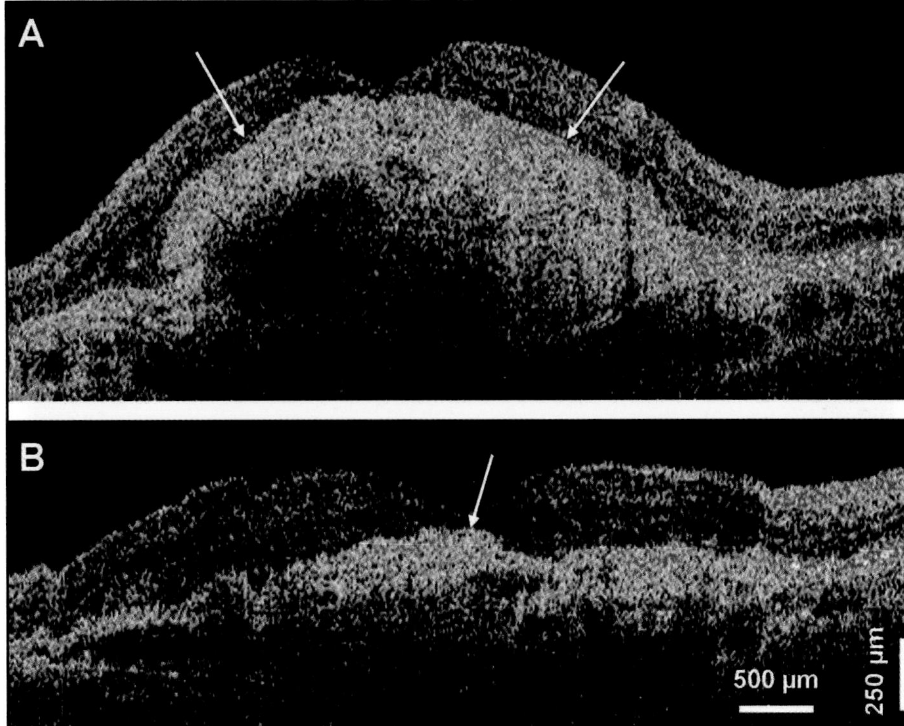

Figure 2-15. Subretinal hemorrhage and fibrovascular proliferation. (A) Hemorrhagic detachment. Blood fills the subretinal space and is evident by its high backscattering. OCT image penetration into the blood is limited, and there is strong shadowing of deeper structures. (B) Fibrovascular pigment epithelial detachment (PED). The fibrovascular PED exhibits moderate backscattering extending in the RPE/choriocapillaris.

through both the detached RPE and hemorrhage is usually less than 100 μm. Similarly, in cases of hemorrhage into the vitreous, the attenuation of incident light depends on the thickness of the scattering medium. Thin hemorrhages appear as thin, highly reflective bands that have little effect on the underlying tissue. Thick hemorrhages, however, completely attenuate the incident light after more than approximately 200 μm and produce a strong shadowing of underlying structures.

Figure 2-15B shows an example of a fibrovascular PED. OCT images of fibrovascular PEDs are characterized by increased optical backscattering that is visible beneath the RPE, sometimes with adjacent subretinal fluid. However, the fibrovascular tissue has a lower optical backscattering when compared to blood, and the OCT image shows a lower brightness from the fibrovascular proliferation and increased image penetration, which often extends to the choroid. Other lesions, such as a vitelliform lesion, may have a similar appearance of constant mild to moderate backscattering that extends between an elevated RPE and the choroid.

Macular Edema

OCT imaging can be particularly useful in evaluating and quantifying macular edema. The ability to both image and quantitatively measure changes in retinal thickness is especially helpful in assessing and tracking patients with macular edema from diabetic retinopathy or for screening and monitoring patients with macular edema after cataract surgery. Figure 2-16A shows an example of an OCT image of cystoid macular edema. The normal foveal contour is absent and the retinal thickness is increased to approximately 500 μm in the fovea. Large cystic structures in the nuclear layers are present. OCT imaging can clearly identify edema as well as concomitant pathologies such as cysts, lamellar macular holes, exudate, and neovascularization. OCT measurements of changes in central foveal thickness correlate with visual acuity changes.[27,59]

Figure 2-16B shows an example of an OCT image of edema due to a temporal branch retinal vein occlusion. Pronounced retinal edema is observed temporal to the fovea with disruption of the normal foveal contour. Cystoid changes are present and can be seen in the INL and ONL. The retina nasal to the fovea appears largely

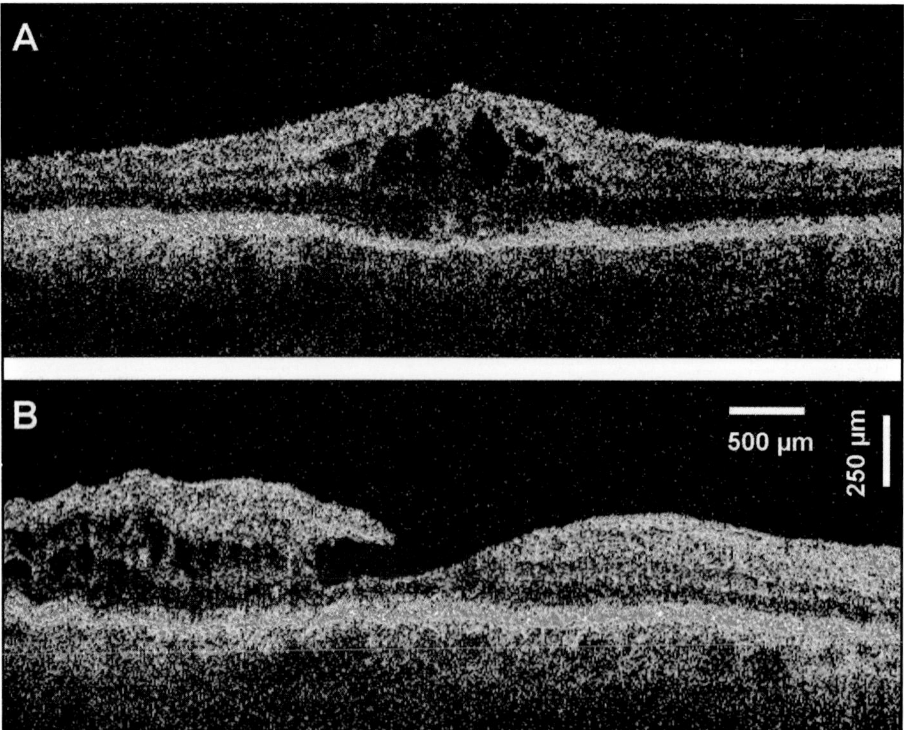

Figure 2-16. (A) Cystoid macular edema. The retina is significantly thickened, with loss of the normal foveal pit contour. Accumulation of intraretinal fluid leads to cystic spaces that are visible as rounded, low scattering areas, which typically occur in the INL or ONL. (B) Branch retinal vein occlusion. Edema with the formation of cysts in the INL and ONL is evident.

normal. In venous occlusive diseases, OCT is especially useful in quantitatively monitoring the development of macular edema and resolution following treatment. OCT imaging can identify macular thickening, cyst formation, lamellar macular holes, subretinal fluid accumulation, and papilledema. Retinal artery obstruction is associated with acute macular edema followed by retinal atrophy. These changes in morphology can be visualized by OCT. As noted previously, OCT imaging can be used to quantitatively assess retinal thickness, thus providing an objective assessment of disease progression or resolution.[59-61]

Retinal Pigment Epithelium and Choriocapillaris

OCT imaging can be used to assess abnormalities in the RPE that are associated with disease.[62,63] The RPE and choriocapillaris are usually not separately resolvable on OCT images, and they appear as a thin, highly backscattering band at the posterior boundary of the retina. The junction between the photoreceptor IS and OS also produces a thin, highly reflective band that is anterior to the RPE and choroid. These features define the posterior boundary of the neurosensory retina and the photoreceptor OS on OCT images. Alterations in these features provide useful information on chorioretinal pathologies such as age-related macular degeneration and choroidal neovascularization.

Hyperpigmentation of the RPE leads to increased reflectivity, mild thickening of the posterior reflective boundary, and concomitant shadowing of the backscattering from the choroid. Detachments of the RPE also produce shadowing of the choroid, as discussed previously. Disciform scars and other fibrosis appear as a severely thickened posterior reflection, due to the high reflectivity and extension of fibrotic structures into the retina. Hypopigmentation or pigment epithelial atrophy results in decreased reflection and an associated window defect, thus enabling increased penetration of the OCT beam to the choroid and increased signals from the deeper layers.

Figure 2-17A shows an example of pigmentary abnormalities resulting from nonexudative age-related macular degeneration. Irregularities in the RPE and the IS and OS of the photoreceptors (white arrows) can be observed. The RPE and choriocapillaris have a roughened and disrupted appearance with evidence of disruption or irregu-

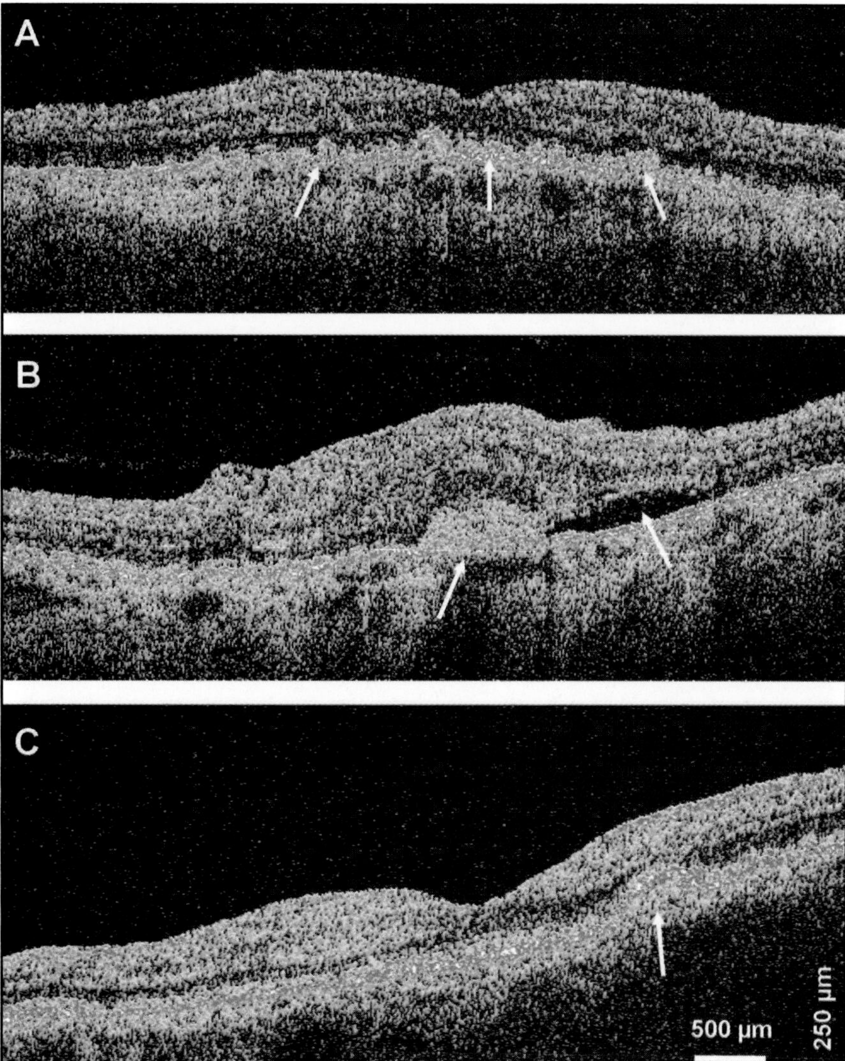

Figure 2-17. (A) Age-related macular degeneration. Disruption of the RPE is evident by its irregular or roughened appearance. (B) Choroidal neovascularization. Choroidal neovascular membrane appears as a localized disruption of the RPE/choriocapillaris and photoreceptor OS. Edema with subretinal or intraretinal fluid or hemorrhage is often visible above the membrane. (C) Soft drusen is evident as a modulation or wavy appearance in the RPE and choriocapillaris. The RPE may appear elevated, and these features sometimes appear similar to small PEDs, except that drusen have lower and less localized backscattering.

larity in the outer segments of the photoreceptors. The inner retinal layers appear to have normal architectural morphology at this stage in the disease.

Figure 2-17B shows an example of choroidal neovascularization. There is a disruption of the RPE, the choriocapillaris, and photoreceptor OS. The ingrowth of new blood vessels through Bruch's membrane results in a fragmented and thickened appearance of the RPE, choriocapillaris, and photoreceptor OS. There is edema of the overlying retina due to intraretinal or subretinal fluid leakage from the neovascularization. This is manifest as a thickening and deviation from the normal retinal contour with an increase in thickness of the layers of the retina. An epiretinal membrane is manifest at the inner retinal boundary with the formation of small cystic spaces and the irregular, contracted appearance of the inner retina.

In cases of chronic edema, there can be a loss of contrast between the layers of the retina, resulting in a smeared-out and homogenous appearance.

Figure 2-17C shows an example of soft drusen. Soft drusen are visible as an apparent modulation or waviness in the thin, highly backreflecting and backscattering bands from the boundary of the photoreceptor IS and OS and the RPE and choroid. This is consistent with accumulation of material within or beneath Bruch's membrane. The elevated appearance of the RPE appears similar to a serous PED. However, soft drusen have shallow margins and lower backscattering with less shadowing.

Atrophy of the Nerve Fiber Layer and Retina: Glaucoma and Dystrophy

The ability of OCT to visualize and quantitatively measure retinal microstructure makes it a powerful tool for diagnosing and tracking neurodegenerative diseases such as glaucoma. Alterations in the thickness of the retinal NFL have been shown to be an important diagnostic of glaucoma and a measure of disease progression. The NFL appears in OCT images as a distinct, highly backscattering layer in the superficial retina. As discussed previously, NFL thickness may be assessed at individual points on a cylindrical or linear tomogram in the peripapillary region. Computer image-processing algorithms can be used to evaluate both retinal and NFL thickness. Figure 2-18 shows a circumpapillary OCT image around the optic disc from a patient with glaucoma. Corresponding measurements of the NFL are also shown. The use of automated algorithms greatly facilitates the interpretation of OCT images. Reduction in NFL thickness can be readily detected by examining the NFL thickness graphs.

OCT images through the optic disc are useful for assessing disc and cup parameters and for evaluating glaucoma. Figure 2-18C shows an OCT of the optic disc, which exhibits cupping with atrophy of the neuroretinal rim and may be compared with the normal image of the optic disc in Figure 2-11. As described previously, automated algorithms can also be applied to OCT images of the optic nerve head in order to perform quantitative measurements of disc parameters.

Since OCT can provide detailed images of retinal layers, it can be applied to a wide range of other retinal diseases that are associated with atrophy of the retina. Figure 2-19 shows an example of OCT imaging of the normal retina versus retinitis pigmentosa. Retinitis pigmentosa is evident as abnormal thinning of the photoreceptor layer outside the fovea manifests as a reduction in the thickness of the ONL when compared to the normal retina shown in Figure 2-19A. In Stargardt's dystrophy, shown in Figure 2-19C, the ONL is abnormally thin and is absent within the fovea. Although many of these degenerative retinal disorders do not yet have effective treatments, OCT may prove useful in clinical research because it enables direct visualization and measurement of changes in retinal architecture that would be useful in elucidating disease pathogenesis or assessing future therapies.

The ability of OCT to perform quantitative measurements of retinal morphology, or morphometry, is especially powerful because it provides a means for comparing imaging measurements to the normal population in order to assess the probability of a diagnosis. Morphometry can also provide an objective measurement of disease progression and the efficacy of treatment.

Quality, Artifacts, and Errors in Optical Coherence Tomography Images

In order to realize the full diagnostic potential of OCT imaging and to avoid diagnostic errors, high-quality OCT images are required. Since optical backreflection and backscattering from retinal structures are very weak, reduction in the signal level of images can occur as the result of operator error during imaging. Although OCT imaging can be performed in patients with ocular opacities, care is required to ensure that images have sufficient quality. Signal-to-noise, or the brightness of retinal features when compared to background noise, is an important indicator of OCT image quality.

Figure 2-20A shows an example of a normal OCT image. Figure 2-20B shows an OCT image with a low signal. The image has a washed-out and dim appearance, with loss of signal and reduced dynamic range. Structures such as the low backscattering GCL and the INL and ONL of the retina have a blue-black appearance in false-color images, indicating that their signal level is close to the background noise level. If there is sufficient loss of signal, then even the higher scattering layers such as the RPE, NFL, and plexiform layers can have reduced intensities. Although scattering from cataracts produces a reduction in image intensity, it usually does not degrade image quality, except in cases of severe opacity. However, care must be taken with these patients, and careful imaging technique must be used to ensure that images have sufficient signal levels.

Figure 2-20C shows an example of an OCT image that has vignetting. Vignetting occurs when the OCT imaging beam is blocked by the iris during a portion of the beam scan and is characterized by loss of signal over a specific portion of the OCT image. This problem is the result of improper alignment of the OCT imaging beam, which should be centered along the axis of the eye during the

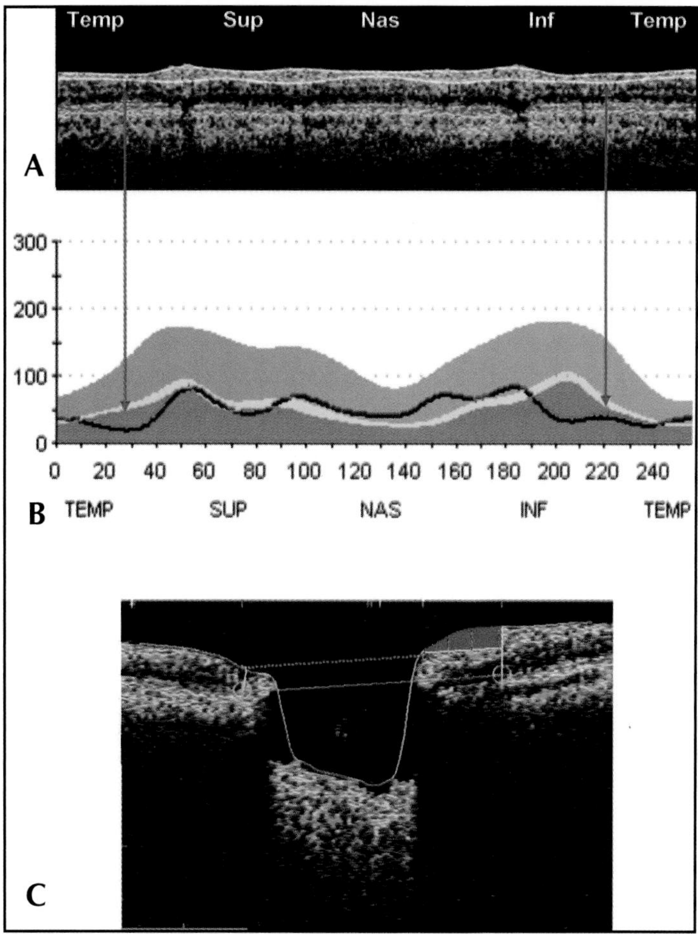

Figure 2-18. Glaucoma. (A) Circumpapillary OCT image in glaucoma. The NFL is markedly thinner in the entire temporal half of the disc. This can be seen from the OCT image and can be quantitatively measured by using image-processing. The subject had paracentral and nasal visual field defects. (B) NFL analysis plot. Comparison to the normative NFL values shows significant loss of nerve fibers in the temporal half of the disc. (C) OCT of the optic nerve head. The neuroretinal rim in most of the temporal half of the disc was significantly atrophied. An increase in the cup-to-disc ratio is evident.

imaging procedure. The OCT instrument is designed so that the OCT imaging beam pivots about the pupil when the beam is scanned on the retina. However, the instrument must be positioned at the correct distance from the eye in order for this beam pivot point to coincide with the pupil. Finally, special care is required when imaging undilated patients because of their small pupil diameter.

Figure 2-20D shows an OCT image with unstable patient fixation. The OCT image exhibits sharp discontinuity of retinal features that are associated with changes in the patient's fixation that occur during the middle of the OCT scan. While motion-correcting algorithms can correct for longitudinal eye motion during the scan, changes in the transverse position of the OCT imaging beam, which occur if the patient shifts gaze, cannot be corrected. Special care, therefore, must be exercised in imaging patients with compromised central vision who have difficulty in maintaining fixation or in patients who have reduced compliance. Since the OCT imaging instrument provides a view of the fundus during imaging, changes in fixation often can be noted by the operator and the scan repeated, if necessary.

OCT imaging is powerful because a wide range of image-processing algorithms can be used to obtain quan-

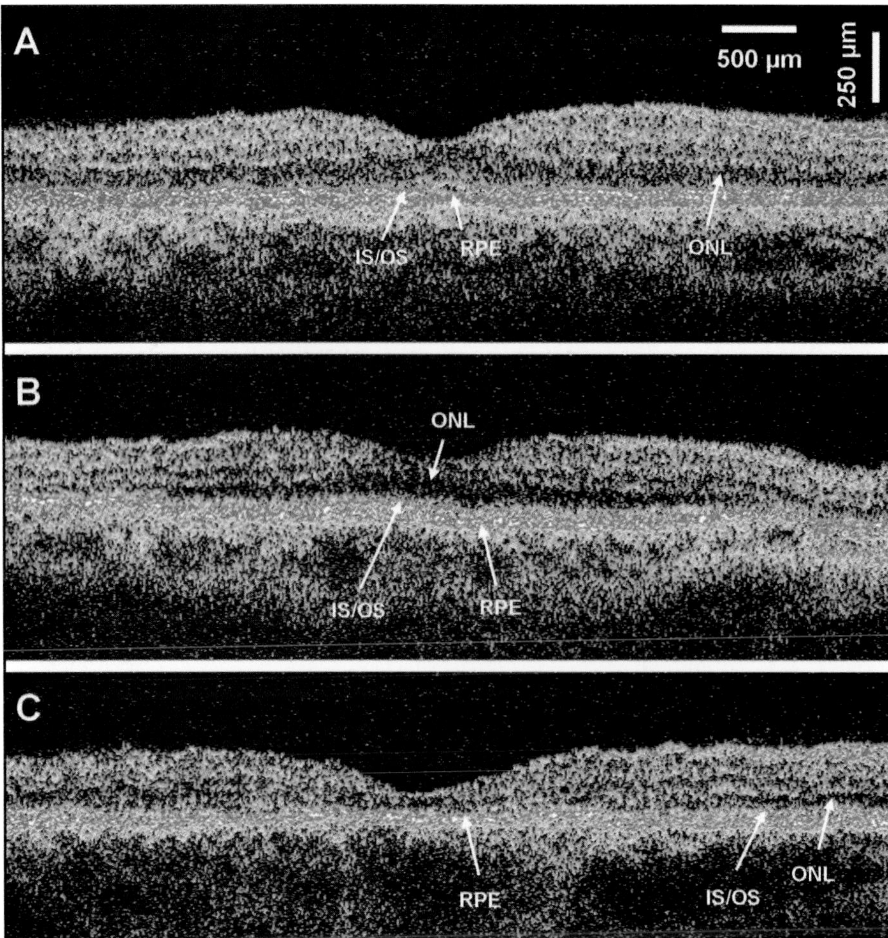

Figure 2-19. Degenerative diseases producing atrophy. OCT imaging can visualize detailed retinal architecture and atrophy. (A) OCT image of a normal macula for baseline comparison. (B) Retinitis pigmentosa. Degeneration of the photoreceptor layer is evident peripheral to the fovea. The ONL is significantly thinner than normal. Degeneration of the photoreceptor OS can also be observed. The fovea appears normal. (C) Stargardt's dystrophy. Degeneration of the photoreceptor layer in the fovea is evident. The ONL is thinner than normal in the foveal region.

titative information from OCT images. However, care is required to ensure that the initial image data are of sufficient quality before these image-processing and measurement algorithms are applied. Even the most robust methods for image-processing will generate incorrect measurements if the initial image is of low quality. Figure 2-21 shows an example of a retinal thickness measurement error due to insufficient signal to noise. In this case, the OCT image of the retina is too dim and the boundary detection in the retinal thickness measurement algorithm fails to detect the correct retinal layer, resulting in an anomalously thin retinal thickness measurement. Figure 2-22 shows an example of a NFL measurement error occurring on a circumpapillary OCT image that has low signal to noise. The algorithm fails to detect the correct retinal NFL boundary in a part of the image and results in an anomalously thin measurement. Generally, it is more difficult to measure the NFL than the overall retinal thickness because the NFL measurement depends upon reliable detection of the posterior boundary of the NFL, which has lower contrast than the anterior or posterior retinal boundaries. It is important to ensure that the original OCT images have sufficient signal to noise. The performance of the algorithms can be checked by a quick visual inspection of the boundaries that they detect to confirm that the software-drawn boundary lines match the boundaries in the OCT image.

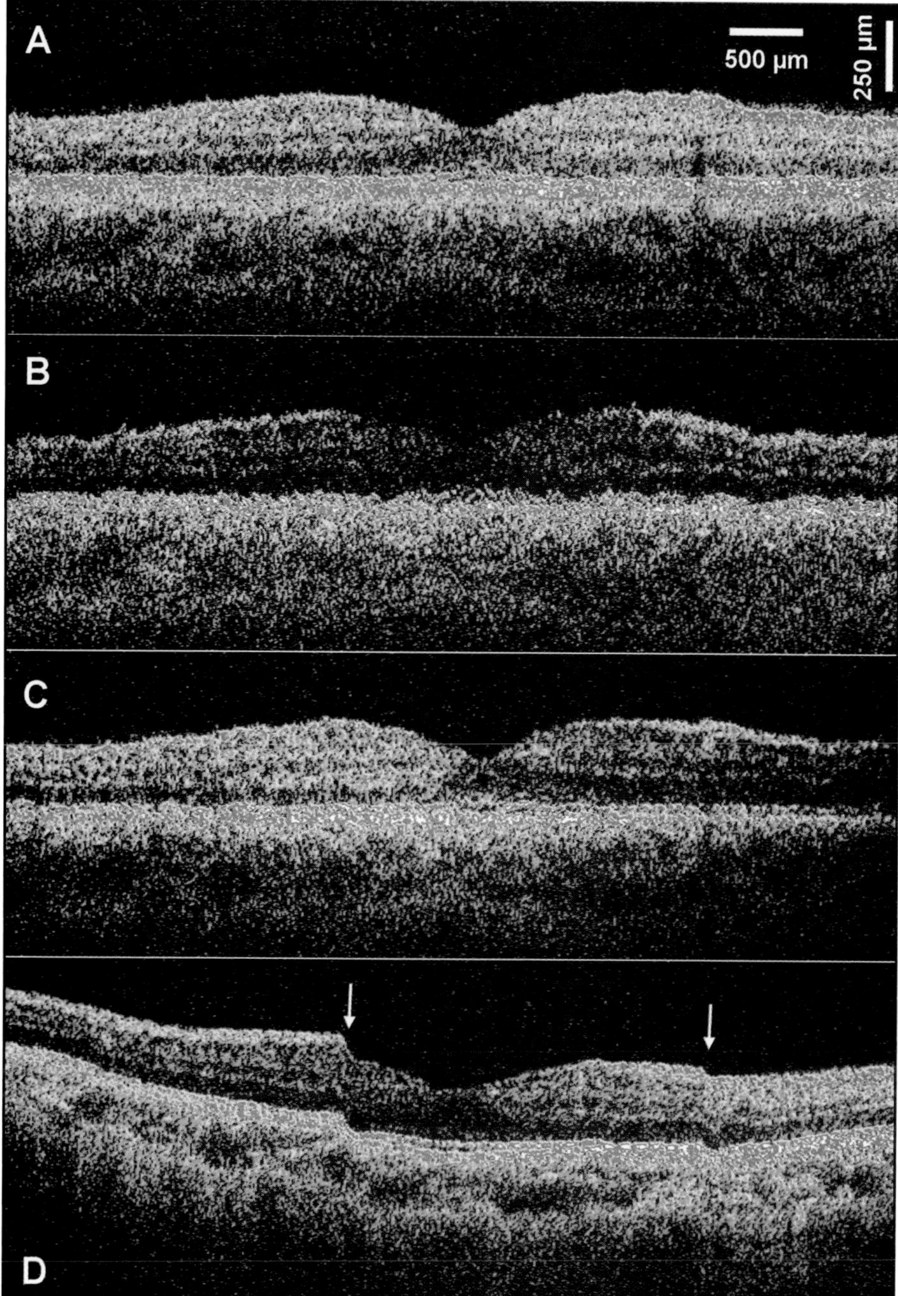

Figure 2-20. In order to realize the full diagnostic potential, as well as to minimize artifacts and misdiagnosis, OCT images must be of good quality. (A) OCT image of good quality without artifacts. (B) Out-of-focus OCT image. The image has low signal to noise and appears dim. Weakly backscattering structures, such as nuclear layers of the GCL, appear blue-black and near the detection limit. With more severe focus error, even highly scattering structures such as the NFL and plexiform layers are dim. Similar effects can be observed with ocular opacity. (C) Vignetted image. A portion of the image has low signal to noise and appears dim because the OCT beam was blocked by the iris during part of the scan. (D) Fixation error. The image has discontinuities that were generated when the patient's fixation point changed during the scan. Since eye motion may not be evident in the OCT image, special attention is required during image acquisition to ensure stable fixation.

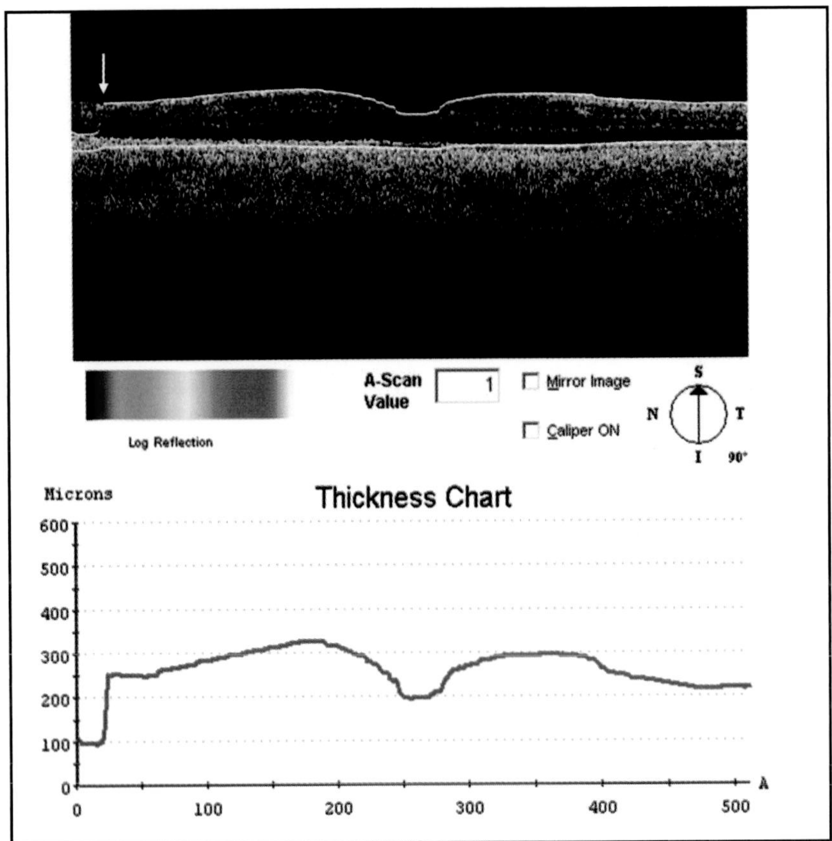

Figure 2-21. OCT images with low signal to noise can produce errors in image analysis. Error in retinal thickness measurement algorithm. The algorithm gives an incorrectly low thickness where the OCT image has low signal (left side). Note that the algorithm is robust and it correctly determines the retinal thickness over most of the image, despite the low signal.

Summary

This chapter described the interpretation of normal OCT images, as well as provided the basic principles of interpreting OCT images of retinal pathology. OCT enables cross-sectional imaging of the retina at unprecedented resolutions, thus enabling the visualization of gross retinal features such as retinal thickness, as well as fine details such as individual retinal layers. The ability to detect abnormalities in retinal architecture can be a powerful and definitive diagnostic tool for many retinal diseases. Automated image-processing techniques enable quantitative measurements of retinal morphology that can be compared with a normative database in order to enhance diagnostic performance. OCT provides a powerful adjunct to conventional fundus examination and fluorescein angiography that can function not only as a sensitive disease diagnostic, but also to track disease progression and monitor treatment. In this context, OCT may be the most powerful and definitive single diagnostic that can be performed next to fundus examination.

References

1. Huang D, Swanson EA, Lin CP, et al. Optical coherence tomography. *Science*. 1991;254(5035):1178-1181.
2. Hee MR, Izatt JA, Swanson EA, et al. Optical coherence tomography of the human retina. *Arch Ophthalmol*. 1995;113(3):325-332.
3. Izatt JA, Hee MR, Swanson EA, et al. Micrometer-scale resolution imaging of the anterior eye in vivo with optical coherence tomography. *Arch Ophthalmol*. 1994;112(12):1584-1589.
4. Puliafito CA, Hee MR, Lin CP, et al. Imaging of macular diseases with optical coherence tomography. *Ophthalmology*. 1995;102(2):217-229.
5. Fujimoto JG, Pitris C, Boppart SA, Brezinski ME. Optical coherence tomography: an emerging technology for biomedical imaging and optical biopsy. *Neoplasia*. 2000;2(1-2):9-25.
6. Patterson MS, Chance B, Wilson BC. Time resolved reflectance and transmittance for the non-invasive measurement of tissue optical properties. *Appl Opt*. 1989;28(12):2331-2336.

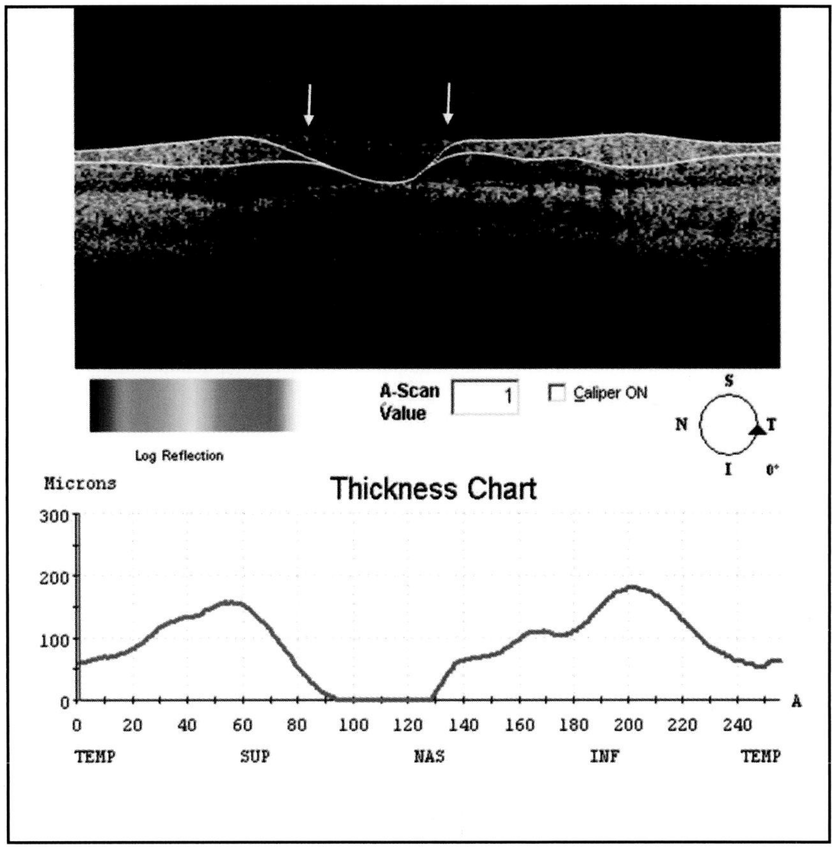

Figure 2-22. Error in NFL thickness algorithm. The NFL thickness algorithm incorrectly measures a zero thickness from the portion of the OCT image that has low signal. In order to avoid these artifacts, it is important to ensure that OCT images are of sufficient quality before they are used for image-processing.

7. Flock ST, Patterson MS, Wilson BC, Wyman DR. Monte Carlo modeling of light propagation in highly scattering tissues. I. Model predictions and comparison with diffusion theory. *IEEE Transactions on Biomedical Engineering.* 1989;36(12):1162-1168.
8. Flock ST, Wilson BC, Patterson MS. Monte Carlo modeling of light propagation in highly scattering tissues. II. Comparison with measurements in phantoms. *IEEE Transactions on Biomedical Engineering.* 1989;36(12):1169-1173.
9. Cheong WF, Prahl SA, Welch AJ. A review of the optical properties of biological tissues. *IEEE Journal of Quantum Electronics.* 1990;26(12):2166-2185.
10. Fujimoto JG, Brezinski ME, Tearney GJ, et al. Optical biopsy and imaging using optical coherence tomography. *Nat Med.* 1995;1(9):970-972.
11. Schmitt JM, Knuttel A, Yadlowsky M, Eckhaus MA. Optical-coherence tomography of a dense tissue: statistics of attenuation and backscattering. *Phys Med Biol.* 1994;39(10):1705-1720.
12. Hogan H, Alvarado JA, E. WJ. *Histology of the Human Eye: An Atlas and Textbook.* Philadelphia, Pa: WB Saunders; 1971.
13. Gass JDM. *Stereoscopic Atlas of Macular Diseases: Diagnosis and Treatment.* Vol 1. 3rd ed. St. Louis, Mo: CV Mosby; 1987:46-65.
14. Krebs W, Krebs I. *Primate Retina and Choroid—Atlas of Fine Structure in Man and Monkey.* New York: Springer Verlag; 1991.
15. Spalton DJ, Hitchings RA, Hunter PA. *Anatomy of the retina. Atlas of clinical ophthalmology.* 2nd ed. St. Louis, Mo: Mosby; 1994.
16. Toth CA, Narayan DG, Boppart SA, et al. A comparison of retinal morphology viewed by optical coherence tomography and by light microscopy. *Arch Ophthalmol.* 1997;115(11):1425-1428.
17. Huang Y, Cideciyan AV, Papastergiou GI, et al. Relation of optical coherence tomography to microanatomy in normal and rd chickens. *Invest Ophthalmol Vis Sci.* 1998;39(12):2405-2416.

18. Li Q, Timmers AM, Hunter K, et al Noninvasive imaging by optical coherence tomography to monitor retinal degeneration in the mouse. *Invest Ophthalmol Vis Sci.* 2001; 42(12):2981-2989.
19. Drexler W, Morgner U, Kartner FX, et al. In vivo ultrahigh-resolution optical coherence tomography. *Optics Letters*. 1999;24(17):1221-1223.
20. Drexler W, Sattmann H, Hermann B, et al. Enhanced visualization of macular pathology with the use of ultrahigh-resolution optical coherence tomography. *Arch Ophthalmol.* 2003;121(5):695-706.
21. Sidman R. The structure and concentration of solids in photoreceptor cells studied by refractometry and interference microscopy. *J Biophys Biochem Cytol.* 1957;3:1530.
22. Schuman JS, Hee MR, Arya AV, et al. Optical coherence tomography: a new tool for glaucoma diagnosis. *Curr Opin Ophthalmol.* 1995;6(2):89-95.
23. Schuman JS, Hee MR, Puliafito CA, et al. Quantification of nerve fiber layer thickness in normal and glaucomatous eyes using optical coherence tomography. *Arch Ophthalmol.* 1995;113(5):586-596.
24. Schuman JS, Pedut-Kloizman T, Hertzmark E, et al. Reproducibility of nerve fiber layer thickness measurements using optical coherence tomography. *Ophthalmology.* 1996;103(11):1889-1898.
25. Radhakrishnan S, Rollins AM, Roth JE, et al. Real-time optical coherence tomography of the anterior segment at 1310 nm. *Arch Ophthalmol.* 2001;119(8):1179-1185.
26. Brezinski ME, Tearney GJ, Bouma BE, et al. Optical coherence tomography for optical biopsy. Properties and demonstration of vascular pathology. *Circulation.* 1996; 93(6):1206-1213.
27. Hee MR, Puliafito CA, Duker JS, et al. Topography of diabetic macular edema with optical coherence tomography. *Ophthalmology.* 1998;105(2):360-370.
28. Blumenthal EZ, Williams JM, Weinreb RN, Girkin CA, Berry CC, Zangwill LM. Reproducibility of nerve fiber layer thickness measurements by use of optical coherence tomography. *Ophthalmology.* 2000;107(12):2278-2282.
29. Bowd C, Weinreb RN, Williams JM, Zangwill LM. The retinal nerve fiber layer thickness in ocular hypertensive, normal, and glaucomatous eyes with optical coherence tomography. *Arch Ophthalmol.* 2000;118(1):22-26.
30. Zangwill LM, Williams J, Berry CC, Knauer S, Weinreb RN. A comparison of optical coherence tomography and retinal nerve fiber layer photography for detection of nerve fiber layer damage in glaucoma. *Ophthalmology.* 2000;107(7):1309-1315.
31. Zangwill LM, Bowd C, Berry CC, et al. Discriminating between normal and glaucomatous eyes using the Heidelberg Retina Tomograph, GDx Nerve Fiber Analyzer, and optical coherence tomograph. *Arch Ophthalmol.* 2001;119(7):985-993.
32. Bowd C, Zangwill LM, Berry CC, et al. Detecting early glaucoma by assessment of retinal nerve fiber layer thickness and visual function. *Invest Ophthalmol Vis Sci.* 2001;42(9):1993-2003.
33. Bowd C, Zangwill LM, Blumenthal EZ, et al. Imaging of the optic disc and retinal nerve fiber layer: the effects of age, optic disc area, refractive error, and gender. *J Opt Soc Am A Opt Image Sci Vis.* 2002;19(1):197-207.
34. Williams ZY, Schuman JS, Gamell L, et al. Optical coherence tomography measurement of nerve fiber layer thickness and the likelihood of a visual field defect. *Am J Ophthalmol.* 2002;134(4):538-546.
35. Aydin A, Wollstein G, Price LL, Fujimoto JG, Schuman JS. Optical coherence tomography assessment of retinal nerve fiber layer thickness changes after glaucoma surgery. *Ophthalmology.* 2003;110(8):1506-1511.
36. Guedes V, Schuman JS, Hertzmark E, et al. Optical coherence tomography measurement of macular and nerve fiber layer thickness in normal and glaucomatous human eyes. *Ophthalmology.* 2003;110(1):177-189.
37. Schuman JS, Wollstein G, Farra T, et al. Comparison of optic nerve head measurements obtained by optical coherence tomography and confocal scanning laser ophthalmoscopy. *Am J Ophthalmol.* 2003;135(4):504-512.
38. Hee MR, Puliafito CA, Wong C, et al. Optical coherence tomography of macular holes. *Ophthalmology.* 1995;102(5): 748-756.
39. Gaudric A, Haouchine B, Massin P, Paques M, Blain P, Erginay A. Macular hole formation: new data provided by optical coherence tomography. *Arch Ophthalmol.* 1999;117(6):744-751.
40. Takahashi H, Kishi S. Optical coherence tomography images of spontaneous macular hole closure. *Am J Ophthalmol.* 1999;128(4):519-520.
41. Takahashi H, Kishi S. Tomographic features of a lamellar macular hole formation and a lamellar hole that progressed to a full-thickness macular hole. *Am J Ophthalmol.* 2000;130(5):677-679.
42. Takahashi H, Kishi S. Tomographic features of early macular hole closure after vitreous surgery. *Am J Ophthalmol.* 2000;130(2):192-196.
43. Massin P, Vicaut E, Haouchine B, Erginay A, Paques M, Gaudric A. Reproducibility of retinal mapping using optical coherence tomography. *Arch Ophthalmol.* 2001;119(8): 1135-1142.
44. Polito A, Shah SM, Haller JA, et al. Comparison between retinal thickness analyzer and optical coherence tomography for assessment of foveal thickness in eyes with macular disease. *Am J Ophthalmol.* 2002;134(2):240-251.
45. Strøm C, Sander B, Larsen N, Larsen M, Lund-Andersen H. Diabetic macular edema assessed with optical coherence tomography and stereo fundus photography. *Invest Ophthalmol Vis Sci.* 2002;43(1):241-245.
46. Imai M, Iijima H, Gotoh T, Tsukahara S. Optical coherence tomography of successfully repaired idiopathic macular holes. *Am J Ophthalmol.* 1999;128(5):621-627.
47. Mikajiri K, Okada AA, Ohji M, et al. Analysis of vitrectomy for idiopathic macular hole by optical coherence tomography. *Am J Ophthalmol.* 1999;128(5):655-657.

48. Ip MS, Baker BJ, Duker JS, et al. Anatomical outcomes of surgery for idiopathic macular hole as determined by optical coherence tomography. *Arch Ophthalmol*. 2002;120(1):29-35.
49. Wilkins JR, Puliafito CA, Hee MR, et al. Characterization of epiretinal membranes using optical coherence tomography. *Ophthalmology*. 1996;103(12):2142-2151.
50. Munuera JM, García-Layana A, Maldonado MJ, Aliseda D, Moreno-Montañés J. Optical coherence tomography in successful surgery of vitreomacular traction syndrome. *Arch Ophthalmol*. 1998;116(10):1388-1389.
51. Azzolini C, Patelli F, Codenotti M, Pierro L, Brancato R. Optical coherence tomography in idiopathic epiretinal macular membrane surgery. *Eur J Ophthalmol*. 1999;9(3):206-211.
52. Gallemore RP, Jumper JM, McCuen BW 2nd, Jaffe GJ, Postel EA, Toth CA. Diagnosis of vitreoretinal adhesions in macular disease with optical coherence tomography. *Retina*. 2000;20(2):115-120.
53. Massin P, Allouch C, Haouchine B, et al. Optical coherence tomography of idiopathic macular epiretinal membranes before and after surgery. *Am J Ophthalmol*. 2000;130(6):732-739.
54. Hee MR, Puliafito CA, Wong C, et al. Optical coherence tomography of central serous chorioretinopathy. *Am J Ophthalmol*. 1995;120(1):65-74.
55. Giovannini A, Amato G, Mariotti C, Scassellati-Sforzolini B. Optical coherence tomography in the assessment of retinal pigment epithelial tear. *Retina*. 2000;20(1):37-40.
56. Azzolini C, Pierro L, Codenotti M, Brancato R. OCT images and surgery of juvenile macular retinoschisis. *Eur J Ophthalmol*. 1997;7(2):196-200.
57. Ip M, Garza-Karren C, Duker JS, et al. Differentiation of degenerative retinoschisis from retinal detachment using optical coherence tomography. *Ophthalmology*. 1999;106(3):600-605.
58. Takano M, Kishi S. Foveal retinoschisis and retinal detachment in severely myopic eyes with posterior staphyloma. *Am J Ophthalmol*. 1999;128(4):472-476.
59. Hee MR, Puliafito CA, Wong C, et al. Quantitative assessment of macular edema with optical coherence tomography. *Arch Ophthalmol*. 1995;113(8):1019-1029.
60. Otani T, Kishi S, Maruyama Y. Patterns of diabetic macular edema with optical coherence tomography. *Am J Ophthalmol*. 1999;127(6):688-693.
61. Rivellese M, George A, Sulkes D, Reichel E, Puliafito C. Optical coherence tomography after laser photocoagulation for clinically significant macular edema. *Ophthalmic Surg Lasers*. 2000;31(3):192-197.
62. Hee MR, Baumal CR, Puliafito CA, et al. Optical coherence tomography of age-related macular degeneration and choroidal neovascularization. *Ophthalmology*. 1996;103(8):1260-1270.
63. Giovannini A, Amato GP, Mariotti C, Scassellati-Sforzolini B. OCT imaging of choroidal neovascularization and its role in the determination of patients' eligibility for surgery. *Br J Ophthalmol*. 1999;83(4):438-442.

SECTION II

OPTICAL COHERENCE TOMOGRAPHY IN RETINAL DISEASES

Chapter 3

Vitreoretinal Interface Disorders

Elias C. Mavrofrides, MD; Adam H. Rogers, MD;
Steven Truong, MD; Carmen A. Puliafito, MD; and James G. Fujimoto, PhD

- Idiopathic Epiretinal Membrane
- Vitreomacular Traction Syndrome
- Idiopathic Macular Hole
- Full-Thickness Macular Hole
- Lamellar Macular Hole

Abnormalities of the vitreoretinal interface are involved in the pathogenesis of several macular conditions. In idiopathic epiretinal membrane (ERM) formation, a layer of abnormal tissue develops on the surface of the retina usually following posterior vitreous detachment. Contraction of this membrane can result in retinal distortion and/or vascular leakage with associated vision loss. In other conditions, such as vitreomacular traction syndrome or idiopathic macular hole, there are abnormal attachments between the vitreous and retina. The resulting traction exerted on the retina causes alterations in retinal anatomy and subsequent loss of vision.

Optical coherence tomography (OCT) has become a powerful tool in the evaluation of these conditions. The vitreoretinal changes that characterize these conditions are often subtle and difficult to distinguish on biomicroscopic examination. By providing a high resolution cross-sectional image of the retina and vitreoretinal interface, OCT can provide valuable information not visible on biomicroscopy. In addition, OCT can provide a more objective means to monitor the natural history and therapeutic response of these conditions.

Idiopathic Epiretinal Membrane

Idiopathic ERMs occur in approximately 6% of patients over the age of 60 with the incidence increasing with age.[1] Symptoms vary from minimal to severe depending on the location, density, and contraction of the membrane. On slit-lamp biomicroscopy, a mild ERM appears as a glistening layer on the retinal surface. Denser membranes may be seen as a gray sheet overlying the retina. Contraction of these membranes can result in retinal distortion, often affecting the course of adjacent retinal vessels. Traction on the vessels may also cause increased permeability and associated retinal edema. Fluorescein angiography highlights the retinal vascular distortion and leakage.

OCT has become a useful diagnostic technique in evaluating ERMs. ERMs are visible on the OCT image as a highly reflective layer on the inner retinal surface. In most patients, the membrane is globally adherent to the retina. In approximately 25% of patients, the membrane is separated from the inner retina, enhancing visibility.[2] In this situation, the ERM must be distinguished from a detached posterior hyaloid face, which can also appear as a reflective band above the retinal surface. The posterior hyaloid usually has a thin, patchy reflection compared to the denser reflection of an ERM. Additionally, the degree of separation from the inner retina is usually greater for the posterior hyaloid.

By providing qualitative and quantitative information about retinal anatomy, OCT can identify factors contributing to vision loss in patients with ERMs. Quantitative measurements of membrane thickness and reflectivity can be used to establish the degree of membrane opacity. Loss of the normal foveal contour is an early sign of retinal distortion from mild membrane formation. More advanced membranes can result in variable retinal thickening that can be quantified on the OCT image. Studies have shown that OCT measurements of retinal thickness correlate with visual acuity in patients with ERMs.[3,4]

ERMs also frequently cause retinal distortion that creates a pseudohole appearance. OCT can effectively distinguish macular pseudohole from lesions that may appear similar on clinical exam. ERM with macular pseudohole displays a steep foveal pit contour with thickening of the macular edges on the OCT image. Although this may simulate a full-thickness hole, the presence of retinal tissue at the base of the pit establishes this as a pseudohole.

Many studies have attempted to establish prognostic indicators of operative success after ERM surgery.[2,4,5-7] Potential indicators include preoperative vision, duration of symptoms, membrane location, membrane thickness, pseudohole formation, retinal thickness, and cystoid macular edema. Studies have been able to establish some predictive significance of preoperative vision and duration of symptoms. Since studies investigating the other characteristics have relied on subjective assessments, the results are controversial. Quantitative measurement with the OCT may provide a new means for investigating the significance of these factors.

Preoperative OCT imaging can also help direct the operative approach. In cases with separation between the membrane and retina, the surgeon may be directed to these areas to initiate membrane peeling. When the membrane is globally attached to the inner retina, the surgeon may anticipate more difficulty peeling the membrane. The surgeon may also proceed with particular caution when extensive intraretinal edema leaves a thin, friable inner retinal layer beneath the membrane.

Postoperative OCT imaging can be used to document surgical response. The completeness of ERM removal can often be assessed by comparing preoperative and postoperative images. Recent studies have used OCT measurements to monitor changes in retinal thickness after surgery. These studies have shown that retinal thickness decreases following successful ERM peeling.[3,4] Azzolini and others have shown a correlation between this decrease in retinal thickness and improved visual acuity after surgery.[3]

Vitreomacular Traction Syndrome

Vitreomacular traction syndrome refers to conditions in which retinal changes develop from incomplete posterior vitreous detachment with persistent vitreous adhesion to the macula. A broad area of vitreous attachment around the optic nerve and macula is often seen ophthalmoscopically. In rare cases, thin vitreous strands attaching to the fovea may be identified.[8] Traction on the retina frequently causes retinal distortion and subsequent cystoid macular edema (CME). These changes result in central vision loss and metamorphopsia.

Although the vitreous attachment to the macula usually appears broad on clinical exam, OCT typically shows a perifoveal vitreous detachment with focal adhesion to the fovea. This configuration appears identical to the vitreous attachment identified in idiopathic macular hole. Why some patients with this progress toward CME (vitreomacular traction syndrome) while others develop macular holes remains unclear. Variations in the location, density, and diameter of the vitreoretinal adhesion may explain these differences. Qualitative and quantitative studies using OCT imaging may clarify this issue in the future.

As with other vitreoretinal interface abnormalities, OCT is extremely useful in monitoring the progression of patients with vitreomacular traction syndrome. Spontaneous resolution of vitreoretinal traction with normalization of the retinal contour has been documented with OCT.[9,10] On the other hand, persistent traction can lead to progressive retinal edema and thickening. Quantifying such changes with the OCT can be valuable in determining the need and/or timing of surgical intervention. After surgery, OCT can be used to evaluate the anatomic response. Cases in the literature have documented improved retinal anatomy in association with increased visual acuity following vitrectomy surgery.[11,12]

Idiopathic Macular Hole

Idiopathic macular holes typically occur in the sixth to seventh decade of life with a 2:1 female preponderance. Symptoms include decreased visual acuity, metamorphopsia, and central scotoma. Bilateral involvement occurs in 15% to 20% of patients.

Lesions that can ophthalmoscopically resemble various stages of macular hole development are relatively common.[13] These lesions include ERM with pseudohole, lamellar hole, macular cysts, and foveal detachment. OCT imaging can effectively distinguish between these conditions. Full-thickness macular holes show complete loss of retinal tissue in the fovea extending to the retinal pigment epithelium (RPE) layer. In contrast, ERM with pseudohole shows a steepened foveal pit contour with persistent retinal tissue at the base of the pit. Lamellar holes show partial thickness loss or separation of retinal tissue with a thin layer of persistent outer retina above the RPE. Macular cysts are identified by clear, signal-free areas that are within the retina. A similar clear space under the fovea characterizes a foveal detachment.

Gass has most completely described the stages of macular hole formation based on biomicroscopic findings.[14] In describing these stages, he emphasized the role of vitreomacular traction in macular hole development. A Stage 1 impending hole is characterized by a foveal detachment that is seen as a yellow spot or ring in the fovea. Approximately half of the impending holes will resolve spontaneously at the time of posterior vitreous detachment, while half will progress to more advanced stages. Stage 2 macular holes have a full-thickness dehiscence of the retina that measures less than 400 microns (μm). A small dehiscence may not be visible biomicroscopically. Stage 3 holes develop with further enlargement of the hole to greater than 400 μm. Stage 4 holes are characterized by complete posterior vitreous detachment regardless of hole size.

OCT has enhanced our understanding of the pathogenesis of macular holes. OCT imaging of the vitreoretinal interface has confirmed the role of vitreomacular traction in macular hole development. Hee and associates were the first to identify a perifoveal vitreous detachment with persistent vitreous traction on the fovea in the fellow eye of patients with unilateral macular hole.[13] Although this configuration was clearly identified on OCT, these changes could not be seen biomicroscopically.

Several subsequent studies looking at fellow eyes have confirmed the importance of this configuration in hole development.[15-19] Some patients maintain a normal visual acuity and foveal contour despite this abnormal foveal attachment. In other patients, progressive traction results in retinal distortion and Stage 1 impending hole formation. Spaide et al have shown that the diameter of vitreous attachment measured on OCT may correlate with the changes induced in foveal anatomy.[20] In this study, narrow attachments were more likely to induce foveal changes than broader attachments. As a result, OCT may become important in identifying patients at increased risk for hole formation.

The anatomic changes identified on OCT have also been correlated with the various stages of macular hole formation. Some patients with persistent foveal traction have developed foveal detachment consistent with a Stage 1 impending hole as described by Gass.[14] Several studies have subsequently shown the development of a pseudocyst as the initial stage of macular hole formation.[15,17,18] This appears as a minimally reflective cavity within the fovea beneath the area of persistent vitreal attachment. Spontaneous resolution of these changes has been documented on OCT with complete detachment of the vitreous. Enlargement of this pseudocyst with loss of the outer retinal layers and dehiscence of the inner retinal layers characterizes progression to a Stage 2 hole. An operculum with vitreous attachment may remain connected to one edge of the hole. Stages 3 holes show further enlargement of the full-thickness defect with variable amounts of subretinal and intraretinal edema at the edges of the hole. An operculum may still be visualized but is now completely separated and suspended above the hole. Because the vitreous has completely detached from the optic nerve and macula, Stage 4 macular holes show large full-thickness defects in the retina without visualization of the posterior hyaloid.

Vitrectomy surgery has become an effective treatment in achieving anatomic closure and improved visual acuity in patients with full-thickness macular holes. One of the quickly expanding roles for OCT is in the perioperative assessment of macular hole patients. Postoperative anatomic changes can be documented with OCT. The fovea can demonstrate one of four distinct patterns after macular hole surgery: open, closed, thin, and foveolar detachment.[21] Closed holes have reapproximation of the hole edges with a relatively normal foveal contour and thickness. Thin cases will have closure of the hole but a central foveal thickness of less than 100 μm. In foveolar detachment, the reapproximated edges of the hole remain detached from the underlying RPE. Over time, the subretinal fluid may be resorbed with resolution of the detachment. These anatomic changes on OCT often correlate with visual improvement, providing useful information about the patient's response to surgery.

Quantitative information about the macular hole can also be obtained from the OCT tomogram. Measurements of minimum hole diameter, base diameter, and retinal edge thickness may be useful in predicting surgical success. Ip and associates were the first to show that preoperative minimum hole diameter determined by OCT has prognostic significance for postoperative success.[22] Macular holes less than 400 μm on OCT had a significantly higher rate of anatomic closure compared to larger holes. There was also a trend for greater visual improvement in patients with smaller holes. Ullrich has subsequently shown that both preoperative minimum hole diameter and base diameter are prognostic factors for visual outcome and anatomic success.[23] The preoperative base diameter, which can only be measured by OCT, showed the strongest correlation with these outcomes.

References

1. Pearstone AD. The incidence of idiopathic preretinal macular gliosis. *Ann Ophthalmol*. 1985;17:378.
2. Wilkins JR, Puliafito CA, Hee MR, et al. Characterization of epiretinal membranes using optical coherence tomography. *Ophthalmology*. 1996;103:2142-2151.
3. Azzolini C, Patelli F, Codenotti M, Pierro L, Brancato R. Optical coherence tomography in idiopathic epiretinal membrane surgery. *Eur J Ophthalmol*. 1999;9:206-211.
4. Massin P, Allouch C, Haouchine B, et al. Optical coherence tomography of idiopathic epiretinal membrane before and after surgery. *Am J Ophthalmol*. 2000;130:732-739.
5. Trese MT, Chandler DB, Machemer R. Macular pucker I. Prognostic criteria. *Graefes Arch Clin Exp Ophthalmol*. 1983;221:12-15.

6. Rice TA, De Bustros S, Michels RG, et al. Prognostic factors in vitrectomy for epiretinal membranes of the macula. *Ophthalmology*. 1986;93:602-610.
7. Pesin SR, Olk RJ, Grand MG, et al. Vitrectomy for premacular fibroplasias. Prognostic factors, long-term follow-up, and time course of visual improvement. *Ophthalmology*. 1991;98:1109-1114.
8. Smiddy WE, Michels RG, Glaser BM, De Bustros S. Vitrectomy for macular traction caused by incomplete vitreous separation. *Arch Ophthalmol*. 1988;106:624-628.
9. Sulkes DJ, Ip MS, Baumal CR, Wu HK, Puliafito CA. Spontaneous resolution of vitreomacular traction documented by optical coherence tomography. *Arch Ophthalmol*. 2000;118:286-287.
10. Kusaka S, Saito Y, Okada AA, et al. Optical coherence tomography in spontaneously resolving vitreomacular traction syndrome. *Ophthalmologica*. 2001;215:139-141.
11. Munuera JM, Garcia-Layana A, Maldonado MJ, et al. Optical coherence tomography of successful surgery of vitreomacular traction syndrome. *Arch Ophthalmol*. 1998;116:1388-1389.
12. Uchino E, Uemura A, Doi N, Ohba N. Postsurgical evaluation of idiopathic vitreomacular traction syndrome by optical coherence tomography. *Am J Ophthalmol*. 2001;132:122-123.
13. Hee MR, Puliafito CA, Wong C, et al. Optical coherence tomography of macular holes. *Ophthalmology*. 1995;102:748-756.
14. Gass JDM. Reappraisal of biomicroscopic classification of stages of development of macular hole. *Arch Ophthalmol*. 1995;119:752-759.
15. Gaudric A, Haouchine B, Massin P, Paques M, Blain P, Erginay A. Macular hole formation. *Arch Ophthalmol*. 1999;117:744-751.
16. Spiritus A, Dralands L, Stalmans I, Spileers W. OCT studies of fellow eyes of macular holes. *Bull Soc Belge Ophthalmol*. 2000;275:81-84.
17. Azzolini C, Patelli F, Brancato R. Correlation between optical coherence tomography data and biomicroscopic interpretation of idiopathic macular hole. *Am J Ophthalmol*. 2001;132:348-355.
18. Haouchine B, Massin P, Gaudric A. Foveal pseudocyst as the first step in macular hole formation. *Ophthalmology*. 2001;108:15-22.
19. Tanner V, Chauhan S, Jackson TL, Williamson TH. Optical coherence tomography of the vitreoretinal interface in macular hole formation. *Br J Ophthalmol*. 2001;85:1092-1097.
20. Spaide RF, Wong D, Fisher Y, Goldbaum M. Correlation of vitreous attachment and foveal deformation in early macular hole states. *Am J Ophthalmol*. 2002;133:226-229.
21. Desai VN, Hee MR, Puliafito CA. Optical coherence tomography of macular holes. In: Madreperla SA, McCuen BW, eds. *Macular Hole*. Boston, Mass: Butterworth-Heinemann; 1999:37-47.
22. Ip MS, Baker BJ, Duker JS, et al. Anatomical outcomes of surgery for idiopathic macular hole as determined by optical coherence tomography. *Arch Ophthalmol*. 2002;120:29-35.
23. Ullrich S, Haritoglou C, Gass C, Schaumberger M, Ulbig MW, Kampik A. Macular hole size as a prognostic factor in macular hole surgery. *Br J Ophthalmol*. 2002;86:390-393.

Case 3-1.
Mild Epiretinal Membrane

Clinical Summary

A 74-year-old female notes mildly decreased visual acuity in the left eye for 6 months duration. The patient's visual acuity in the left eye is 20/30. Dilated fundus examination of this eye (A) shows a posterior vitreous detachment with a mild ERM formation. There is no apparent retinal distortion or macular edema on exam.

Optical Coherence Tomography

OCT examination (B) shows a reflective band on the surface of the retina corresponding to the ERM. Adjacent to the fovea, contraction of the ERM has caused distortion of the inner retinal layers. The membrane also extends over the fovea, resulting in loss of the normal foveal contour. Central retinal thickness is increased to 290 μm, reflecting this change in foveal contour.

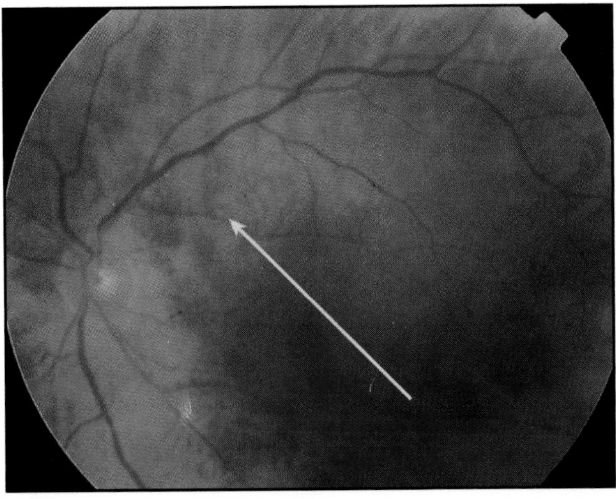

A

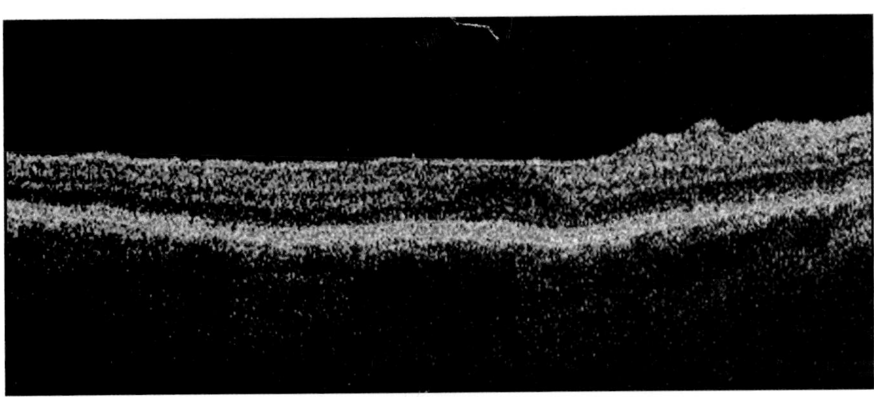

B

Case 3-2. Epiretinal Membrane With Pseudohole

Clinical Summary

A 74-year-old male is referred for evaluation of a macular hole in the left eye. His visual acuity is 20/30 in this eye. Dilated fundus examination (A) shows evidence of an ERM that is most dense temporal to the fovea with apparent pseudohole formation.

Optical Coherence Tomography

OCT examination (B) shows an abnormally deep and wide foveal pit contour. The thin layer of retinal tissue at the base of the fovea confirms that this is a pseudohole configuration. On the left side of the image there are small irregularities in the inner retina that correspond to retinal striae from membrane traction. The ERM itself is tightly adherent to the inner retinal surface and can not be readily distinguished on the OCT image. A faint and patchy linear density suspended above the retina represents the detached posterior hyaloid.

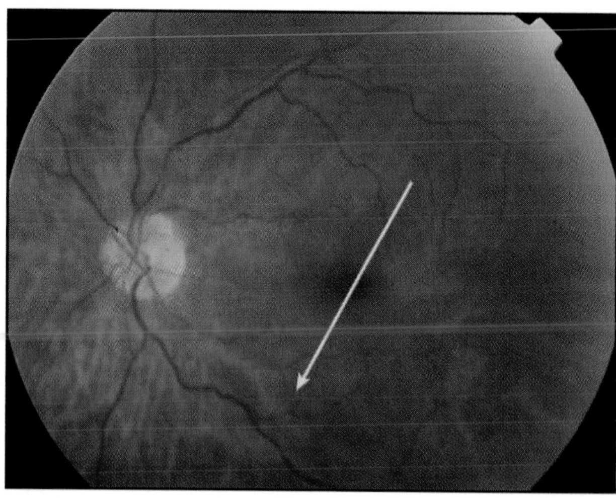

A

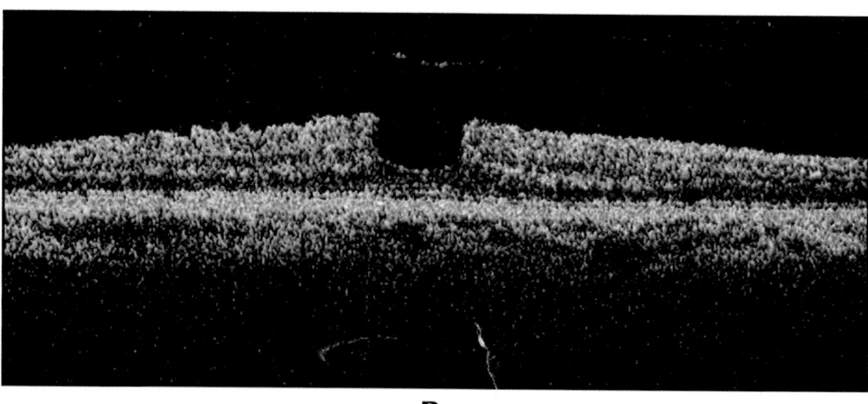

B

Case 3-3. Epiretinal Membrane With Pseudohole

Clinical Summary

A 68-year-old female reports mild distortion of the central vision in her left eye. Her visual acuity is 20/30 in this eye. Dilated fundus examination (A) shows a dense ERM around the fovea with retinal distortion and pseudohole formation. Fluorescein angiography does not show evidence of significant leakage in the late frames.

Optical Coherence Tomography

OCT examination (B) shows the ERM as a hyper-reflective band on the inner retinal surface. The membrane is most clearly seen on the right side of the scan where there are focal areas of separation between the membrane and the retina. An edge of the membrane can also be identified in this area. On the left side of the scan, the membrane is less distinct because it is closely adhered to the retina. Secondary effects of the membrane are evident in this area, however, as small irregularities of the retinal surface. The steep and wide foveal pit contour suggests a macular hole, but the reflective retinal tissue at the base of the fovea confirms a pseudohole configuration.

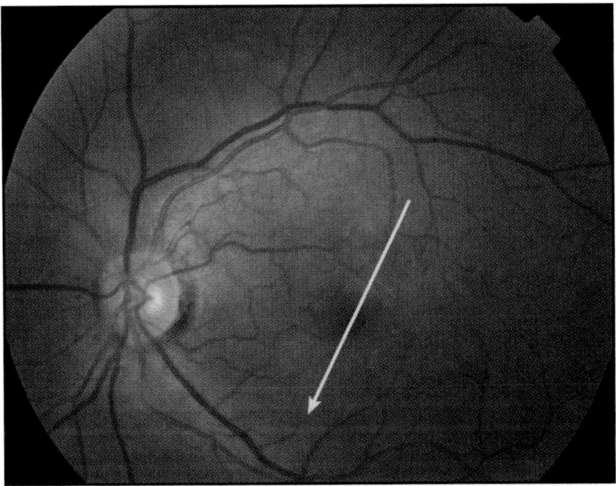

A

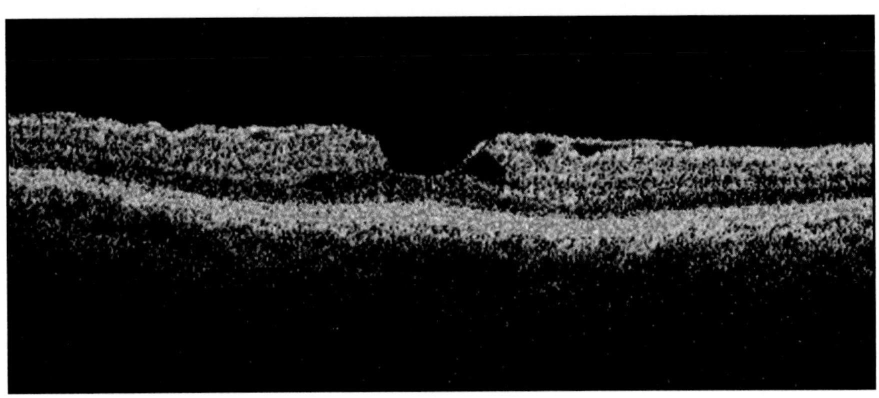

B

Case 3-4A. Epiretinal Membrane With Macular Edema in Both Eyes

Clinical Summary

A 69-year-old male is referred for evaluation of macular pucker. He has a history of glaucoma and has undergone combined cataract extraction and filtering surgery in both eyes. His vision is 20/70 in the right eye. Dilated fundus examination (A) shows an ERM with mild retinal distortion. Fluorescein angiography (B) shows very mild late hyperfluorescence.

Optical Coherence Tomography

OCT examination (C) clearly shows the ERM as a thin band of increased signal on the retinal surface. The membrane is separated from the inner retinal surface in multiple areas enhancing visibility. The retina underlying this membrane is diffusely thickened with loss of the normal foveal contour. Central retinal thickness measures 458 µm on the thickness map (D).

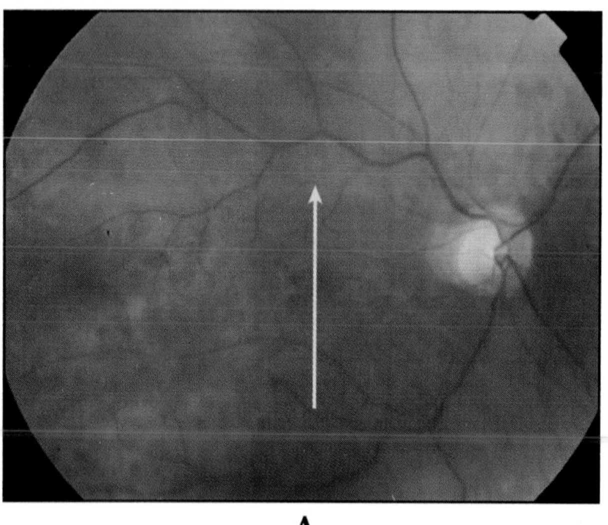

A

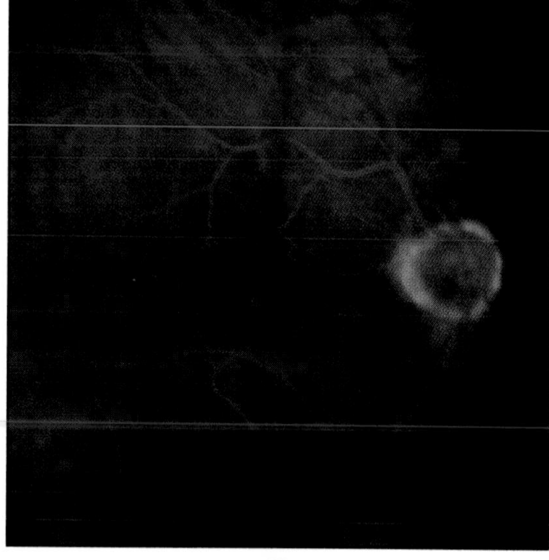

B

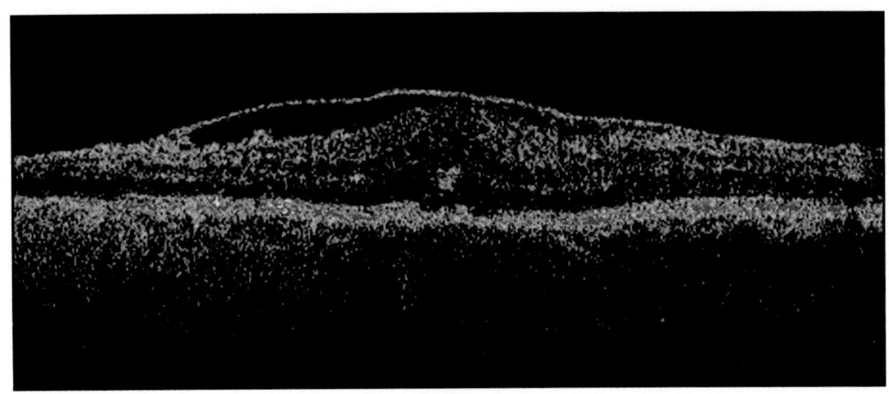

C

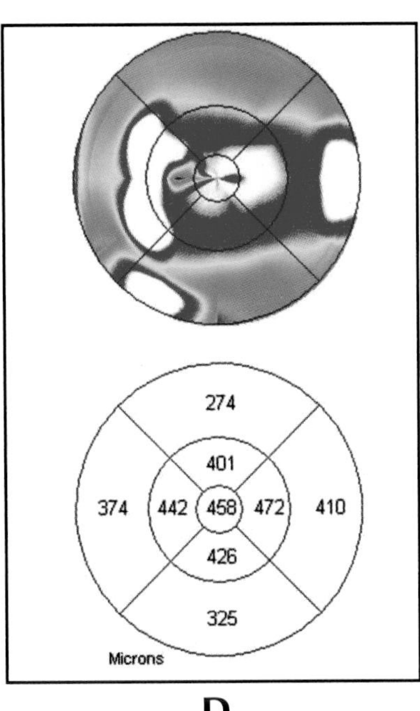

D

Case 3-4B. Epiretinal Membrane With Macular Edema in Both Eyes

Clinical Summary

His visual acuity in the left eye is 20/70. Dilated fundus examination (E) shows a dense ERM with extensive retinal distortion. Membrane traction has resulted in straightening of the retinal vessels off the temporal edge of the optic disc. Fluorescein angiography (F) reveals late hyperfluorescence consistent with macular edema.

Optical Coherence Tomography

In this eye, the membrane is globally adherent to the inner retina on the OCT image (G). Despite this close adherence, this dense ERM can still be seen as a highly reflective band on the retinal surface. The retina is extensively thickened beneath the membrane. An area of decreased reflectivity in the outer retina represents intraretinal fluid. The thickness map (H) confirms retinal thickening in the area of the membrane with a maximum of 551 µm at the fovea.

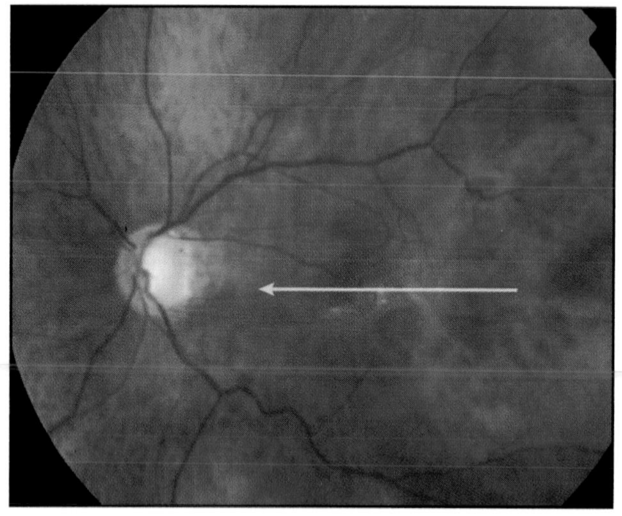

E

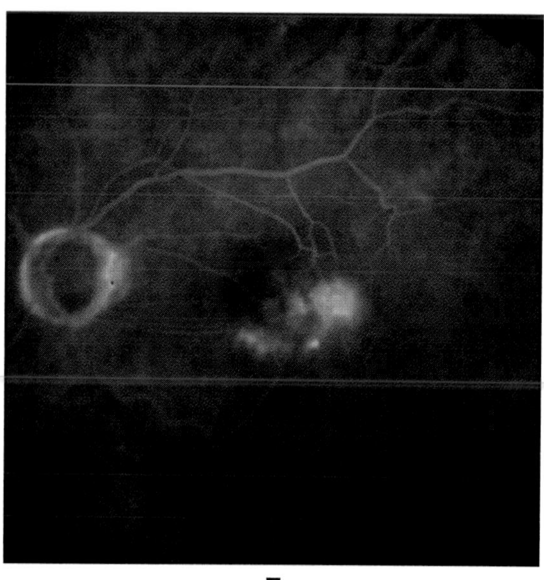

F

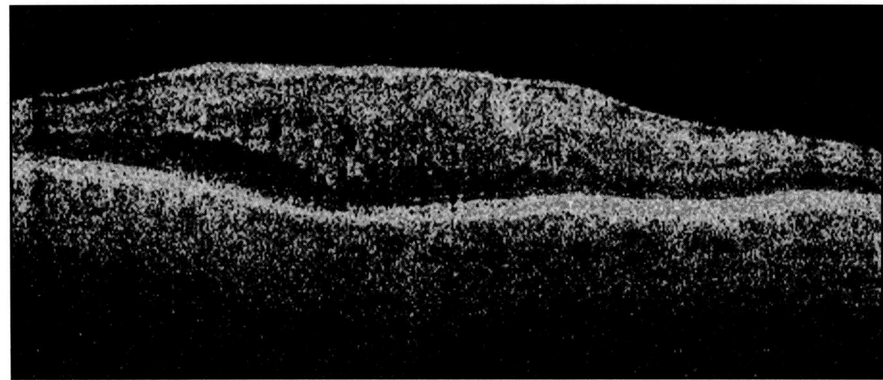

G

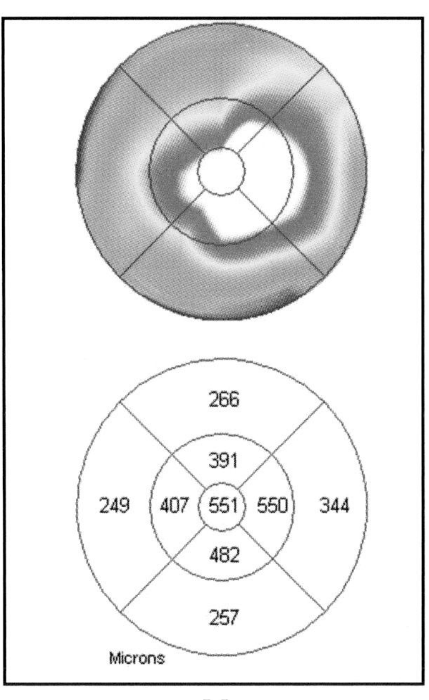

H

Case 3-5. Epiretinal Membrane With Macular Edema

Clinical Summary

A 74-year-old female is referred for evaluation of an ERM in her right eye. Her vision in this eye is 20/400. Dilated fundus examination (A) shows a dense ERM with associated retinal distortion and thickening. Fluorescein angiography (B) shows straightening of the vessels off the temporal edge of the disc, with increased tortuosity of the vessels under the membrane. In the late frames, there is mild hyperfluorescence.

Optical Coherence Tomography

OCT examination (C) clearly shows the ERM as a highly reflective band on the inner retinal surface. Temporal to the fovea, the membrane is only slightly separated from the retina, while nasally the degree of separation is greater. The fovea is extensively thickened from intraretinal edema with loss of the foveal depression. The thickness map (D) shows extensive retinal thickening throughout the central macula, reaching a peak of 468 μm just superior to the fovea.

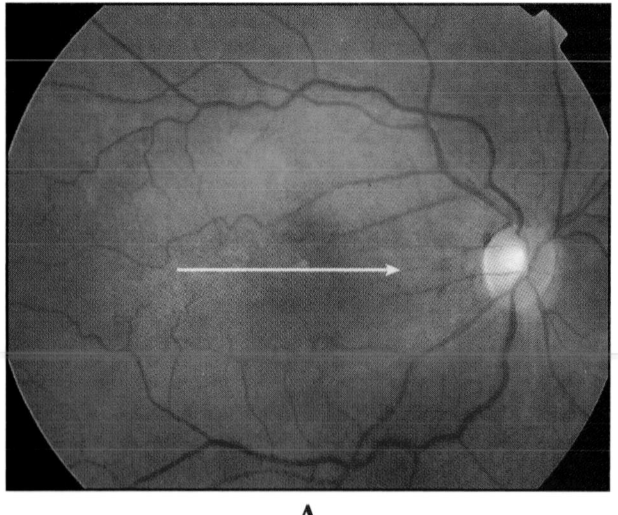

A

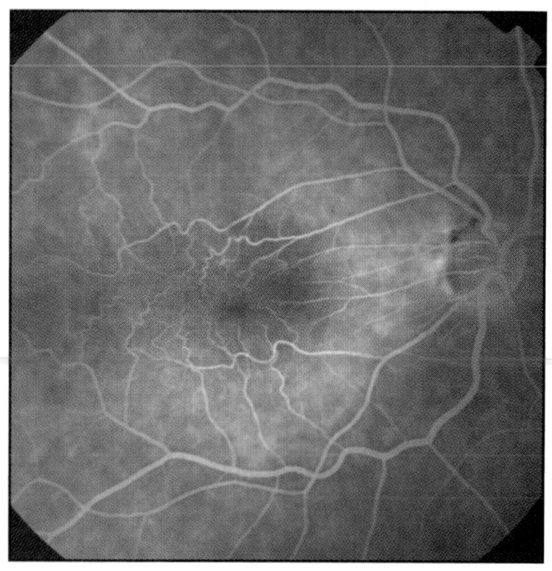

B

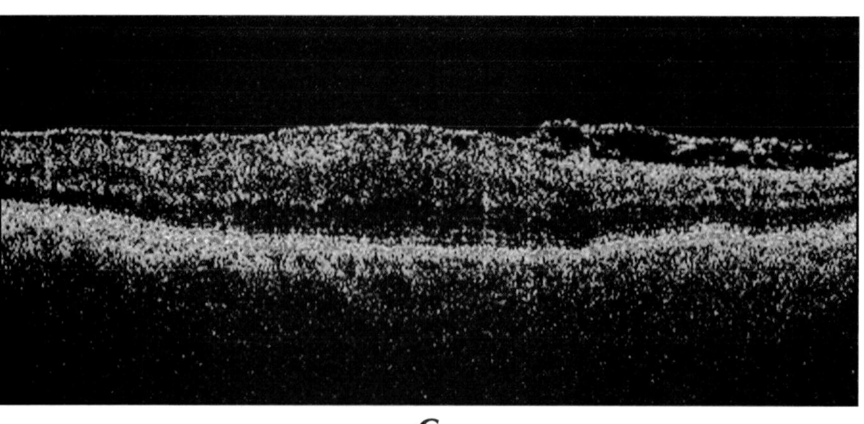

C

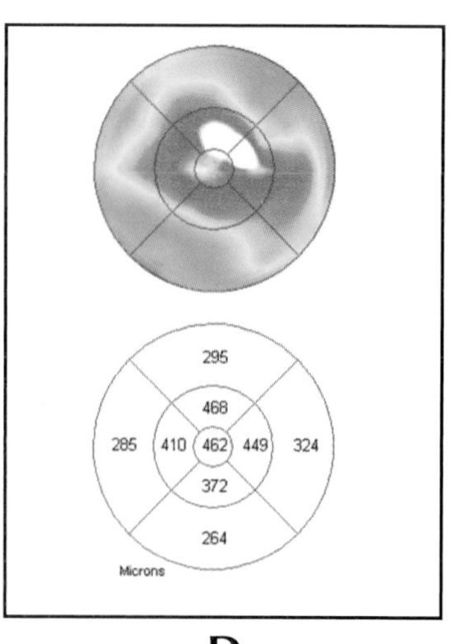

D

Case 3-6. *Epiretinal Membrane With Macular Edema*

Clinical Summary

A 72-year-old female is referred for evaluation of ERM in the right eye. Her visual acuity in this eye is 20/400. Dilated fundus examination (A) shows a dense ERM in the foveal region. Traction exerted by this membrane has altered the course of the retinal vessels in this area.

Optical Coherence Tomography

OCT examination (B) clearly shows the hyperreflective membrane on the surface of the retina. Small areas of separation between the retina and membrane enhance visualization. In the fovea, there appears to be a discontinuity in the ERM. The abnormally thickened retina protrudes above the plane of the membrane through this discontinuity. The retinal thickness map (C) highlights this abnormal configuration. Foveal thickness measures 591 μm, which is more than 100 μm greater than the adjacent retina.

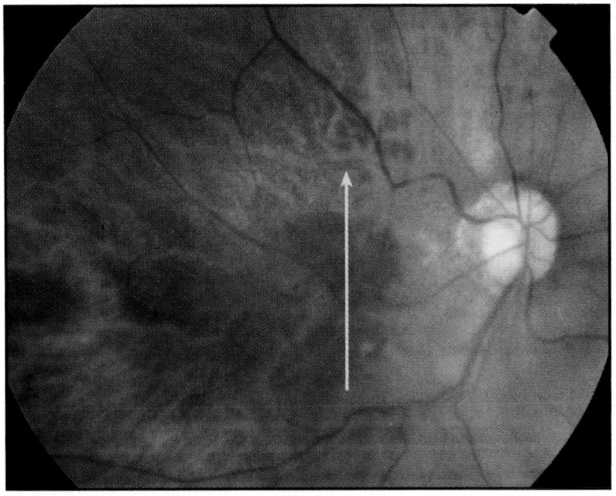

A

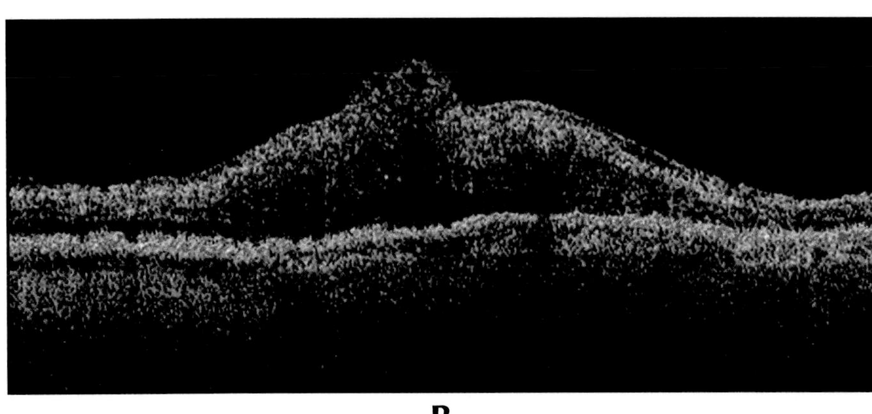

B

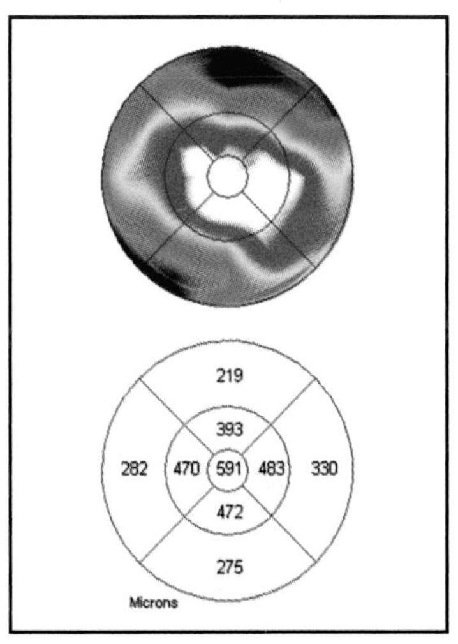

C

Case 3-7. Epiretinal Membrane With Extensive Macular Edema

Clinical Summary

A 52-year-old male with prior trauma and counting fingers visual acuity in the right eye is referred for evaluation of metamorphopsia and decreased visual acuity in the left eye. His visual acuity in the left eye is 20/30. Clinical examination demonstrates an ERM with macular edema. Given that the patient is functionally monocular with adequate visual acuity in the left eye, he continues to be conservatively managed with observation.

Optical Coherence Tomography

OCT (A) of the left eye identifies macular edema as intraretinal, hyporeflective, black spaces. The ERM is a thin, yellow-red reflective line at the vitreoretinal interface inserting into the retina at the area of the fovea. The tension of the ERM separates it from the retina, as visualized by the hyporeflective black space on either side of the fovea. The retina is thrown into folds secondary to the traction placed in the retina.

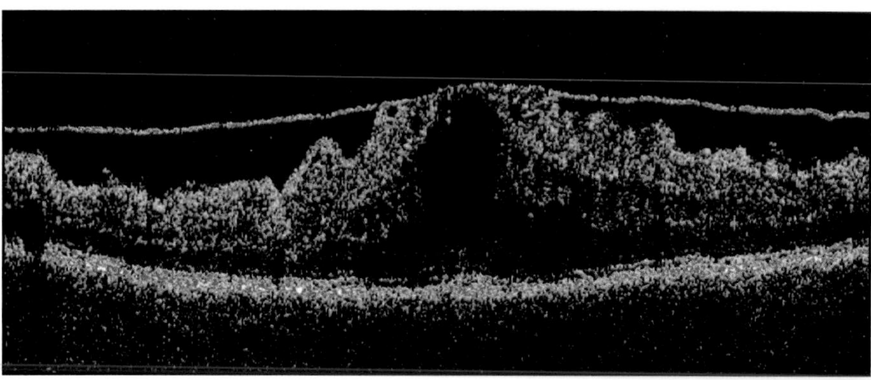

A

Case 3-8. Epiretinal Membrane With Macular Edema Improved After Vitrectomy Surgery

Clinical Summary

A 64-year-old female with a history of retinal detachment in the left eye repaired with scleral buckle surgery 1 year prior returns with 20/70 visual acuity. Clinical examination reveals good buckling effect peripherally with an attached retina. CME is visible with a pigmented ERM. A petalloid pattern of hyperfluorescence is present on fluorescein angiography consistent with CME (A). Medical treatment with topical and periocular steroids is not effective in treating the CME. Pars plana vitrectomy is performed with removal of the pigmented membrane. Despite an initial decline in visual acuity to 20/200, visual acuity improves to 20/50 3 months postoperatively.

Optical Coherence Tomography

Initial OCT (B) shows intraretinal hyporeflective black spaces consistent with CME. The images of the retina outside of the fovea are normal. There is mild hyperreflectivity of the inner retina near the vitreoretinal interface. However, there is no obvious ERM delineated by the OCT. Three months postoperatively (C) there is near complete resolution of the CME with restoration of a foveal contour. A central foveal cyst is still present.

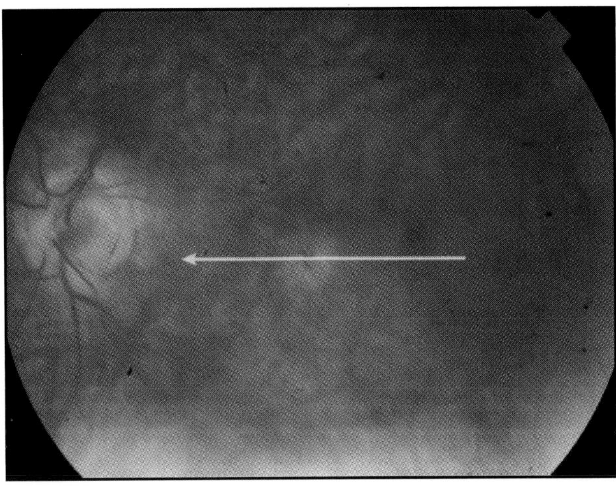

A

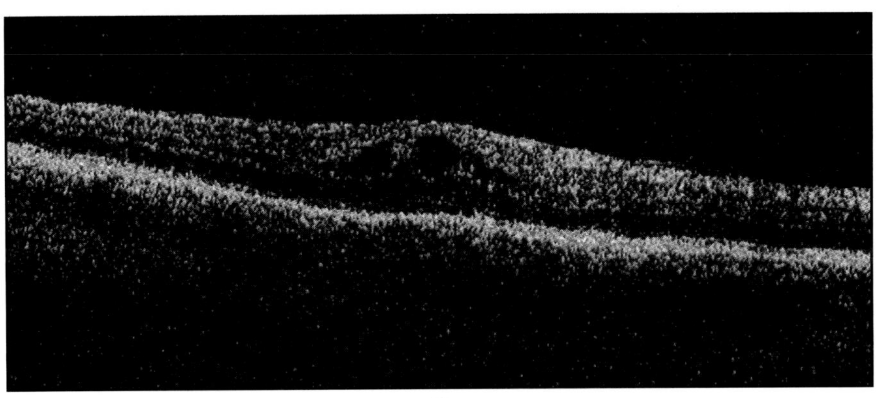

B

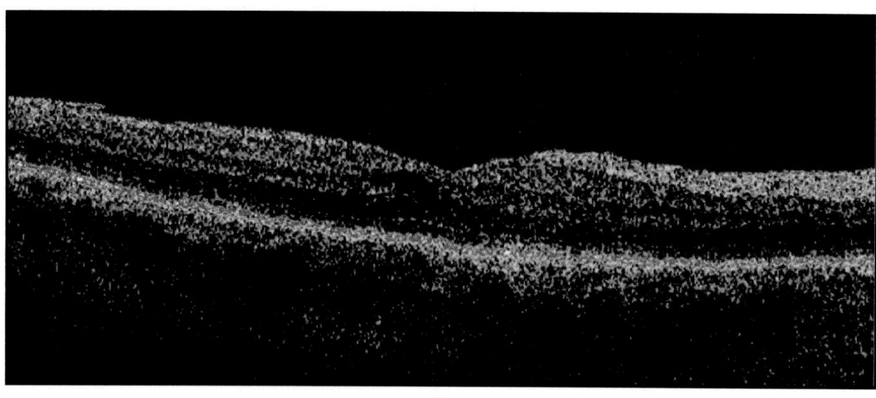

C

Case 3-9. Dense Epiretinal Membrane With Extensive Macular Edema

Clinical Summary

A 60-year-old male complains of worsening vision in the right eye over the past year. He has not noticed any improvement after cataract extraction 2 months ago. His visual acuity in this eye is 20/100. On dilated fundus examination (A), there is evidence of a dense ERM that has resulted in retinal distortion and pseudohole formation. There is extensive intraretinal edema in the area of this membrane. Fluorescein angiography (B) shows a large area of hyperfluorescent leakage extending from the fovea to the superior temporal arcade.

Optical Coherence Tomography

The OCT scan (C) is off set slightly to include more of the superior macula. This scan shows persistent attachment of the vitreous to the fovea. The detached portions of the posterior vitreous appear as discrete bands above the surface of the retina. At the fovea, there is a relatively broad attachment of the vitreous to the inner retinal layers. The ERM is best identified superior to the fovea, where there is a small amount of separation between the highly reflective membrane and the inner retinal surface. There is extensive fluid accumulation within the retina with the development of large intraretinal cysts. The retinal thickness is greatly increased throughout the macular region with the fovea measuring 731 μm.

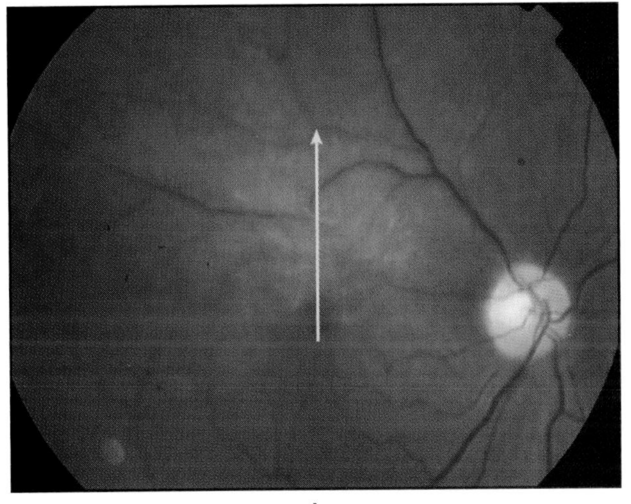

A

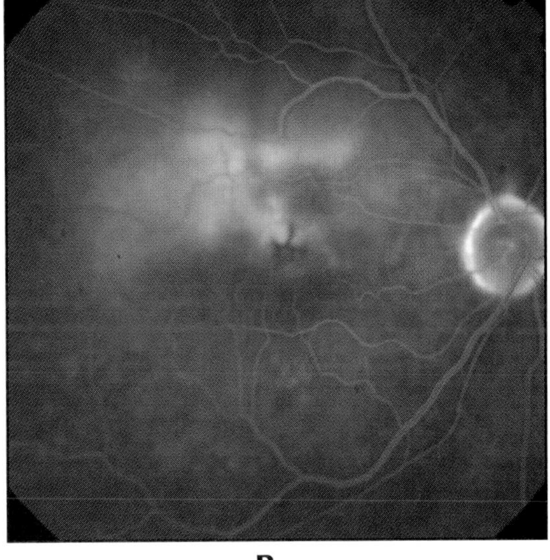

B

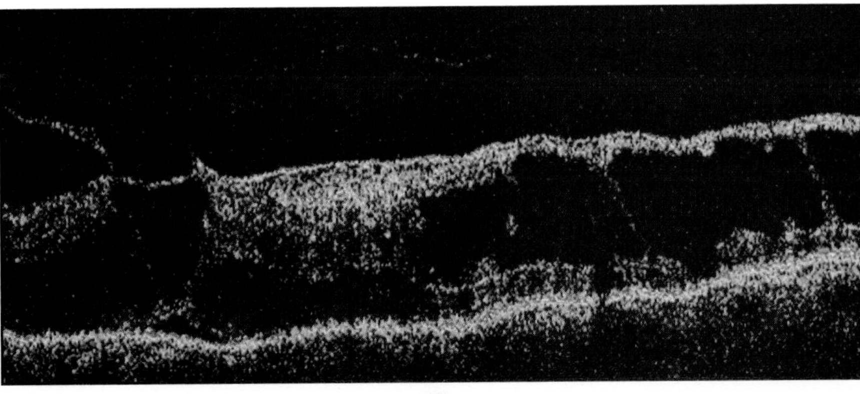

C

Case 3-10. Vitreomacular Traction and Epiretinal Membrane With Macular Edema

Clinical Summary

An 83-year-old female complains of decreased visual acuity in the right eye over the past year. Her vision did not significantly improve after neodymium:yttrium:aluminum:garnet (Nd:YAG) laser posterior capsulotomy 5 months earlier. Her visual acuity in the right eye is 20/200, and dilated fundus examination (A) shows an ERM with mild retinal edema. The fluorescein angiogram (B) shows late hyperfluorescent leakage in the fovea consistent with macular edema.

Optical Coherence Tomography

OCT examination (C) shows two linear densities suspended above the retinal surface and inserting into the foveal region. This corresponds to an incomplete separation of the posterior vitreous with persistent foveal attachment. An ERM can be seen adjacent to the fovea as a hyperreflective band on the inner retinal surface. Small areas of separation from the retina enhance visualization of the membrane. The underlying retina is thickened with loss of the normal foveal contour. There are small cystic changes in the inner retina near the area of persistent vitreal attachment. Foveal thickness is increased to 374 μm, and retinal thickness reaches a peak of 411 μm in the inferior macula.

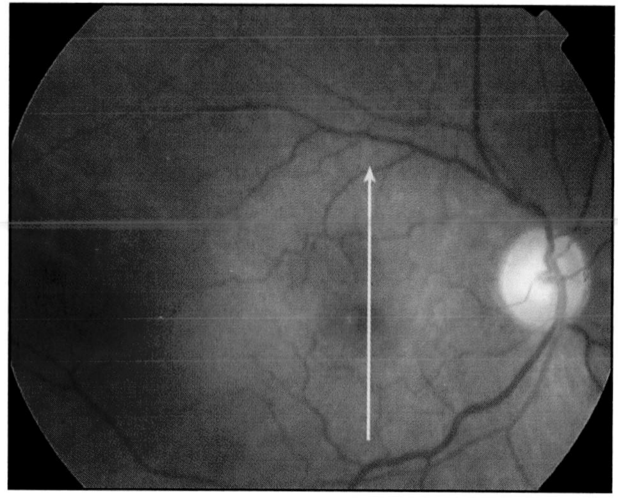

A

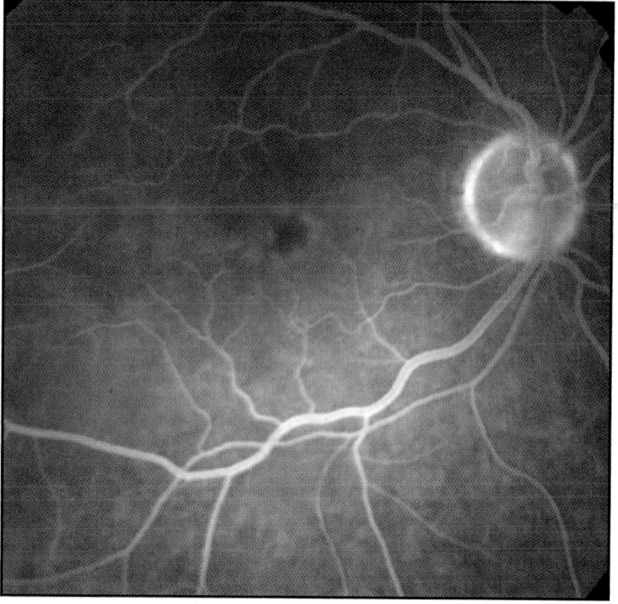

B

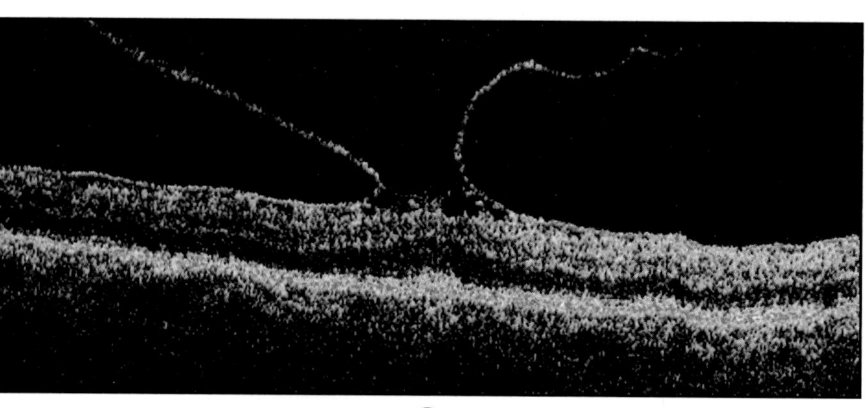

C

Case 3-11. Vitreomacular Traction and Epiretinal Membrane Successfully Treated With Vitrectomy Surgery

Clinical Summary

A 67-year-old notes a progressive decrease in vision of the left eye over the past 6 months. The visual acuity in this eye is 20/200. Fundus examination (A) demonstrates macular edema and retinal folds associated with a glistening ERM. Pars plana vitrectomy with membrane peeling is performed. Three months postoperatively, the macular edema resolved with improvement in visual acuity to 20/40.

Optical Coherence Tomography

Preoperative OCT (B) defines vitreomacular traction with attachment of the posterior hyaloid (two low reflective lines in the vitreous cavity) directly to the fovea. The tractional forces from the vitreous lead to the formation of CME, visible as the large, hyporeflective, black circular spaces in the fovea. Increased linear reflectivity along the anterior retina represents ERM formation. The central foveal thickness measures 415 µm. Postoperative OCT (C) demonstrates relief of the vitreomacular traction with removal of the ERM, resulting in a normal foveal contour. Foveal thickness measures 235 µm.

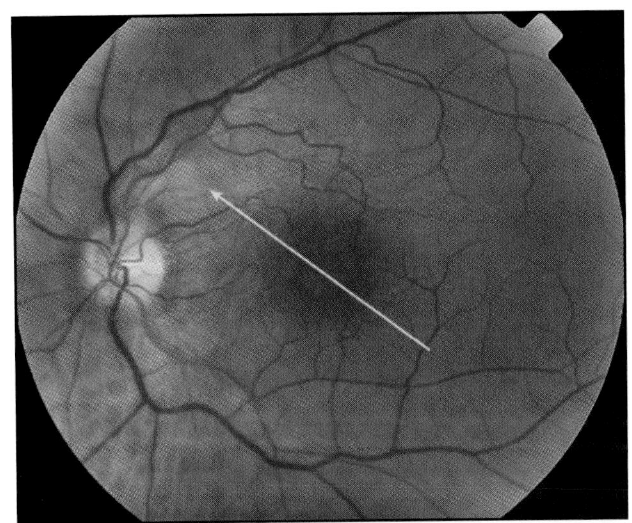

A

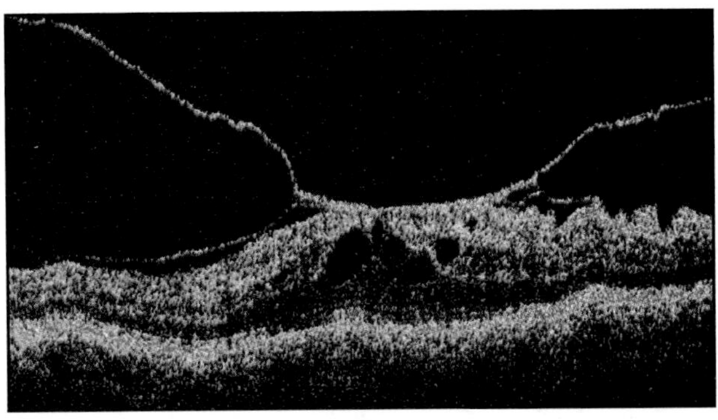

B

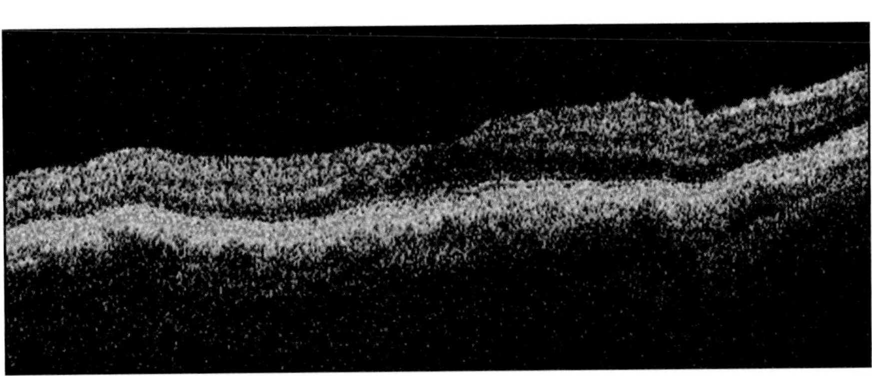

C

Case 3-12. Vitreomacular Traction and Epiretinal Membrane Successfully Treated With Vitrectomy Surgery

Clinical Summary

A 73-year-old female is referred following cataract surgery for failure of her vision to improve. Visual acuity at presentation measures 20/40. Clinical examination of the left eye (A) demonstrates an ERM with CME. The CME is delineated on fluorescein angiography with late leakage (B). Staining of the optic nerve is also observed. Pars plana vitrectomy with membrane peeling is performed without complication. During surgery, the posterior hyaloid was found to be tightly adherent to the fovea. One month postoperatively, the visual acuity improves to 20/30.

Optical Coherence Tomography

On initial OCT (C), the blue-yellow reflective lines represent the posterior vitreous hyaloid inserting to the fovea. A reflective line along the anterior surface of the retina represents an ERM. The traction induced from the vitreous inserting into the fovea has resulted in retinal cysts represented by low reflective black spaces in the fovea. OCT (D) 6 days postoperatively demonstrates relief of the vitreous traction with persistent CME. One month postoperatively (E), the foveal contour is visible with resolution of the CME.

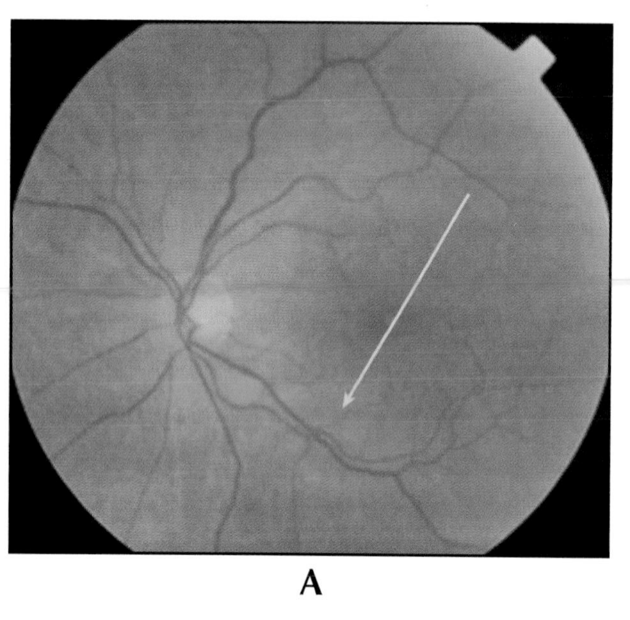

A

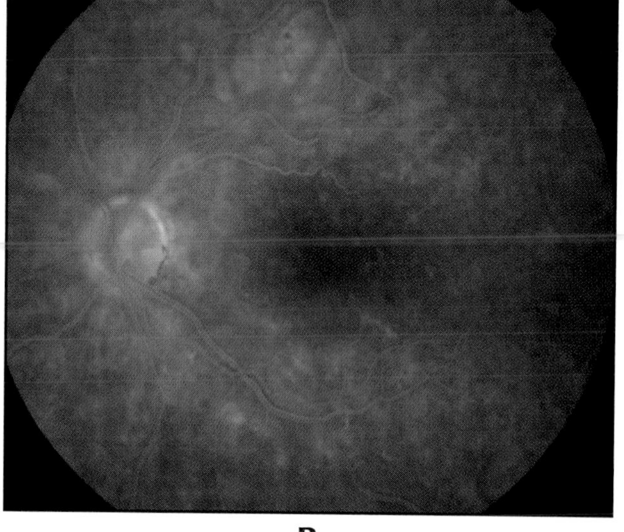

B

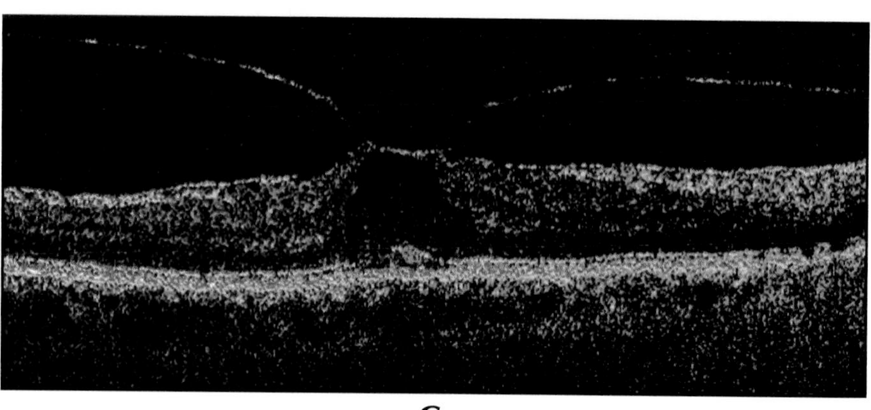

C

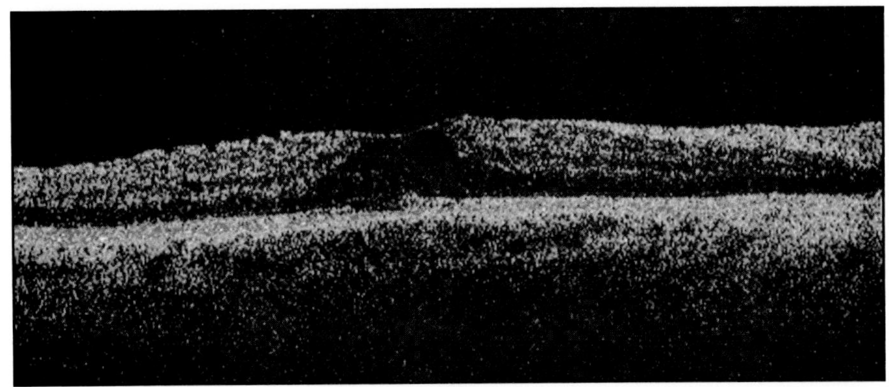

D

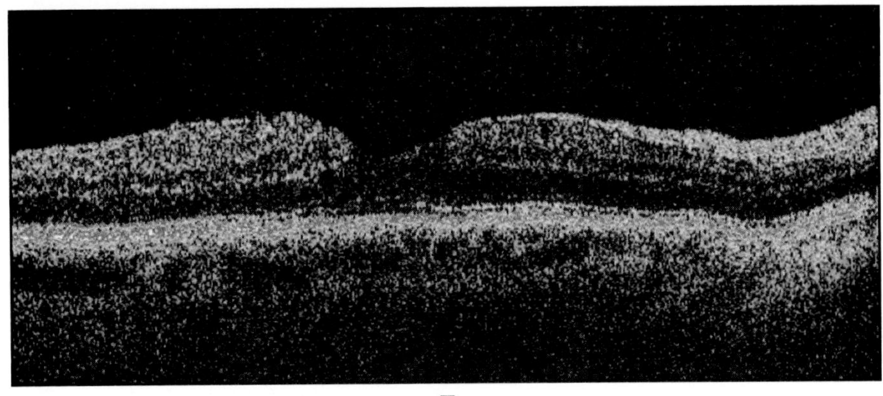

E

Case 3-13. Stage 1A Macular Hole

Clinical Summary

A 60-year-old man presents with a 3-month history of distortion in his right eye. The visual acuity measures 20/40. Clinical examination reveals a central yellow reflection and trace ERM without evidence of subretinal fluid.

Optical Coherence Tomography

OCT (A) reveals separation of the retina from the RPE layer in the fovea defining a Stage 1A macular hole. The dome-shaped area of separation is represented by a hyporeflective, black space. A foveal contour is still present in contrast to a Stage 1B hole. An ERM is visible to the left of the fovea as a thin linear reflection at the vitreoretinal interface. The tangential traction from the ERM creates mild undulations of the retinal surface. Repeat OCT 3 months later remains unchanged (B).

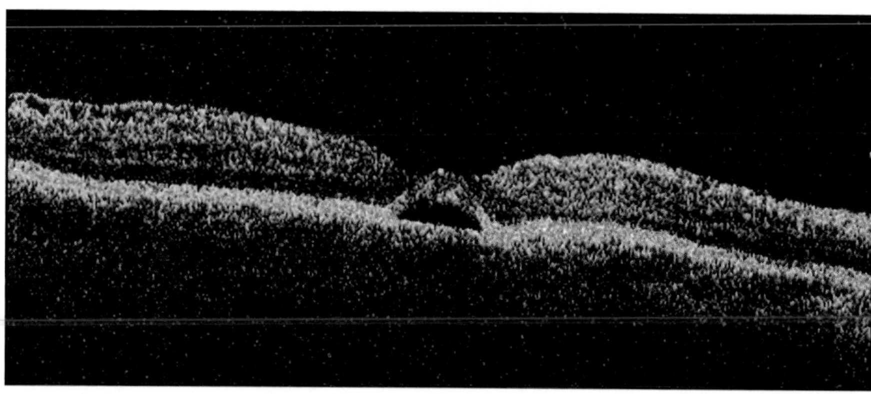

A

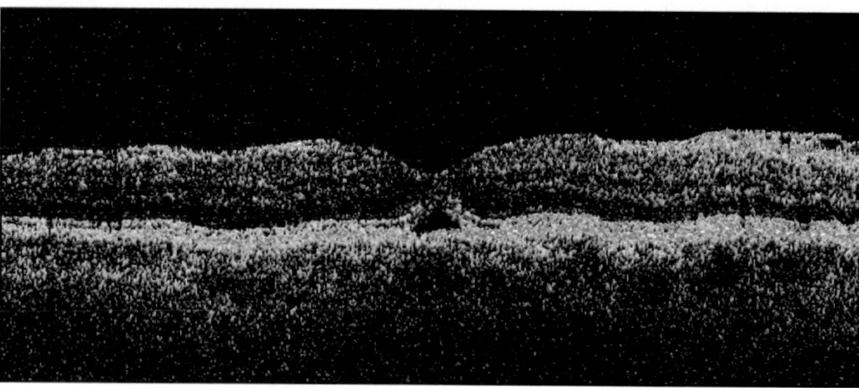

B

Case 3-14A.
Impending Macular Hole With Spontaneous Resolution

Clinical Summary

A 75-year-old male complains of decreased vision with central distortion in the right eye for 3 weeks. Visual acuity in this eye is 20/25. Dilated fundus examination (A) shows a yellow spot in the fovea that measures approximately 300 μm. There is no evidence of posterior vitreous detachment. Fluorescein angiography (B) reveals a faint hyperfluorescent spot in the fovea without associated leakage. The patient returns 2 months later and reports slight worsening of his vision with increased central distortion. The vision has decreased one line to 20/30. Dilated fundus exam is unchanged.

Optical Coherence Tomography

On OCT examination (C), there is a perifoveal vitreous detachment with persistent vitreous traction on the fovea. The posterior hyaloid face can be seen as discrete liner bands above the retina that insert into the fovea. There is a relatively broad area of attachment between the vitreous and retina. The foveal retina is elevated and distorted from traction exerted by the adherent vitreous. Decreased reflectivity within this area indicates intraretinal edema. There is a shallow detachment of the neurosensory retina and underlying RPE in the fovea. On OCT examination (D) 2 months later, there is persistent vitreomacular traction. The vitreous continues to be broadly attached to the inner retina at the fovea. Intraretinal cystic changes are still present. The retinal elevation and distortion appear slightly worse than on previous exam.

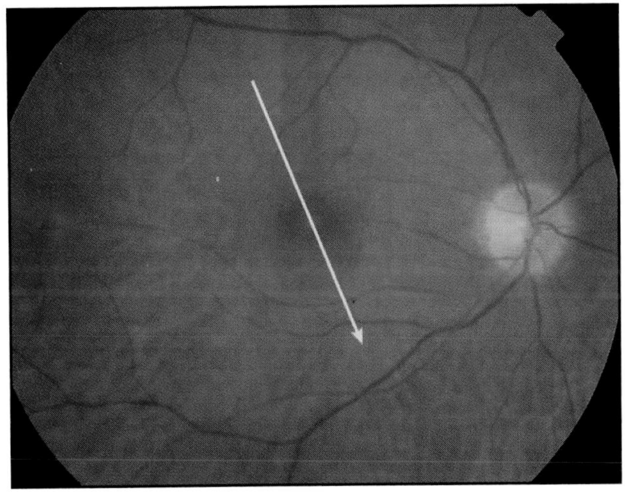

A

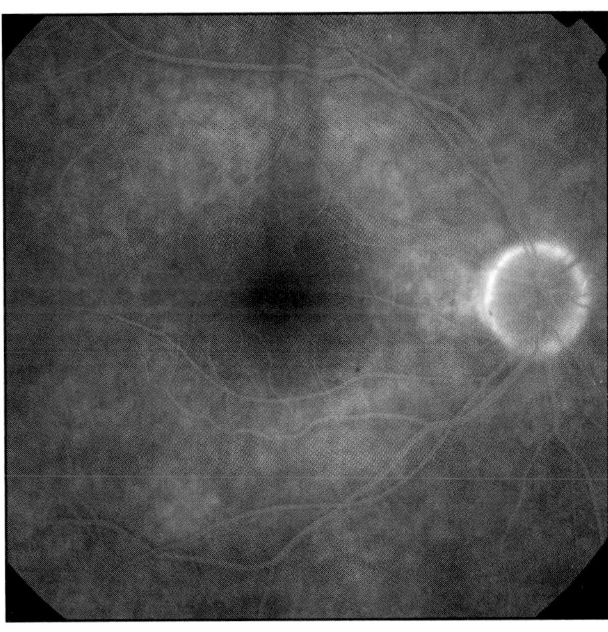

B

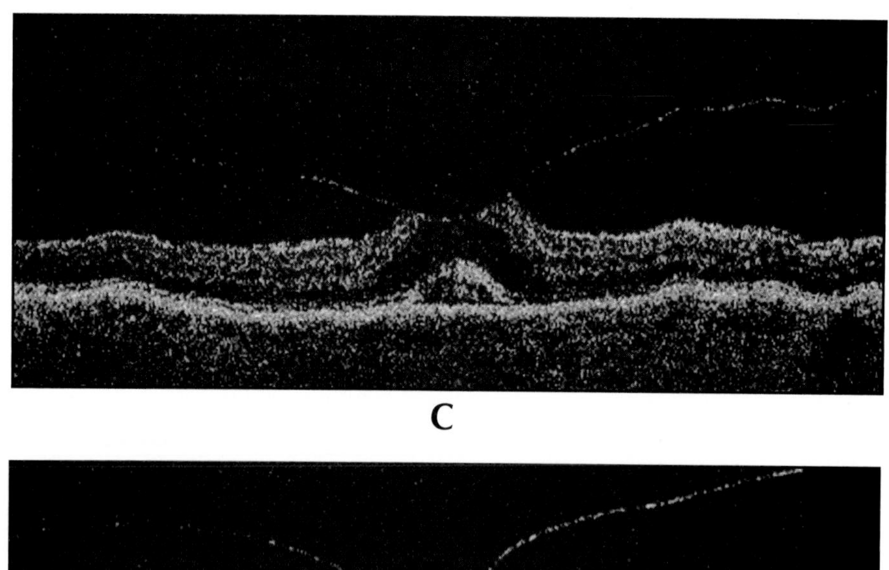

C

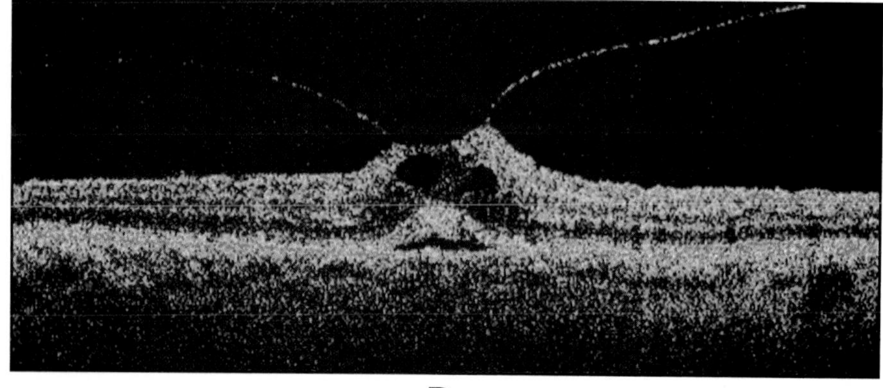

D

Case 3-14B.
Spontaneous Resolution

Continuation of Clinical Summary

The patient returns 1 month later and describes sudden resolution of his central distortion with normalization of his vision. His visual acuity is now 20/20. Fundus examination shows evidence of a posterior vitreous detachment and normal foveal coloration. The previously seen yellow spot is no longer evident.

Follow-Up Optical Coherence Tomography

On OCT examination (E), the vitreomacular traction has spontaneously resolved. The posterior hyaloid face is no longer visible in the OCT cuts. The foveal contour is now normal without evidence of persistent elevation or edema.

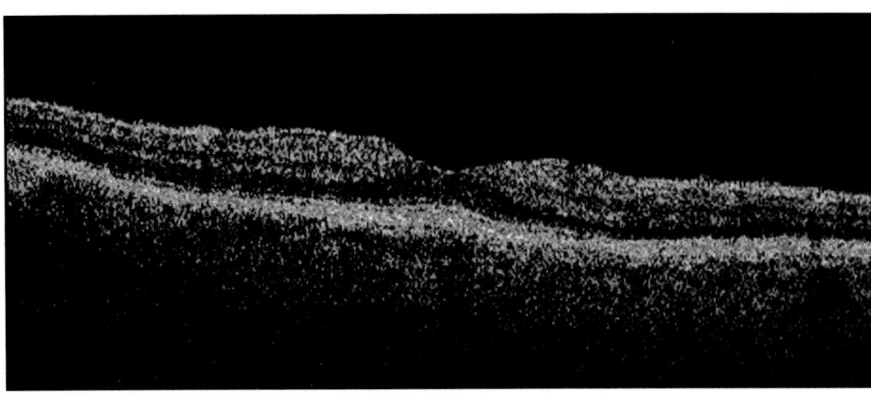

E

Case 3-15. Macular Hole Formation and Surgical Management

Clinical Summary

A 64-year-old male reports decreased central vision in his left eye for 2 weeks. His visual acuity is 20/50 in this eye, and dilated fundus exam shows a yellow spot in the fovea. There is no evidence of posterior vitreous detachment on clinical exam. Over the next 3 weeks he notices increasing central distortion and decreasing vision. His visual acuity declines to 20/70, and dilated fundus exam now shows a small full-thickness macular hole. He undergoes pars plana vitrectomy, membrane peel, and C3F8 injection for management of this macular hole. Five weeks after surgery, his visual acuity is 20/70 with mild cataract formation. Dilated fundus exam shows mottling in the fovea but no evidence of macular hole.

Optical Coherence Tomography

Initial OCT examination (A) shows loss of the normal foveal contour with retinal thinning and a small nonreflective space under the fovea consistent with a foveal detachment. There was no evidence of a full-thickness retinal defect on multiple OCT scans through this area. The posterior hyaloid can be seen shallowly detached from the perifoveal retina but appears to be persistently attached in the foveal region. This configuration corresponds to a Stage I macular hole with persistent vitreomacular traction. Three weeks later, OCT examination (B) now confirms the full-thickness defect in the retina with an operculum attached to one edge. The posterior hyaloid can again be seen as a faint membrane above the perifoveal retina that continues to be attached to this operculum. This configuration is consistent with a Stage 2 macular hole and highlights the role of vitreomacular traction in hole development. Postoperative OCT examination (C) confirms complete closure of the macular hole with resolution of the previously identified vitreomacular traction. The retina is still mildly thickened and has not yet regained the normal foveal contour.

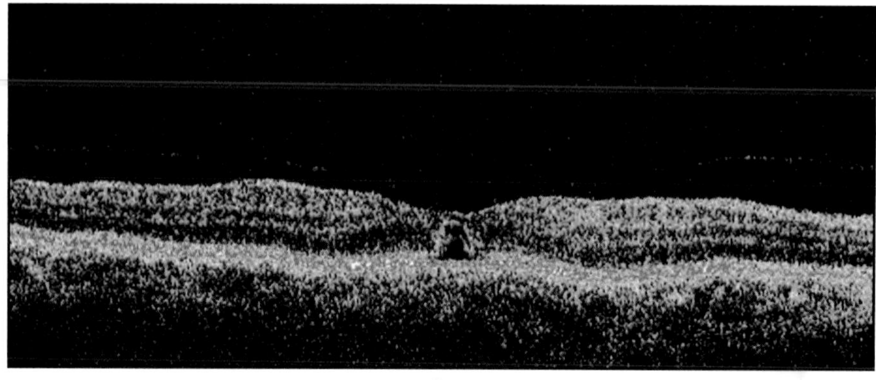

A

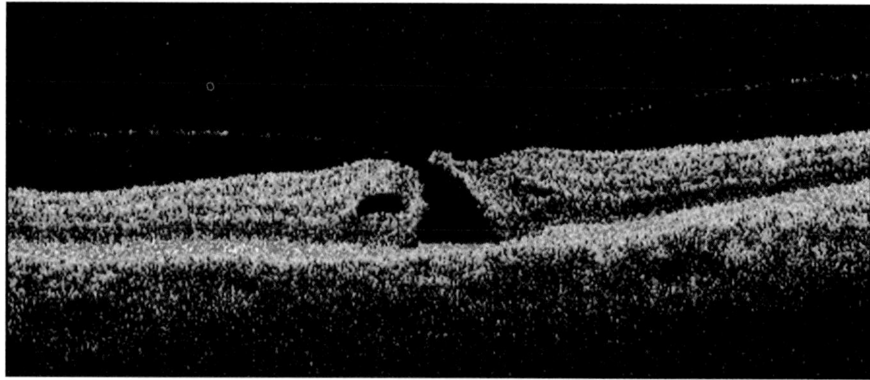

B

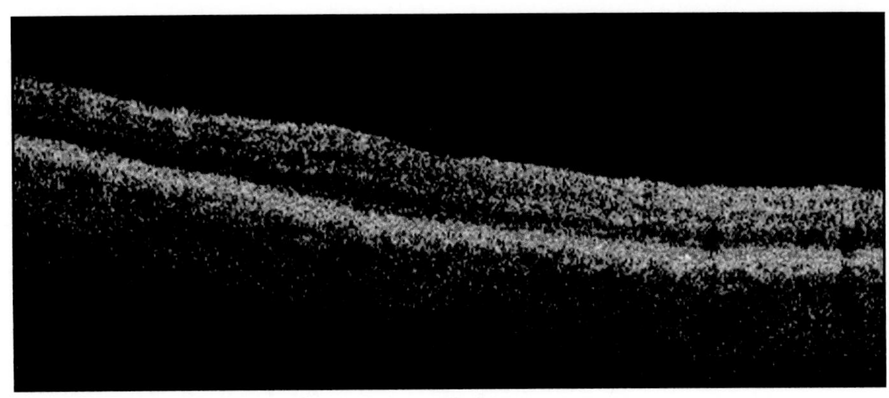

C

Case 3-16. Stage 1B Macular Hole Successfully Treated With Vitrectomy Surgery

Clinical History

A 62-year-old female is referred for a 3-week history of decreased vision. On examination, the visual acuity measures 20/50 OD with a normal anterior segment examination. Retinal examination demonstrates a cystic foveal change consistent with a Stage 1 macular hole without evidence of a PVD (A). The Stage 1B macular hole is confirmed by OCT and the patient is followed. Three weeks later, the visual acuity declines to 20/70 without any change in clinical exam or OCT. Pars plana vitrectomy is performed with creation of a posterior vitreous detachment. Follow-up 2 months postoperatively demonstrates closure of the macular hole with improvement in visual acuity to 20/40.

Optical Coherence Tomography

Initial OCT (B) demonstrates a Stage 1B macular hole with elevation of the foveal retina to the level of the vitreoretinal interface. The remaining foveal retina bridges over the hole. No obvious strands of vitreous are visible inserting to the retinal surface. The RPE layer is intact without any overlying adherent retinal tissue. Postoperative OCT (C) demonstrates restoration of foveal contour with closure of the macular hole. A small foveal cyst, evident as a hyporeflective, black circle, is visible just anterior to the thinned yellow-red RPE layer. OCT obtained 5 months postoperatively demonstrates a normal foveal contour with resolution of the foveal cyst (D).

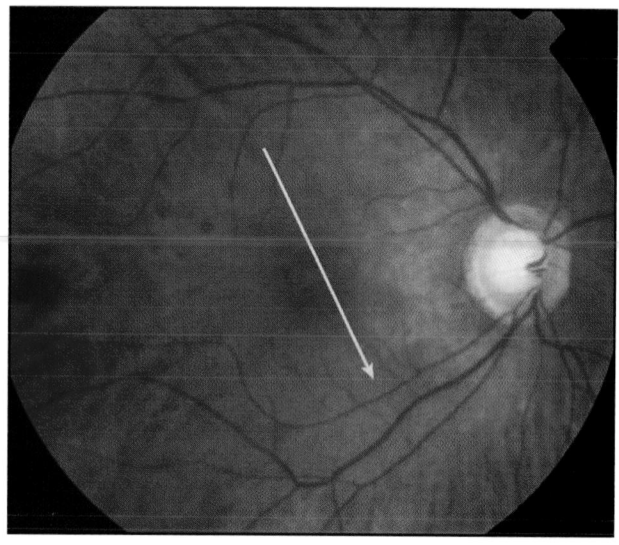

A

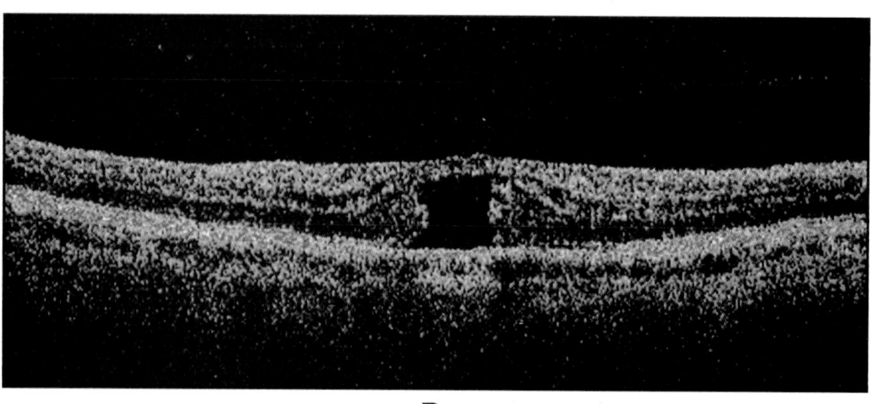

B

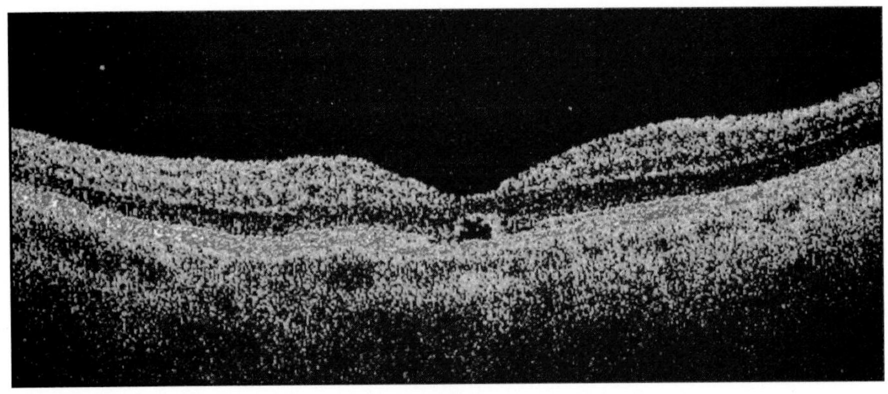

C

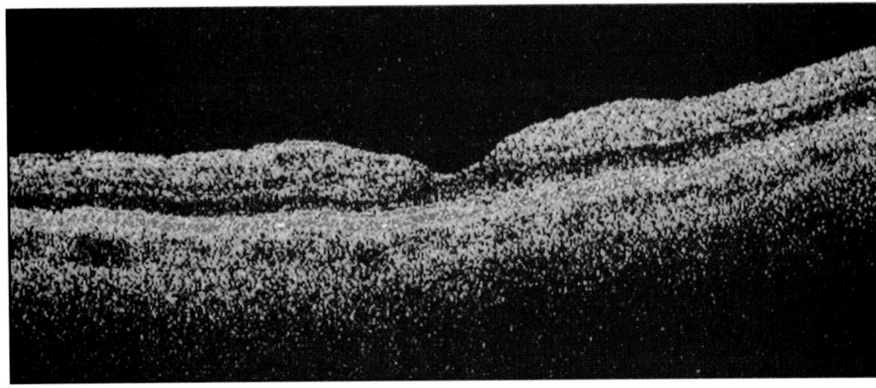

D

Case 3-17A. Impending Macular Hole With a Stage 2 Full-Thickness Macular Hole in the Fellow Eye

Clinical Summary

A 64-year-old female with a history of poor visual acuity in the left eye for 5 years complains of central distortion in the right eye for 1 month. Her visual acuity in the right eye is 20/40. Dilated fundus exam (A) shows a large cyst in the fovea.

Optical Coherence Tomography

OCT examination (B) shows a perifoveal vitreous detachment with persistent vitreous attachment to the fovea. There is a relatively broad area of vitreous attachment to the thin inner retinal layers. Traction from this vitreous attachment has elevated the inner retina and created large nonreflective cysts within the retina. The inner retina layer is elevated to 640 µm above the underlying RPE signal. Outer retinal tissue persists at the base of the fovea and can be seen as reflective material beneath this nonreflective cavity.

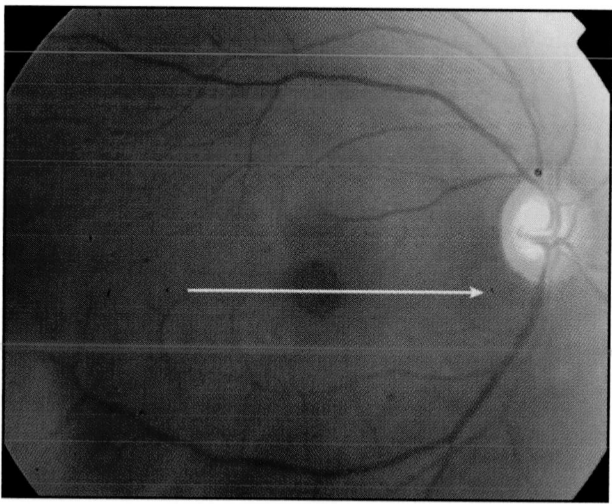

A

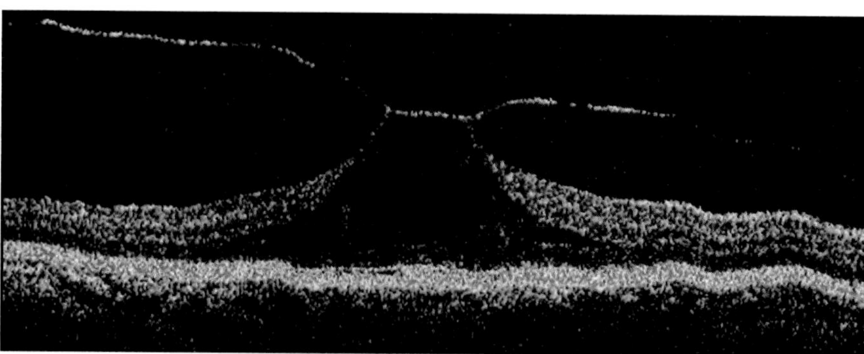

B

Case 3-17B. Impending Macular Hole With a Stage 2 Full-Thickness Macular Hole in the Fellow Eye

Clinical Summary

Her visual acuity in the left eye is 20/400. Dilated fundus exam (C) shows a full-thickness macular hole with a partial operculum attached to the inferior edge of the hole.

Optical Coherence Tomography

OCT examination (D) of this eye shows a full-thickness defect in the retina at the fovea. An operculum can be seen on one edge of the retinal defect consistent with a Stage 2 classification. The partially detached posterior hyaloid, a thin reflective layer suspended above the retina, can be seen inserting onto the operculum. Traction from this attachment has resulted in a dehiscence of the inner retinal layers and subsequent hole formation. The retinal edges are thickened, with cystoid changes indicating intraretinal edema.

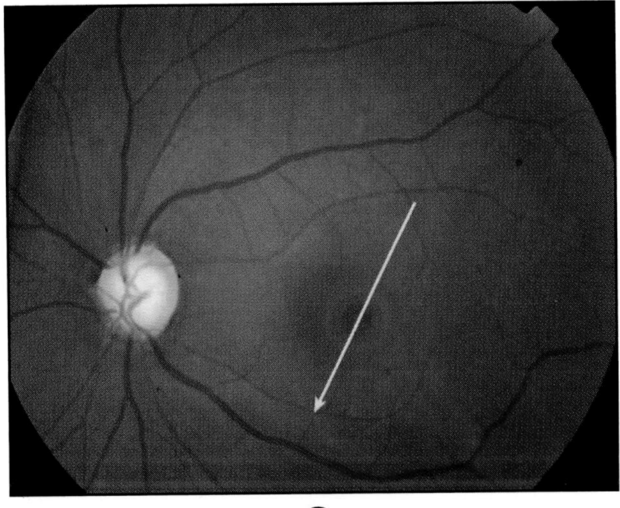

C

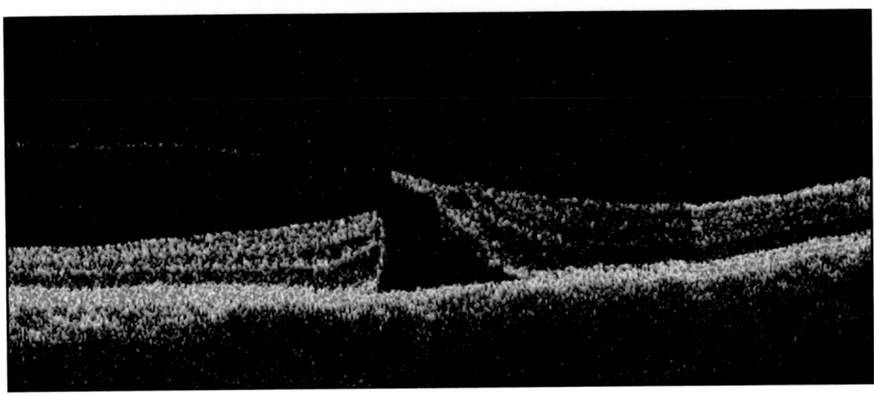

D

Case 3-18.
Stage 2 Full-Thickness Macular Hole

Clinical Summary

A 68-year-old female is referred for evaluation of a macular hole in her left eye. Her visual acuity is 20/200, and dilated fundus exam (A) shows a full-thickness macular hole with an apparent cuff of subretinal fluid.

Optical Coherence Tomography

OCT examination (B) shows a full-thickness defect in the fovea. There is an operculum attached to one edge of the hole consistent with a Stage 2 classification. The detached posterior hyaloid can be seen in the left-hand portion of the image, but the signal fades near the foveal region. As a result, it is unclear whether the vitreous remains attached to the retinal operculum. The edges of the hole are thickened with areas of reduced optical reflectivity resulting from fluid accumulation. The retinal thickness reaches a maximum of 455 μm in this area.

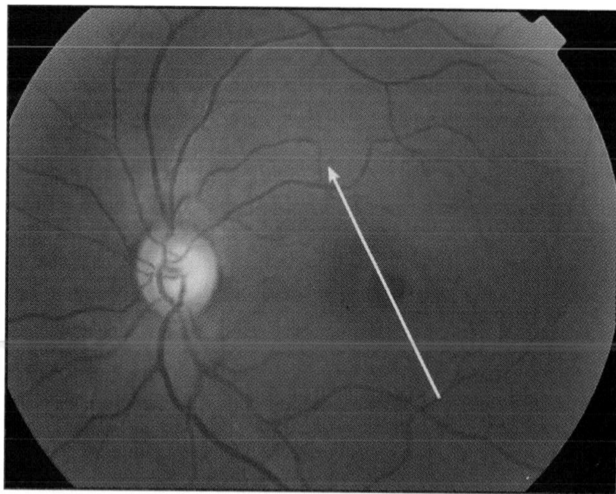

A

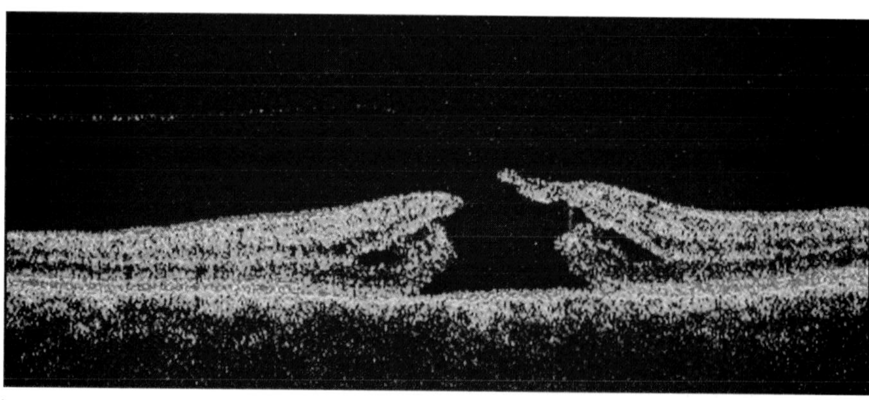

B

Case 3-19.
Stage 3 Full-Thickness Macular Hole

Clinical Summary

A 68-year-old male complains of deceasing visual acuity in his left eye over the last 4 to 5 months. His visual acuity in this eye is 20/200. Dilated fundus exam (A) shows a full-thickness macular hole with surrounding fluid. There is no evidence of an operculum or posterior vitreous detachment on clinical exam.

Optical Coherence Tomography

OCT examination (B) confirms a full-thickness loss of retinal tissue in the fovea. The minimum inner diameter of this hole measures 325 µm, while the base diameter measures 487 µm. The posterior vitreous can be seen shallowly detached from the retina as a thin linear density 265 µm above the retinal surface. The edges of the hole are slightly thickened, with areas of reduced optical reflectivity resulting from fluid accumulation. The retinal thickness reaches a maximum of 287 µm in this area.

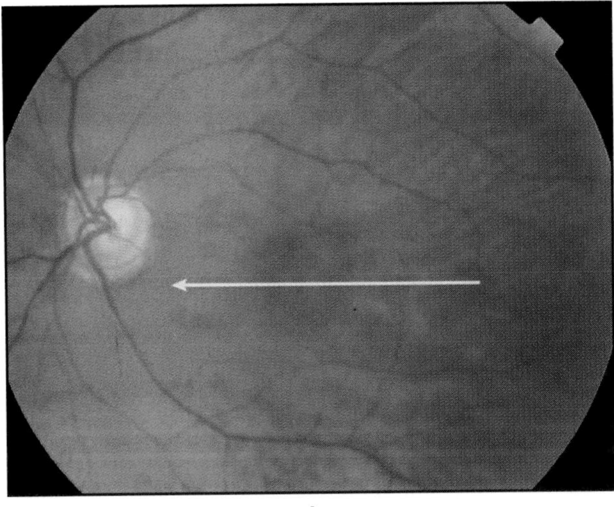

A

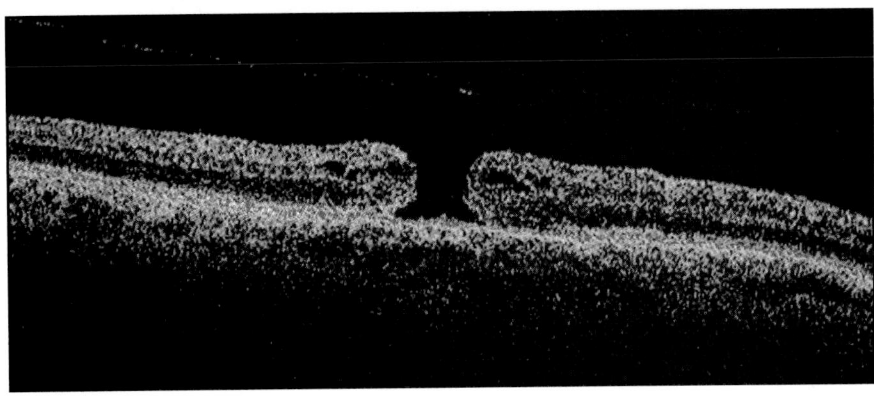

B

Case 3-20. Stage 3 Full-Thickness Macular Hole

Clinical Summary

A 68-year-old male complains of decreased visual acuity in the left eye for 2 months. Six months earlier his visual acuity was 20/30 with a normal retinal exam. His current visual acuity is 20/200, and dilated fundus exam shows a full-thickness macular hole with a cuff of subretinal fluid.

Optical Coherence Tomography

OCT examination (A) shows a full-thickness defect in the retina consistent with a Stage 3 classification. The inner retinal diameter measures 300 μm while the base diameter is 675 μm. The detached posterior hyaloid sits 250 μm above the temporal edge of the hole and 150 μm above the nasal edge. The small circular density suspended above the hole by the posterior hyaloid represents an operculum. The retina at the edge of the hole is shallowly detached and demonstrates large nonreflective spaces from intraretinal fluid accumulation. The retinal edge reaches a maximum thickness of 490 μm on this tomogram.

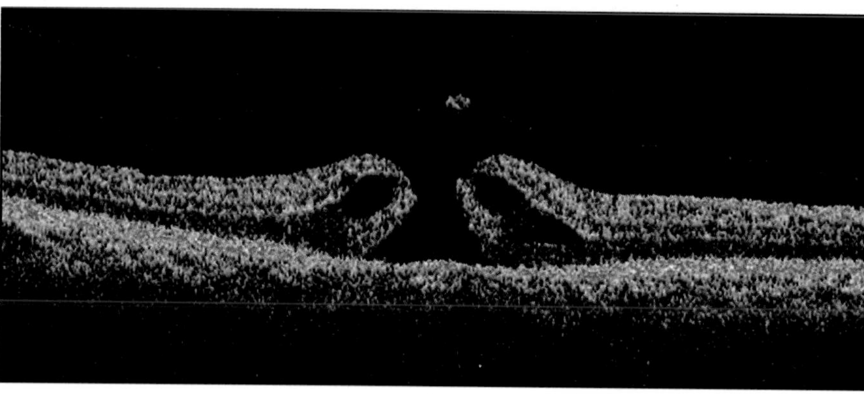

A

Case 3-21A. *Bilateral Full-Thickness Macular Holes*

Clinical Summary

A 61-year-old female complains of decreased visual acuity worse in the right eye than the left over the past several months. Her visual acuity in the right eye is 20/200, and dilated fundus examination (A) shows evidence of a full-thickness macular hole. A posterior vitreous detachment could not be seen on exam.

Optical Coherence Tomography

OCT examination (B) confirms a full-thickness loss of retinal tissue in the fovea consistent with a Stage 3 macular hole. The shallowly detached posterior hyaloid can be seen as a thin linear density approximately 325 µm above the retinal surface. An operculum can be seen as a small density suspended above the hole by the vitreous. The inner diameter of the hole measures 625 µm, while the base diameter is slightly larger at 825 µm. There is extensive edema with cystoid changes within the retina at the edge of the hole. As a result, the retinal thickness is significantly increased to maximum of 400 µm. Small, nodular elevations in the RPE signal at the base of the hole correspond to drusen-like deposits seen clinically.

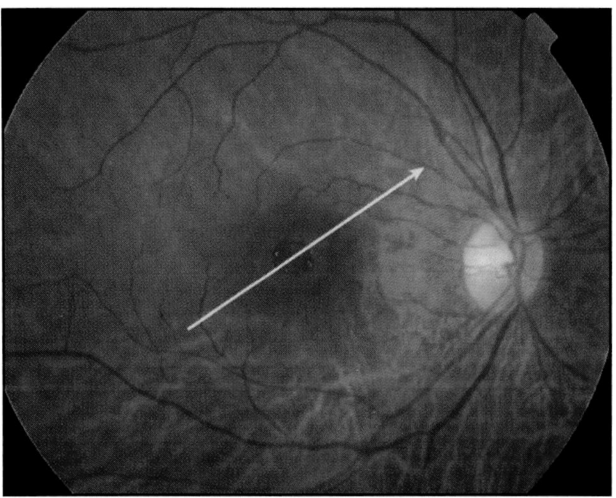

A

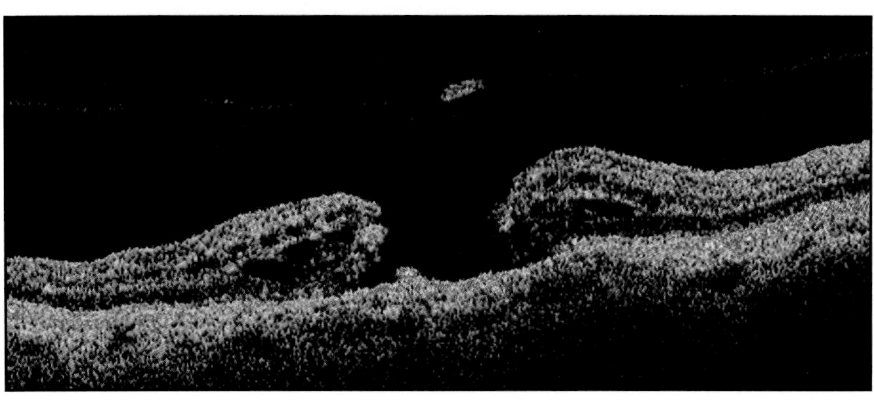

B

Case 3-21B. Bilateral Full-Thickness Macular Holes

Clinical Summary

The vision in the left eye is 20/70, and dilated fundus exam (C) shows a slightly smaller full-thickness macular hole in this eye.

Optical Coherence Tomography

OCT examination (D) demonstrates a full-thickness dehiscence of the retina at the fovea with a thin operculum attached to one edge of the hole. This appearance is consistent with a Stage 2 classification. The vitreous is detached around the fovea, but remains focally attached to this operculum. The inner diameter of the hole measures 380 μm. Retinal thickening and cystoid changes are again evident at the edges of the hole. Retinal thickness at the edge of the hole measures 390 μm.

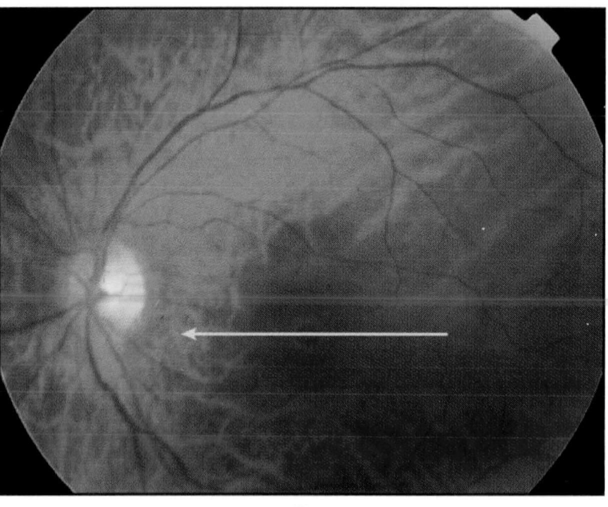

C

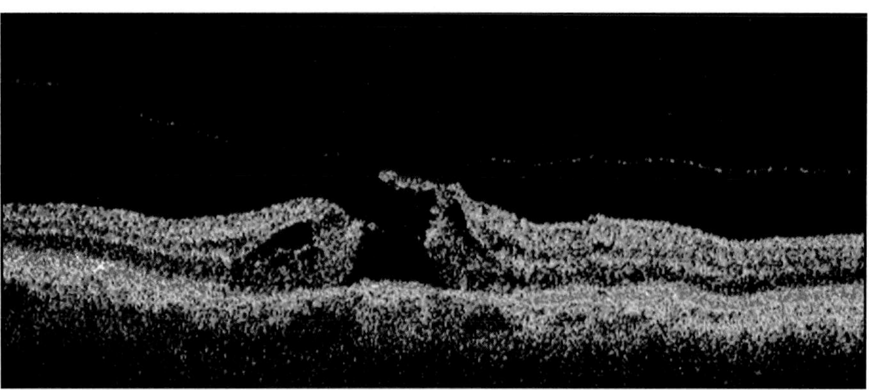

D

Case 3-22. Myopic Degeneration With a Full-Thickness Macular Hole

Clinical Summary

A 60-year-old female with a history of myopic degeneration has poor visual acuity in the right eye after developing choroidal neovascularization 2 years earlier. She now complains of worsening visual acuity in her left eye over the past 2 months. Her current visual acuity in the left eye is 20/200. Dilated fundus exam (A) shows a tilted optic nerve with peripapillary atrophy. There is extensive pigmentary mottling in the macular region that limits visualization of the macular hole on clinical exam.

Optical Coherence Tomography

A horizontal OCT image (B) taken through the macula confirms the presence of a full-thickness macular hole. The posterior hyaloid face is not identified on the OCT cuts, and there is no evidence of persistent vitreous traction on the retina. The macular hole and adjacent retina appear similar on the OCT to cases of idiopathic macular hole formation. The myopic pigmentary atrophy, however, allows greater penetration and reflectivity of the signal, resulting in a thicker and brighter RPE/choroidal band. Choroidal vessels can be seen as nonreflective spaces within this highly reflective band.

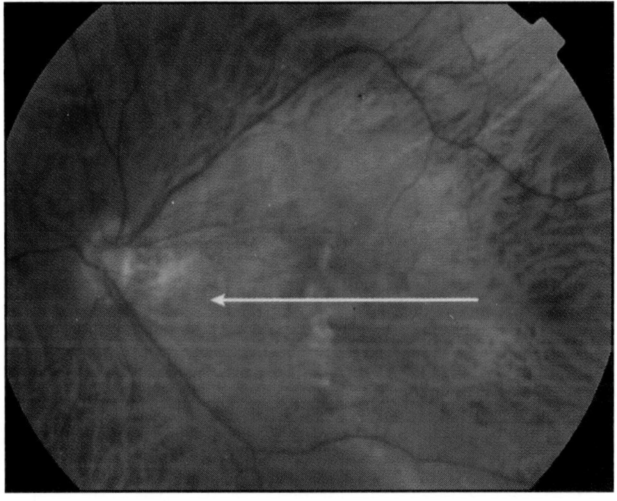

A

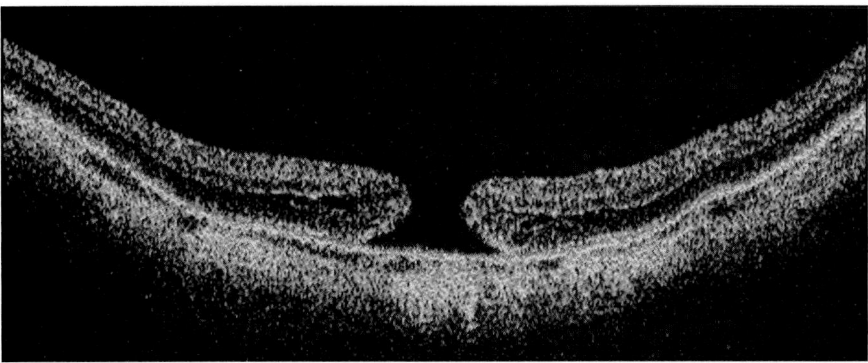

B

Case 3-23. Full-Thickness Macular Hole Successfully Closed With Vitrectomy Surgery

Clinical Summary

A 74-year-old male is referred for management of a macular hole in his right eye. He has noticed decreased central vision in this eye for 6 months, and his current visual acuity is 20/80. Dilated fundus exam shows a small full-thickness macular hole with a cuff of fluid. A pars plana vitrectomy with membrane peel and C3F8 injection is performed. One month after surgery, his visual acuity has improved to 20/40. Dilated fundus examination shows mild mottling in the fovea but no macular hole. Four months after surgery, his visual acuity has improved to 20/25, and the fundus exam is unchanged.

Optical Coherence Tomography

The initial OCT image (A) confirms a full-thickness defect in the retina at the fovea. The edges of the hole show mild thickening and intraretinal cystoid changes. There is no evidence of vitreous traction or operculum on the OCT images. The postoperative OCT image (B) now shows closure of the hole with reapposition of the retinal edges. Retinal edema has decreased, and there is a fairly normal foveal contour. A small amount of persistent foveal elevation is indicated by a clear space beneath the fused edges. Four months after surgery, OCT image (C) shows continued closure of the hole with a normal foveal contour and retinal thickness. The clear space beneath the fovea is no longer present, confirming resolution of the small foveal detachment.

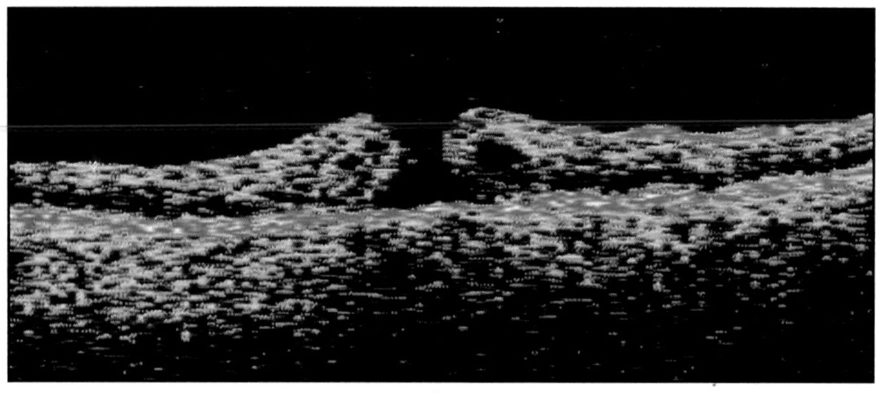

A

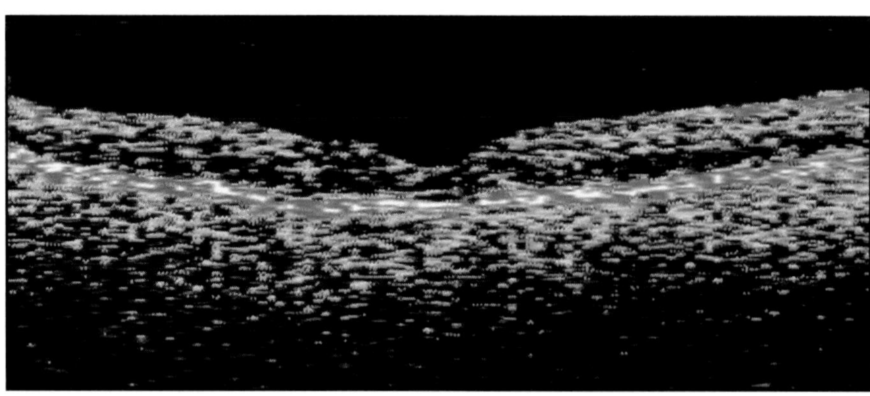

B

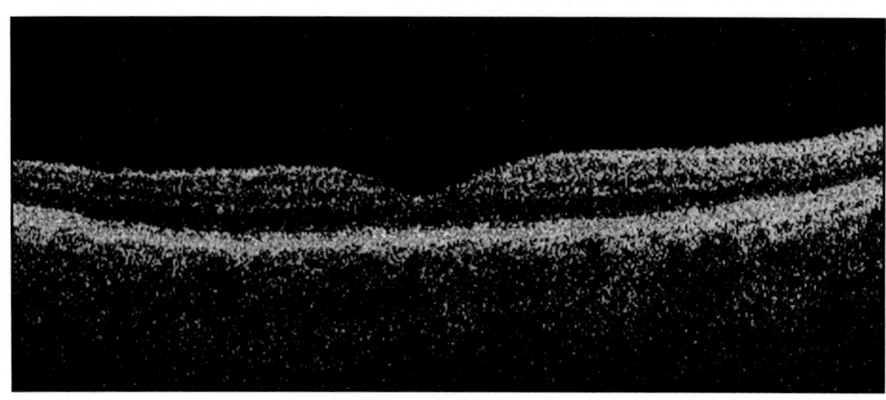

C

Case 3-24A. Full-Thickness Macular Hole With a Lamellar Macular Hole in the Fellow Eye

Clinical Summary

A 69-year-old female complains of decreased visual acuity in the right eye for 3 months. Her visual acuity in this eye is 20/200. On dilated fundus exam (A and B), there appears to be a large full-thickness macular hole with breadcrumb deposits at the base. A posterior vitreous detachment is not seen on the exam

Optical Coherence Tomography

OCT images (C) through the center of this lesion show persistent vitreous attachment to a thin inner retinal membrane at the fovea. There is loss of the outer retinal layers underneath this thin inner layer. There is a small amount of retinal schisis at the edge of this lesion. The base diameter of this lesion is 812 μm. Small excrescences in the RPE signal at the base of this lesion correspond to breadcrumbs seen clinically.

Vertical OCT imaging (D) at the temporal edge of this lesion shows a small dehiscence of the inner retinal layer creating a full-thickness retinal defect. The incompletely detached posterior vitreous remains attached to the operculum, and the associated traction appears to have caused this dehiscence.

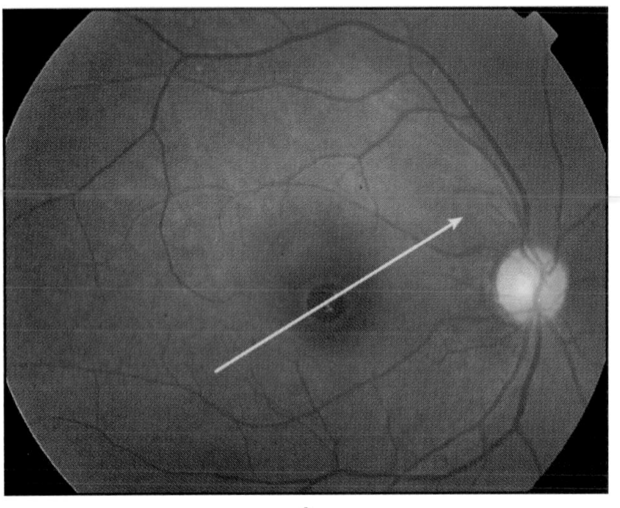

A

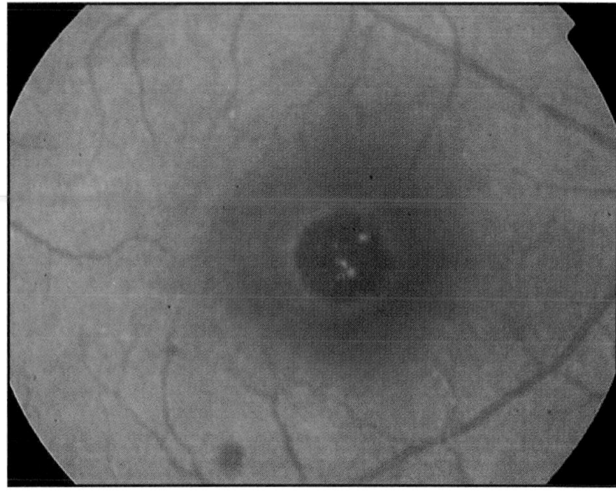

B

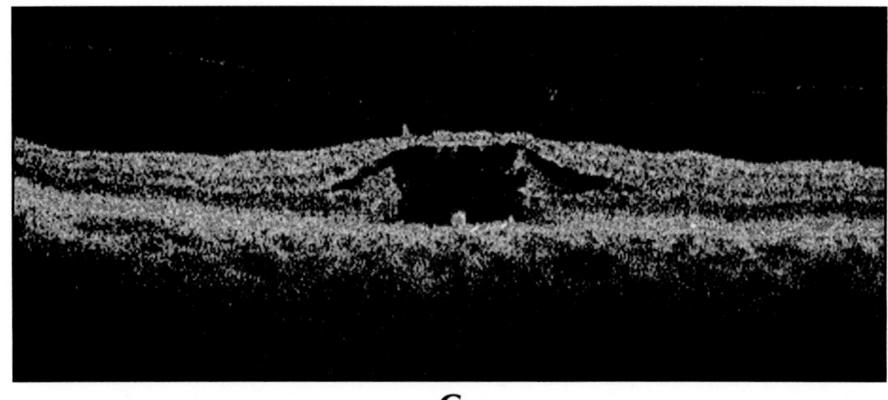

C

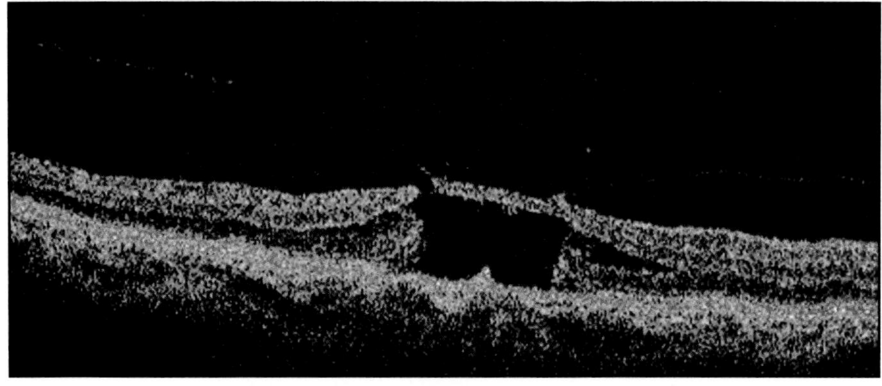

D

Case 3-24B. Full-Thickness Macular Hole With a Lamellar Macular Hole in the Fellow Eye

Clinical Summary

Her visual acuity in the left eye has been stable at 20/25. There appears to be a lamellar macular hole with a small overlying operculum on dilated fundus exam (E).

Optical Coherence Tomography

OCT images (F) a small reflective operculum suspended above the fovea by the detached posterior hyaloid face. The foveal contour is abnormal with only a thin layer of outer retinal tissue at the center of the fovea. This configuration is most consistent with a lamellar or partial thickness macular hole.

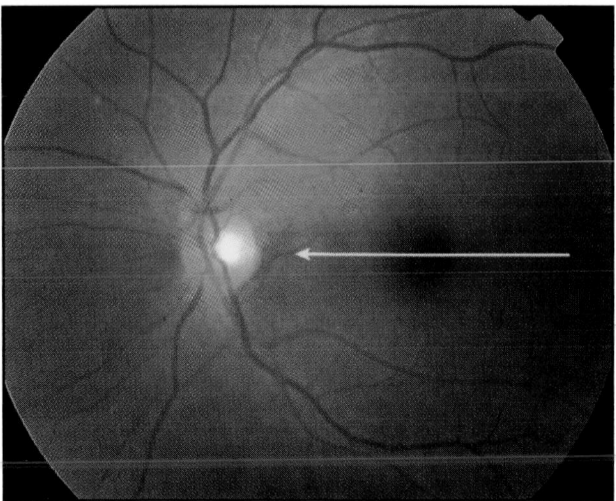

E

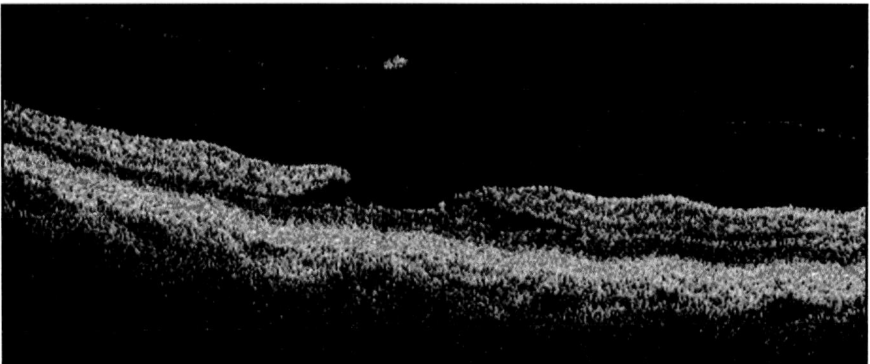

F

Case 3-25. Lamellar Macular Hole

Clinical Summary

A 60-year-old male is examined for decreased central visual acuity of 1-month duration. Floaters were noted at the time of the initial decrease in vision, but visual acuity has since remained stable at 20/50. Clinical examination (A) demonstrates a posterior vitreous detachment with an ERM and lamellar hole. Faint fluorescence is visible during the late phase of the fluorescein angiogram with apparent delineation of the lamellar hole (B).

Optical Coherence Tomography

OCT (C) demonstrates partial absence of retinal tissue in the fovea. Retinal tissue is present at the base of the hole defining this as a lamellar hole compared with full-thickness retinal tissue loss in a macular hole. There is a slight increase in the reflectivity of inner retina at the vitreoretinal interface. However, an ERM is not well-delineated by the scan.

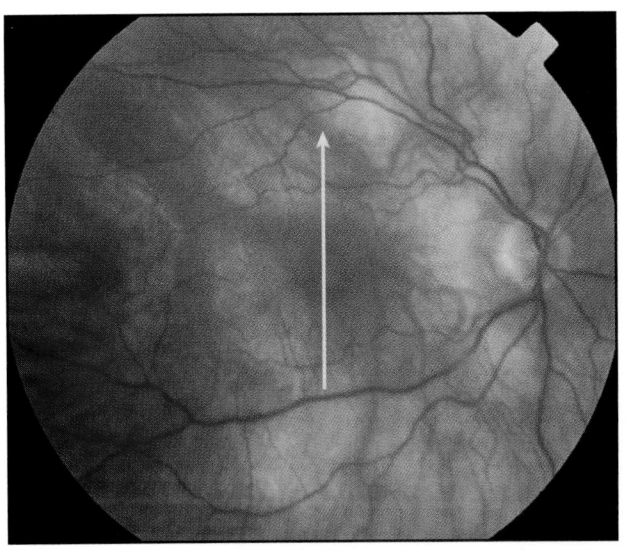

A

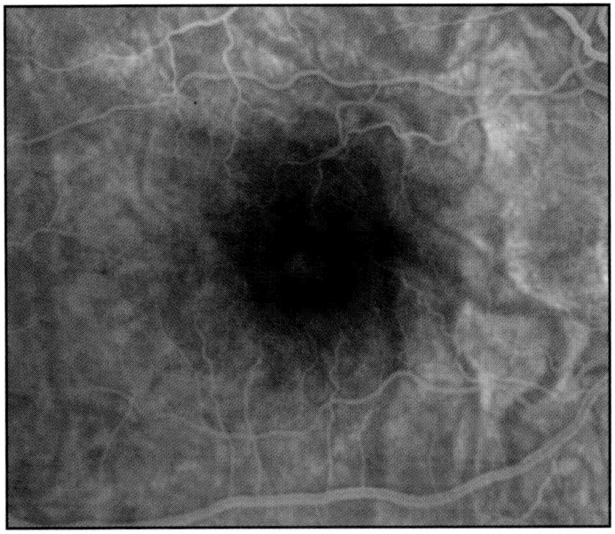

B

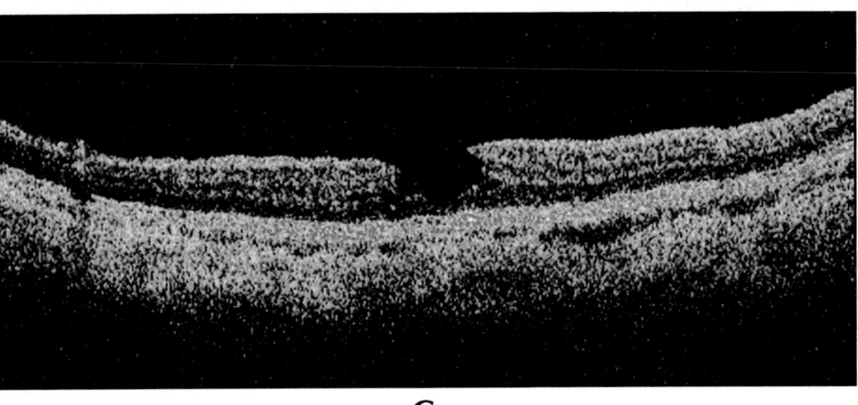

C

Case 3-26. Lamellar Macular Hole

Clinical Summary

A 61-year-old male is referred for evaluation of macular pigmentary changes. He has noted a mild decrease in the visual acuity of the right eye over the past year. His vision in this eye is 20/60. Dilated fundus exam (A) shows patchy pigmentary changes in the central and inferior macula. The fovea shows evidence of a possible macular hole versus pseudohole. Fluorescein angiography (B) displays mottled hyperfluorescence corresponding to areas of pigmentary alteration without evidence of late leakage. Angiography does not help differentiate between a true hole and a lamellar hole.

Optical Coherence Tomography

OCT imaging (C) shows an abnormal contour to the fovea with separation of the inner retinal layers. The reverse anvil configuration to the central clear space suggests the formation of a macular hole. However, since outer retinal tissue persists at the base of the fovea, this actually represents a partial thickness or lamellar hole. There is also some nonspecific irregularity to the RPE/choroid signal corresponding to the pigmentary changes on the exam.

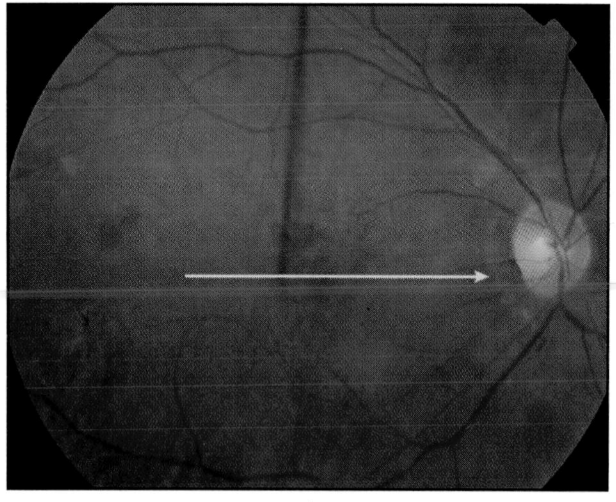

A

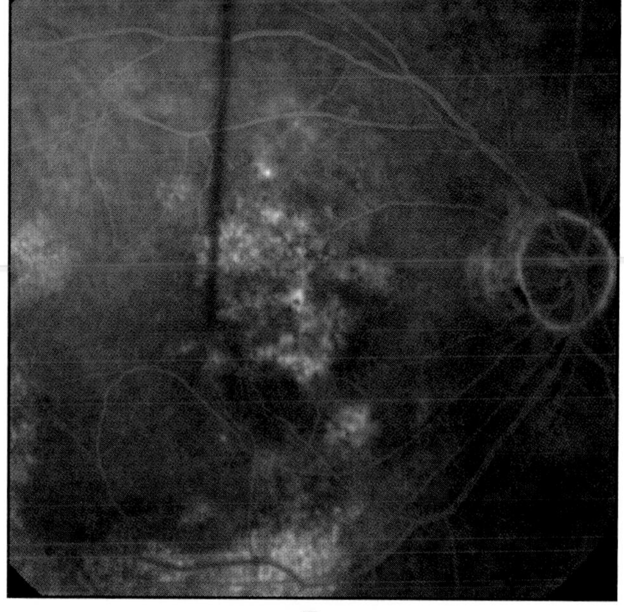

B

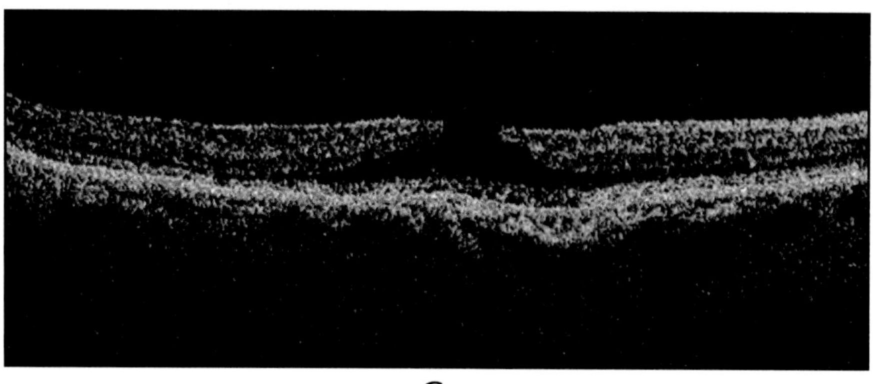

C

Case 3-27. Lamellar Macular Hole

Clinical Summary

A 60-year-old female with a history of peripheral retinal degeneration complains of decreasing central vision in both eyes. Her vision in the right eye is 20/30. Dilated fundus exam shows patchy pigmentary atrophy in the retinal periphery. The fovea shows evidence of a possible macular hole versus pseudohole.

The vision in her left eye is 20/60. Dilated fundus exam shows similar pigmentary changes in the retinal periphery. The fovea again shows evidence of a possible macular hole versus pseudohole.

Optical Coherence Tomography

OCT image (A) of the right eye shows an abnormal contour to the fovea with separation of the inner retinal layers. Reflectivity is clearly present from the outer retinal layers at the base of this defect. This configuration corresponds to a partial thickness or lamellar hole. The retina at the base of this lamellar hole measures approximately 135 μm thick, while the inner edges of this lesion are separated by 712 μm.

The OCT (B) shows that a lamellar hole is also present in this eye. There is again separation of the inner retinal layers with a dumbbell-shaped area of central clearing. Outer retinal tissue remains at the base of the fovea beneath this central clearing. The configuration of the inner retinal layers suggests that this may have developed from the rupturing of a central cyst.

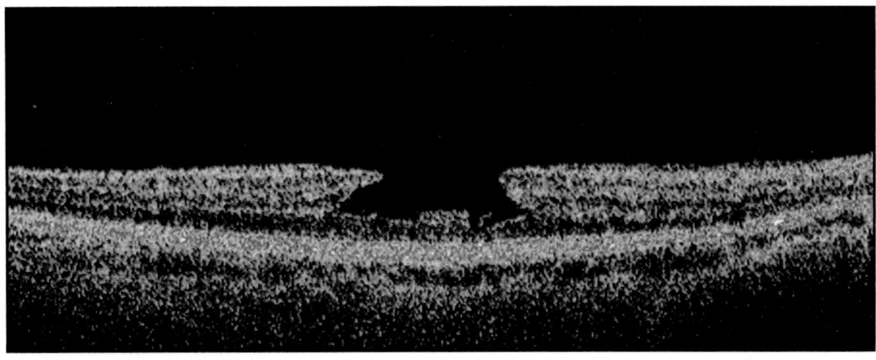

A

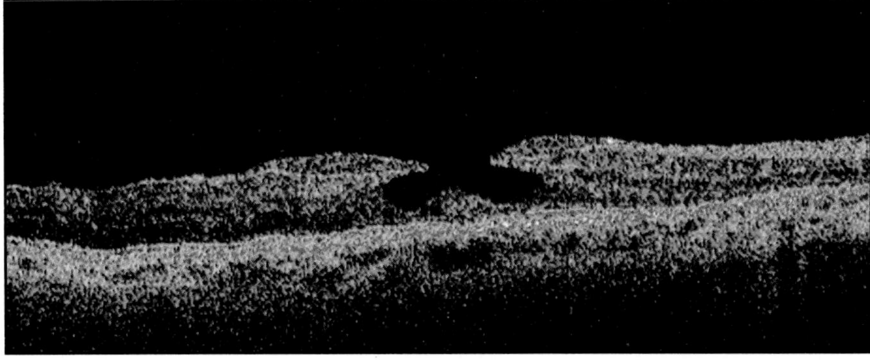

B

Chapter 4

Retinal Vascular Diseases

Vanessa Cruz-Villegas, MD; Carmen A. Puliafito, MD; and James G. Fujimoto, PhD

- Branch Retinal Artery Occlusion
- Central Retinal Artery Occlusion
- Branch Retinal Vein Occlusion
- Central Retinal Vein Occlusion
- Bilateral Idiopathic Juxtafoveal Retinal Telangiectasis
- Retinal Arterial Macroaneurysm

Retinal vascular diseases are common etiologies for central visual loss. Optical coherence tomography (OCT) complements the information obtained from clinical examination and angiographic studies on these conditions. Furthermore, OCT provides objective information in a reproducible way such that monitoring the natural course of evolution of these conditions as well as assessing response to therapeutic interventions are feasible.

Branch Retinal Artery Occlusion

Branch retinal artery occlusion (BRAO) is usually characterized by sudden visual field loss or vision decrease. The mechanism of occlusion usually involves embolization or thrombosis of the affected vessel. Superficial retinal whitening occurs in the distribution of the occluded arteriole. Fluorescein angiography confirms a delay or lack of perfusion of the involved branch retinal artery. Histopathologic studies of acute retinal artery occlusions reveal intracellular edema and ischemia of the inner retinal layers. The findings of acute BRAO on OCT correlates with the aforementioned histopathologic reports. The area affected by the obstructed vessel shows increased retinal thickness without cystic spaces of low reflectivity. This finding probably correlates with the fact that the edema that occurs in retinal artery occlusions is in the intracellular instead of the extracellular space. Also, the inner retinal layers tend to be more highly reflective in OCT, probably due to ischemia or coagulative necrosis of these layers. This high reflectivity of the inner retinal layers causes shadowing of the optical signal of the outer retinal layers and retinal pigment epithelium (RPE)/choriocapillaris complex beneath.

Central Retinal Artery Occlusion

Central retinal artery occlusion (CRAO) shares the same thromboembolic etiologic mechanism with BRAO. Patients with CRAO experience sudden severe visual loss unless sparing of the fovea occurs due to the presence of a patent cilioretinal artery. The clinical picture of an acute CRAO is characterized by retinal whitening with a central cherry red spot in the foveola. On intravenous fluorescein angiography, delayed filling of the central retinal artery with boxcarring of the blood column is observed. This lack of adequate perfusion results in ischemia of the inner retinal layers as reported in histopathologic studies.[1,2] OCT makes an understanding of the pathophysiology of this condition possible. The inner retinal layers typically show enhanced reflectivity, which may represent ischemic cellular damage and accumulation of by-products. The increased thickness of the inner retina typically seen in acute artery occlusions corresponds to the intracellular edema. Histopathologic studies report the presence of edema in the intracellular instead of the extracellular compartment in acute occlusions.[1,2] This accounts for the usual lack of low reflective intraretinal fluid spaces in OCT with artery occlusions. Blocking of the optical reflections from the outer retinal layers and RPE/choriocapillaris complex occurs secondarily to the presence of a thickened, highly reflective inner retina. OCT images of chronic CRAO are characterized by thinning and atrophy of the inner retinal layers as described in histopathologic reports. A patient with a chronic CRAO usually presents with a featureless retinal appearance, but by performing an OCT scan, the diagnosis may be established.

Branch Retinal Vein Occlusion

Branch retinal vein occlusion (BRVO) may produce decreased vision and metamorphopsia. Clinical signs include intraretinal hemorrhages, dilated tortuous retinal veins, cotton wool spots, and retinal thickening in the sector drained by the obstructed vein. Macular edema may be responsible for central visual loss. OCT is very valuable in diagnosing, monitoring, and managing macular edema secondary to retinal vein occlusions.[3,4] By furnishing objective qualitative and quantitative information in a noninvasive way, detecting and monitoring the effect of therapeutic interventions such as focal laser photocoagulation, intravitreal triamcinolone acetonide injection, adventitial sheathotomy, and pars plana vitrectomy are possible.[5,6] Macular edema due to BRVO is represented by an increase in the retinal thickness and areas of intraretinal reduced reflectivity on OCT. Usually, this fluid accumulation has a cystic appearance. It is not unusual to observe subretinal fluid accumulation and neurosensory detachment in these cases.[7] BRVO OCT findings may also include epiretinal membranes, pseudoholes, lamellar holes, and subhyaloid or preretinal hemorrhages. Subhyaloid hemorrhages are visualized as high reflective areas underneath a reflective band (posterior hyaloid). See Chapter 3 for information on epiretinal membranes, pseudoholes, and lamellar holes.

Central Retinal Vein Occlusion

Central retinal vein occlusion (CRVO) is also a common retinal vascular condition usually affecting individuals older than 50 years. Patients typically experience visual loss and present with dilated tortuous retinal veins and scattered intraretinal hemorrhages in all four quadrants. Cotton wool spots, optic disc swelling, and macular edema may be appreciated. Intravenous fluorescein angiography (IVFA) may show areas of blocked fluorescence from the intraretinal blood, staining of the vessel walls, a delayed arteriovenous phase, nonperfused areas, and perifoveal leakage. However, perifoveal leakage sometimes may not be visualized on IVFA despite the presence of macular edema due to the presence of a marked hemorrhagic component or because of the lack of intact perifoveal vessels. OCT detects macular edema in spite of these circumstances. Recent studies have shown the efficacy of intravitreal triamcinolone injection in macular edema secondary to CRVO.[8,9] OCT plays a pivotal role in quantitatively monitoring changes in retinal thickness after this treatment modality.

Bilateral Idiopathic Juxtafoveal Retinal Telangiectasis

Idiopathic juxtafoveal retinal telangiectasis is a bilateral retinal vascular disorder consisting of an incompetent and ectatic capillary bed in the juxtafoveal temporal region. Central vision may become affected due to exudation. Gass described a classification of three subgroups.[10,11] Group I A (unilateral congenital parafoveolar telangiectasis) is characterized by telangiectatic capillaries temporal to the fovea often associated with a circinate ring of exudation. Group I B (unilateral, idiopathic, focal juxtafoveolar telangiectasis) consists of a small focal area of incompetent capillaries next to the foveal avascular zone. Exudative alterations may be present. Group II A (bilateral idiopathic acquired parafoveolar telangiectasis) is characterized by bilateral regions of retinal thickening temporal to the fovea. Right-angled venules, retinal pigment epithelial hyperplastic plaques, subretinal neovascularization, and crystalline deposits may be observed. Gass described retinal telangiectasis in two siblings.[10,11] He described this group as II B, or juvenile occult familial idiopathic juxtafoveolar retinal telangiectasis. Patients with group III A (occlusive idiopathic juxtafoveolar retinal telangiectasis) may experience visual loss due to obliteration of perifoveal capillaries. Patients with group III B (occlusive idiopathic juxtafoveolar retinal telangiectasis associated with central nervous system vasculopathy) share the same findings from group III A plus central nervous system involvement.[10,11] OCT depicts clearly the involvement of the intraretinal and subretinal spaces in this condition. This vascular disorder may show low reflective intraretinal areas of macular edema and highly reflective lipid exudates in OCT. Plaques of retinal pigment hyperplasia appear as intraretinal hyperreflective spots associated with shadowing of the reflections from the tissues below.[12] For details about OCT findings of subretinal neovascularization associated with juxtafoveal telangiectasis, refer to Chapter 8.

Retinal Arterial Macroaneurysm

Retinal artery macroaneurysms (RAM) are vascular dilations that may present in association with macular edema, retinal lipid exudation, or hemorrhage. Visual loss may result if the macula becomes involved. Hemorrhage may occur in different levels: vitreous, subhyaloid or preretinal, intraretinal or subretinal. OCT depicts clearly the hemorrhagic component of ruptured RAM. Subhyaloid hemorrhages are represented as regions of high backscattering below the reflective posterior hyaloid band. Hemorrhagic lesions beneath the internal limiting membrane also can be appreciated by OCT. The internal limiting membrane tends to be more reflective than the posterior hyaloid. Subretinal hemorrhages appear as dense highly reflective bands below the neurosensory retina. Shadowing of the optical reflections from the tissues under those hemorrhagic lesions is usually observed. In the case of subhyaloid or preretinal blood, blocking of the neurosensory retina and RPE/choriocapillaris reflections is observed. Subretinal blood blocks the reflections from the RPE/choriocapillaris only. Other morphological findings associated with RAM seen in OCT are hard lipid exudates, which appear as intraretinal dots or areas of increased reflectivity, and low reflective intraretinal fluid accumulation and edema. The natural course of this condition can be followed with OCT as well as the response to therapeutic interventions.

References

1. Dahrling BE II. The histopathology of early central retinal artery occlusion. *Arch Ophthalmol*. 1965;73:506-510.
2. Kroll AJ. Experimental central retinal artery occlusion. *Arch Ophthalmol*. 1968;79:453-469.
3. Lerche RC, Schaudig U, Scholz F, Walter A, Richard G. Structural changes of the retina in retinal vein occlusion—imaging and quantification with optical coherence tomography. *Ophthalmic Surg Lasers*. 2001;32(4):272-280.
4. Imasawa M, Iijima H, Morimoto T. Perimetric sensitivity and retinal thickness in eyes with macular edema resulting from branch retinal vein occlusion. *Am J Ophthalmol*. 2002; 133:428-429.
5. Saika S, Tanaka T, Miyamoto T, Ohnishi Y. Surgical posterior vitreous detachment combined with gas/air tamponade for treating macular edema associated with branch retinal vein occlusion: retinal tomography and visual outcome. *Graefes Arch Clin Exp Ophthalmol*. 2001;239(10):729-732.
6. Fujii GY, De Juan E Jr, Humayun MS. Improvements after sheathotomy for branch retinal vein occlusion documented by optical coherence tomography and scanning laser ophthalmoscope. *Ophthalmic Surg Lasers Imaging*. 2003;34(1): 49-52.
7. Spaide RF, Lee JK, Klancnik JM Jr, Gross NE. Optical coherence tomography of branch retinal vein occlusion. *Retina*. 2003;23(3):343-347.
8. Jonas JB, Kreissig I, Degenring RF. Intravitreal triamcinolone acetonide as treatment of macular edema in central retinal vein occlusion. *Graefe's Arch Clin Exp Ophthalmol*. 2002;240(9):782-783.
9. Greenberg PB, Martidis A, Rogers AH, Duker JS, Reichel E. Intravitreal triamcinolone acetonide for macular edema due to central retinal vein occlusion. *Br J Ophthalmol*. 2002;86(2):247-248.
10. Gass JDM, Blodi BA. Idiopathic juxtafoveolar retinal telangiectasis; update of classification and follow-up study. *Ophthalmology*. 1993;100:1536-1546.
11. Gass JDM. *Stereoscopic Atlas of Macular Diseases*. 4th ed. St. Louis: CV Mosby; 1997:374-376.
12. Trabucchi G, Brancato R, Pierro L, Introini U, Sannace C. Idiopathic juxtafoveolar retinal telangiectasis and pigment epithelial hyperplasia: an optical coherence tomographic study. *Arch Ophthalmol*. 1999;117(3):405-406.

Case 4-1.
Acute Branch Retinal Artery Occlusion

Clinical Summary

An 80-year-old woman noticed the sudden onset of a superior visual field defect in her left eye. Her visual acuity was 20/30 in this eye. Slit-lamp biomicroscopy revealed the presence of retinal opacification in the distribution of an inferotemporal retinal arteriole. A fibrin-platelet embolus was appreciated on the origin of the retinal arteriole next to the optic nerve head (A). Fluorescein angiography (B) showed delayed perfusion of the obstructed branch retinal artery with segmentation of the blood column.

Optical Coherence Tomography

OCT (C) illustrated increased thickness and reflectivity of the inner retinal layers consistent with neuronal cell edema and ischemia. The enhanced reflectivity of the inner retinal layers accounts for the reduced backscattering of the outer retinal layers by shadowing the optical signal of the outer retina as well as the RPE/choriocapillaris complex.

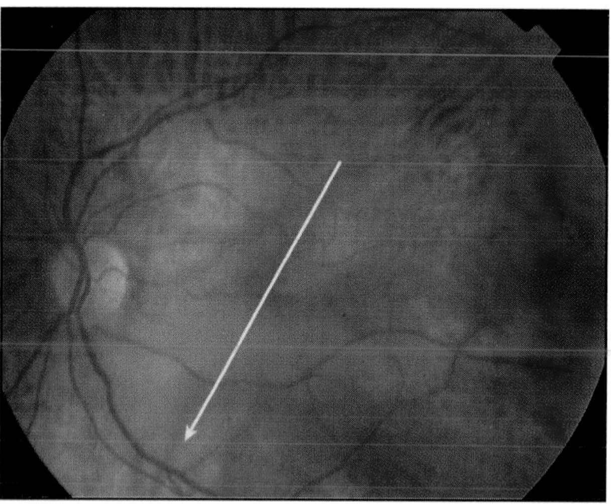

A

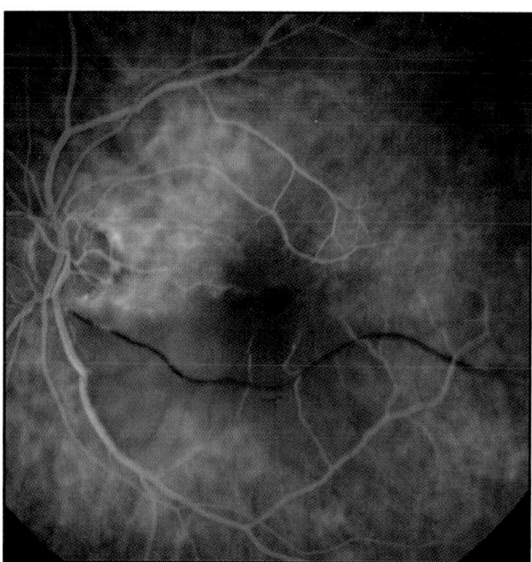

B—Early

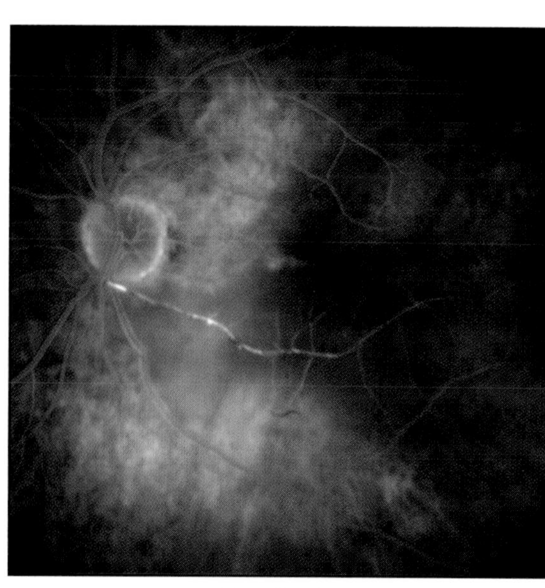

B—Late

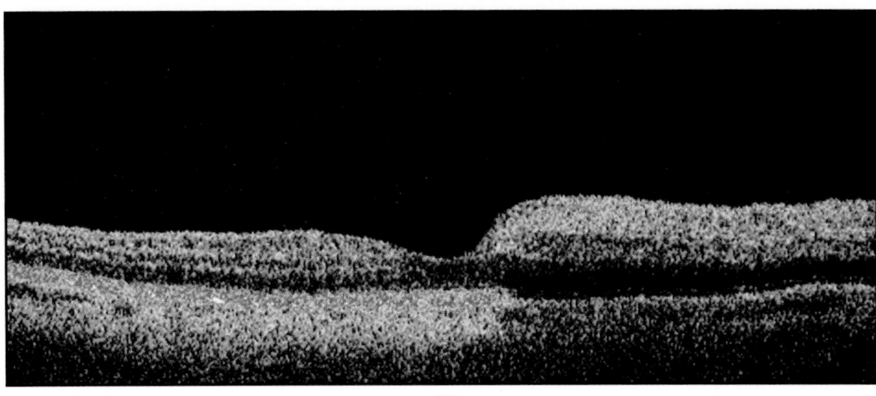

C

Case 4-2. Acute Branch Retinal Artery Occlusion

Clinical Summary

A 51-year-old man experienced loss of the superior visual field in his left eye. The visual acuity in this eye was 20/25. Dilated fundus examination showed retinal whitening in the distribution of an inferotemporal branch retinal artery (A). Fluorescein angiography (B) revealed delayed filling of the involved branch retinal artery.

Optical Coherence Tomography

OCT (C) showed increased reflectivity and thickness of the inner retinal layers compatible with the acute ischemic tissue insult. Shadowing of the outer retinal layers and RPE/choriocapillaris optical signals was appreciated.

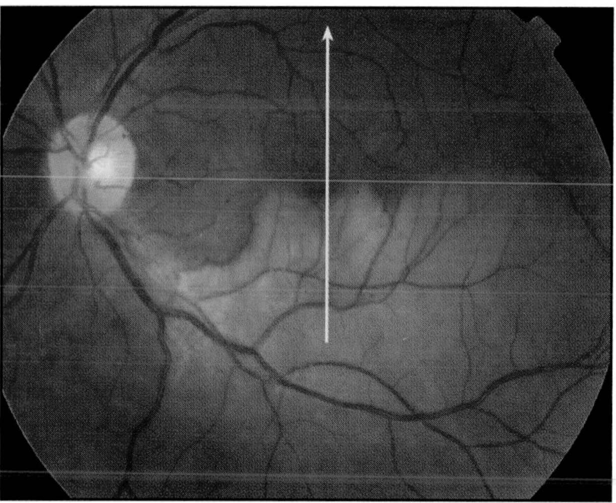

A

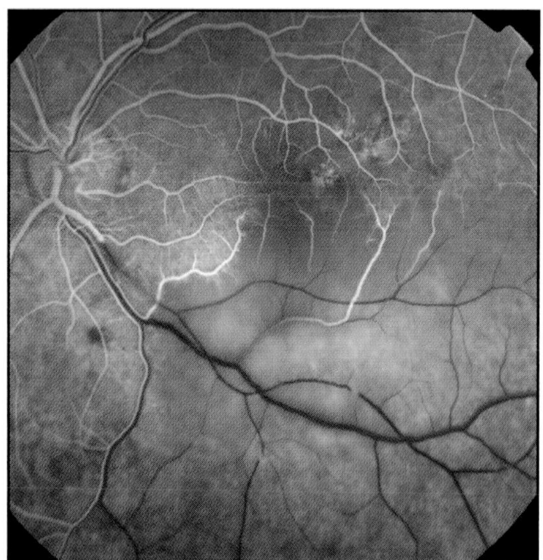

B—Early

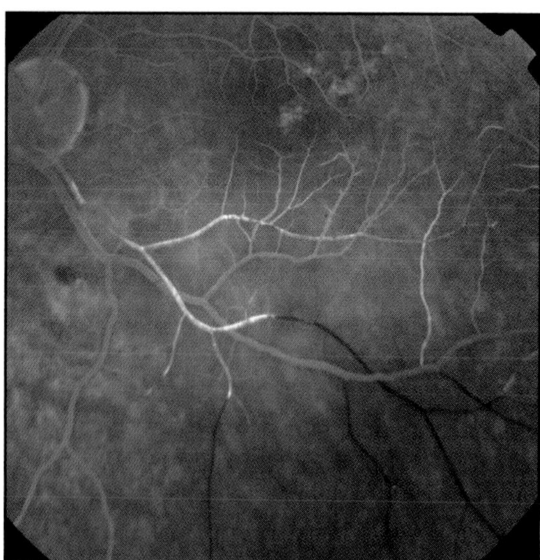

B—Late

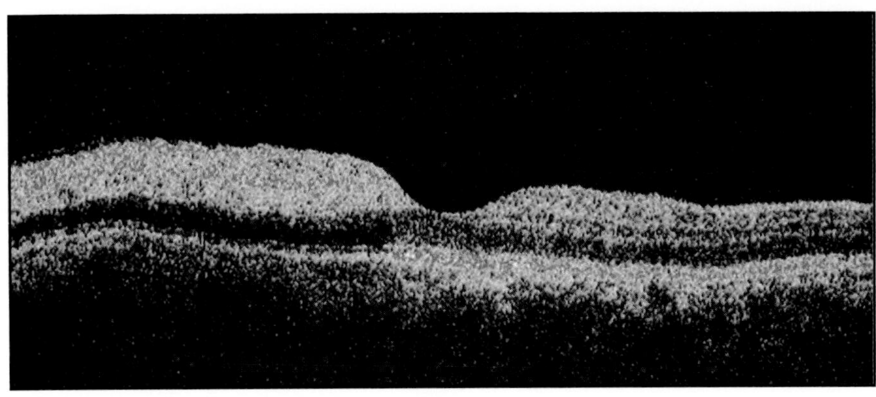

C

Case 4-3. Central Retinal Artery Occlusion

Clinical Summary

A 69-year-old woman reported sudden decrease of her vision in the right eye approximately 3 days earlier. Her visual acuity was counting fingers in this eye. Dilated fundus examination was remarkable for retinal opacification in the macular area and a cherry red spot in the foveola (A).

Optical Coherence Tomography

OCT (B) illustrated a slight increase in retinal thickness and reflectivity of the inner layers in the area corresponding to the opaque macula. This correlates with the histopathological findings of intracellular edema and ischemia described in the literature. The optical signals of the outer retina and RPE/choriocapillaris complex were slightly shadowed by the inner layers.

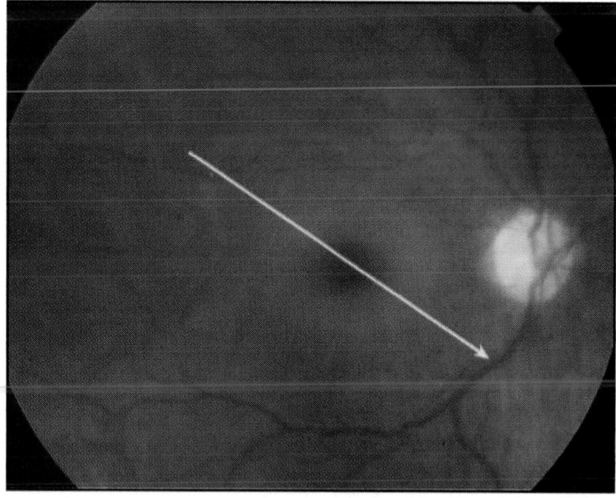

A

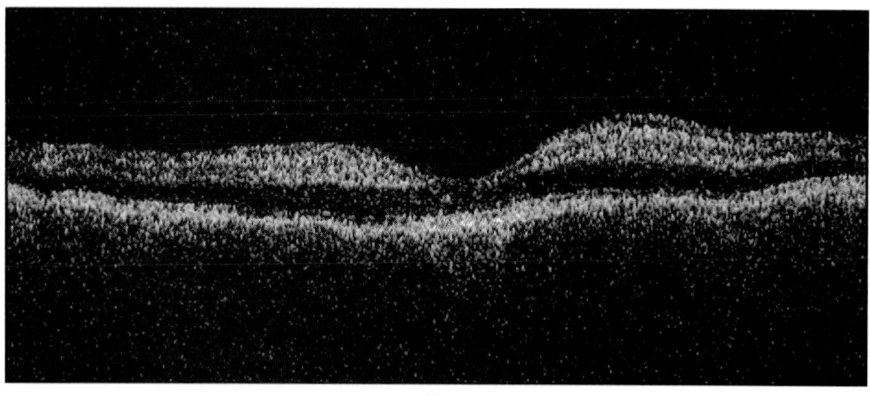

B

Case 4-4.
Branch Retinal Vein Occlusion

Clinical Summary

A 55-year-old man noticed central distortion in his left eye over the past 6 months. His visual acuity measured 20/70 in this eye. Slit-lamp biomicroscopy showed a sclerotic superotemporal branch retinal vein associated with telangiectatic vessels and retinal thickening involving the superior fovea (A). Fluorescein angiography (B) confirmed the presence of telangiectatic vessels and late leakage consistent with edema.

Optical Coherence Tomography

OCT (C) illustrated loss of the normal foveal contour and a central space of reduced reflectivity just beneath the fovea representing a cyst. Smaller cysts were evident superonasal to the fovea (right side of the scan). The foveal thickness measured 445 μm (D). The patient underwent an intravitreal injection of triamcinolone acetonide (4 mg/0.1 cc). An OCT scan (E) performed 1 month following the procedure showed disappearance of the cystic macular edema (CME). The foveal thickness measured 190 μm (F). The visual acuity improved to 20/40.

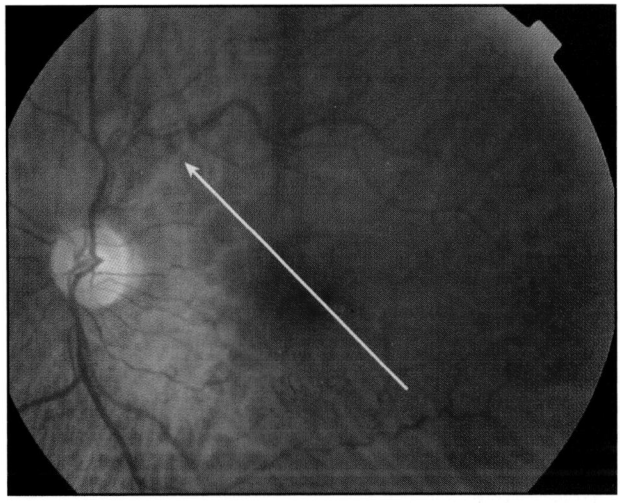

A

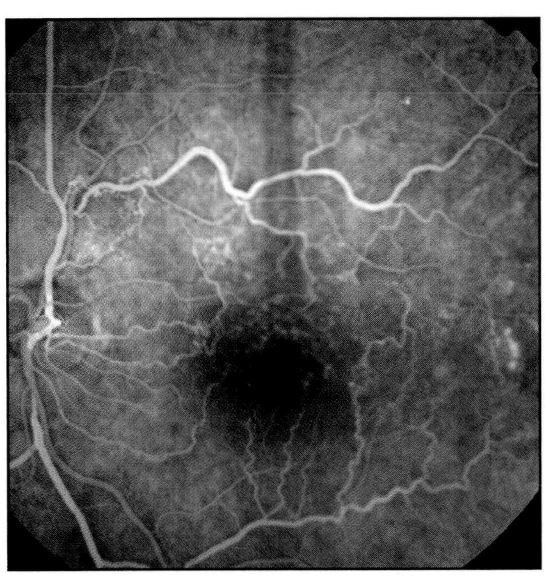

B—Early

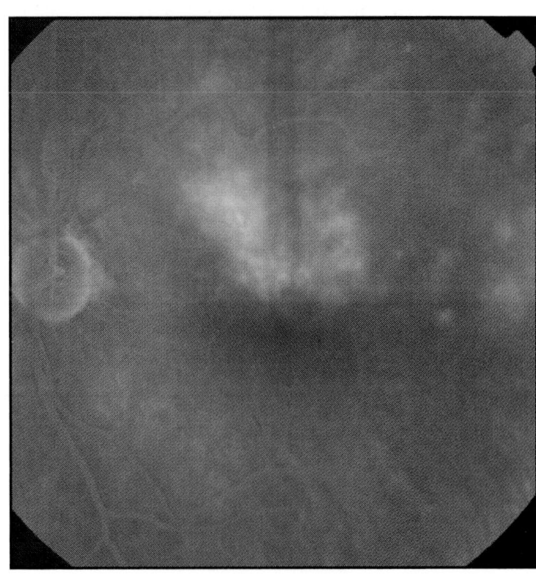

B—Late

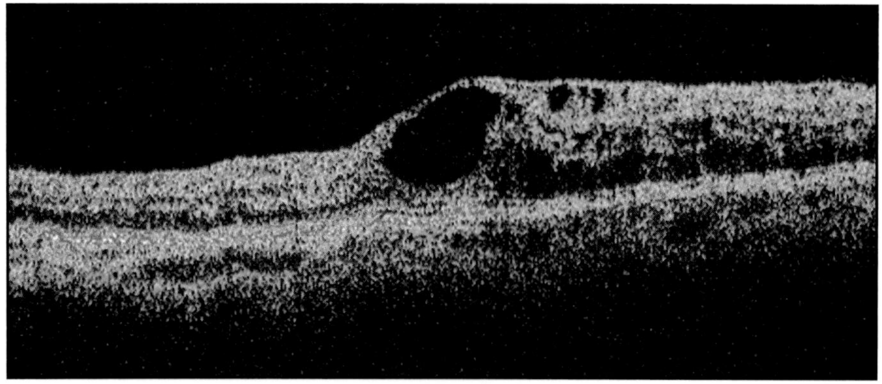

C

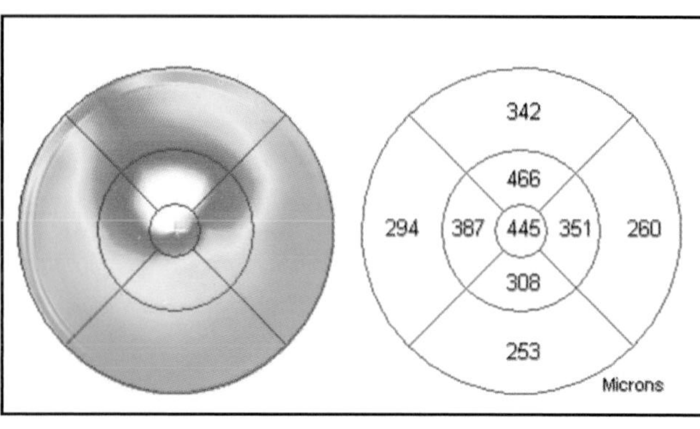
342
466
294
387
445
351
260
308
253
Microns

D

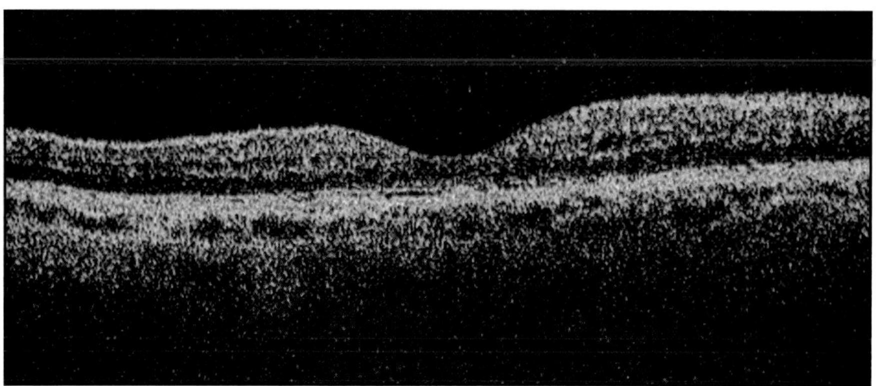

E

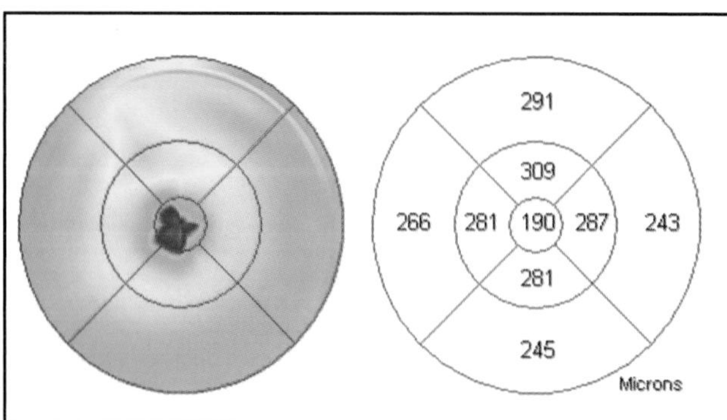
291
309
266
281
190
287
243
281
245
Microns

F

Case 4-5. *Branch Retinal Vein Occlusion*

Clinical Summary

A 59-year-old man had a 6-month history of decreased vision and distortion in his left eye. His visual acuity in this eye measured 20/60. Dilated fundus examination showed intraretinal hemorrhages, cotton wool spots, microaneurysms, and retinal thickening in the posterior pole along the superotemporal arcade extending to the fovea (A). Fluorescein angiography (B) showed telangiectatic vessels, dots of hyperfluorescence consistent with microaneurysms, extensive areas of capillary nonperfusion, and late leakage.

Optical Coherence Tomography

An OCT scan (C) obtained through fixation revealed diffuse retinal thickening from the foveal center toward the superotemporal portion of the posterior pole. Low reflective spaces separated by septae were identified corresponding to cystic fluid accumulation. An area of reduced backscattering was present beneath the neurosensory retina representing subretinal fluid accumulation. The foveal thickness measured 587 μm (D). Laser photocoagulation was not advisable due to the extensive nature of the capillary nonperfusion. An intravitreal injection of triamcinolone acetonide (4 mg/0.1 cc) was done. Two months later, obtained OCT images (E) confirmed a complete resolution of the intraretinal and subretinal fluid. The foveal thickness decreased to 176 μm (F) and the vision improved to 20/20.

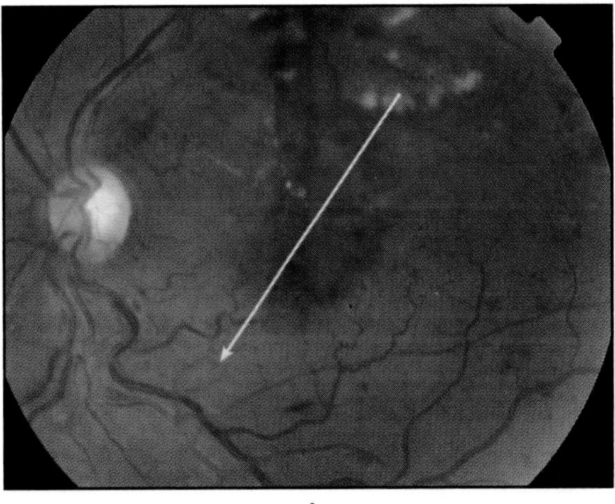

A

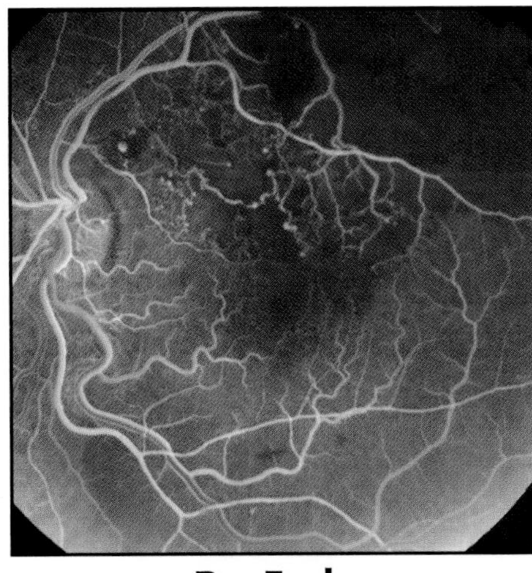

B—Early

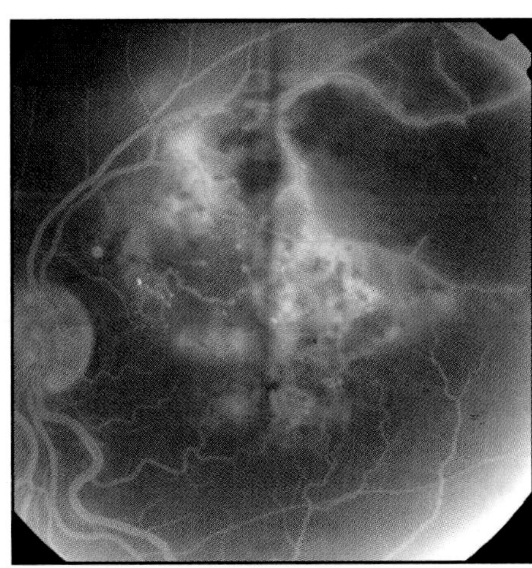

B—Late

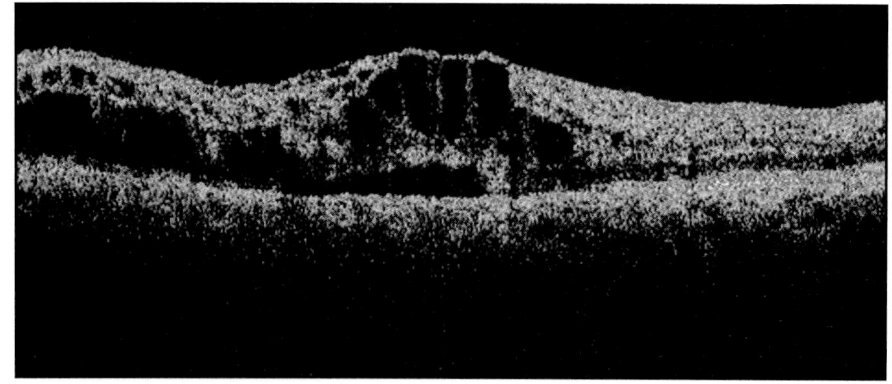

C

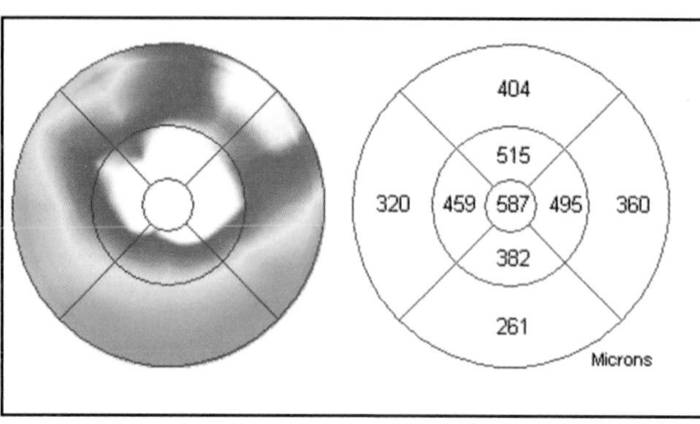
404
515
320
459
587
495
360
382
261
Microns

D

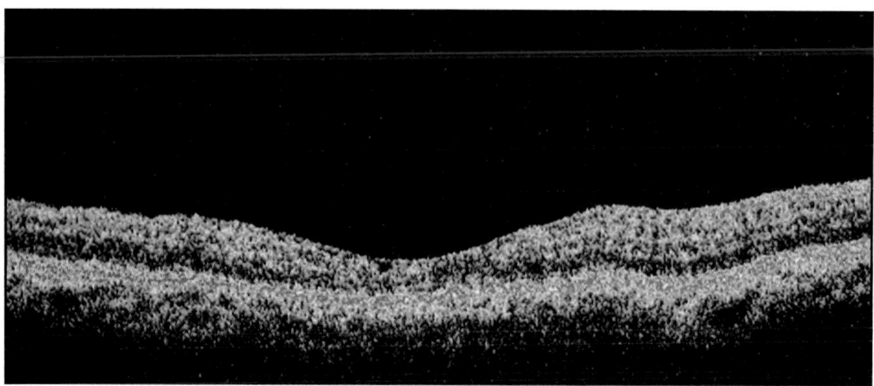

E

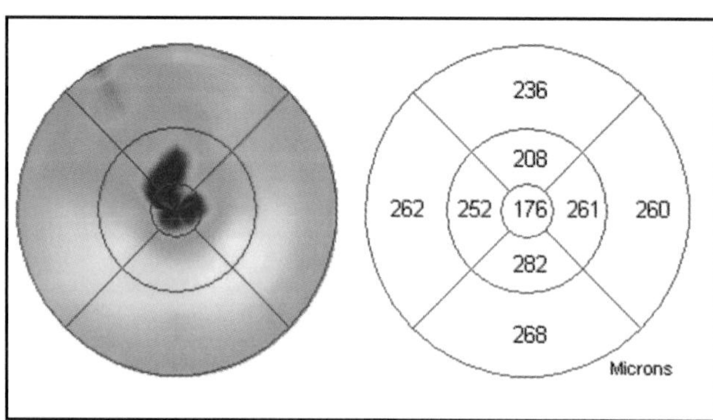
236
208
262
252
176
261
260
282
268
Microns

F

Case 4-6. Branch Retinal Vein Occlusion

Clinical Summary

A 62-year-old woman experienced vision loss in her right eye 4 months earlier. Her visual acuity was 20/300 in this eye. Examination revealed flame-shaped hemorrhages and retinal thickening in an arcuate configuration in the distribution of a superotemporal branch retinal vein. Also, sheathing of the involved venule as well as macular edema were appreciated (A). Early frames of an intravenous fluorescein angiography showed delayed filling of the obstructed vein and significant areas of capillary nonperfusion affecting the foveal avascular zone. As the angiogram progressed, staining of the occluded venule wall and leakage involving the macular area were noted (B).

Optical Coherence Tomography

An OCT scan (C) obtained through the fovea revealed marked retinal thickening superotemporally involving the foveal center. Spaces of reduced reflectivity were identified preferentially in the outer plexiform layer consistent with cystic fluid accumulation. An elevation of the neurosensory retina, representing subretinal fluid accumulation just beneath the fovea, was observed. The retinal map analysis showed a foveal thickness of 482 μm (D). Due to the presence of perifoveal capillary drop out, an intravitreal injection of triamcinolone acetonide (4 mg/0.1 cc) was offered to the patient. One month after the procedure, an OCT scan (E) obtained through foveal fixation showed resolution of the intraretinal and subretinal fluid accumulation. The foveal thickness had decreased to 195 μm (F) and the visual acuity improved to 20/50. A retinal examination performed 4 months after the injection revealed clearing of the intraretinal hemorrhages and resolution of the retinal thickening (G). A follow-up fluorescein angiography showed a significant decrease in the amount of leakage (H). An OCT scan (I) obtained through the fovea confirmed the complete resolution of the macular edema as well as the neurosensory detachment. The foveal thickness measured 175 μm (J). Vision improved to 20/40.

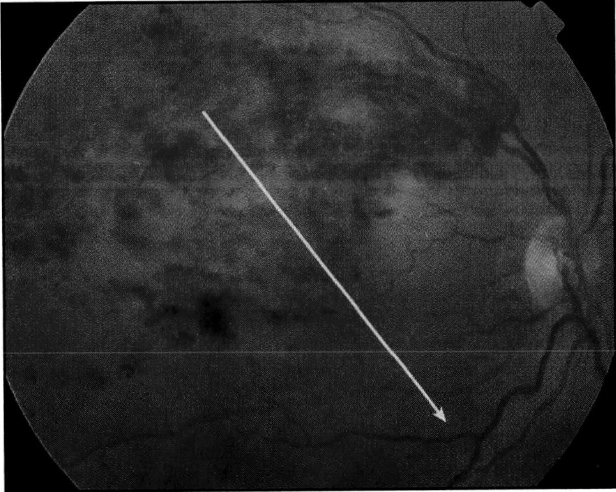

A

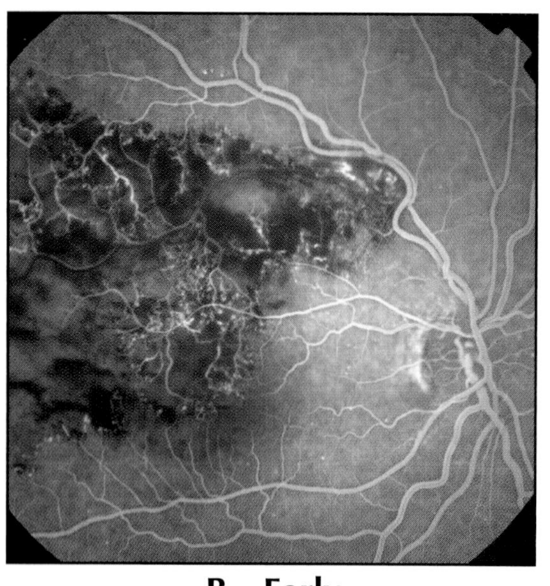

B—Early

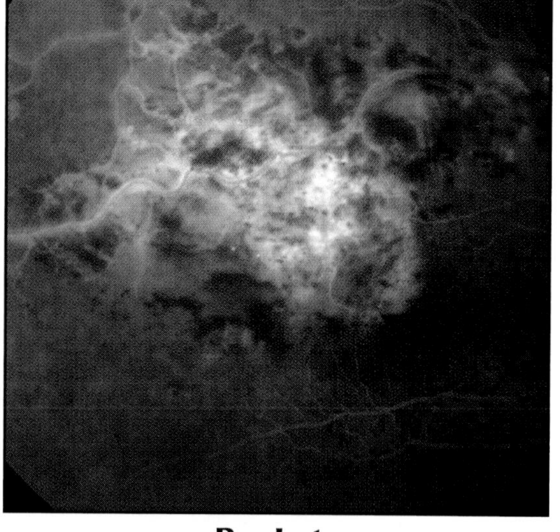

B—Late

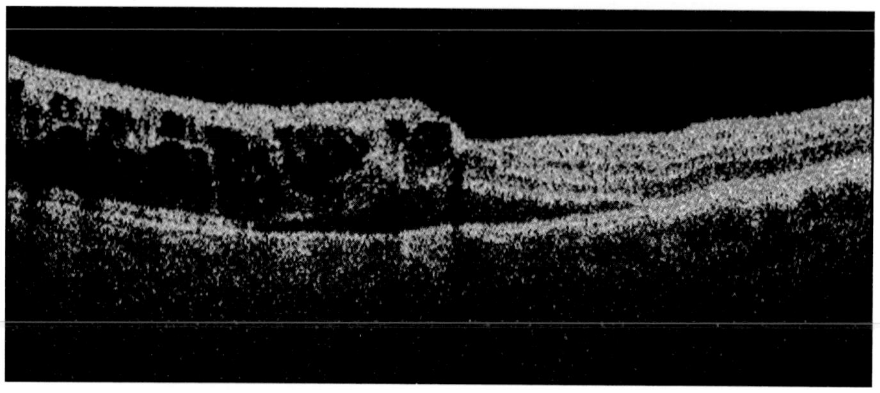

C

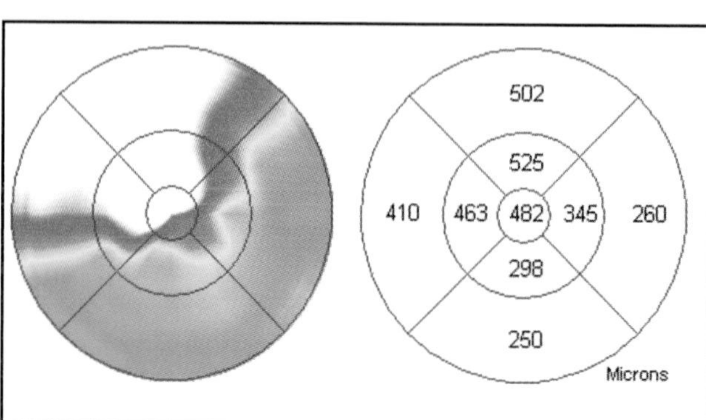

D

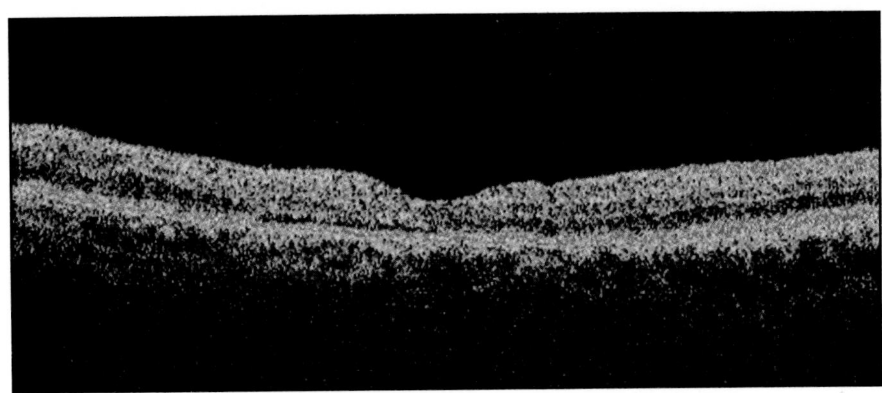

E

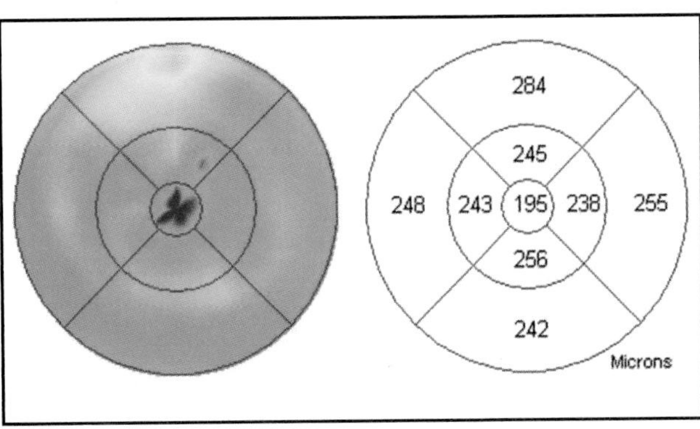

F

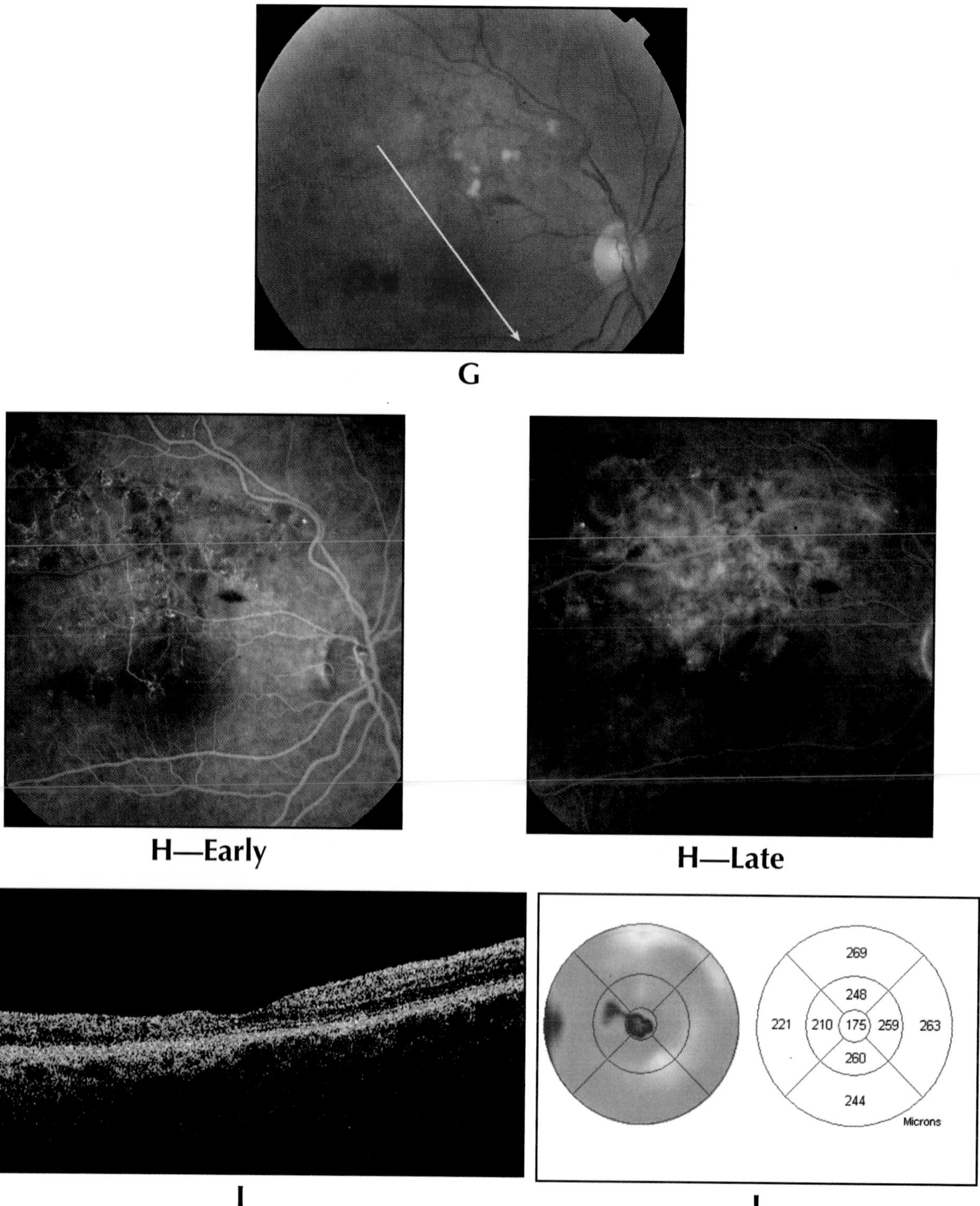

G

H—Early

H—Late

I

J

Case 4-7. Branch Retinal Vein Occlusion

Clinical Summary

A 56-year-old woman experienced sudden decrease of her vision in the left eye 3 days earlier. The visual acuity measured 6/200. Clinical examination showed cotton wool spots, intraretinal and flame-shaped hemorrhages, as well as edema in the superior aspect of the macula (A). Fluorescein angiography (B) showed blocked fluorescence from the hemorrhage and late leakage consistent with edema.

Optical Coherence Tomography

A vertical OCT scan (C) revealed marked thickening in the superior macula associated with high reflectivity in the inner layers from the intraretinal blood. Reduced backscattering was observed in the retinal layers below due to edema as well as blocked reflections from the RPE/choriocapillaris/choroid. The central retinal thickness measured 448 μm (D). The patient was re-evaluated 3 months later. At that time, her visual acuity was 20/200. The extensive hemorrhagic component precluded from laser photocoagulation. A vertical OCT scan (E) obtained at that time again showed increased retinal thickness and highly reflective inner layers blocking the reflections of the RPE/choriocapillaris/choroid complex. The foveal thickness was 521 μm (F). An intravitreal injection of triamcinolone acetonide (4 mg/0.1 cc) was offered to her. OCT images (G) obtained 1 month after the procedure depicted a marked decrease of thickness and intraretinal fluid. The reflections of the RPE/choriocapillaris/choroid were significantly less shadowed. The central thickness had decreased to 278 μm (H). Visual acuity improved to 20/20. An OCT scan (I) performed 3 months following the procedure looked similar with a central thickness of 297 μm (J). Vision remained at the same level.

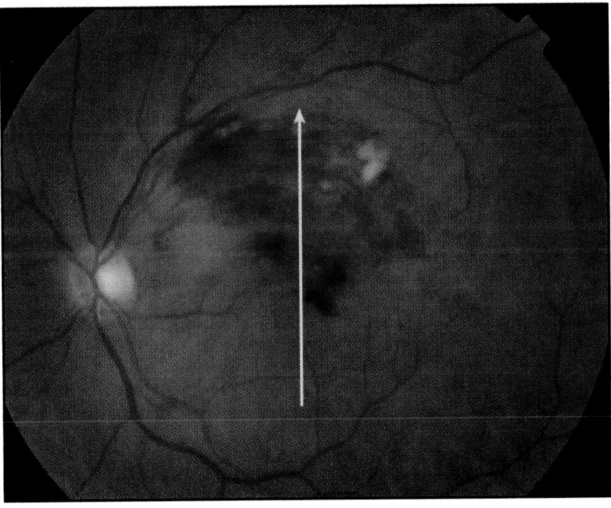

A

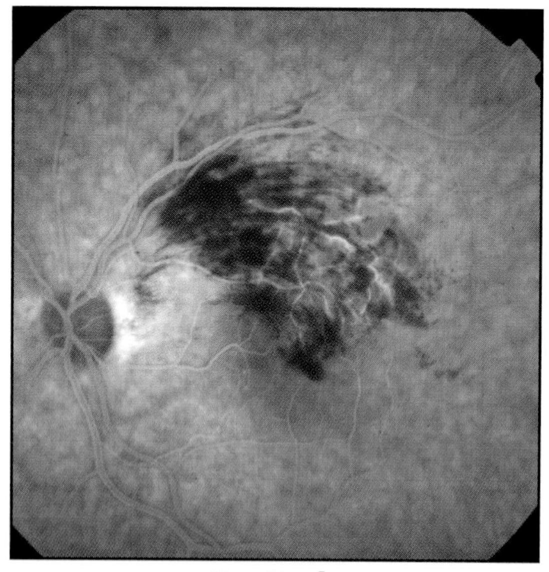

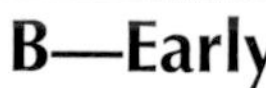

B—Early

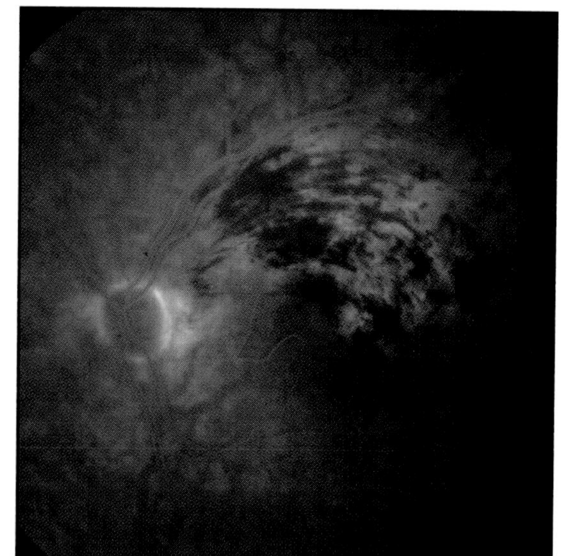

B—Late

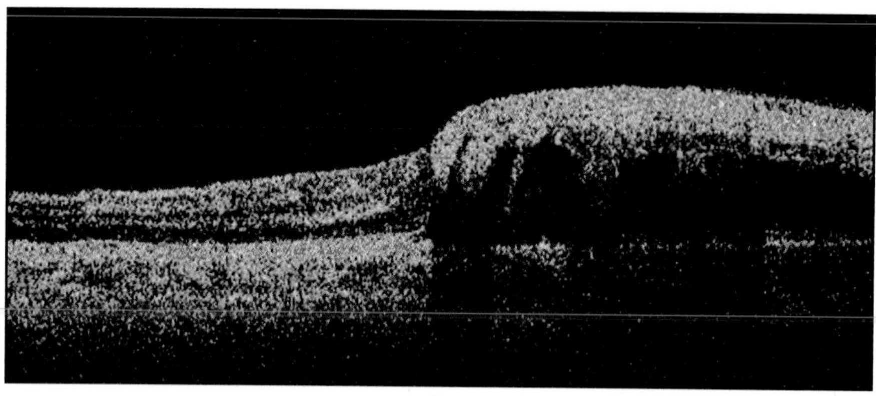

C

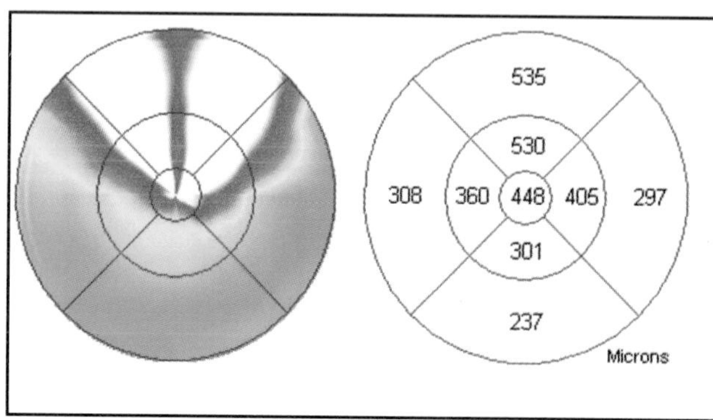

D

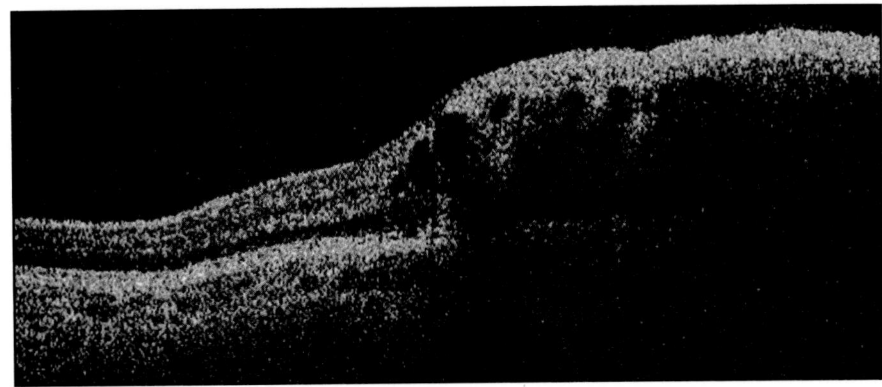

E

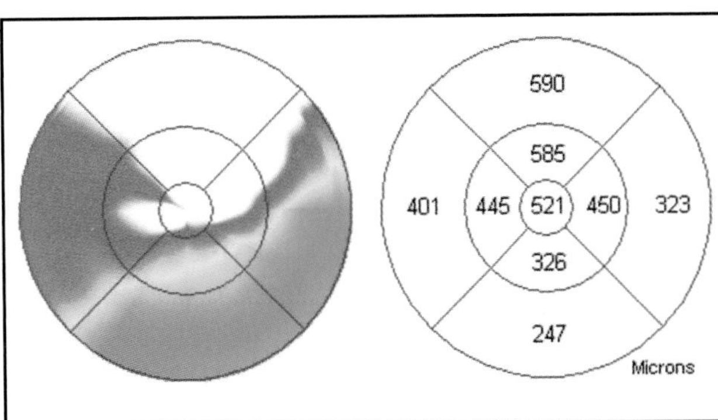
590
585
401
445
521
450
323
326
247
Microns

F

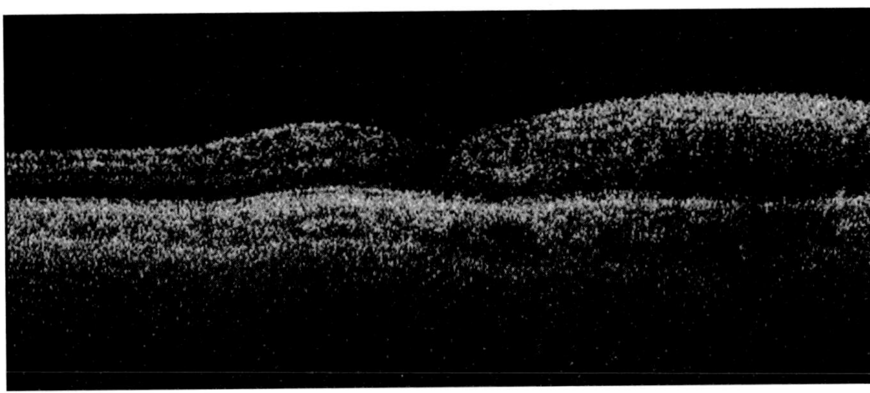

G

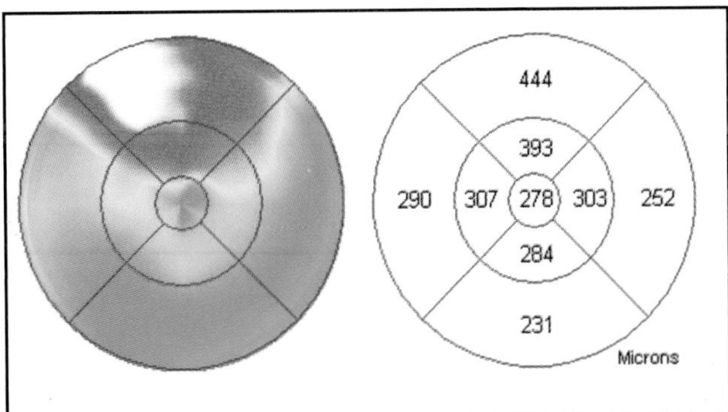
444
393
290
307
278
303
252
284
231
Microns

H

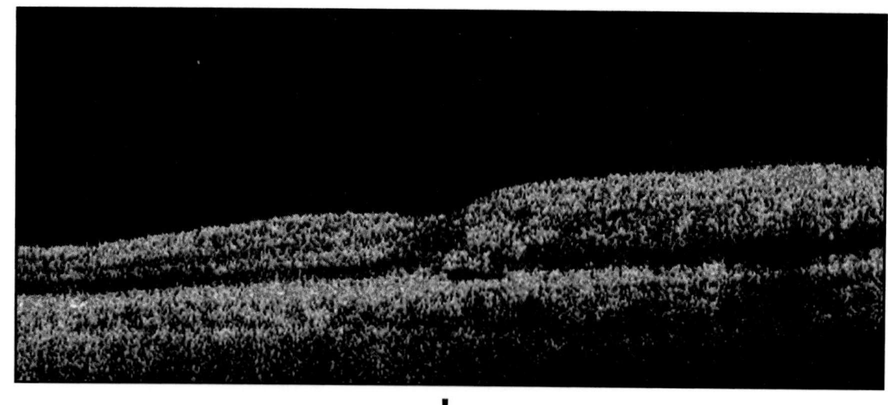

I

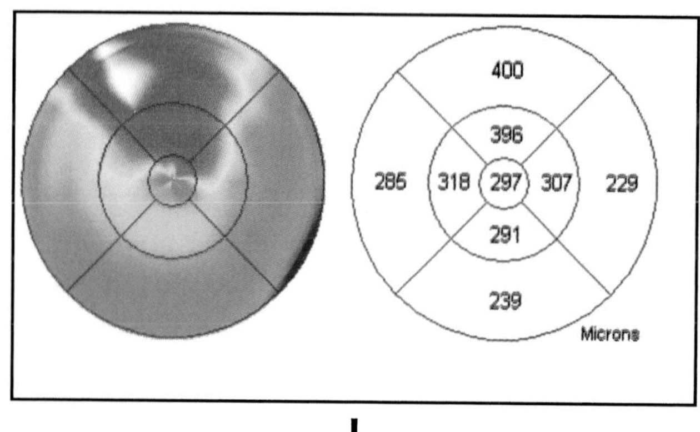

J

Case 4-8. *Branch Retinal Vein Occlusion*

Clinical Summary

A 48-year-old man with a history of a BRVO in the left eye was examined. His visual acuity was 20/20 in this eye. Dilated fundus examination showed a sclerotic superonasal branch retinal vein associated with telangiectatic vessels and old dehemoglobinized subhyaloid blood superior to the optic nerve (A). Fluorescein angiography (B) showed a delayed filling of the involved vein and minimal leakage from the telangiectatic vessels.

Optical Coherence Tomography

OCT scan (C) acquired through the subhyaloid blood showed an area of high reflectivity, which shadowed the optical signals from the retinal, RPE, and choriocapillaris layers underneath. Superiorly (right side of the scan), a reflective band was appreciated consistent with the posterior hyaloid. The subhyaloid space was visualized as a low reflective area beneath that reflective band.

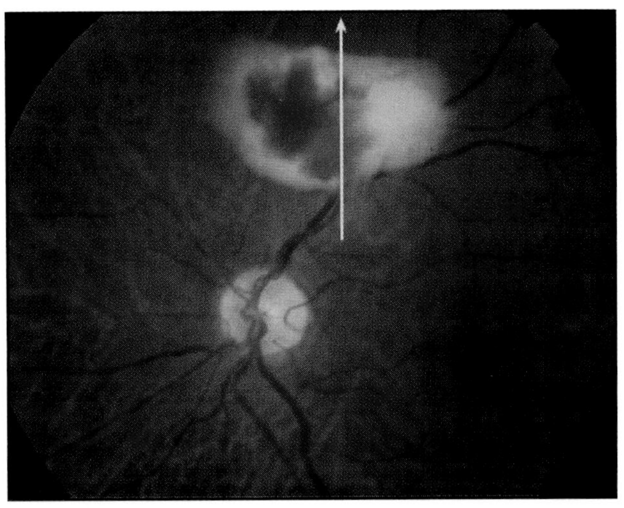

A

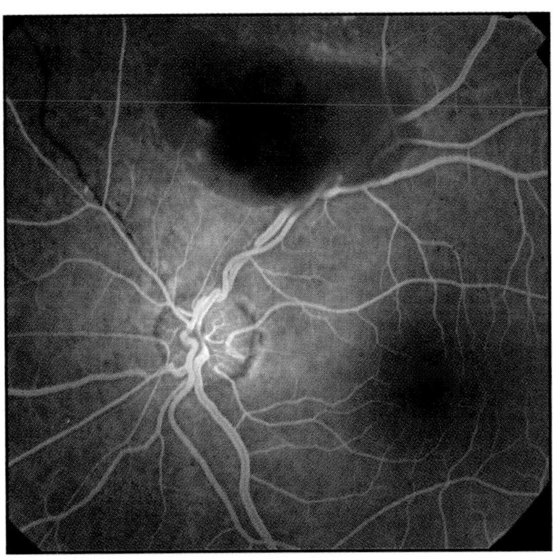

B—Early

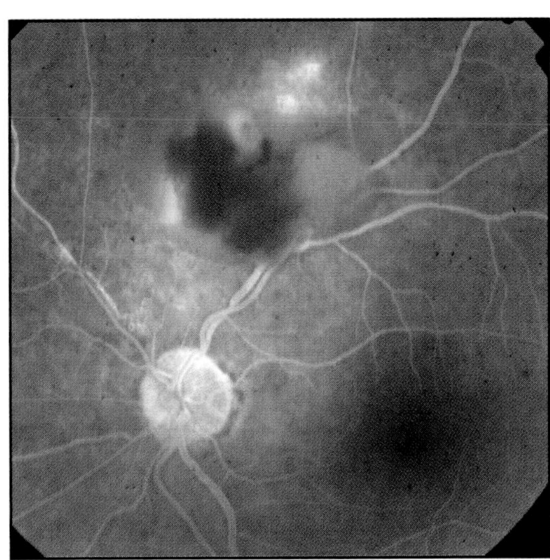

B—Late

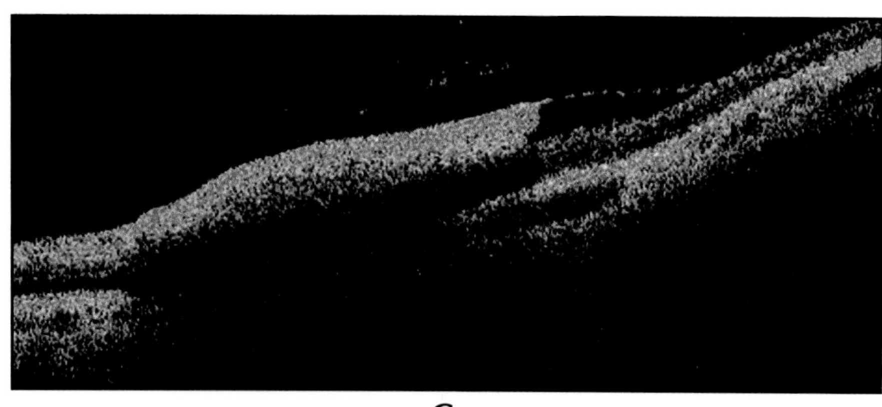

C

Case 4-9A.
Central Retinal Vein Occlusion

Clinical Summary

An 81-year-old man experienced sudden vision loss in his right eye. His visual acuity was 20/400 in this eye. Examination revealed optic nerve head edema, dilated tortuous retinal veins, scattered intraretinal hemorrhages in all quadrants, and macular edema (A). Fluorescein angiography (B) showed delayed perfusion of the veins and a prolonged arteriovenous transit time with staining of the vessel walls.

Optical Coherence Tomography

An OCT scan (C) obtained through the fovea illustrated loss of the normal foveal contour and marked retinal thickening. Large areas of low intraretinal reflectivity consistent with cystic fluid accumulation and edema were seen preferentially in the outer retinal layers. Also a detachment of the neurosensory retina with subretinal fluid accumulation was detected below the fovea. The retinal map analysis showed a foveal thickness of 789 μm (D).

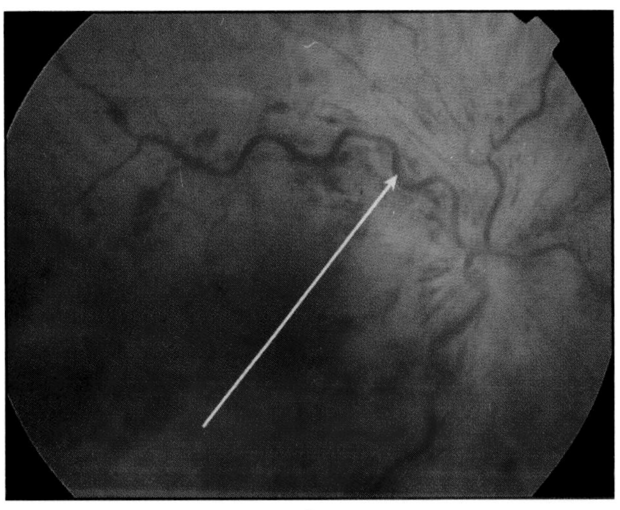

A

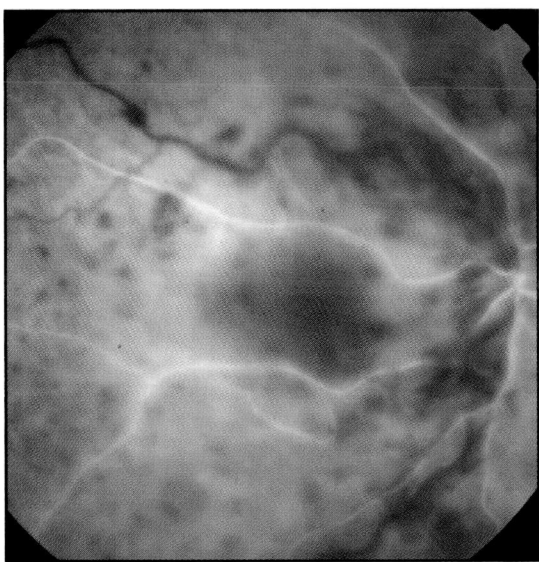

B—Early

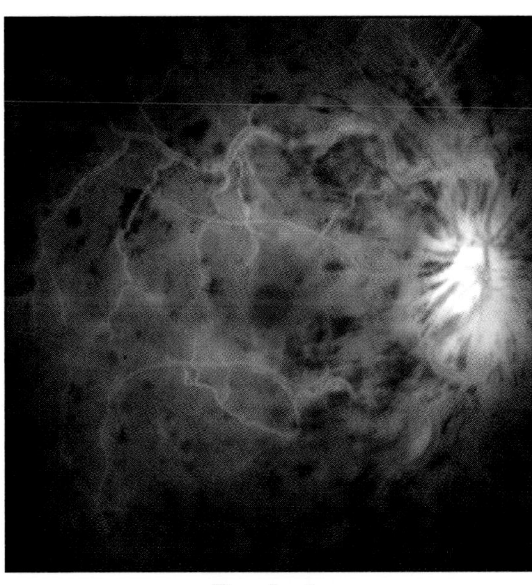

B—Late

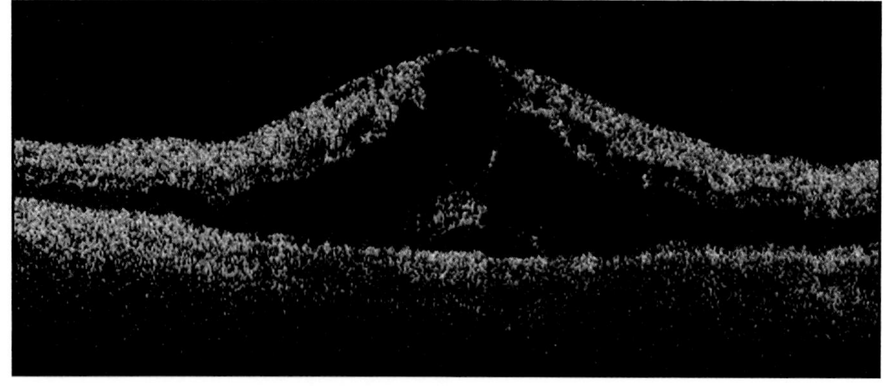

C

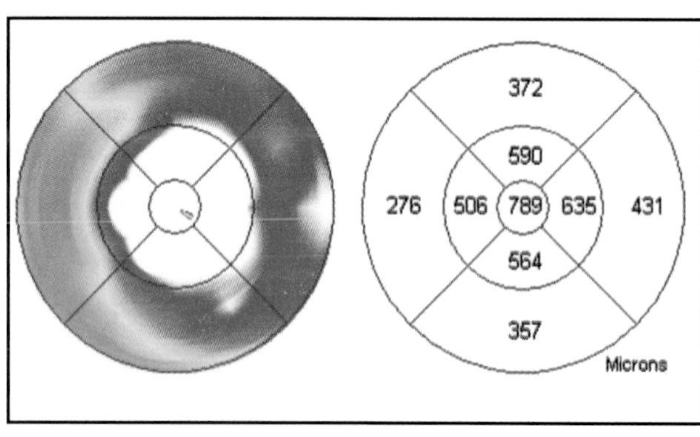

D

Case 4-9B. Central Retinal Vein Occlusion

Clinical Summary

The same patient had a CRVO in his left eye 3 months earlier. The visual acuity was counting fingers in this eye. On examination, dilated tortuous retinal veins, cotton wool spots, and scattered intraretinal hemorrhages were appreciated (E). Fluorescein angiography (F) revealed widespread areas of capillary nonperfusion, staining of vessel walls, and leakage from telangiectatic vessels.

Optical Coherence Tomography

An OCT scan (G) acquired through the fovea showed diffuse retinal thickening and low intraretinal reflectivity consistent with intraretinal fluid accumulation and edema. The foveal thickness measured 545 μm (H).

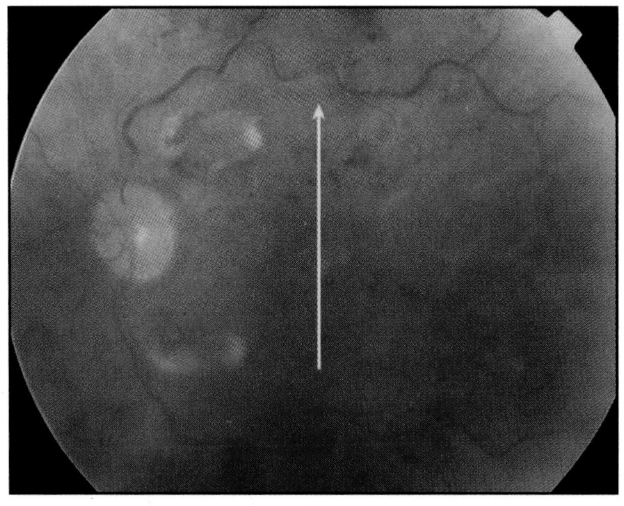

E

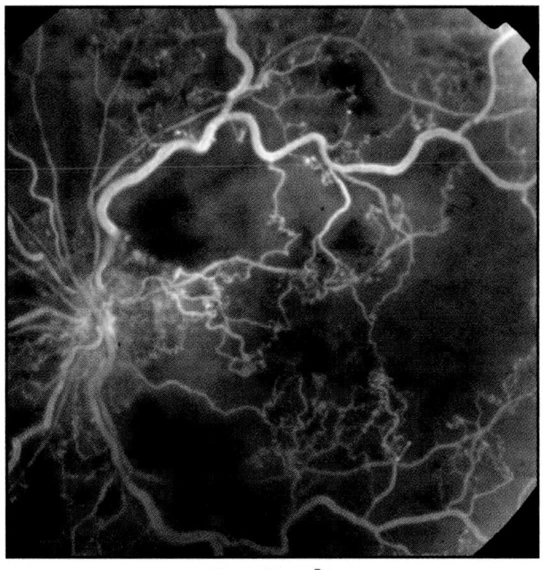

F—Early

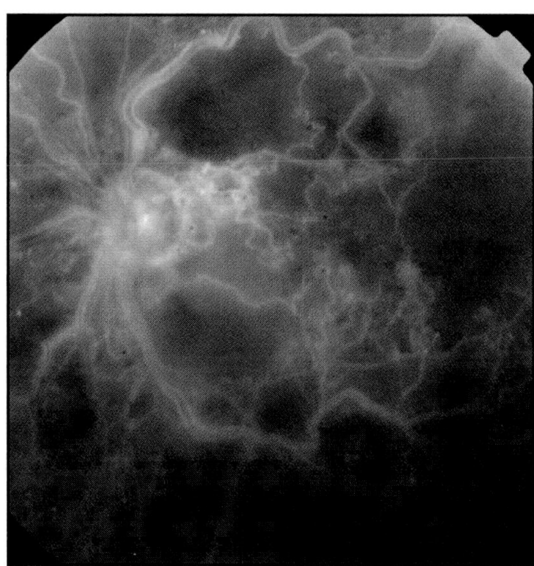

F—Late

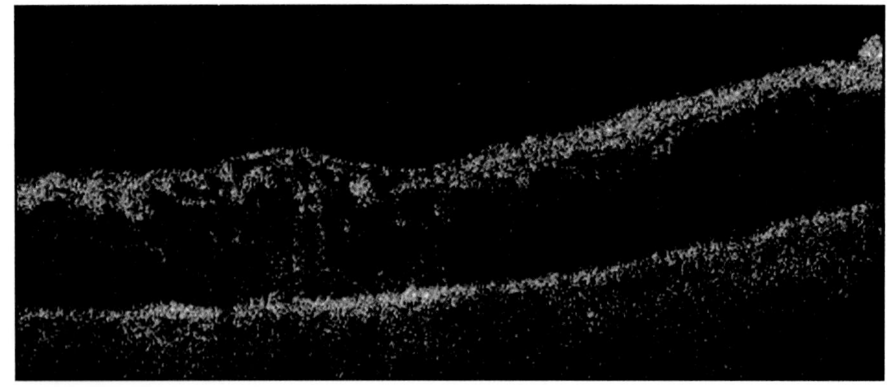

G

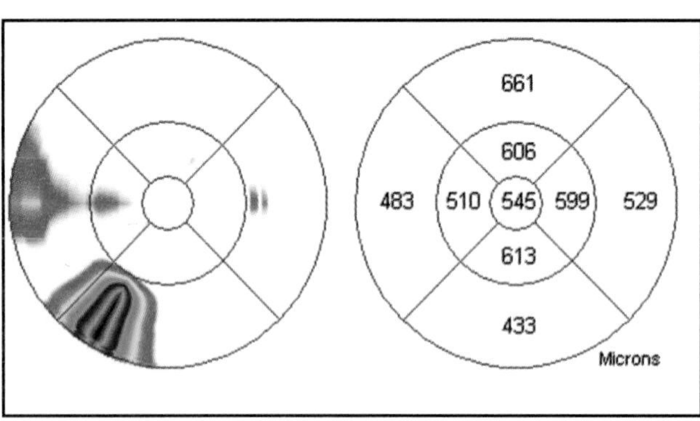

H

Case 4-10. Central Retinal Vein Occlusion

Clinical Summary

A 74-year-old man noticed decreased vision in his left eye 8 months earlier. His visual acuity was 20/300 in this eye. Retinal examination revealed peripapillary flame-shaped hemorrhages, macular edema, and scattered intraretinal hemorrhages in all four quadrants (A).

Optical Coherence Tomography

An OCT scan (B) obtained through the fovea confirmed the presence of macular edema with loss of the normal foveal contour. Large areas of low reflectivity in the outer retinal layers were seen consistent with cystic fluid accumulation. A detachment of the neurosensory retina with subretinal fluid accumulation was observed underneath the fovea. The retinal map analysis showed a foveal thickness of 494 µm (C). An intravitreal injection of triamcinolone acetonide (4 mg/0.1 cc) was offered to the patient. One month later, a follow-up OCT scan (D) revealed resolution of the intraretinal cystic fluid accumulation as well as of the subretinal fluid. The foveal thickness decreased to 210 µm (E) and the visual acuity improved to 20/60.

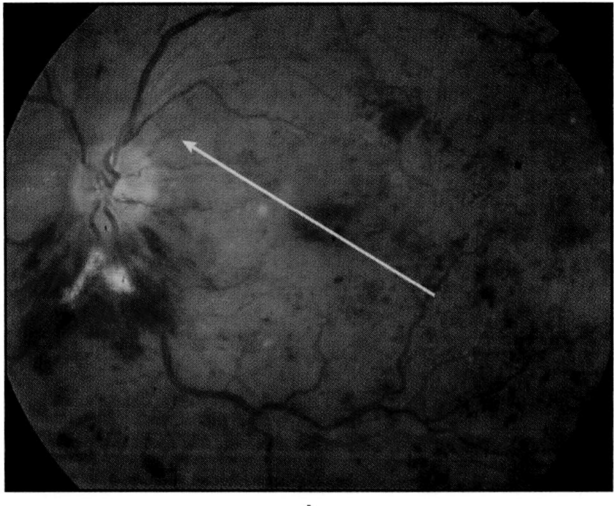

A

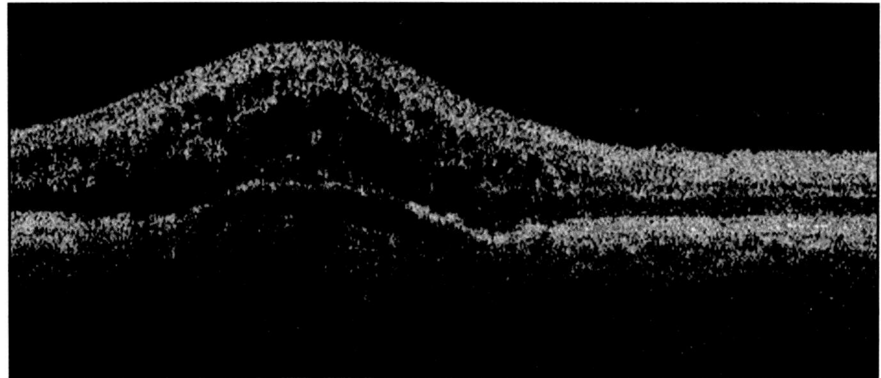

B

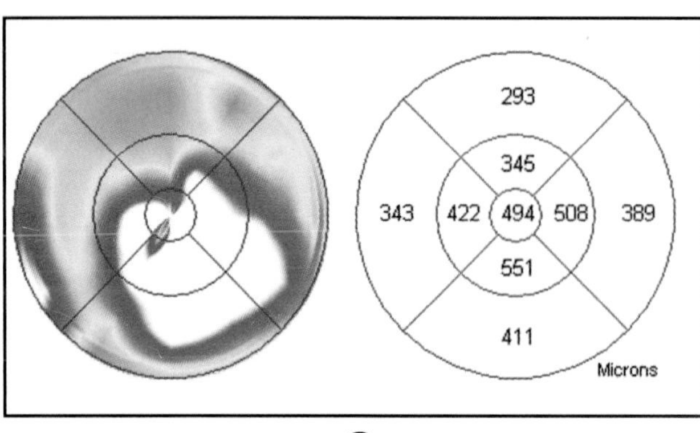
293
345
343
422
494
508
389
551
411
Microns

C

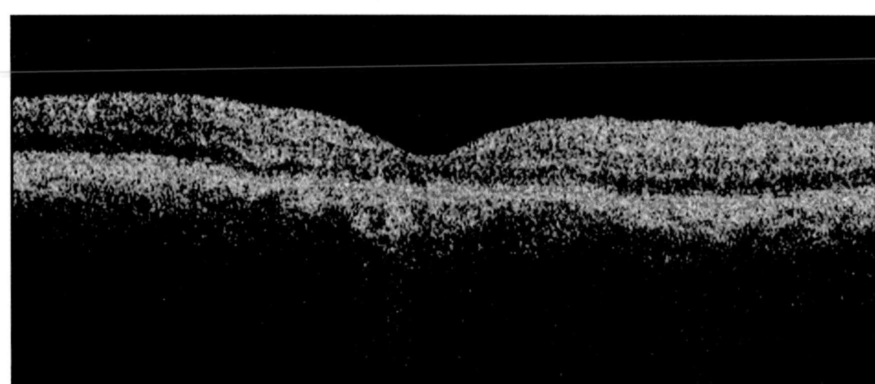

D

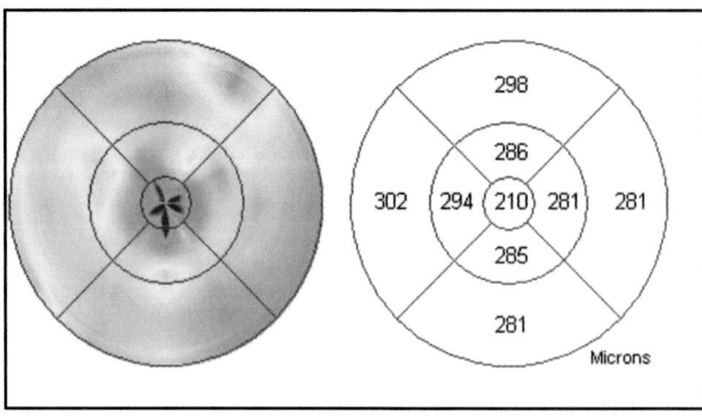
298
286
302
294
210
281
281
285
281
Microns

E

Case 4-11. Central Retinal Vein Occlusion

Clinical Summary

A 45-year-old man reported vision loss in his right eye. His visual acuity was 20/400 in this eye. Examination revealed optic disc edema, dilated and tortuous retinal veins, scattered intraretinal hemorrhages, and macular edema (A).

Optical Coherence Tomography

OCT scan (B) through the fovea showed diffuse retinal thickening and numerous low reflective cystic spaces preferentially in the outer retinal layers representing fluid accumulation. A striking neurosensory detachment with significant subretinal fluid accumulation was detected. The retinal map analysis showed a foveal thickness of 958 µm (C). The patient underwent an intravitreal injection of triamcinolone acetonide (4 mg/0.1 cc) in this eye. An OCT scan (D) was obtained through the fovea 2 weeks later and showed resolution of the cystic retinal edema and a remarkable decrease in the neurosensory detachment. The foveal thickness had decreased to 310 µm (E). The visual acuity improved to 20/40. The patient was evaluated 10 weeks after the procedure. An OCT scan (F) obtained at that time depicted a normal foveal contour and complete resolution of the edema and subretinal fluid. The retinal map analysis revealed a foveal thickness of 226 µm (G) and the visual acuity measured 20/30.

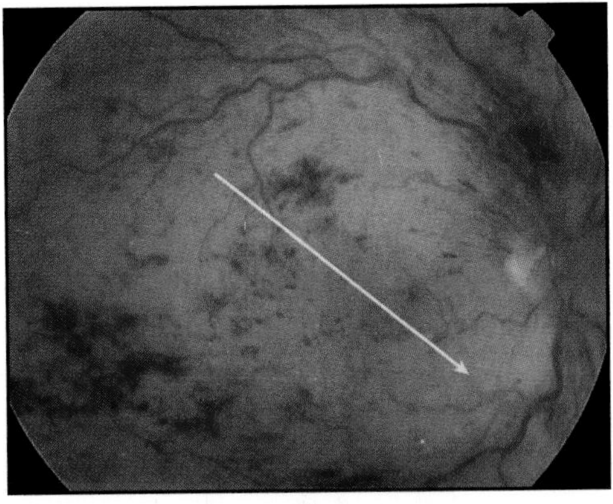

A

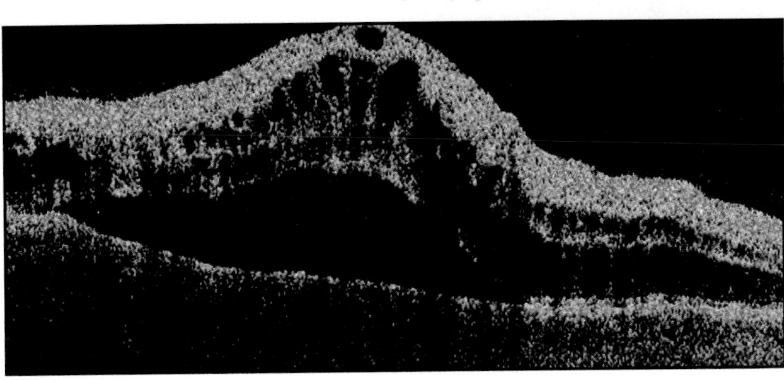

B

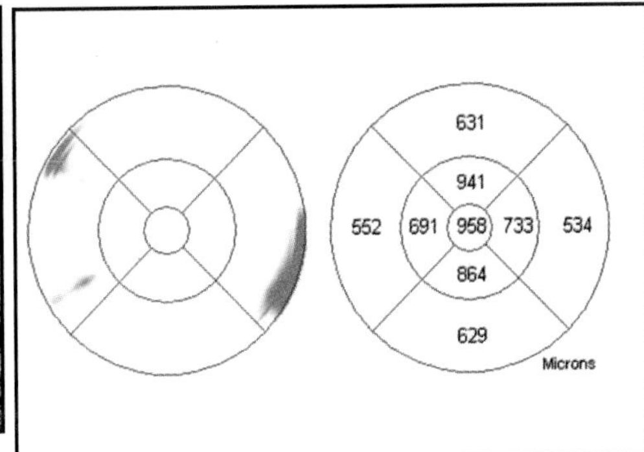

C

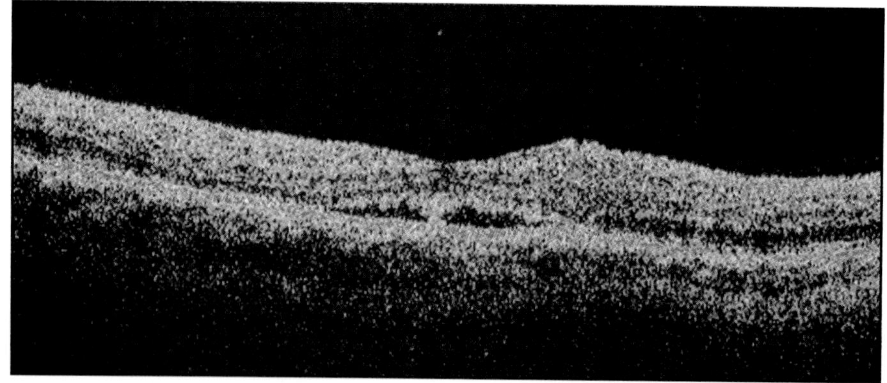

D

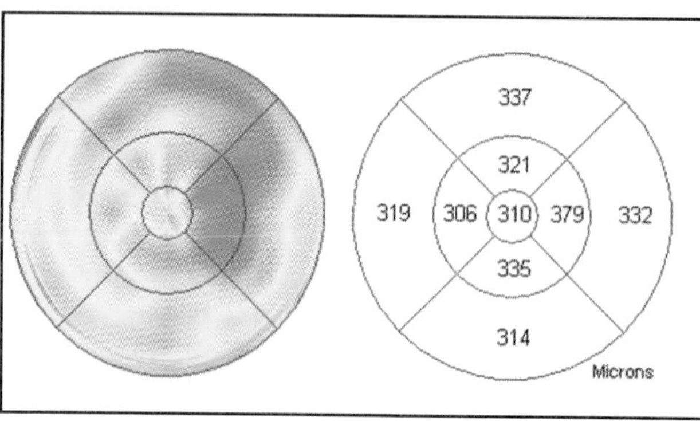
337
321
319
306
310
379
332
335
314
Microns

E

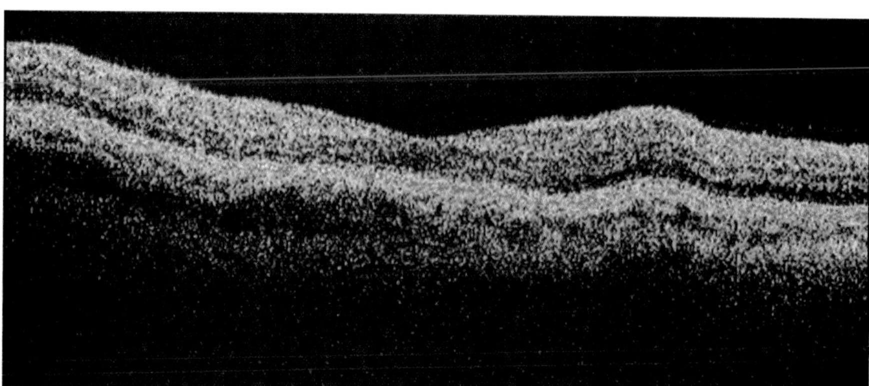

F

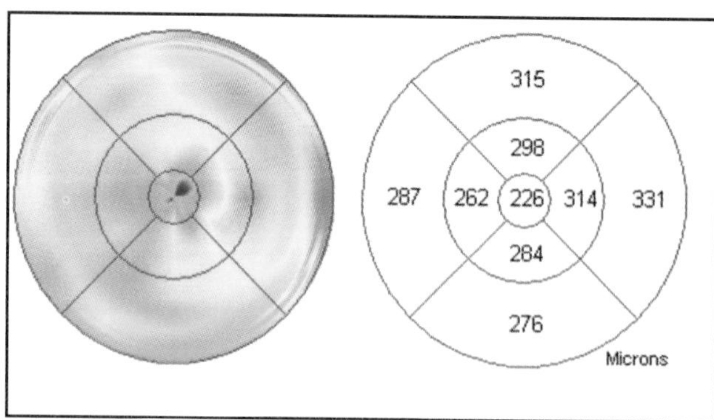
315
298
287
262
226
314
331
284
276
Microns

G

Case 4-12. Central Retinal Vein Occlusion

Clinical Summary

A 67-year-old woman reported an abrupt visual acuity decrease in her right eye 1 month earlier. The visual acuity was 20/400 in this eye. Dilated fundus examination showed optic nerve head edema, peripapillary flamed-shaped hemorrhages, dilated tortuous retinal veins, scattered dot and blot intraretinal hemorrhages, and macular edema (A). Fluorescein angiography (B) revealed a prolonged arteriovenous transit time, staining of the vessel walls, and perifoveal leakage consistent with macular edema.

Optical Coherence Tomography

A vertical OCT scan (C) obtained through the fovea revealed diffuse retinal thickening and reduced optical backscattering consistent with macular edema. A large low reflective space, representing an intraretinal cyst, was visualized just in the foveal center. A detachment of the neurosensory retina was identified beneath the fovea. The retinal thickness measured 478 µm directly in the fovea (D). An intravitreal injection of triamcinolone acetonide (4 mg/0.1 cc) was administered. A horizontal OCT scan (E) obtained 1 month later through foveal fixation illustrated a marked decrease in retinal thickness and disappearance of the subretinal fluid. The visual acuity was still 20/400. Three months later, a follow-up OCT scan (F) confirmed resolution of the CME. The foveal thickness measured 233 µm (G). The visual acuity was 20/200.

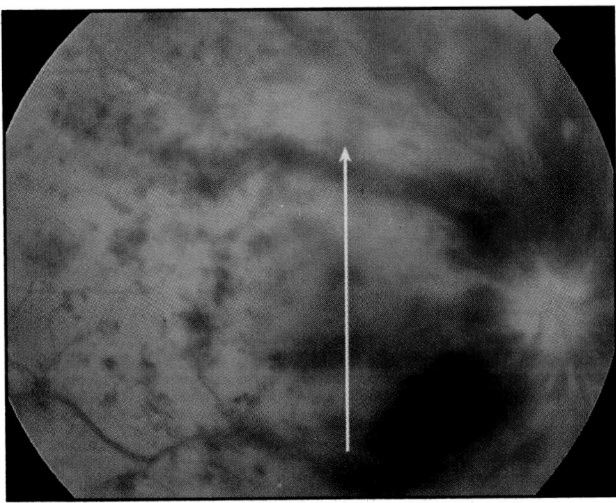

A

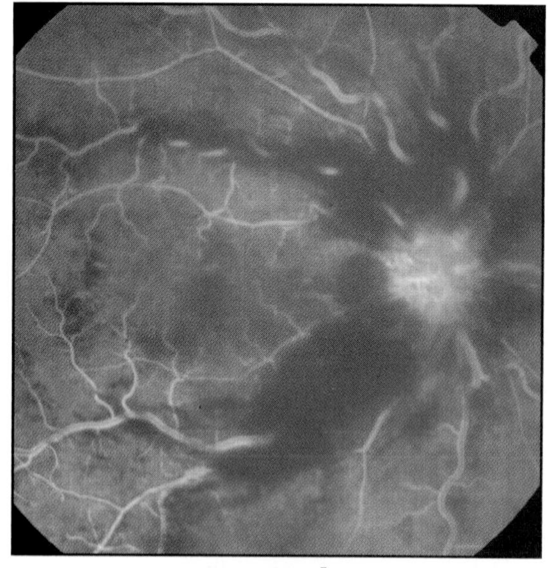

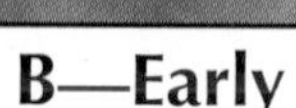

B—Early

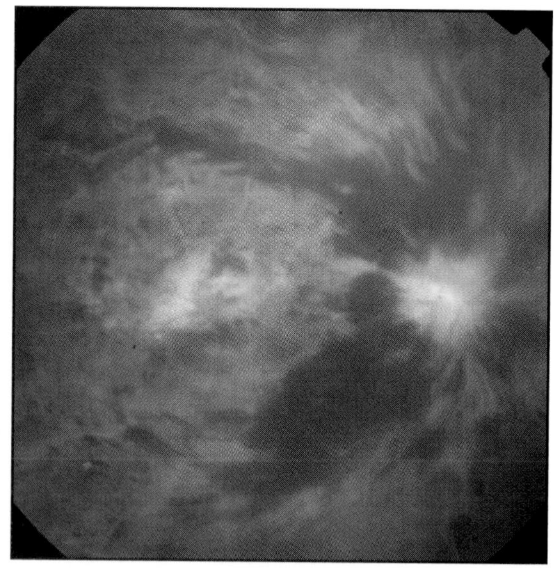

B—Late

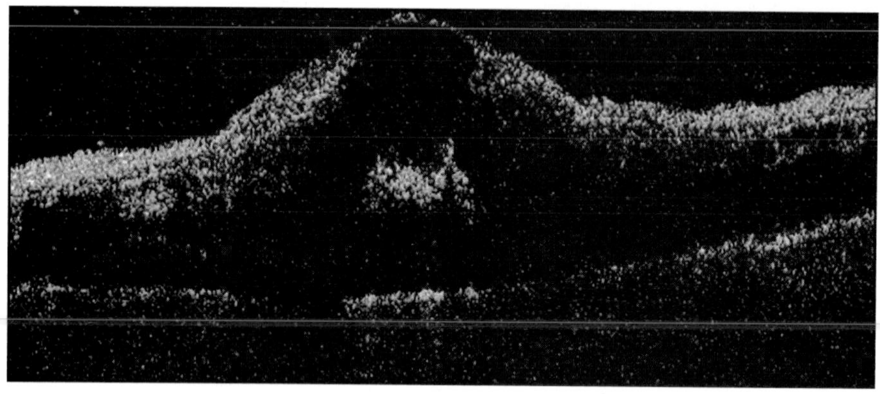

C

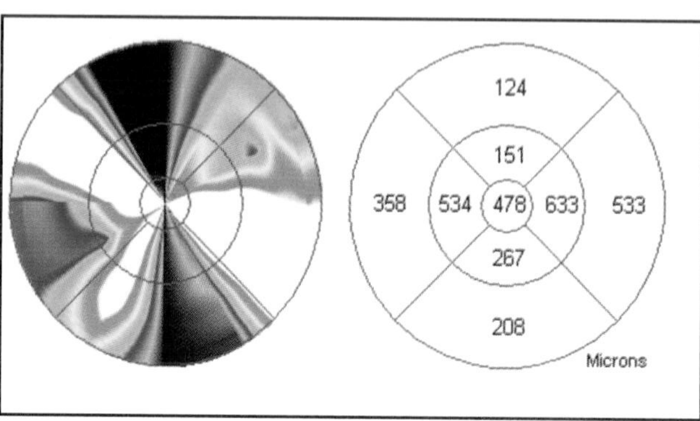

D

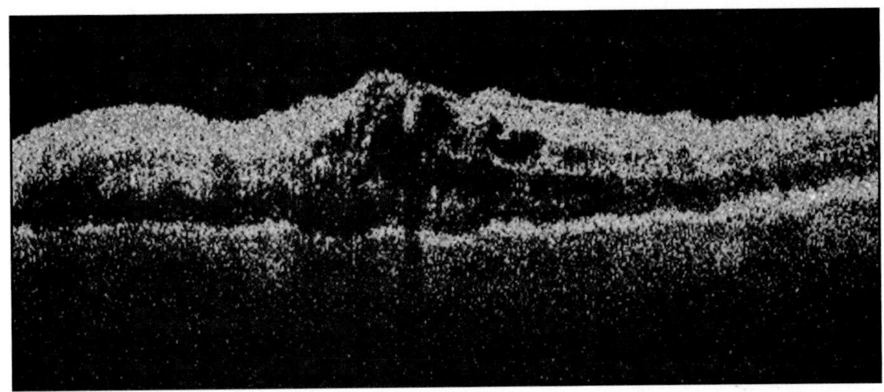

E

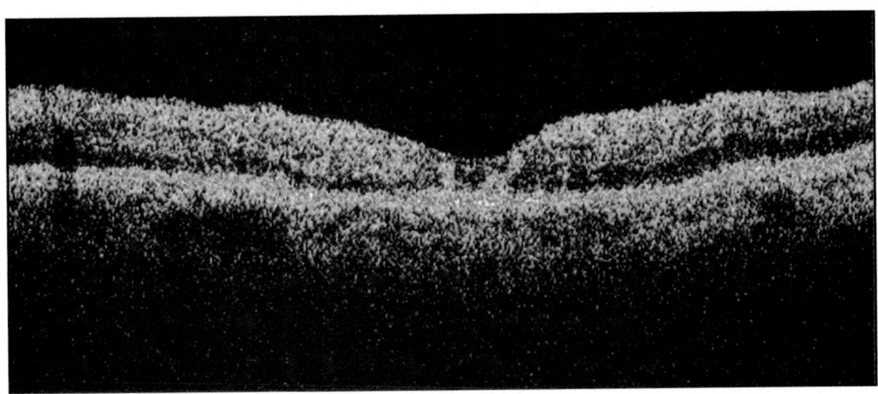

F

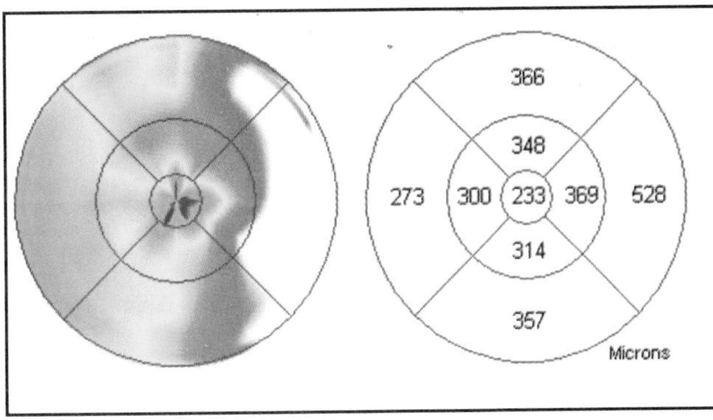

G

Case 4-13A. Central Retinal Vein Occlusion

Clinical Summary

A 52-year-old woman presented with a 3-month history of decreased vision in her right eye. The visual acuity measured 10/200 in this eye. Clinical examination revealed intraretinal hemorrhages in all four quadrants, cotton wool spots, and macular edema (A).

Optical Coherence Tomography

OCT scan (B) acquired through the fovea showed a thickened elevated macula with marked decreased reflectivity of the outer retinal layers from the fluid accumulation. Enhanced reflectivity of the inner retinal layers was observed superonasal to the fovea probably related to ischemia. The optical signal of the RPE/choriocapillaris complex appeared to be shadowed by the marked edema and highly reflective inner layers. Central retinal thickness measured 580 μm (C). The patient underwent an intravitreal injection of triamcinolone acetonide (4 mg/0.1 cc) in this eye. One month later, a follow-up OCT scan (D) revealed a remarkable decrease in the retinal thickness as well as resolution of the cystic fluid. Central retinal thickness decreased to 265 μm (E). The visual acuity measured 20/400.

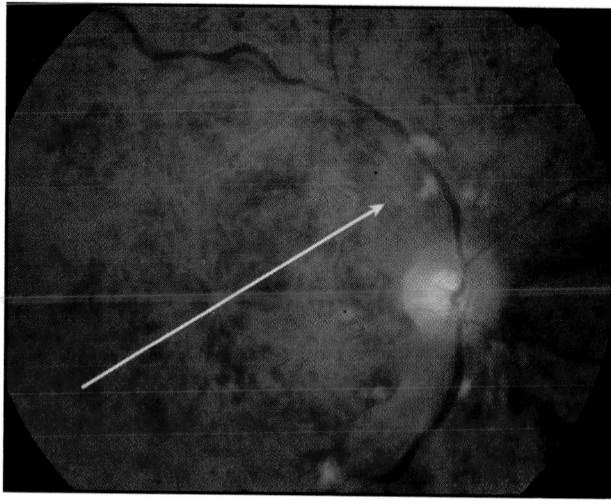

A

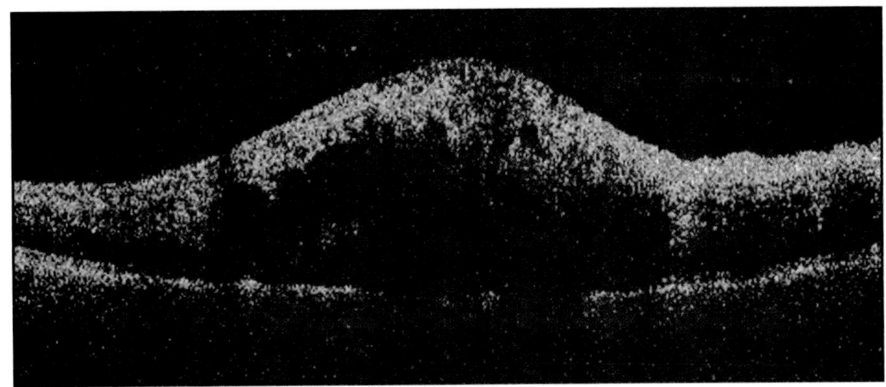

B

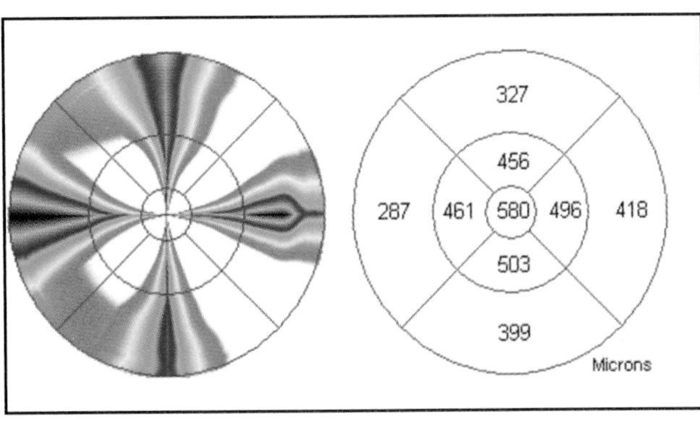
327
456
287
461
580
496
418
503
399
Microns

C

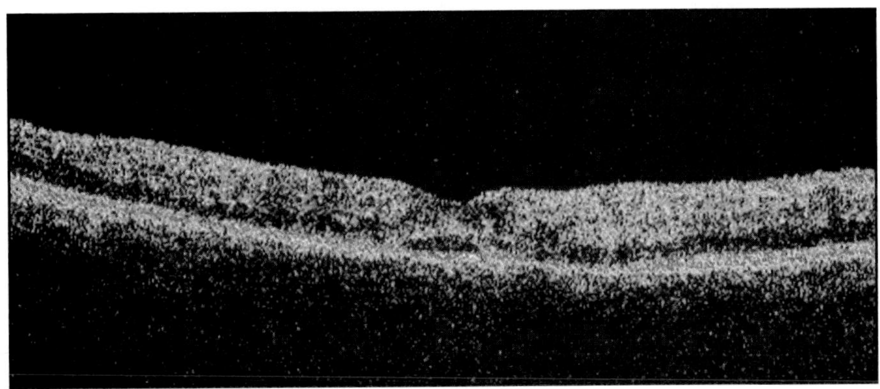

D

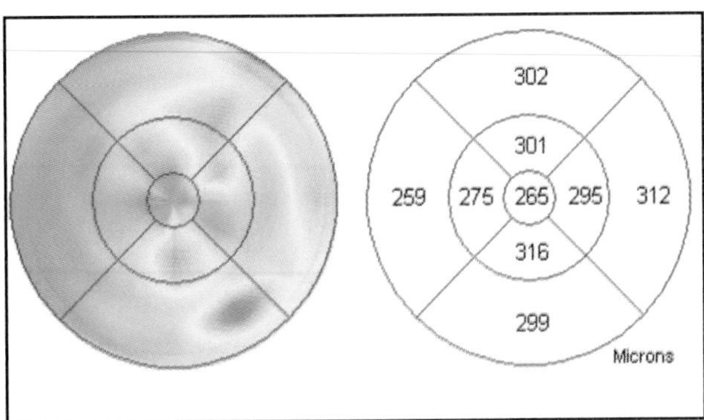
302
301
259
275
265
295
312
316
299
Microns

E

Case 4-13B. Central Retinal Vein Occlusion

Clinical Summary

The patient had a 1-year history of a CRVO in her left eye. The visual acuity was counting fingers at 6 feet in this eye. Fundus examination was hampered by the presence of a dense vitreous hemorrhage (F).

Optical Coherence Tomography

Despite the presence of a dense vitreous hemorrhage, the macular status was assessed by OCT examination. A vertical scan (G) obtained through the fovea illustrated an abnormal contour of the foveal pit with outer retinal tissue remaining at the base of the fovea. Cystic areas of reduced reflectivity were identified in the outer retinal layers consistent with edema. This configuration corresponds to a lamellar hole developing from ruptured central cysts. Central retinal thickness measured 249 μm (H).

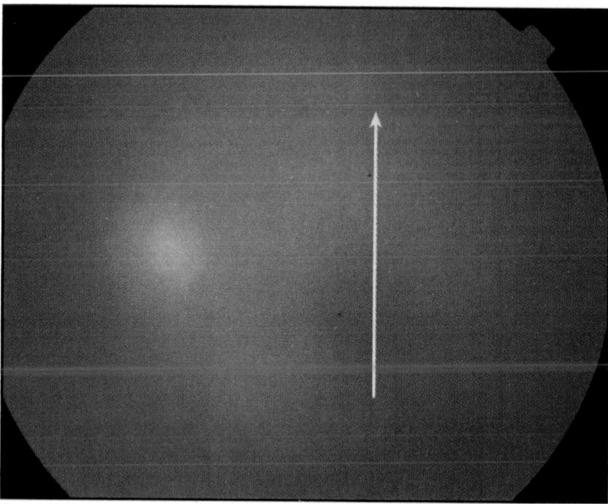

F

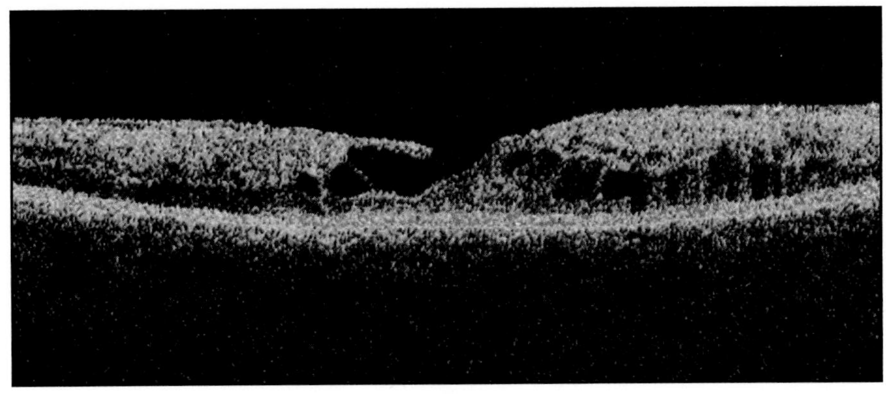

G

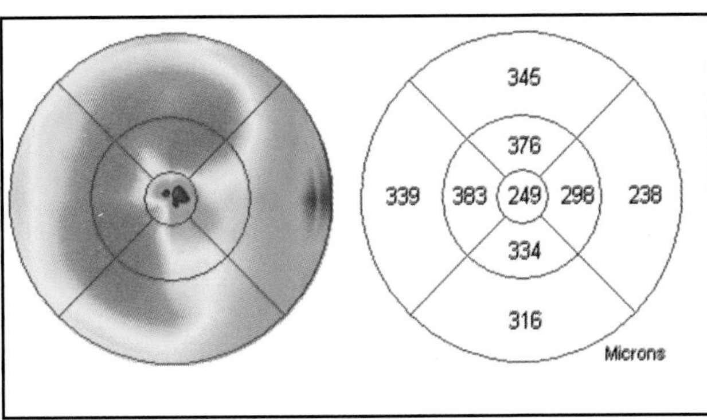

H

Case 4-14A. Bilateral Idiopathic Juxtafoveal Retinal Telangiectasis

Clinical Summary

A 60-year-old woman with a history of bilateral idiopathic juxtafoveal retinal telangiectasis was examined. Her visual acuity in the right eye measured 20/80. Slit-lamp biomicroscopy of this eye showed mild retinal thickening and right-angle venules with adjacent stellate pigment plaques in the temporal fovea (A). Fluorescein angiography (B) illustrated staining and mild leakage in the temporal macular area.

Optical Coherence Tomography

OCT (C) showed thinning preferentially of the outer retina. A focal area of high backscattering representing the aforementioned pigment plaques shadowed the reflection from the RPE/choriocapillaris layers underneath. The central retinal thickness measured 161 μm (D).

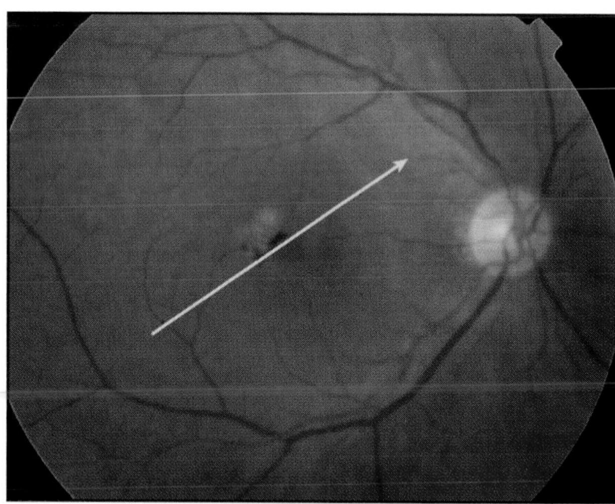

A

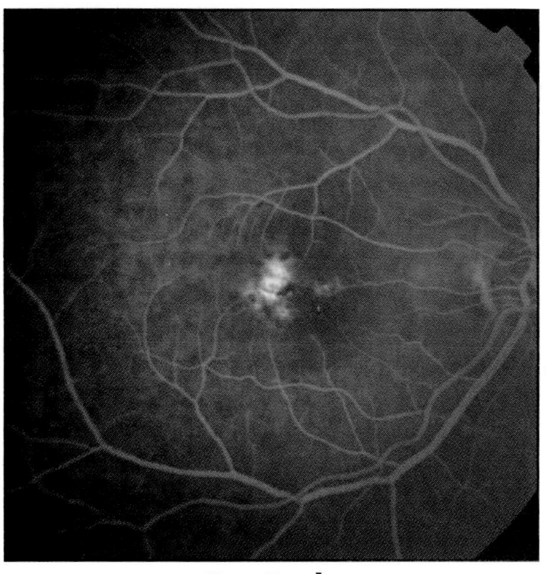

B—Early

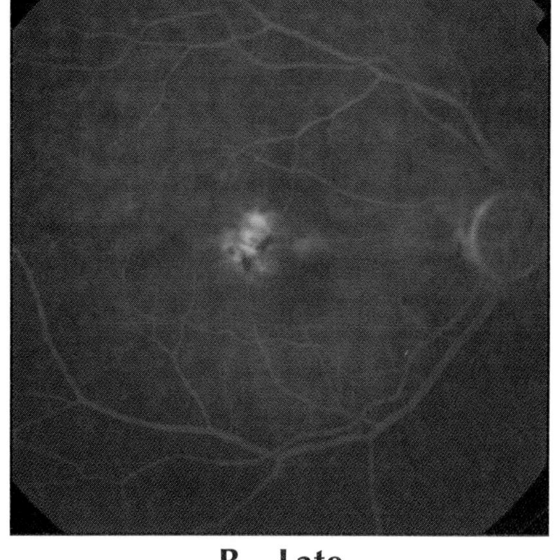

B—Late

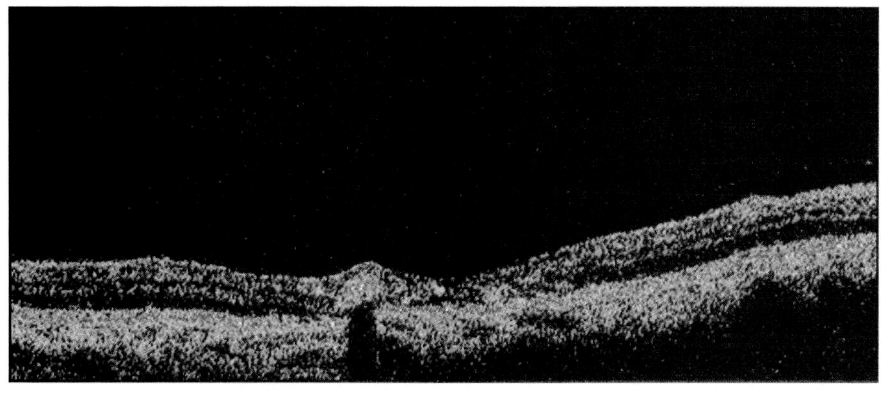

C

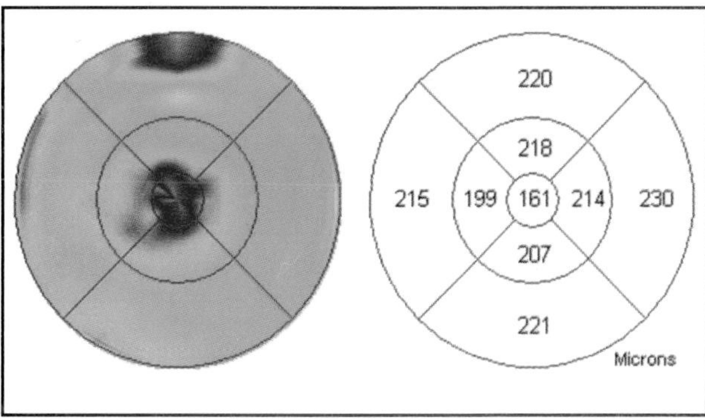

D

Case 4-14B. Bilateral Idiopathic Juxtafoveal Retinal Telangiectasis

Clinical Summary

The vision in her left eye was 20/60. Slit-lamp biomicroscopy again revealed mild retinal thickening, grayish discoloration, right-angle venules, and pigment metaplasia in the temporal fovea (E). Fluorescein angiography (F) showed staining and mild intraretinal leakage in the temporal portion of the macula.

Optical Coherence Tomography

A horizontal OCT (G) depicted a highly reflective area temporal to the fovea consistent with pigment metaplasia, which blocked the reflections of the tissues below. There was also retinal atrophic changes mainly centrally and temporal to the fovea (left side of the scan). The central retinal thickness measured 195 μm (H).

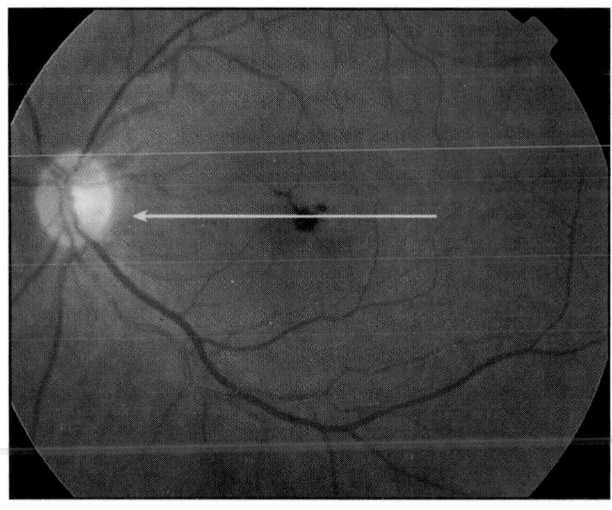

E

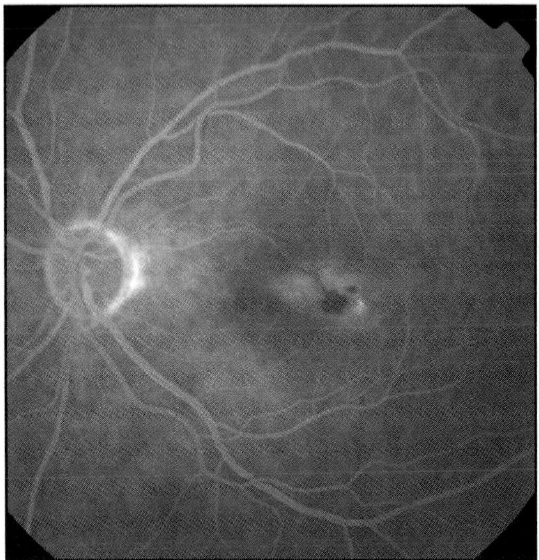

F—Early

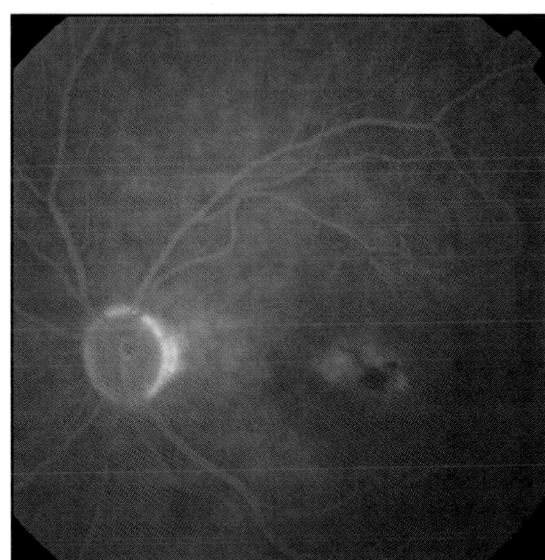

F—Late

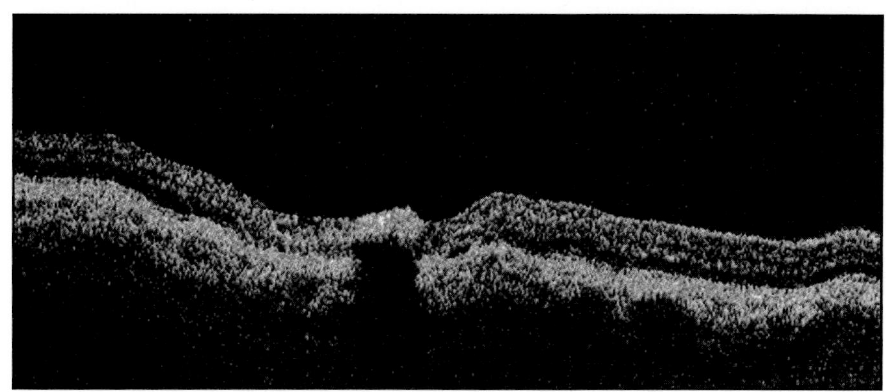

G

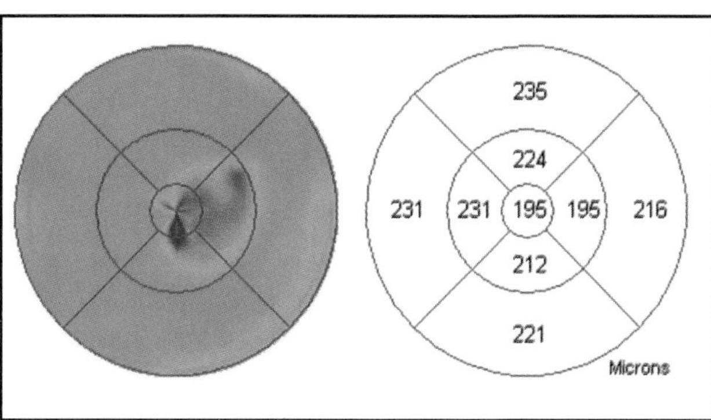

H

Case 4-15A. Bilateral Idiopathic Juxtafoveal Retinal Telangiectasis

Clinical Summary

A 64-year-old man reported central distortion in his right eye over the past year. His visual acuity in this eye was 20/50. On examination, there was evidence of a grayish discoloration and retinal thickening in the temporal portion of the fovea (A). Fluorescein angiography (B) showed telangiectatic vessels and late leakage of dye.

Optical Coherence Tomography

A vertical OCT scan (C) obtained through fixation revealed a small central area of low intraretinal reflectivity in a slit configuration consistent with fluid accumulation. No other pockets or spaces of low reflectivity were identified. In spite of that area of fluid accumulation, the central retinal thickness measured 193 μm (D).

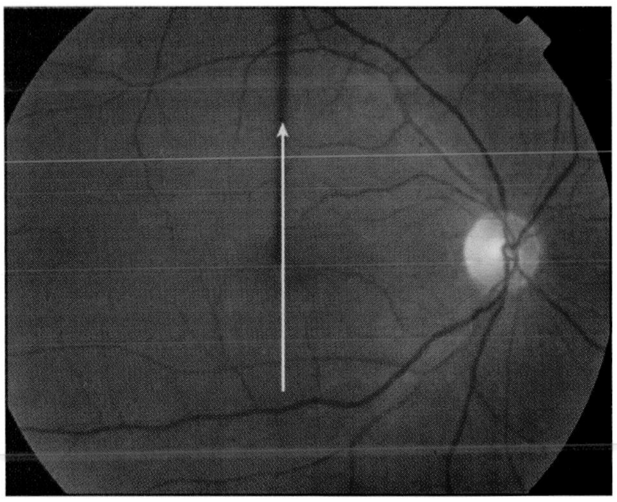

A

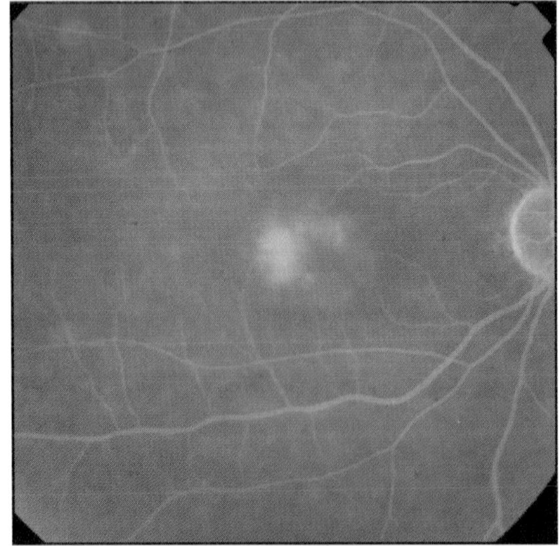

B—Early

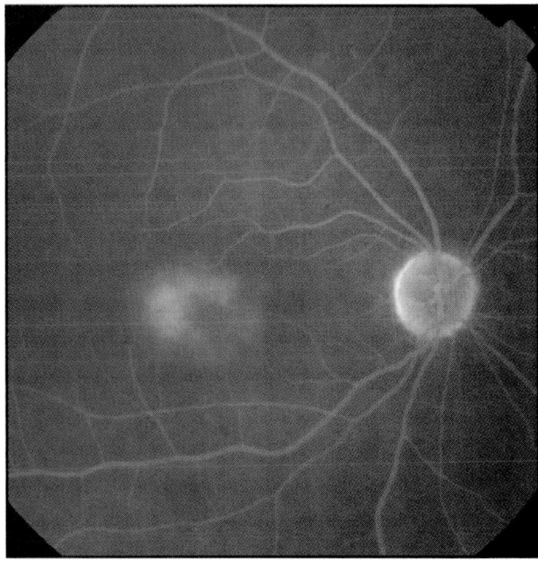

B—Late

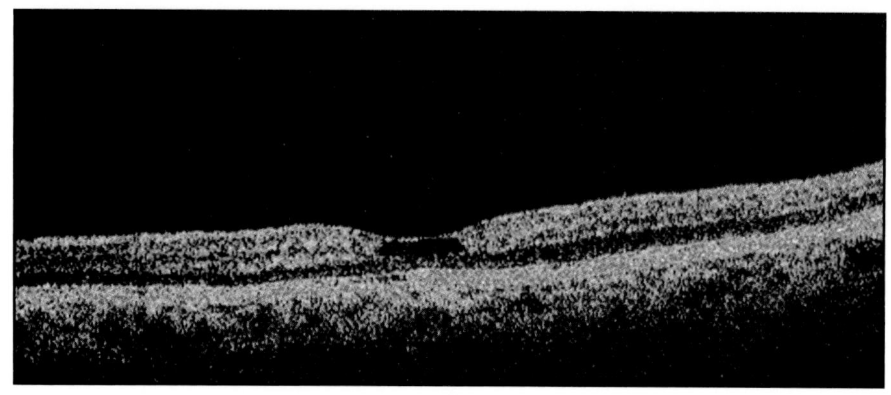

C

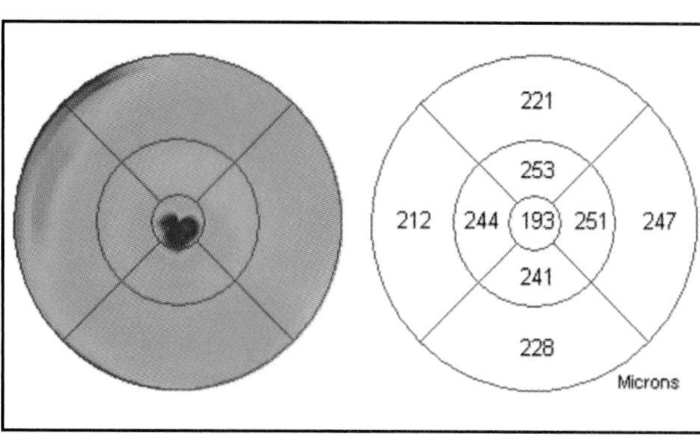

D

Case 4-15B. Bilateral Idiopathic Juxtafoveal Retinal Telangiectasis

Clinical Summary

Examination of the patient's left eye revealed subretinal fibrosis, right-angle venules, intraretinal pigment migration, and lipid exudates temporal to the fovea (E). The visual acuity in this eye measured 20/200. Fluorescein angiography (F) showed staining.

Optical Coherence Tomography

OCT (G) revealed a region of increased optical reflectivity in the macular area at the level of RPE/choriocapillaris complex consistent with subretinal fibrosis. The central retinal thickness measured 195 μm (H).

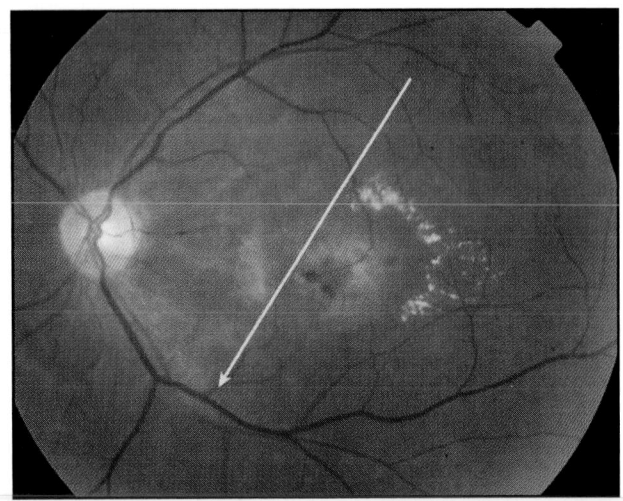

E

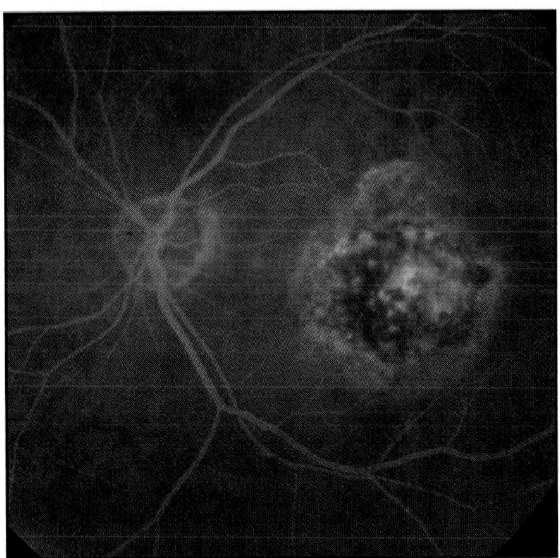

F—Early

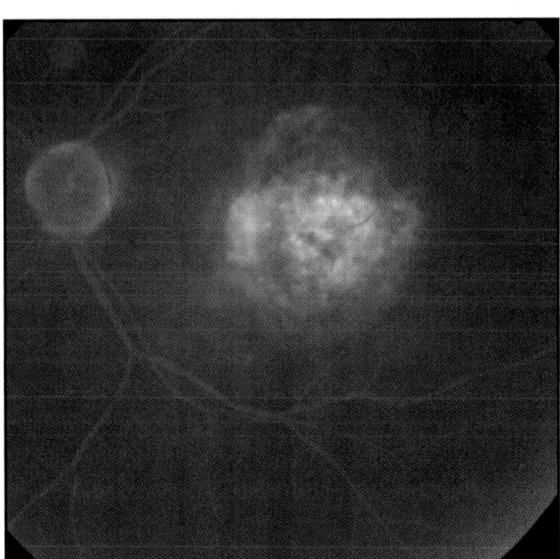

F—Late

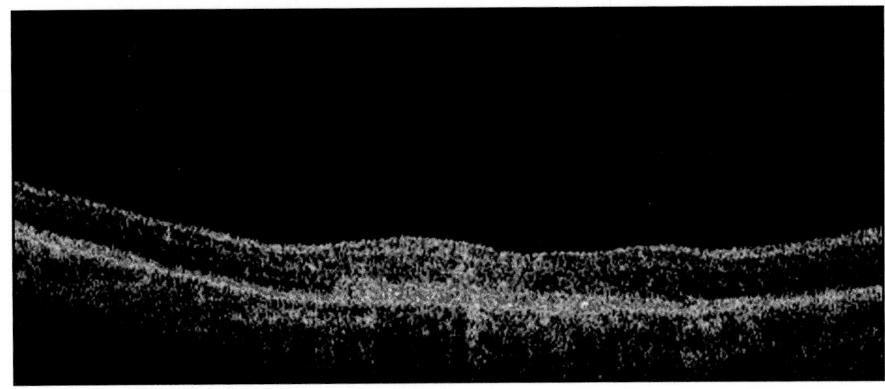

G

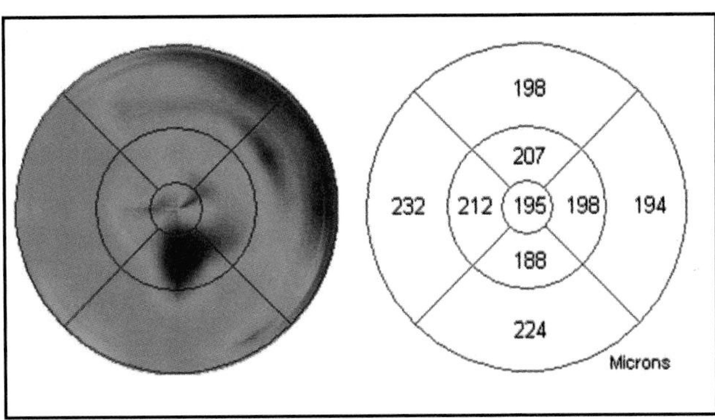

H

Case 4-16. Retinal Arterial Macroaneurysm

Clinical Summary

A 72-year-old man had a 3-day history of vision loss in his left eye. His vision measured 1/200 in this eye. On examination, intraretinal and subretinal hemorrhages were evident in the macular region extending toward the inferior arcade. An arterial macroaneurysm was visualized along the course of an arteriole inferotemporally (A). Fluorescein angiography (B) showed early filling of the macroaneurysm with late staining. Blocked fluorescence of the choroidal vasculature from the intraretinal and subretinal blood was appreciated.

Optical Coherence Tomography

An OCT scan (C) obtained through fixation showed marked elevation of the macula with cystic spaces of low reflectivity at the level of the outer plexiform layer corresponding to fluid accumulation. High backscattering was appreciated in the subretinal space as well as intraretinally, which shadowed the optical reflections from the choriocapillaris and choroid layers underneath. A horizontal OCT scan (D) depicted that much of the hemorrhagic component lay in the sub-RPE space. Six weeks later, vision measured 8/200. On examination, dehemoglobinized blood was still present (E). An OCT scan (F) obtained at that time revealed resolution of the intraretinal fluid accumulation. The blood looked more organized in the sub-RPE space. The macroaneurysm was visualized in one of the images (G) as a round focal area of enhanced reflectivity that blocked the optical signals from the tissues below.

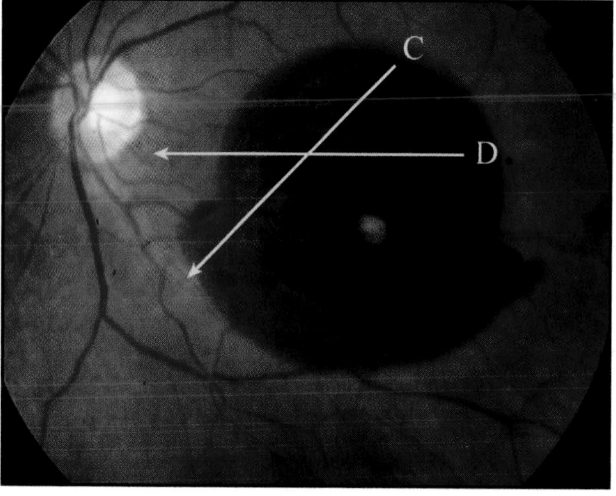

A

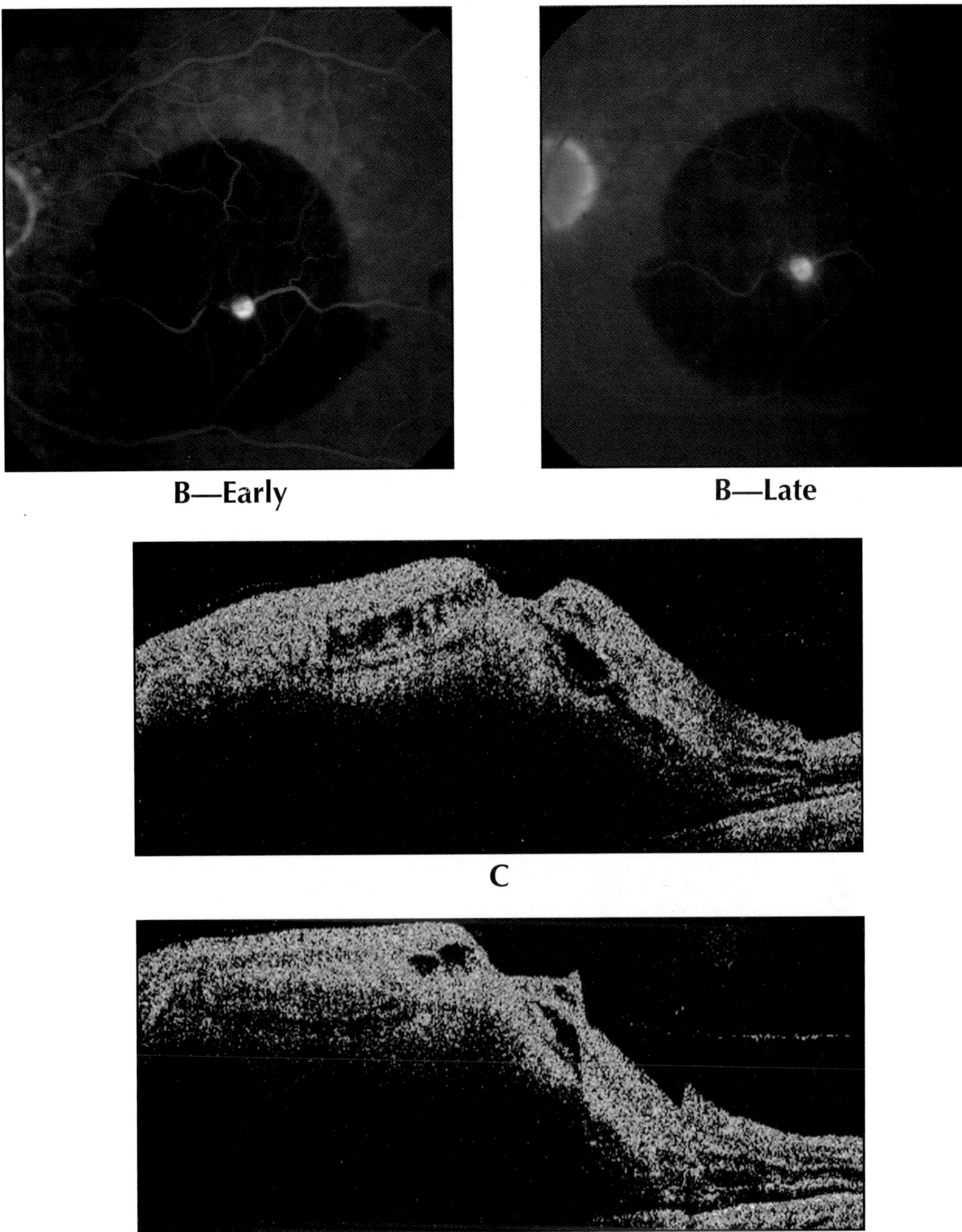

B—Early

B—Late

C

D

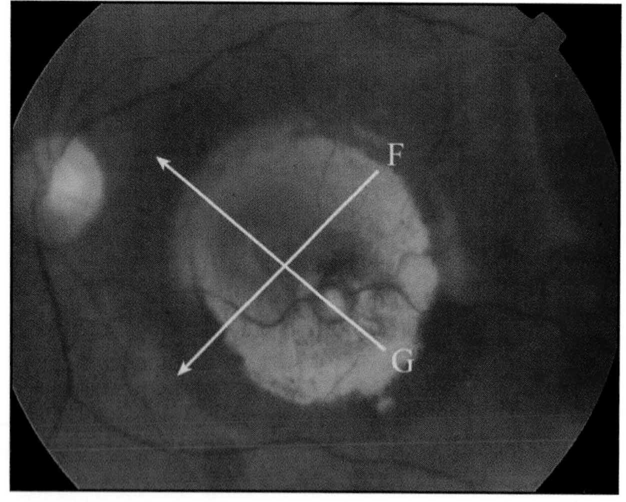

E

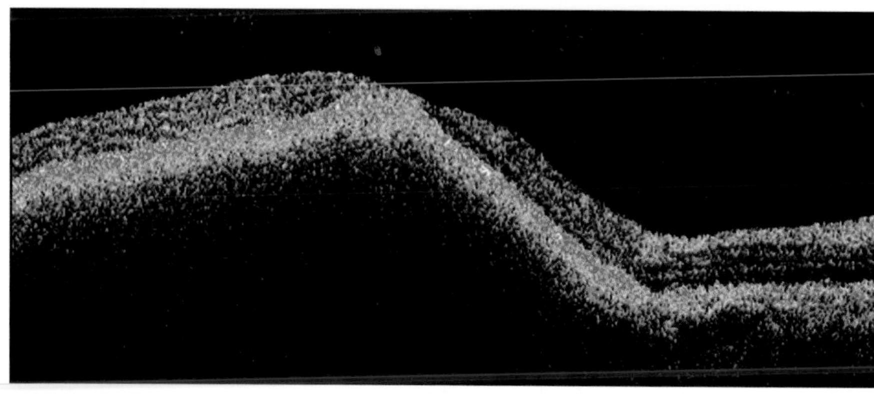

F

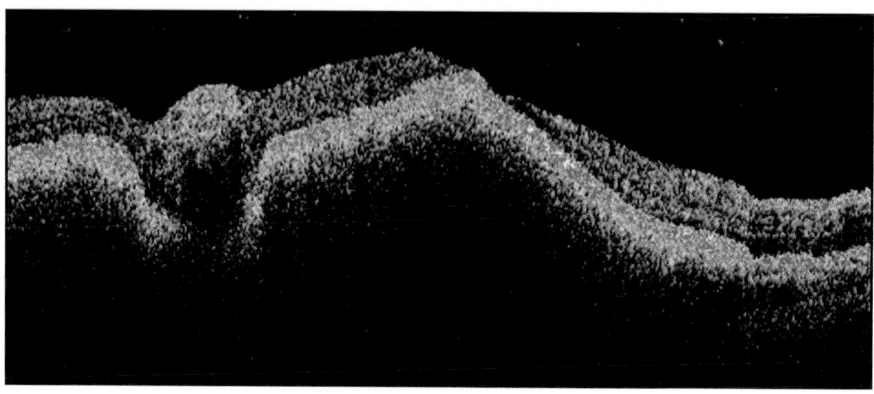

G

Case 4-17.
Retinal Arterial Macroaneurysm

Clinical Summary

A 69-year-old woman experienced vision loss in her left eye. On examination, the visual acuity was 20/400 in this eye. Dilated fundus examination showed an arterial macroaneurysm along the course of a superotemporal arteriole associated with subretinal and preretinal hemorrhage involving the foveal center (A). Fluorescein angiography (B) showed early filling of the macroaneurysm with late staining. The subretinal hemorrhage blocked the choroidal vasculature fluorescence and the preretinal blood blocked the retinal vessels.

Optical Coherence Tomography

An OCT scan (C) was obtained through the preretinal hemorrhage. It showed a dome-shaped, elevated, highly reflective space beneath the internal limiting membrane (ILM), which was visualized as a reflective band (left side of the scan). The presence of the preretinal blood blocked the optical reflections from the retina below. Scan D was obtained through both preretinal and subretinal blood. In the center of the scan, a brightly reflective area was seen beneath the posterior hyaloid (reflective band), which shadowed the reflections from the retina underneath corresponding to the preretinal hemorrhage. The preretinal blood merged imperceptibly with the neurosensory retina (right side of the scan). Another region of high backscattering was noticeable below the neurosensory retina consistent with the subretinal blood (right side of the scan). It blocked the reflections from the RPE and choroid below. Scan E confirmed the presence of the preretinal and subretinal components of the hemorrhage. A small, highly reflective area was appreciated in the central top region of the scan representing the scant amount of preretinal blood adjacent to the ruptured macroaneurysm. This blood was present beneath the ILM, which was characterized by a highly reflective band. A slightly less reflective band was seen anterior to the ILM consistent with the posterior hyaloid face. Subretinal blood was visualized beneath the retinal tissue. Optical reflections from the tissues underneath were shadowed.

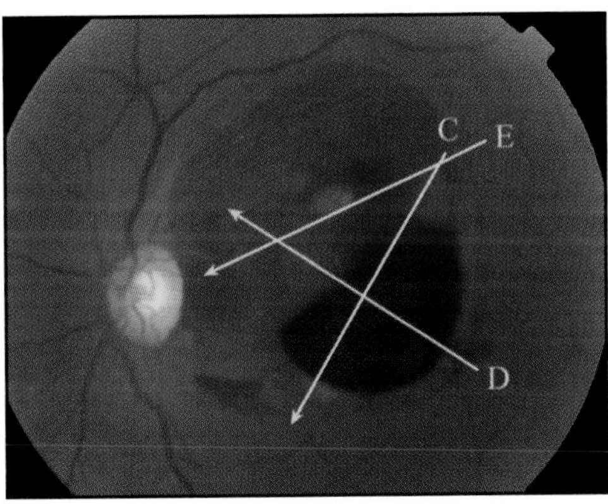

A

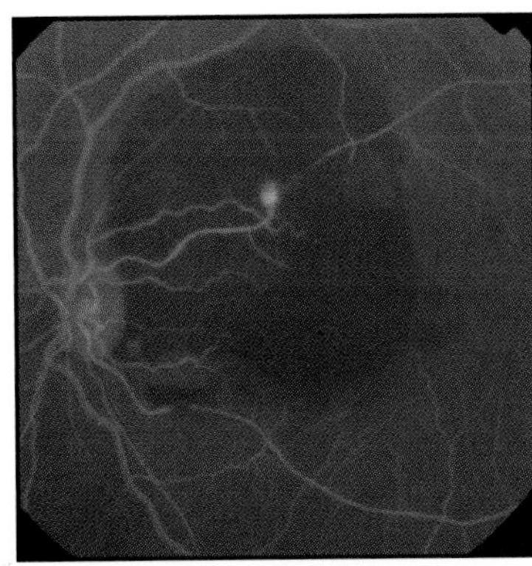

B—Early

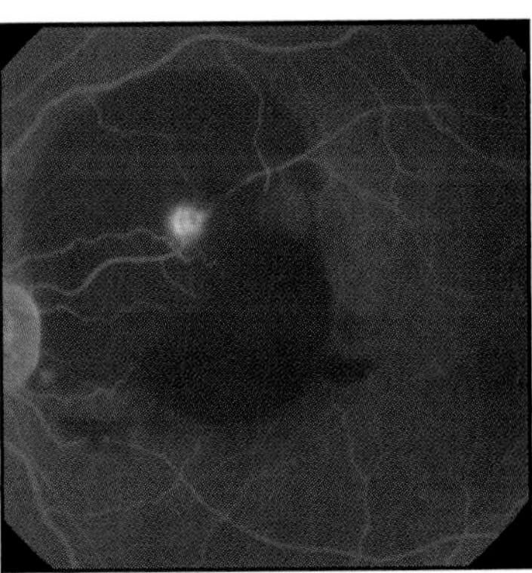

B—Late

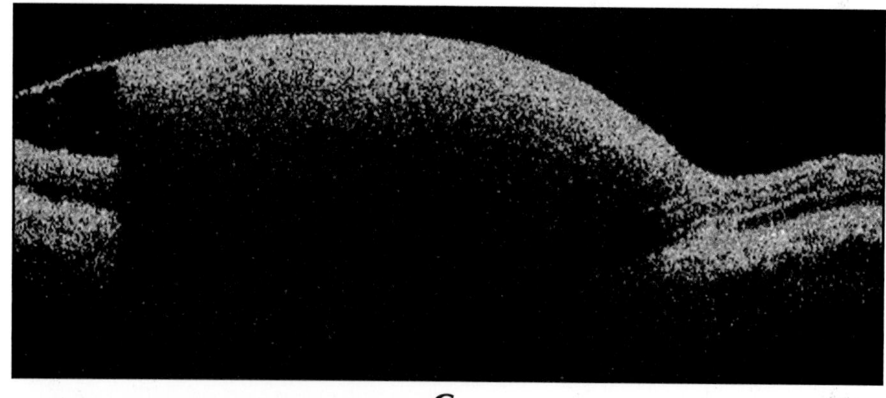

C

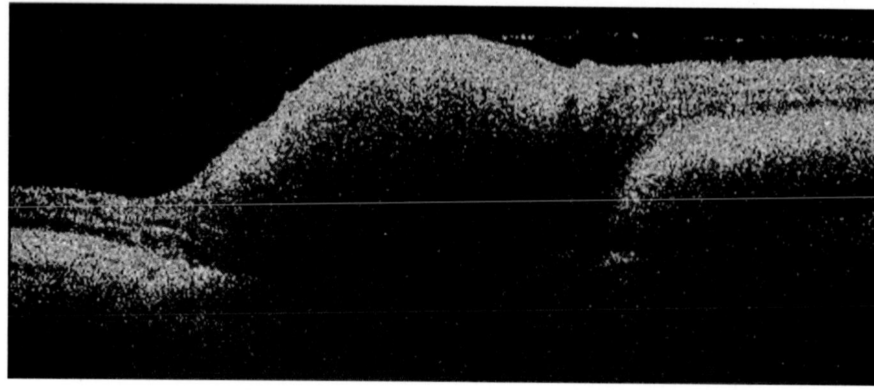

D

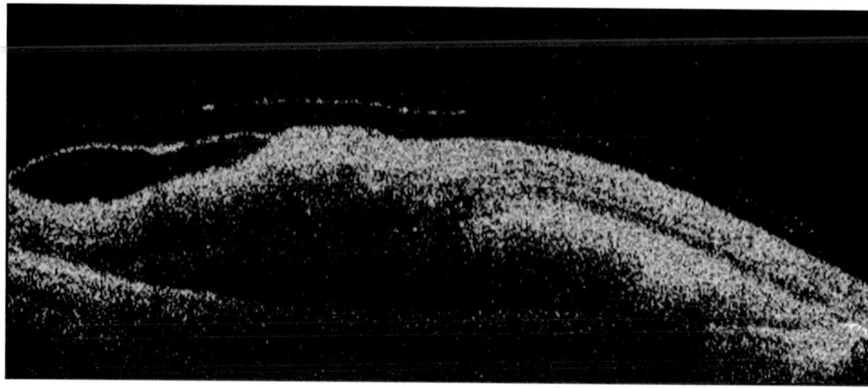

E

Case 4-18. Retinal Arterial Macroaneurysm

Clinical Summary

A 78-year-old woman presented with a 2-month history of decreased vision in her right eye. On examination, the visual acuity was 20/100 in this eye. Slit-lamp biomicroscopy revealed macular thickening with hard lipid exudates. An arterial macroaneurysm was seen along the course of the inferotemporal artery associated with intraretinal hemorrhages and retinal thickening (A). Fluorescein angiography (B) showed blocked fluorescence corresponding to the presence of intraretinal blood and late staining of the macroaneurysm with faint perifoveal leakage.

Optical Coherence Tomography

OCT (C) confirmed the increase in the retinal thickness. Loss of the normal foveal contour was observed in addition to a diffuse region of low reflectivity in the outer plexiform layer consistent with edema. Hard lipid exudates were characterized by tiny, round, brightly reflective structures. The retinal thickness measured 485 μm centrally (D).

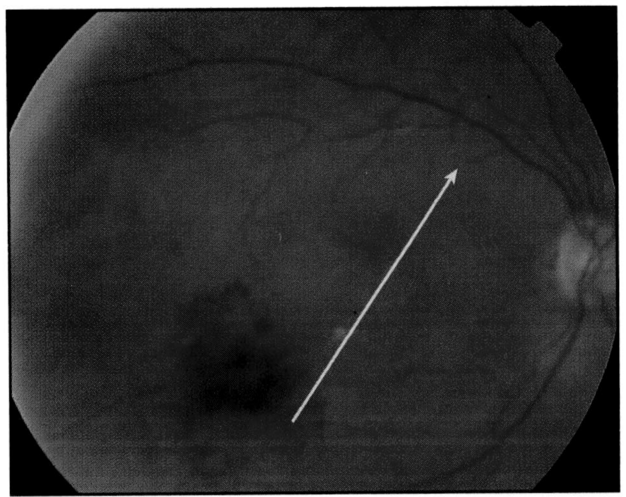

A

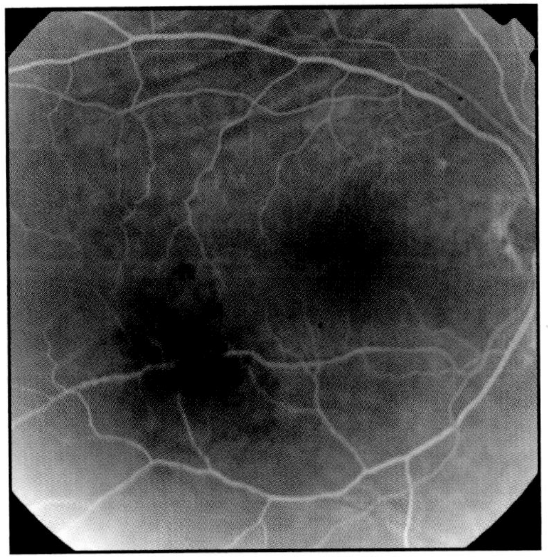

B—Early

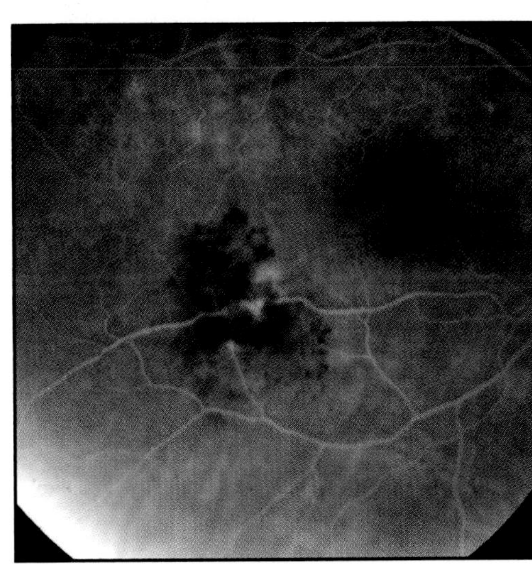

B—Late

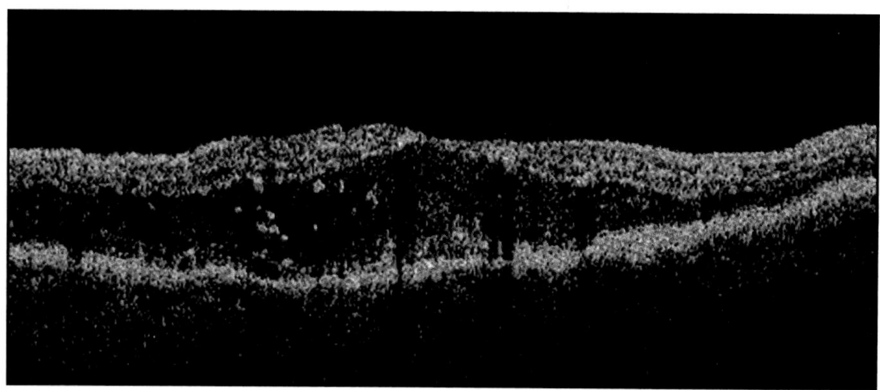

C

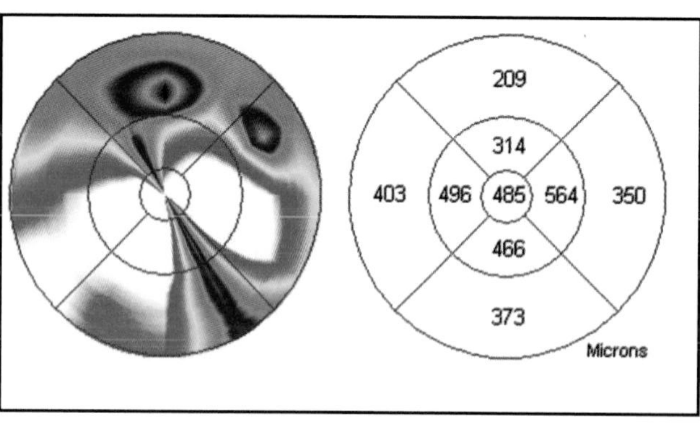

D

Chapter 5

Diabetic Retinopathy

Vanessa Cruz-Villegas, MD and Harry W. Flynn Jr, MD

- Nonproliferative Diabetic Retinopathy
- Diabetic Macular Edema
- Proliferative Diabetic Retinopathy

Diabetic retinopathy is the leading cause of new blindness in individuals under 65 years of age in the United States. Diabetic retinopathy can be classified into nonproliferative diabetic retinopathy (NPDR) and proliferative diabetic retinopathy (PDR). The clinical features of NPDR include microaneurysms, intraretinal hemorrhages, hard exudates, nerve fiber layer infarcts or cotton wool exudates, and intraretinal microvascular abnormalities (IRMA). The clinical picture of PDR includes the features from NPDR in addition to proliferating new vessels on the optic nerve head, retina, or iris.

Diabetic macular edema is a principal cause of visual loss in diabetic patients.[1,2] It can occur at any stage of diabetic retinopathy. The role of optical coherence tomography (OCT) in the assessment and management of diabetic retinopathy has become significant in understanding the vitreoretinal relationships and the internal architecture of the retina. The macular thickness can be accurately measured due to the characteristic and well-defined optical reflectivity of the anterior and posterior margins or boundaries of the neurosensory retina.[3] Studies have shown that OCT may be more sensitive in evaluating diabetic macular edema than slit-lamp examination.[3,4] In addition, central macular thickness correlates with visual acuity even better than fluorescein leakage.[3,5] OCT also allows quantification of macular thickness in a reproducible manner.[6,7] With this capability, the acquisition of reliable documentation of the progression of retinal thickness is possible. The response of macular edema to focal grid laser treatment as well as new treatments, such as intravitreal triamcinolone acetonide injections or intravitreal steroid devices, can be documented accurately by OCT imaging.[8-10]

OCT images of macular edema depict the presence of low intraretinal reflectivity, which corresponds to intraretinal fluid accumulation. This reduced reflectivity or backscattering tends to be more apparent in the outer retinal layers. Cystic spaces of decreased intraretinal reflectivity are evident on OCT, consistent with a cystoid macular edema (CME) configuration shown by fluorescein angiography. In addition to increased retinal thickness and CME, diabetic eyes can show neurosensory retinal detachments with subretinal fluid accumulation.[11] Other morphological features of diabetic retinopathy that can be appreciated by OCT are intraretinal hard lipid exudates and intraretinal hemorrhages. Hard exudates are represented as highly reflective intraretinal areas. Shadowing of the optical reflection from the retinal tissue and choroid beneath the exudate is sometimes observed. Hemorrhages also appear as areas of high backscattering with shadowing of the reflection of deeper tissue layers.

OCT also helps to distinguish those patients with diabetic macular edema, which has a component of vitreous traction or retinoschisis. Vitreoretinal adhesions are detected more precisely by OCT than with slit-lamp examination.[12] A taut posterior hyaloid or vitreoretinal adhesion is seen as a reflective membrane with persistent focal attachment to the fovea. Moreover, a shallow traction macular detachment or retinoschisis may be present but only visualized by OCT.[13] Studies have shown a benefit from pars plana vitrectomy in those patients with diabetic macular edema and vitreomacular traction.[14-17] Diabetic patients with macular retinoschisis generally have a poor visual prognosis. Thus, OCT is effective in determining the necessity of, as well as the response to, surgical management.[17-19]

PDR could be visualized in OCT as highly reflective preretinal bands anterior to the retinal surface consistent with preretinal fibrovascular or fibroglial proliferation. Diffuse retinal thickening, distortion, and irregularity of the retinal contour can also occur as a result of the contraction of these preretinal membranes. An associated retinal traction detachment may be observed. OCT is valuable in determining the extent of the tractional component as well as the presence of foveal involvement. Again, OCT assists in the decision-making process of surgical intervention.

References

1. Moss SE, Klein R, Klein BE. Ten-year incidence of visual loss in a diabetic population. *Ophthalmology*. 1994;101(6):1061-1070.
2. Moss SE, Klein R, Klein BE. The 14-year incidence of visual loss in a diabetic population. *Ophthalmology*. 1998;105(6):998-1003.
3. Hee MR, Puliafito CA, Wong C, et al. Quantitative assessment of macular edema with optical coherence tomography. *Arch Ophthalmol*. 1995;113(8):1019-1029.
4. Yang CS, Cheng CY, Lee FL, Hsu WM, Liu JH. Quantitative assessment of retinal thickness in diabetic patients with and without clinically significant macular edema using optical coherence tomography. *Acta Ophthalmol Scand*. 2001;79(3):266-270.
5. Hee MR, Puliafito CA, Duker JS, et al. Topography of diabetic macular edema with optical coherence tomography. *Ophthalmology*. 1998;105(2):360-370.
6. Massin P, Vicaut E, Haouchine B, Erginay A, Paques M, Gaudric A. Reproducibility of retinal mapping using optical coherence tomography. *Arch Ophthalmol*. 2001;119(8):1135-1142.
7. Goebel W, Kretzchmar-Gross T. Retinal thickness in diabetic retinopathy: a study using optical coherence tomography (OCT). *Retina*. 2002;22(6):759-767.
8. Rivellese M, George A, Sulkes D, Reichel E, Puliafito CA. Optical coherence tomography after laser photocoagulation for clinically significant macular edema. *Ophthalmic Surg Lasers*. 2000;31(3):192-197.
9. Lattanzio R, Brancato R, Pierro L, et al. Macular thickness measured by optical coherence tomography (OCT) in diabetic patients. *Eur J Ophthalmol*. 2002;12(6):482-487.
10. Martidis A, Duker JS, Greenberg PB, et al. Intravitreal triamcinolone for refractory diabetic macular edema. *Ophthalmology*. 2002;109(5):920-926.
11. Otani T, Kishi S, Maruyama Y. Patterns of diabetic macular edema with optical coherence tomography. *Am J Ophthalmol*. 1999;127(6):688-693.
12. Gallemore RP, Jumper JM, McCuen BW II, Jaffe GJ, Postel EA, Toth CA. Diagnosis of vitreoretinal adhesions in macular disease with optical coherence tomography. *Retina*. 2000;20(2):115-120.
13. Kaiser PK, Rieman CD, Sears JE, Lewis H. Macular traction detachment and diabetic macular edema associated with posterior hyaloidal traction. *Am J Ophthalmol*. 2001;131(1):44-49.
14. Lewis H, Abrams GW, Blumenkranz MS, Campo RV. Vitrectomy for diabetic macular traction and edema associated with posterior hyaloidal traction. *Ophthalmology*. 1992;99(5):753-759.
15. Harbour JW, Smiddy WE, Flynn HW Jr, Rubsamen PE. Vitrectomy for diabetic macular edema associated with a thickened and taut posterior hyaloid membrane. *Am J Ophthalmol*. 1996;121(4):405-413.
16. Pendergast SD, Hassan TS, Williams GA, et al. Vitrectomy for diffuse macular edema associated with a taut premacular posterior hyaloid. *Am J Ophthalmol*. 2000;130(2):178-186.
17. Massin P, Duguid G, Erginay A, Haouchine B, Gaudric A. Optical coherence tomography for evaluating diabetic macular edema before and after vitrectomy. *Am J Ophthalmol*. 2003;135(2):169-177.
18. Otani T, Kishi S. Tomographic assessment of vitreous surgery for diabetic macular edema. *Am J Ophthalmol*. 2000;129(4):487-494.
19. Giovannini A, Amato G, Mariotti C, Scassellati-Sforzolini B. Optical coherence tomography findings in diabetic macular edema before and after vitrectomy. *Ophthalmic Surg Lasers*. 2000;31(3):187-191.

Case 5-1. Nonproliferative Diabetic Retinopathy and Diabetic Macular Edema

Clinical Summary

A 70-year-old man with history of NPDR complained of decreased vision in his left eye. His visual acuity in this eye was 20/80. Retinal examination showed dot and blot hemorrhages throughout the posterior pole in addition to retinal thickening. A hard lipid exudate was appreciated in the foveal center (A).

Optical Coherence Tomography

OCT (B) depicted diffuse thickening with blunting of the normal foveal contour. A spot of high reflectivity was noted in the foveal center representing the aforementioned foveal hard exudate. Shadowing of the optical reflection from the retina and choroid was observed below the exudate. The retinal map analysis showed a foveal thickness of 336 microns (μm) in this eye (C).

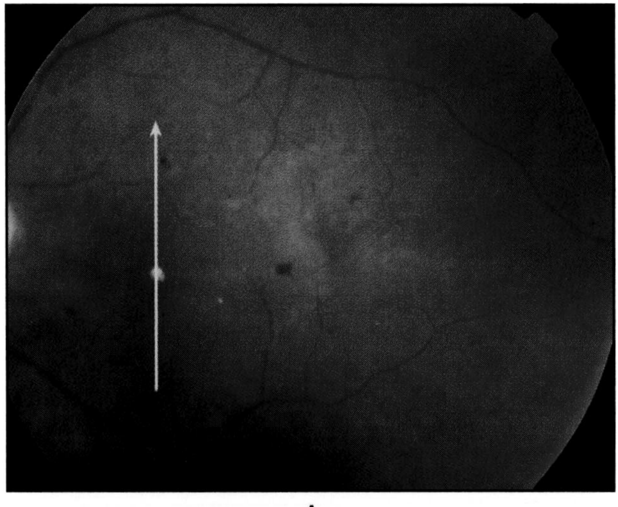

A

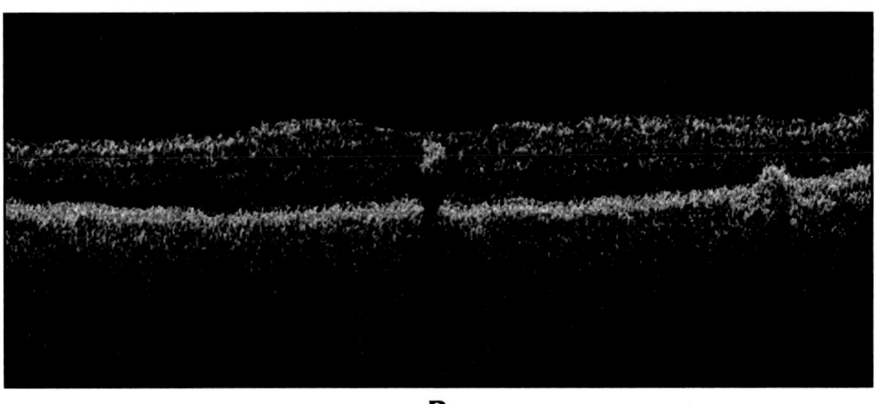

B

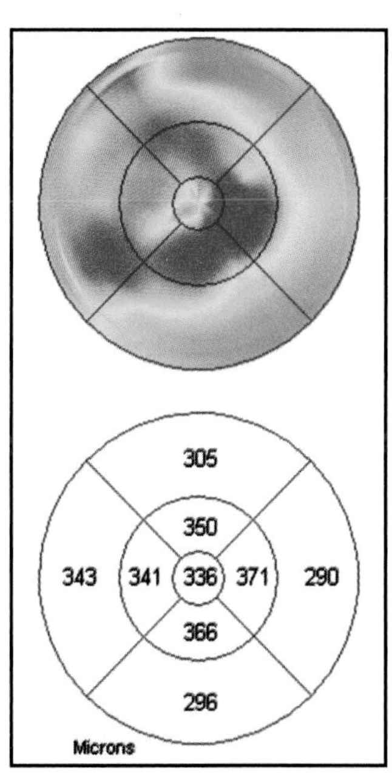

C

Case 5-2. Nonproliferative Diabetic Retinopathy and Diabetic Macular Edema

Clinical Summary

A 71-year-old man with NPDR received focal/grid laser photocoagulation in his left eye 3 months earlier for clinically significant macular edema. On examination, intraretinal hemorrhages, hard exudates, as well as retinal thickening were appreciated (A). His visual acuity in this eye was 20/60. Fluorescein angiography (B) revealed the presence of retinal pigment epithelium (RPE) window defects consistent with previous laser scars, perifoveal dots of hyperfluorescence consistent with microaneurysms, and late leakage consistent with macular edema.

Optical Coherence Tomography

A horizontal OCT scan (C) obtained through the fovea revealed loss of the normal foveal contour, diffuse macular thickening, and large areas of low intraretinal reflectivity consistent with intraretinal cysts and fluid accumulation. Also, a detachment of the neurosensory retina with subretinal fluid accumulation was detected in the fovea. The retinal map analysis revealed a foveal thickness of 592 µm (D). The patient underwent an intravitreal injection of triamcinolone acetonide (4 mg/0.1 cc) in this eye. One month after the injection, a follow-up OCT scan showed that the foveal thickness had decreased to 289 µm. The cystic spaces resolved and the subretinal fluid accumulation flattened (E and F). His visual acuity improved to 20/40. A follow-up OCT (G) was obtained 4 months after the injection and showed a normal foveal contour. Complete resolution of the intraretinal and subretinal fluid was observed. His visual acuity improved to 20/25 and the foveal thickness decreased to 192 µm (H).

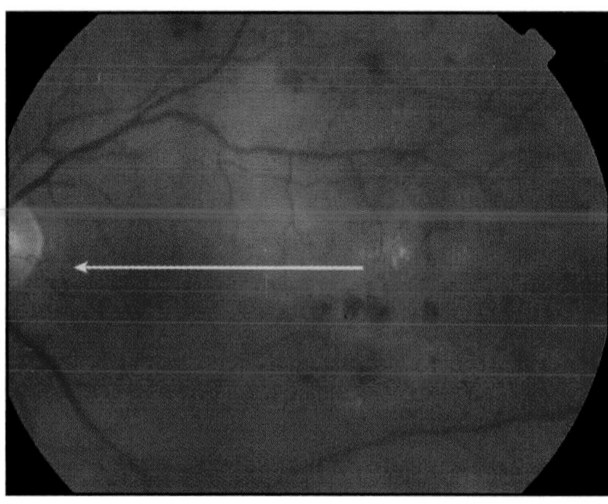

A

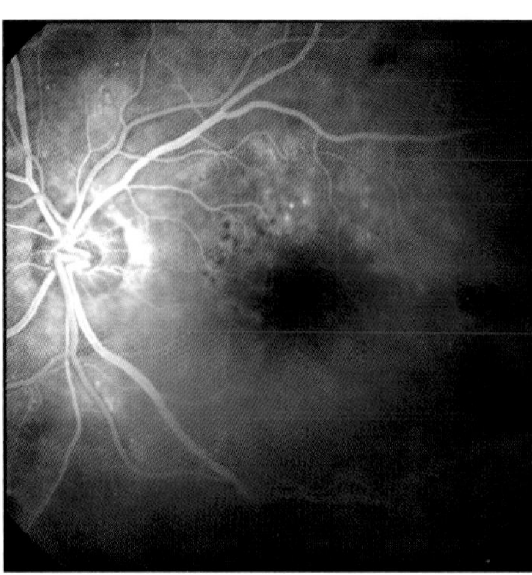

B—Early

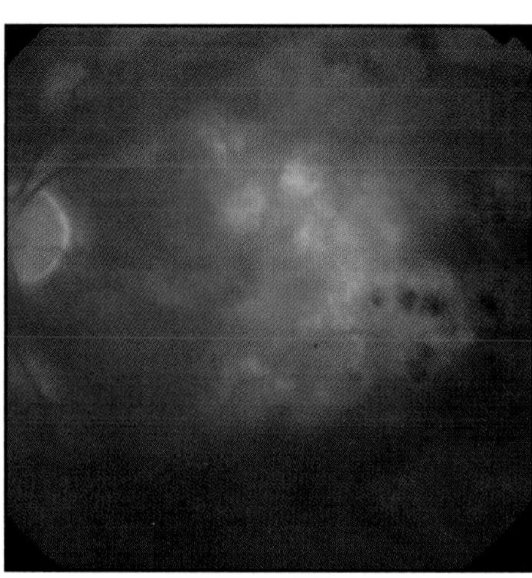

B—Late

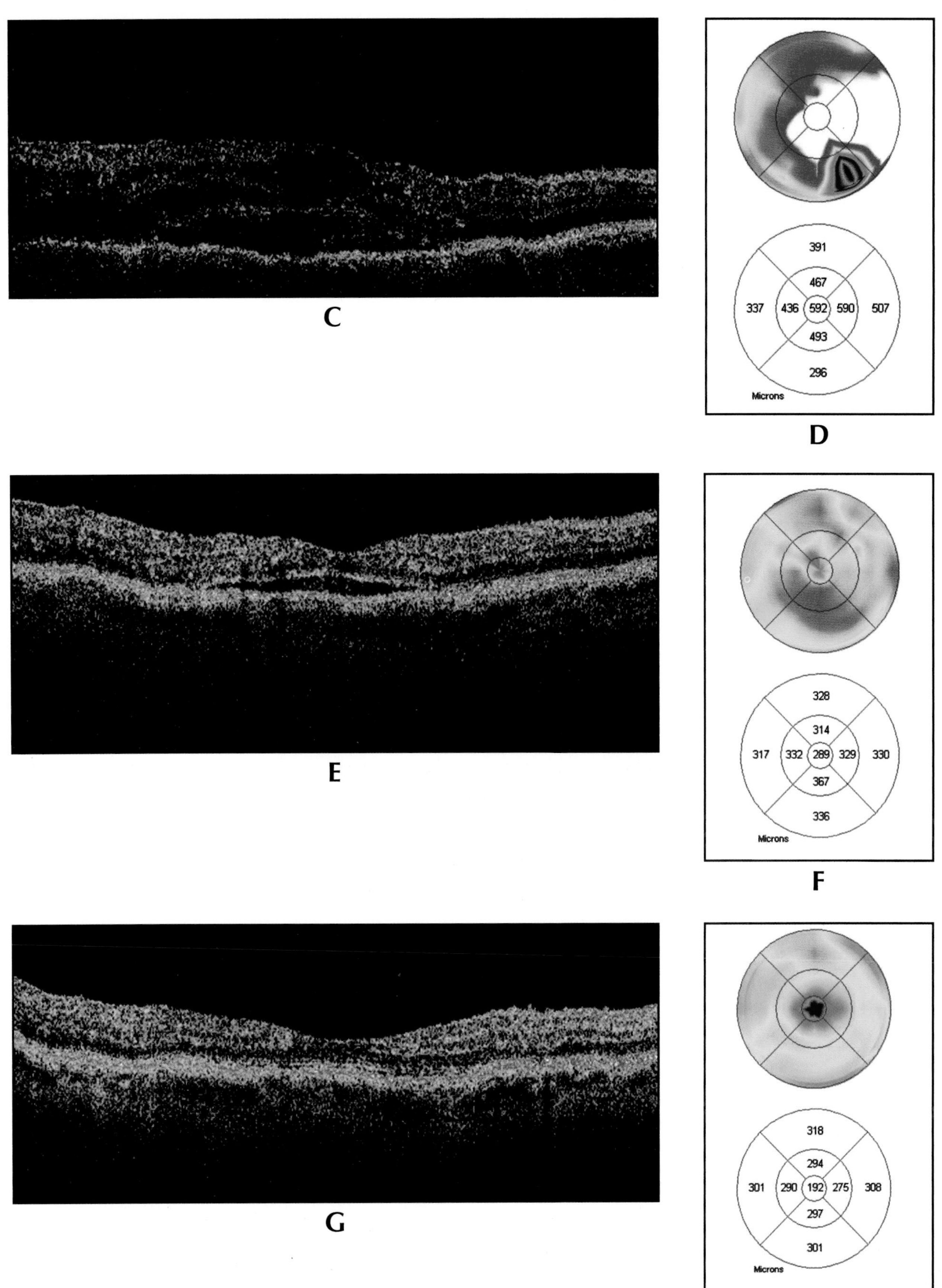
391
467
337 436 592 590 507
493
296
Microns
328
314
317 332 289 329 330
367
336
Microns
318
294
301 290 192 275 308
297
301
Microns

C

D

E

F

G

H

Case 5-3A. Nonproliferative Diabetic Retinopathy and Diabetic Macular Edema

Clinical Summary

A 57-year-old man with a diagnosis of NPDR and macular edema was examined. On examination, the visual acuity of the right eye was 20/50. Dilated fundus examination of this eye showed scattered dot and blot hemorrhages throughout the posterior pole and midperiphery. Evaluation of the macula revealed the presence of microaneurysms, hard exudates, and retinal thickening consistent with clinically significant macular edema (A). Fluorescein angiography (B) demonstrated the presence of focal areas of hyperfluorescence consistent with microaneurysms and late leakage.

Optical Coherence Tomography

OCT (C) revealed loss of the normal foveal contour, macular thickening, and low reflective spaces consistent with intraretinal cysts and fluid accumulation. The retinal map analysis revealed a foveal thickness of 386 μm (D). Focal/grid laser photocoagulation was performed. Two months after the procedure, a follow-up OCT scan showed that the foveal thickness had decreased to 337 μm and the cystic changes had flattened (E and F). Visual acuity improved to 20/30.

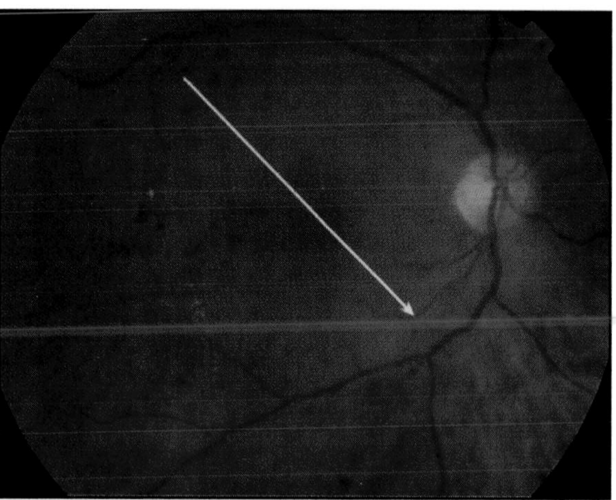

A

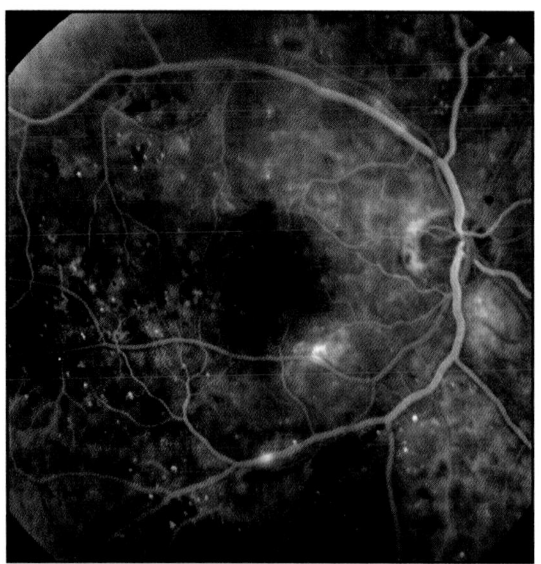

B—Early

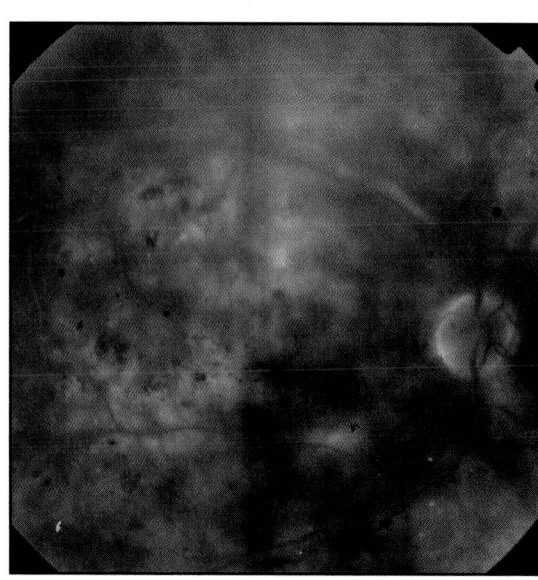

B—Late

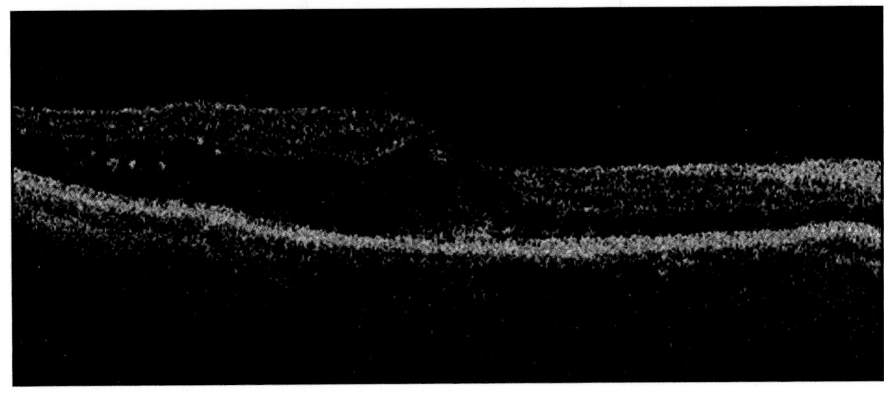

C

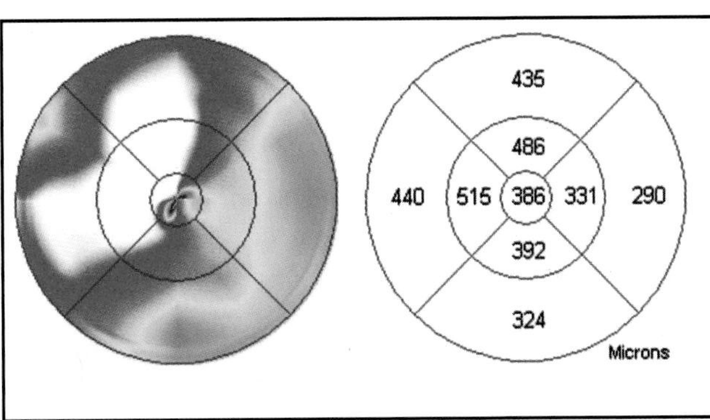
435
486
440
515
386
331
290
392
324
Microns

D

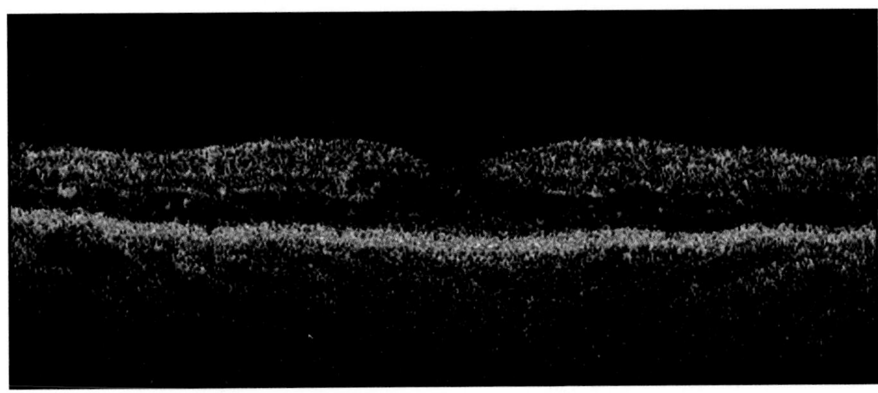

E

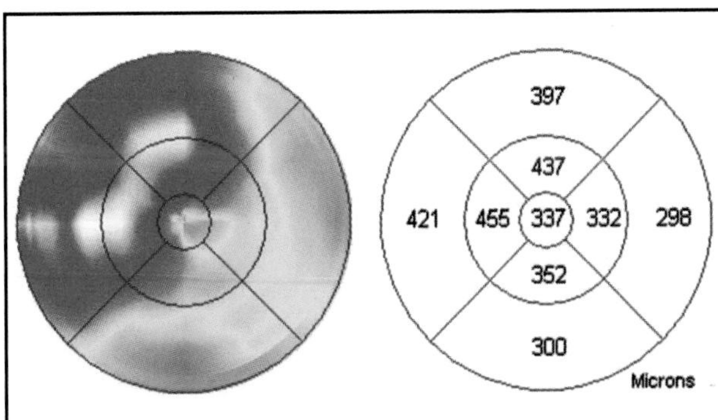
397
437
421
455
337
332
298
352
300
Microns

F

Case 5-3B. Nonproliferative Diabetic Retinopathy and Diabetic Macular Edema

Clinical Summary

Slit-lamp biomicroscopy of the patient's left eye revealed dot and blot hemorrhages, numerous microaneurysms, hard exudates, and extensive retinal thickening in the macular region consistent with clinically significant macular edema (G). The visual acuity in this eye was 20/400. Fluorescein angiography (H) showed perifoveal hyperfluorescent dots consistent with microaneurysms and late leakage.

Optical Coherence Tomography

OCT (I) revealed marked retinal thickening and extensive areas of low intraretinal reflectivity consistent with fluid accumulation and macular cysts. Highly reflective intraretinal dots (right side of the scan) representing hard lipid retinal exudates were noted. The foveal thickness measured 621 μm (J). The patient elected to receive an intravitreal injection of triamcinolone acetonide (4 mg/0.1 cc). Two months later, a follow-up OCT scan demonstrated a reduction in foveal thickening to 363 μm (K and L). The visual acuity improved to 20/200.

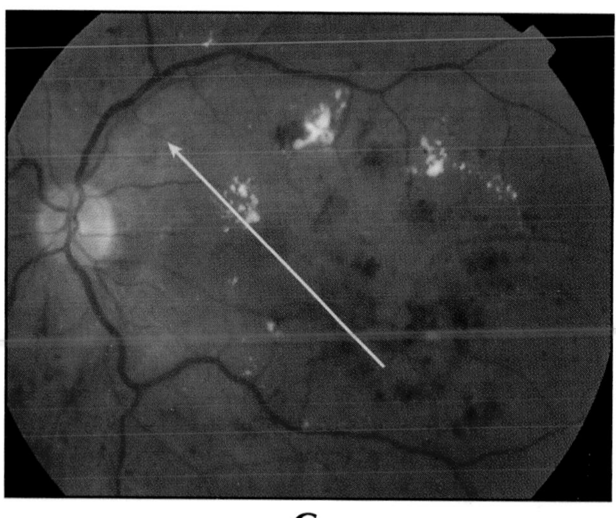

G

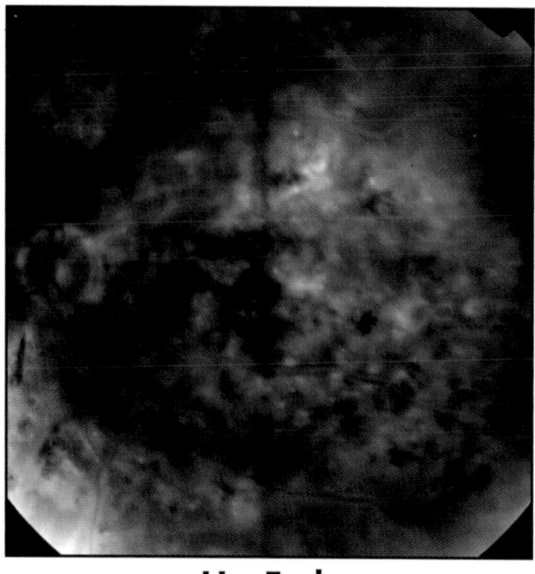

H—Early

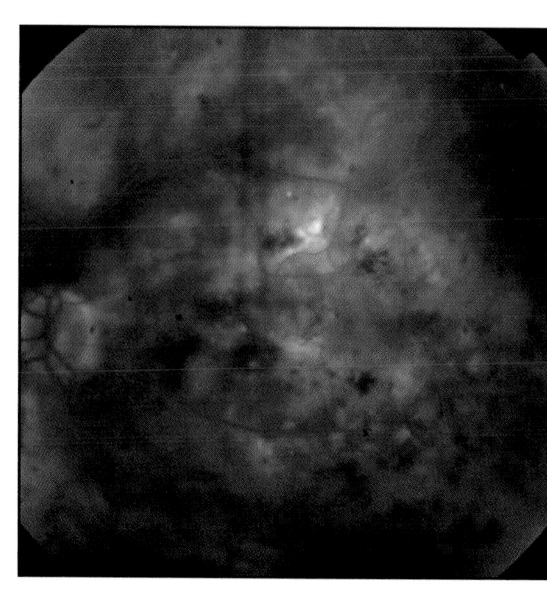

H—Late

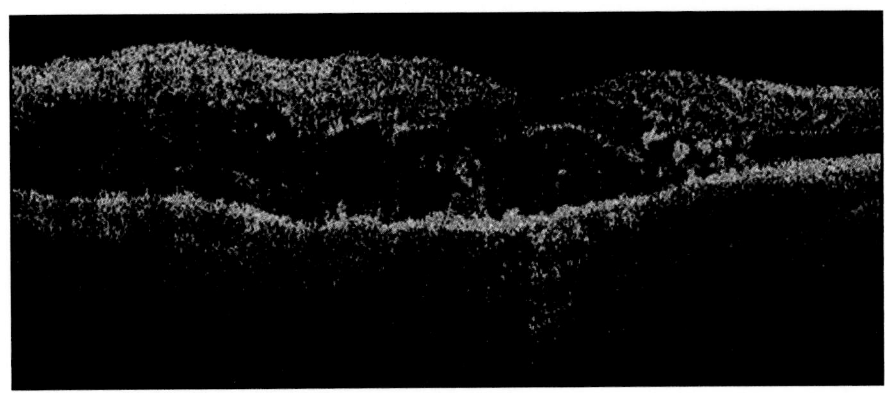

I

418
550
361 521 621 682 578
582
492
Microns

J

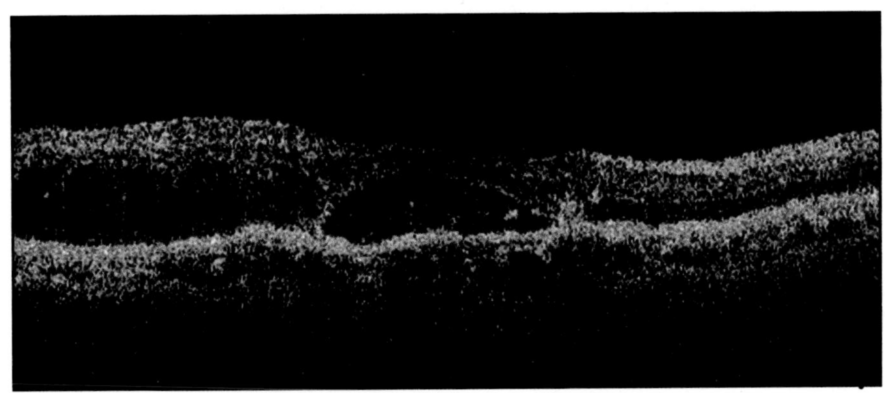

K

328
355
313 312 363 482 450
397
375
Microns

L

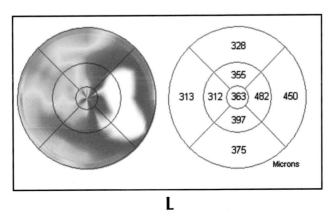

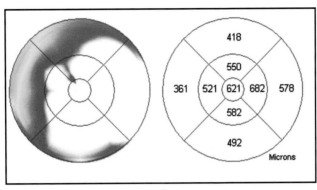

Case 5-4. Nonproliferative Diabetic Retinopathy and Diabetic Macular Edema

Clinical Summary

A 69-year-old woman with NPDR presented with a visual acuity of 20/400 in the left eye. Retinal examination of this eye showed scattered dot and blot hemorrhages, microaneurysms, and clinically significant macular edema (A). Fluorescein angiography (B) revealed focal areas of blocked fluorescence consistent with intraretinal hemorrhages, hyperfluorescent spots corresponding to microaneurysms, and late leakage.

Optical Coherence Tomography

OCT (C) revealed diffuse macular thickening and low reflective spaces consistent with intraretinal fluid accumulation. The retinal map analysis revealed a foveal thickness of 558 μm (D). Focal/grid laser photocoagulation was performed.

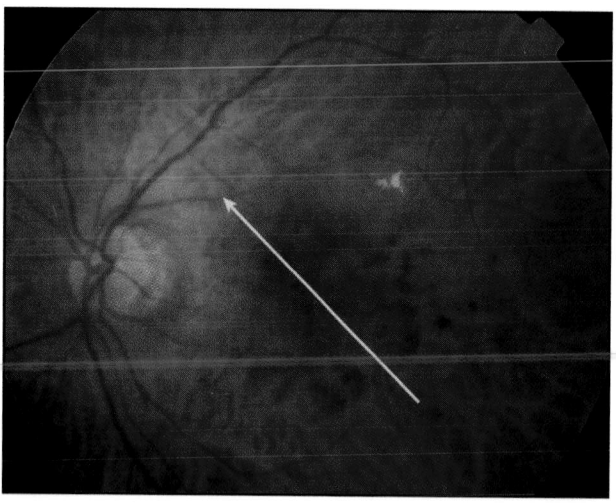

A

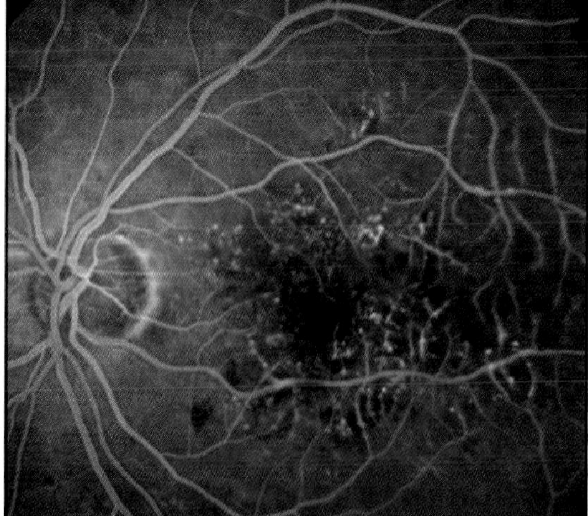

B—Early

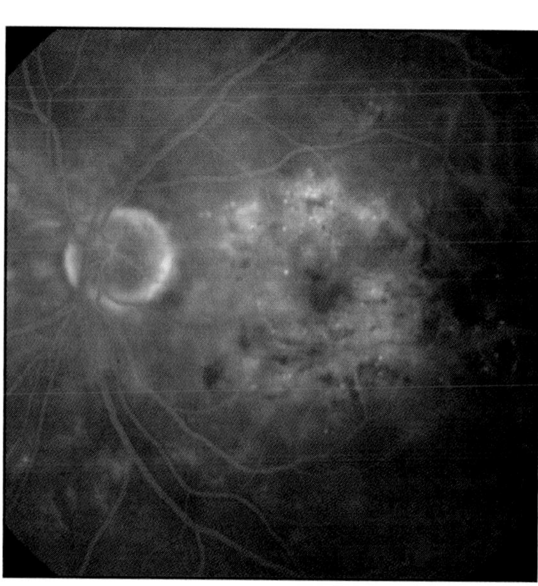

B—Late

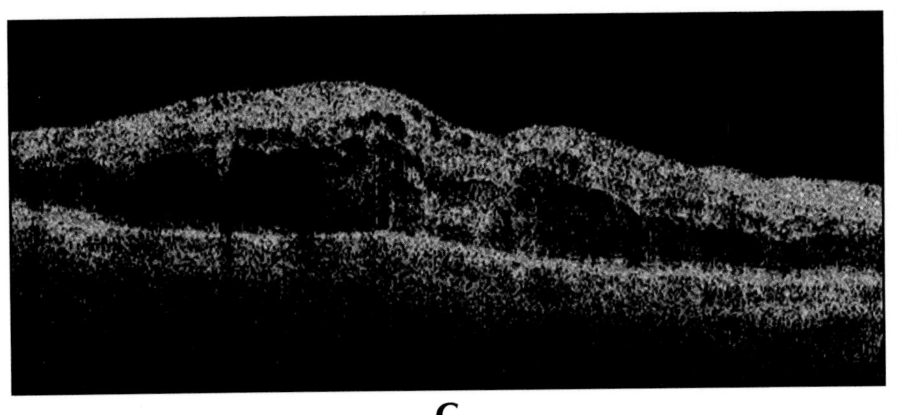

C

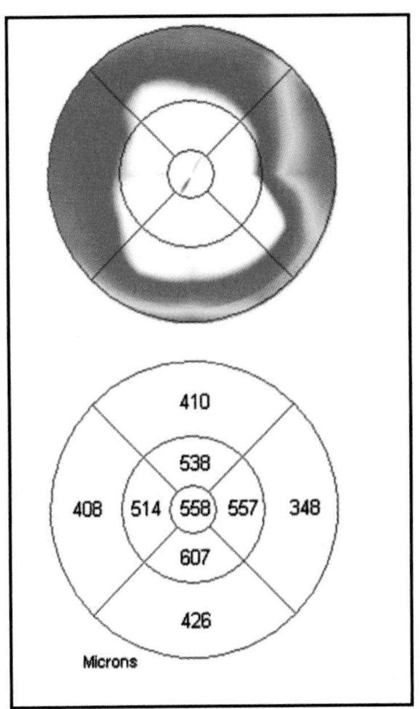

D

Case 5-5. Nonproliferative Diabetic Retinopathy and Diabetic Macular Edema

Clinical Summary

A 77-year-old woman with NPDR was examined 10 months after focal/grid laser photocoagulation for clinically significant macular edema in both eyes. Fundus examination of her left eye showed scattered dot and blot hemorrhages and numerous microaneurysms. Laser scars were noted in the macular area. In addition, hard exudates and retinal thickening were appreciated in the macular region consistent with clinically significant macular edema (A). The visual acuity in this eye was 20/100. Fluorescein angiography (B) showed laser scars, dots of perifoveal hyperfluorescence consistent with microaneurysms, and late leakage consistent with macular edema.

Optical Coherence Tomography

OCT (C) revealed loss of the normal foveal contour, retinal thickening, and a central cystic space of low intraretinal reflectivity surrounded by smaller cysts consistent with fluid accumulation. A small detachment of the neurosensory retina with subretinal fluid accumulation was detected in the fovea. Small regions of high intraretinal backscattering were evident corresponding to hard lipid exudates. The retinal map analysis revealed a foveal thickness of 457 µm (D). The patient elected to receive an intravitreal injection of triamcinolone acetonide (4 mg/0.1 cc) in this eye. Three weeks after the injection, a follow-up OCT scan showed that the foveal thickness had decreased to 269 µm (E and F). The cystic spaces and the subretinal fluid accumulation resolved. His visual acuity improved to 20/60. A follow-up OCT (G), obtained 2 months after the injection, showed a normal foveal contour and resolution of the intraretinal and subretinal fluid. The foveal thickness had decreased to 236 µm (H). The visual acuity in this eye was 20/70.

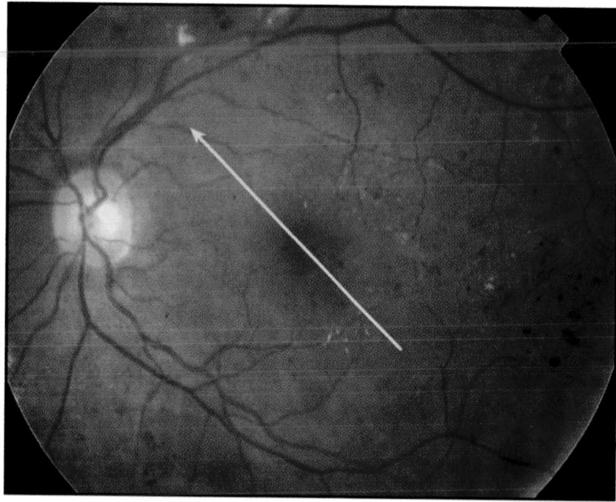

A

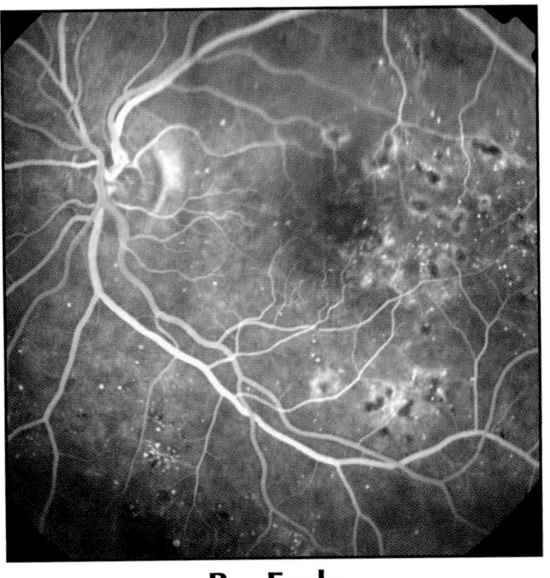

B—Early

B—Late

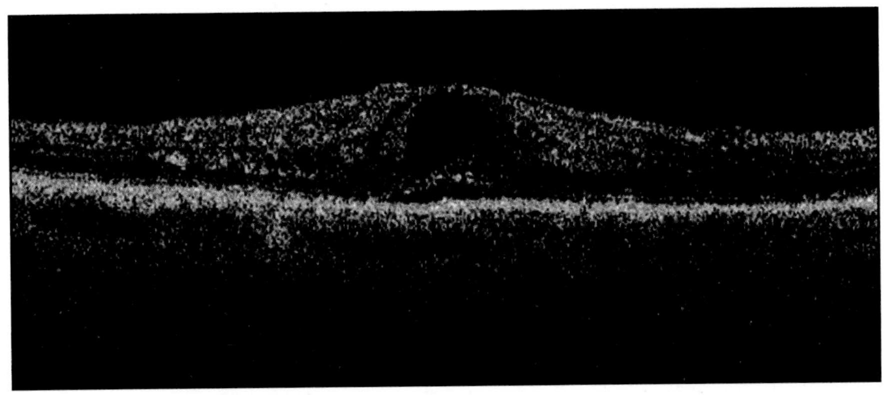

C

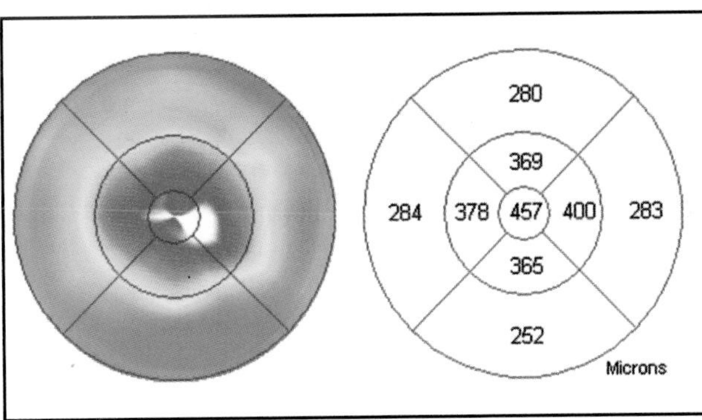

D

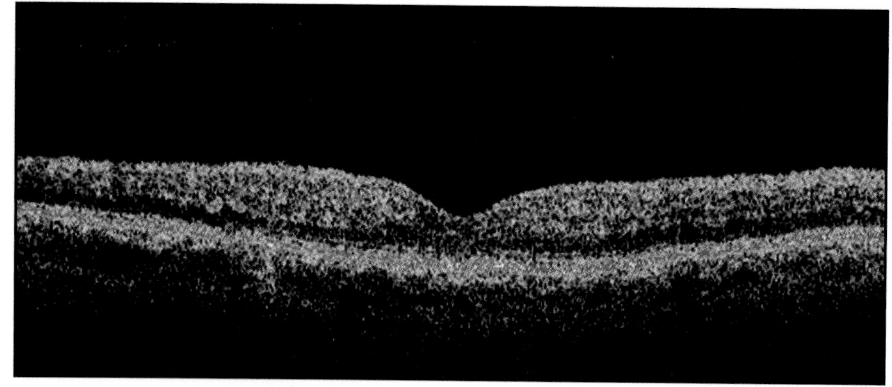

E

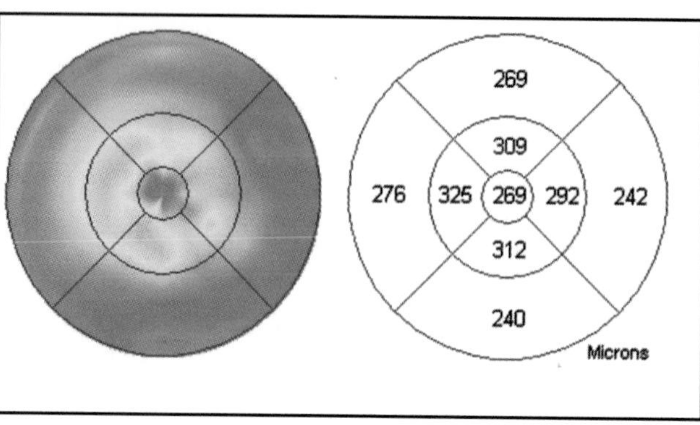
269
309
276
325
269
292
242
312
240
Microns

F

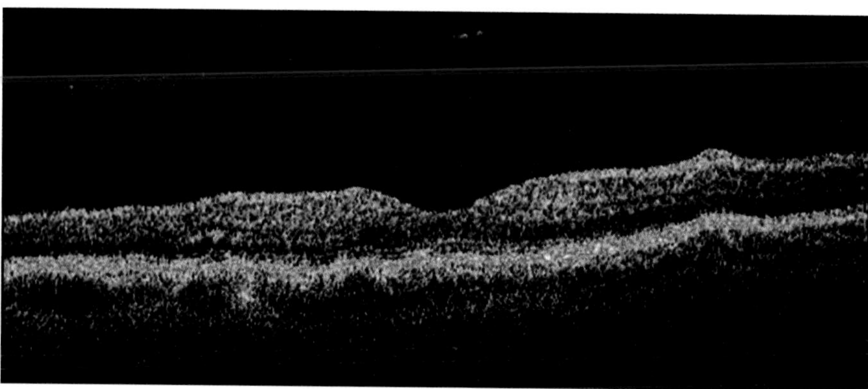

G

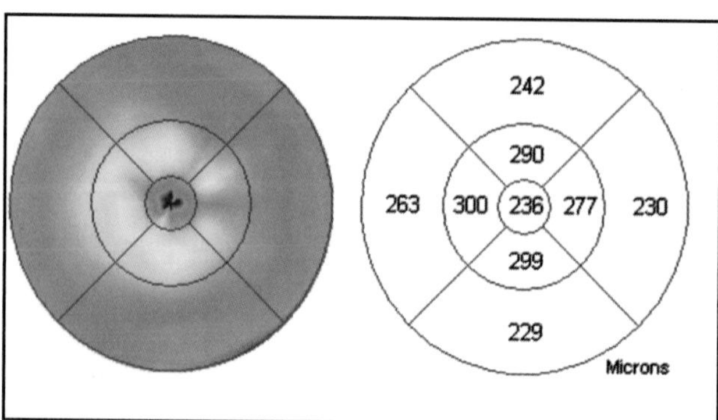
242
290
263
300
236
277
230
299
229
Microns

H

Case 5-6. Nonproliferative Diabetic Retinopathy and Diabetic Macular Edema

Clinical Summary

A 66-year-old woman with NPDR received focal/grid laser photocoagulation in her left eye 4 months earlier for clinically significant edema. Her visual acuity in this eye was 20/200. Dilated fundus examination revealed laser scars, retinal thickening, microaneurysms, and hard exudates throughout the macular region (A). Fluorescein angiography (B) revealed perifoveal late leakage consistent with macular edema.

Optical Coherence Tomography

A vertical OCT scan (C) obtained through the fovea revealed loss of the normal foveal contour, increased retinal thickness, and spaces of reduced optical reflectivity consistent with intraretinal cystic fluid accumulation. Focal areas of high reflectivity were evident representing hard lipid exudates. The foveal thickness was 445 μm (D). The patient elected to receive an intravitreal injection of triamcinolone acetonide (4 mg/0.1 cc). Six weeks after the injection, a follow-up OCT scan showed that the foveal thickness had decreased to 215 μm (E and F). Complete resolution and flattening of the cystic spaces were observed. The hard exudates with their characteristic high reflective appearance were still evident. Her visual acuity improved to 20/80.

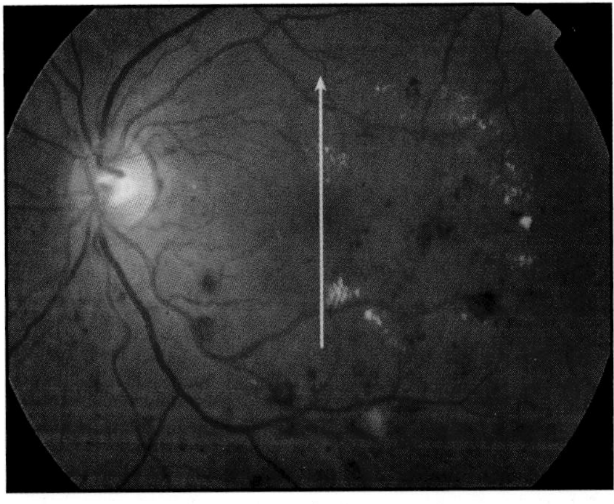

A

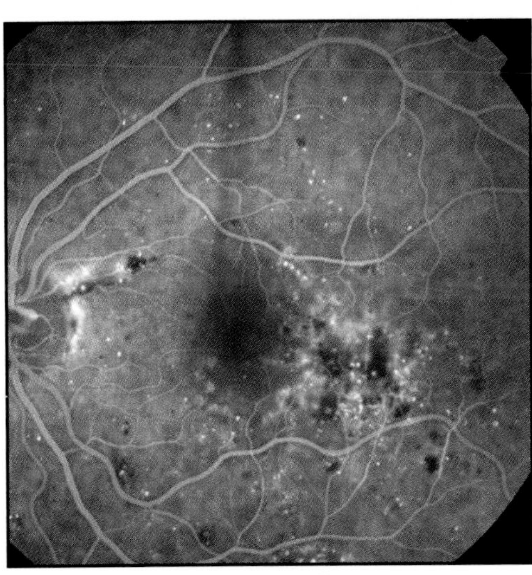

B—Early

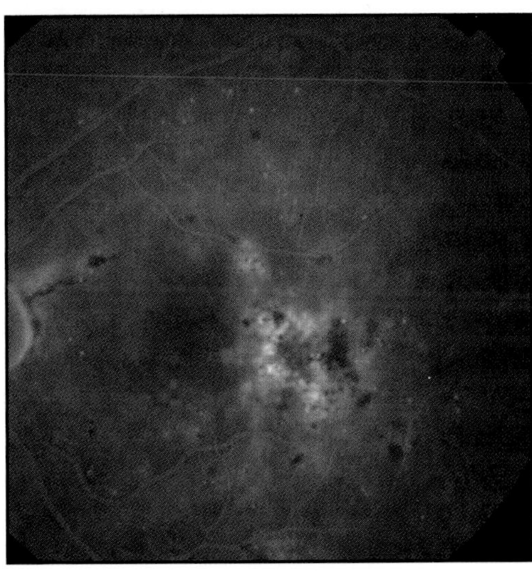

B—Late

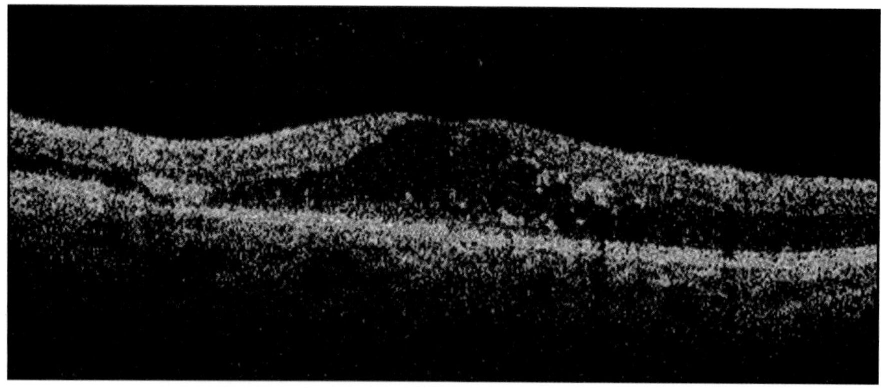

C

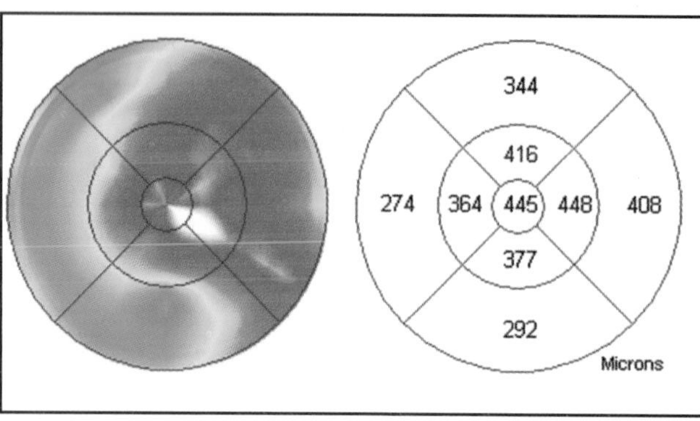
344
416
274
364
445
448
408
377
292
Microns

D

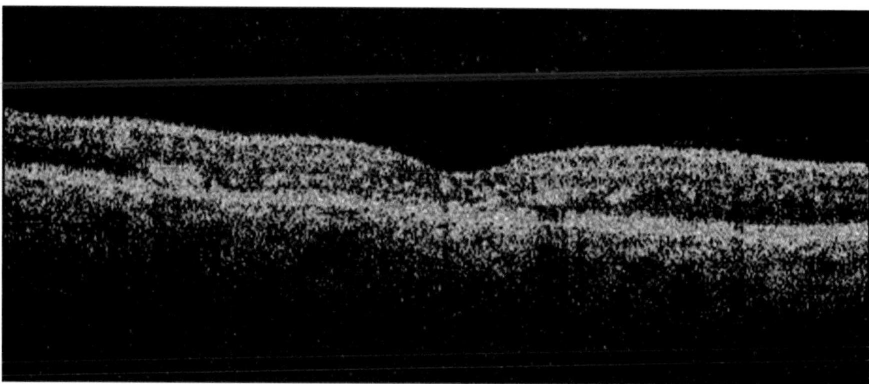

E

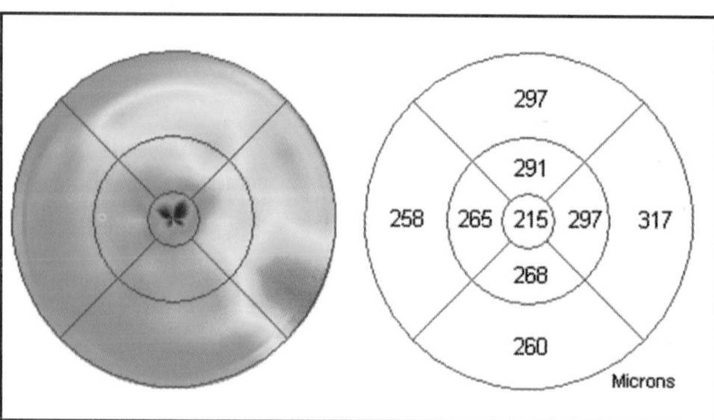
297
291
258
265
215
297
317
268
260
Microns

F

Case 5-7. Nonproliferative Diabetic Retinopathy and Macular Edema

Clinical Summary

A 77-year-old woman, who underwent focal/grid laser photocoagulation for clinically significant macular edema in her left eye 4 months earlier, reported blurred vision. Her visual acuity in this eye was 20/60. Slit-lamp biomicroscopy of this eye revealed focal/grid photocoagulation laser scars, hard lipid exudates, and retinal thickening in the macular area consistent with clinically significant macular edema (A). Fluorescein angiography (B) showed perifoveal late leakage, confirming the presence of macular edema.

Optical Coherence Tomography

A vertical OCT scan (C) showed loss of the normal foveal contour and a large cystic area of low intraretinal reflectivity in the foveal center surrounded by smaller cysts. Areas of high intraretinal reflectivity, representing hard exudates, were seen more conspicuously superior to the fovea (right side of the scan). The foveal thickness measured 372 μm (D).

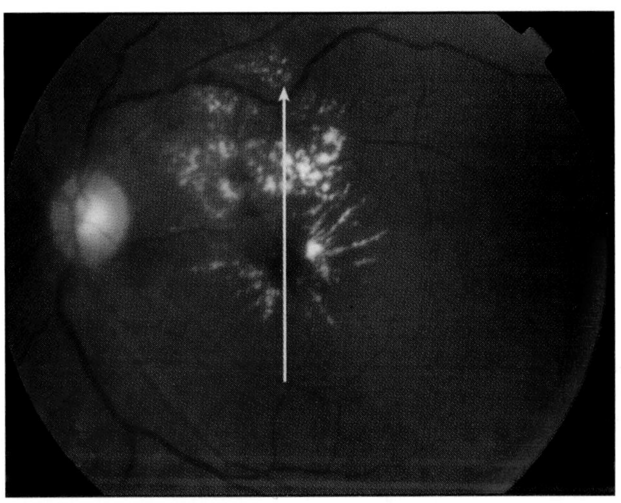

A

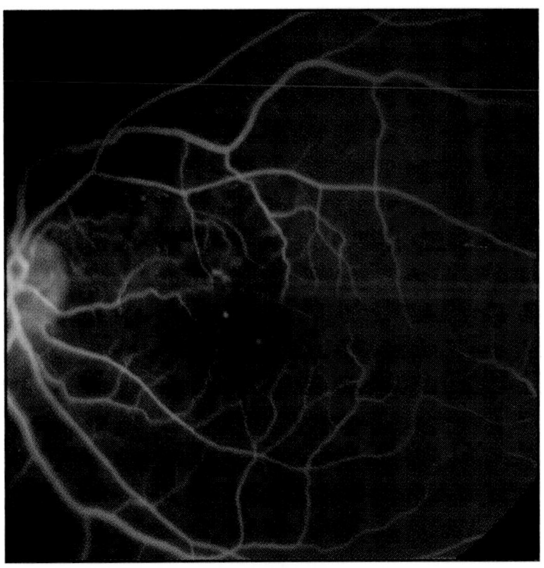

B—Early

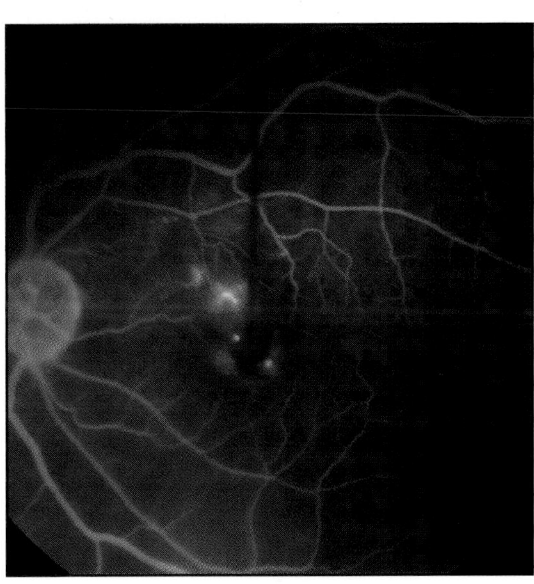

B—Late

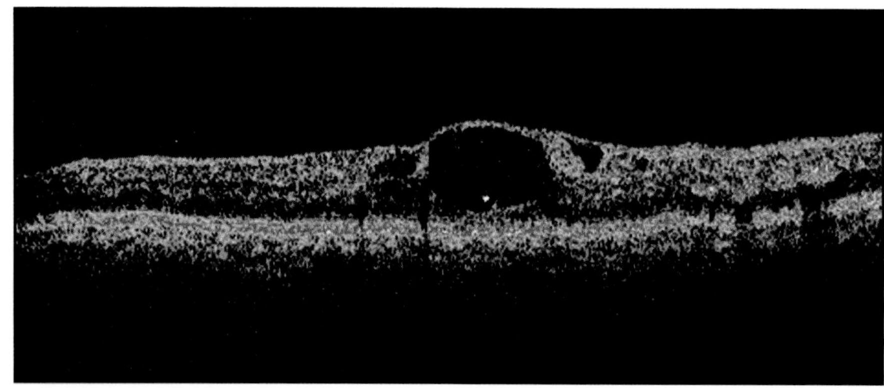

C

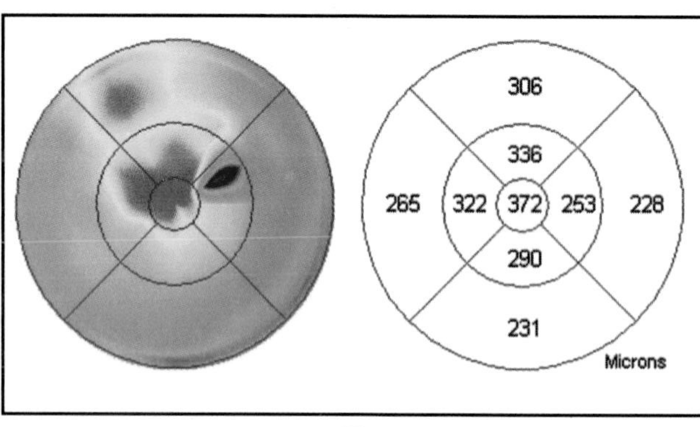

D

Case 5-8A. Nonproliferative Diabetic Retinopathy and Diabetic Macular Edema

Clinical Summary

A 68-year-old woman with NPDR was examined. She underwent bilateral focal/grid laser photocoagulation for clinically significant macular edema 1 year earlier. Slit-lamp biomicroscopy of the right eye showed scattered dot and blot hemorrhages throughout the posterior pole, hard exudates temporal to the fovea, and diffuse macular thickening (A). The visual acuity in this eye was 20/80. Intravenous fluorescein angiography revealed telangiectatic vessels and areas of pinpoint hyperfluorescence consistent with microaneurysms. As the angiogram progressed, perifoveal leakage in a petalloid fashion was evident (B).

Optical Coherence Tomography

OCT (C) demonstrated macular thickening and cystic areas of low intraretinal reflectivity consistent with intraretinal fluid accumulation. A detachment of the neurosensory retina with subretinal fluid accumulation was detected in the fovea. The retinal map analysis revealed a foveal thickness of 718 µm (D). An intravitreal injection of triamcinolone acetonide (4 mg/0.1 cc) was performed in this eye. OCT images (E) obtained 1 week after the injection demonstrated a significant decrease in the macular thickness and resolution of the cystic changes. The foveal thickness measured 300 µm (F). Also, the neurosensory detachment flattened. Hard exudates were visualized as highly reflective intraretinal areas. Her visual acuity improved to 20/70. Further resolution of the macular edema was appreciated 6 weeks after the procedure. Disappearance of the cystic spaces and subretinal fluid was observed (G). The foveal thickness decreased to 136 µm (H). Her vision remained at the same level. Her macula remained stable at the 4-month examination with a central thickness of 134 µm (I and J). No further vision improvement occurred.

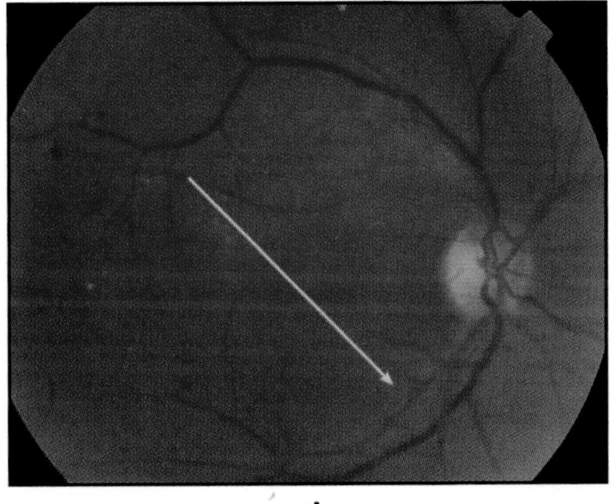

A

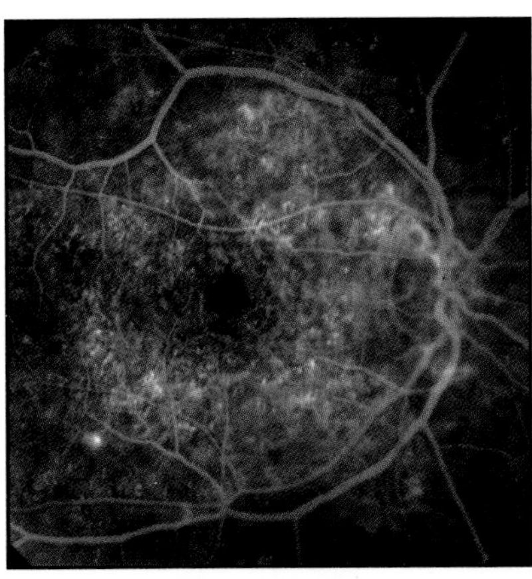

B—Early

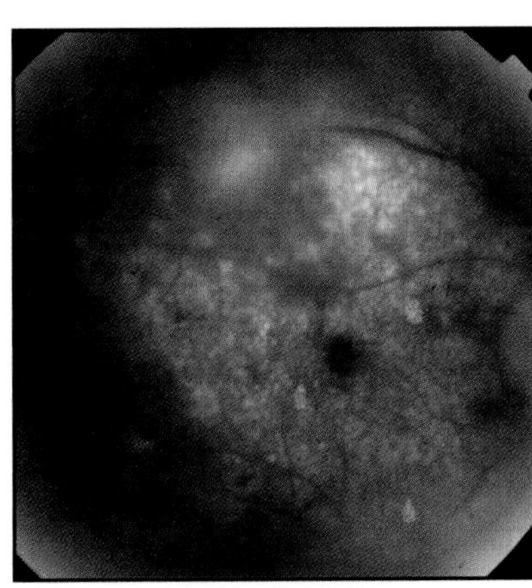

B—Late

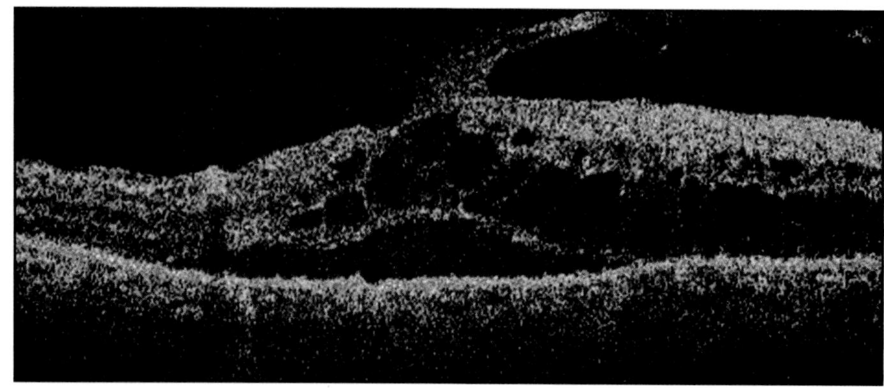

C

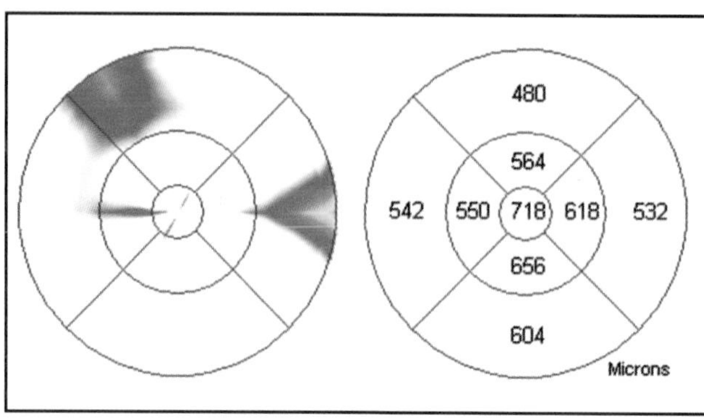
480
564
542
550
718
618
532
656
604
Microns

D

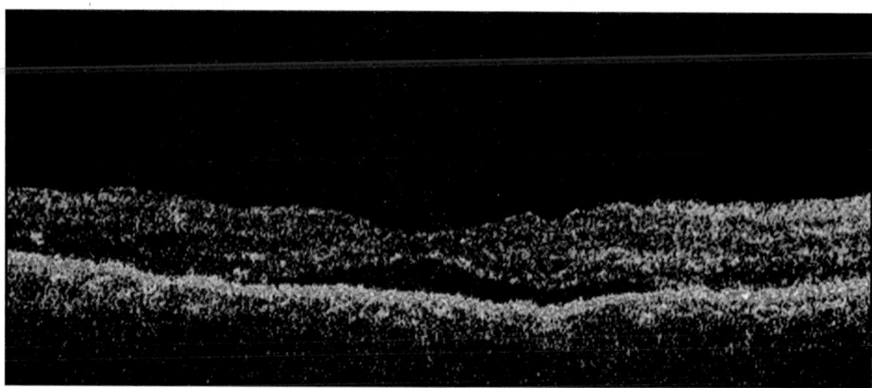

E

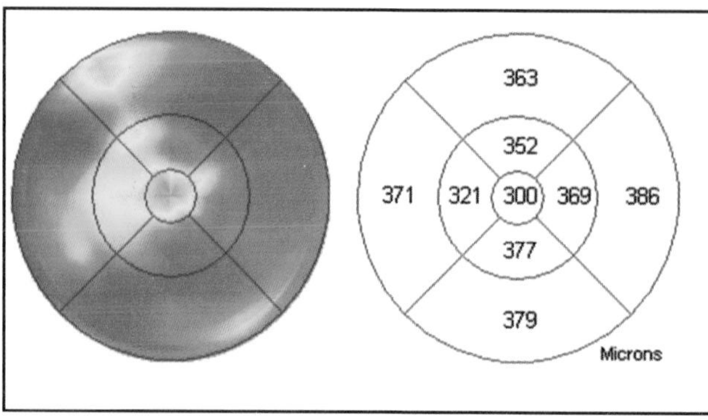
363
352
371
321
300
369
386
377
379
Microns

F

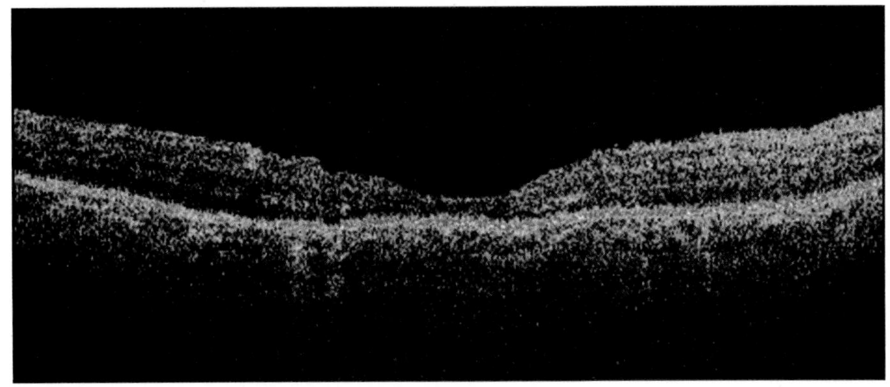

G

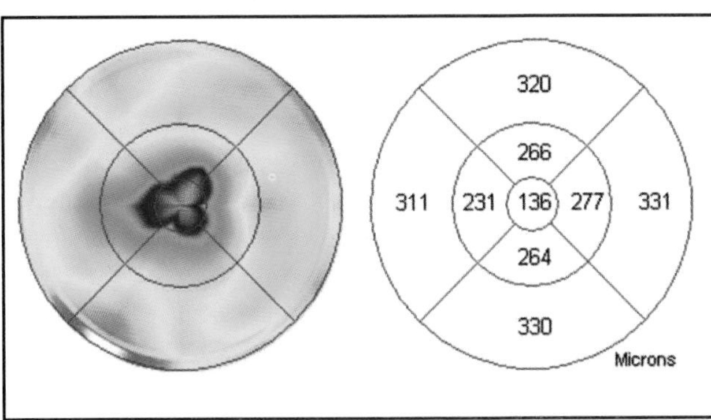
320
266
311
231
136
277
331
264
330
Microns

H

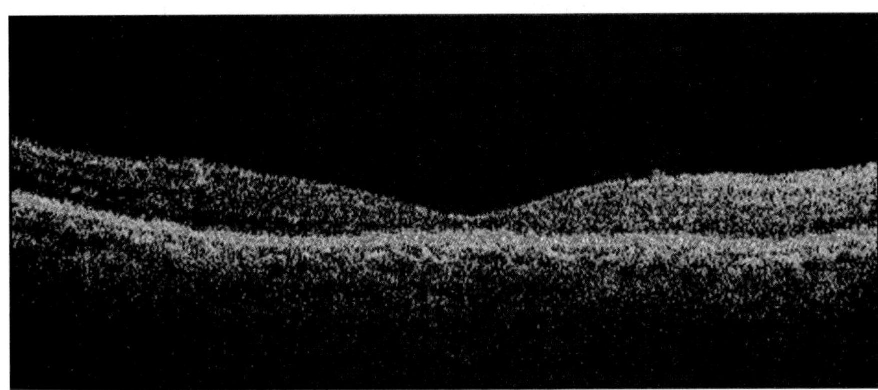

I

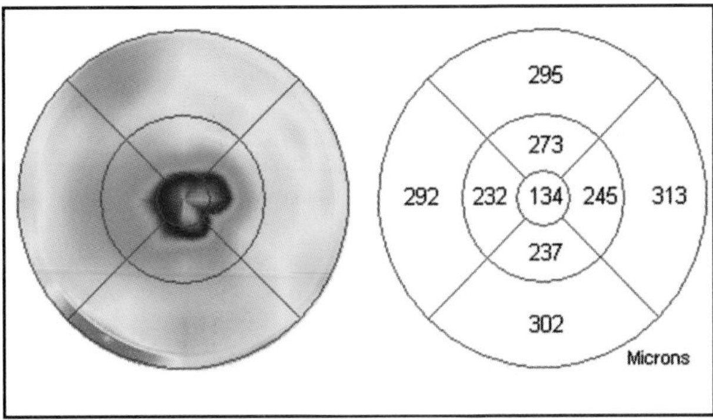
295
273
292
232
134
245
313
237
302
Microns

J

Case 5-8B. Nonproliferative Diabetic Retinopathy and Diabetic Macular Edema

Clinical Summary

Examination of the left eye showed focal laser scars, hard lipid exudates, microaneurysms, and retinal thickening in the macular region consistent with macular edema (K). The visual acuity of this eye was 20/300. Fluorescein angiography (L) revealed perifoveal leakage in a petalloid fashion consistent with CME.

Optical Coherence Tomography

OCT (M) illustrated diffuse retinal thickening and cystic spaces of reduced reflectivity consistent with intraretinal fluid accumulation and macular edema. Subretinal fluid accumulation was evident beneath the fovea. The foveal thickness was 699 μm (N). The patient underwent an intravitreal injection of triamcinolone acetonide (4 mg/0.1 cc). One week after the injection, acquired OCT images showed a significant decrease in the foveal thickness and disappearance of the cysts. The neurosensory detachment looked smaller (O). The foveal thickness measured 341 μm (P). Her visual acuity improved to 20/60. Four weeks later, a follow-up OCT (Q) revealed resolution of the subretinal and intraretinal fluid accumulation. Hard exudates were visualized as highly reflective spots. The foveal thickness decreased to 187 μm (R). The vision did not show further improvement at that time. Three months after the procedure, the retina remained stable without further accumulation of fluid (S). Foveal thickness measured 160 μm (T) and visual acuity improved to 20/50.

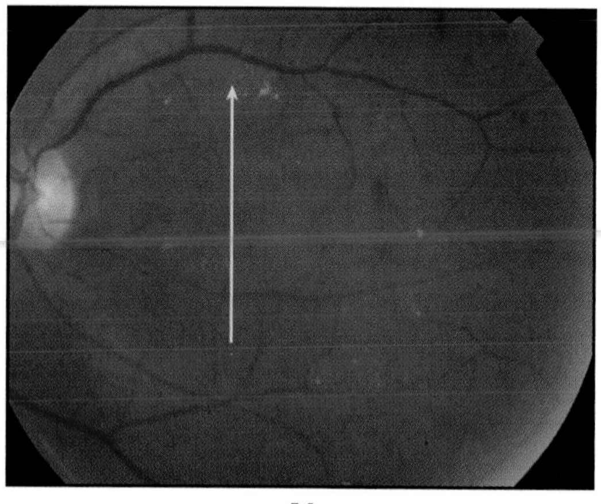

K

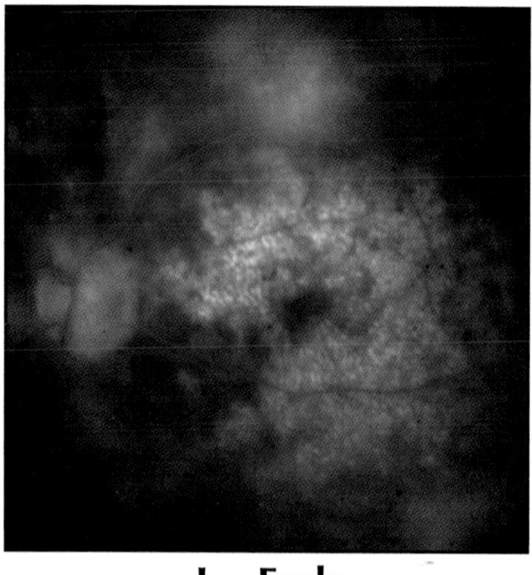

L—Early

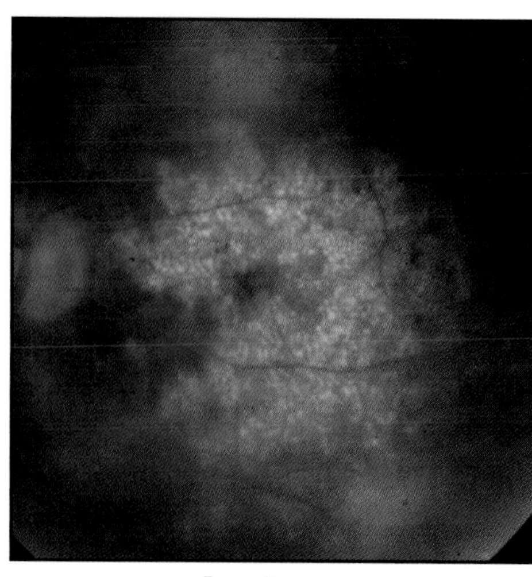

L—Late

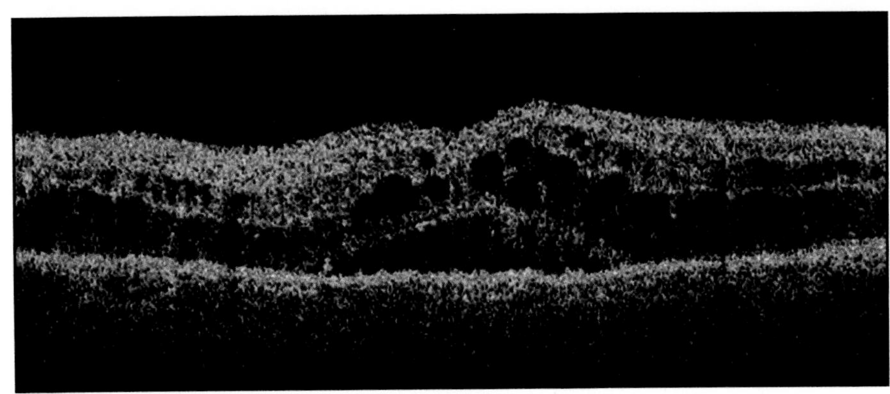

M

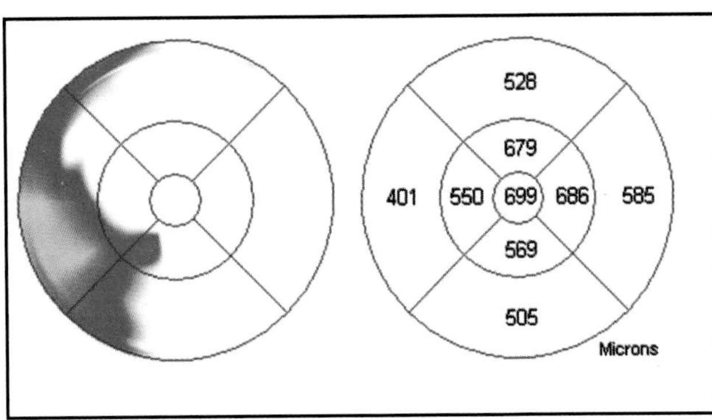
528
679
401
550
699
686
585
569
505
Microns

N

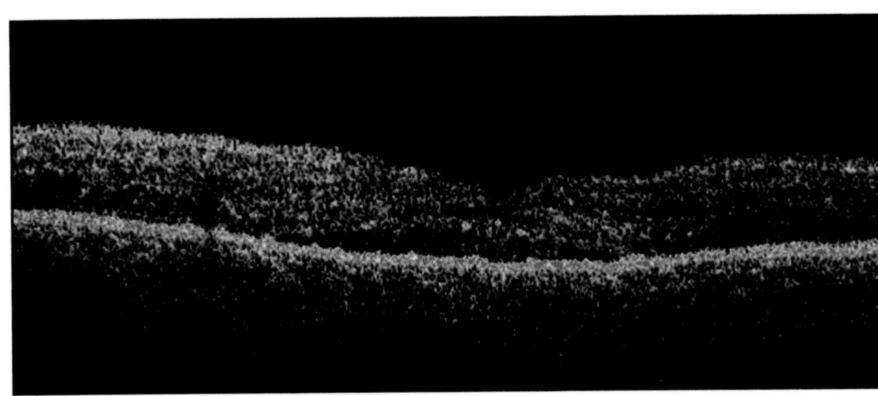

O

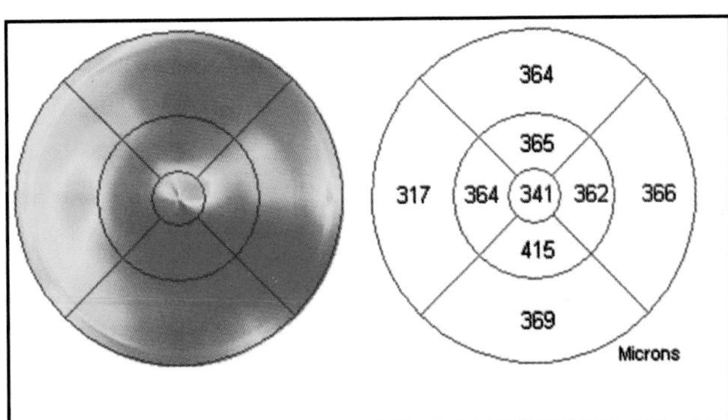
364
365
317
364
341
362
366
415
369
Microns

P

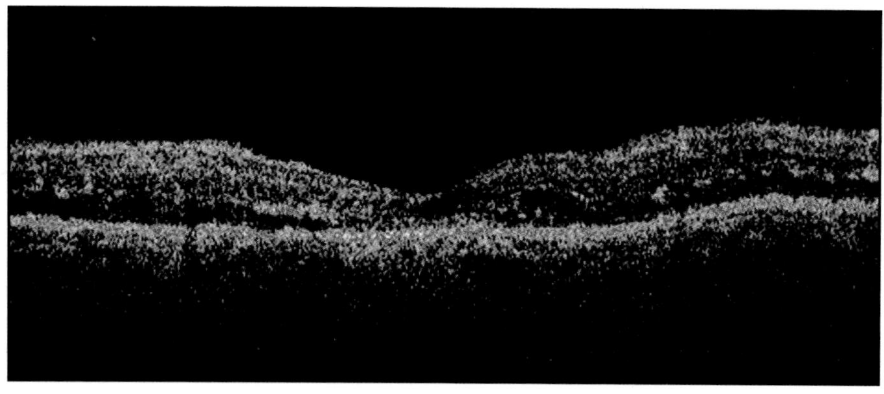

Q

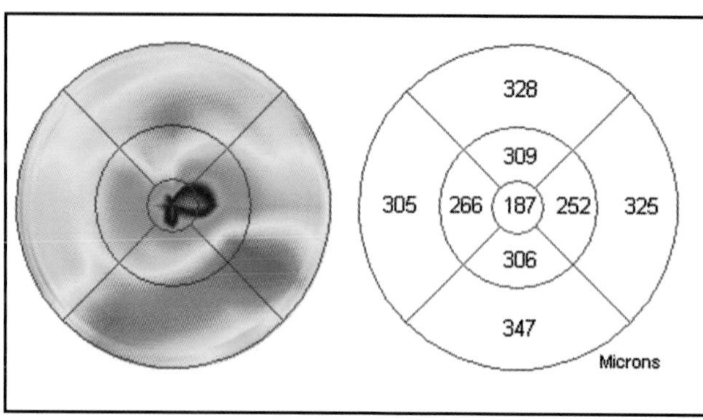
328
309
305
266
187
252
325
306
347
Microns

R

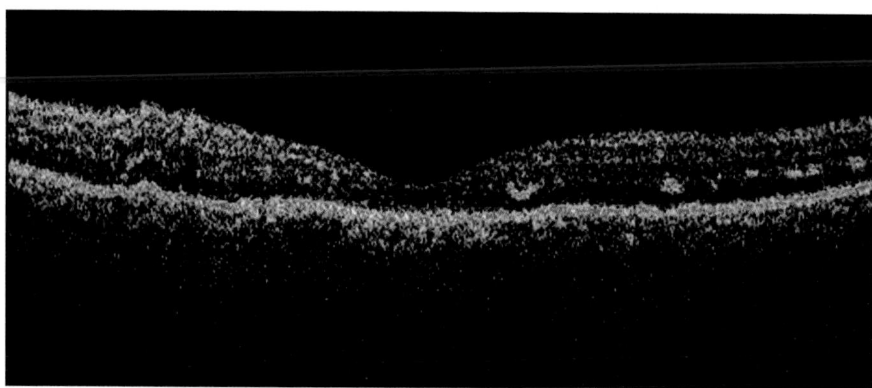

S

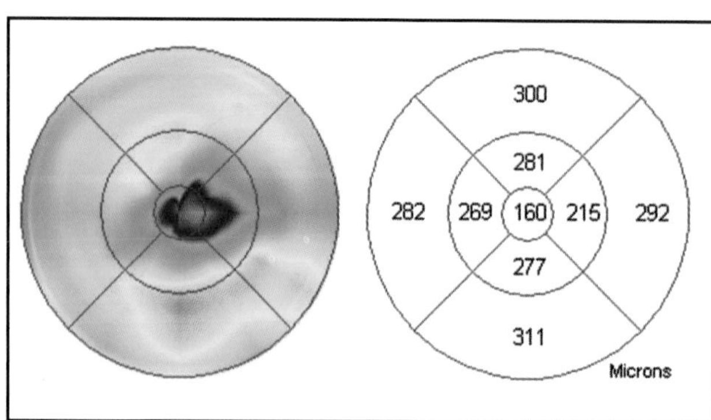
300
281
282
269
160
215
292
277
311
Microns

T

Case 5-9. Nonproliferative Diabetic Retinopathy With Epiretinal Membrane Formation and Macular Edema

Clinical Summary

A 67-year-old man with a history of NPDR underwent focal/grid laser photocoagulation approximately 10 months earlier for clinically significant macular edema in his left eye. His visual acuity in this eye was 20/50. Dilated fundus examination of this eye showed laser scars, micro-aneurysms, hard lipid exudates, and retinal thickening temporal to the fovea consistent with clinically significant macular edema. An epiretinal membrane was also observed (A). Fluorescein angiography (B) demonstrated laser scars, dots of hyperfluorescence corresponding to microaneurysms, and perifoveal late leakage.

Optical Coherence Tomography

OCT (C) illustrated loss of the normal foveal contour and retinal thickening. Areas of reduced optical backscattering corresponded to intraretinal fluid accumulation. Hard retinal exudates were visible as highly reflective intraretinal dots (left side of the scan). A highly reflective band corresponding to the epiretinal membrane was seen in the retinal surface. This membrane was slightly separated from the retina superotemporally (left side of the scan) and more adherent inferonasally (right side of the scan). The central macular thickness measured 519 μm (D). Focal/grid laser photocoagulation was performed.

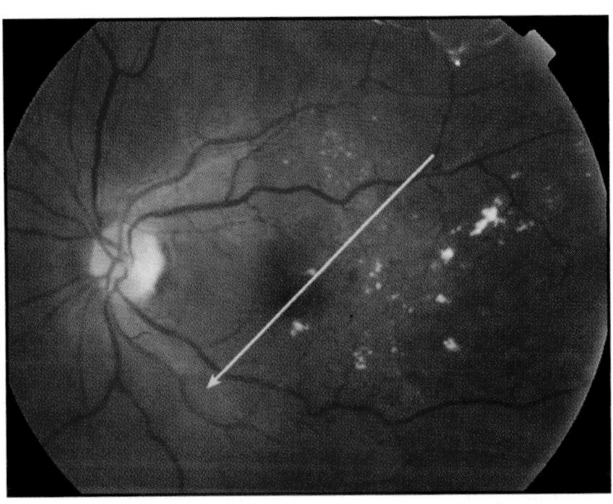

A

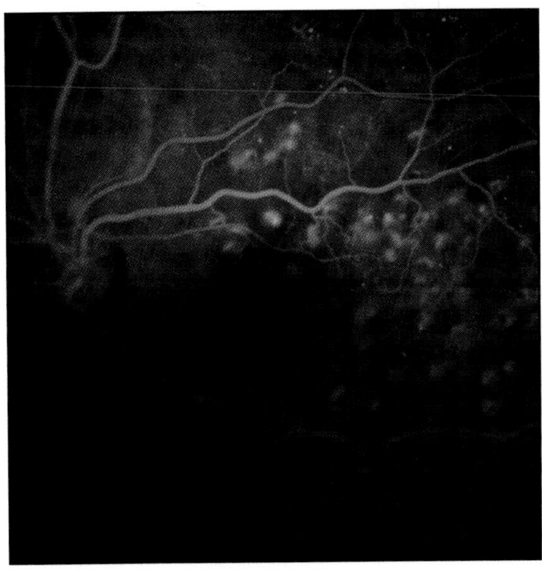

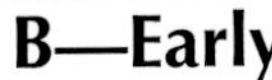

B—Early

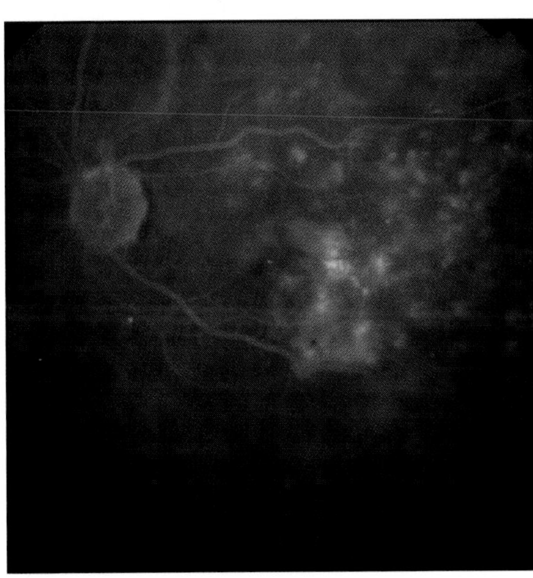

B—Late

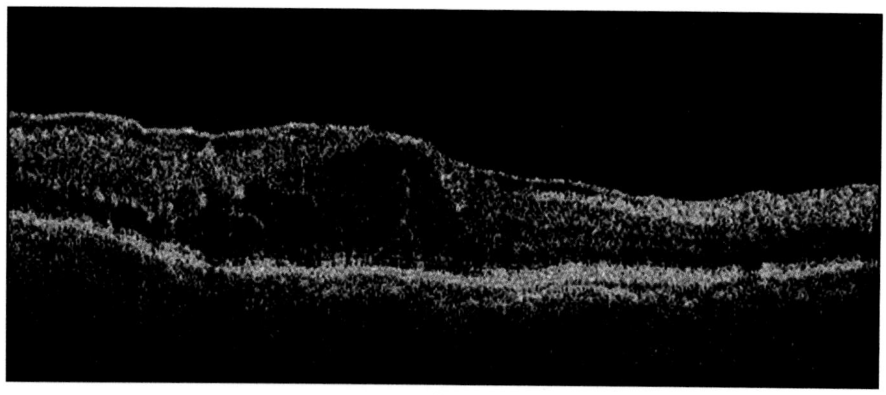

C

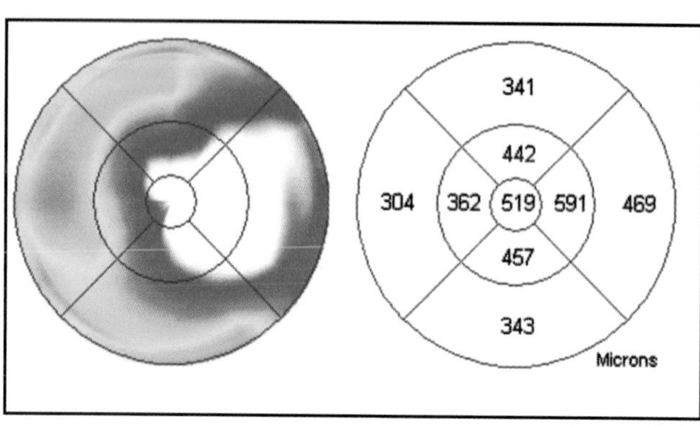

D

Case 5-10. Nonproliferative Diabetic Retinopathy and Diabetic Macular Edema With Lamellar Hole

Clinical Summary

A 71-year-old diabetic woman complained of decreased vision in her left eye. The visual acuity was 20/100 in this eye. Dilated fundus examination showed scattered dot and blot hemorrhages throughout the posterior pole and midperiphery, in addition to hard exudates and retinal thickening temporal to the fovea consistent with clinically significant edema (A). Fluorescein angiography (B) demonstrated focal areas of hyperfluorescence associated with late leakage in a petalloid fashion consistent with macular edema.

Optical Coherence Tomography

A vertical OCT scan (C) showed diffuse retinal thickening and low reflective spaces consistent with macular cysts. The central macular thickness measured 292 μm (D). The patient underwent focal/grid laser photocoagulation. Four months later, a follow-up OCT (E) scan demonstrated a steep and irregular foveal pit with retinal tissue remaining at the base consistent with a lamellar hole. The configuration of the foveal contour suggests rupture of the macular cysts. Retinal thickening and areas of low intraretinal reflectivity corresponding to fluid accumulation were still present. Central macular thickness measured 339 μm (F). The visual acuity was 20/70 at that time. The patient elected to receive an intravitreal injection of triamcinolone acetonide (4 mg/0.1 cc). Three months after this procedure, an OCT scan (G) illustrated complete resolution of the lamellar hole as well as the cystic changes. Foveal thickness measured 160 μm (H) and the visual acuity improved to 20/60.

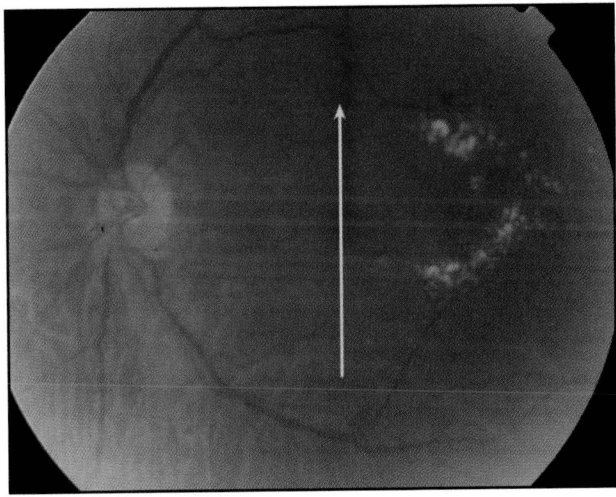

A

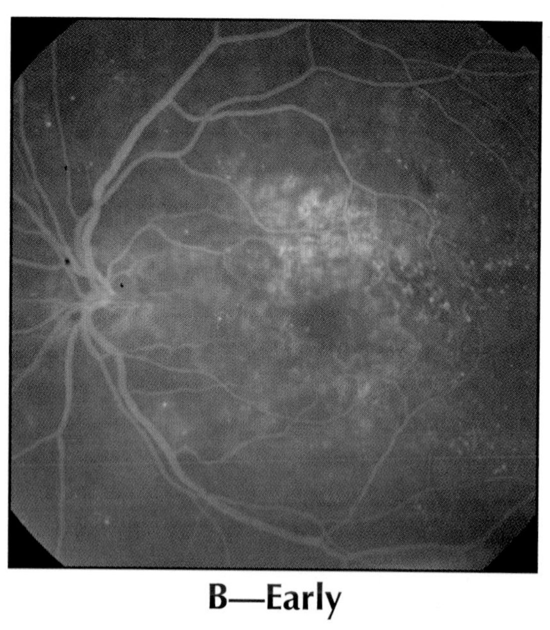

B—Early

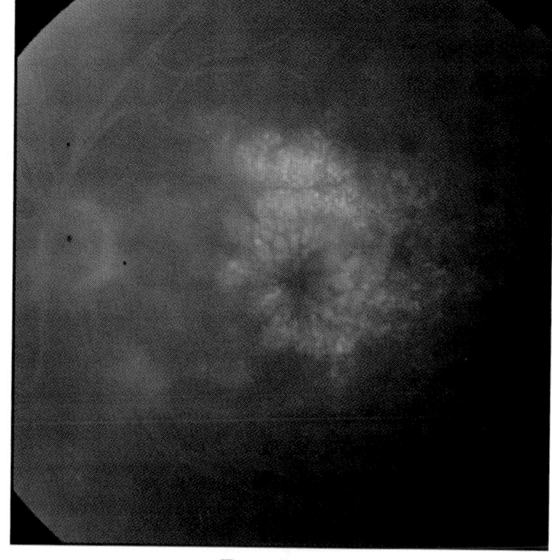

B—Late

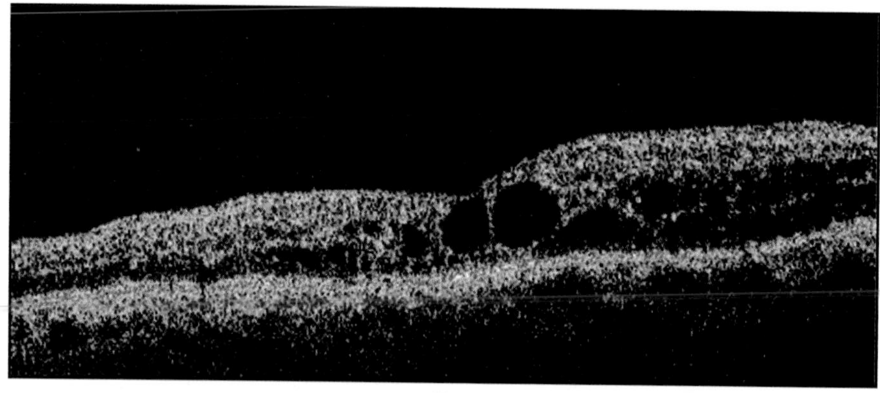

C

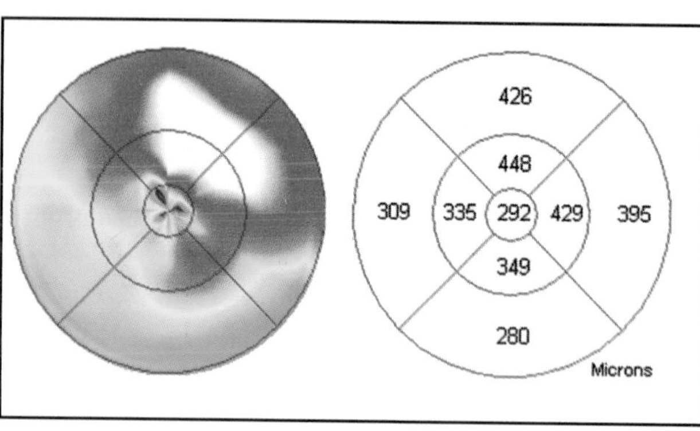

D

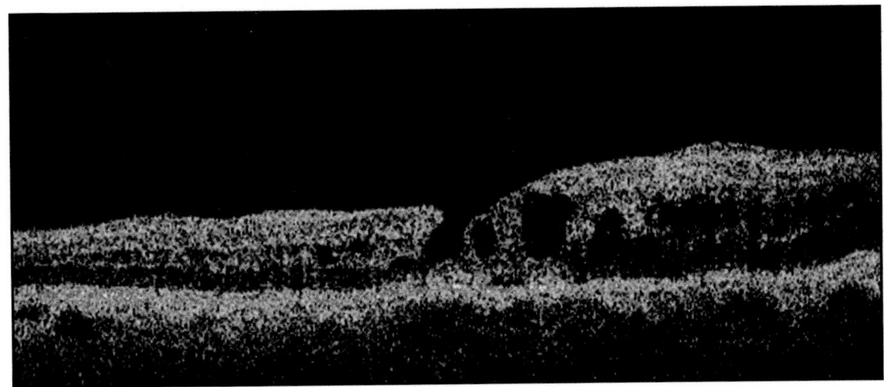

E

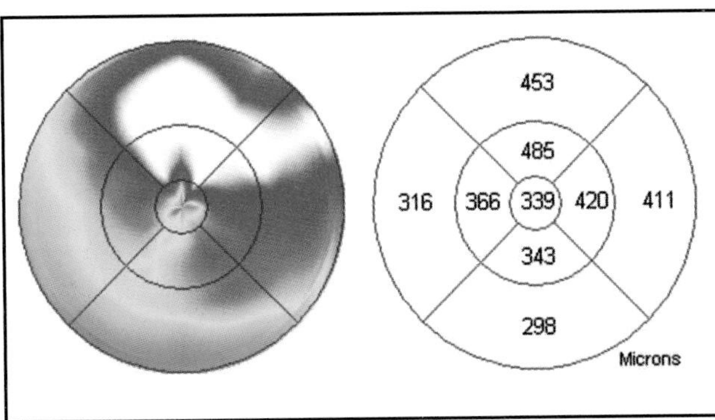
453
485
316
366
339
420
411
343
298
Microns

F

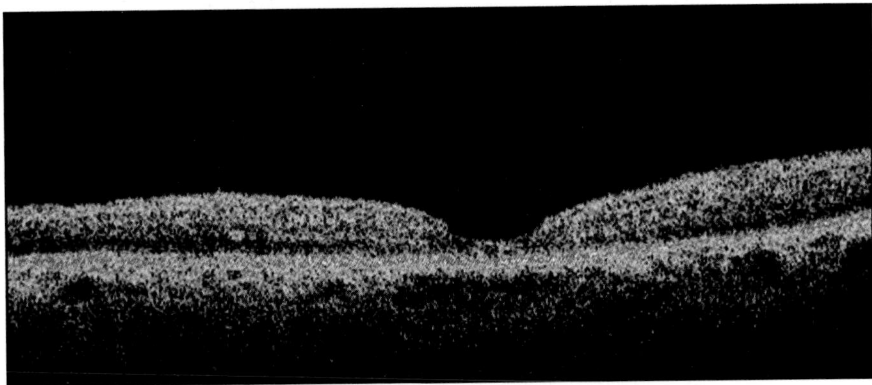

G

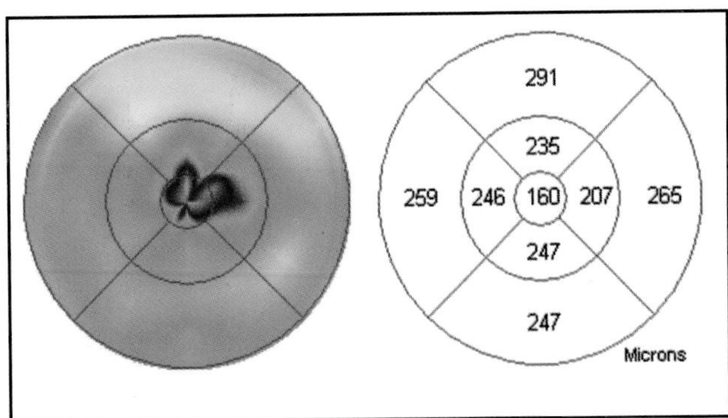
291
235
259
246
160
207
265
247
247
Microns

H

Case 5-11. Proliferative Diabetic Retinopathy With Macular Edema

Clinical Summary

A 63-year-old woman with PDR previously received panretinal laser photocoagulation. On examination, panretinal laser scars as well as macular thickening with hard lipid exudates were evident in the right eye. Her visual acuity in this eye was 20/200 (A). Fluorescein angiography (B) disclosed laser scars and perifoveal late leakage.

Optical Coherence Tomography

OCT (C) obtained through the fovea revealed loss of the normal foveal contour, increased retinal thickness, and spaces of reduced optical reflectivity corresponding to intraretinal fluid accumulation. A focal area of high backscattering was appreciated corresponding to a retinal hard exudate located superotemporal to the fovea (left side of the scan). This highly reflective spot shadowed the optical reflections from the tissues underneath. The retinal map analysis revealed a foveal thickness of 377 μm (D). The patient underwent focal/grid laser photocoagulation.

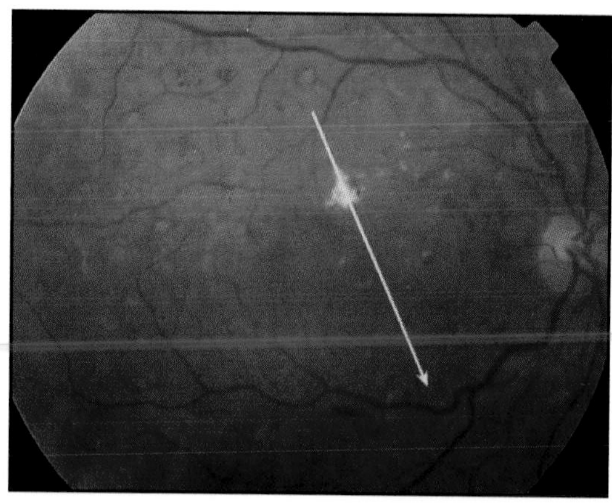

A

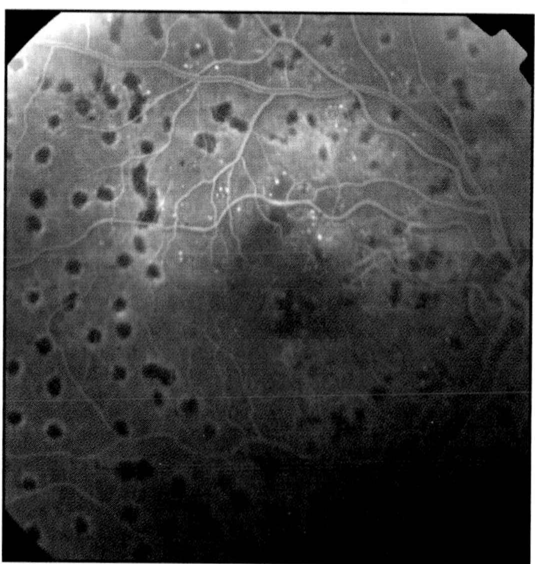

B—Early

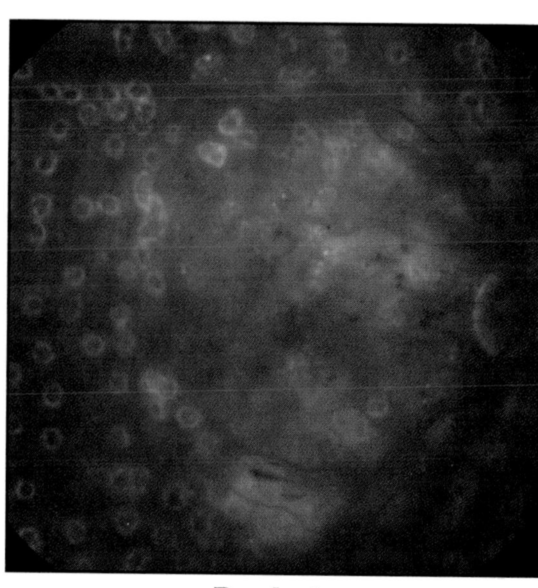

B—Late

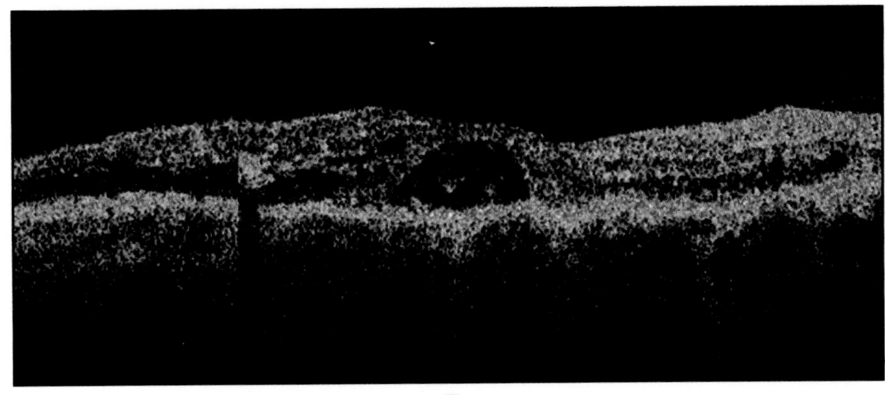

C

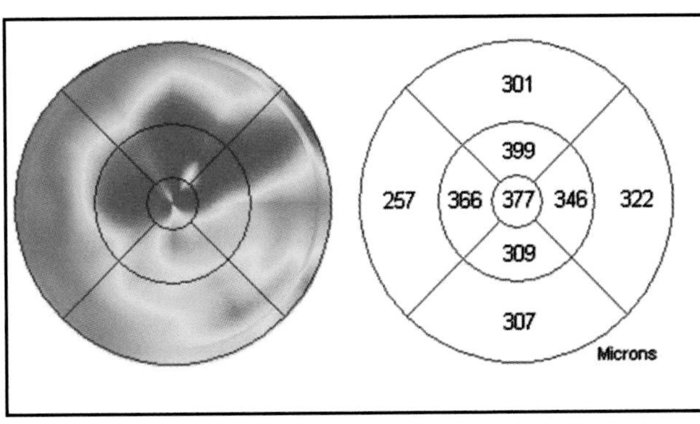

D

Case 5-12A. Proliferative Diabetic Retinopathy and Macular Edema

Clinical Summary

A 67-year-old man with PDR had focal laser photocoagulation in both eyes 5 months earlier for clinically significant edema. His visual acuity in the right eye was 4/200. On examination, his right eye showed scattered hemorrhages, laser scars, diffuse retinal thickening, and microaneurysms throughout the macular region (A). Fluorescein angiography (B) revealed areas of capillary nonperfusion and perifoveal late leakage consistent with macular edema.

Optical Coherence Tomography

A horizontal OCT scan (C) revealed loss of the normal foveal contour, marked diffuse macular thickening, and large spaces of reduced optical reflectivity consistent with intraretinal cystic fluid accumulation. The retinal map analysis revealed a foveal thickness of 764 μm (D). An intravitreal injection of triamcinolone acetonide (4 mg/0.1cc) was performed. Six weeks after the procedure, a follow-up OCT scan (E) revealed complete flattening of the cystic areas and resolution of the macular edema. The central foveal thickness measured 170 μm (F). The visual acuity improved to 20/400. Three months later, the macula remained stable without recurrence of edema (G). The visual acuity and the central macular thickness stayed the same (H).

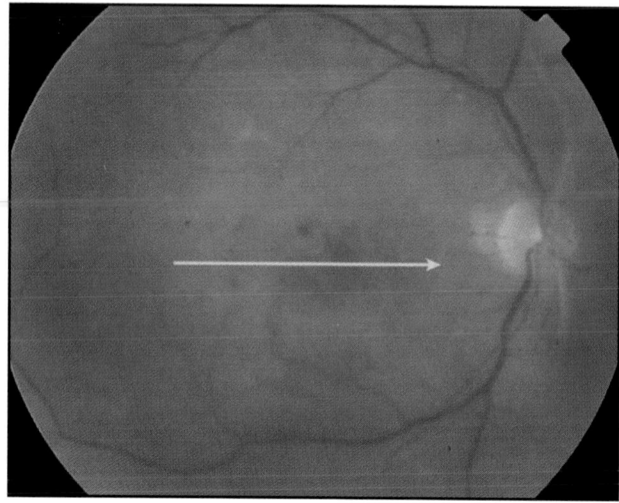

A

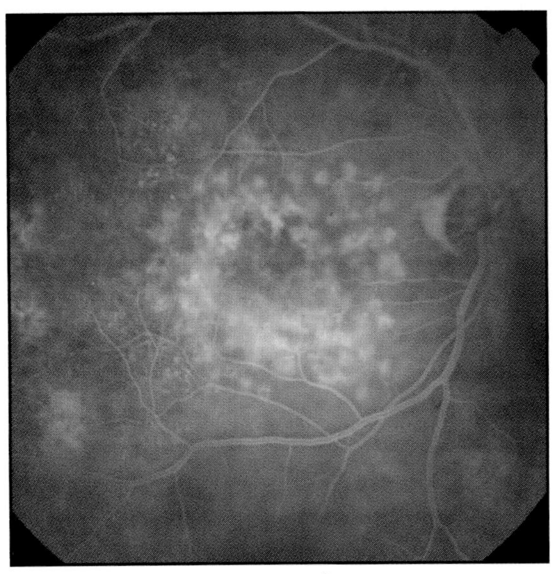

B—Early

B—Late

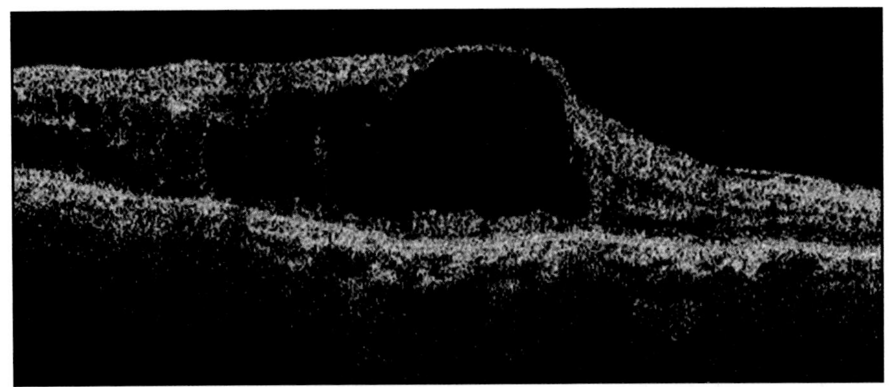

C

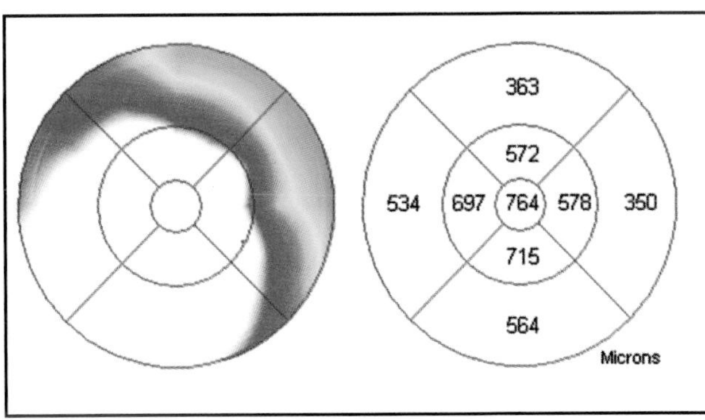

D

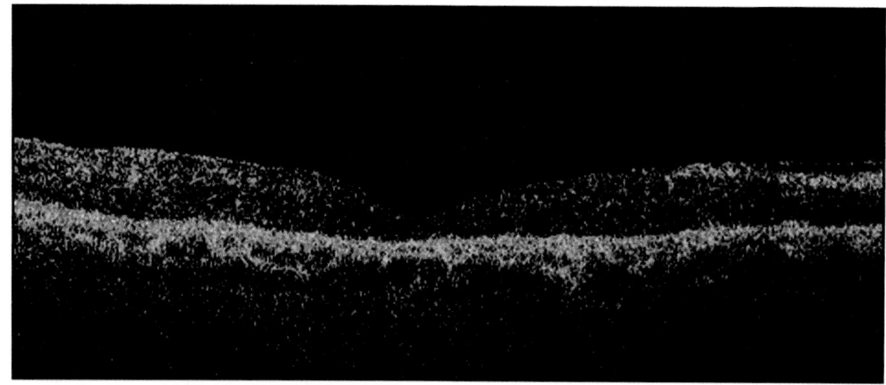

E

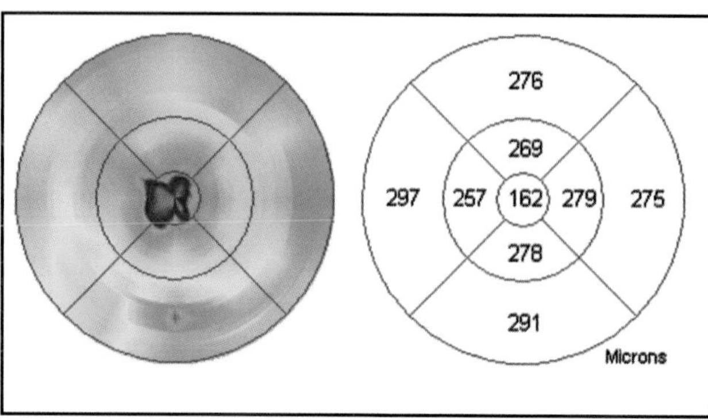
276
269
297
257
162
279
275
278
291
Microns

F

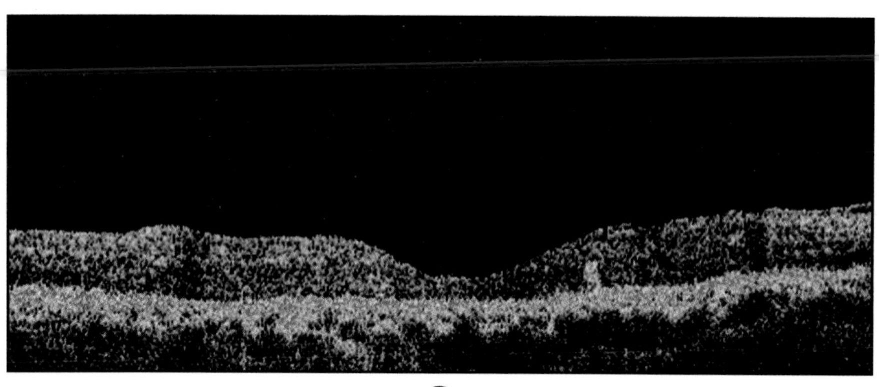

G

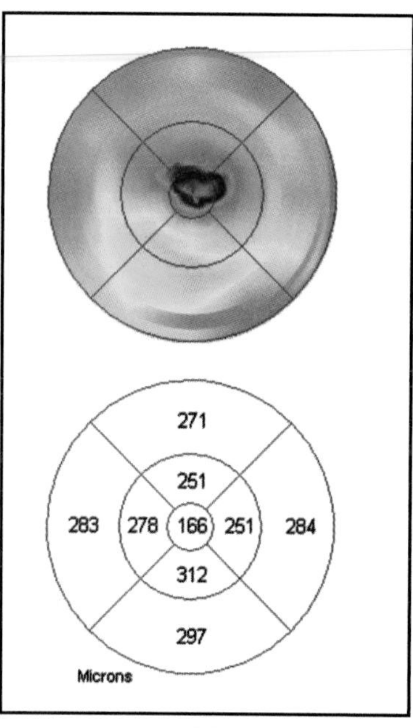
271
251
283
278
166
251
284
312
297
Microns

H

Case 5-12B. Proliferative Diabetic Retinopathy and Macular Edema

Clinical Summary

Examination of the patient's left eye also showed laser scars, scattered hemorrhages, and retinal thickening with hard exudates throughout the macular region (I). The visual acuity in this eye was 20/200. Fluorescein angiography (J) revealed perifoveal late leakage consistent with macular edema.

Optical Coherence Tomography

OCT scan obtained through the fovea (K) displayed a space of low intraretinal reflectivity corresponding to a cyst. The posterior hyaloid face—represented as a hyperreflective band—is adherent to this cystic area, suggesting a traction component. Also, there was evidence of retinal thickening in the perifoveal area. The retinal map analysis revealed a foveal thickness of 336 μm (L). A follow-up OCT scan (M) obtained 6 weeks later still showed a taut posterior hyaloid with an increase in the size of the cyst. Foveal thickness measured 351 μm (N). Vision stayed at the same level. A posterior vitreous detachment occurred 3 months later with release of the tractional component and resolution of the cystic changes in the foveal center. The perimacular area still was thickened (O and P). The visual acuity did not improve.

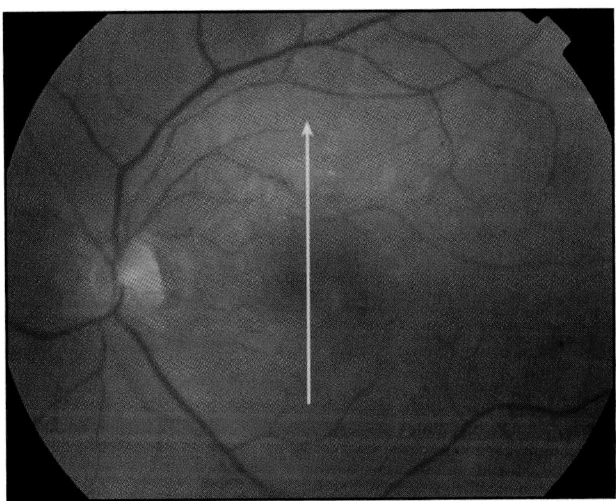

I

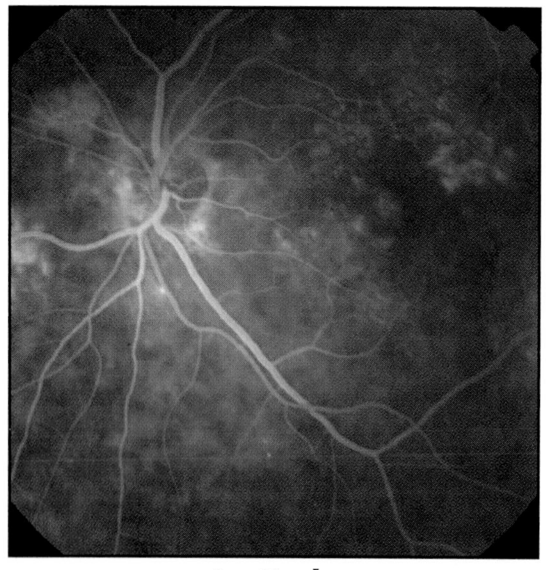

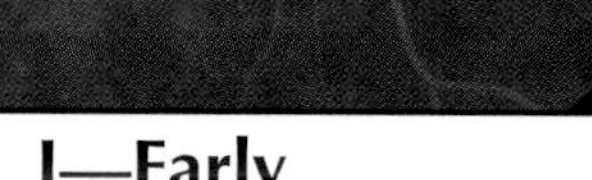

J—Early

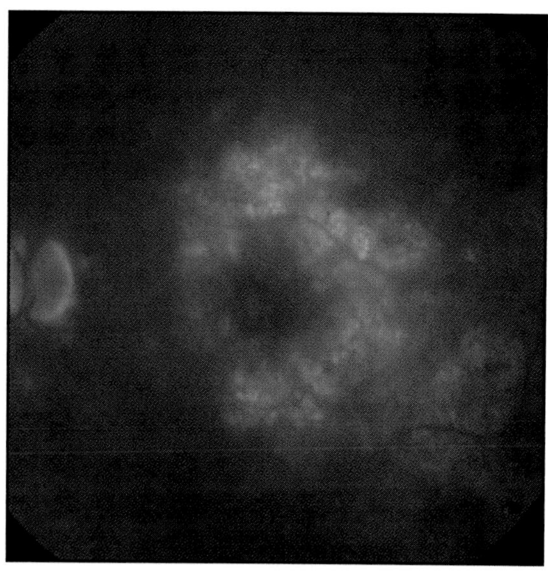

J—Late

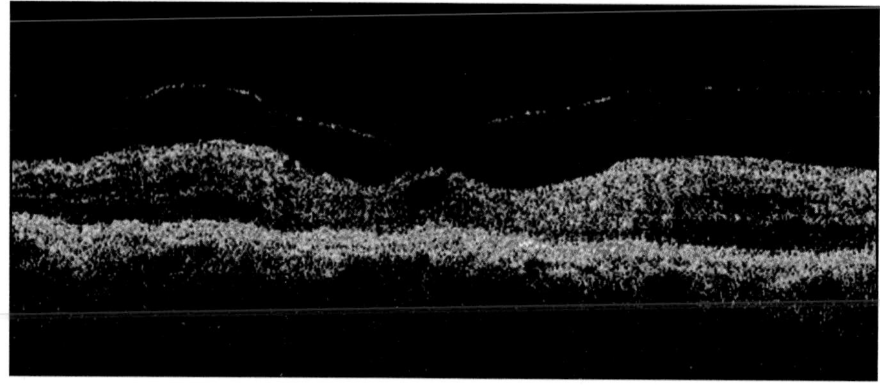

K

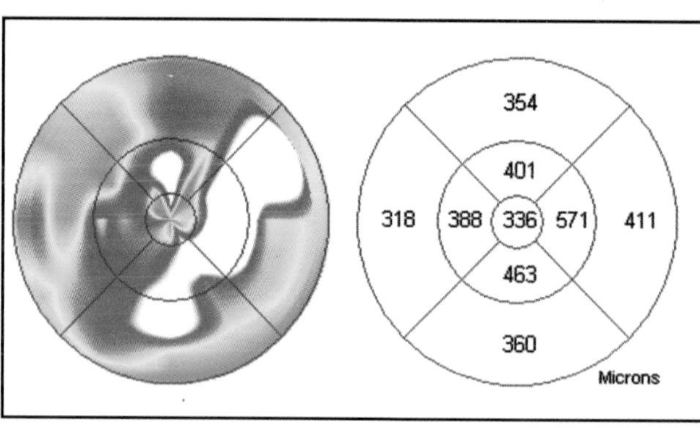

L

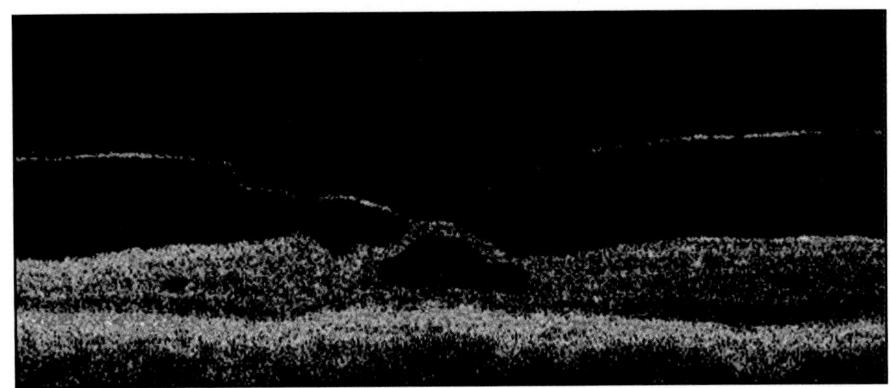

M

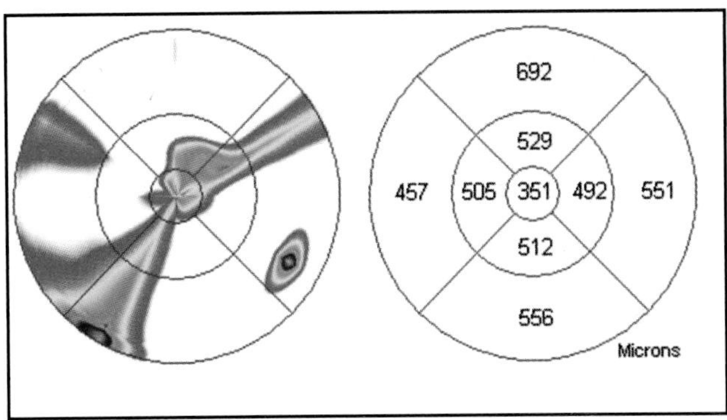
692
529
457
505
351
492
551
512
556
Microns

N

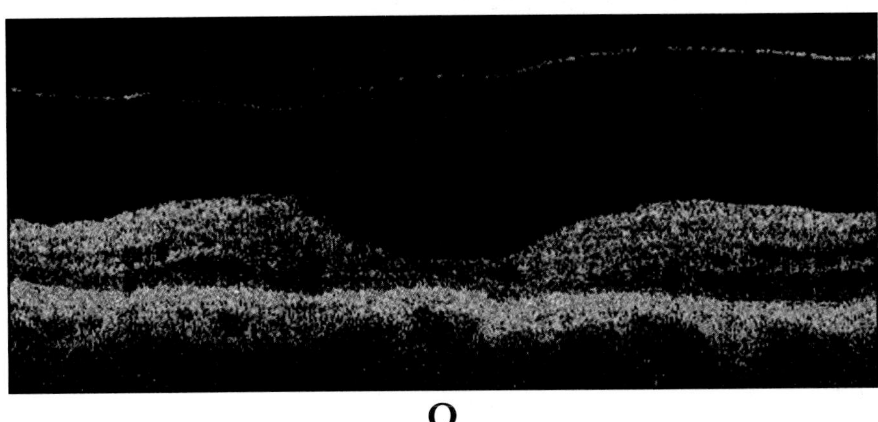

O

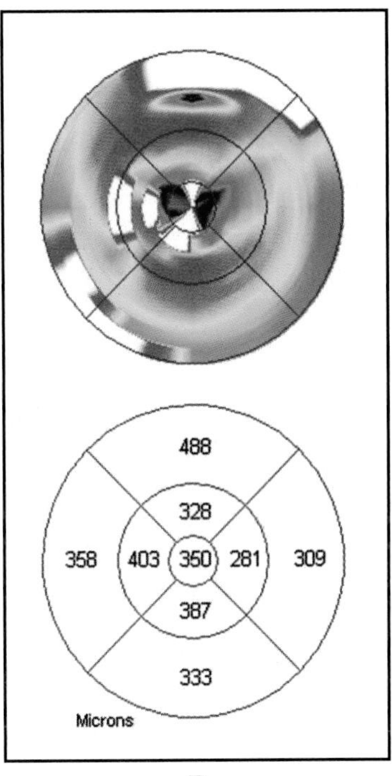
488
328
358
403
350
281
309
387
333
Microns

P

Case 5-13A. Proliferative Diabetic Retinopathy and Macular Edema With Epiretinal Membrane Formation

Clinical Summary

A 64-year-old man with a history of PDR undergoing panretinal laser photocoagulation noted decreased vision in both eyes. His visual acuity in the right eye was 20/300. Dilated fundus examination of the right eye revealed a hazy media due to the presence of a vitreous hemorrhage. Panretinal laser scars, scattered hemorrhages, and hard exudates were noted (A). Fluorescein angiography (B) showed diffuse perifoveal late leakage.

Optical Coherence Tomography

Despite the presence of a hazy media, which precludes from adequate visualization of the macula, a vertical OCT scan (C) clearly illustrated marked diffuse thickening with loss of the normal foveal contour. Reduced optical backscattering, consistent with intraretinal fluid accumulation and edema, was observed. A highly reflective band was noticed extending from the foveal center to the superior macular area (right side of the scan). This band represented an epiretinal membrane that was tightly adherent to the retinal surface in the foveal center and superiorly but more loose between those regions. The central macular thickness measured 582 μm (D). The patient underwent focal/grid laser photocoagulation. No clinical response was observed 4 months after the procedure, and an intravitreal injection of triamcinolone acetonide (4 mg/0.1 cc) was performed at that time. One month later, a follow-up OCT scan showed a remarkable decrease in retinal thickness as well as increased optical reflectivity in the neurosensory retina, which correlates with less fluid accumulation (E). The central macular thickness decreased to 336 μm (F). The vision improved to 20/200.

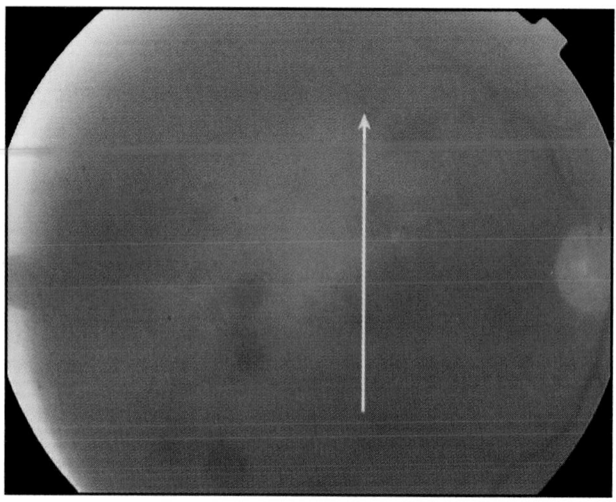

A

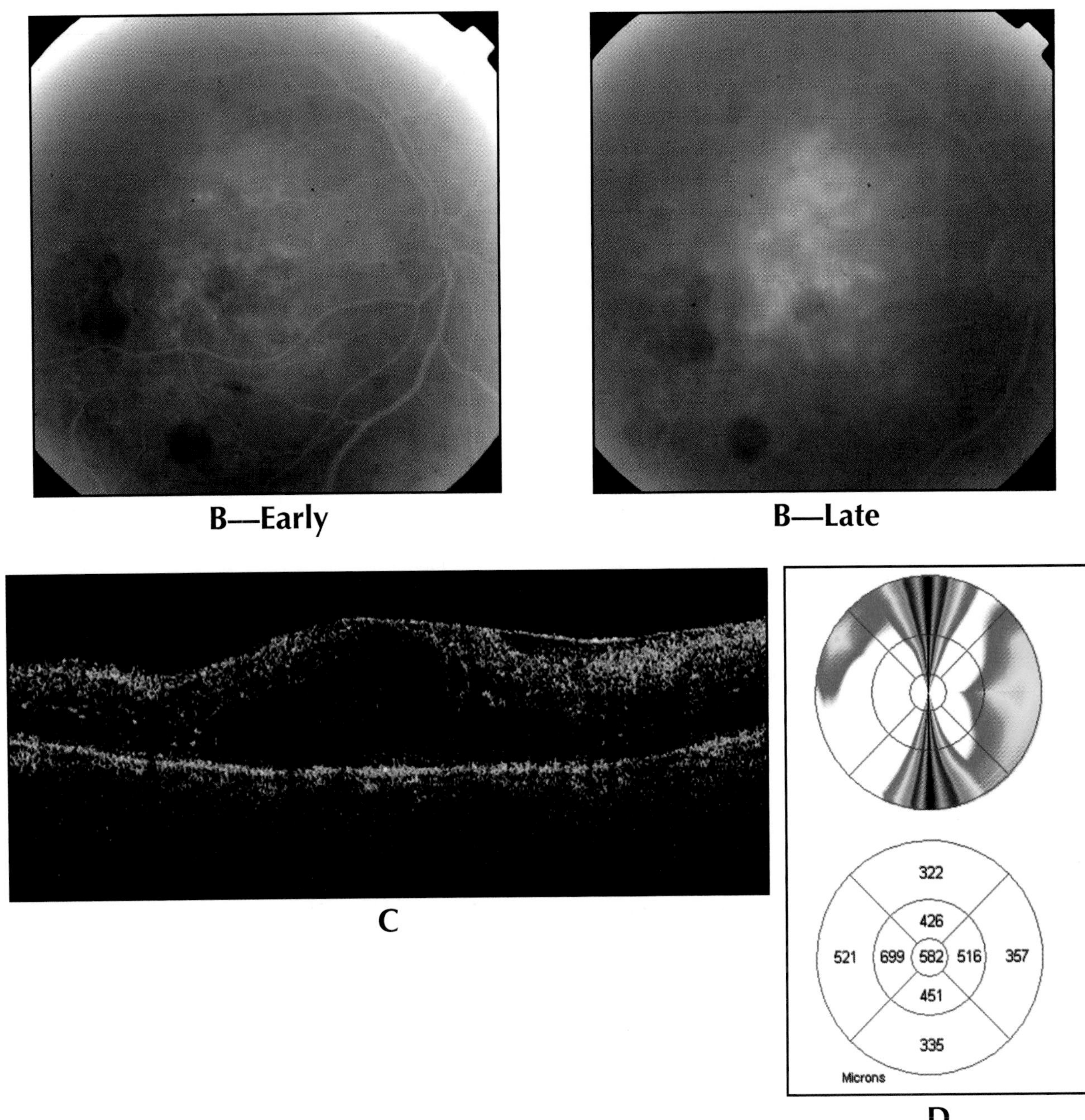

B—Early

B—Late

C

D

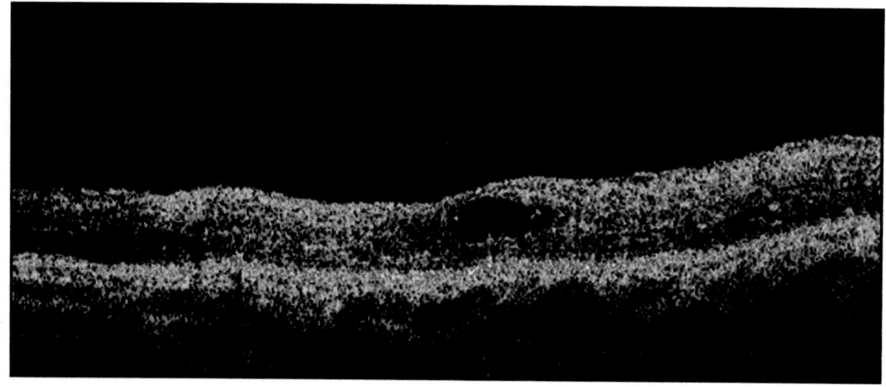

E

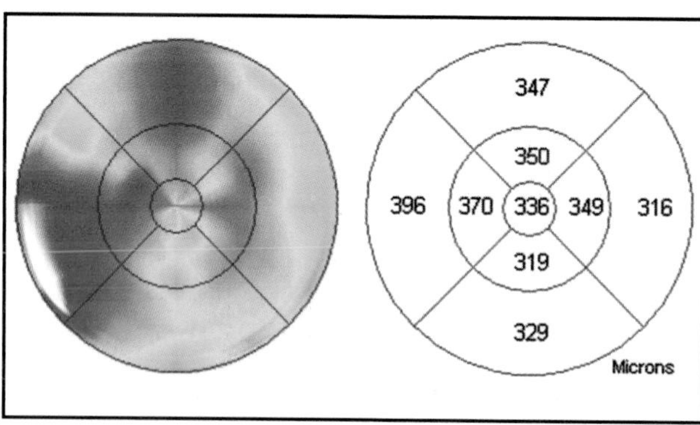

F

Case 5-13B. Proliferative Diabetic Retinopathy and Macular Edema With Epiretinal Membrane Formation

Clinical Summary

Examination of the left eye showed panretinal laser scars and hemorrhages throughout the posterior pole and midperiphery. The macular region revealed hard exudates temporal to the fovea and retinal thickening consistent with clinically significant macular edema (G). The visual acuity in this eye was 20/100. Fluorescein angiography (H) showed numerous dots of hyperfluorescence, representing microaneurysms, and perifoveal late leakage in a cystoid petalloid fashion.

Optical Coherence Tomography

A vertical OCT scan (I) pictured intraretinal areas of reduced reflectivity consistent with intraretinal cystic fluid accumulation. Also, a small detachment of the neurosensory retina representing subretinal fluid accumulation was appreciated. The foveal thickness measured 630 µm (J). The patient underwent focal/grid laser photocoagulation and was re-evaluated 5 months later. The foveal thickness decreased to 395 µm and a reduction in the cystic component of the edema was appreciated (K and L). The vision improved to 20/80.

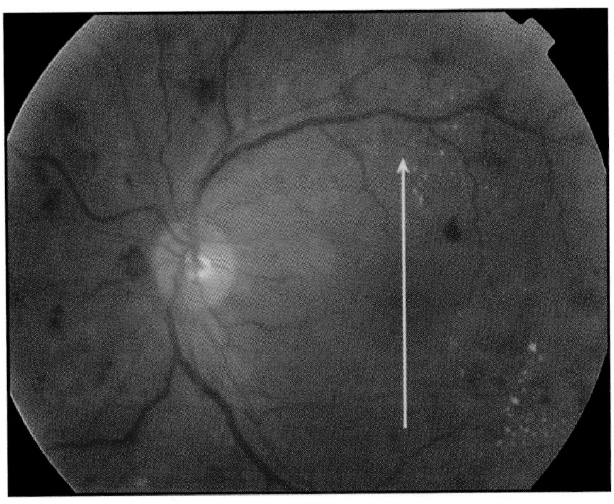

G

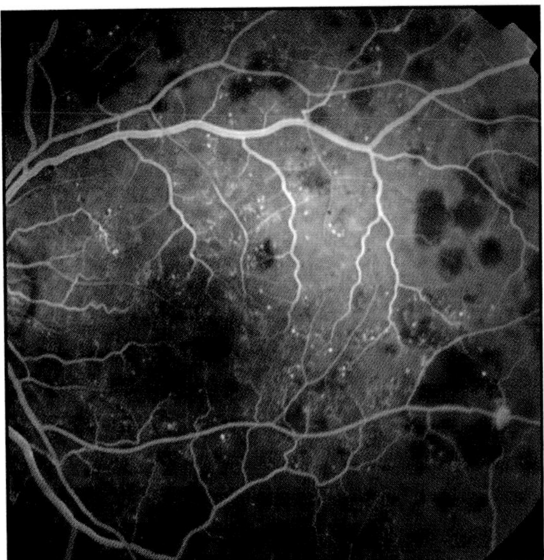

H—Early

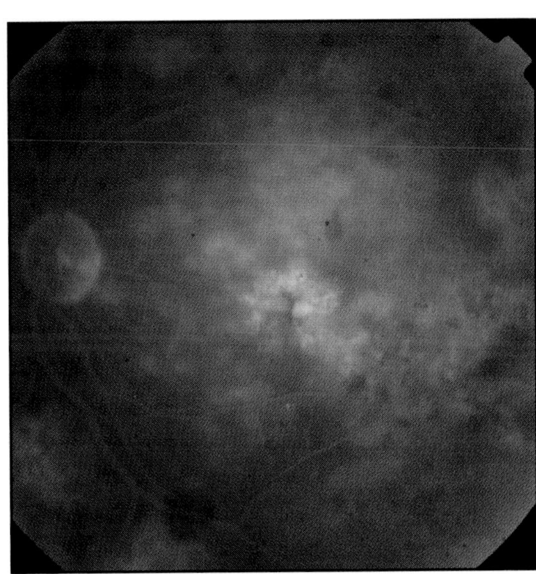

H—Late

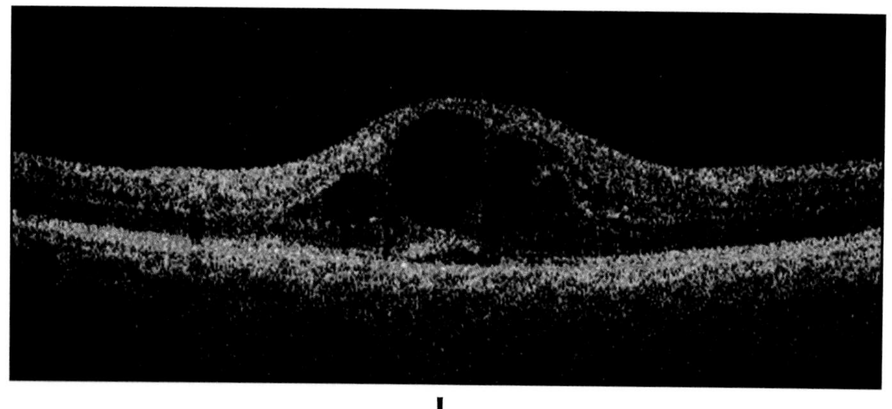

I

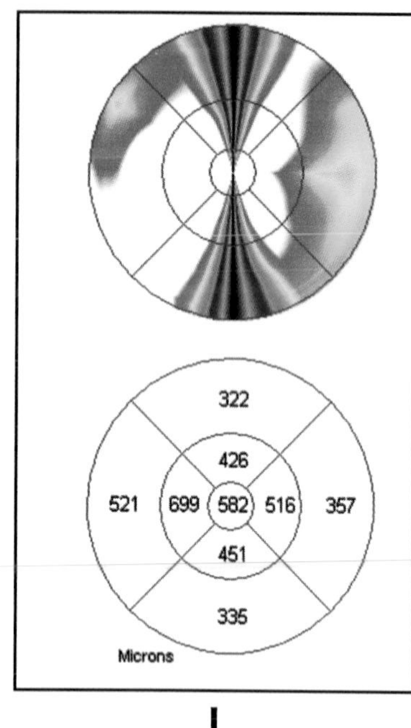
322
426
521
699
582
516
357
451
335
Microns

J

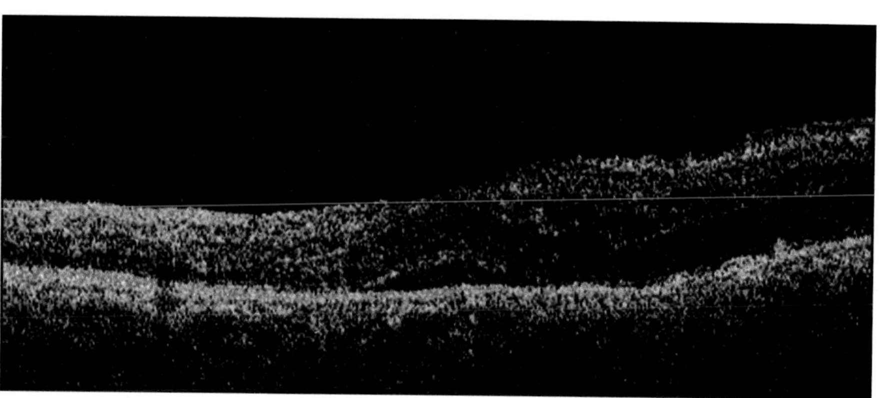

K

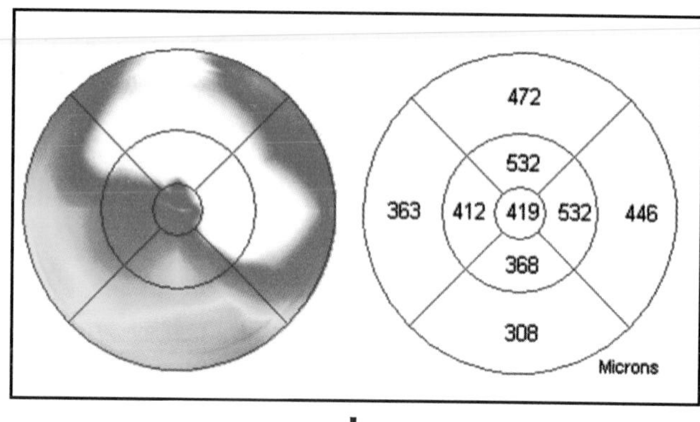
472
532
363
412
419
532
446
368
308
Microns

L

Case 5-14A. Proliferative Diabetic Retinopathy and Macular Edema

Clinical Summary

A 53-year-old man with a history of PDR noted blurred vision in both eyes. He underwent bilateral panretinal laser photocoagulation and focal/grid laser treatment 5 months earlier. His visual acuity in the right eye was 20/400. Fundus examination of this eye showed panretinal and focal/grid photocoagulation laser scars. Scattered hemorrhages, hard exudates, and retinal thickening were observed in the macular region (A). Fluorescein angiography (B) showed diffuse late leakage consistent with macular edema.

Optical Coherence Tomography

A vertical OCT scan (C) illustrated diffuse retinal thickening, loss of the normal foveal contour, and low intraretinal reflectivity consistent with fluid accumulation. Small highly reflective areas visualized in the intraretinal space corresponded to hard retinal exudates. The foveal thickness measured 517 µm (D). An intravitreal injection of triamcinolone acetonide (4 mg/0.1 cc) was offered to the patient. Seven weeks after the injection, a follow-up OCT (E and F) scan showed a striking reduction in the macular thickness to 222 µm. His visual acuity improved to 20/60.

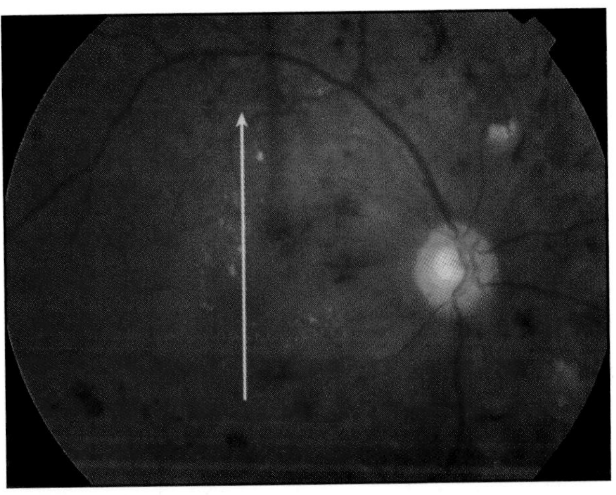

A

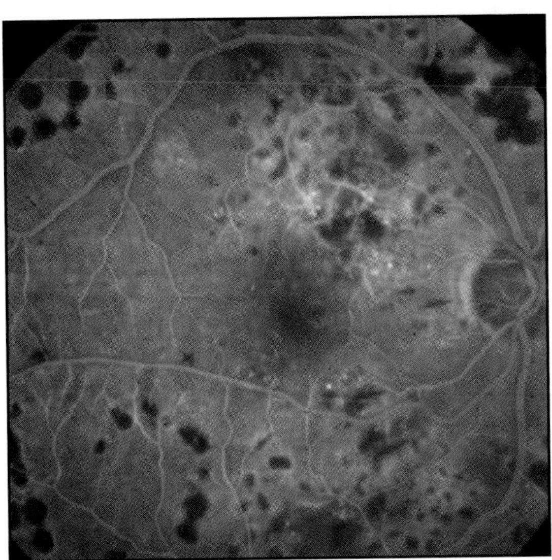

B—Early

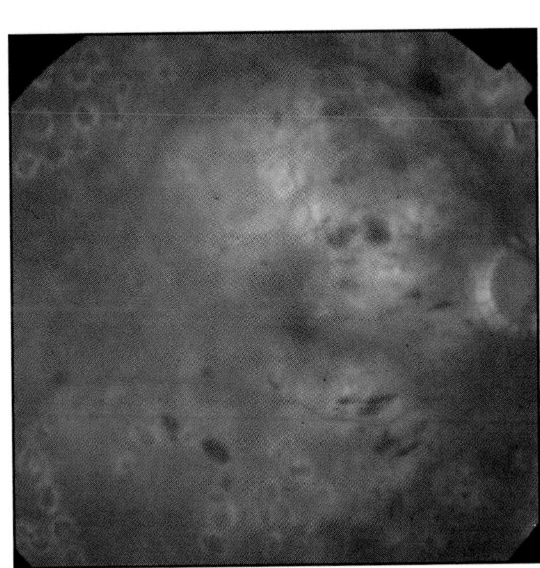

B—Late

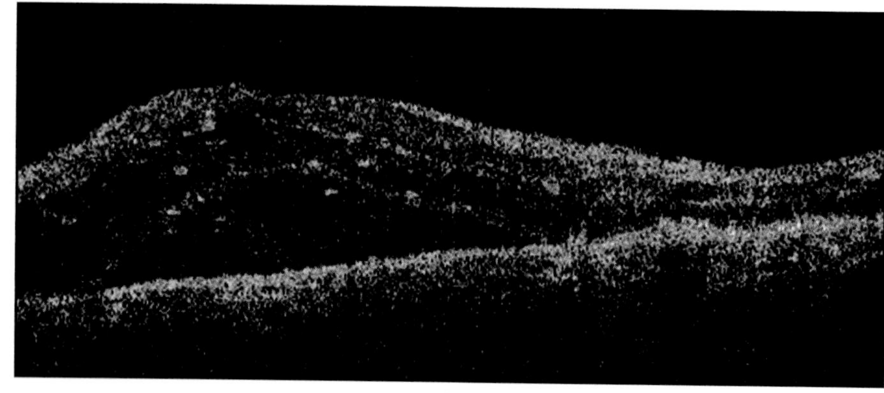

C

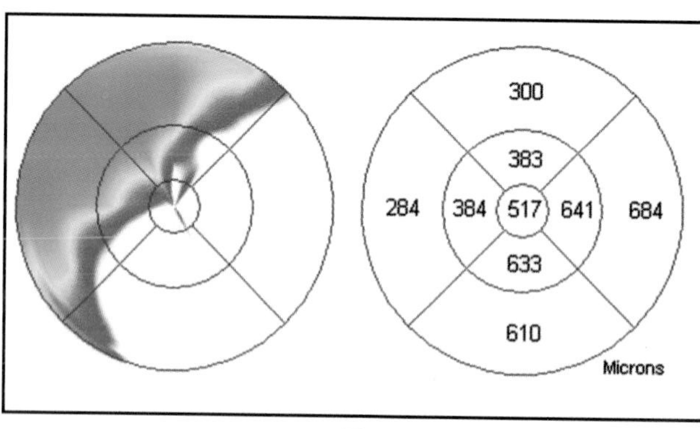
300
383
284
384
517
641
684
633
610
Microns

D

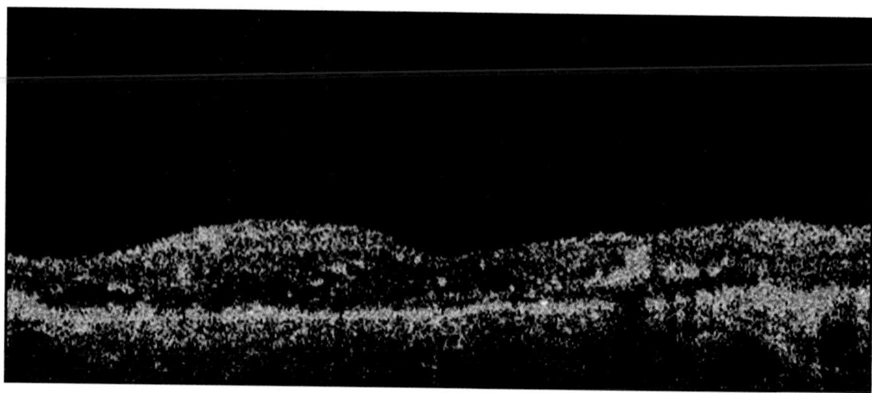

E

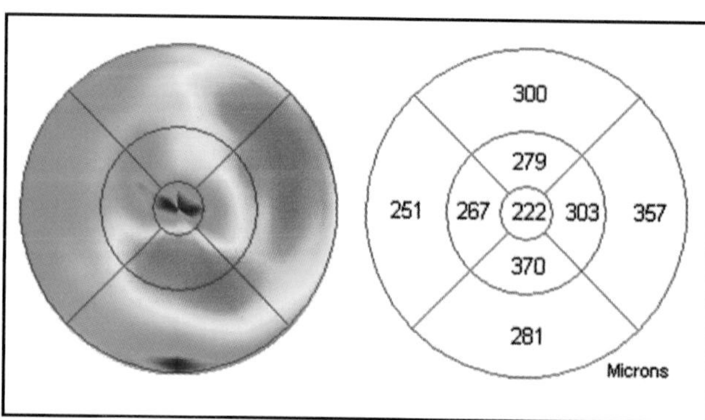
300
279
251
267
222
303
357
370
281
Microns

F

Case 5-14B. Proliferative Diabetic Retinopathy and Macular Edema

Clinical Summary

His visual acuity in the left eye was 20/100. On examination, hard lipid exudates and macular thickening were evident consistent with clinically significant macular edema. Laser scars and intraretinal hemorrhages were also observed (G). Fluorescein angiography (H) showed diffuse late leakage, confirming the presence of macular edema.

Optical Coherence Tomography

A vertical OCT scan (I) demonstrated loss of the normal foveal contour with diffuse macular thickening and low intraretinal reflectivity consistent with macular edema. Hard retinal exudates were depicted as areas of high reflectivity. The foveal thickness measured 421 µm (J). The patient underwent an intravitreal injection of triamcinolone acetonide (4 mg/0.1cc). A follow-up OCT scan (K) was performed 6 weeks after the injection. It clearly showed a remarkable reduction in the macular thickness. The foveal thickness measured 240 µm (L). His visual acuity improved to 20/40.

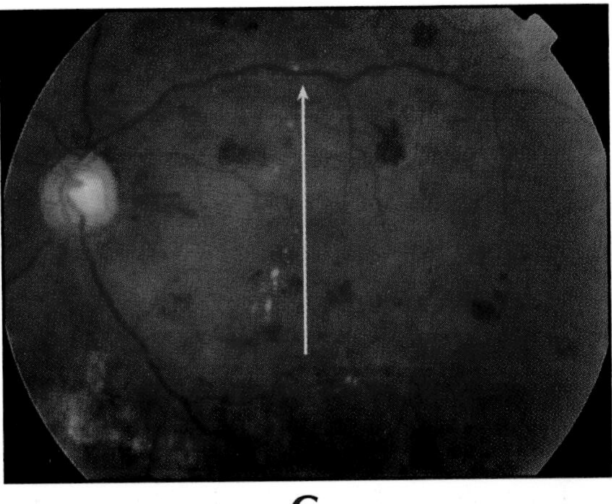

G

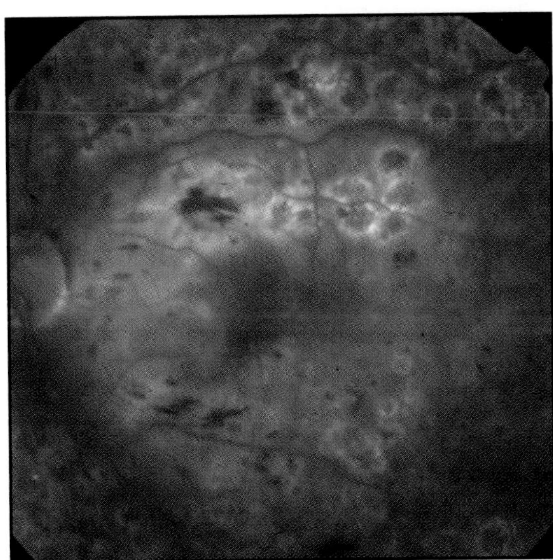

H—Early

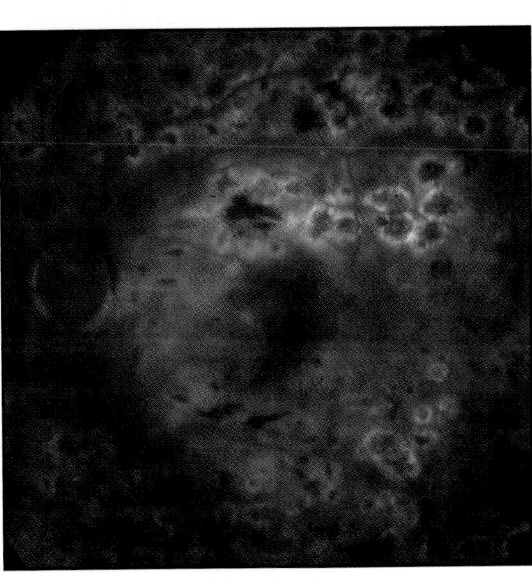

H—Late

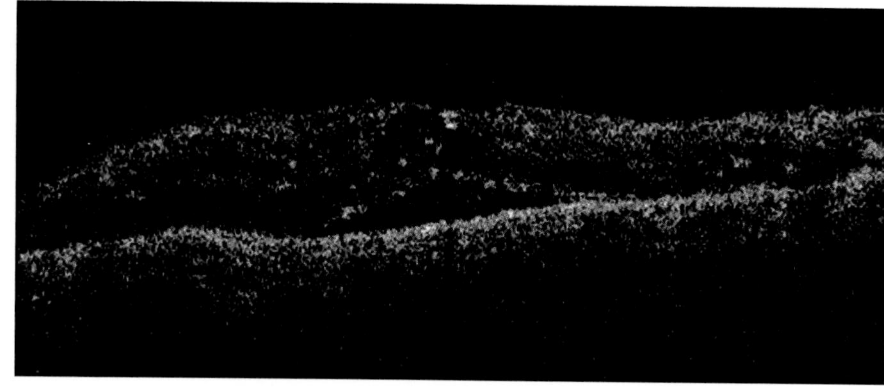

I

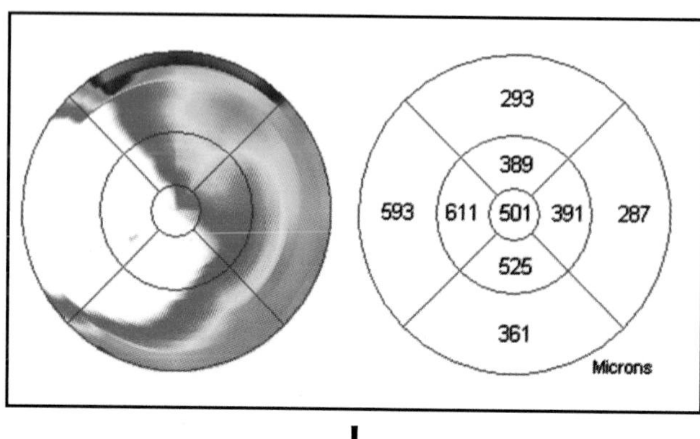
293
389
593
611
501
391
287
525
361
Microns

J

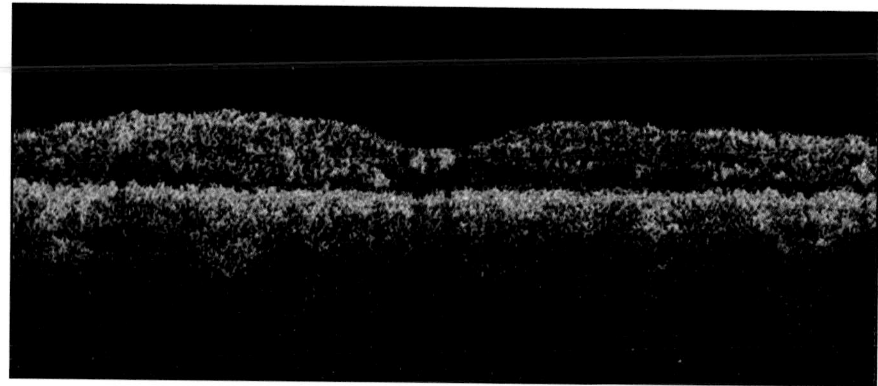

K

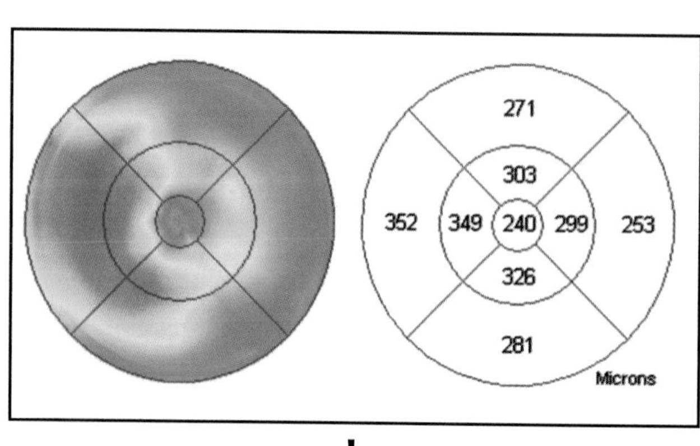
271
303
352
349
240
299
253
326
281
Microns

L

Case 5-15. Proliferative Diabetic Retinopathy and Taut Posterior Hyaloid

Clinical Summary

A 59-year-old woman with PDR had received panretinal laser photocoagulation 12 months earlier. Her visual acuity in the right eye was 20/200. Dilated fundus examination revealed panretinal laser scars, retinal thickening in the macular region, and no evidence of active neovascularization (A). Fluorescein angiography (B) revealed perifoveal leakage in a petalloid fashion consistent with CME.

Optical Coherence Tomography

A vertical OCT scan (C) through the fovea revealed a taut posterior hyaloid represented as hyperreflective bands exerting traction on the macular region. Macular thickening and large areas of low intraretinal reflectivity, corresponding to intraretinal cysts and fluid accumulation, were also appreciated. The retinal map analysis revealed a foveal thickness of 503 μm (D). Pars plana vitrectomy was offered to the patient.

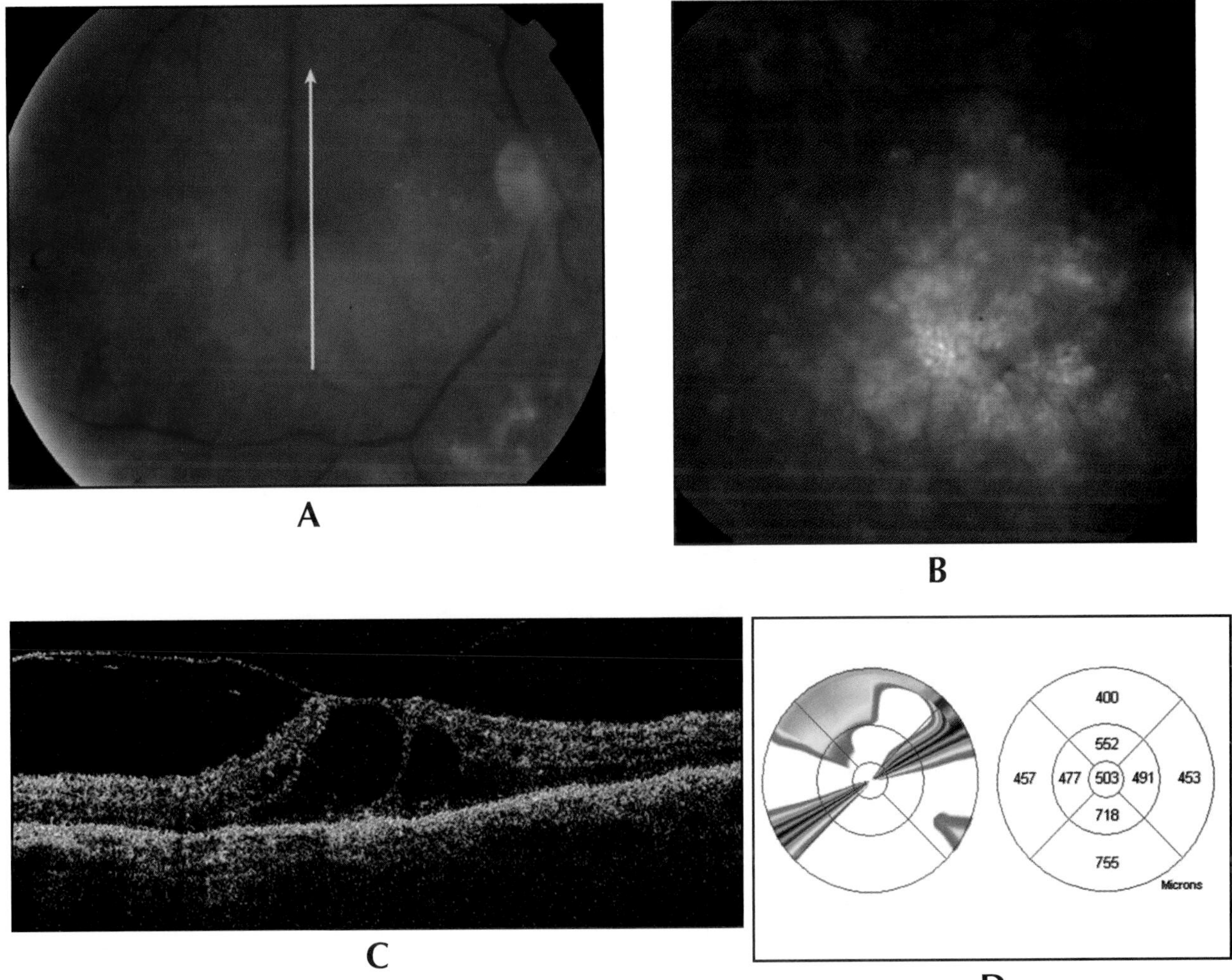

A

B

C

D

Case 5-16. Proliferative Diabetic Retinopathy With Taut Premacular Posterior Hyaloid

Clinical Summary

A 71-year-old man with PDR was examined. The right eye had a visual acuity of 20/400. Dilated fundus examination (A) revealed focal laser scars, hard exudates, and retinal thickening in the macular area. Scattered dot and blot hemorrhages were evident throughout the posterior pole. Panretinal photocoagulation laser scars were noted in the periphery. Intravenous fluorescein angiography (B) showed areas of early pinpoint hyperfluorescence consistent with micro-aneurysms associated with perifoveal late leakage.

Optical Coherence Tomography

OCT (C) demonstrated marked macular thickening and low intraretinal reflectivity consistent with intraretinal fluid accumulation. Two reflective bands were adherent to the retinal surface, representing a taut posterior hyaloid face. The retinal map analysis revealed a foveal thickness of 630 μm (D).

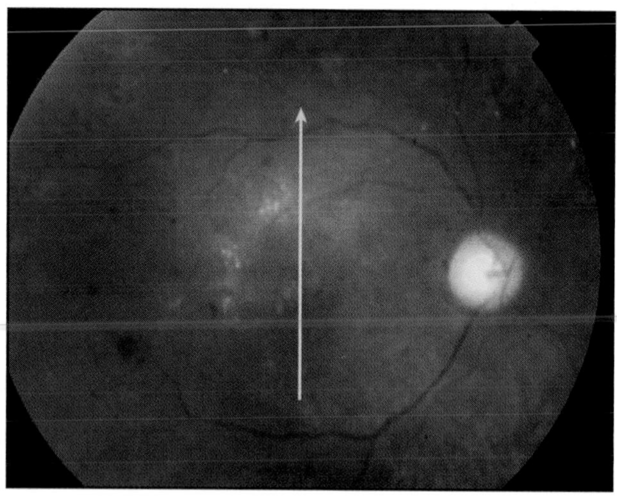

A

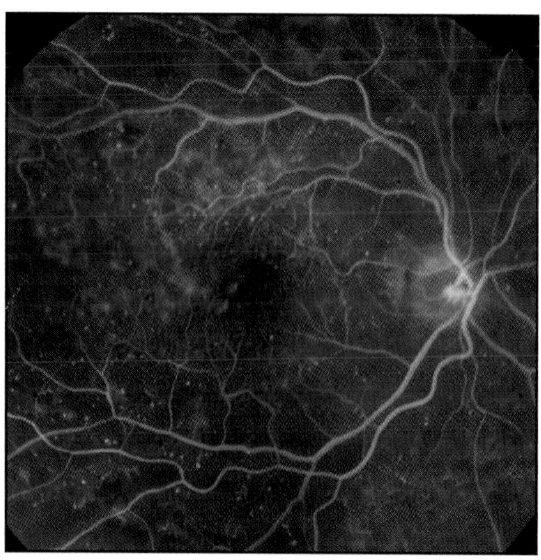

B—Early

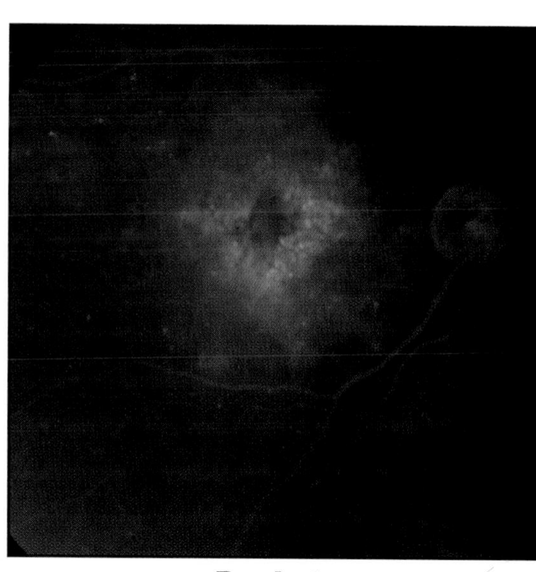

B—Late

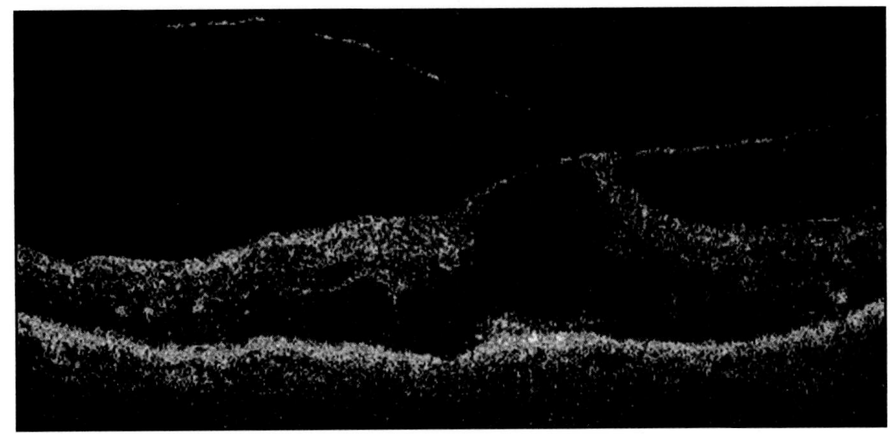

C

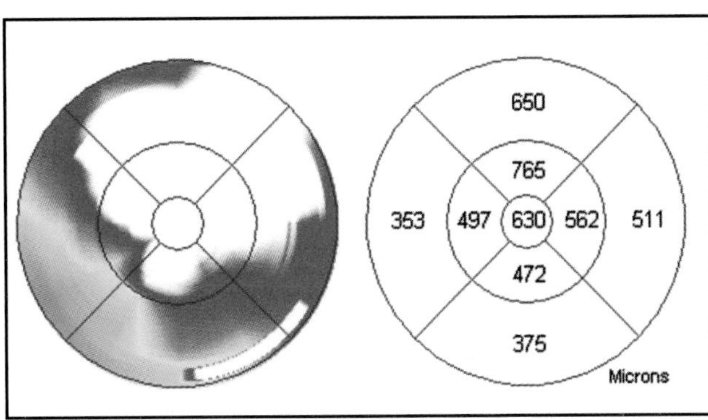

D

Case 5-17. Proliferative Diabetic Retinopathy With Preretinal Fibroglial Tissue

Clinical Summary

A 55-year-old woman with a history of PDR and macular ischemia was evaluated. The left eye had a visual acuity of 20/300. Dilated fundus examination (A) revealed scattered dot and blot hemorrhages throughout the posterior pole and fibroglial tissue extending from the superotemporal arcade toward the inferior peripapillary area. Panretinal photocoagulation laser scars were noted in the periphery.

Optical Coherence Tomography

OCT images (B) illustrated loss of the normal foveal contour and a preretinal hyperreflective band adherent to the retinal surface. This preretinal membrane is separated from the retina inferonasally (right side of the scan). The retinal map analysis revealed a foveal thickness of 317 μm (C).

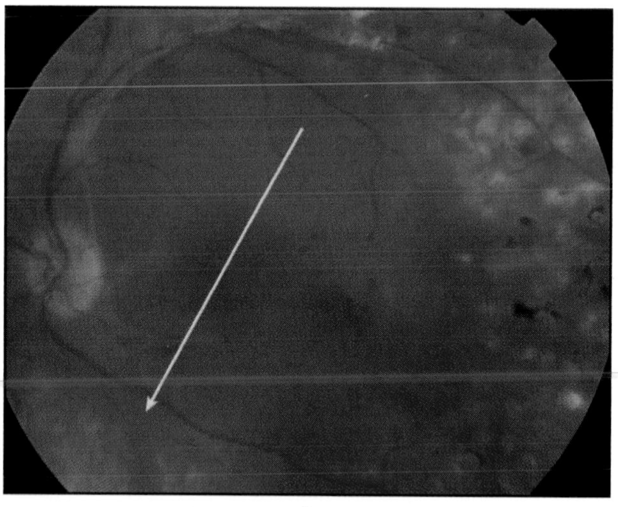

A

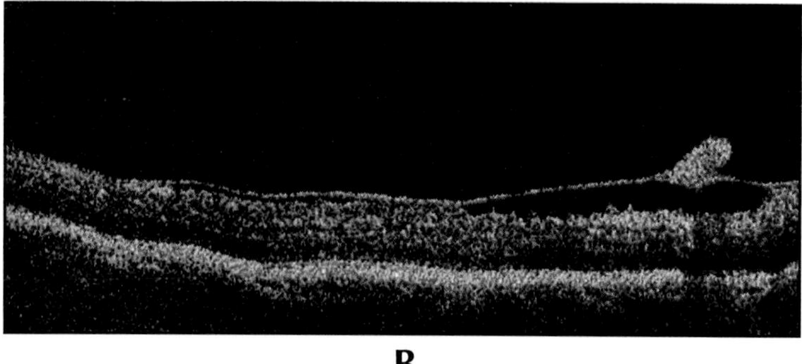

B

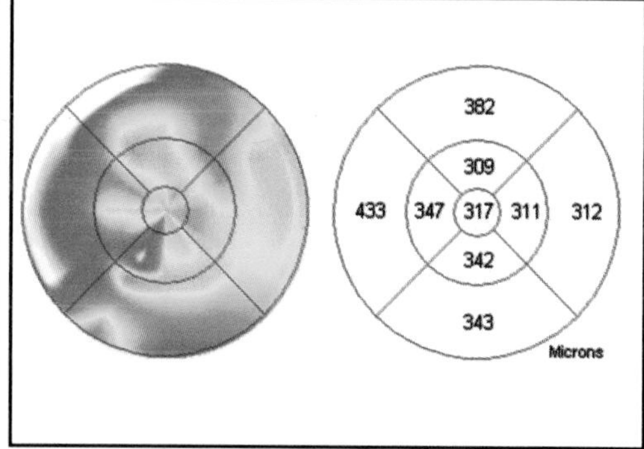

C

Case 5-18. Proliferative Diabetic Retinopathy With Macular Schisis Formation

Clinical Summary

A 77-year-old woman with a history of PDR and poor vision in the right eye was examined. Her visual acuity was HM in this eye. Clinical examination revealed sclerotic retinal vessels and diffuse pigmentary and cystic alterations in the macular region (A). Fluorescein angiography (B) showed staining and diffuse leakage in the posterior pole.

Optical Coherence Tomography

A vertical OCT scan (C) illustrated a splitting at the level of the outer retinal layers forming a schisis. An opening of the inner retina was observed. Another OCT image (D) showed cystic low reflective intraretinal spaces. Again, the hole or opening of the inner retina was visualized reminiscent of a giant lamellar hole with a schitic configuration. Probably rupture of the macular cysts created this configuration. The central foveal thickness measured 434 μm (E).

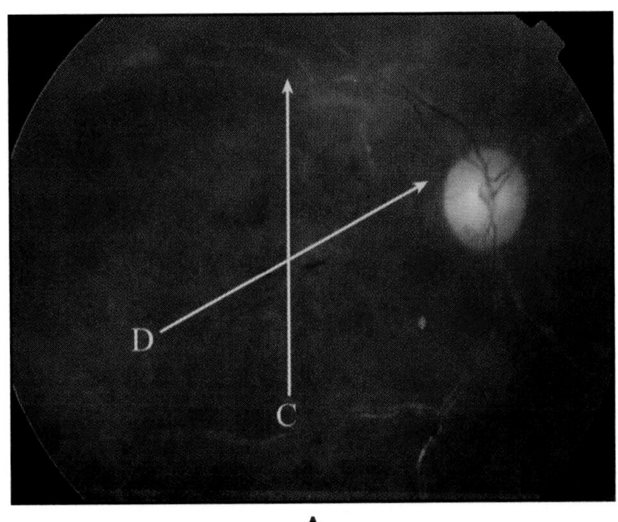

A

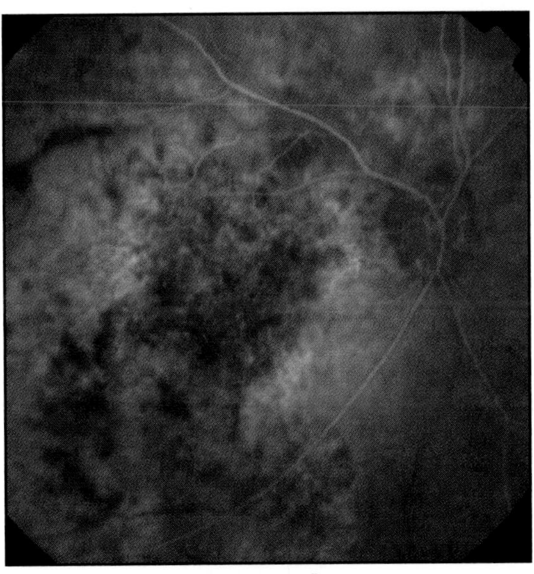

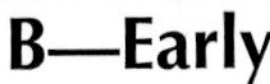

B—Early

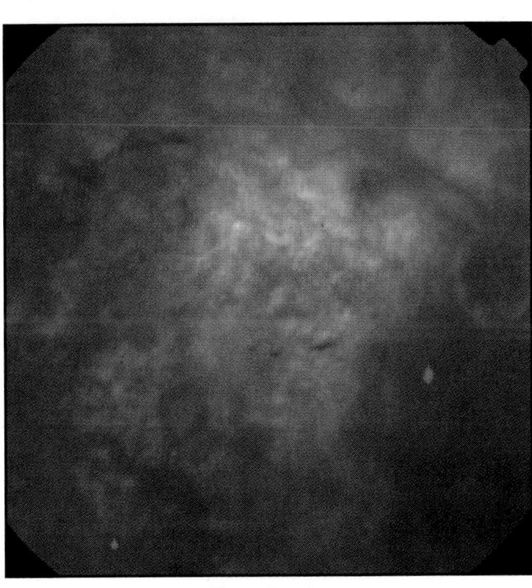

B—Late

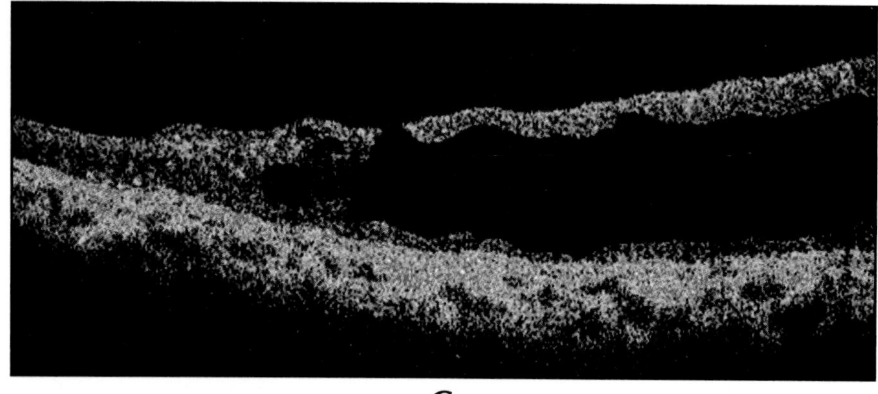

C

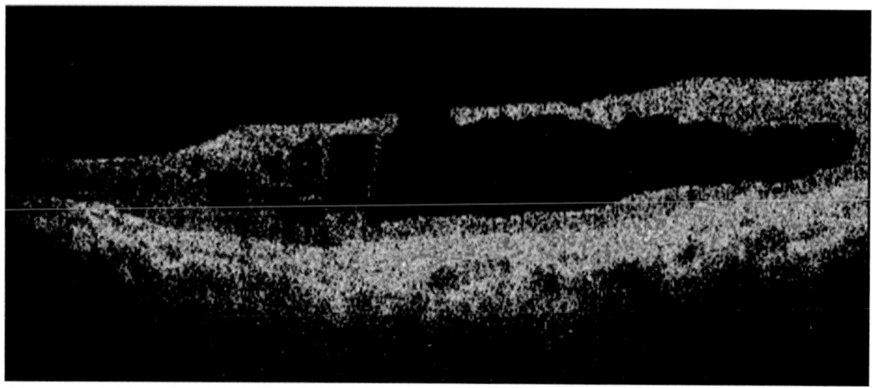

D

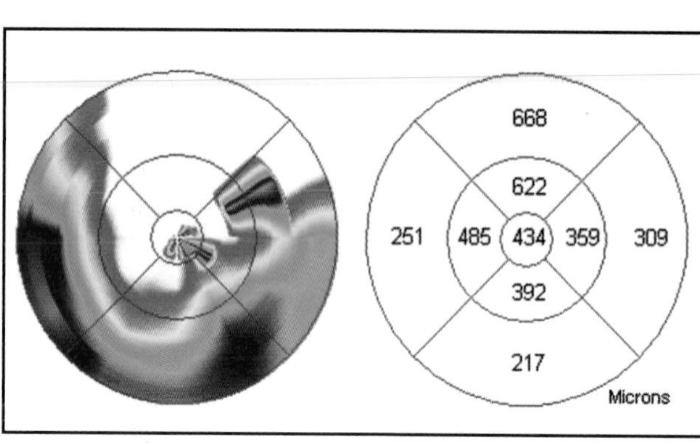

E

Case 5-19. Proliferative Diabetic Retinopathy With Tractional Retinal Detachment

Clinical Summary

A 55-year-old man with PDR was examined 1 year after receiving panretinal laser photocoagulation in his left eye. His visual acuity in this eye was 20/100. On examination, preretinal fibroglial tissue extending from the optic nerve head toward the superior and inferior arcades was evident. A localized tractional retinal detachment was observed encroaching into the nasal macula (A).

Optical Coherence Tomography

A horizontal OCT scan (B), acquired through the fovea, illustrated loss of the normal foveal contour and an area of retinal elevation nasal to the fovea (right side of the scan). A highly reflective band was noted anterior to the retina. This band or preretinal membrane was thicker nasally (right side of the scan) and associated with focal elevation and irregularity of the retina consistent with a traction retinal detachment. The band was thinner temporally (left side of the scan). This part of the band probably represented the posterior hyaloid. There was also shadowing or attenuation of the RPE/choroid reflection signal beneath the preretinal membrane. The fovea appeared intact and not elevated. Scan C showed a focal elevation of the retina inferonasal to the fovea associated with retinal thickening and a highly reflective band (right side of the scan). The band corresponded to a posterior hyaloid/preretinal gliotic membrane complex. The posterior hyaloid component of the membrane was evident as the thinner band and the preretinal membrane component was dense and tightly adherent to the retinal surface at several focal points. Areas of high optical backscattering were observed corresponding to hard lipid intraretinal exudates. Also, a small detachment of the neurosensory retina with subretinal fluid accumulation was detected. Scan D, acquired nasal to the fovea, showed retinal thickening and cystic areas of low reflectivity, at the level of the outer plexiform layer, consistent with intraretinal fluid accumulation superior to the fovea (left side of the scan). A neurosensory detachment was present, representing subretinal fluid accumulation. Again, there was thickening, elevation, and distortion of the retina inferonasal to the fovea (right side of the scan) in association with a highly reflective preretinal membrane.

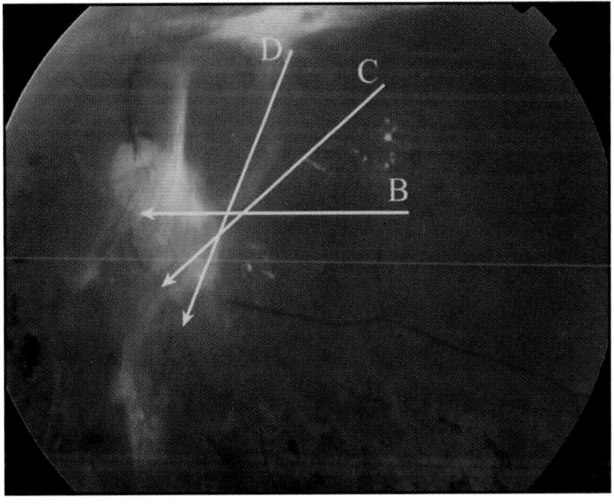

A

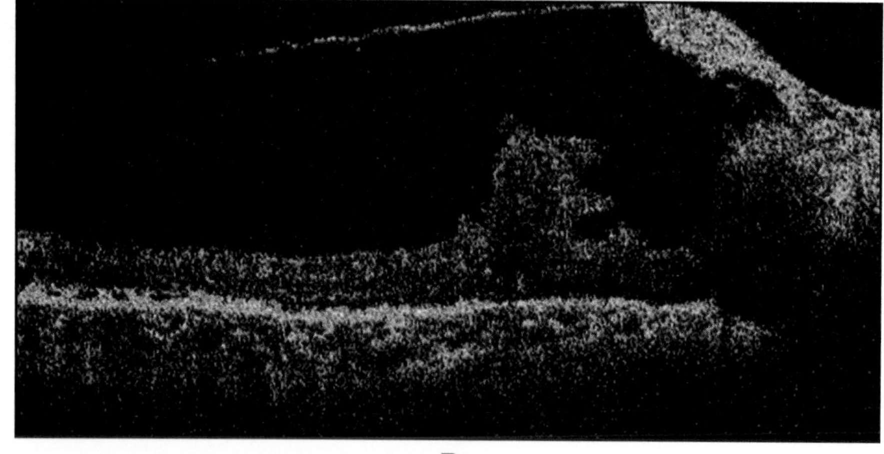

B

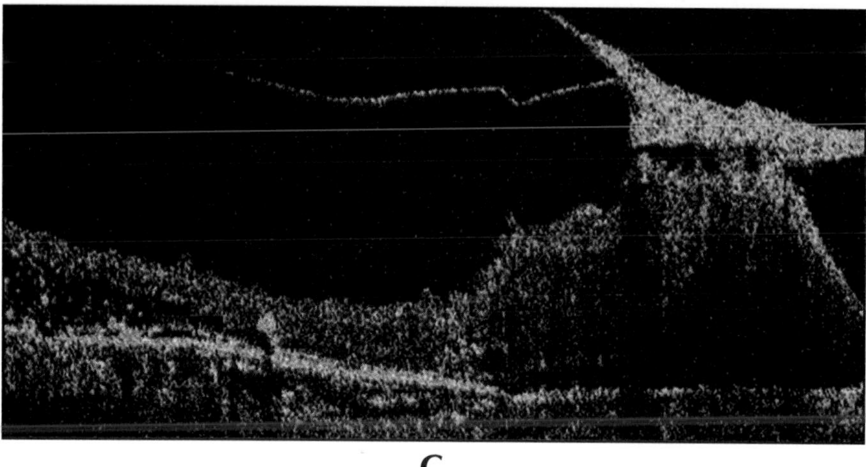

C

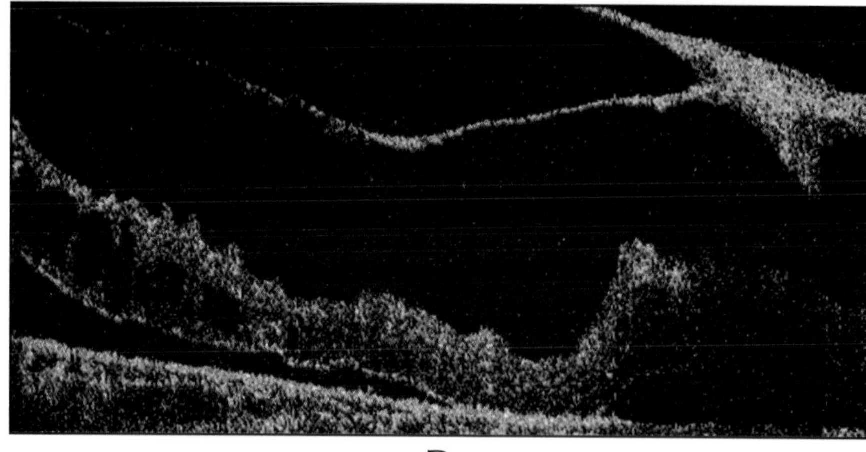

D

Case 5-20. Proliferative Diabetic Retinopathy With Tractional Retinal Detachment

Clinical Summary

A 48-year-old man with PDR undergoing panretinal laser photocoagulation in his left eye was examined. His visual acuity in this eye was 8/200. Dilated fundus examination showed a vitreous hemorrhage and preretinal fibrovascular tissue proliferation extending from the optic nerve head toward the arcades and macular area. A preretinal hemorrhage was observed along the inferotemporal arcade (A).

Optical Coherence Tomography

An OCT scan (B) revealed macular elevation and thickening associated with traction from contracted epiretinal membranes, which appeared as reflective bands attached to the retina. Cystic macular changes were visualized as low reflective spaces, more prominently at the level of the outer retinal layers. Pockets of subretinal fluid accumulation were pictured as low reflective areas beneath the neurosensory retina. A horizontal OCT scan (C) showed a highly reflective band corresponding to fibrovascular tissue inserting at the fovea and nasally (right side of the scan). An OCT scan (D) was obtained through the preretinal hemorrhage, which was characterized as a highly reflective layer in front of the retinal tissue. Shadowing of the optical reflections from the tissues beneath was noticed. The central foveal thickness measured 439 µm (E). The patient underwent pars plana vitrectomy and membrane peel with gas fluid exchange. Two months later, clinical examination revealed a flat retina with no tractional component (F). An OCT scan (G) confirmed resolution of the CME and relief of the traction resulting in a normal foveal contour. The foveal thickness decreased to 175 µm (H). The visual acuity improved to 20/100.

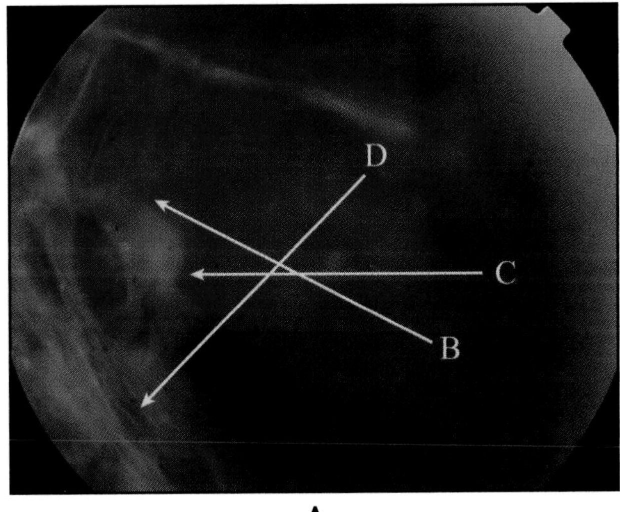

A

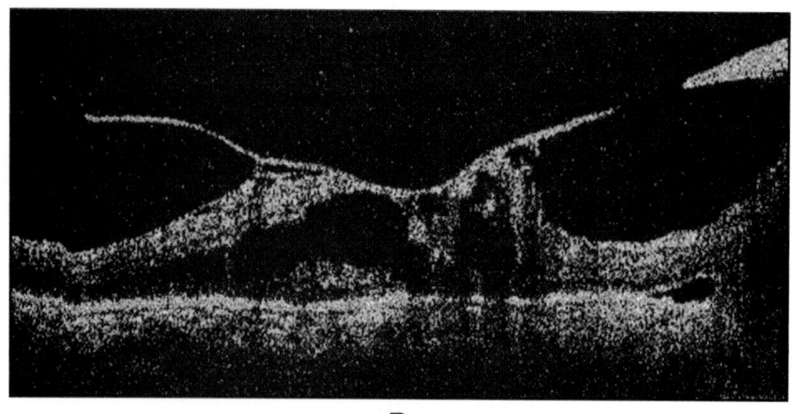

B

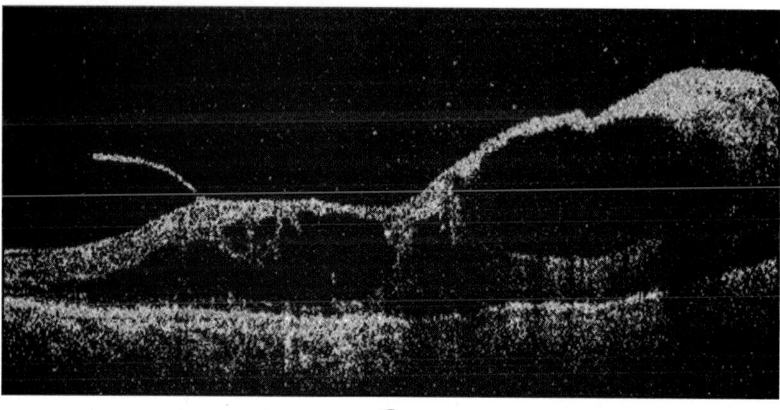

C

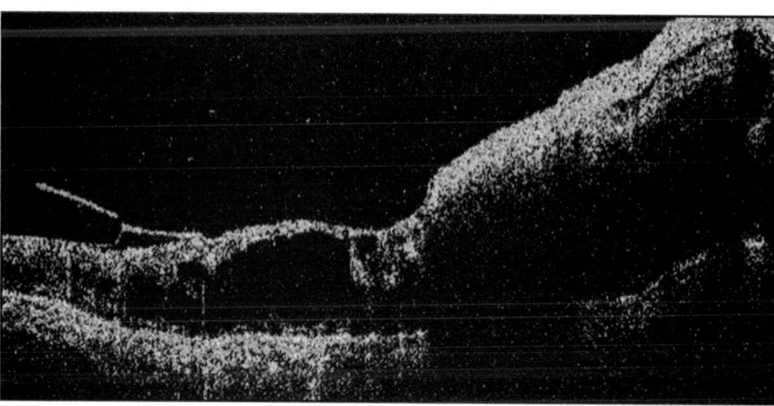

D

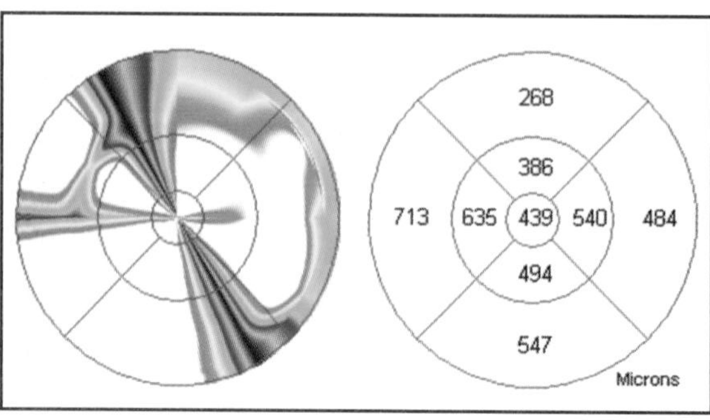

E

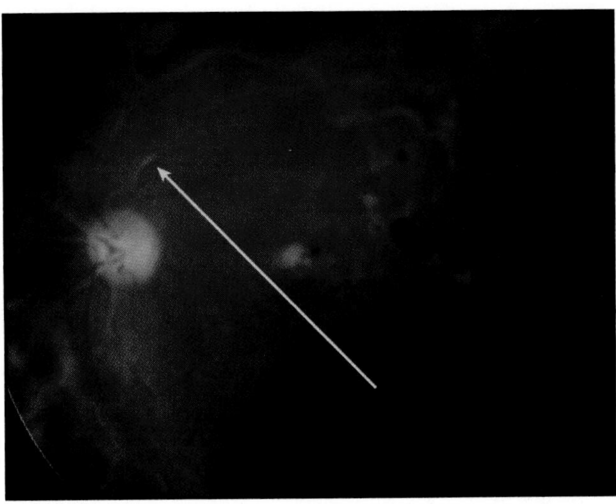

F

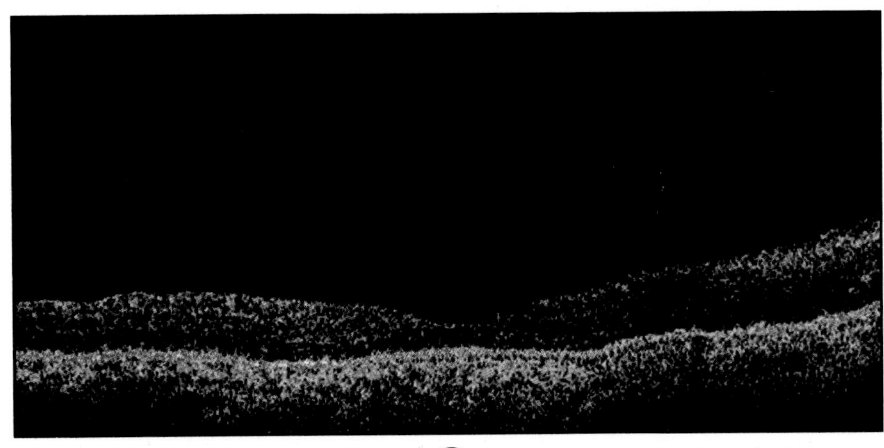

G

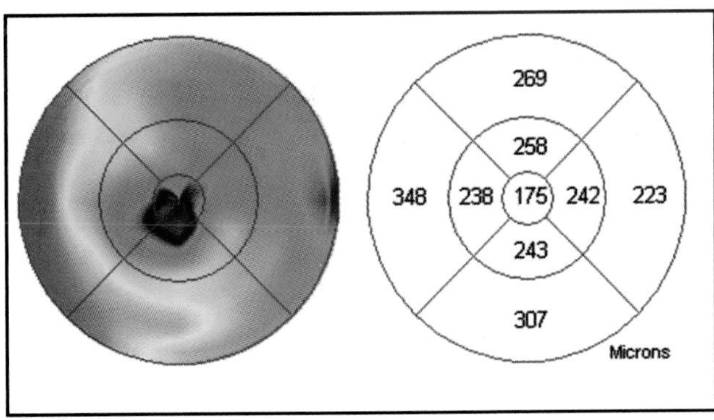

H

Chapter 6

Central Serous Chorioretinopathy

Elias C. Mavrofrides, MD; Carmen A. Puliafito, MD; and James G. Fujimoto, PhD

- Typical Central Serous Chorioretinopathy
- Chronic Central Serous Chorioretinopathy
- Bullous Central Serous Chorioretinopathy
- Laser Treatment for Central Serous Chorioretinopathy
- Photodynamic Therapy Treatment for Central Serous Chorioretinopathy

Central serous chorioretinopathy (CSCR) is characterized by serous detachment of the neurosensory retina in the macular region. This condition occurs most commonly in healthy individuals between 20 to 50 years of age, and there is a strong male predominance.[1,2] Stressful events, "type A" personality, pregnancy, and steroid use are common predisposing factors to this condition.[3-6]

Patients usually present with complaints of decreased and distorted central visual acuity. Micropsia, central scotoma, and decreased color vision are also common complaints. Most patients show evidence of a well-circumscribed neurosensory detachment in the macular region. The fovea is frequently involved, and small associated pigment epithelial detachments are commonly seen.[1,2]

Fluorescein angiography shows one or more focal leaks at the level of the retinal pigment epithelium (RPE) with subsequent pooling of dye in the subretinal space. Indocyanine green (ICG) angiography typically demonstrates large hyperfluorescent patches with late leakage, suggesting abnormal choroidal hyperpermeability as an etiologic factor.[1,2,7]

Optical coherence has become an effective means for both qualitative and quantitative evaluation of patients with CSCR. Serous detachment of the neurosensory retina can be seen on the optical coherence tomography (OCT) image as elevation of the retinal layers above an optically clear fluid-filled cavity. When the underlying pigment epithelium remains attached, this can be seen as a highly reflective band at the base of this clear cavity.

The serous pigment epithelial detachments that frequently accompany elevation of the neurosensory retina are also readily identified on the OCT image. These appear as localized elevations of the highly reflective RPE signal over a clear cavity. The detached RPE causes attenuation of the reflected light, resulting in extensive shadowing of the underlying choroidal signal. This sign can be helpful in distinguishing retinal detachment from larger serous RPE detachments. Occasionally, the reflection from the posterior surface of detached neurosensory retina may be increased and mimic a detachment of the RPE; however, in this case, there is only minimal shadowing of the choroidal signal.[8]

In some cases, diagnosis of CSCR can be difficult due to shallow subretinal fluid. Despite significant visual complaints, there may be minimal changes identified on clinical exam. OCT is highly sensitive in establishing small elevations of the retina because of the clear difference in optical reflectivity between retinal tissue and serous fluid. Wang and associates have recently reported on a series of seven patients with classic symptoms of CSCR in which the presence of subretinal fluid could not be definitely established with biomicroscopy or fluorescein angiography.[9] All of these patients showed shallow elevation of the neurosensory retina on OCT imaging, demonstrating that OCT is superior to these other techniques in identifying such detachments.

OCT imaging can be useful in defining anatomic changes of the detached neurosensory retina. Hee and associates were the first to describe thickening of the detached neurosensory retina with intraretinal cystic changes in a case of CSCR.[8] Iida and associates have subsequently demonstrated thickening of the detached retina in 23 patients during the acute phase of CSCR. Despite this thickening, most patients maintained some evidence of a foveal pit in the area of detachment. All patients showed a statistically significant decrease in foveal thickness following resolution of the neurosensory detachment.[10]

Although CSCR typically occurs in young patients, this condition can be seen in the elderly. In these cases, it may be difficult to differentiate this condition clinically from age-related macular degeneration (ARMD) and subretinal neovascularization.[11] In addition, occult choroidal neovascularization may have a similar angiographic appearance to CSCR when a focal leakage point is present. OCT can provide additional information to distinguish these conditions by confirming the presence of a serous neurosensory detachment versus the abnormalities in the RPE and choriocapillaris that result from neovascular membranes (see Chapter 7).

One of the most important applications of OCT in CSCR is quantitative monitoring of the clinical course over time. Most cases of CSCR will resolve spontaneously over 4 to 6 months. Therapeutic interventions such as focal laser or photodynamic therapy are considered when there is persistence of fluid, recurrence of fluid, and/or significant visual dysfunction.[1,2]

Quantitative measurements of subretinal fluid on OCT can be used to identify changes on follow-up examinations. This can be extremely useful in determining proper management. Small improvements may not be recognized by the patient and may be difficult to establish on clinical exam alone. Quantitatively establishing even small reductions in subretinal fluid may indicate the need for further observation. Conversely, documenting persistent or increased subretinal fluid after a period of observation can provide the impetus for intervention.

References

1. Gass JDM. Pathogenesis of disciform detachment of the neuroepithelium, II: idiopathic central serous chorioretinopathy. *Am J Ophthalmol*. 1976;63:587-615.
2. Ciardella AP, Guyer DR, Spitznas M, Yannuzzi LA. *Central serous chorioretinopathy*. In: Ryan SA, ed. *Retina*. St. Louis, Mo: Mosby; 2001:1169-1170.
3. Gelber GS, Schatz H. Loss of vision due to central serous chorioretinopathy following psychological stress. *Am J Psychiatry*. 1987;144:46-50.
4. Yannuzzi LA. Type-A behavior and central serous chorioretinopathy. *Retina*. 1987;7:111-131.
5. Gass JDM. Central serous chorioretinopathy and white subretinal exudation during pregnancy. *Arch Ophthalmol*. 1991;109:677-681.
6. Gass JD, Little H. Bilateral bullous exudative retinal detachment complicating idiopathic central serous chorioretinopathy during systemic corticosteroid therapy. *Ophthalmology*. 1995;102:737-747.
7. Piccolino FC, Borgia L. Central serous chorioretinopathy and indocyanine green angiography. *Retina*. 1994;14:231-242.
8. Hee MR, Puliafito CA, Wong C, et al. Optical coherence tomography (OCT) of central serous chorioretinopathy. *Am J Ophthalmol*. 1995;120:65-74.
9. Wang M, Sander B, Lund-Anderson H, Larsen M. Detection of shallow detachments in central serous chorioretinopathy. *Acta Ophthalmol Scand*. 1999;77:402-405.
10. Iida T, Norikazu H, Sato T, Kishi S. Evaluation of central serous chorioretinopathy with optical coherence tomography. *Ophthalmology*. 2000;129:16-20.
11. Schatz H, Madeira D, Johnson RN, McDonald HR. Central serous chorioretinopathy occurring in patients 60 years of age and older. *Ophthalmology*. 1992;99:63-67.

Case 6-1. Central Serous Chorioretinopathy

Clinical Summary

A 38-year-old male is referred for evaluation of distorted central vision in the right eye for the past week. His best-corrected visual acuity (BCVA) is 20/25 in this eye. Dilated fundus examination (A) shows a well-defined, circular area of retinal elevation. The fluorescein angiogram (B) shows a small hyperfluorescent spot under this area of retinal elevation that progressively leaks throughout the study.

Optical Coherence Tomography

The vertical OCT tomogram (C) confirms detachment of the neurosensory retina involving the fovea. The optically clear space beneath the detached retina indicates serous subretinal fluid. This subretinal fluid cavity measures 220 microns (μm) in maximum height. Mild intraretinal edema has resulted in slight thickening of the detached fovea and blunting of the foveal pit contour. The high-intensity RPE signal is uniform in appearance and remains in its normal anatomic position.

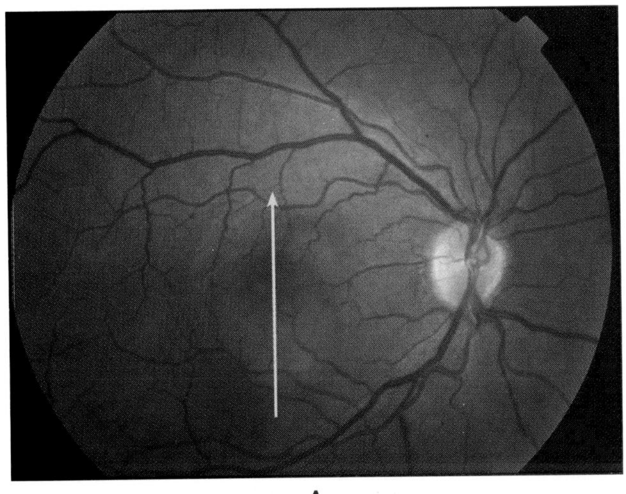

A

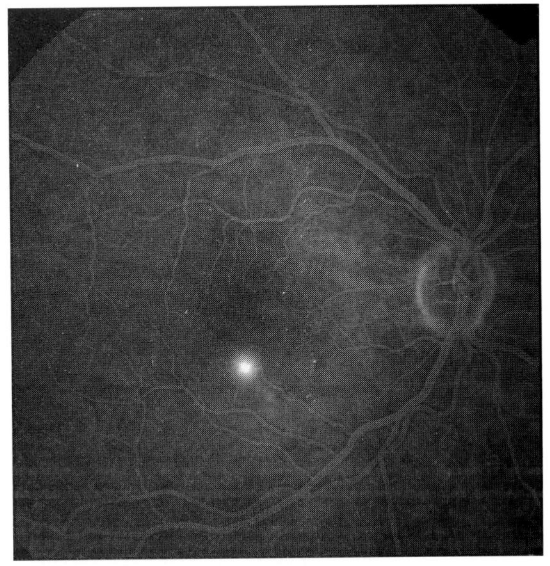

B

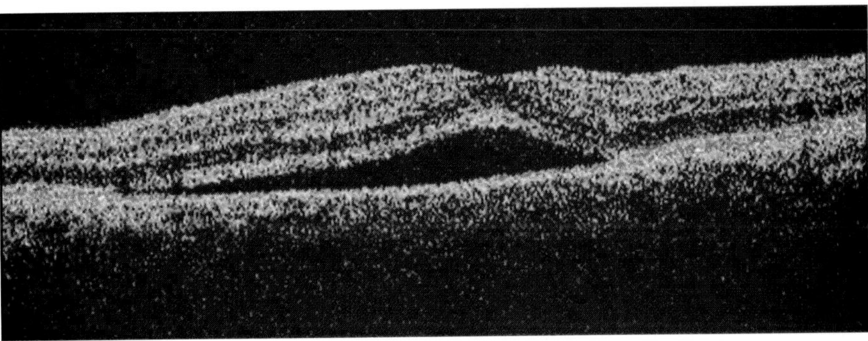

C

Case 6-2. Central Serous Chorioretinopathy

Clinical Summary

A 42-year-old male complains of painless, progressive loss of his central vision in the right eye over the past month. His BCVA is 20/40 in this eye. On dilated fundus examination (A), there is blunting of the foveal reflex with questionable shallow. The fluorescein angiogram (B) shows a single pinpoint leak inferior to the fovea but does not delineate the area of subretinal fluid.

Optical Coherence Tomography

Radial OCT cuts through the fovea (C to F) can be used to define the area of neurosensory detachment. There is a large area of subretinal fluid in the inferonasal macula over the area of leakage seen on the angiogram. The fluid extends under the fovea, but the neurosensory retina superior to the fovea remains attached. The detached retina shows preservation of the foveal pit contour with minimal anatomic alteration.

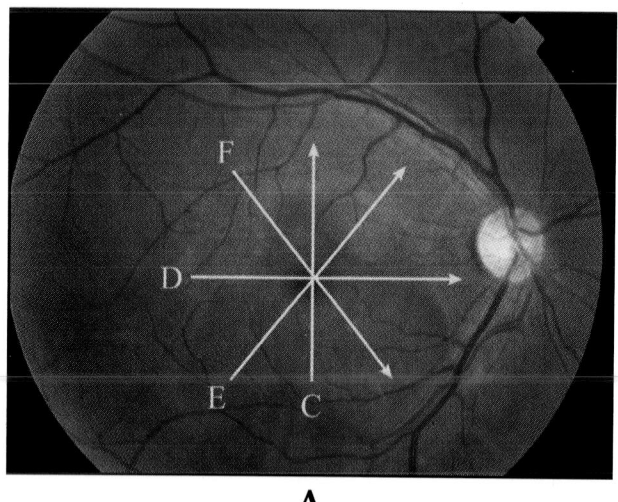

A

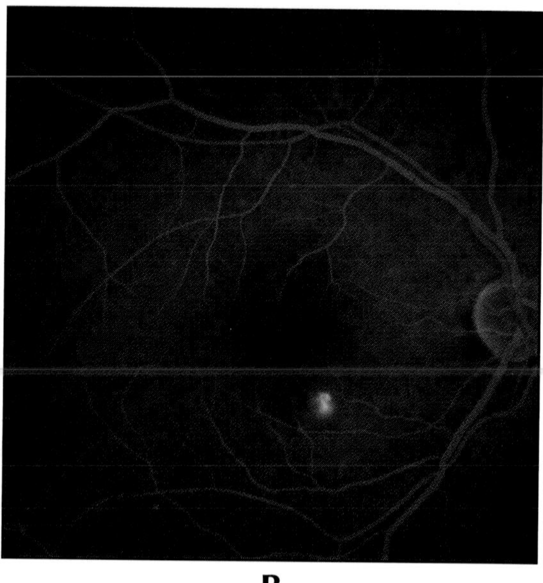

B

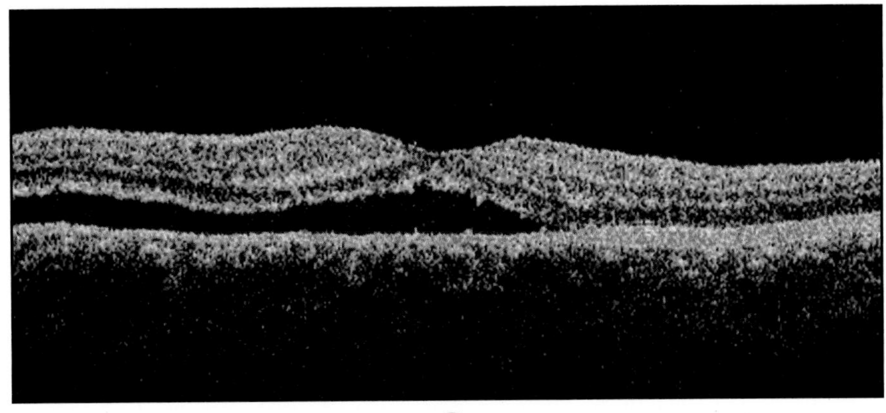

C

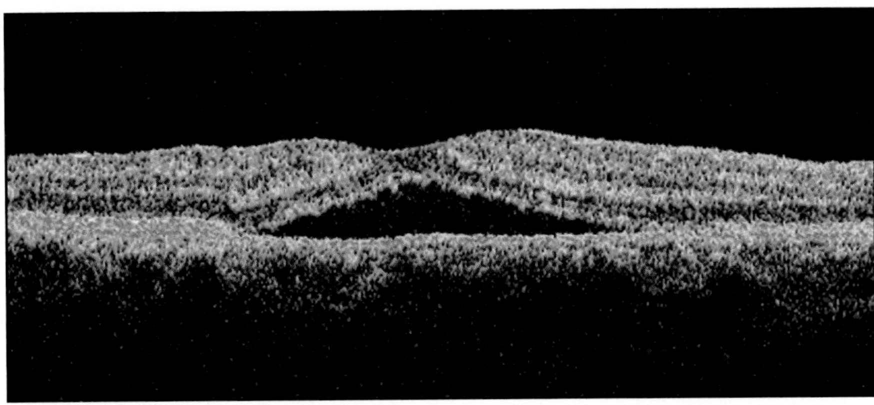

D

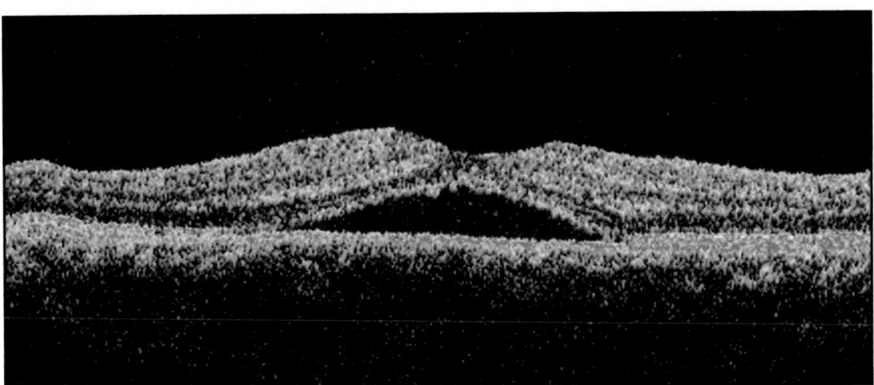

E

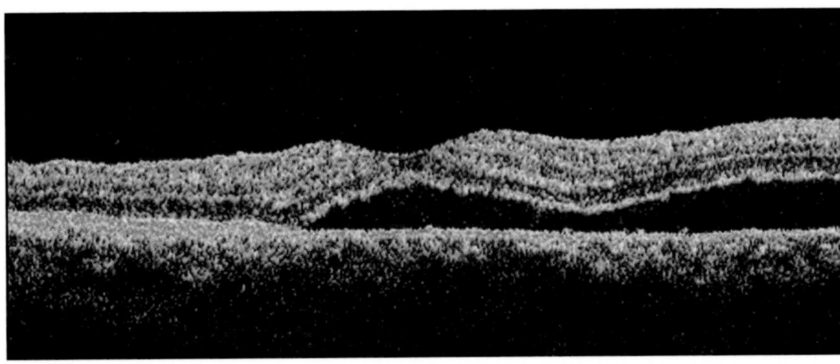

F

Case 6-3. Central Serous Chorioretinopathy

Clinical Summary

A 48-year-old male complains of a dark spot in the center of his vision in the right eye. This spot has fluctuated in size over the past 3 weeks. His visual acuity in this eye is 20/25. Dilated fundus examination (A) shows subtle elevation of the fovea. The fluorescein angiogram (B) shows two well-defined hyperfluorescent spots adjacent to the fovea and mottled hyperfluorescence around the disc. The presence of subretinal fluid cannot be confirmed on the angiogram.

Optical Coherence Tomography

The OCT (C) demonstrates a pocket of serous fluid elevating the neurosensory retina. At the edge of this neurosensory detachment, there is a focal elevation of the RPE signal over a clear space. This corresponds to the small serous pigment epithelial detachment seen on angiography. The subretinal fluid cavity reaches a maximum height of 220 µm under the fovea, while the RPE detachment has a maximum height of 115 µm.

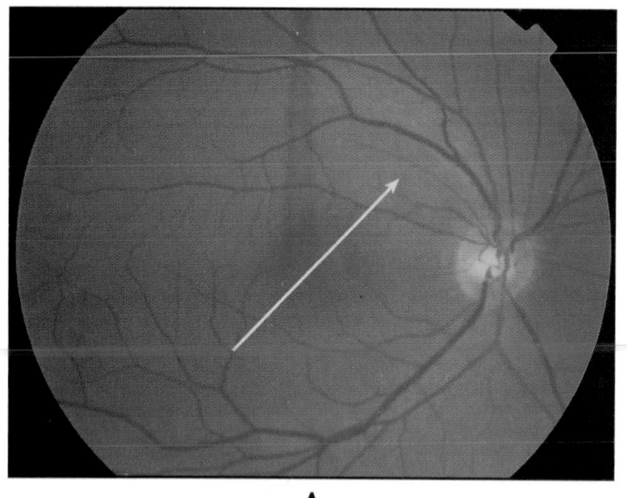

A

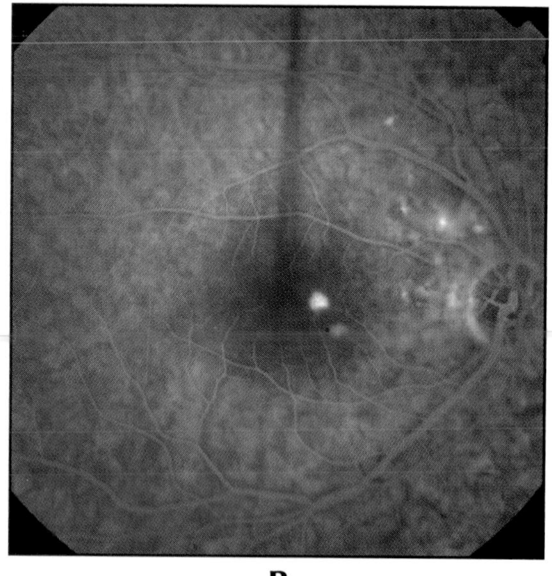

B

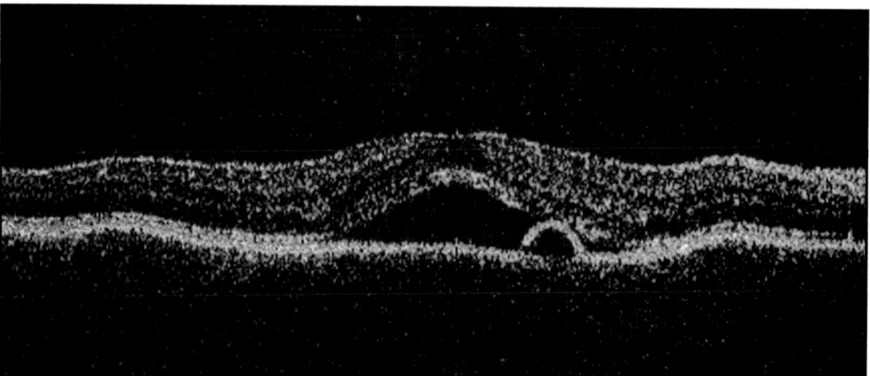

C

Case 6-4. Central Serous Chorioretinopathy

Clinical Summary

A 61-year-old male presents with worsening central vision in his right eye over the past 2 weeks. His visual acuity in this eye is 20/200 but improves to 20/40 with a more hyperopic refraction. Dilated fundus examination (A) shows a circular area of subretinal fluid involving the fovea without associated subretinal hemorrhage or exudates. The fluorescein angiogram (B) reveals a localized area of leakage just superior to the fovea.

Optical Coherence Tomography

The OCT (C) confirms a serous detachment of the neurosensory retina extending through the fovea. There is focal elevation of the RPE signal, suggesting a localized serous RPE detachment, as the scan passes through the area of leakage identified on the angiogram. Abnormal thickening or disruption of the reflective band that corresponds to the RPE and choriocapillaris is not observed, which provides evidence against the diagnosis of choroidal neovascularization.

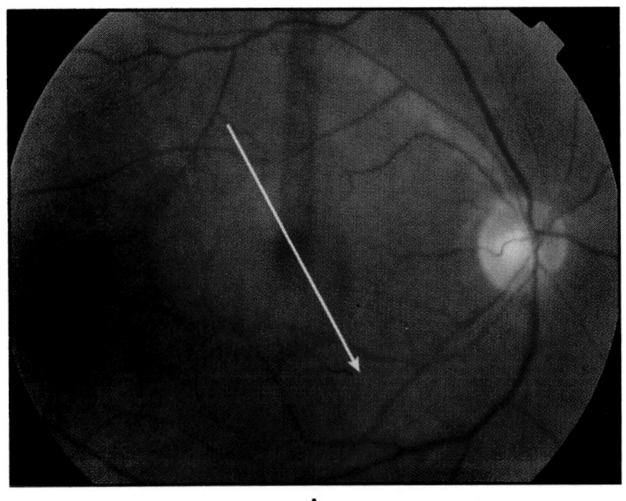

A

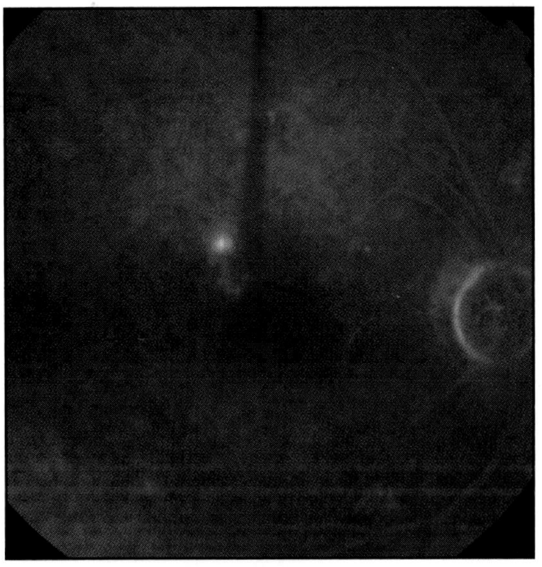

B

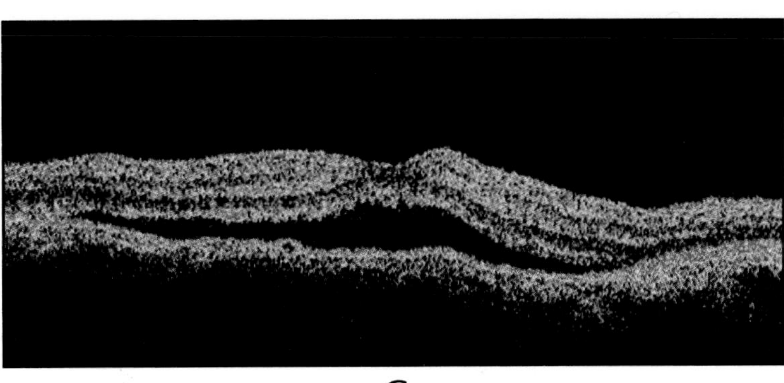

C

Case 6-5A. Chronic Central Serous Chorioretinopathy

Clinical Summary

A 64-year-old male presents for a second opinion regarding his poor central visual acuity in both eyes. He has noticed fluctuating vision in the right eye over the past year. His current visual acuity is 20/60 in this eye. Dilated fundus examination (A) shows elevation of the retina in the central macula with underlying pigmentary mottling. Fluorescein angiography (B) reveals multiple hyperfluorescent spots in the posterior pole that leak in the late frames of the study.

Optical Coherence Tomography

The horizontal OCT image (C) demonstrates elevation of the neurosensory retina involving the fovea. There is a localized elevation of the RPE signal adjacent to the fovea that corresponds to an area of leakage on the fluorescein angiogram. Additional irregularities of the RPE signal reflect the pigmentary alterations identified on exam. The detached fovea does not appear to be thickened, but there is thickening and cystic spaces in the retinal tissue nasal to the fovea.

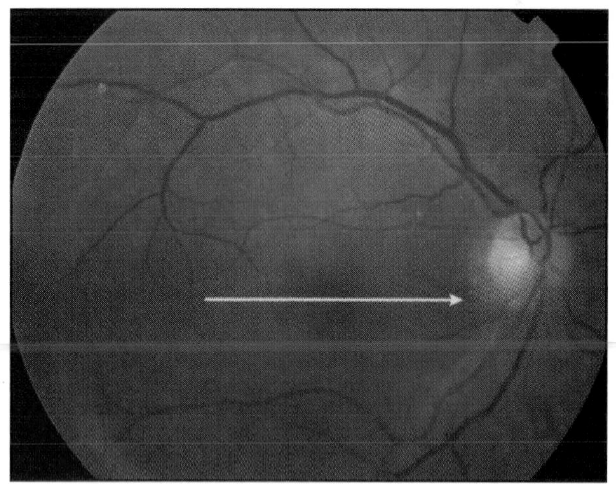

A

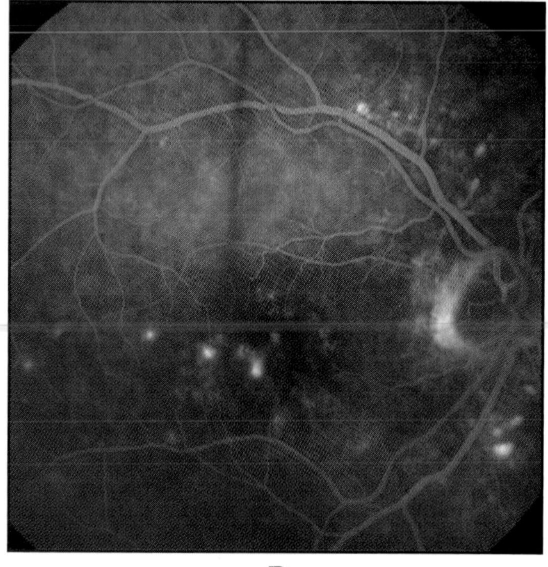

B

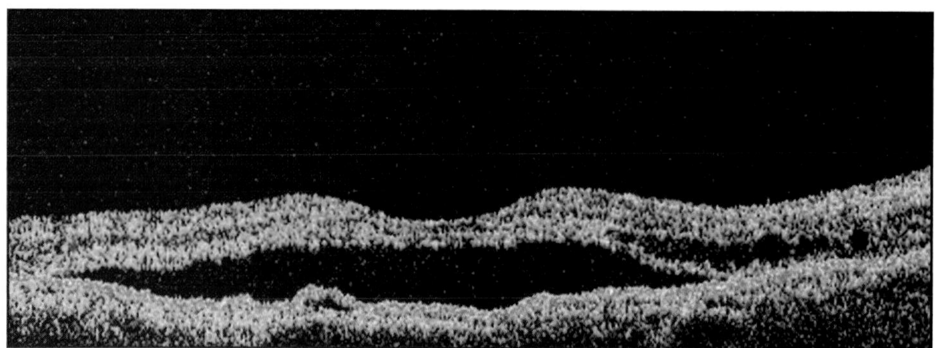

C

Case 6-5B. Chronic Central Serous Chorioretinopathy

Clinical Summary

His vision has been poor in the left eye for 2 years with progressive worsening over the past year. His visual acuity in this eye is 20/300. On dilated fundus exam (D), there is subretinal fluid in the macula with associated pigmentary mottling and exudates. The fluorescence angiogram (E) shows mottled hyperfluorescence in the macula with a prominent area of leakage beneath the fovea.

Optical Coherence Tomography

The horizontal OCT image (F) confirms detachment of the neurosensory retina in this eye. The elevated retinal tissue has an irregular contour with foveal thinning. There are also mild irregularities in the contour of the underlying RPE/choroidal signal consistent with the chronic pigmentary alterations.

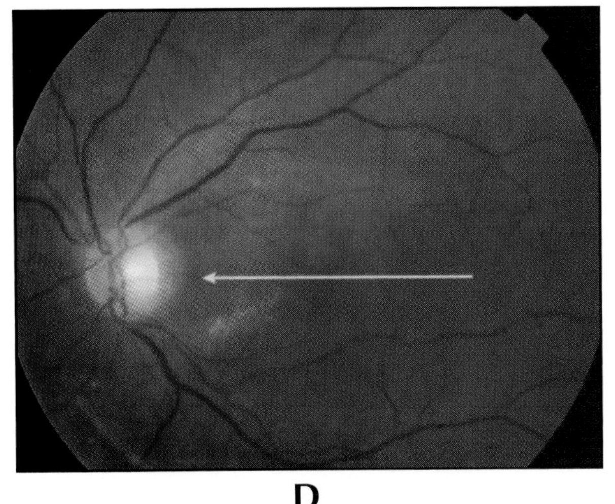

D

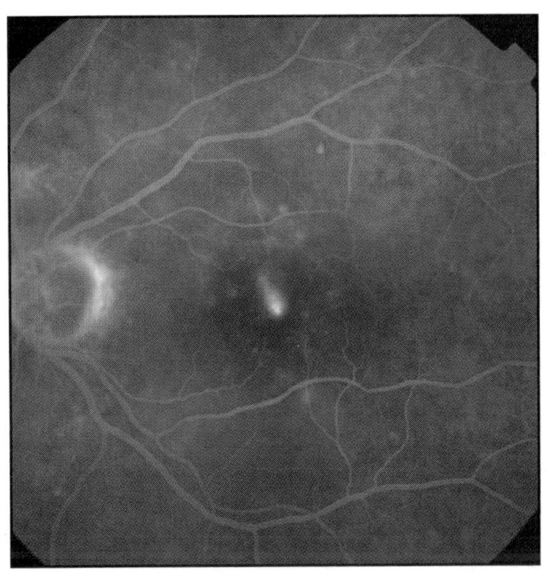

E

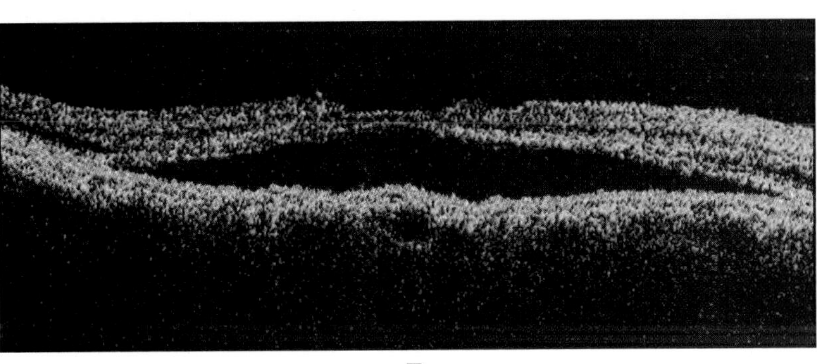

F

Case 6-6A. Bullous Central Serous Chorioretinopathy

Clinical Summary

A 38-year-old Asian female complains of decreased visual acuity in her left eye for 2 to 3 weeks. She has not noticed any problems with her right eye, and her visual acuity in this eye is 20/20. Dilated fundus examination of the right eye (A) shows mild pigmentary mottling in the foveal region and a large pigment epithelial detachment in the temporal macula. Fluorescence and indocyanine green (ICG) angiography (B and C) show multiple small areas of leakage in the posterior pole and filling of the large pigment epithelial defect (PED).

Optical Coherence Tomography

The OCT image through the fovea of the right eye (D) reveals a normal foveal contour without evidence of subretinal fluid. An image taken through the temporal macula (E) confirms the presence of a PED. The neurosensory retina and the RPE (seen as a bright orange band adjacent to the outer retina) are highly elevated above the faint choroidal signal. The choroidal signal is reduced due to attenuation of the reflected light by the highly elevated pigment epithelial detachment.

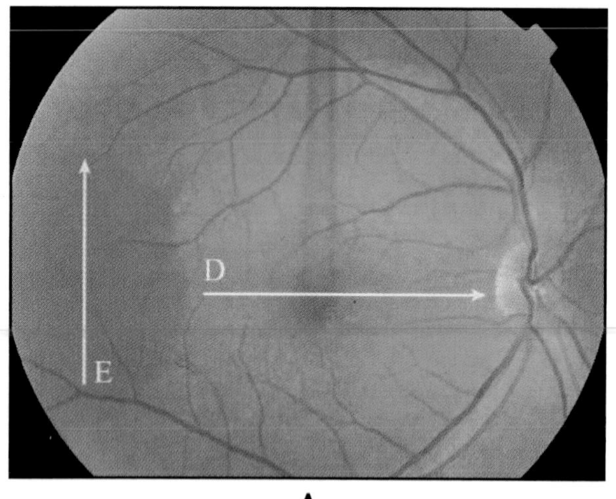

A

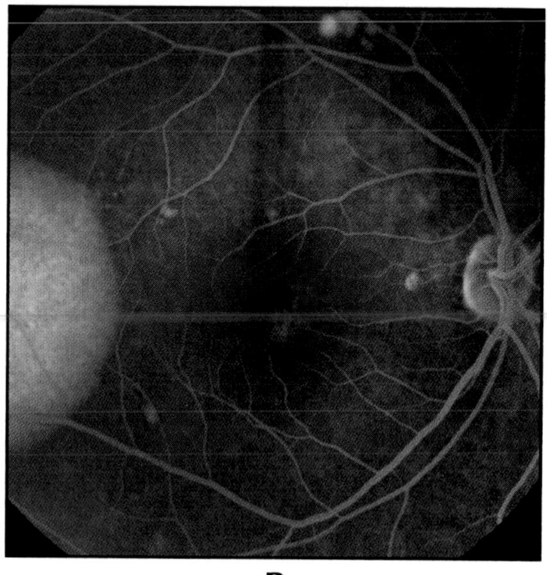

B

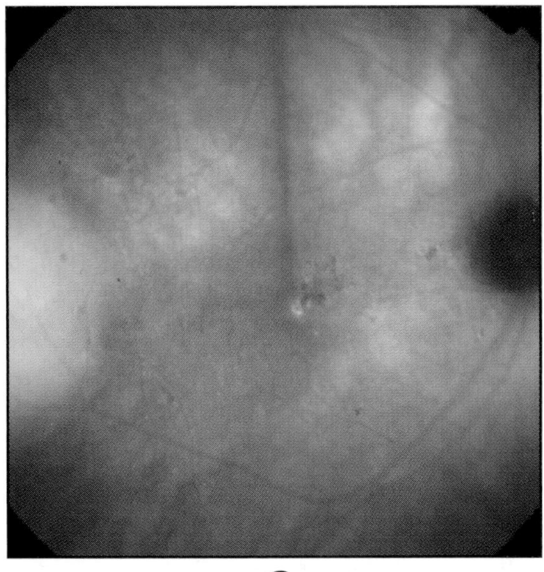

C

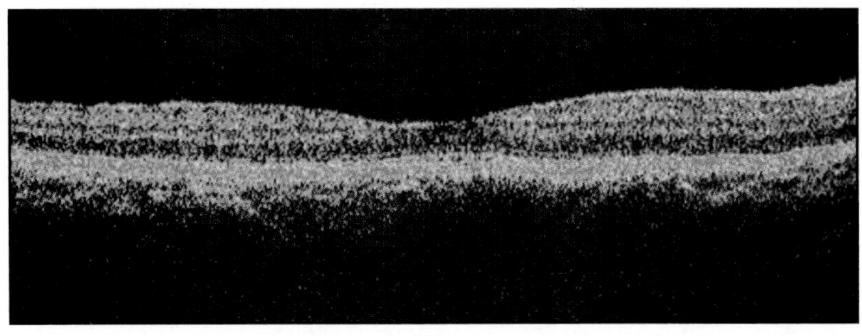

D

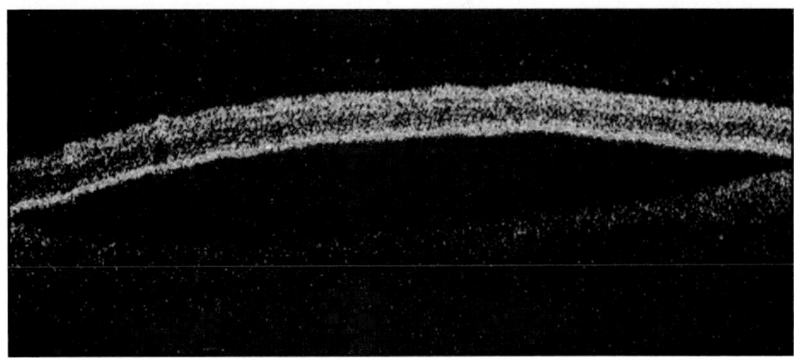

E

Case 6-6B. Bullous Central Serous Chorioretinopathy

Clinical Summary

Her BCVA is 20/80 in the left eye. Dilated fundus examination of the left eye (F) shows a large area of subretinal fluid centered in the macula. Fluorescence and ICG angiography (G and H) outline the area of macular subretinal fluid and reveal several small hyperfluorescent pigment epithelial detachments.

Optical Coherence Tomography

A vertical OCT image (I) through the fovea shows a large detachment of the neurosensory retina with an underlying clear cavity of subretinal fluid. The bright orange band that represents the RPE is shallowly elevated in the center of this tomogram and more highly elevated on the right side of the image. These pigment epithelial detachments correspond to areas of hyperfluorescence seen on angiography.

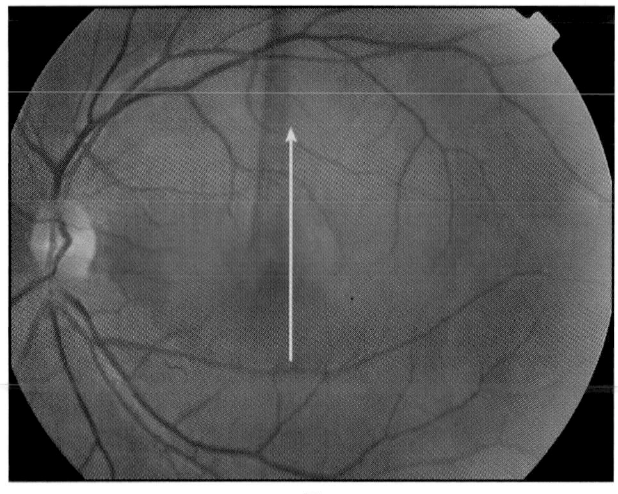

F

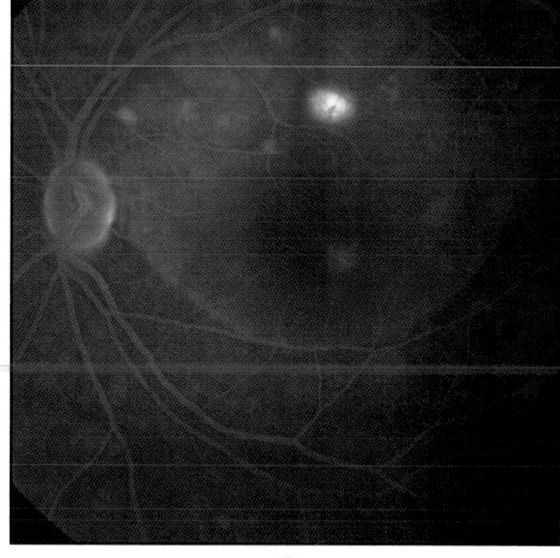

G

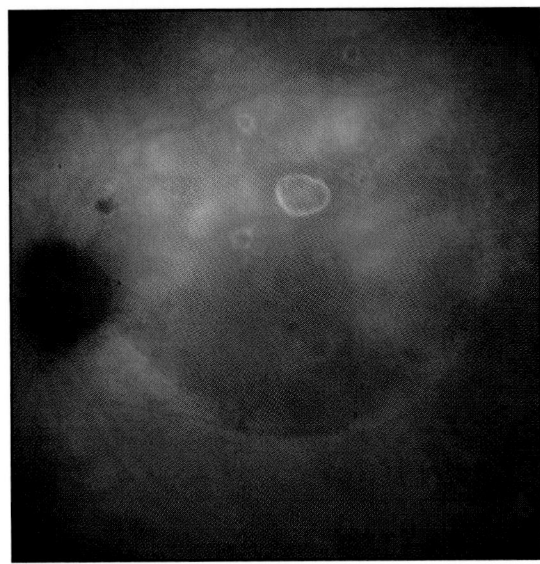

H

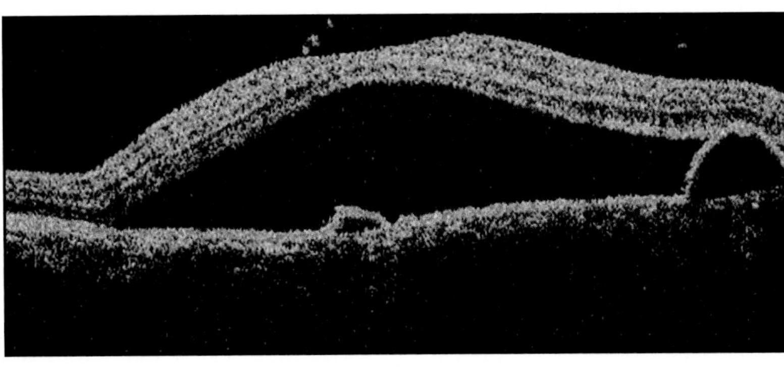

I

Case 6-7A. Central Serous Chorioretinopathy That Resolves Spontaneously

Clinical Summary

A 45-year-old male presents with a 1-week history of distorted central vision in his right eye. His BCVA is 20/400 in this eye. Dilated fundus examination (A) shows a well-defined, circular area of subretinal fluid in the right macula. Fluorescein angiography (B) shows an area of hyperfluorescence just superior to the fovea with "smoke-stack" leakage from the temporal edge. A second area of hyperfluorescence is seen superior to the optic nerve.

Optical Coherence Tomography

The vertical OCT imaging (C) acquired through the fovea illustrates elevation of the neurosensory retina above an optically clear, fluid-filled cavity. As the scan proceeds superiorly (right side of the scan), there is shallow elevation of the RPE signal. This RPE detachment corresponds to the area of hyperfluorescence seen on the angiogram just superior to the fovea. Attenuation of the choroidal signal beneath the PED is an expected finding. The subretinal fluid cavity has a maximum height of 715 µm, while the RPE detachment measures 175 µm in height.

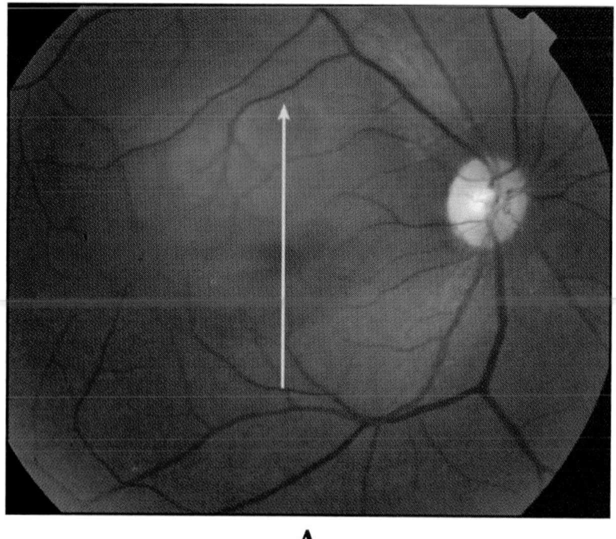

A

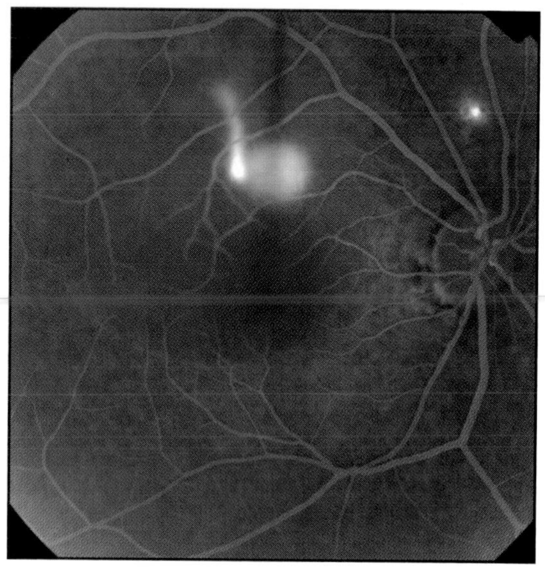

B

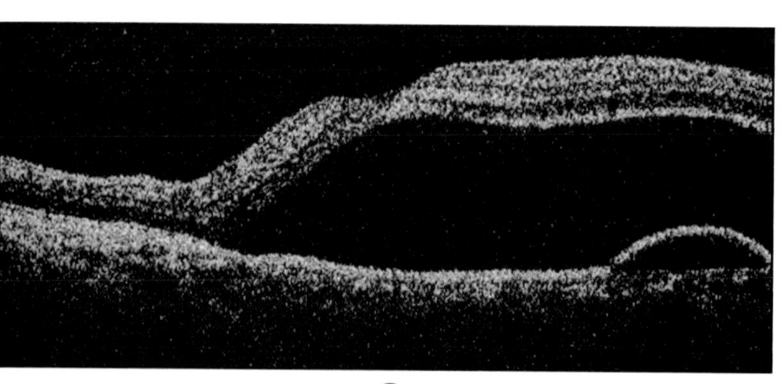

C

Case 6-7B. Spontaneous Resolution

Continuation of Clinical Summary

After 4 months of observation, the patient reports resolution of his visual distortion. His visual acuity has improved to 20/20, and fundus examination shows the retina to be flat throughout the macular region.

Follow-Up Optical Coherence Tomography

The vertical OCT tomogram (D) taken through the fovea confirms resolution of the neurosensory and RPE detachments. The retinal thickness and foveal contour are relatively normal in appearance, and the underlying high-intensity RPE/choroidal signal shows minimal irregularity.

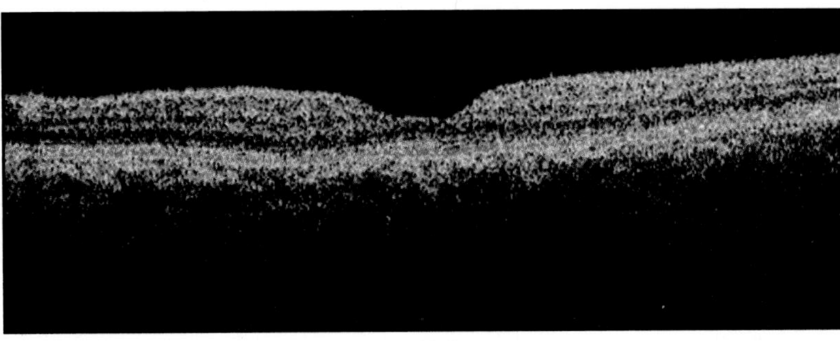

D

Case 6-8A. Central Serous Chorioretinopathy That Improves Spontaneously

Clinical Summary

A 42-year-old male complains of a gray circle in the center of his vision for the past 2 weeks. His BCVA is 20/30 in this eye. Dilated fundus examination (A) shows a shallow elevation of the fovea. The fluorescein angiogram (B) identifies a pinpoint area of leakage with late pooling of dye in the subretinal space.

Optical Coherence Tomography

The OCT image (C) illustrates elevation of the neurosensory retina. The serous subretinal fluid reaches a maximum height of 300 μm directly under the fovea. The elevated retina shows mild thickening with small intraretinal cysts consistent with intraretinal edema. The high-intensity RPE signal shows minimal irregularity and remains flat beneath the subretinal fluid cavity.

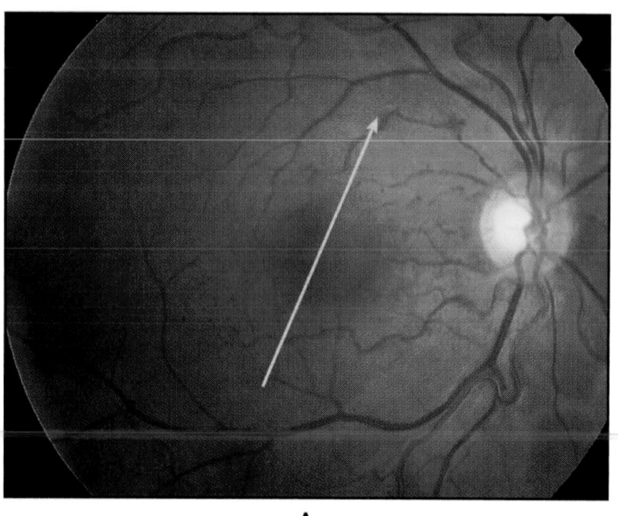

A

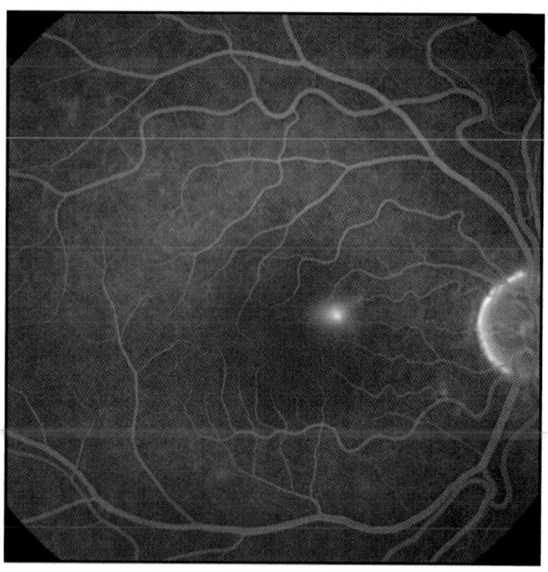

B

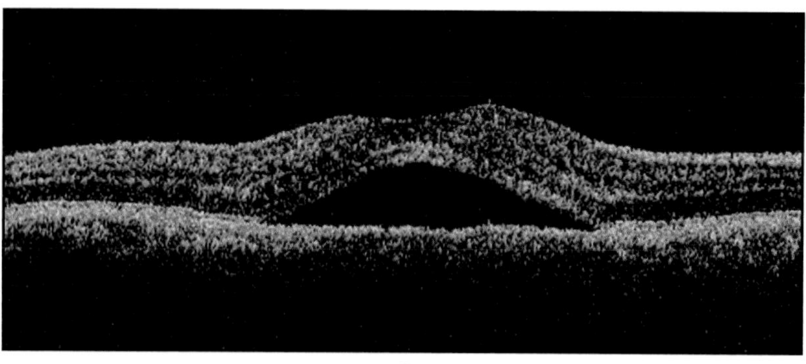

C

Case 6-8B. Spontaneous Resolution

Continuation of Clinical Summary

The patient returns 4 months later and reports improvement of his vision with mild persistent metamorphopsia. His visual acuity has improved to 20/20, and there is no evidence of retinal elevation on fundus exam.

Follow-Up Optical Coherence Tomography

The OCT tomogram (D) now shows a significant decrease in the amount of subretinal fluid. The fovea is reattached with restoration of the foveal pit, but there is still a small pocket of residual subretinal fluid adjacent to the fovea. The reattached fovea has decreased in thickness to 150 μm, while the subretinal fluid now measures only 75 μm in height. This small amount of fluid, which explains his persistent visual symptoms, cannot be identified on clinical exam.

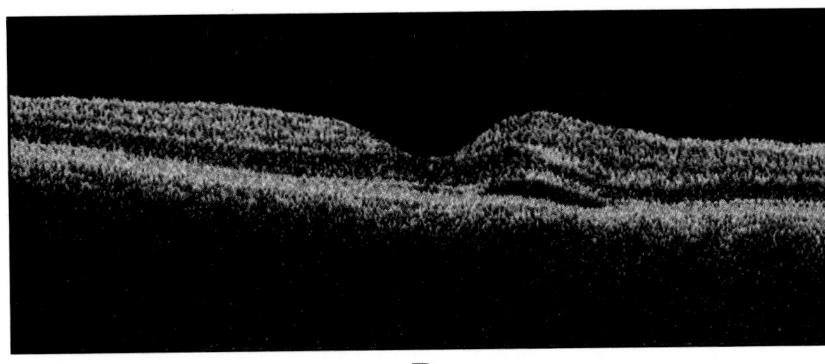

D

Case 6-9A. Fluctuating Subretinal Fluid in Central Serous Chorioretinopathy

Clinical Summary

A 28-year-old male complains of a dark spot in the center of his vision in the left eye that began 1 day earlier. His visual acuity is 20/25 in this eye, and dilated fundus examination (A) shows a circular area of retinal elevation in the superior macula adjacent to the fovea. The fluorescein angiogram (B) confirms an area of leakage beneath the elevated retina.

Optical Coherence Tomography

The initial OCT image (C) shows shallow elevation of the neurosensory retina nasal to the fovea. The fovea remains attached with a relatively normal foveal contour. The RPE signal does show mild irregularity, but there is no evidence of elevation in this image.

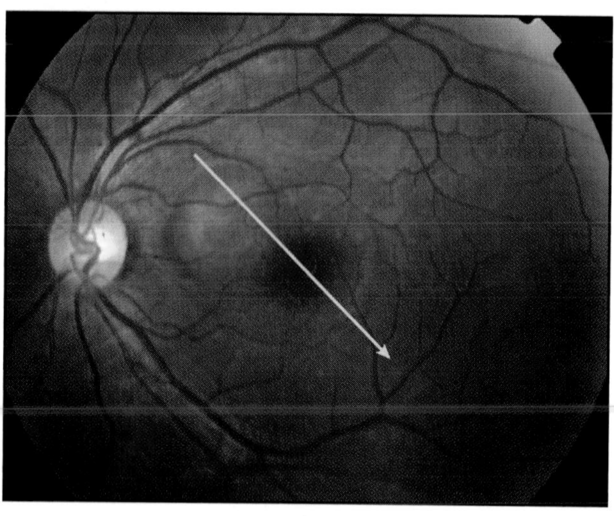

A

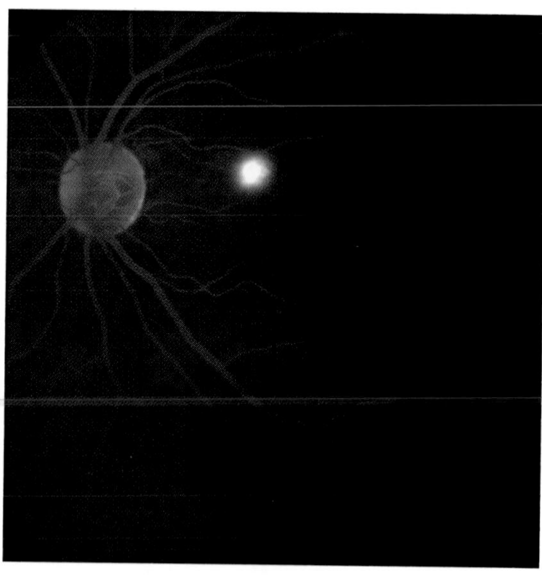

B

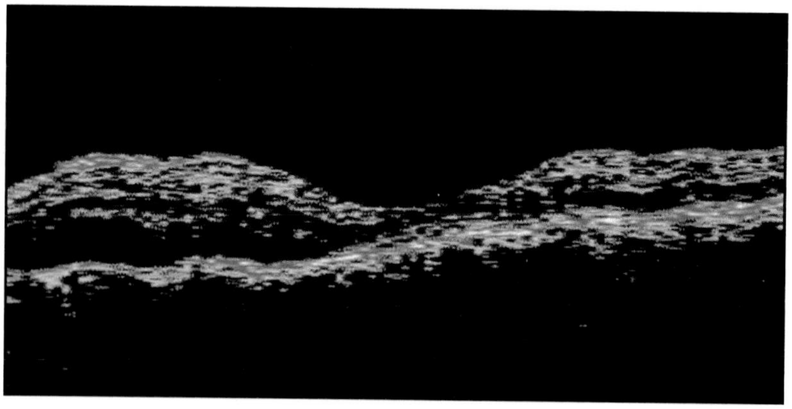

C

Case 6-9B. Fluctuating Subretinal Fluid in Central Serous Chorioretinopathy

Follow-Up Examination and Optical Coherence Tomography

Observation was recommended, and the patient's course was monitored with serial OCT imaging. One week after initial presentation, he complains of worsening distortion and his vision decreases to 20/30. The OCT image (D) now shows an increase of subretinal fluid with extension under the fovea. One month later, his visual acuity improves to 20/25, and the OCT image (E) reveals minimal residual fluid with only a thin layer of decreased reflectivity beneath the fovea. The previously identified subretinal fluid adjacent to the fovea has now resolved. Four months later, the patient returns complaining of recurrent visual distortion. BCVA declines to 20/40, and the OCT image (F) confirms reaccumulation of serous fluid beneath the fovea. After more 6 weeks of observation, the vision again normalizes with complete resolution of the neurosensory detachment (G).

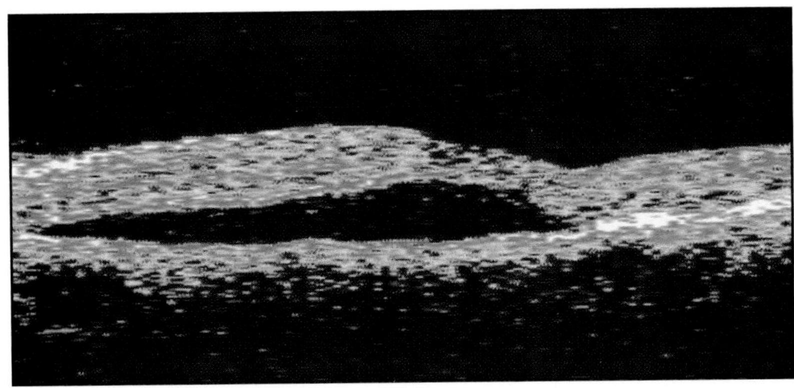

D

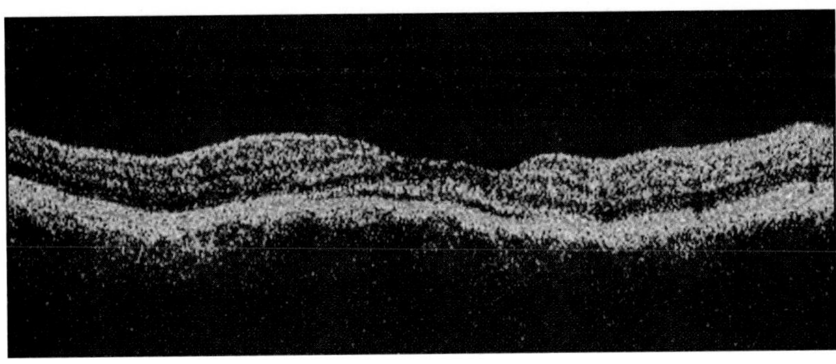

E

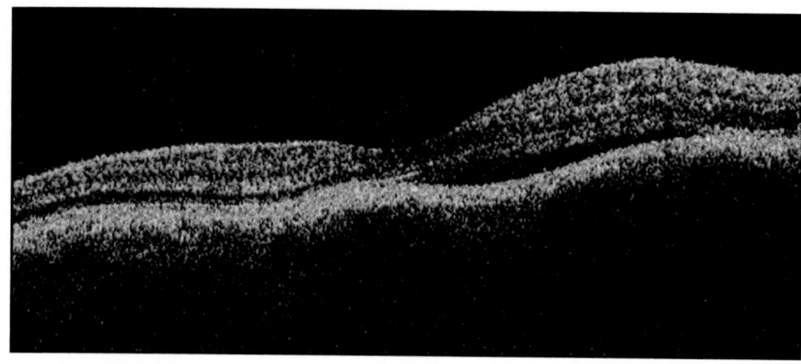

F

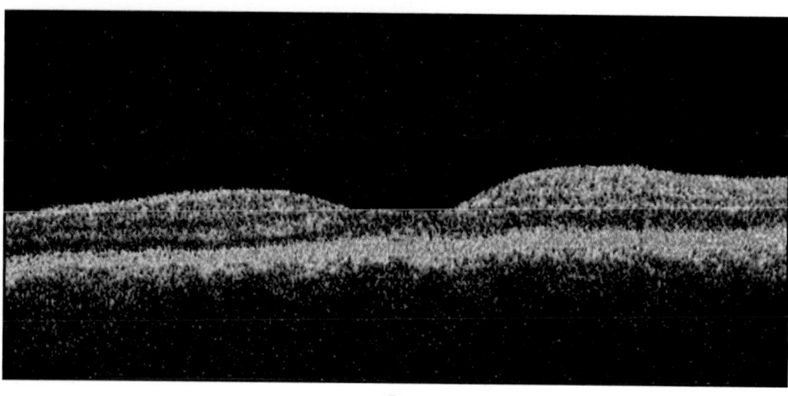

G

Case 6-10A. Central Serous Chorioretinopathy Treated With Focal Laser

Clinical Summary

A 35-year-old male complains of decreased central visual acuity in the left eye for 1 month. His visual acuity is 20/200 in this eye, and dilated fundus examination (A) shows a large area of subretinal fluid in the macula extending through the fovea. Fluorescein angiography (B) shows an area of hyperfluorescent leakage temporal to the fovea with gradual pooling of dye in the area of serous detachment.

Optical Coherence Tomography

The horizontal OCT tomogram (C) through the fovea shows a large detachment of the neurosensory retina. The optically clear cavity beneath the detached retina represents subretinal fluid and measures 600 μm in height. The detached retinal tissue is mildly thickened, measuring 195 μm in the fovea and 320 μm adjacent to the fovea. There is a small pigment epithelial detachment in the area of leakage temporal to the fovea.

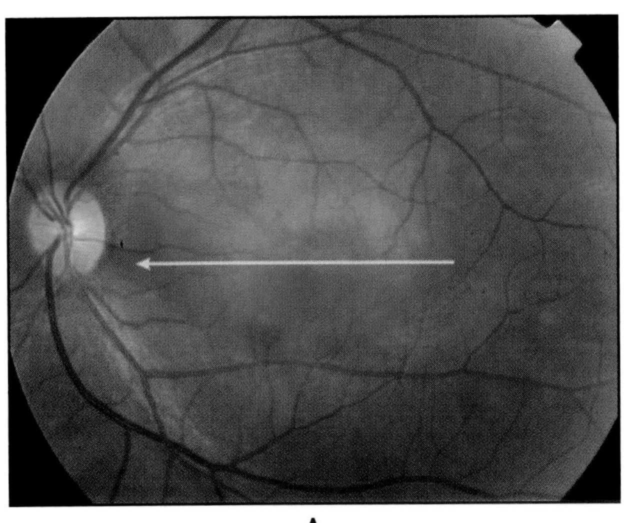

A

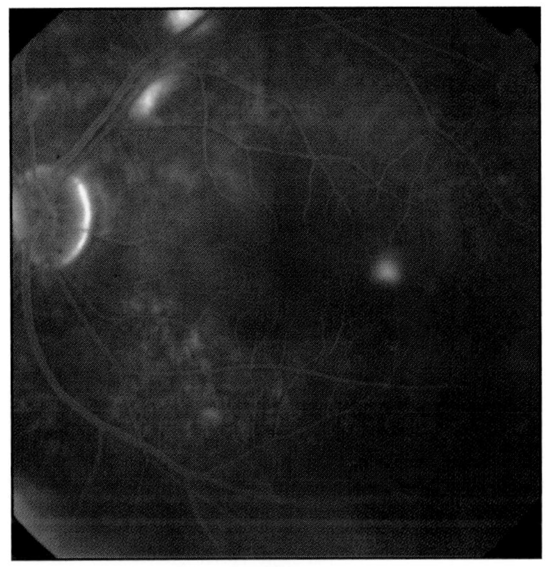

B

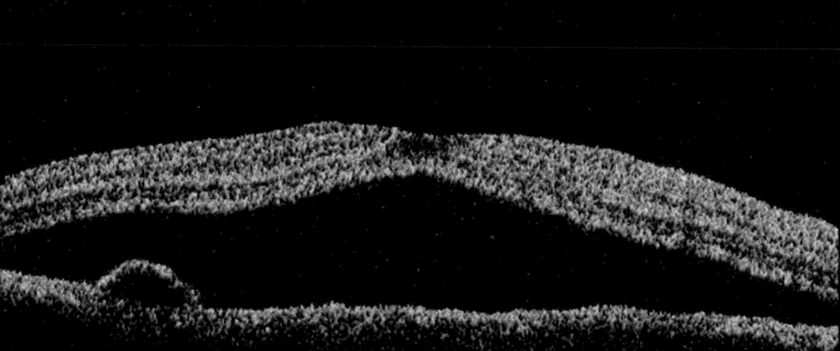

C

Case 6-10B. Focal Laser Treatment

Follow-Up Examination

The patient underwent focal laser treatment to the area of leakage temporal to the fovea. One week after treatment, he notes some visual improvement and his vision measures 20/80. Dilated fundus exam (D) shows persistent subretinal fluid in the macula and a hypopigmented area from the laser treatment temporal to the fovea. Fluorescein angiography (E) shows hypofluorescence without persistent leakage in the area of laser treatment. One month later, the visual acuity has improved to 20/25, and there is no evidence of residual subretinal fluid.

Follow-Up Optical Coherence Tomography

The 1-week postlaser OCT image (F) now shows a shallower detachment of the neurosensory retina with a decrease in the height of the subretinal fluid cavity to 465 µm. The retinal thickness has remained mostly unchanged. The previously seen RPE detachment is no longer present, but there is mild irregularity of the signal in this area from the laser treatment. One month after treatment, the OCT image (G) confirms the complete resolution of the subretinal fluid. There is irregularity adjacent to the fovea from the laser, but the foveal contour is relatively normal. Central foveal thickness now measures 150 µm.

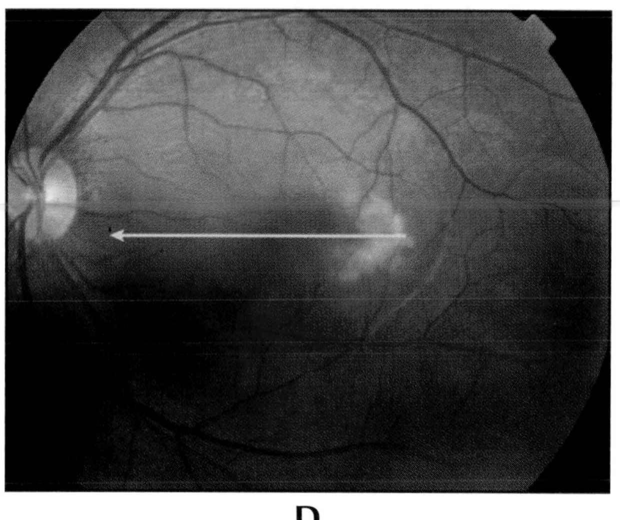

D

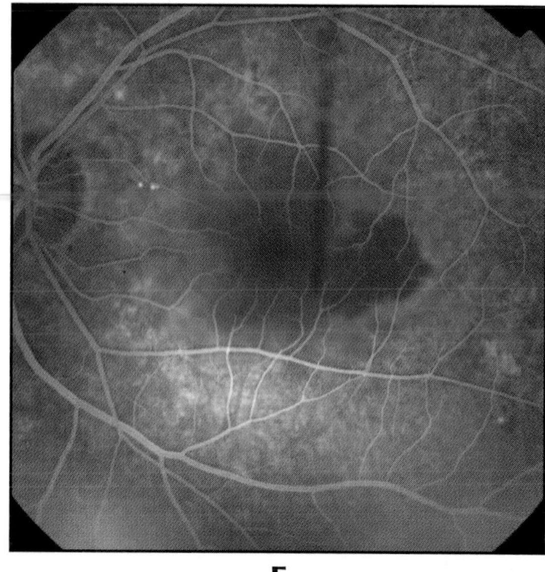

E

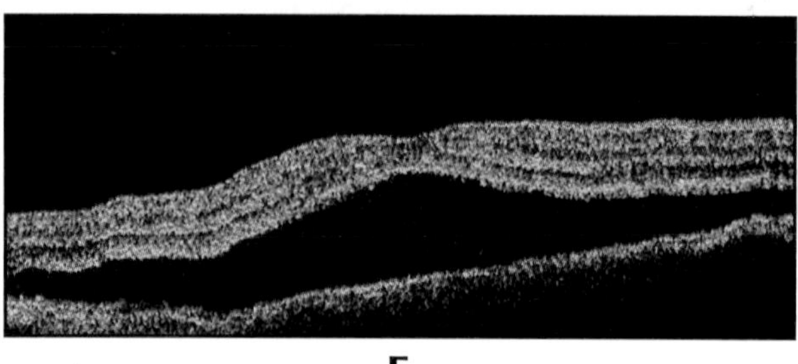

F

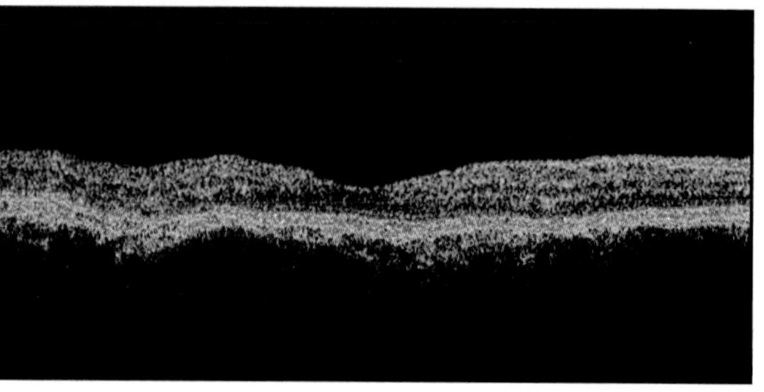

G

Case 6-11A. Central Serous Chorioretinopathy Treated With Photodynamic Therapy

Clinical Summary

A 43-year-old truck driver is referred for evaluation of chronic CSCR in the left eye. His visual acuity has remained 20/70 for the past 6 months due to persistent neurosensory detachment involving the fovea (A). Fluorescein angiogram (B) shows an area of leakage just superior to the fovea. ICG angiography (C) demonstrates a placoid area of hyperfluorescence under the fovea.

Optical Coherence Tomography

OCT imaging (D) acquired through the fovea confirms detachment of the neurosensory retina. The high-intensity signal beneath the fluid cavity corresponds to the RPE, indicating neurosensory detachment without RPE detachment.

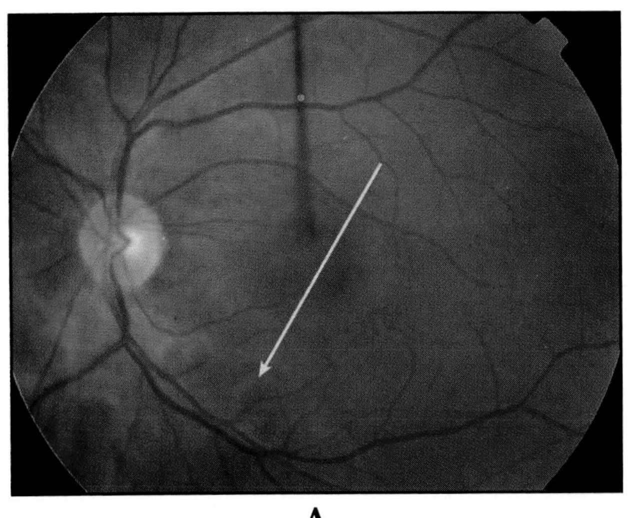

A

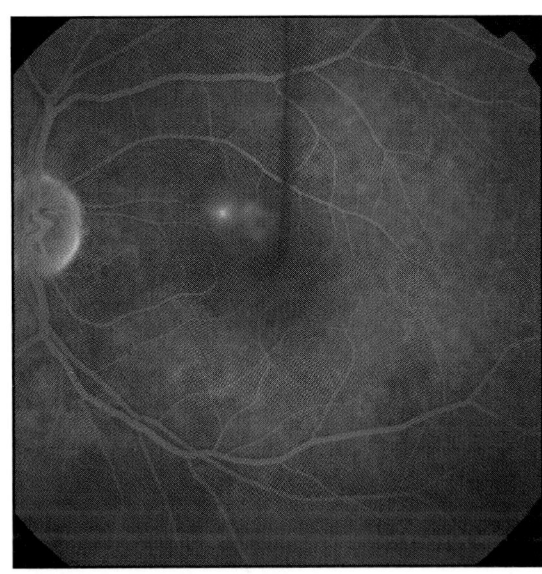

B

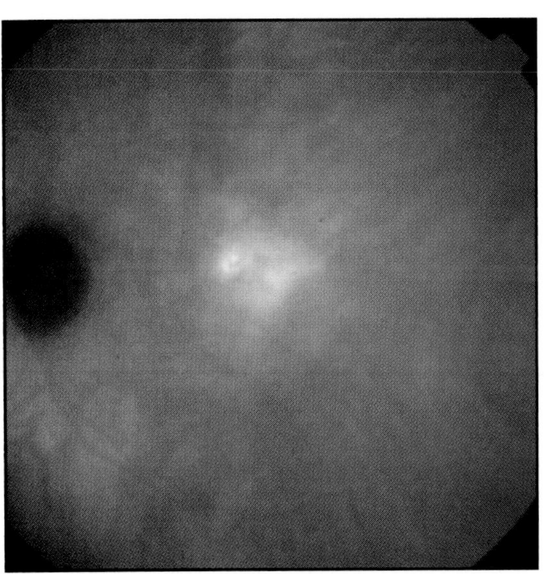

C

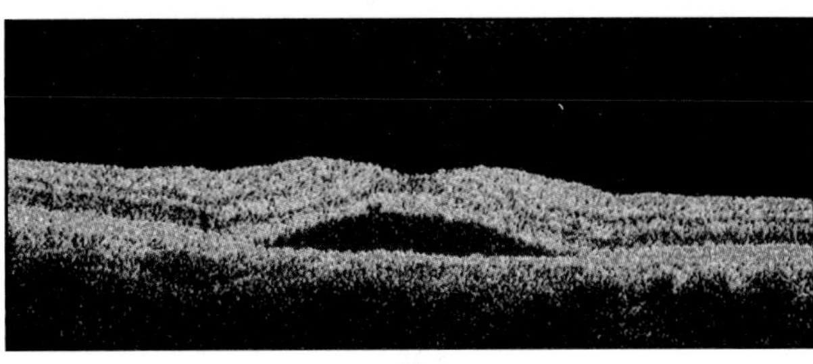

D

Case 6-11B. Treatment With Photodynamic Therapy

Continuation of Clinical Summary

Because this condition was chronic and creating significant visual dysfunction, intervention was indicated. There were concerns about proceeding with focal laser to the leakage site because of the proximity to the fovea. The patient, therefore, underwent photodynamic therapy to the area hyperfluorescence identified on ICG angiography. The patient noticed normalization of his vision within 3 weeks of the treatment. At the return visit 2 months after treatment, his vision was 20/20. Dilated fundus exam (E) showed mild pigmentary mottling but no subretinal fluid. Fluorescein angiography (F) showed mottled fluorescence but no evidence of leakage.

Follow-Up Optical Coherence Tomography

The post-treatment OCT tomogram (G) taken through the fovea shows resolution of the neurosensory detachment with normalization of the foveal contour. There is mild irregularity of the RPE signal consistent with the pigmentary changes on exam.

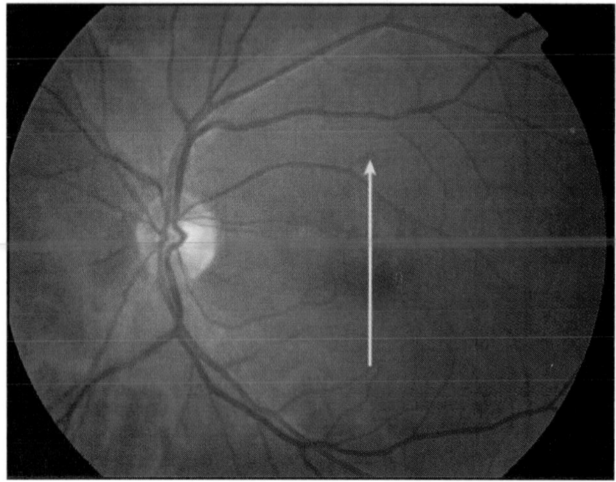

E

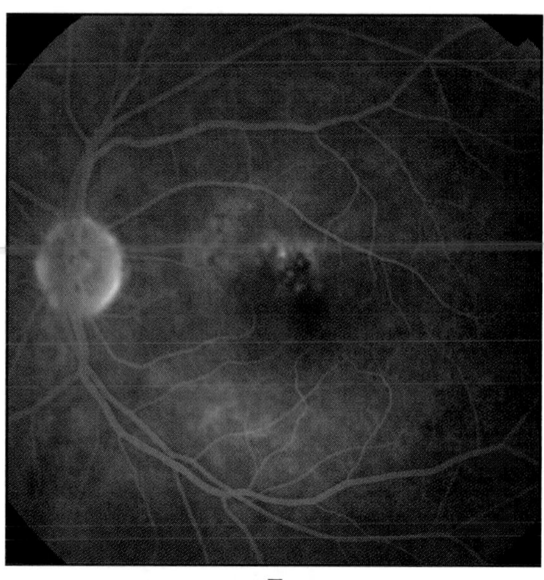

F

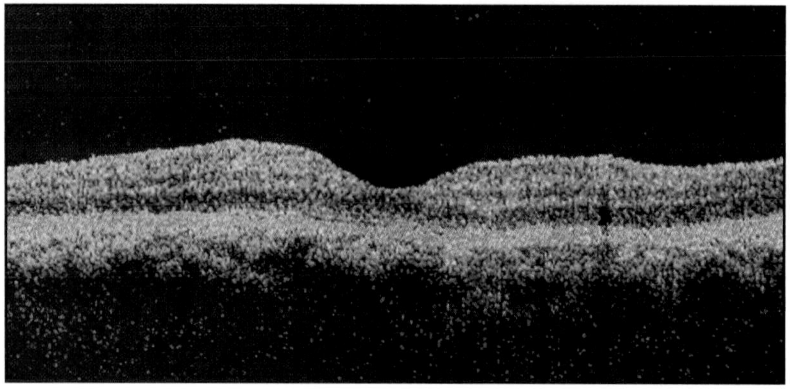

G

Case 6-12A. Central Serous Chorioretinopathy Treated With Photodynamic Therapy

Clinical Summary

A 35-year-old male with a history of CSCR is referred for evaluation of decreased visual acuity and persistent subretinal fluid in the left eye. His central visual distortion has not improved after 4 months of observation, and his visual acuity has remained 20/50 over this time. Dilated fundus exam (A) reveals a shallow serous detachment of the fovea. The fluorescein angiogram (B) confirms leakage of dye from a focal point under the fovea. A placoid area of hyperfluorescence beneath the fovea is seen in the late phase of the ICG angiogram (C).

Optical Coherence Tomography

The OCT (D) clearly demonstrates elevation of the fovea over a small pocket of subretinal fluid. The elevated retina is thickened at the fovea with loss of the foveal pit. The high-intensity reflection from the posterior surface of the detached retina mimics detachment of the RPE. However, the presence of a second high-intensity signal at the base of the fluid cavity and the lack of significant choroidal shadowing indicate that this is an isolated neurosensory detachment without RPE detachment.

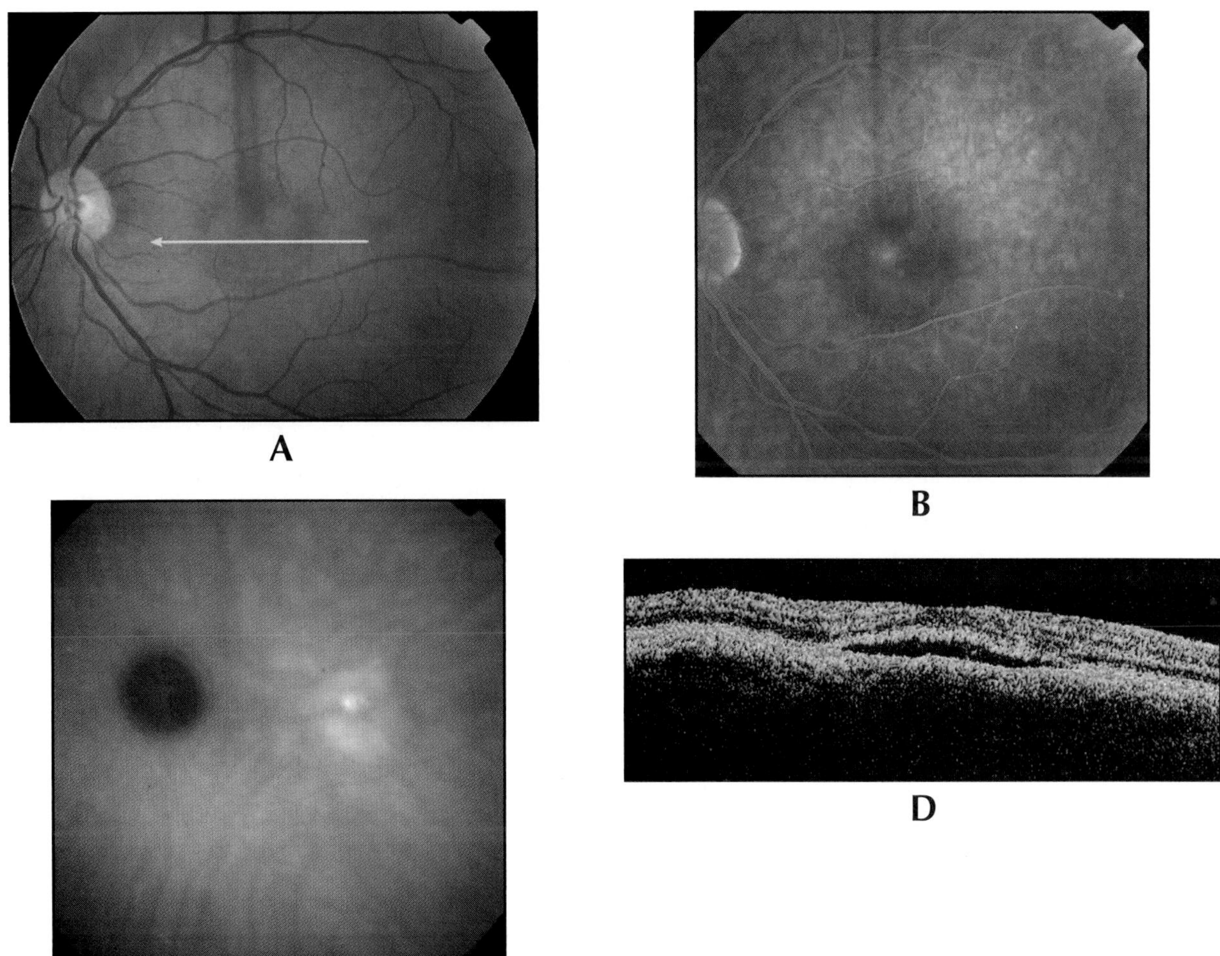

Case 6-12B. Treatment With Photodynamic Therapy

Continuation of Clinical Summary

Because the leakage was beneath the foveal center, focal laser treatment is prohibited. Therefore, photodynamic therapy to the area hyperfluorescence identified on ICG angiography is recommended. The patient reports improvement of his symptoms within 2 weeks of the treatment, and his visual acuity returns to 20/20 at his 2-month follow-up. He remains asymptomatic 4 months after the treatment.

Follow-Up Optical Coherence Tomography

The OCT image (E) taken 2 months after treatment shows complete resolution of the subretinal fluid. The foveal thickness has decreased to normal with reformation of the foveal pit. The OCT image remains stable 4 months after treatment (F) without evidence of recurrent subretinal fluid.

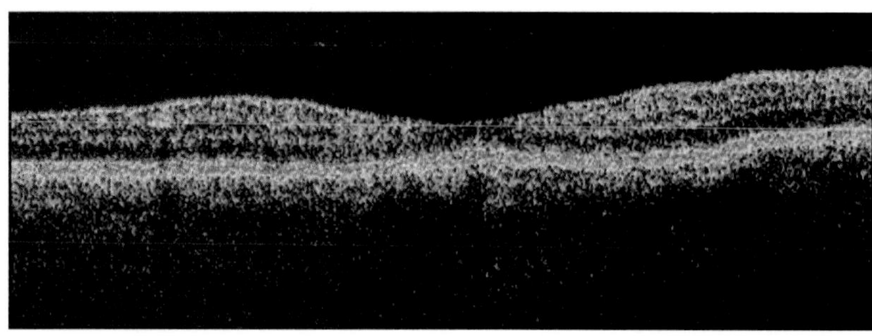

E

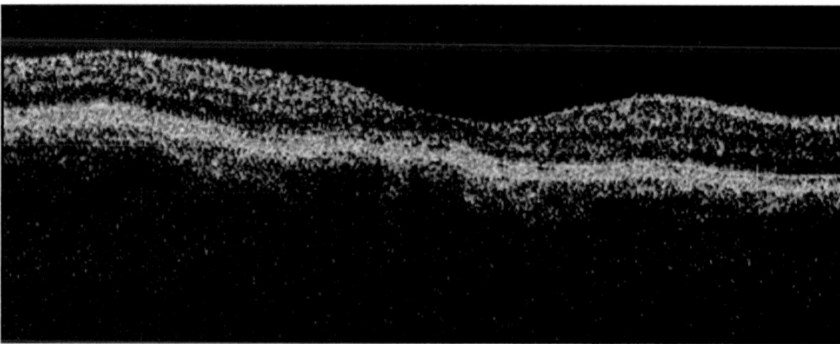

F

Chapter 7

Age-Related Macular Degeneration

Elias C. Mavrofrides, MD; Natalia Villate, MD;
Philip J. Rosenfeld, MD; and Carmen A. Puliafito, MD

- Drusen
- Vitelliform Macular Degeneration
- Geographic Atrophy
- Choroidal Neovascularization
- Retinal Angiomatous Proliferation
- Retinal Pigment Epithelial Tear
- Subretinal Hemorrhage
- Disciform Scarring

Age-related macular degeneration (ARMD) is the leading cause of irreversible severe vision loss among the elderly in Western populations.[1] The cause of ARMD remains elusive and complex, with both environmental and genetic contributions.[2,3] ARMD has two distinct forms known as "dry," or non-neovascular, ARMD and "wet," or neovascular, ARMD. Neovascular ARMD evolves from non-neovascular ARMD and represents a late stage of the disease. Neovascular ARMD gets its name from the formation of choroidal neovascularization (CNV) under the macula or the formation of intraretinal neovascularization or a combination of both processes. Most of the severe vision loss in ARMD is caused by neovascular ARMD, but neovascular ARMD represents only a minority of ARMD cases. The only proven therapies for ARMD treat the neovascular form of the disease and include both thermal laser photocoagulation and verteporfin photodynamic therapy (PDT).

Optical coherence tomography (OCT) allows cross-sectional imaging of the retina with an axial resolution of approximately 10 microns (μm), providing images that permit identification and differentiation of detailed structures within the neurosensory retina, the underlying retinal pigment epithelium (RPE)/Bruch's/choriocapillaris complex, and, in some cases, even the deeper choroid. When performed by an experienced technician, OCT provides both qualitative and quantitative information about these structures and allows for the examination of these structures over time to assess disease progression.[4-7] OCT is a noninvasive, dynamic technology ideal for observing the natural course of ARMD. The structural information provided by OCT is becoming a valuable diagnostic adjunct to fluorescein angiography (FA) and indocyanine green angiography (ICGA). The goal of using OCT is to correlate these observed structural changes to changes in visual acuity, not only to better understand the mechanism of vision loss associated with ARMD, but also to understand the mechanism of visual acuity benefits attributed to various treatments. In particular, OCT is a valuable tool for probing the treatment effects associated with PDT as well as periocular and intraocular pharmacologic therapy in neovascular ARMD.

Drusen are a characteristic fundus finding associated with non-neovascular or dry ARMD.[8] Soft drusen are observed as modulations in the external, highly reflective band consistent with the accumulation of material within or beneath Bruch's membrane. The localized elevation of the external band associated with drusen is shallow compared to the more pronounced scatter-free elevation observed with a serous pigment epithelial detachment (PED). Within the elevation associated with drusen, there is a mild backscatter of the signal probably resulting from the accumulated material that forms the drusen.

Geographic atrophy is a late-stage of dry ARMD devoid of drusen and resulting from the loss of RPE and underlying choriocapillaris. This stage has a distinctive appearance on OCT,[4,9] with thinning of the overlying retina and the external band, which represents the RPE/Bruch's/choriocapillaris complex. The loss of the choriocapillaris and the resulting scatter caused by the circulating red blood cells permit increased penetration of the light deeper into the choroid, significantly enhancing the reflections from this layer.

Serous PEDs present as localized, dome-shaped elevations of the external high reflective band that appear optically empty with sharp margins. Reflections from the deeper choroid can be appreciated. This ability to visualize the deeper choroid can be attributed to increased penetration of the probe light through the decompensated RPE, a PED containing low-reflective serous fluid, and diminished circulation within the choriocapillaris.

Hemorrhagic PEDs are notable for the absence of reflectance from the choroid with loss of the choroidal image due to the scattering of light from the blood under the RPE. The loss of choroidal detail correlates with the thickness of the blood.

Neovascular lesions have a distinct appearance on FA and ICGA, and these imaging modalities have served as the standards for assessing lesion types and disease progression or regression.[8] While OCT cannot predict with certainty the angiographic appearance of neovascular lesions, there are characteristic features observed on OCT that complement angiography and may even serve as better predictors of disease status. OCT has the advantage of discriminating small changes in the structure of the retinal layers and subretinal space, allowing for precise anatomic detection of structural changes that may signal progression or regression of the lesions.

Classic CNV is defined by FA as early bright, lacy hyperfluorescence associated with late leakage that typically obscures the initial boundaries of the CNV on the angiogram.[8] OCT imaging of classic CNV lesions may reveal a fusiform enlargement of the RPE/Bruch's/choriocapillaris reflective band with defined borders. The highly reflective band may appear irregular and duplicated, with high backscattering material between the two bands. Occasionally, it may be possible to image the membrane above the RPE (Type 2 CNV).

Subretinal fluid appears on OCT imaging as an optically clear space adjacent to the presumed CNV. This space represents a collection of fluid that can be evaluated quantitatively with the OCT. Visual acuity may be reduced by causes other than the presence of subretinal fluid, such as macular edema.

Macular edema can be focal, such as cystoid macular edema (CME), or diffuse macular edema, and can be easily missed when interpreting FA images alone due to the overwhelming fluorescence arising from the CNV. OCT has demonstrated the presence of macular edema in 46% of eyes with subfoveal CNV from ARMD, and there is a strong association between CME and classic CNV.[5] In contrast to FA, OCT is a reliable technique for distinguishing between macular edema, persistent leakage from CNV, or fibrotic scarring as the cause of vision loss. In the future, the ability to distinguish between these causes of vision loss may help in determining which treatment may be beneficial, when treatment should be initiated, and when retreatment should be offered. In particular, OCT may prove to be a valuable tool in assessing patients for retreatment with PDT, but it should be emphasized that the decision to retreat with verteporfin therapy should be based on the fluorescein angiographic findings alone until a formal clinical study using OCT alone is performed.

Occult CNV is defined by FA as a fibrovascular PED or as late leakage of an undetermined source.[8] A fibrovascular PED is described as an irregular elevation of the RPE that corresponds on FA with early stippled hyperfluorescence (usually within the first 1 to 2 minutes) going on to fluorescein leakage from CNV in the late phase. OCT imaging of fibrovascular PEDs includes a well-defined RPE elevation of the external band with a deeper area of mild backscattering corresponding to fibrous proliferation. Late leakage of undetermined source represents speckled fluorescein leakage at the RPE level in the late phase of the angiogram without a corresponding source of leakage in the early phase. The choroidal reflection may be enhanced on the OCT image due to increased light penetration secondary to degenerative changes in the RPE/Bruch's/choriocapillaris complex. During the natural course of macular degeneration, or as the result of treatment, the configuration of the neovascular complex can change over time.

RPE tears can be identified early in their evolution by observing a PED with an undulating or corrugated external band. This may signal the development of an evolving RPE tear that may or may not be obvious on FA. This appearance may evolve so that the PED appears more elevated, less dome-shaped with a steeper contour, and discontinuous along the highly reflective external band at the edge of the RPE tear. OCT can image the evolution of a tear and often identifies the site of separation and the rolling edge of the tear.

Blood in the subretinal or sub-RPE space can be distinguished using OCT imaging. Blood in the subretinal space shows an elevated and often edematous retina with a highly reflective underlying layer that is the blood. This blood causes shadowing of the underlying RPE/Bruch's/choriocapillaris complex, and this external band is not visualized. Blood in the sub-RPE space shows an elevated and intact external band with an underlying area of high reflectivity and shadowing corresponding to the blood. Choroidal details are not observed.

Subretinal fibrosis or disciform scarring is the end stage of neovascular ARMD. This area of scarring consists of white, fibrous tissue under the retina involving the RPE/Bruch's/choriocapillaris complex. This tissue is highly reflective on OCT and is frequently associated with overlying retinal atrophy.

Retinal lesion anastomoses and retinal angiomatous proliferations (RAPs) appear early as small intraretinal hemorrhages. RAPs often have these intraretinal hemorrhages overlying a serous PED.[10] As RAPs evolve, macular edema is associated with multiple intraretinal hemorrhages and the PED. The small intraretinal hemorrhages often correspond to small interruptions in the layers of the neurosensory retina as seen by OCT, often followed by the formation of an intraretinal or subretinal neovascular complex. Later in the course of the disease, the lesion appears to extend into the sub-RPE space. The clinical course of RAPs is somewhat intermediate between the usually rapid and aggressive course of classic CNV and the more insidious, slowly progressive course of occult CNV. While laser photocoagulation might be useful for the initial intraretinal neovascularization stage (Stage I RAP), thermal laser and verteporfin therapy are not particularly useful for the treatment of later stages (Stage II: subretinal neovascularization and Stage III: CNV). There is no single ideal treatment for RAPs, but encouraging results have been observed using PDT followed by intravitreal steroids and antiangiogenic therapy in selected cases.

Response to therapy is one of the most important clinical uses of OCT. OCT can be used to quantify changes in central retinal thickness and volume, as well as subretinal fluid. OCT currently provides useful information when deciding if patients require additional courses of therapy following their initial treatment with verteporfin therapy.[4] OCT, when used in conjunction with FA, is helpful in characterizing changes following verteporfin therapy and in detecting early accumulation of subretinal fluid associated with recurrence of CNV.

The radial scan pattern centered in the fovea allows for detailed characterization of the choroidal neovascular complex. To assess the entire lesion, all six scans should be reviewed. The appearance of the retina and the presence and location of subretinal fluid can be quantitatively and qualitatively assessed by comparing similar scans.

Reproducibility of the images between follow-up visits in patients with ARMD requires an experienced OCT technician. The vast majority of patients with wet ARMD do not have good fixation and are unable to see the internal fixation device of the OCT with the affected eye. If the other eye has preserved central vision, external fixation with the good eye can usually be obtained. When there is no fixation, careful attention should be given to the anatomic landmarks visualized in the video image to obtain scans that are at a similar location at every visit. Since the video image does not provide the exact location of the scan, there is no reliable method of assuring scan reproducibility other than the expertise of the technician. Often, manual relocation of the scan line during the image acquisition process is necessary.

The topographic map of the central 6 mm gives important information about the shape of the central macula. Remodeling of the central macula is observed following treatment or as the result of natural progression of the disease. The algorithm is designed to identify the boundaries of the neurosensory retina and calculate its thickness and volume. Careful comparative analysis of the maps between visits is helpful in determining if thickened areas are in the same previous location, represent new extensions of the neovascular complex to adjacent areas, or signal the occurrence of other related complications like RPE tears or neurosensory detachments. The central thickness value provided by the map often correlates well with the visual acuity. Reproducibility of the central thickness measure in patients with poor fixation is best obtained using the fast map scan pattern. Parallel raster scans or linear pattern scans can be obtained at different levels of a lesion and off-centered from the macula to document eccentric lesions when indicated. When the anatomy of the central 6 mm is severely distorted, the interpretation of the map should proceed with caution since the displayed thickness may not represent the actual thickness of the neurosensory retina, but include areas of RPE detachment, subretinal fluid, or hemorrhages.

References

1. Klein R. Epidemiology. In: Berger JW, Fine SL, Maguire MG, eds. *Age-Related Macular Degeneration*. St. Louis, Mo: Mosby; 1999:31-56.
2. Rosenfeld PJ, Gorin MB. Genetics of age-related maculopathy. In: Berger JW, Fine SL, Maguire MG, eds. *Age-Related Macular Degeneration*. St. Louis, Mo: Mosby; 1999:69-80.
3. Schick JH, Iyengar SK, Klein BE, et al. A whole-genome screen of a quantitative trait of age-related maculopathy in sibships from the beaver dam eye study. *Am J Hum Genet*. 2003;72(6):1412-1424.
4. Rogers AH, Martidis A, Greenberg PB, Puliafito CA. Optical coherence tomography findings following photodynamic therapy of choroidal neovascularization. *Am J Ophthalmol*. 2002;134(4):566-576.
5. Ting TD, Oh M, Cox TA, Meyer CH, Toth CA. Decreased visual acuity associated with cystoid macular edema in neovascular age-related macular degeneration. *Arch Ophthalmol*. 2002;120(6):731-737.
6. Neubauer AS, Priglinger S, Ullrich S, et al. Comparison of foveal thickness measured with the retinal thickness analyzer and optical coherence tomography. *Retina*. 2001;21(6):596-601.
7. Van Kerckhoven W, Lafaut B, Follens I, De Laey JJ. Features of age-related macular degeneration on optical coherence tomography. *Bull Soc Belge Ophthalmol*. 2001;(281):75-84.
8. Macular diseases. In: Berkow JW, Flower RW, Orth DH, Kelley JS, eds. *Fluorescein and Indocyanine Green Angiography—Technique and Interpretation*. San Francisco, CA:

American Academy of Ophthalmology; 1997:91-103.

9. Hassenstein A, Ruhl R, Richard G. Optical coherence tomography in geographic atrophy—a clinicopathologic correlation. *Klin Monatsbl Augenheilkd.* 2001;218(7):503-509.
10. Yannuzzi LA, Negrao S, Iida T, et al. Retinal angiomatous proliferation in age-related macular degeneration. *Retina.* 2001;21(5):416-434.

Case 7-1. Soft Drusen

Clinical Summary

A 63-year-old man was diagnosed with ARMD. Dilated fundus exam revealed confluent soft drusen in both eyes (A and B). No distortion was present on the Amsler grid. Visual acuity was 20/25 in the right eye and 20/30 in the left eye. No subretinal fluid, hemorrhage, or exudates were present on clinical examination. FA (not shown) displayed multiple, discrete areas of hyperfluorescence corresponding to the drusen without evidence of leakage.

Optical Coherence Tomography

Vertical OCT scans (C and D) through the fovea showed irregular elevation and disruption of the external highly reflective band in the center of both maculae, with material having high reflectivity beneath the band. In the right eye, a duplication of the external highly reflective band was apparent. This sign may indicate localized disruption of the Bruch's membrane. The foveal contour was slightly flattened, but the layers of the neurosensory retina were well preserved.

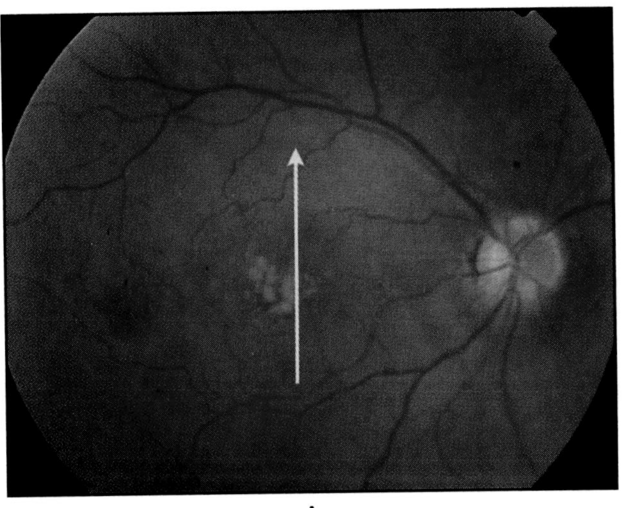

A

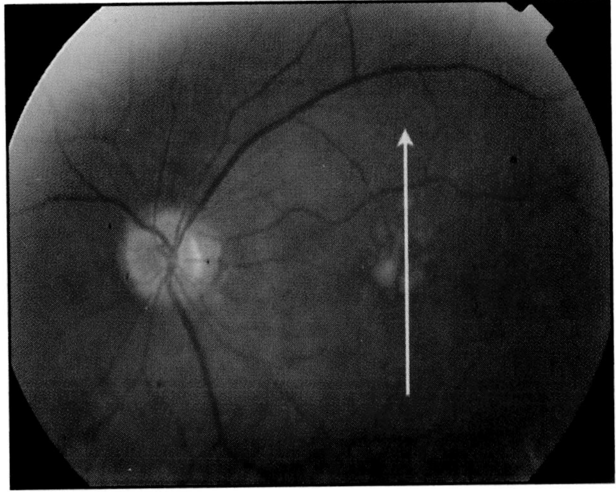

B

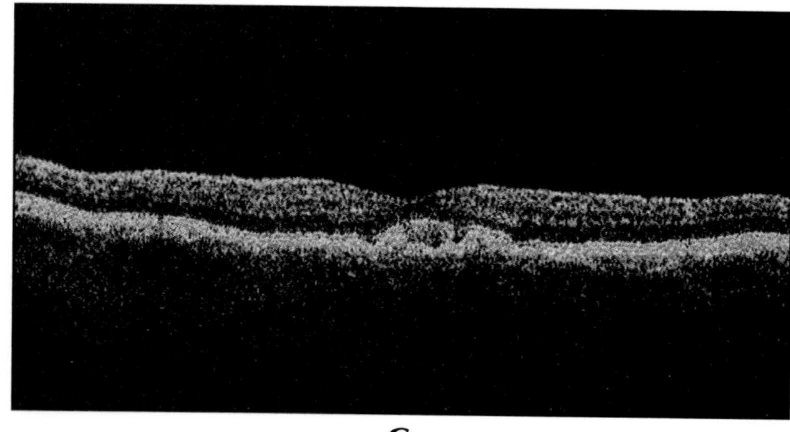

C

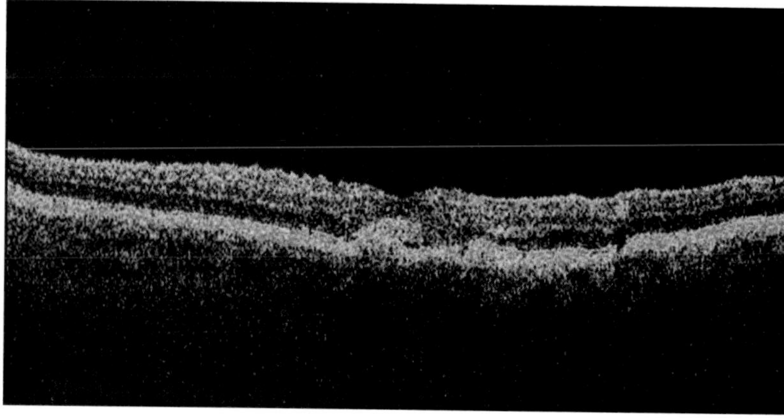

D

Case 7-2A. *Drusen*

Clinical Summary

A 79-year-old man with a clinical diagnosis of ARMD complained of decreased vision with metamorphopsia in the right eye for 1 year with worsening over the past 6 months. The right eye was phakic and had a visual acuity of 20/50. Soft confluent drusen with central pigmentary changes were present within the macula (A). FA (B) showed late staining of drusen.

Optical Coherence Tomography

OCT scan through the fovea (C) showed irregularity in the contour of the external high reflective band are represents the RPE/Bruch's/ choriocapillaris complex. The foveal contour was preserved with a central foveal thickness of 189 μm. Some atrophic changes and localized disorganization within the photoreceptor layer overlying the drusen are observed. There is no evidence of subretinal or intraretinal edema.

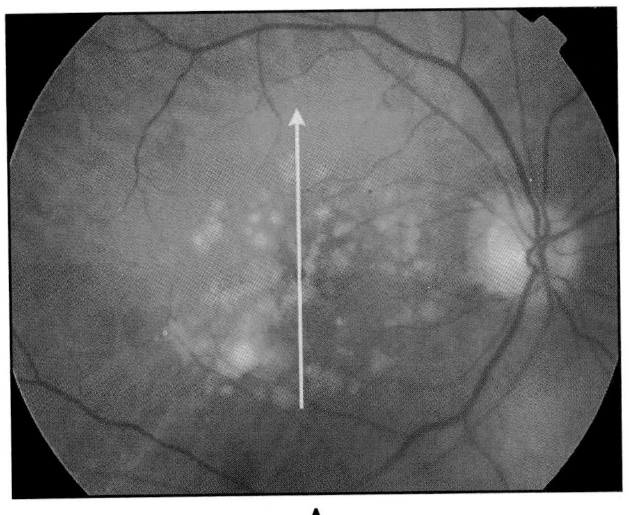

A

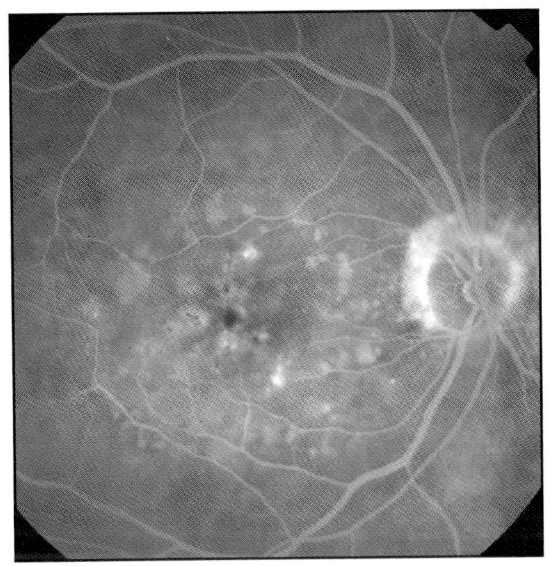

B

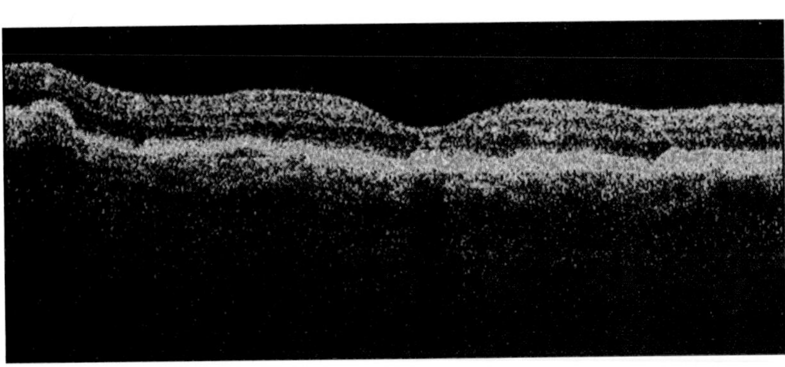

C

Case 7-2B. Drusen

Clinical Summary

The left eye was pseudophakic and had a visual acuity of 20/40. The retinal exam (D) showed multiple soft confluent drusen with central pigmentary changes. FA (E) again showed late staining of drusen with areas of coalescent drusen known as *drusenoid RPE detachments*.

Optical Coherence Tomography

OCT scan of the left eye (F) shows an altered foveal contour with central thinning and marked atrophic changes in the photoreceptor layer. There are focal elevations in the highly reflective band, some of which appear to coalesce under the foveal center with highly reflective material underneath. In some areas, the external band appears thinner and discontinuous. Atrophic changes in the layers comprising the external band result in less attenuation and greater penetration of the light into the deeper choroid, enhancing the reflections from this layer.

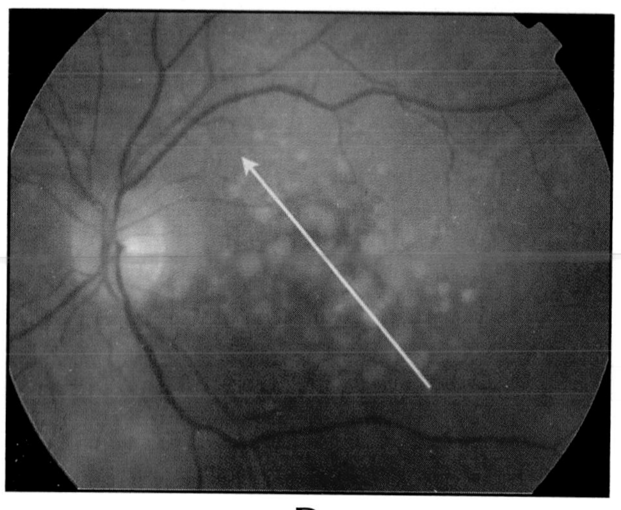

D

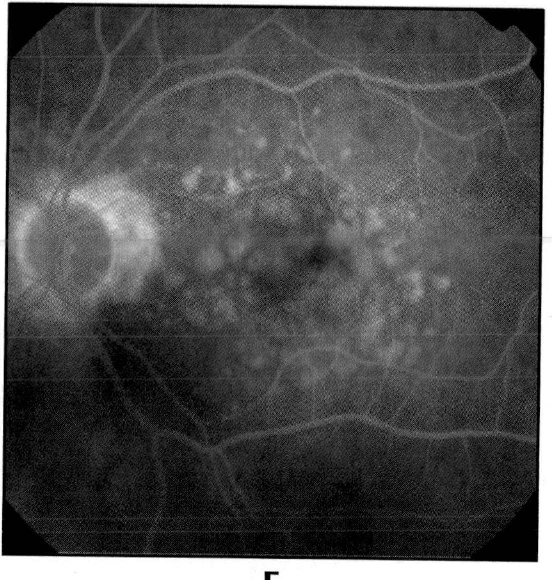

E

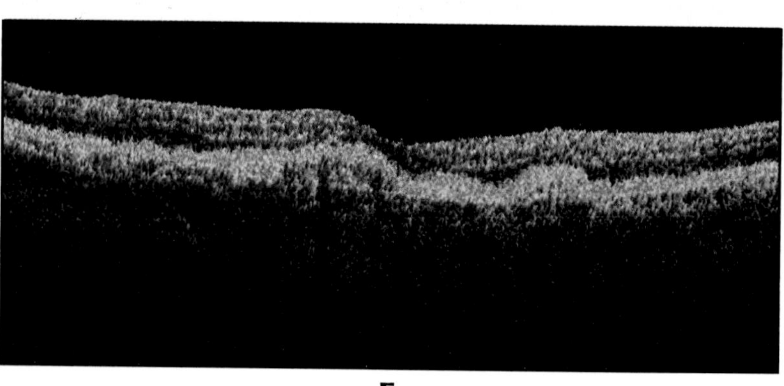

F

Case 7-3.
Basal Laminar Drusen

Clinical Summary

A 57-year-old woman had numerous discrete drusen, with focal areas of confluent drusen in her left macula (A). Visual acuity was 20/20. No subretinal fluid, hemorrhage, or exudates were present on clinical examination. FA (B) revealed multiple focal areas of fluorescein staining corresponding to the drusen. No fluorescein leakage was detected.

Optical Coherence Tomography

A horizontal scan through the macula (C) showed multiple nodules along the RPE/Bruch's/choriocapillaris complex (external band). These discrete elevations were observed beneath the neurosensory retina. The overlying neurosensory retina had normal thickness and contour except focal localized thinning of the photoreceptor layer overlying some of the nodules. There was no retinal thickening (edema) or evidence of subretinal fluid.

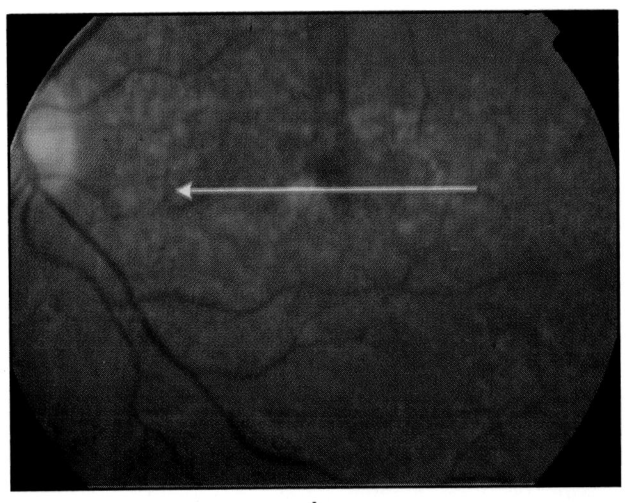

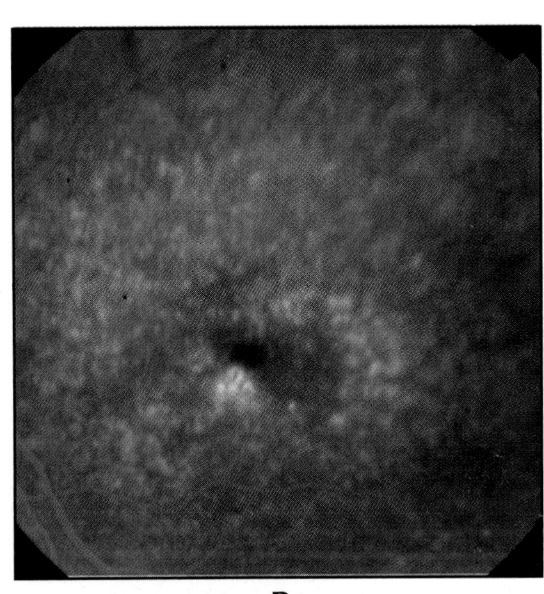

B

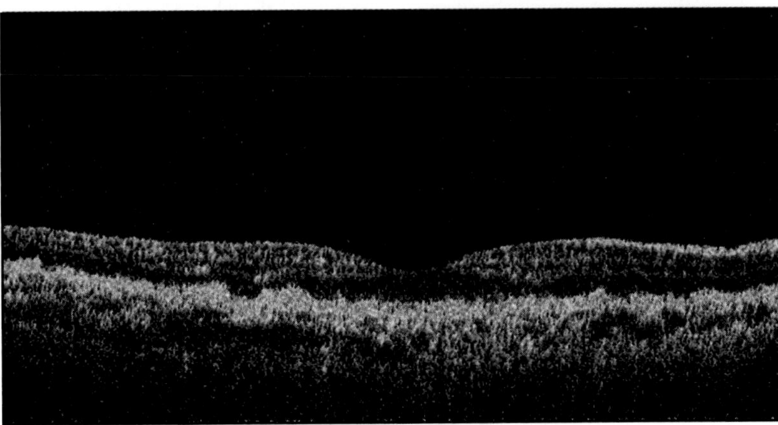

C

Case 7-4. Basal Laminar Drusen With Vitelliform Macular Lesion

Clinical Summary

The right eye of a 57-year-old woman had a visual acuity of 20/40. A vitelliform lesion was evident within the macula (A). FA (B) revealed an early, well-delineated hypofluorescent area corresponding to the vitelliform lesion with late confluent fluorescence within this area (C). ICGA (not shown) did not reveal hot spots or plaques corresponding to the areas of fluorescence.

Optical Coherence Tomography

A vertical scan (D) showed a diminished foveal depression with a normal overlying neurosensory retina. No macular edema was evident. Highly reflective subretinal material was observed inferiorly, which created a shadowing effect that obscured the underlying layers. The linear demarcation between the areas of hyper- and hypofluorescence on the angiogram corresponded to the sharp transition between the areas of high and low reflectivity seen on the OCT. Most likely, the areas of low reflectance represent subretinal fluid. The external band corresponding to the RPE/Bruch's/choriocapillaris complex underlying this area was not well visualized probably due to atrophy. Therefore, the hyperfluorescence seen on FA most likely represented diffuse leakage from the choroidal circulation due to the loss of the RPE and did not represent leakage from CNV. The characteristic nodular thickening of cuticular drusen was observed superiorly (right side of the scan).

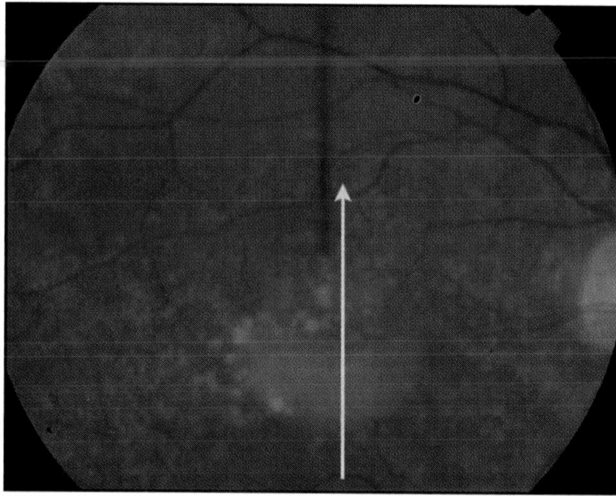

A

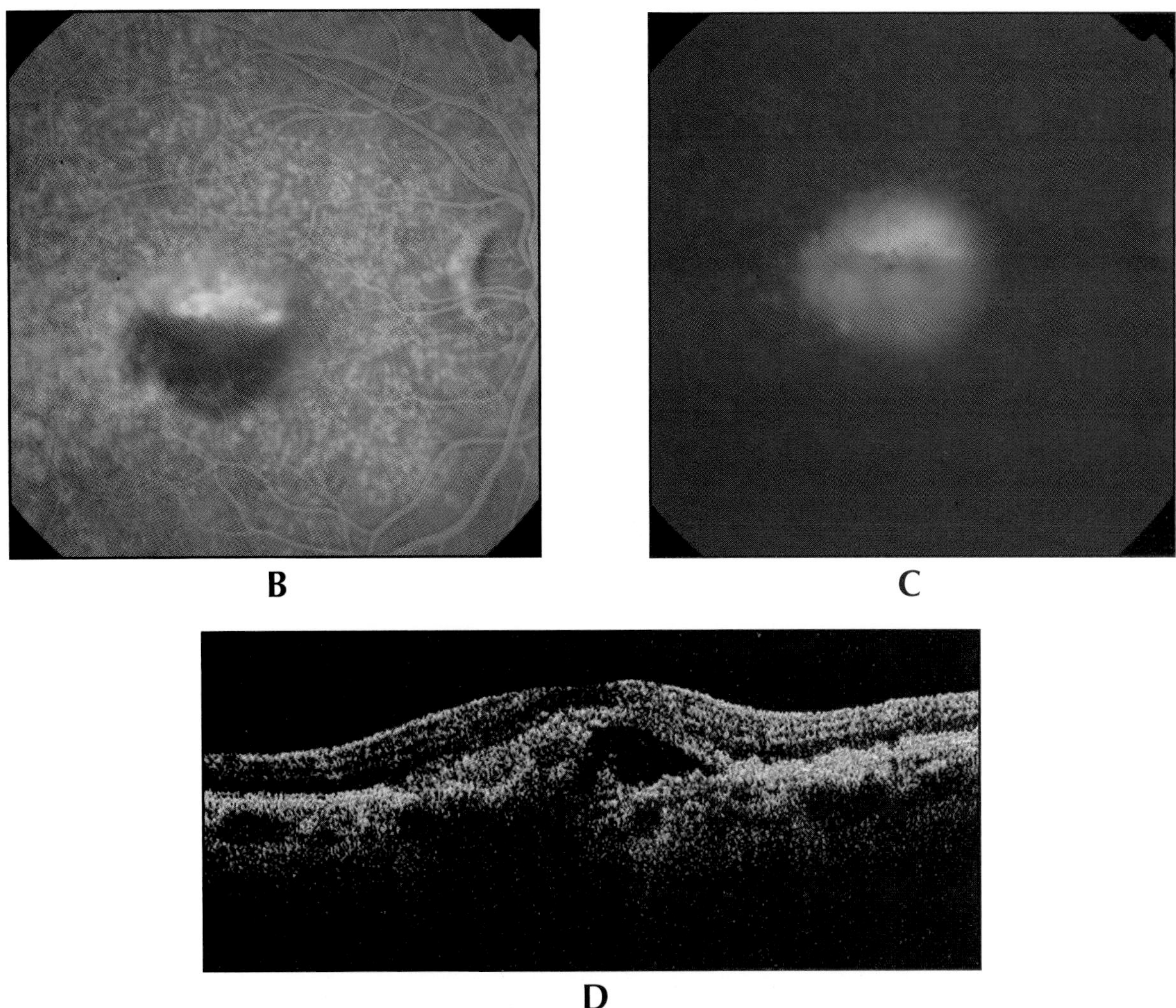
B
C
D

Case 7-5. Basal Laminar Drusen With Vitelliform Macular Lesion

Clinical Summary

A 57-year-old man has been followed for 4 years with a mild decrease in vision. Visual acuity was 20/20 in the right eye and fluctuated between 20/25 and 20/40 in the left eye. Fundus examination revealed basal laminar drusen in both eyes and a vitelliform macular lesion in the right eye (A). Early angiographic images revealed a well-delineated hypofluorescent area corresponding to the vitelliform lesion (B), with late confluent fluorescence within this area (C).

Optical Coherence Tomography

A vertical scan through the foveal center (D) showed elevation of the center with normal appearance of the overlying neurosensory retina. Highly reflective subretinal material was observed inferiorly. This material created a shadowing effect that obscured the layers below. There was a sharp transition between the areas of high and low reflectivity seen on the OCT. The area of low reflectivity most likely represents subretinal fluid. The RPE/Bruch's/choriocapillaris complex underlying this area was not seen probably due to atrophy.

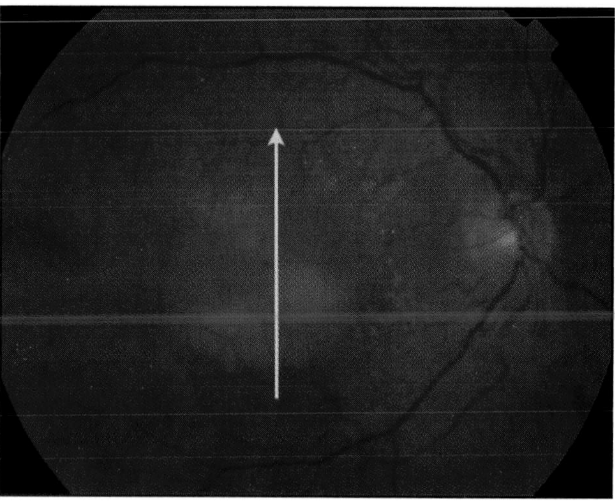

A

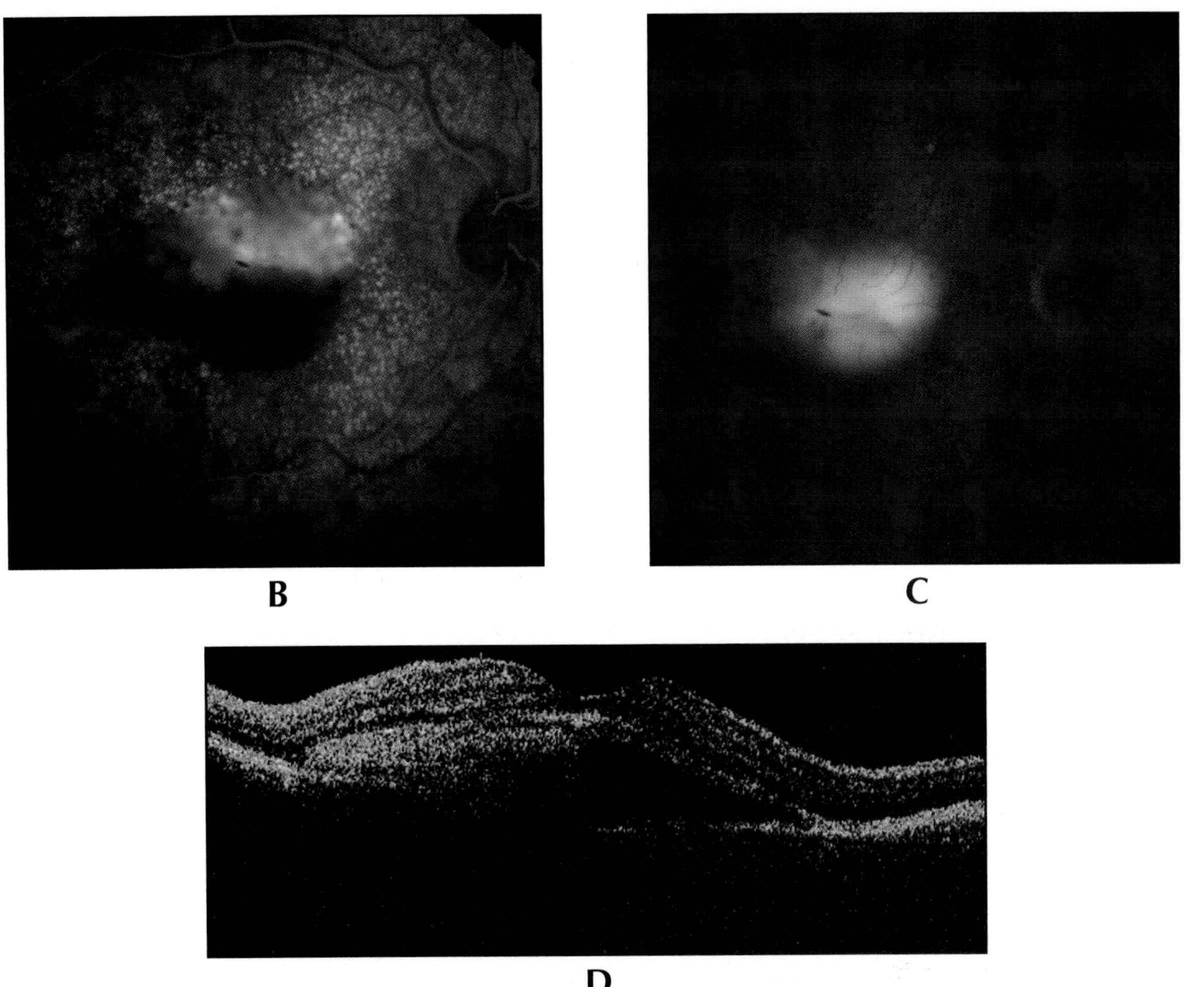
B
C
D

Case 7-6. Foveal Vitelliform Lesion

Clinical Summary

A 70-year-old man complained of blurry vision in his right eye for 2 weeks. Right eye visual acuity was 20/40 while the visual acuity in the left eye was 20/25. Fundus examination of the right eye (A) revealed a round, well-delineated, yellow lesion under the foveal center. Small drusen were observed temporally. A few scattered drusen were observed in the macula of the left eye (B).

Optical Coherence Tomography

A vertical scan through the macula (C) in the right eye showed a flattened foveal contour with a mound of highly reflective material under the fovea elevating the neurosensory retina. No subretinal fluid was observed. A vertical scan through the foveal center in the left eye (D) showed a normal foveal contour and central thickness. Perifoveal vitreoretinal attachments without significant retinal alteration were seen. The external band in this eye was relatively normal in appearance.

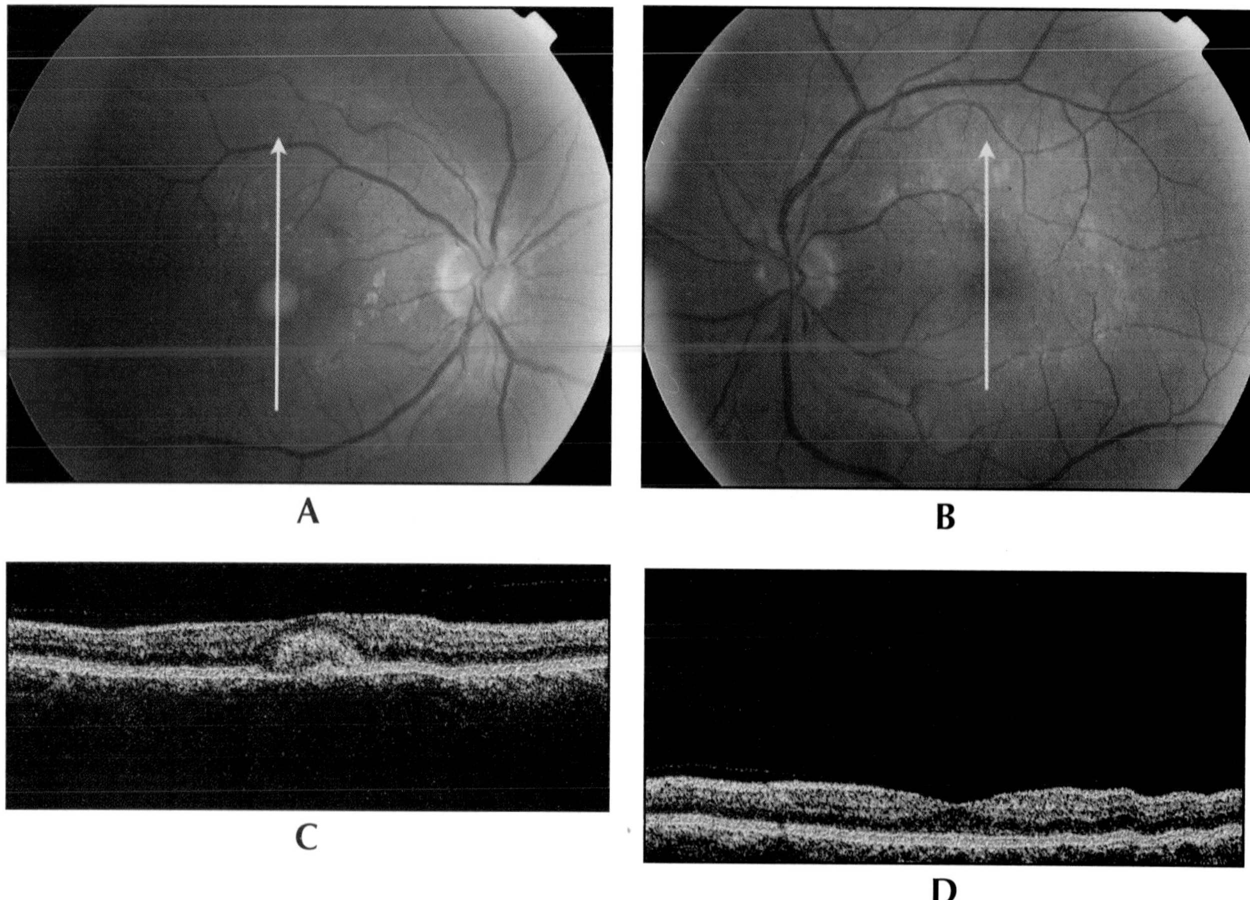

Case 7-7. Geographic Atrophy

Clinical Summary

An 81-year-old woman had a 20-year history of neovascular ARMD with vision loss in her left eye to the 20/400 level. Over the past several months, she noticed worsening vision in her right eye. Visual acuity in this eye was 20/30. Fundus examination of the right eye (A) revealed well-defined areas of geographic atrophy. FA revealed well-defined hyperfluorescence corresponding to these areas of geographic atrophy (B) with late staining but no evidence of leakage (C).

Optical Coherence Tomography

A horizontal scan through the macula (D) showed thinning of the highly reflective external band corresponding to the geographic atrophy nasal to the foveal center. There were deeper reflections observed from the choroid in this area as would be expected in an area of geographic atrophy with corresponding attenuation of the RPE/Bruch's/choriocapillaris complex. The retina overlying this area appeared thinner with loss of the outer layers corresponding to loss of photoreceptors. There is no evidence of subretinal or intraretinal edema, which would indicate the presence of CNV.

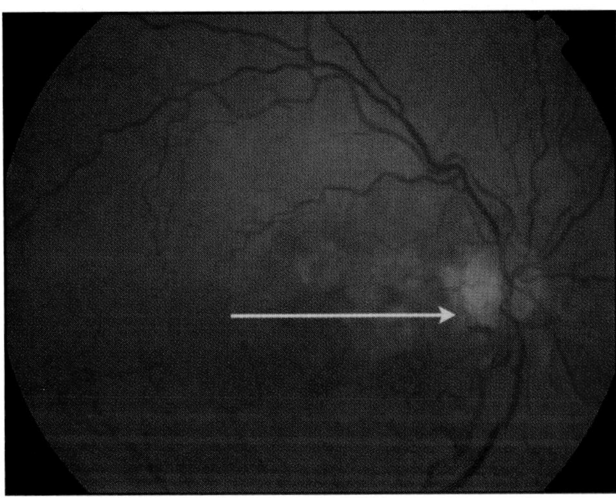

A

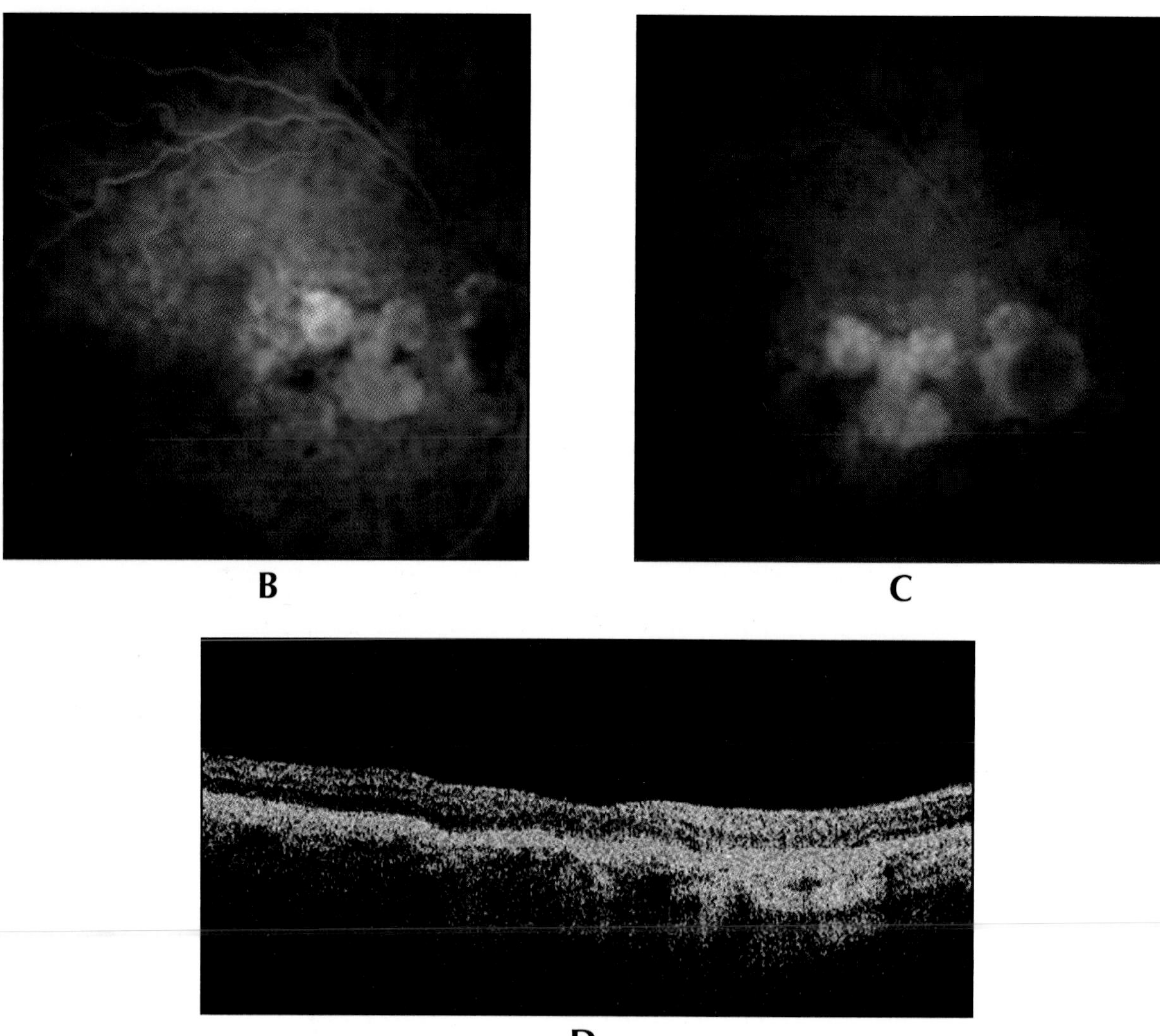
B
C
D

Case 7-8. Geographic Atrophy

Clinical Summary

A 76-year-old woman with a history of chronic vision loss from ARMD had a visual acuity of 20/200 in her left eye. Fundus examination (A) revealed a well-defined area of geographic atrophy compromising the macular area. FA (B) revealed areas of circumscribed fluorescence corresponding to the areas of atrophy with late staining but no evidence of leakage.

Optical Coherence Tomography

A horizontal scan through the macula (C) showed a highly reflective signal from the choroid in the area of geographic atrophy. This results from enhanced penetration and reflection of the signal from the choroid due to the attenuation of the RPE/Bruch's/choriocapillaris complex. The retina overlying this area appeared thinned with loss of the layered structure of the retina. There is no evidence of subretinal or intraretinal fluid accumulation.

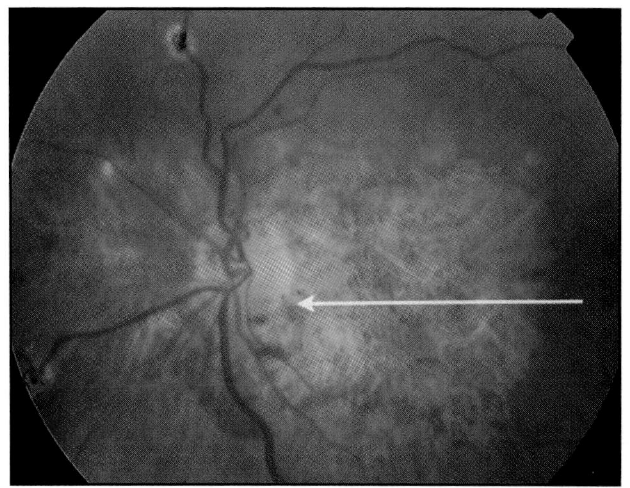

A

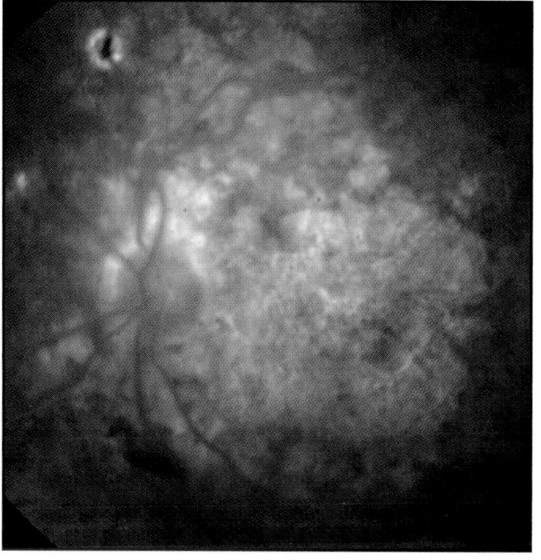

B

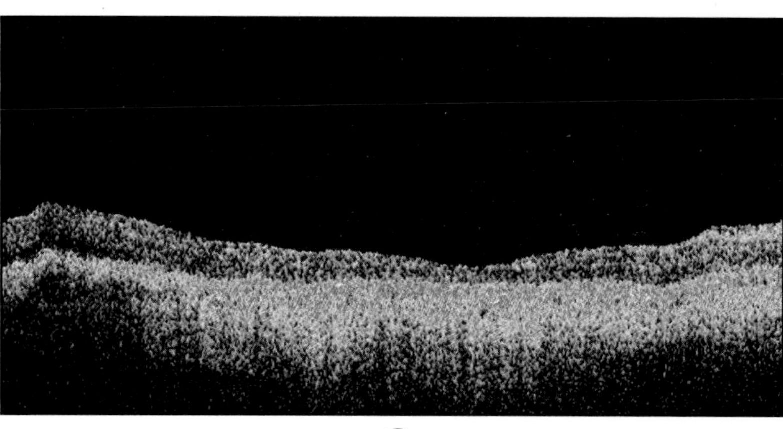

C

Case 7-9. Occult Choroidal Neovascularization—Fibrovascular Pigment Epithelial Detachment

Clinical Summary

A 64-year-old woman with a 4-month history of decreased vision in her right eye has a visual acuity of 20/80. Fundus examination of the right macula (A) revealed soft confluent drusen, pigment mottling, and central retinal thickening. FA revealed early subfoveal stippled hyperfluorescence arising from an elevated and irregular RPE layer (B) associated with late leakage (C), characteristic of occult CNV due to a fibrovascular PED.

Optical Coherence Tomography

An oblique scan through the macula (D) showed an area of decreased reflectivity beneath the neurosensory retina corresponding to subretinal fluid accumulation from the CNV. There did not appear to be significant intraretinal edema, and the foveal contour was mostly preserved. The highly reflective external band under the central macula appeared thickened and irregular. This probably corresponded to the occult CNV, while areas with decreased reflectivity probably represented atrophy.

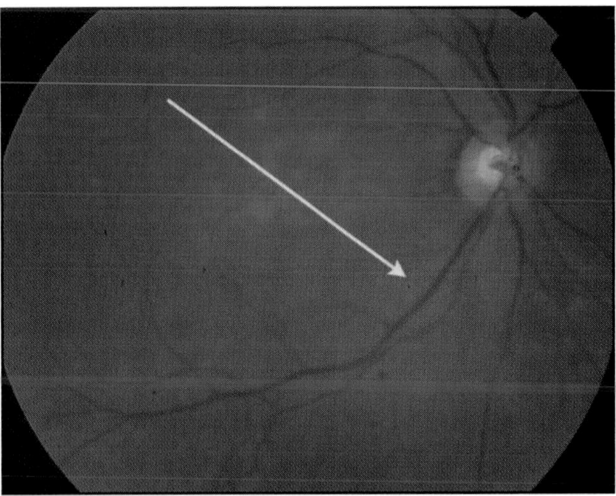

A

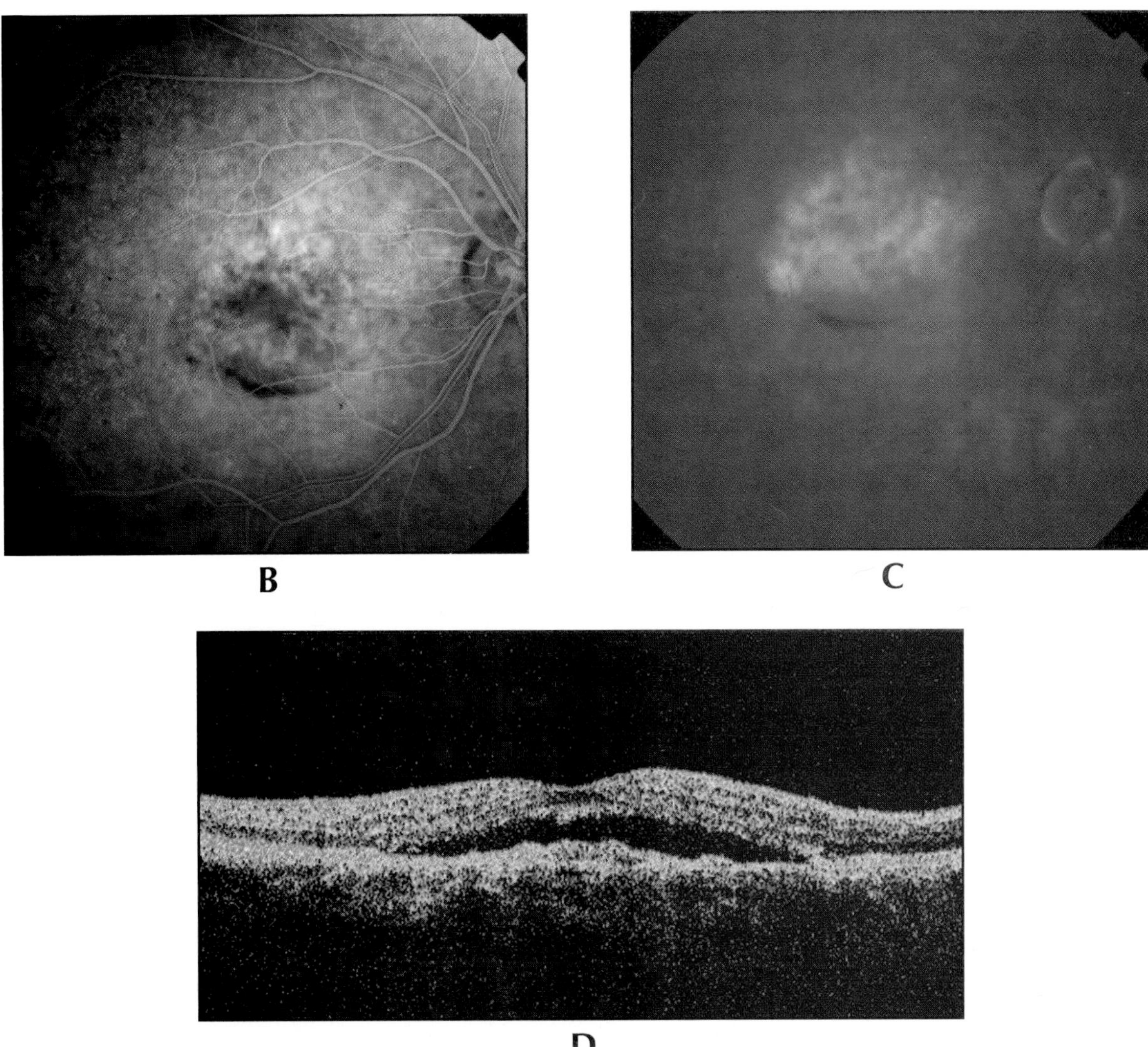
B
C
D

Case 7-10A. Occult Choroidal Neovascularization

Clinical Summary

An 82-year-old woman with a 15-year history of ARMD and stable visual acuity of 20/40 in the right eye complained of distortion and blurry vision for 4 months. Visual acuity in this eye decreased to 20/200. Fundus examination (A) of the right eye revealed retinal thickening, drusen, and pigmentary changes in the central macula. FA showed early stippled hyperfluorescence (B) and diffuse late leakage (C) characteristic of an occult CNV. The patient was observed.

Optical Coherence Tomography

A vertical scan through the macula (D) showed an irregular foveal contour associated with intraretinal and subretinal fluid. The thin layer of subretinal fluid extended beneath the center of the fovea. The highly reflective external band appeared diffusely thickened and irregular.

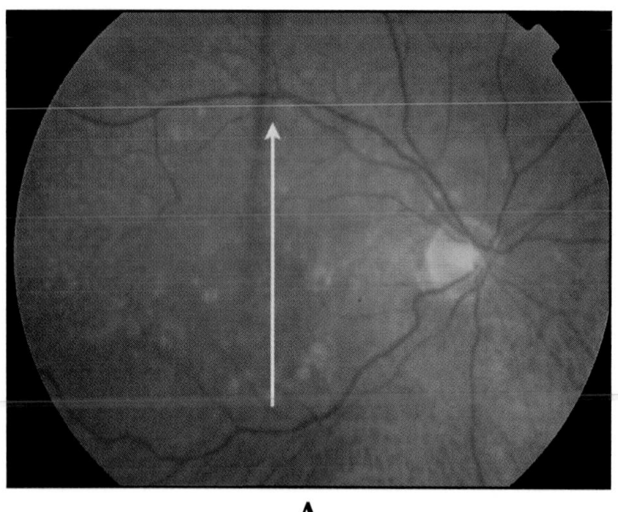

A

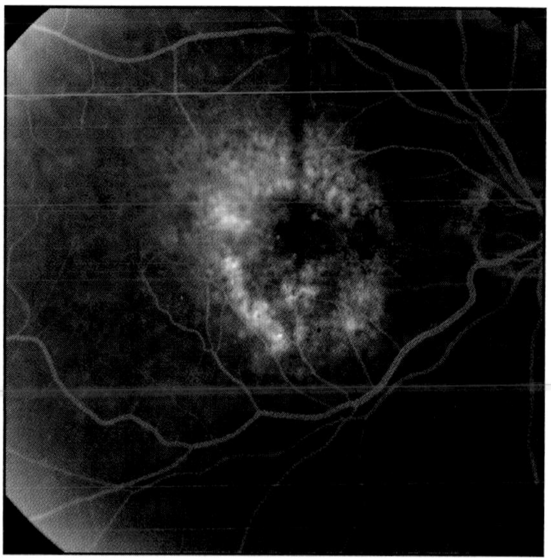

B

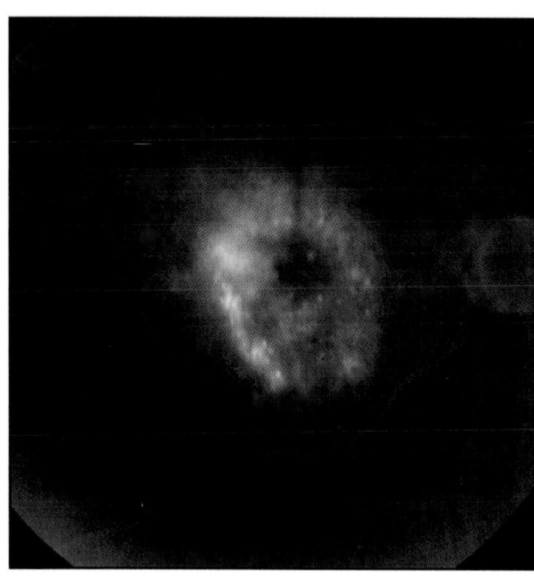

C

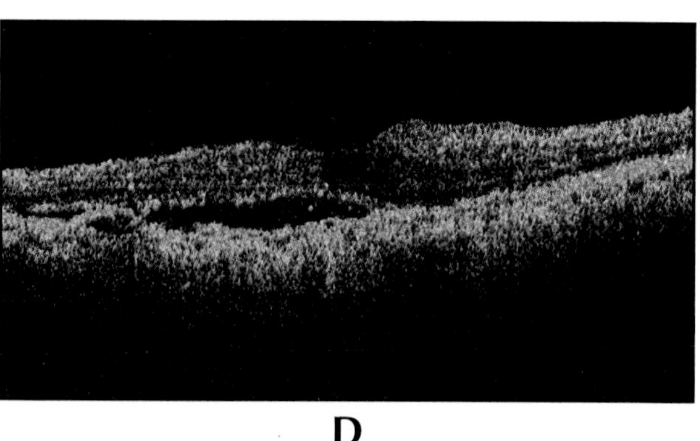

D

Case 7-10B. Occult Choroidal Neovascularization

Continuation of Clinical Summary

Five months later, her vision decreased to 20/300. Fundus examination (E) revealed persistence of the retinal thickening. FA (F) showed a small area of early hyperfluorescence temporal to the foveal center surrounded by stippled fluorescence. In the late phase (G), there was diffuse leakage from these areas.

Follow-Up Optical Coherence Tomography

Repeat vertical scan through the foveal center (H) revealed a diffusely thickened retina. The foveal contour was preserved, but the outer retinal layers appeared highly disorganized likely accounting for the decreased vision. The external highly reflective band appeared diffusely thickened and irregular. There was a small amount of fluid beneath the fovea.

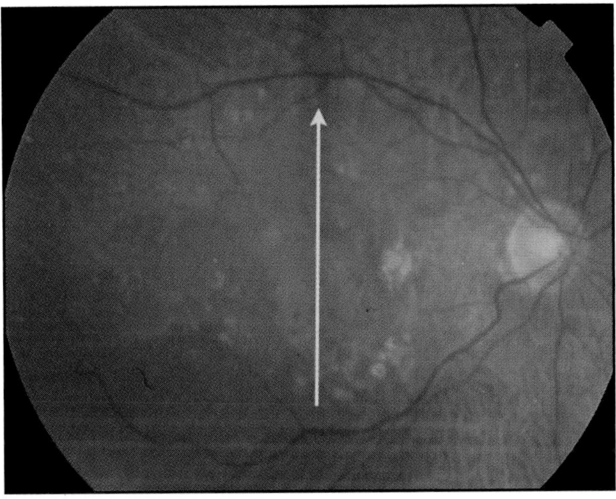

E

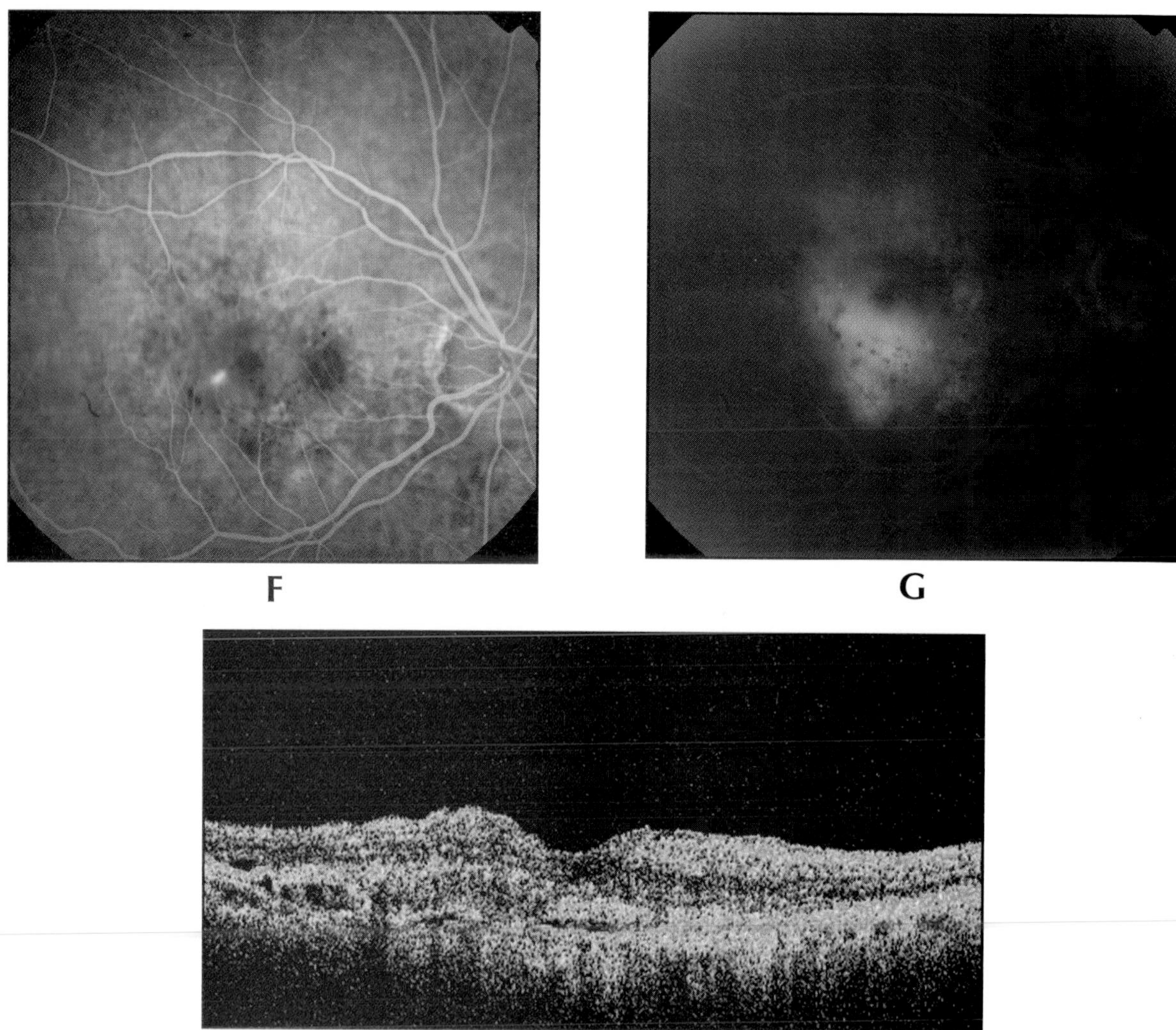
F
G
H

Case 7-11. Minimally Classic Choroidal Neovascularization

Clinical Summary

An 81-year-old woman presented with macular edema, subretinal fluid, and loss of choroidal markings in her left eye (A). Visual acuity was 20/400. FA revealed minimally classic CNV. A central area of classic CNV was surrounded by occult CNV as shown by the early and late frames of the angiogram (B and C).

Optical Coherence Tomography

A horizontal OCT scan through the foveal center (D) revealed disruption of the external band with diminished reflections from the underlying choroid. This optically silent area under the retina was probably caused by light scattering from the fibrovascular tissue seen on angiography. The external highly reflective band appeared thinned and discontinuous with apparent splitting centrally, possibly identifying the CNV within Bruch's membrane. The detailed layered appearance of the neurosensory retina was lost, and there was extensive intraretinal cystic edema.

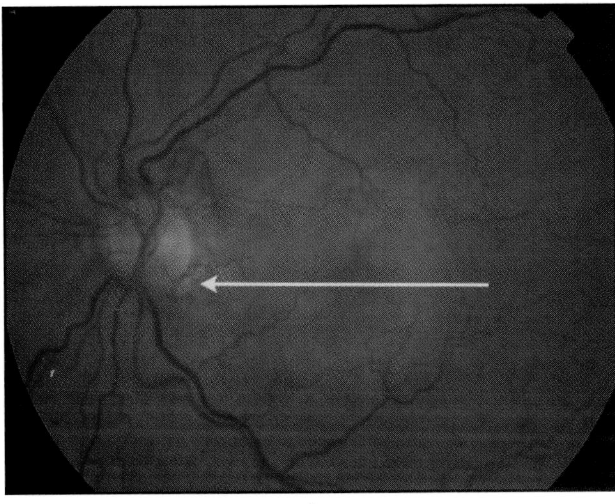

A

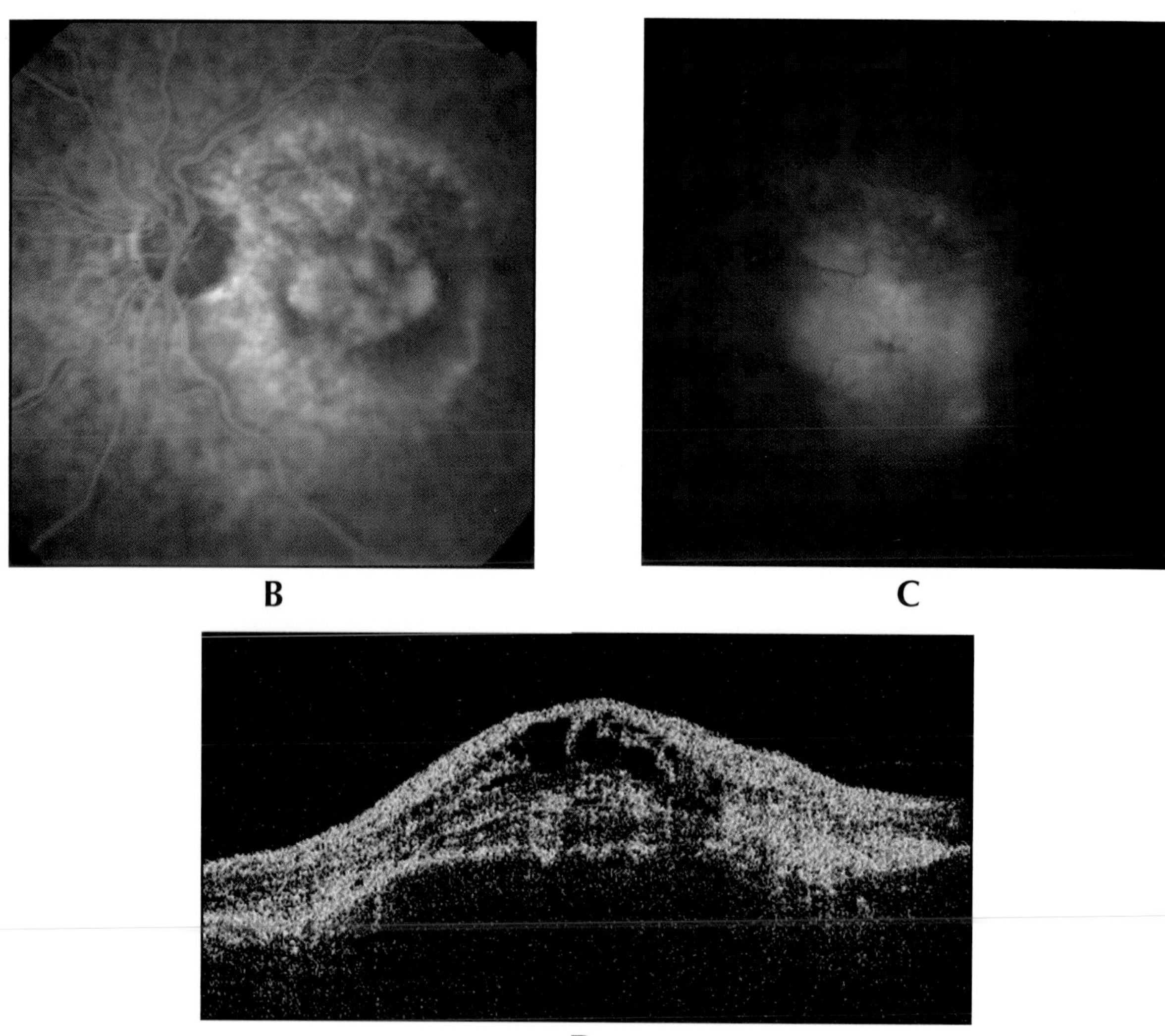
B
C
D

Case 7-12. Minimally Classic Choroidal Neovascularization

Clinical Summary

A 55-year-old woman with a 5-month history of decreased vision had a visual acuity of 20/100 in her left eye. Fundus examination (A) revealed subretinal fluid in the central macula with a rim of subretinal hemorrhage superiorly. The early angiographic image (B) revealed a well-defined area of hyperfluorescence with surrounding stippled fluorescence. There was diffuse leakage on the late angiogram images (C). This pattern was consistent with a minimally classic lesion. The patient was observed.

Optical Coherence Tomography

An oblique OCT scan through the fovea (D) showed an asymmetric foveal contour with evidence of retinal thickening and loss of retinal details extending inferotemporally from the foveal center (left side of the scan). The external highly reflective band appeared thickened and irregular centrally, probably representing the fibrovascular tissue identified angiographically as classic CNV. The areas of low reflectivity under the retina and adjacent to the presumed CNV corresponded to subretinal fluid.

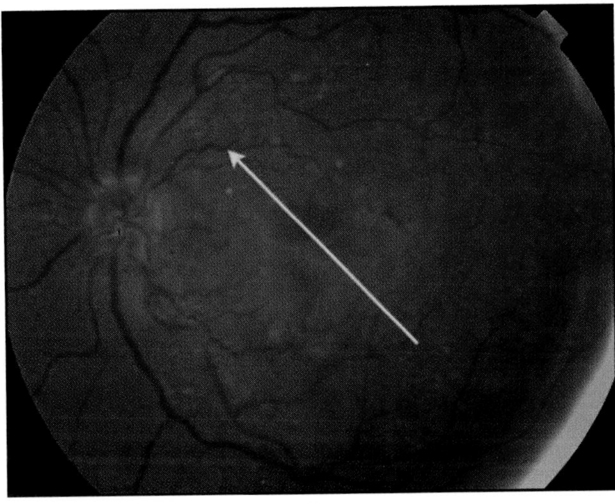

A

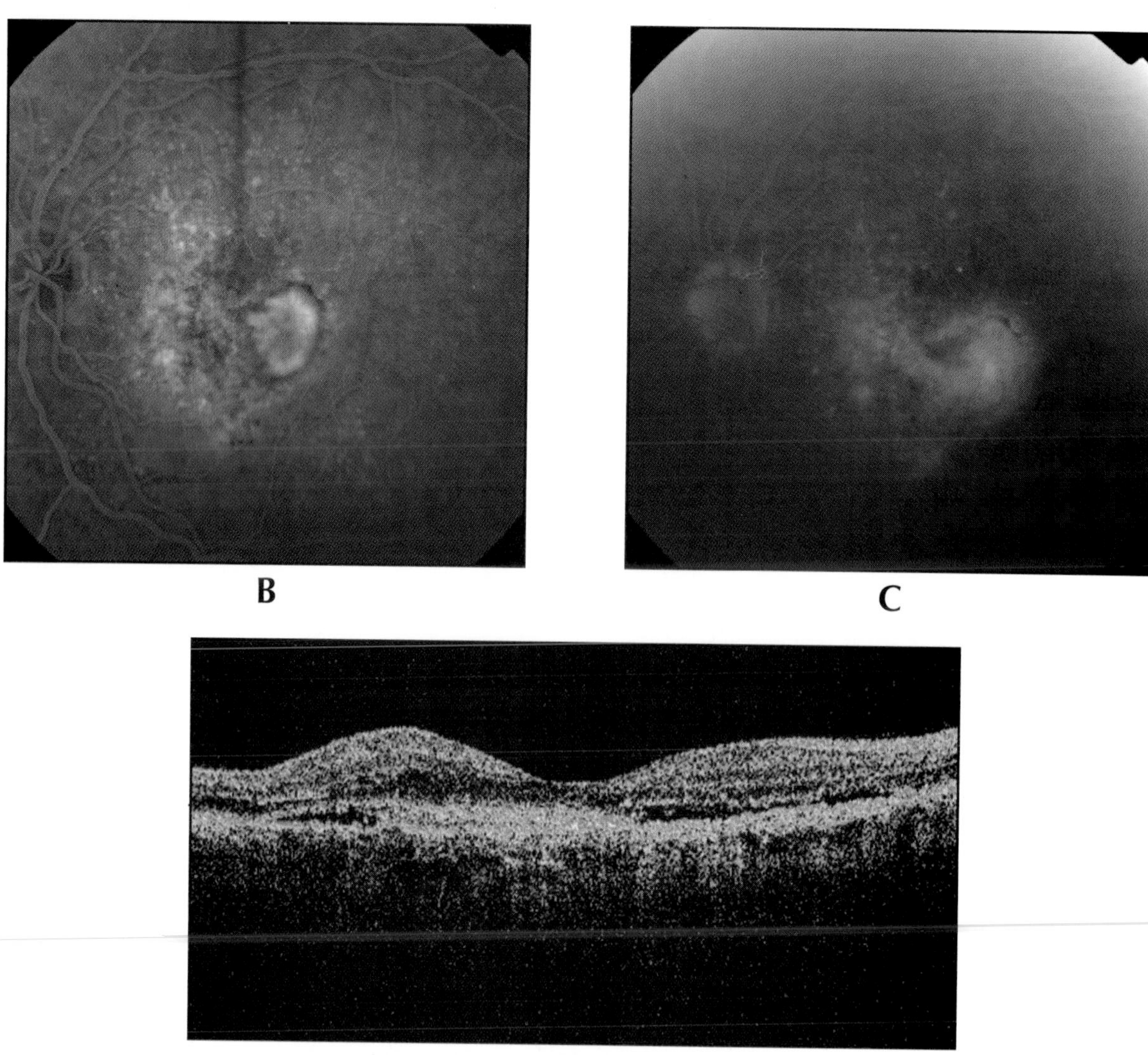
B
C
D

Case 7-13. Minimally Classic Choroidal Neovascularization With an Occult Component Characterized as a Fibrovascular Pigment Epithelial Detachment

Clinical Summary

A 65-year-old man with a 3-year history of decreased vision in his left eye had a visual acuity of 20/200. Fundus examination of the left macula (A) revealed macular edema with evidence of subfoveal fluid. FA (B and C) showed minimally classic CNV with a small area of classic CNV visible nasal to the foveal center surrounded by a larger area of occult CNV. The occult CNV was seen as early stippled fluorescence and late leakage on the angiogram, which is characteristic of a fibrovascular PED.

Optical Coherence Tomography

A vertical scan through the foveal center (D) revealed an irregular highly reflective external band with focal thickening in the area corresponding to the classic CNV component observed on angiography. Areas of mild external band elevation with highly reflective material beneath were observed inferior to the foveal center corresponding to the fibrovascular PED. Subretinal fluid indicating active exudation from the neovascularization was evident as an optically clear space between the neurosensory retina and the external band.

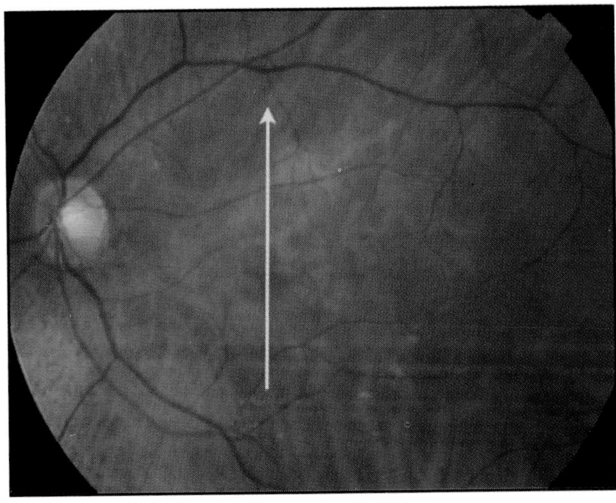

A

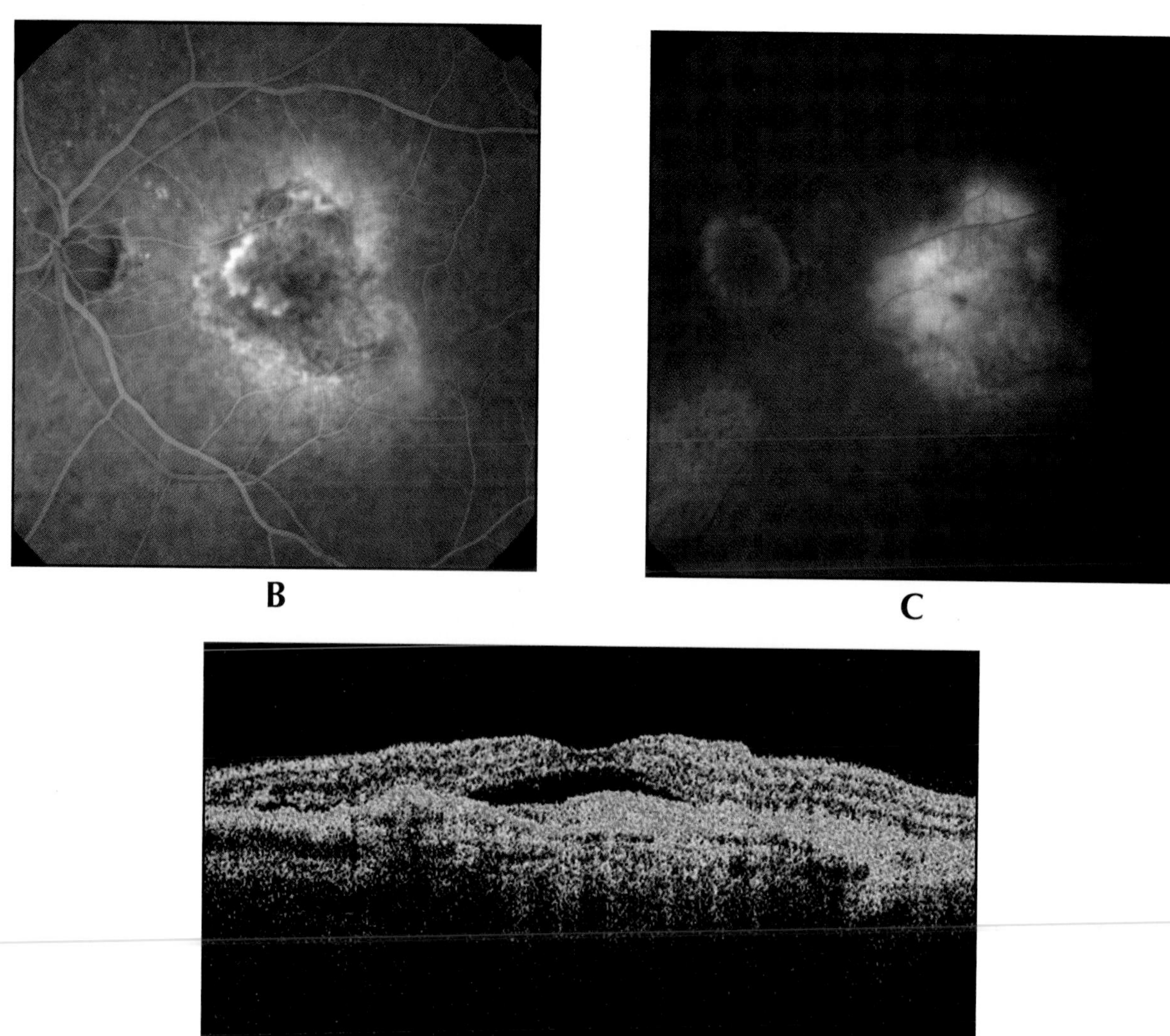
B
C
D

Case 7-14. Minimally Classic Choroidal Neovascularization—Retinal Angiomatous Proliferation

Clinical Summary

A 75-year-old woman was referred for evaluation of occult CNV in the left eye with slowly deteriorating vision over the past 6 months. Visual acuity was 20/60 in the left eye. Fundus examination (A) of the left eye showed a small, dome-shaped PED with a punctate intraretinal hemorrhage. FA (B) showed a pinpoint area of early hyperfluorescence adjacent to the intraretinal hemorrhage. The surrounding PED filled slowly and stained late within the original borders of the lesion (C). The findings were felt to be consistent with a RAP.

Optical Coherence Tomography

An oblique scan through the fovea (D) showed loss of the foveal contour with mild intraretinal cystic edema. There was elevation of the external reflective band consistent with a PED. The elevated external band appeared thickened and irregular. The choroidal reflections under the PED appeared decreased due to shadowing. An area of subretinal fluid could be seen off the edge of the PED.

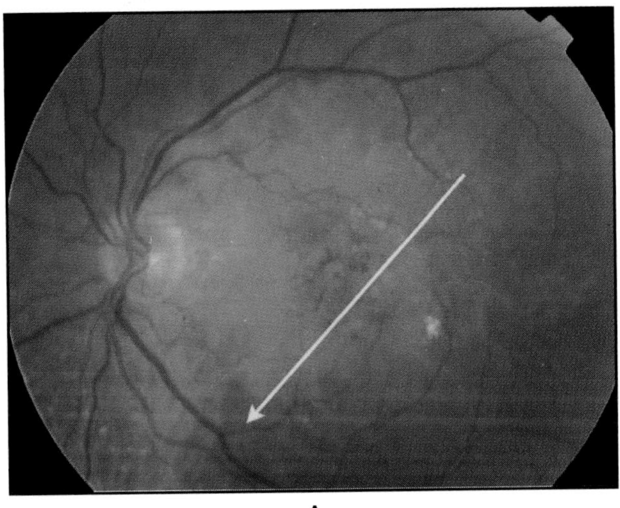

A

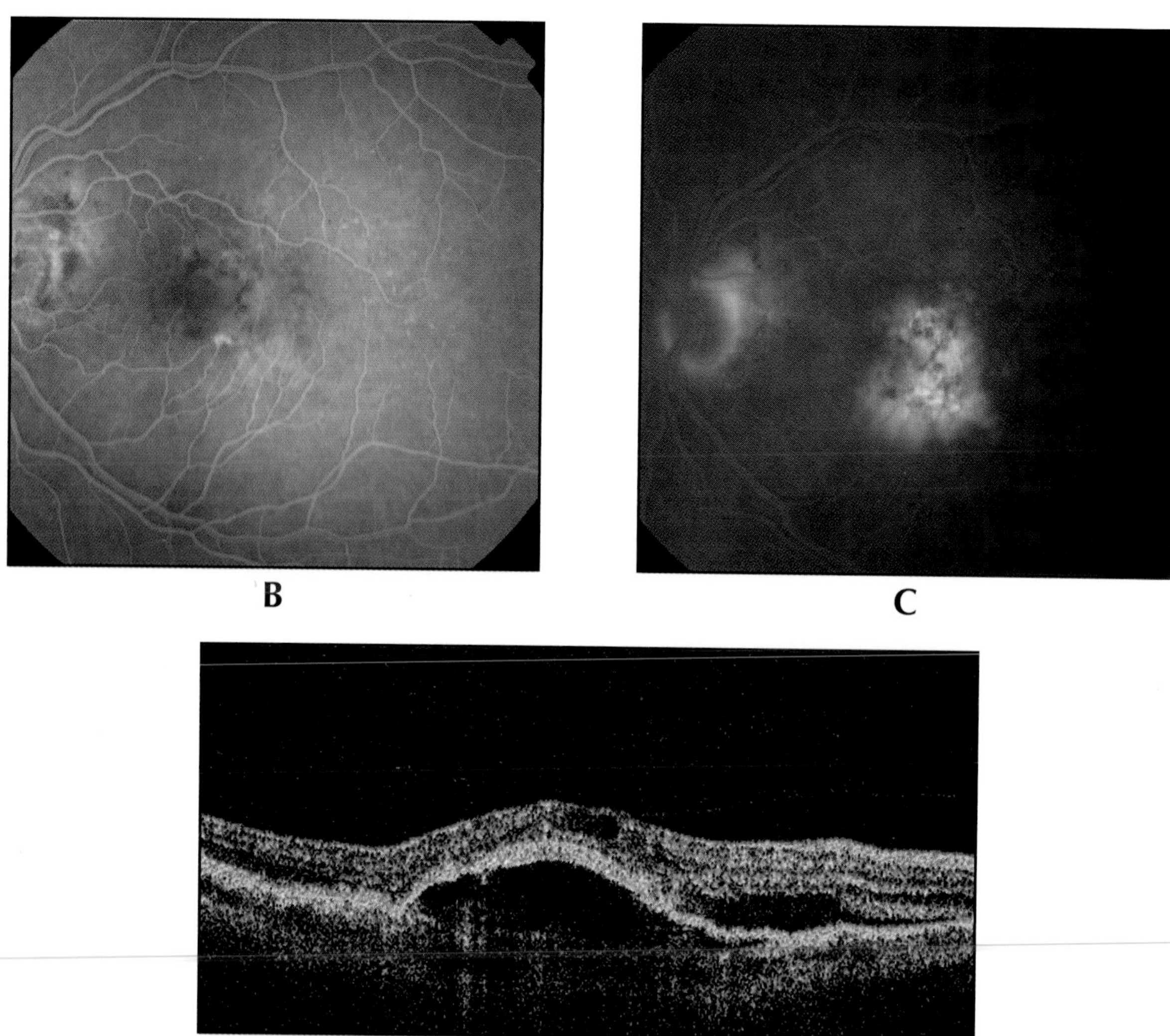
B
C
D

Case 7-15A.
Predominantly Classic Choroidal Neovascularization

Clinical Summary

A 78-year-old man presented with a 5-month history of decreased vision in his right eye and visual acuity of 20/200. Metamorphopsia was present on Amsler grid testing. Fundus examination (A) revealed a centrally elevated gray lesion of approximately 1.5 disc diameters surrounded by small intraretinal hemorrhages, subretinal fluid, and retinal edema. FA (B and C) showed predominantly classic subfoveal CNV. The patient was treated with PDT.

Optical Coherence Tomography

A horizontal scan through the foveal center (D) showed central elevation with loss of the foveal contour. The external highly reflective band appeared diffusely thickened in the area corresponding to the classic CNV. The optically silent areas in the perifoveal region represented fluid leaking from the CNV, although it was unclear whether this was subretinal or intraretinal in location. The central band of reflectivity corresponded to the hypofluorescent center of the CNV lesion, and probably represented a focal area of adherence between the CNV and the retina. The detailed layered appearance of the neurosensory retina was partially lost due to the retinal edema.

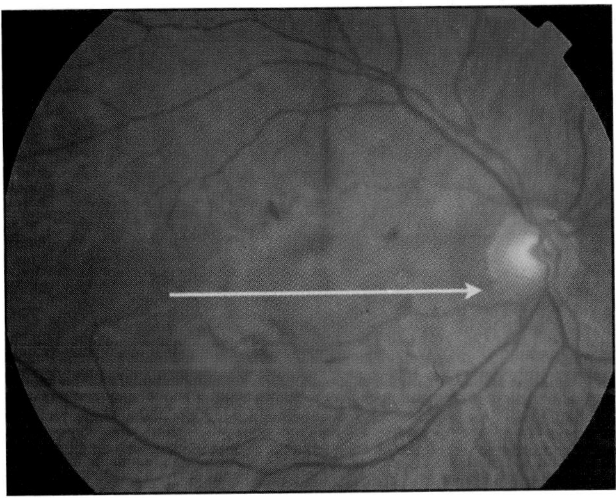

A

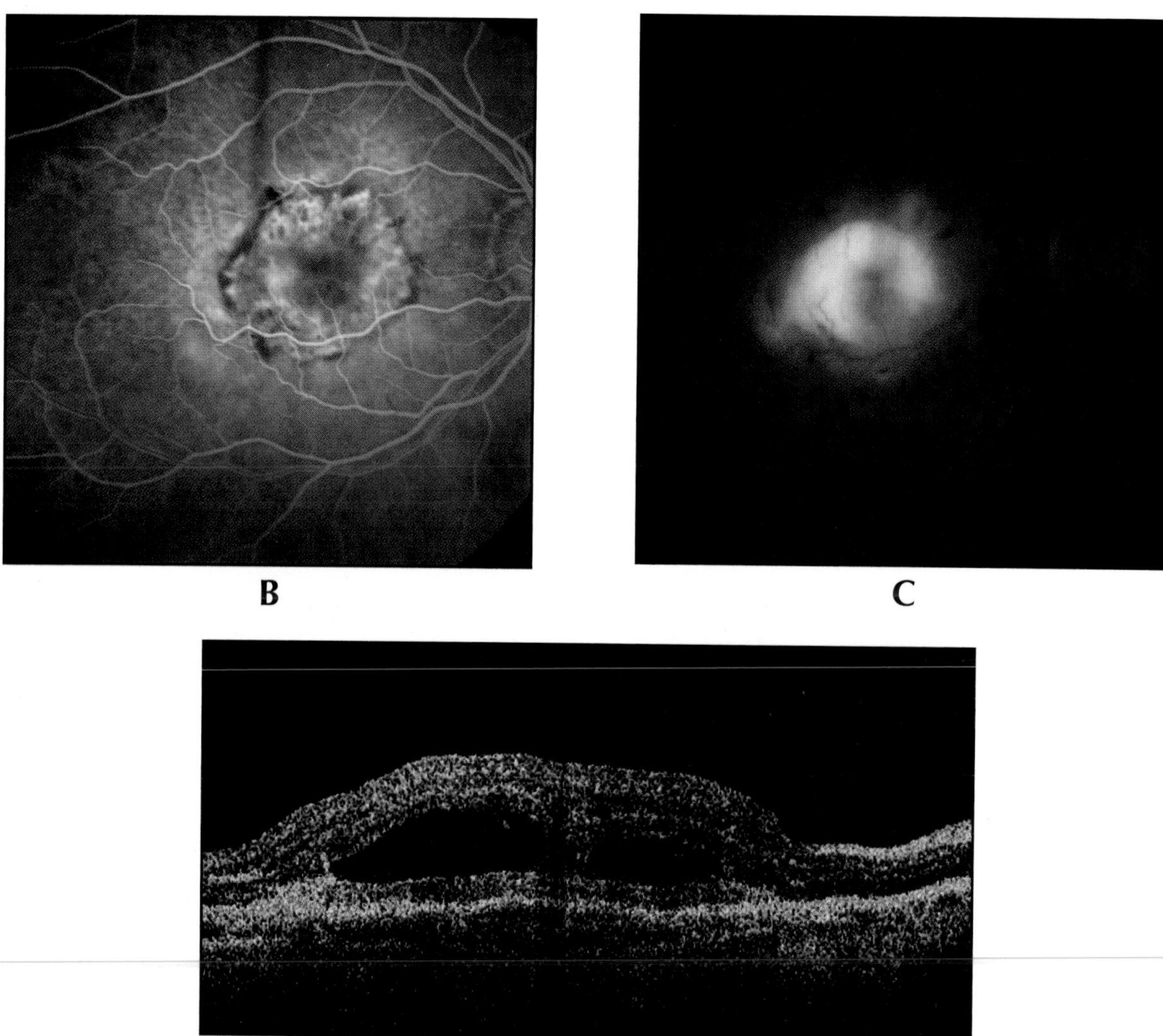
B
C
D

Case 7-15B. Three Months After Photodynamic Therapy

Continuation of Clinical Summary

Three months after PDT, vision in the right eye improved slightly to 20/80. The CNV appeared fibrotic with a persistent hemorrhagic rim inferiorly (E). FA showed a smaller classic component within an area of circular hypofluorescence corresponding to the PDT spot (F). Fluorescein staining with questionable leakage was observed in the late frames of the angiogram (G). Observation was recommended.

Follow-Up Optical Coherence Tomography

A horizontal scan through the foveal center (H) showed reduced retinal edema/subretinal fluid. Only a few small cystic cavities remained within the retina, and the foveal contour was improved. The external highly reflective band showed a central area of fusiform thickening that is better defined at this time. The reduction in exudation indicated good response to treatment.

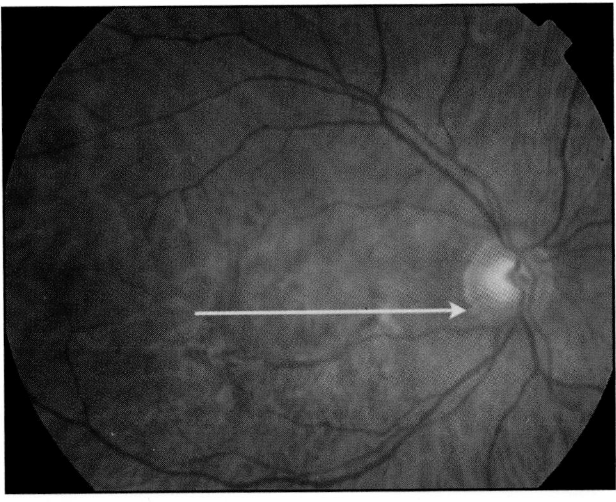

E

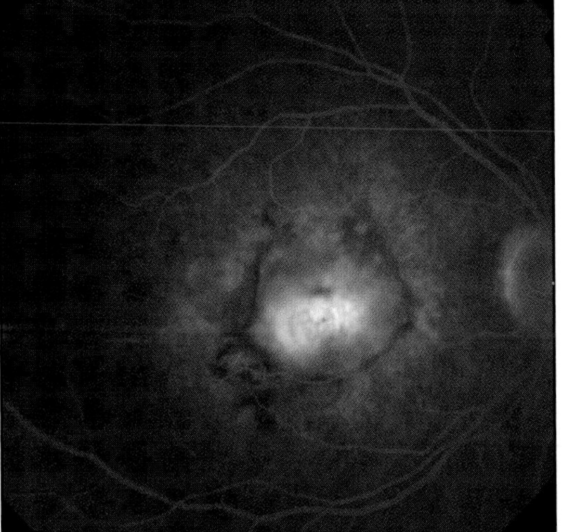

F

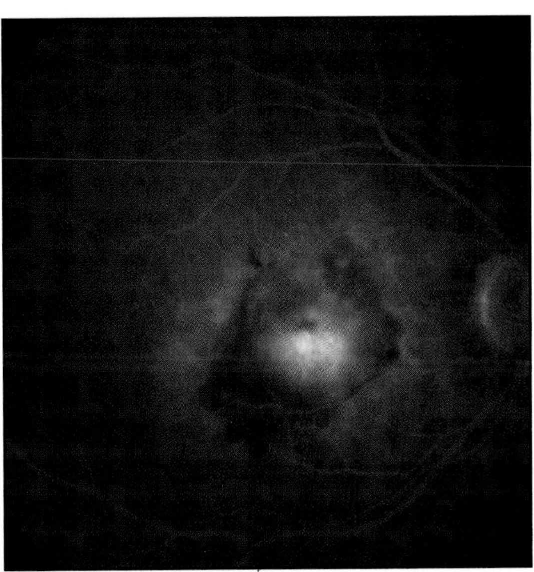

G

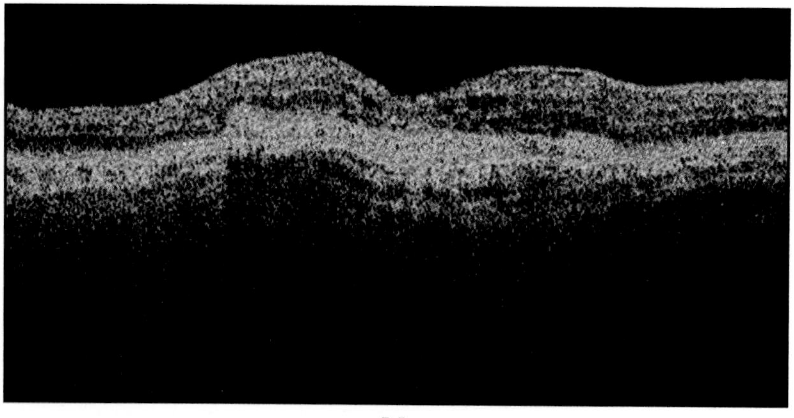

H

Case 7-15C. Additional Monitoring After Photodynamic Therapy

Continuation of Clinical Summary

Six weeks later (4.5 months after PDT), vision in the patient's right eye remained 20/80. The CNV lesion appeared fibrotic surrounded by RPE atrophy and no evidence of hemorrhage (I). FA showed early central hyperfluorescence and late staining (J and K). Continued observation was recommended.

Follow-Up Optical Coherence Tomography

Repeat scan through the fovea (L) showed a single large intraretinal cyst but was otherwise mostly unchanged. There was also stable central thickening of the external highly reflective band. There was still no evidence of subretinal fluid accumulation.

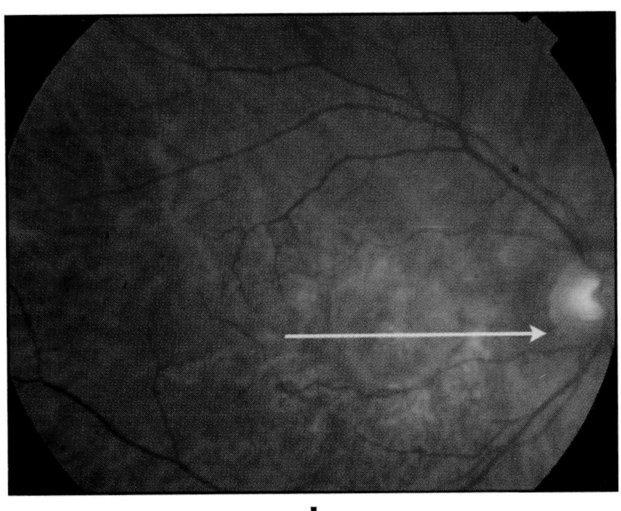

I

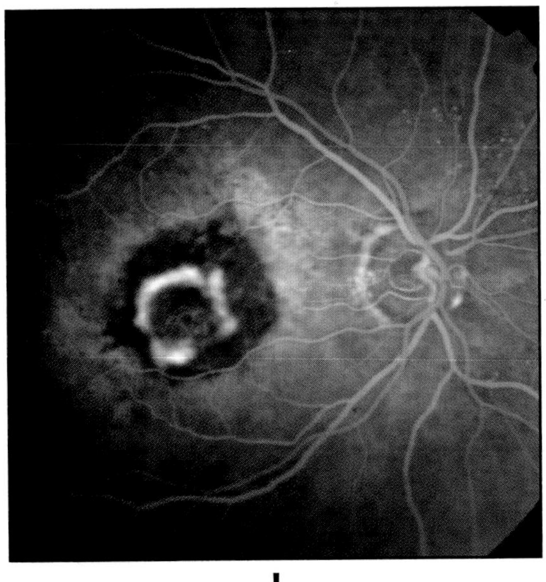

J

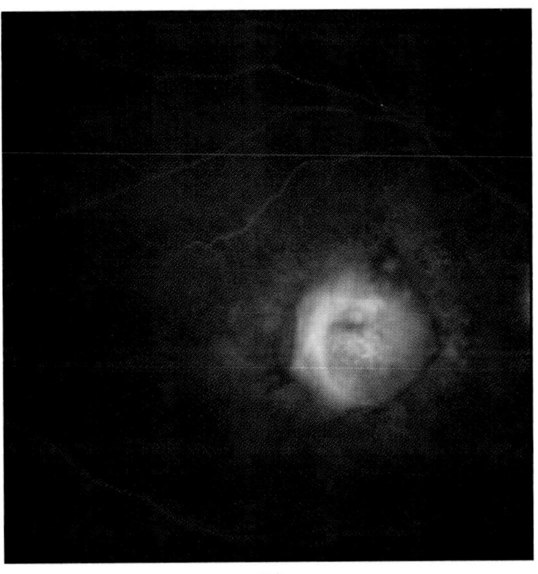

K

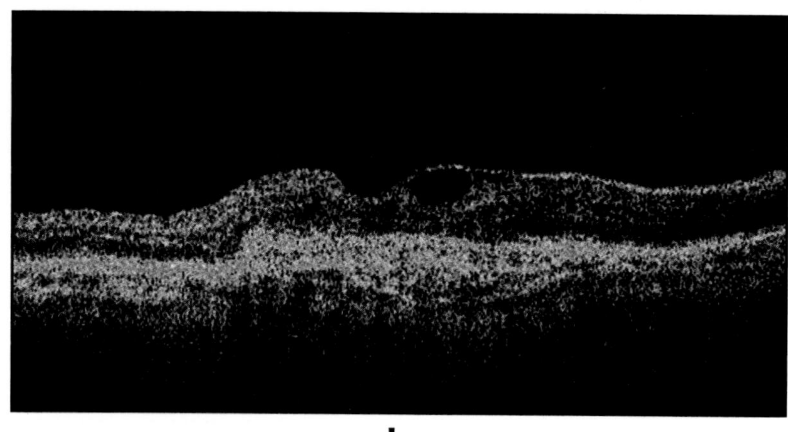

L

Case 7-16A. Classic Choroidal Neovascularization

Clinical Summary

A 73-year-old woman presented with a 4-month history of decreased vision in her right eye. Visual acuity was 20/100. Fundus examination (A) revealed a pigmented lesion extending superiorly from the foveal center with surrounding subretinal fluid. An early angiographic image (B) showed well-delineated lacy subfoveal CNV. Diffuse leakage was evident in a late angiographic image (C). The patient was treated with PDT.

Optical Coherence Tomography

A vertical scan through the foveal center (D) showed retinal thickening with loss of the foveal contour. There was localized thickening and irregularity of the highly reflective external band extending superiorly from the foveal center corresponding to the classic CNV. A small pocket of subretinal fluid was present. The detached posterior hyaloid could be seen as a thin linear opacity suspended above the retina.

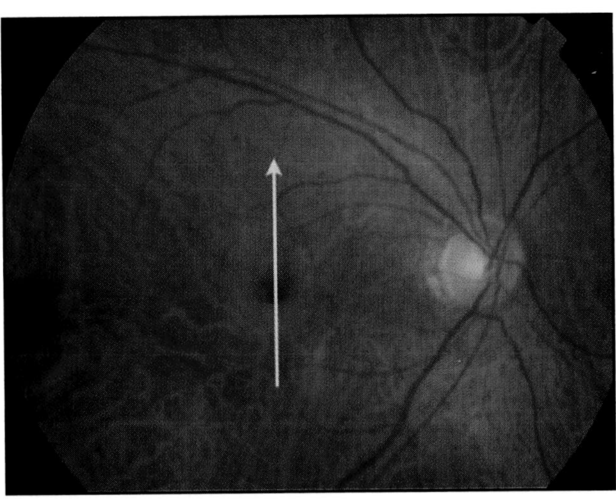

A

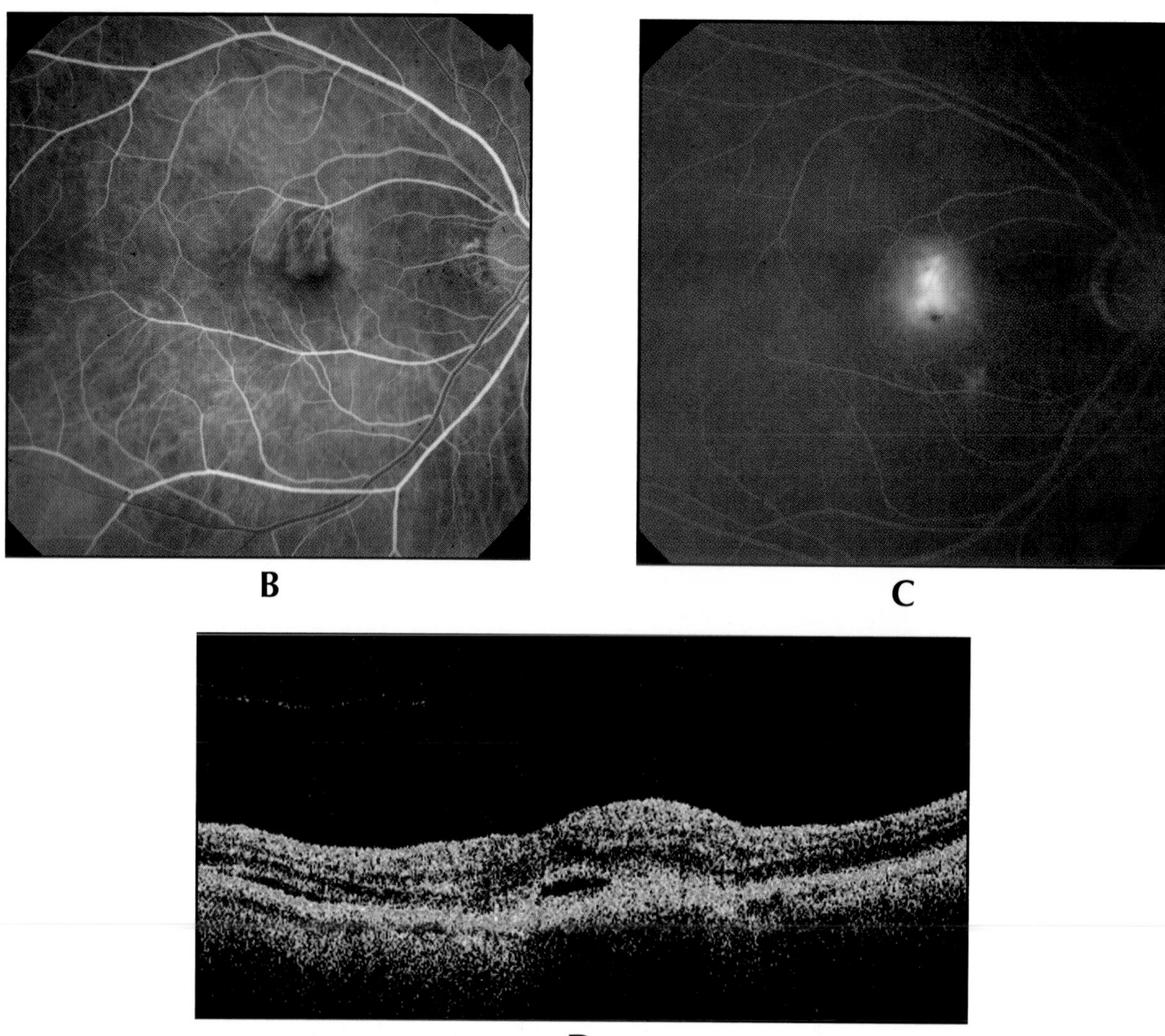

B

C

D

Case 7-16B. Six Weeks After Photodynamic Therapy

Continuation of Clinical Summary

Six weeks after treatment, the patient's vision improved to 20/60. There was less subfoveal fluid present on fundus examination (E). FA (F and G) showed a marked decrease in the size of the lesion and in the amount of leakage. The patient was observed.

Follow-Up Optical Coherence Tomography

Repeat scan through the foveal center (H) showed an improved foveal contour with a decrease in retinal thickening. The layered structure of the inner retina appeared more compact and organized. There was a well-defined area of external band thickening that extends superiorly from the foveal center corresponding to the treated CNV. A thin layer of subretinal fluid persisted under the foveal center.

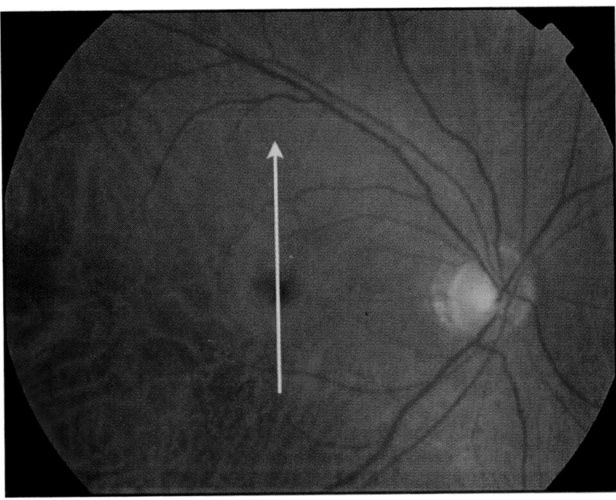

E

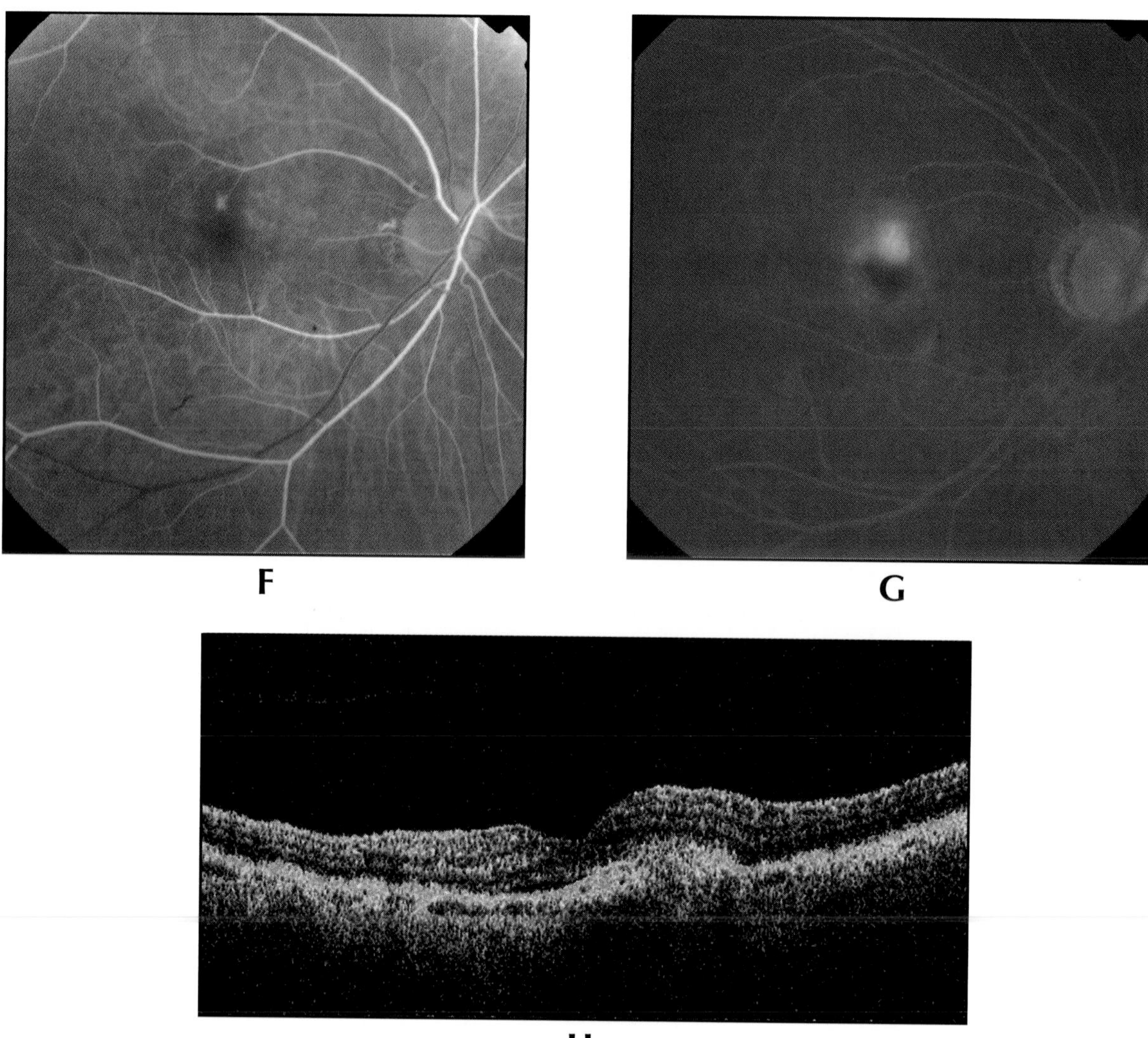
F
G
H

Case 7-16C. Three Months After Photodynamic Therapy

Continuation of Clinical Summary

Three months after PDT, the visual acuity remained 20/60. The lesion extended superiorly from the foveal center (I). Compared to the previous angiogram from the 6-week visit, these angiograms (J and K) showed enlargement of the lesion with increased leakage. The patient was given a second treatment with PDT.

Follow-Up Optical Coherence Tomography

A vertical scan trough the foveal center (L) showed an increase in the amount of subretinal fluid. The area of the external band corresponding to the CNV appeared thicker. The overlying retina showed only mild thickening with some preservation of the foveal contour. Increases in the size of the CNV and amount of subretinal fluid clearly indicate recurrent activity of the CNV.

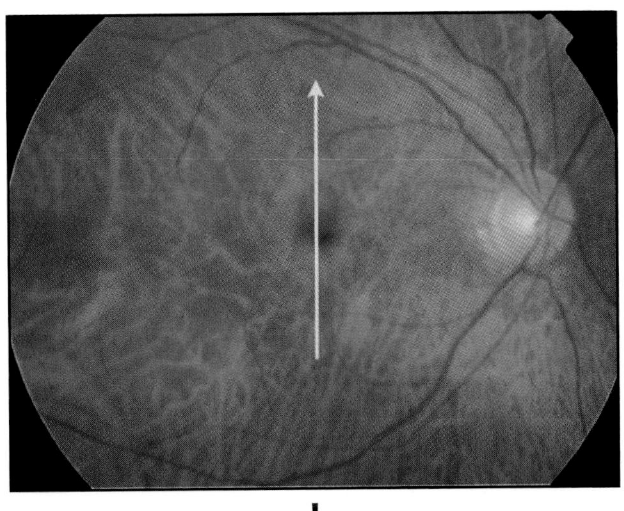

I

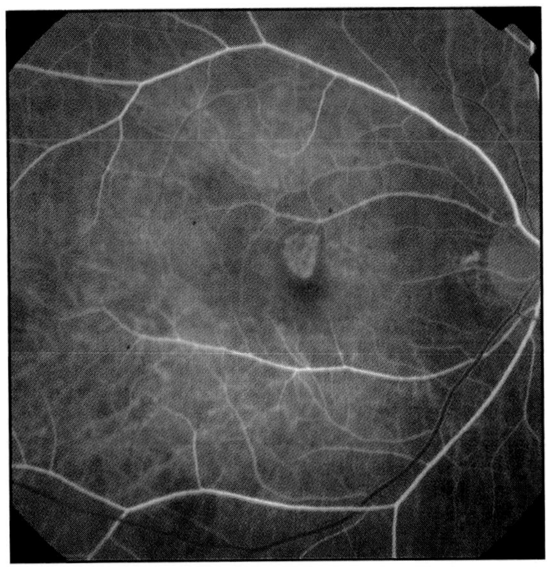

J

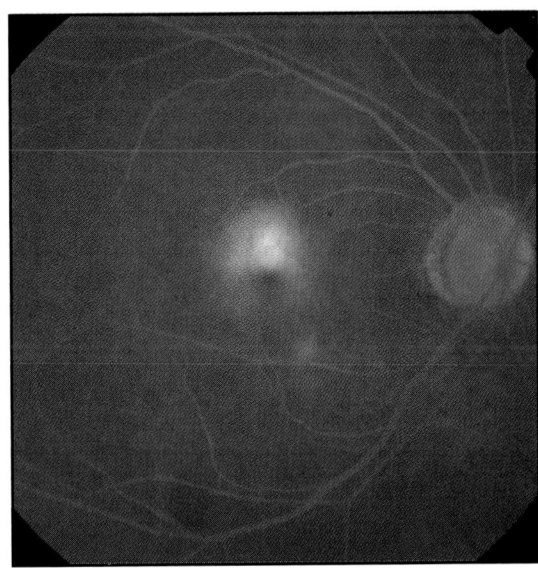

K

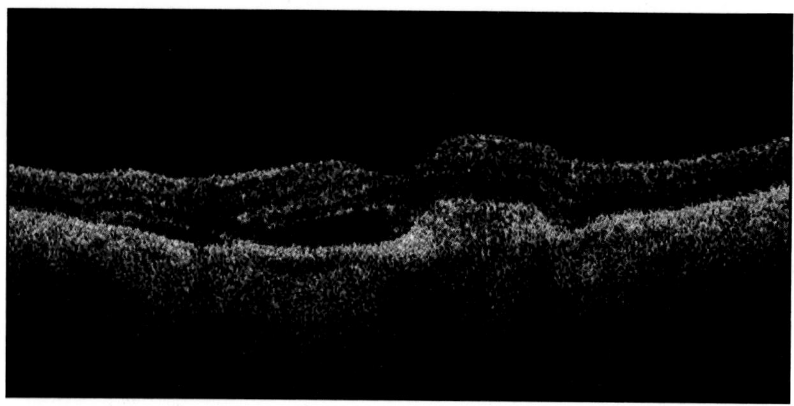

L

Case 7-16D. Three Months After the Second Photodynamic Therapy Treatment

Continuation of Clinical Summary

Three months after the second PDT treatment, the visual acuity was 20/50. The lesion showed persistent edema and was surrounded by small hemorrhages (M). An angiogram showed enlargement of the classic CNV lesion with late leakage (N and O). The patient received a third PDT treatment.

Follow-Up Optical Coherence Tomography

A repeat scan through the foveal center (P) showed further increase in the subretinal fluid inferior to the CNV. A small amount of subretinal fluid was now also evident superior to the CNV. The CNV lesion showed only mild enlargement. The layered architecture of the retina and the foveal contour was preserved.

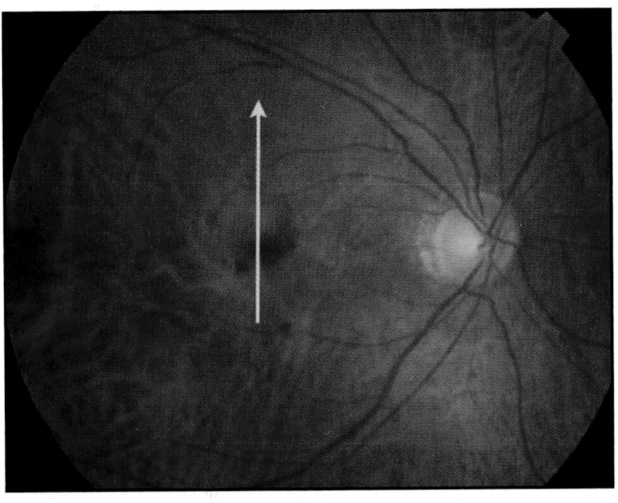

M

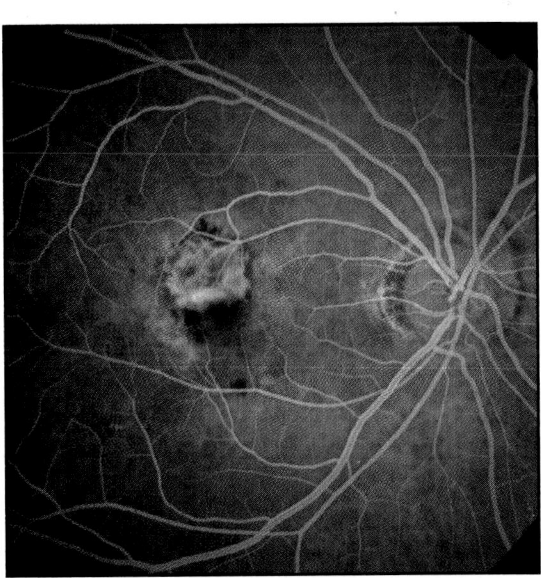

N

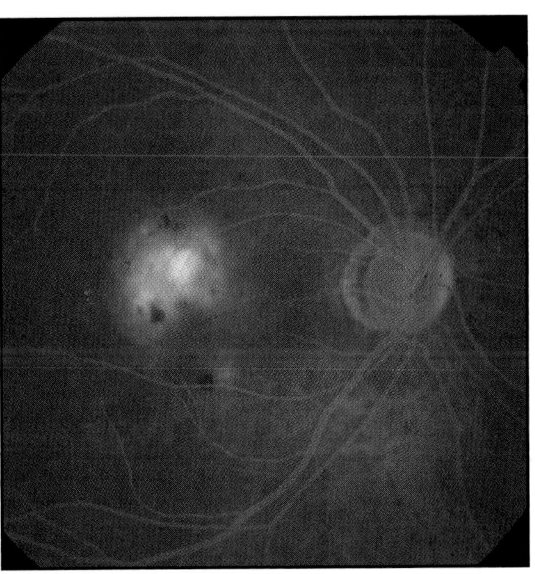

O

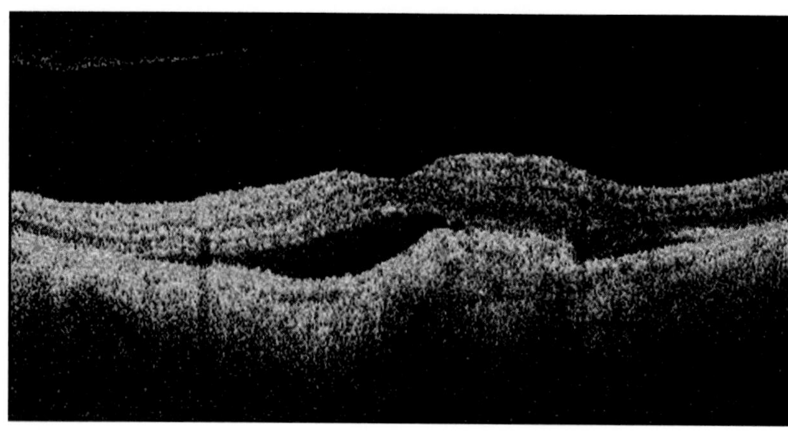

P

Case 7-16E. Three Months After the Third Photodynamic Therapy Treatment

Continuation of Clinical Summary

Three months after the third PDT, the vision was stable at 20/50. The lesion (Q) appeared well demarcated with early fibrosis. A small amount of subretinal fluid was still present around the lesion. An early angiogram showed a well-defined CNV lesion with mild leakage in the late phases (R and S). The patient received a fourth PDT treatment.

Follow-Up Optical Coherence Tomography

A repeat scan through the foveal center (T) showed a decrease in the subretinal fluid inferior to the CNV. The area of thickening that represented the CNV lesion was mostly stable. The retina continued to show minimal thickening with a preserved foveal contour.

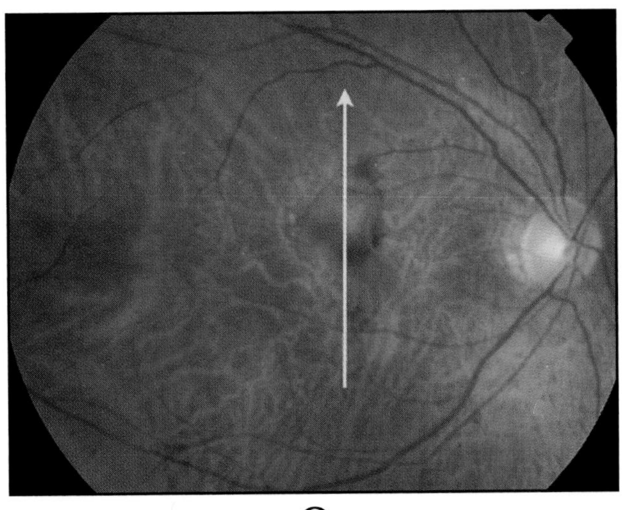

Q

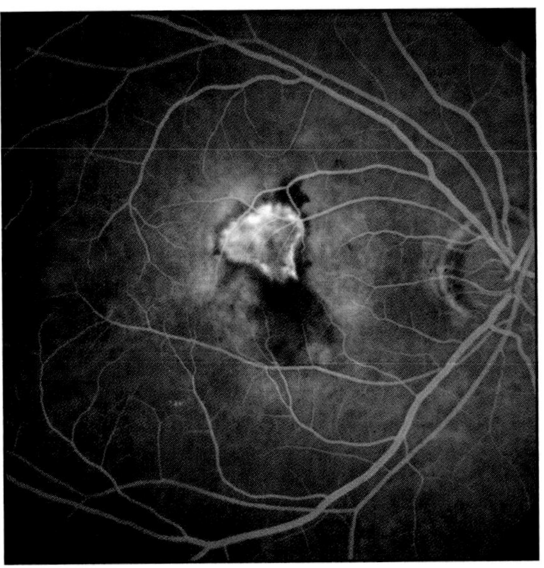

R

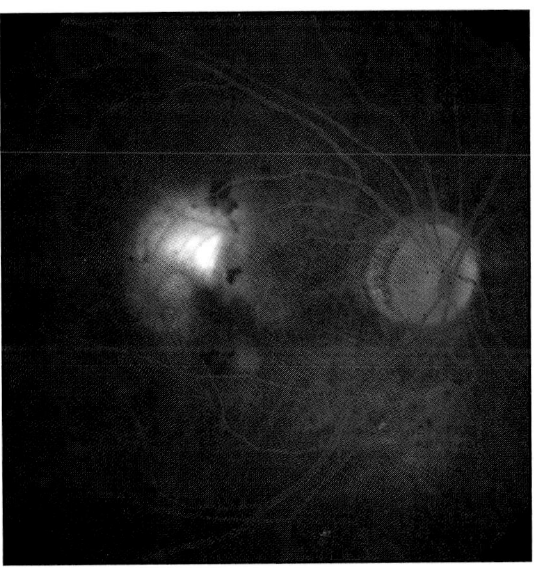

S

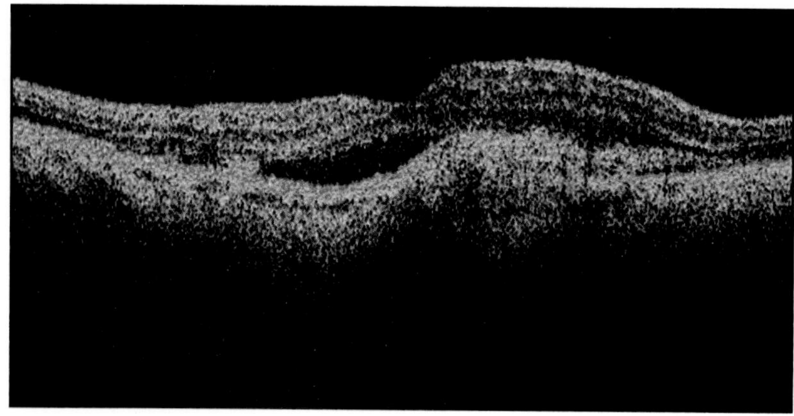

T

Case 7-17A. Classic Choroidal Neovascularization

Clinical Summary

A 79-year-old man complained of decreased vision in his right eye for the last 3 months. Visual acuity was 20/100. Fundus examination (A) revealed loss of the foveal reflex with a pigmented lesion adjacent to the foveal center. There was subretinal fluid and subretinal hemorrhage surrounding this lesion. An early angiographic image (B) showed a well-delineated fluorescent area with late leakage (C) consistent with predominantly classic CNV. The patient was treated with PDT.

Optical Coherence Tomography

A horizontal scan through the foveal center (D) showed loss of the foveal contour. There was a localized fusiform thickening and duplication of the highly reflective external band corresponding to the area of classic CNV observed in the angiogram. Subretinal fluid was present temporal to the CNV lesion (left side of the OCT image). The overlying retina showed mild thickening with loss of the foveal contour.

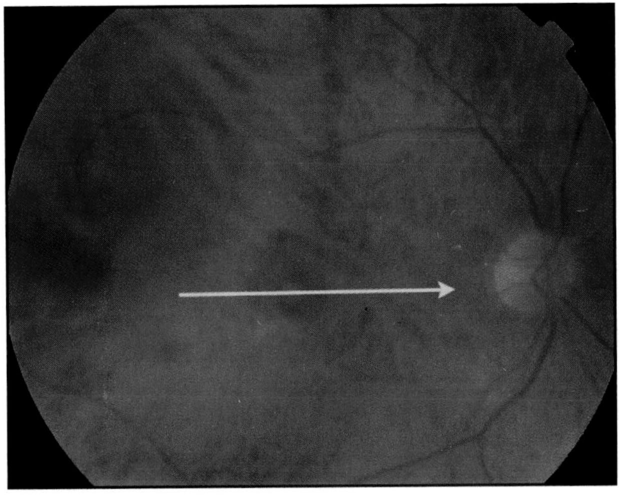

A

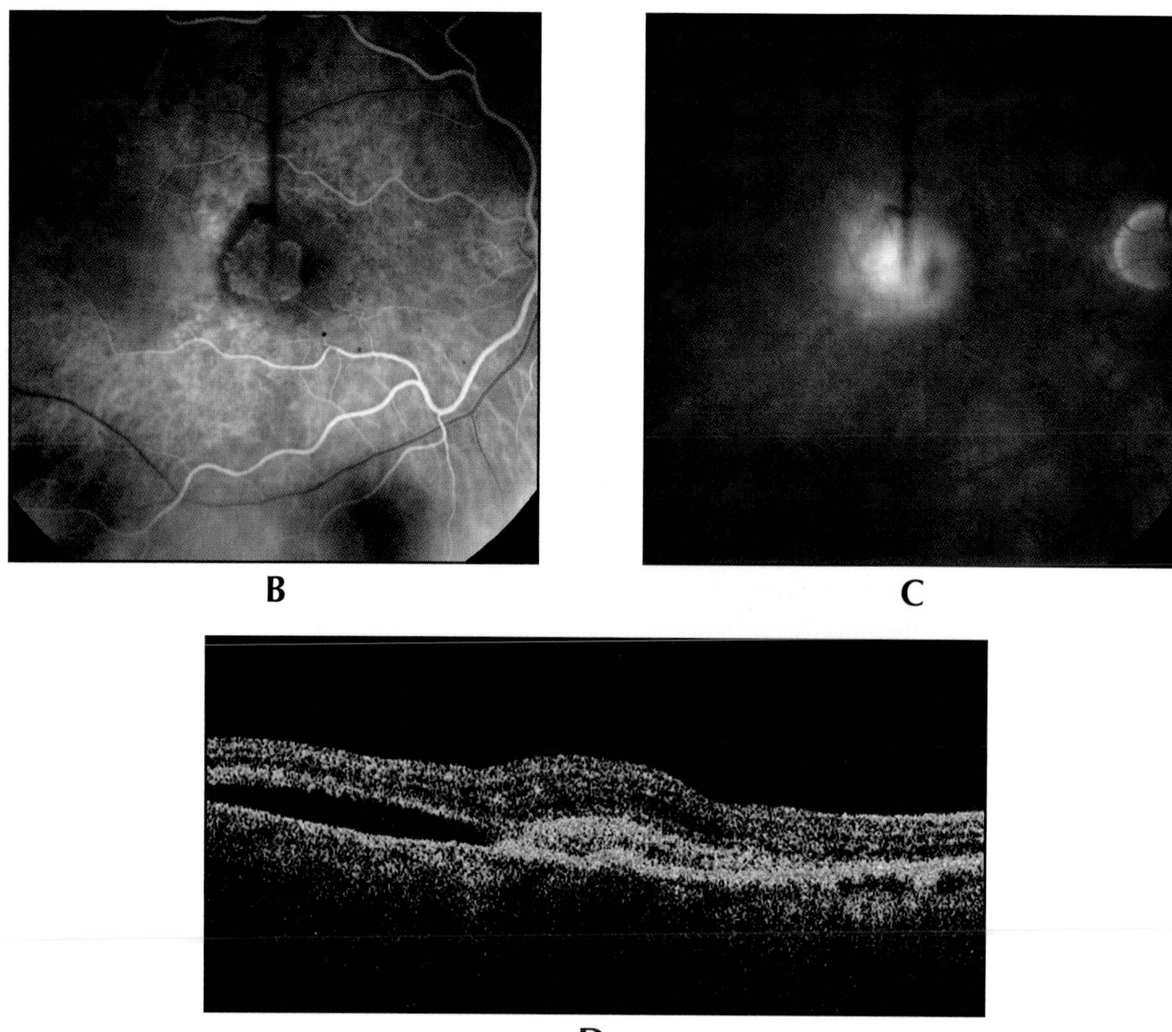
B
C
D

Case 7-17B. Follow-Up After Photodynamic Therapy—Subretinal Hemorrhage

Continuation of Clinical Summary

The visual acuity improved to 20/80 at the 3-month visit. Clinical exam and FA (not shown) showed stabilization of the lesion at that time. Three months later (6 months after PDT), the patient returned complaining of decreased vision and enlargement of the central scotoma. Visual acuity decreased to 20/400. Fundus examination revealed a subretinal hemorrhage superior to the CNV lesion (E). An early angiographic image (F) showed enlargement of the classic CNV adjacent to an area of blocked fluorescence corresponding to the hemorrhage. Late leakage from the classic CNV was observed (G). The patient was retreated with PDT.

Follow-Up Optical Coherence Tomography

A vertical scan through the foveal center (H) revealed persistent thickening of the highly reflective external band in the area of classic CNV. There was a highly reflective material occupying the subretinal space superior to the CNV that corresponded to the blood. Distinction between the blood and CNV lesion was difficult because of similar reflectivity. Subretinal fluid was identified superiorly as a nonreflective cavity beneath the retina.

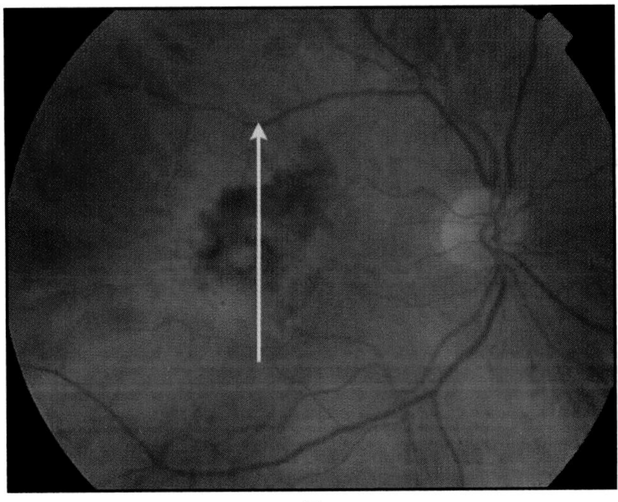

E

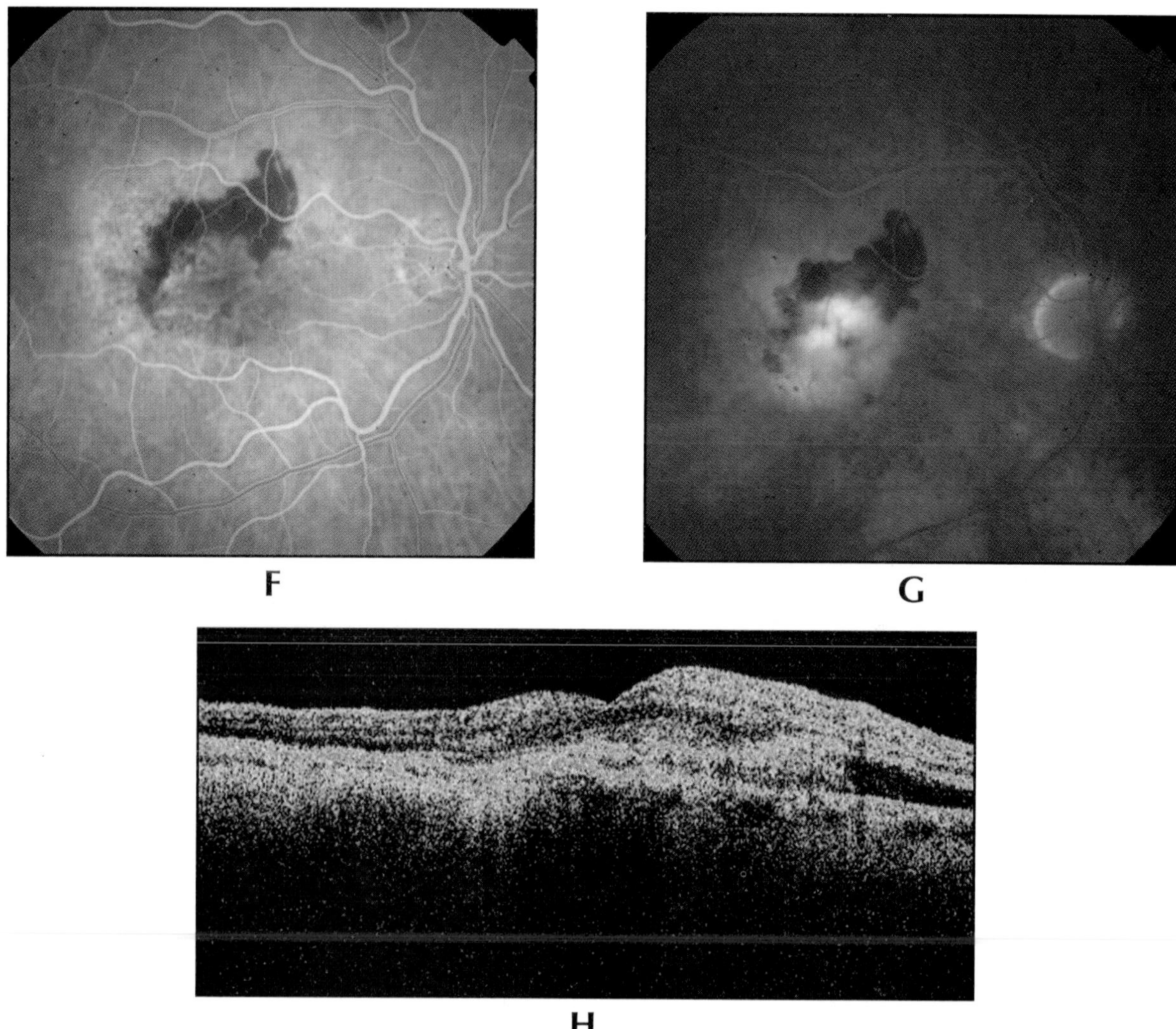
F
G
H

Case 7-17C. Three Months After the Second Photodynamic Therapy Treatment

Continuation of Clinical Summary

Three months after the second PDT treatment, the visual acuity was 20/300. Fundus examination (I) revealed almost complete resolution of the hemorrhage with a decrease in the retinal edema and subretinal fluid around the pigmented lesion. FA showed decrease in the size of the classic CMN with a small area of blockage within the temporal edge and late staining (J and K). Observation was recommended.

Follow-Up Optical Coherence Tomography

A repeat scan through the foveal center (L) revealed a flattened foveal contour with mild cystoid intraretinal edema. The highly reflective external band corresponding with the area of classic CNV appeared thickened and disorganized but more sharply demarcated. No subretinal fluid was observed.

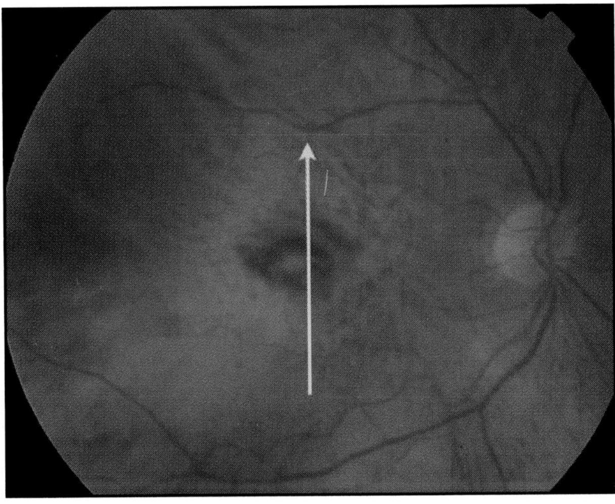

I

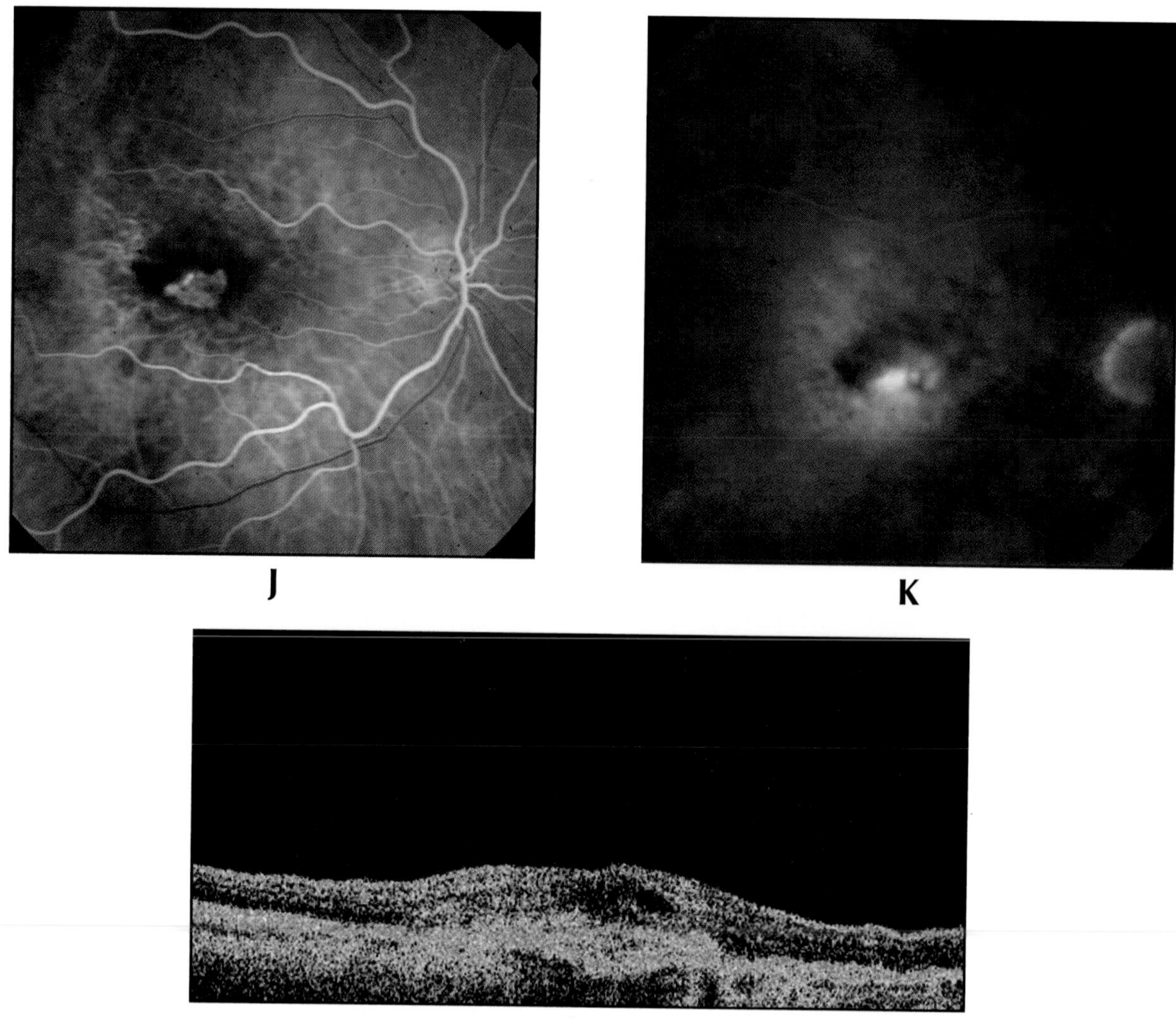
J
K
L

Case 7-18. Classic Choroidal Neovascularization

Clinical Summary

A 75-year-old man complained of decreased vision in his left eye for 2 weeks. Visual acuity was 20/300. Fundus examination (A) revealed loss of the foveal reflex with a pigmented lesion superior to the foveal center surrounded by retinal edema and subretinal fluid. An early angiographic image (B) showed a well-delineated fluorescent area with late leakage consistent with a predominantly classic CNV (C). The patient was treated with PDT.

Optical Coherence Tomography

A vertical scan through the foveal center (D) showed an area of decreased reflectivity in the subretinal space inferior to the foveal center (left side of the scan) corresponding to fluid from the CNV. There was a dome-shaped area of thickening extending from the highly reflective external band in the area of the classic CNV. There was mild retinal thickening with distortion of the foveal contour in this area.

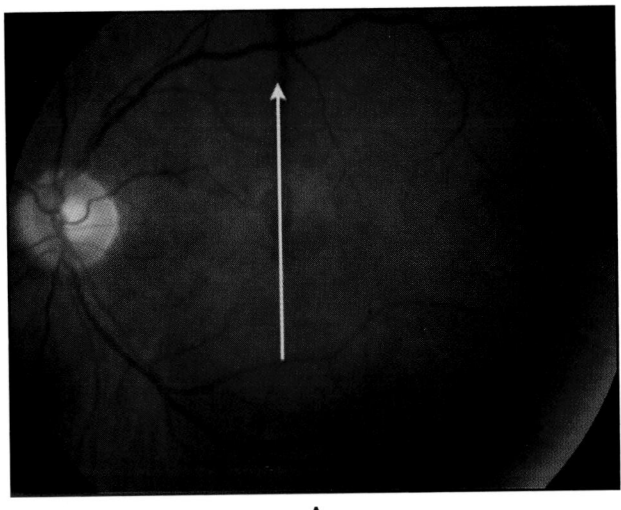

A

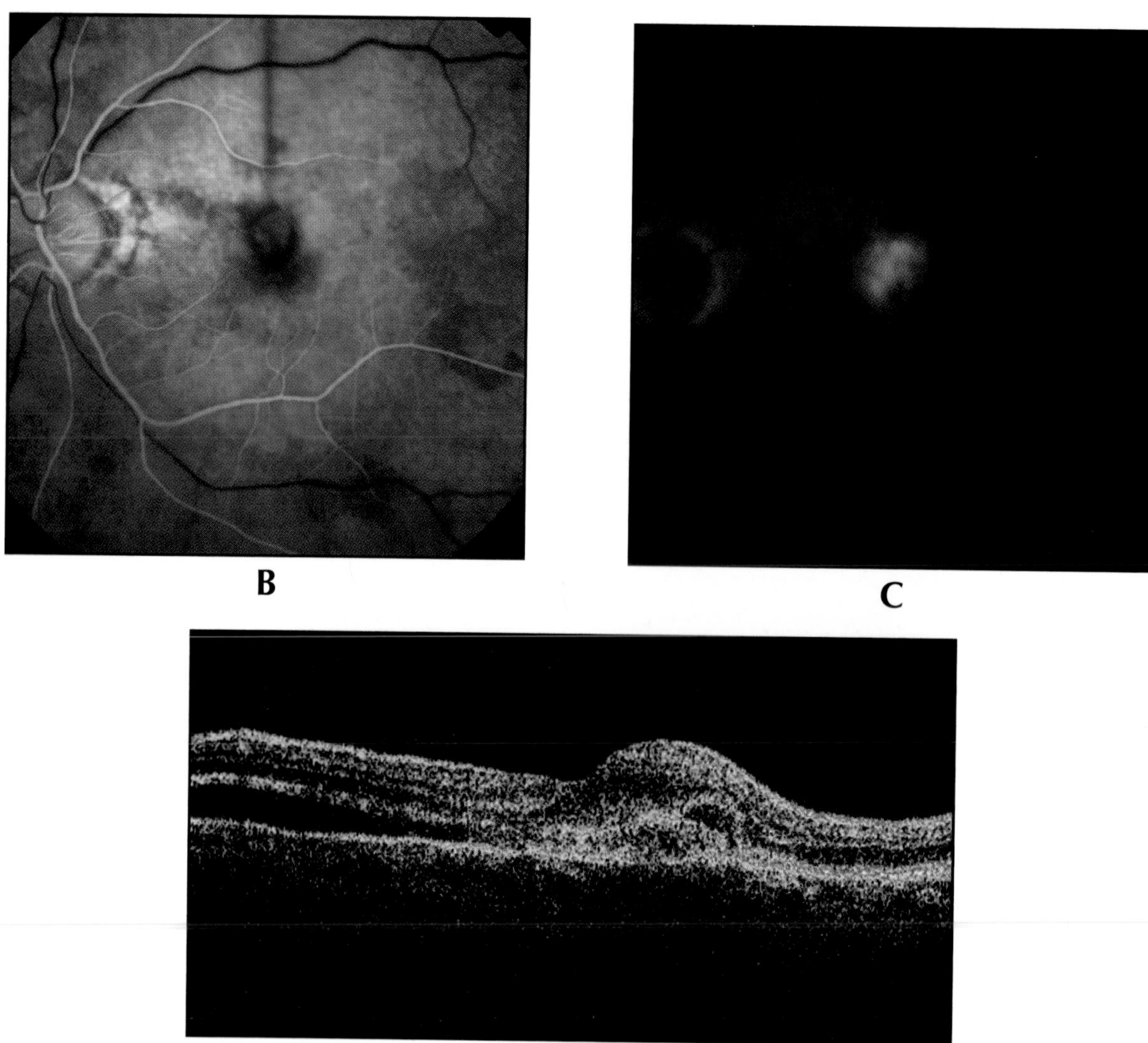
B
C
D

Case 7-18B. Six Weeks After Photodynamic Therapy

Continuation of Clinical Summary

Six weeks after PDT treatment, visual acuity improved to 20/40. Fundus examination (E) revealed a decrease in the subretinal fluid and retinal edema. The angiogram showed decreased size of the classic CNV on the early phases (F). There was mild persistent leakage on the late phase of the angiogram (G). The patient was observed.

Follow-Up Optical Coherence Tomography

A repeat scan through the foveal center (H) showed decreased subretinal fluid inferior to the foveal center. The area of the CNV appeared more distinct but was otherwise unchanged. The photoreceptor layer overlying the CNV continued to be disorganized and indistinct. The foveal contour showed persistent distortion.

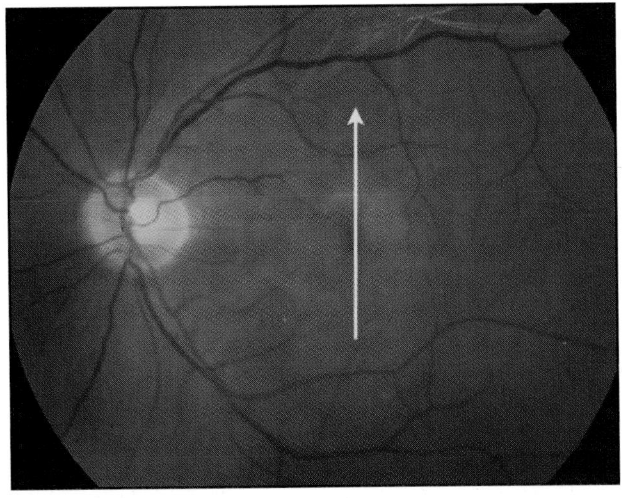

E

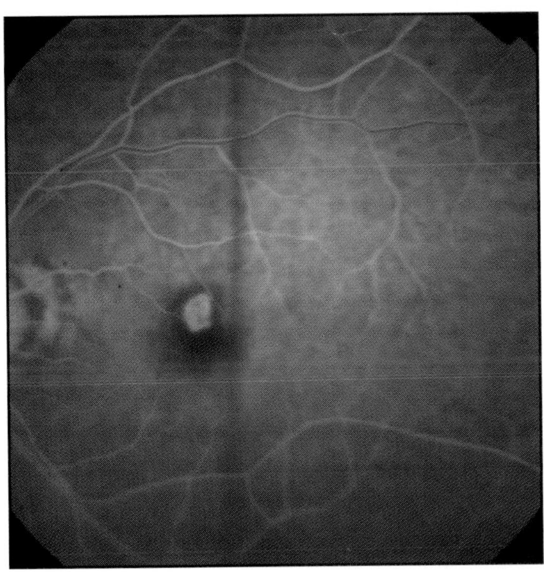

F

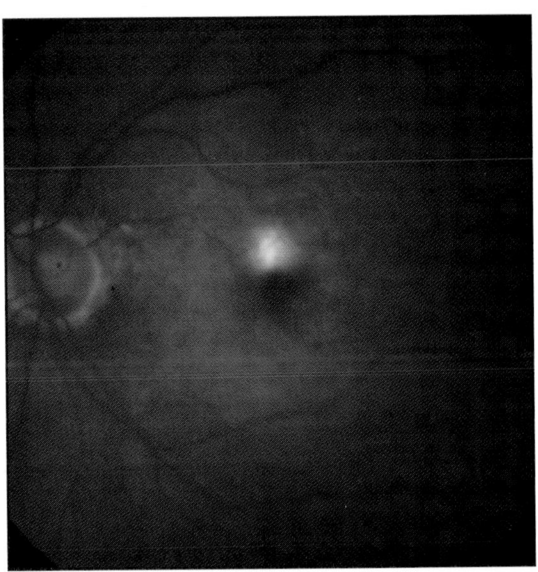

G

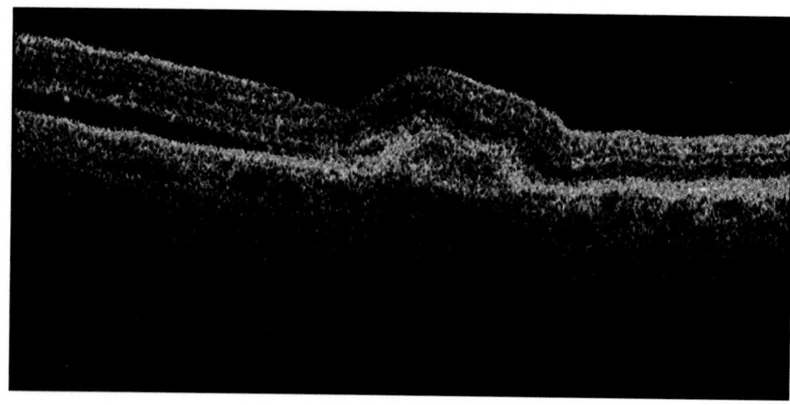

H

Case 7-18C. *Three Months After Photodynamic Therapy*

Continuation of Clinical Summary

Three months after PDT treatment, visual acuity decreased to 20/400. Fundus examination (I) revealed increased exudation with a new area of subretinal hemorrhage superonasal to the foveal center. The angiograms (J and K) showed an increase in the size of the classic component with late leakage. The patient received a second PDT treatment.

Follow-Up Optical Coherence Tomography

A repeat OCT scan through the foveal center (L) showed persistent subretinal fluid inferior to the foveal center. Subretinal fluid was also observed superiorly, adjacent to the new area of bleeding. The area of the external band corresponding to the CNV appeared larger and thicker consistent with the increase in size observed on angiography. This enlargement of the lesion resulted in further distortion of the retinal contour in the foveal region.

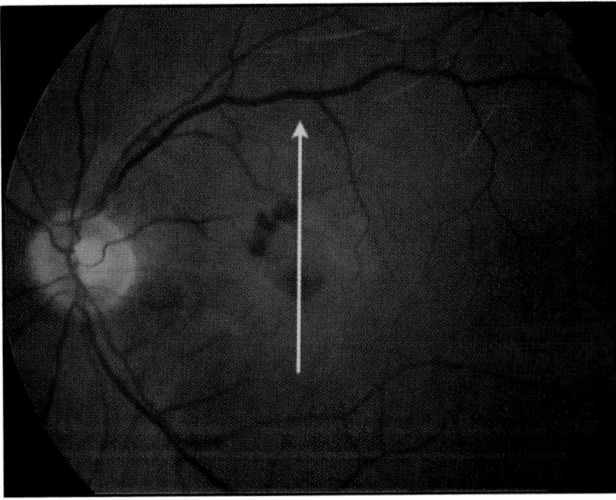

I

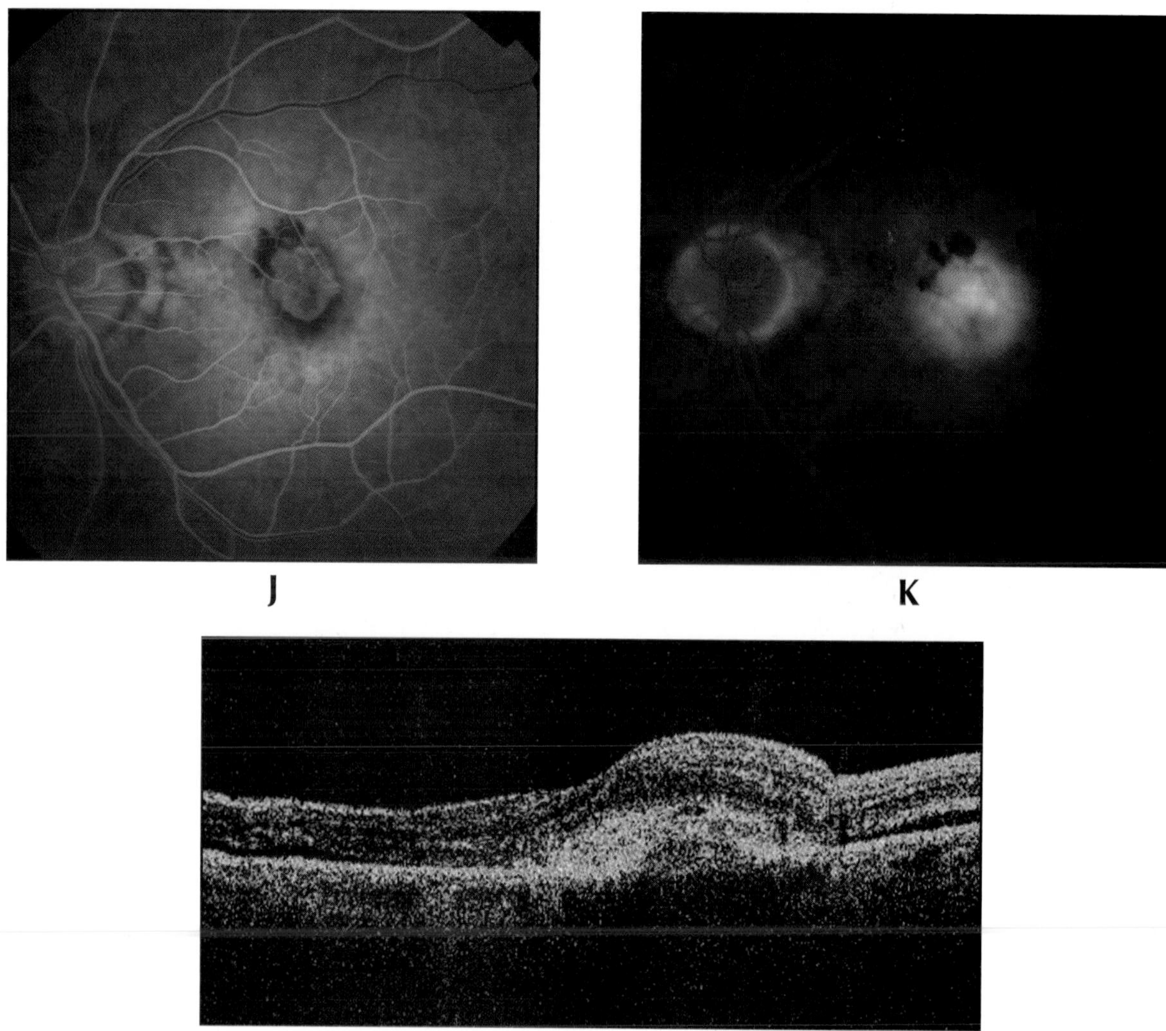
J K L

Case 7-18D. Three Months After the Second Photodynamic Therapy

Continuation of Clinical Summary

Three months after the second PDT, vision was 20/70. Fundus examination (M) revealed persistent thickening around the pigmented lesion with a small rim of blood superiorly. The angiogram showed a decrease in the size of the classic component with persistent leakage (N and O). The patient received a third session of PDT.

Follow-Up Optical Coherence Tomography

A repeat OCT scan through the foveal center (P) showed decreased subretinal fluid. The CNV lesion appears slightly smaller in basal dimension but slightly thicker than on the previous study. The retina continues to be distorted by this elevated lesion, but the foveal contour is slightly more distinct on this image.

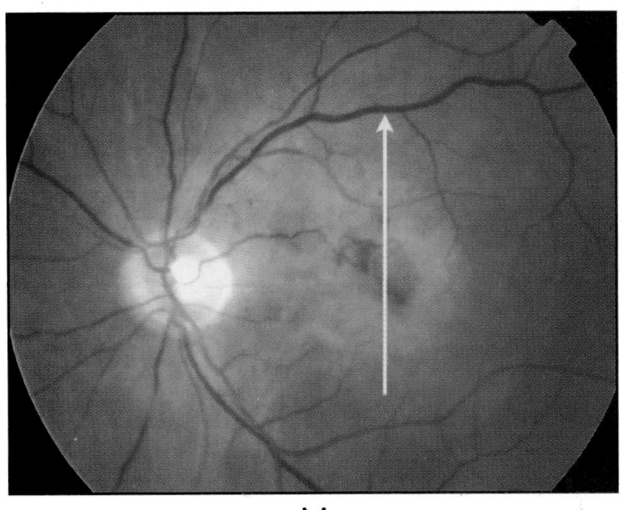

M

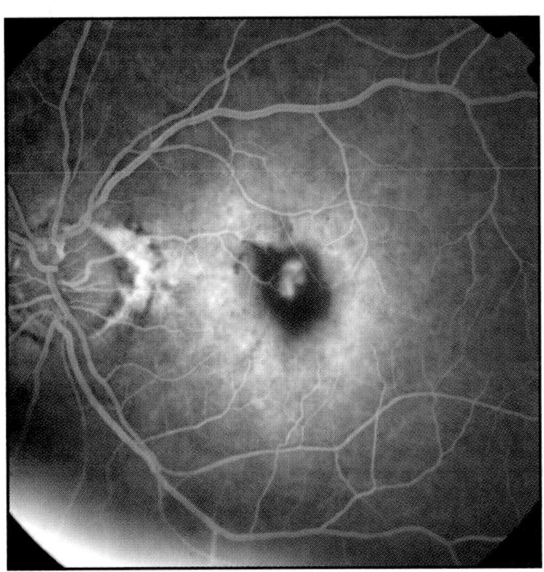

N

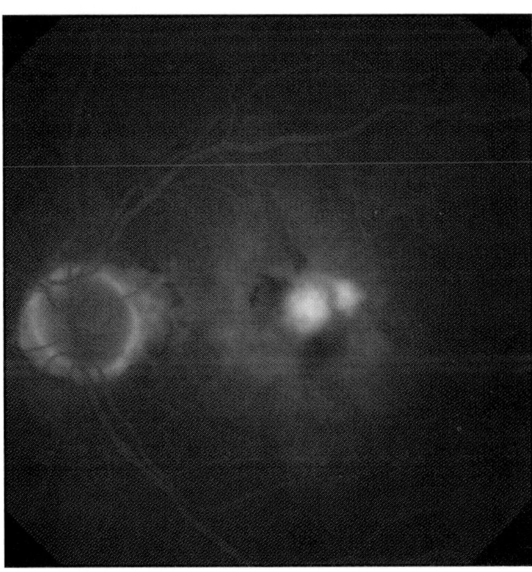

O

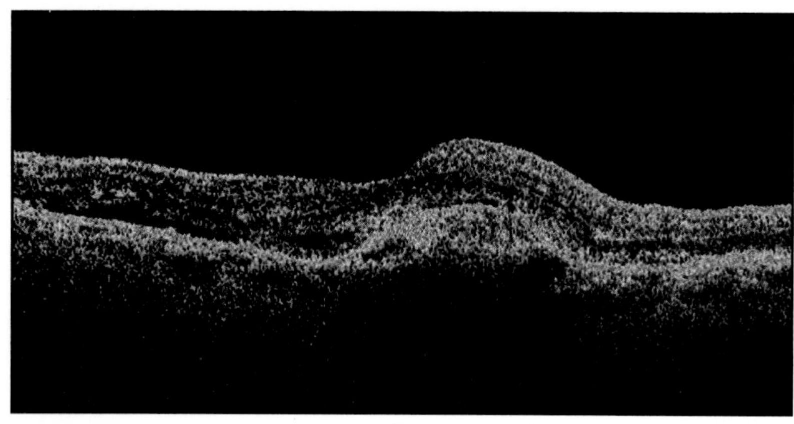

P

Case 7-18E. *Three Months After the Third Photodynamic Therapy*

Continuation of Clinical Summary

Three months after the third PDT, vision decreased to 20/100. Fundus examination (Q) revealed increased subretinal fluid around the CNV lesion and a small amount of blood at the superonasal edge of the lesion. The angiograms showed persistent activity of the lesion (R and S). The patient received a fourth session of PDT.

Follow-Up Optical Coherence Tomography

A repeat OCT scan through the foveal center (T) showed slightly more fluid beneath the retina around the CNV lesion. There was also a small amount of subretinal fluid overlying the lesion. The retinal distortion was slightly worse with further disruption of the foveal contour. The CNV lesion, though, appeared mostly unchanged.

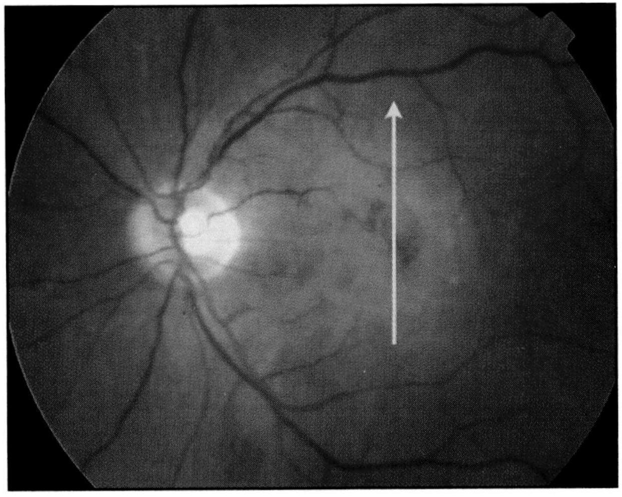

Q

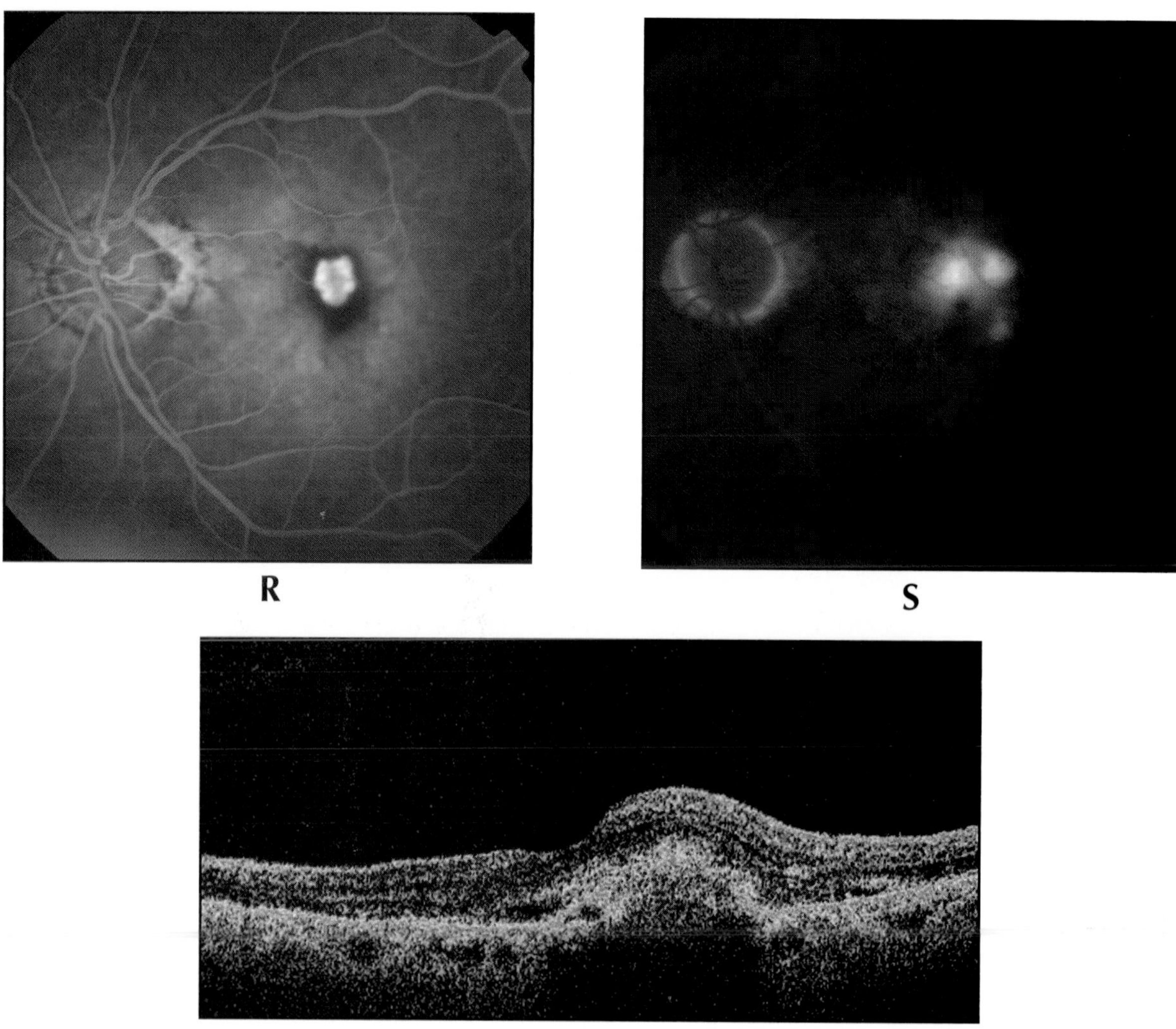
R
S
T

Case 7-18F. Three Months After the Fourth Photodynamic Therapy

Continuation of Clinical Summary

Three months after the fourth PDT session, vision improved again to 20/60. Fundus examination (U) revealed increased pigmentation around the CNV lesion with surrounding RPE atrophy. FA showed early fluorescence with late staining (V and W). The patient was observed.

Follow-Up Optical Coherence Tomography

A repeat OCT scan through the foveal center (X) showed reduced subretinal fluid. The CNV area appeared more sharply demarcated and consolidated. The overlying retina was more organized and less thickened compared with the previous scan. The foveal contour, although still distorted by the lesion, appeared better than before.

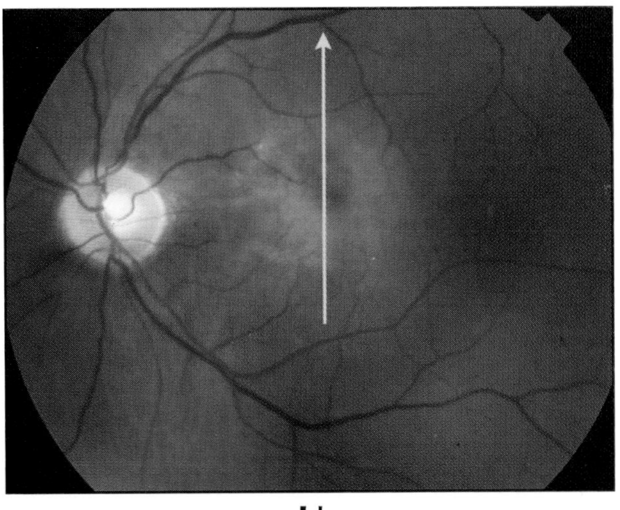

U

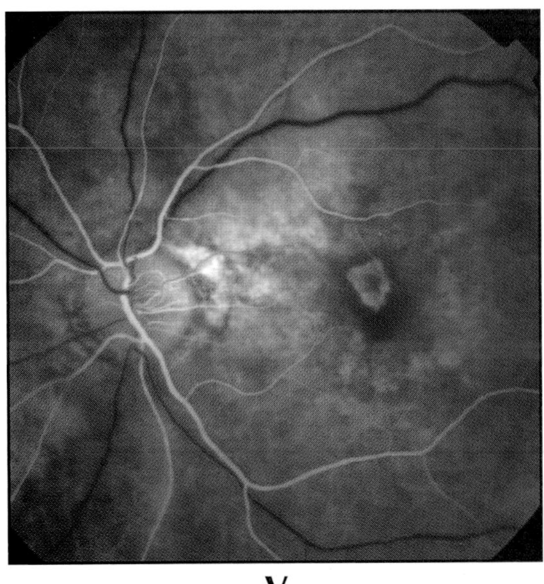

V

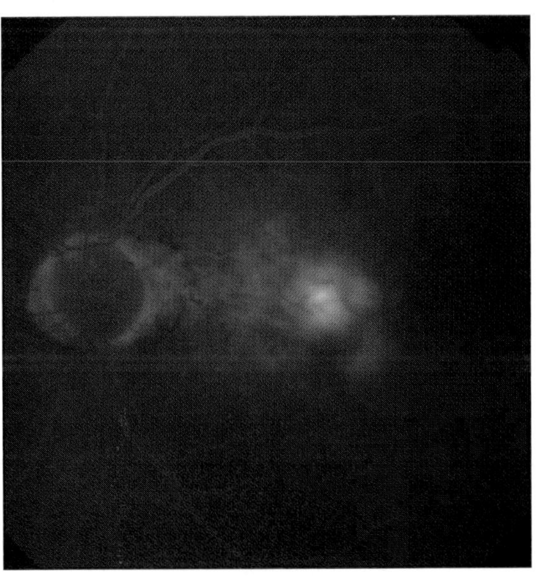

W

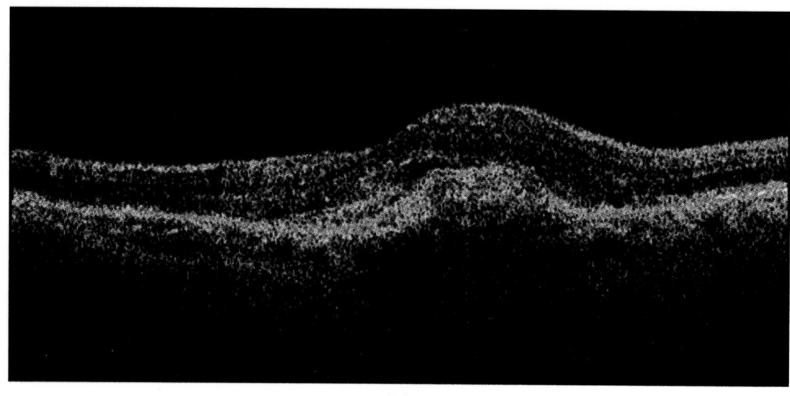

X

Case 7-19A. Classic Choroidal Neovascularization—Acute Vision Loss After Photodynamic Therapy

Clinical Summary

A 65-year-old woman complained of decreased visual acuity in her left eye 6 weeks after cataract surgery. Her visual acuity was 20/70 in this eye. Fundus examination (A) revealed pigmentary mottling in the macular region with shallow subretinal fluid extending to the fovea. FA (B and C) revealed a well-defined area of early hyperfluorescence with late leakage consistent with CNV. The patient was treated with PDT.

Optical Coherence Tomography

A horizontal OCT scan through the foveal center (D) showed serous elevation of the neurosensory retina. Beneath this area of subretinal fluid, the external band was shallowly elevated. The external band in this area also showed abnormal thinning and irregularity. The retina overlying this fluid shows only mild alterations with relative preservation of the foveal contour.

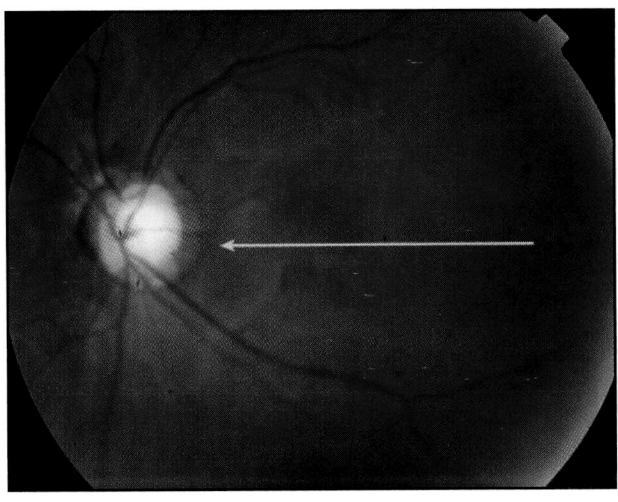

A

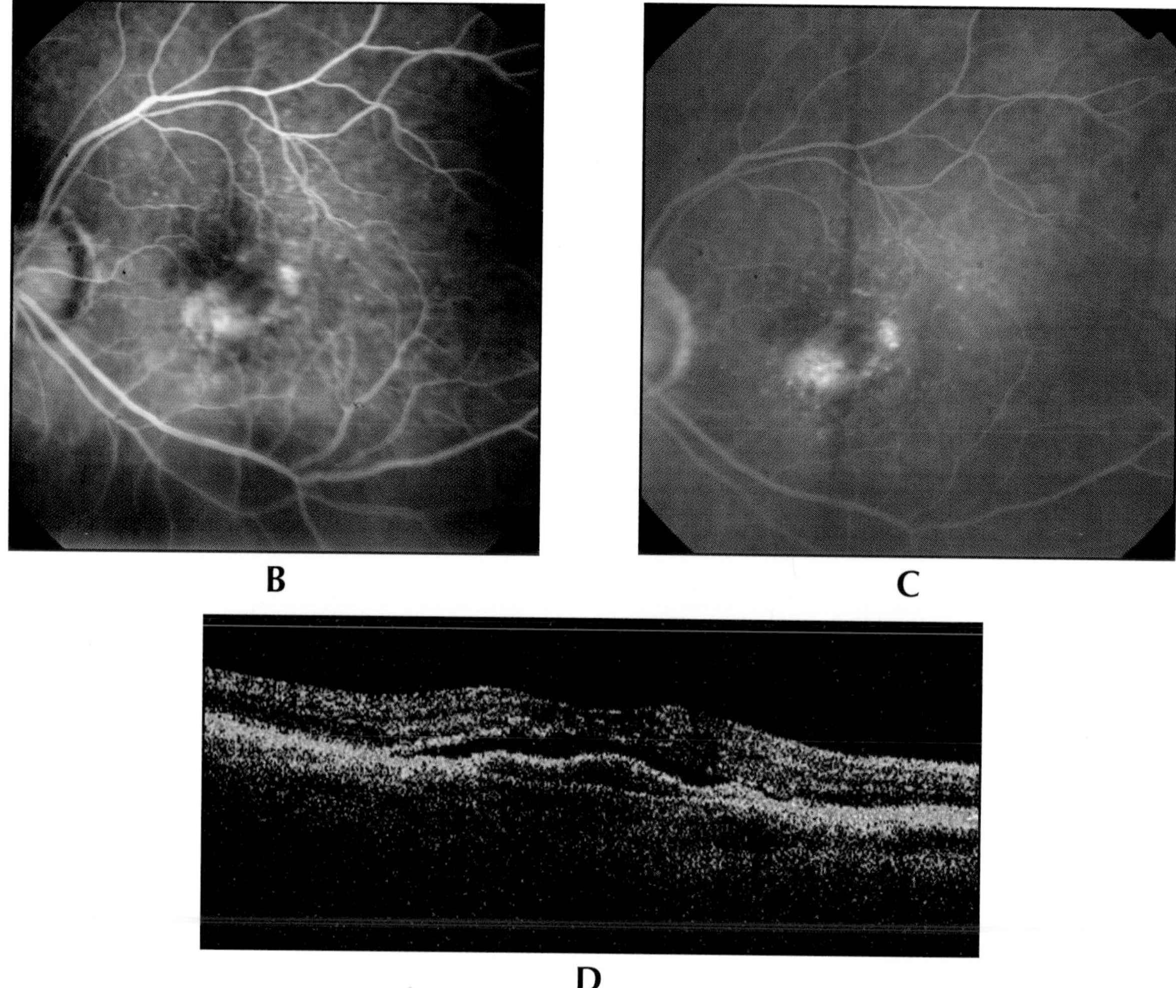
B
C
D

Case 7-19B. Acute Vision Loss After Photodynamic Therapy

Continuation of Clinical Summary

The patient complained of worsening vision after the PDT treatment. She returned for evaluation 1 week after the treatment, and her visual acuity had decreased to 20/200. Examination showed a significant increase in the amount of subretinal fluid. Her vision slowly improved back to 20/70 over the next week. At a 2-month follow-up visit, her vision was maintained at the 20/70 level.

Follow-Up Optical Coherence Tomography

Repeat OCT scan (E) 1 week after PDT confirmed extensive subretinal fluid elevating the neurosensory retina. The retinal stroma showed minimal change from the pretreatment image. The external band showed moderate irregularity, but no longer appeared elevated. The OCT image taken 1 week later (F) showed a decrease in the amount of subretinal fluid. The neurosensory retina remained stable, while the external band appeared thickened and irregular. Two months after treatment (G), there was complete resolution of the subretinal fluid.

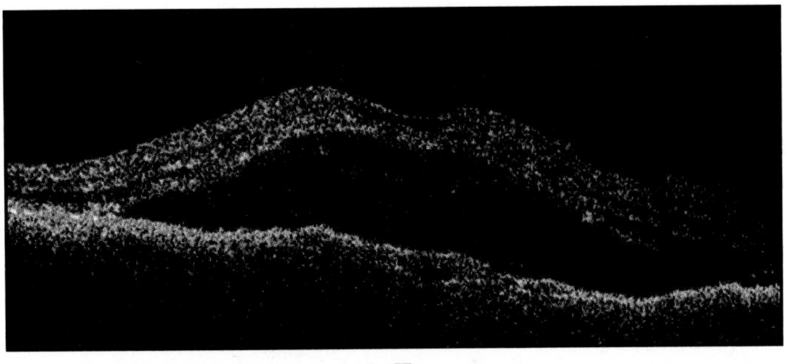

E

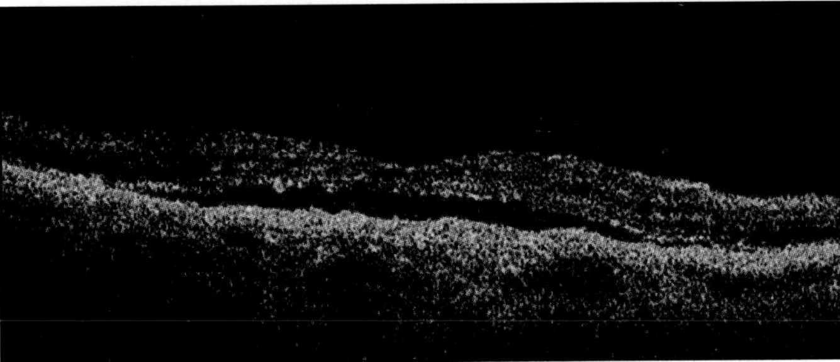

F

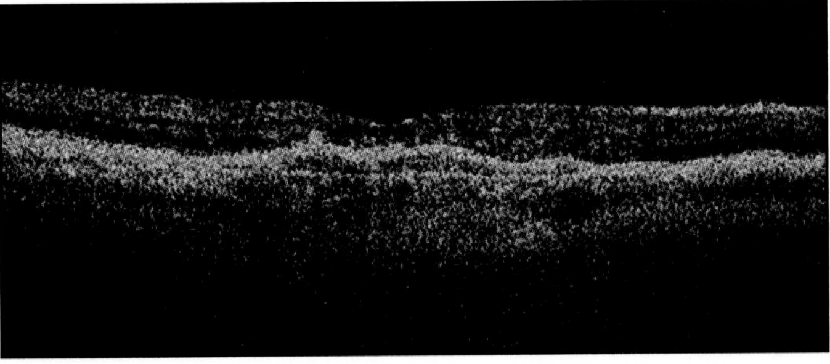

G

Case 7-20. Vascularized Pigment Epithelial Detachment

Clinical Summary

A 79-year-old man with a history of decreased vision had a visual acuity of 20/50 in the left eye. Fundus examination of the left macula (A) reveled pigment mottling and a PED. FA (B and C) showed the outline of a well-demarcated serous PED with a notch in the nasal edge. ICGA (D and E) showed a classic PED with some areas of reticular pigment and a hot spot in the area of the notch.

Optical Coherence Tomography

A horizontal scan through the foveal center (F) showed a dome-shaped elevation of the highly reflective external band with low reflectivity underlying this band consistent with a serous PED. Low reflectance from the choroid underlying the PED was observed secondary to shadowing. The overlying retina appeared relatively normal, and the layered architecture of the neurosensory retina overlying the PED was preserved. A small amount of subretinal fluid was present surrounding the PED.

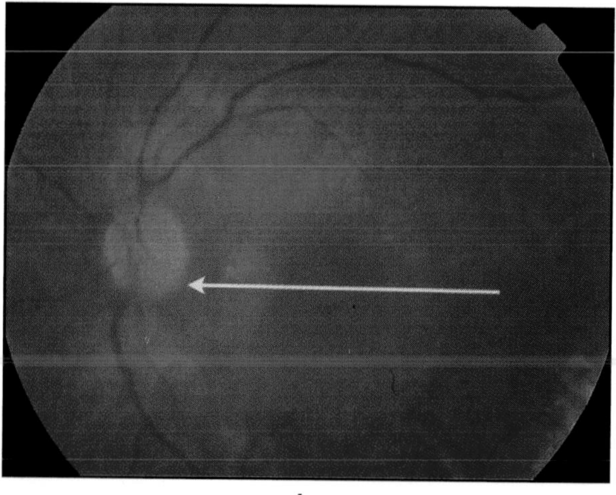

A

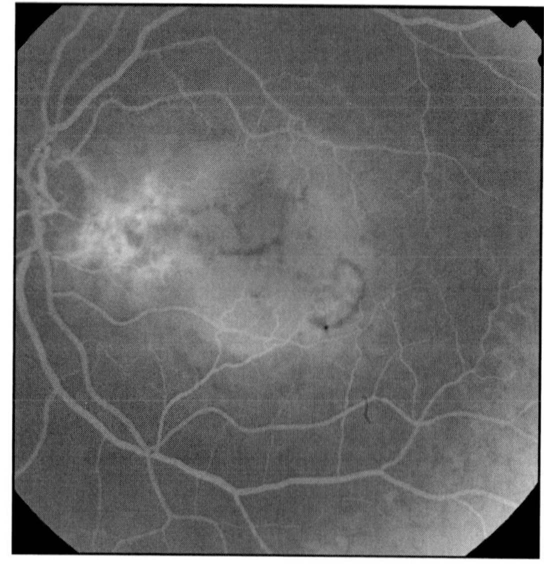

B

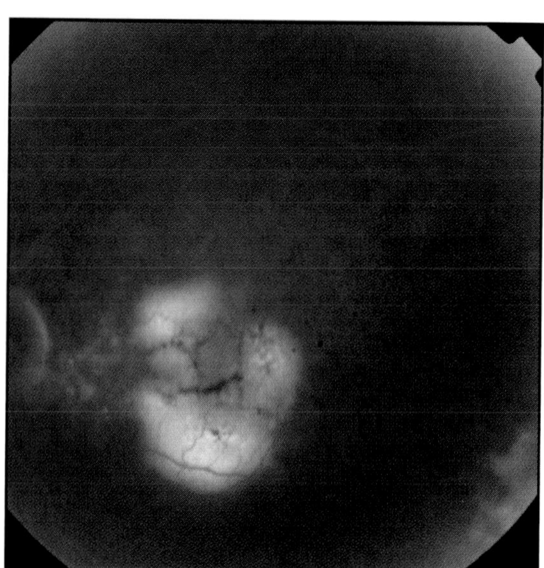

C

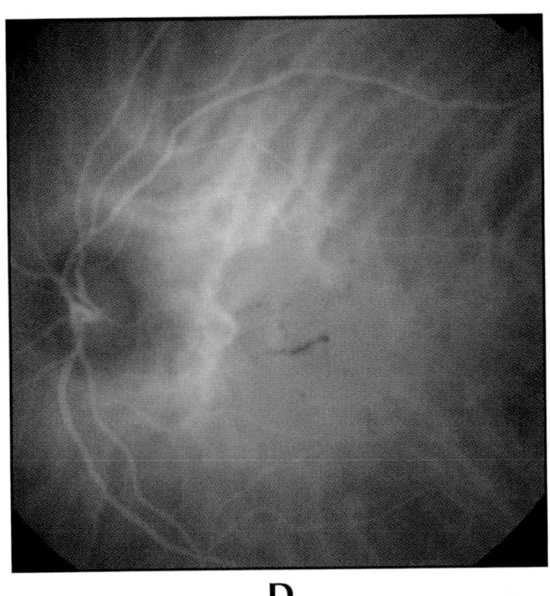

D

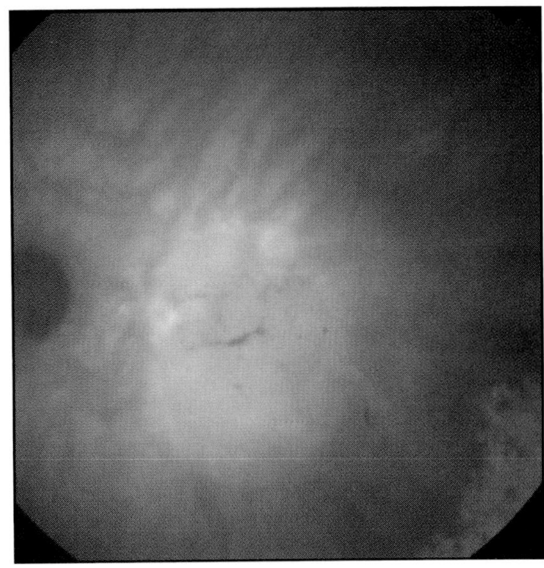

E

F

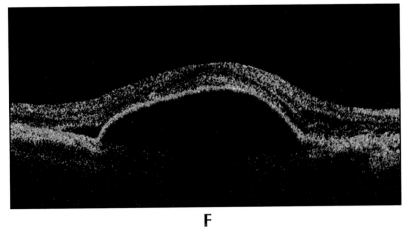

Case 7-21. Retinal Angiomatous Proliferation

Clinical Summary

A 79-year-old man complained of decreased vision in his right eye. Visual acuity was 20/60. Fundus examination (A) of the right eye revealed a large PED centered in the macula with a focal intraretinal hemorrhage inferior to the foveal center. FA (B and C) showed a focal fluorescent area adjacent to the hemorrhage identified as an early retinal angiomatous proliferation with an overlying anastomotic lesion. The PED appeared as an early circular hyperfluorescent area with well-defined borders. ICGA showed a well-defined PED with a hot spot, confirming the subretinal component of the angiomatous proliferation (D and E).

Optical Coherence Tomography

A vertical scan through the foveal center (F) showed elevation of the highly reflective external band in the area of the serous PED. Intraretinal cystic edema was seen overlying the PED. Subretinal fluid was present around the PED inferiorly (left side of the scan).

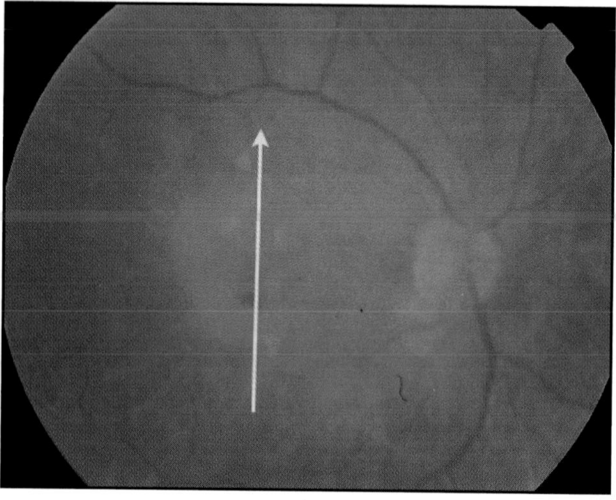

A

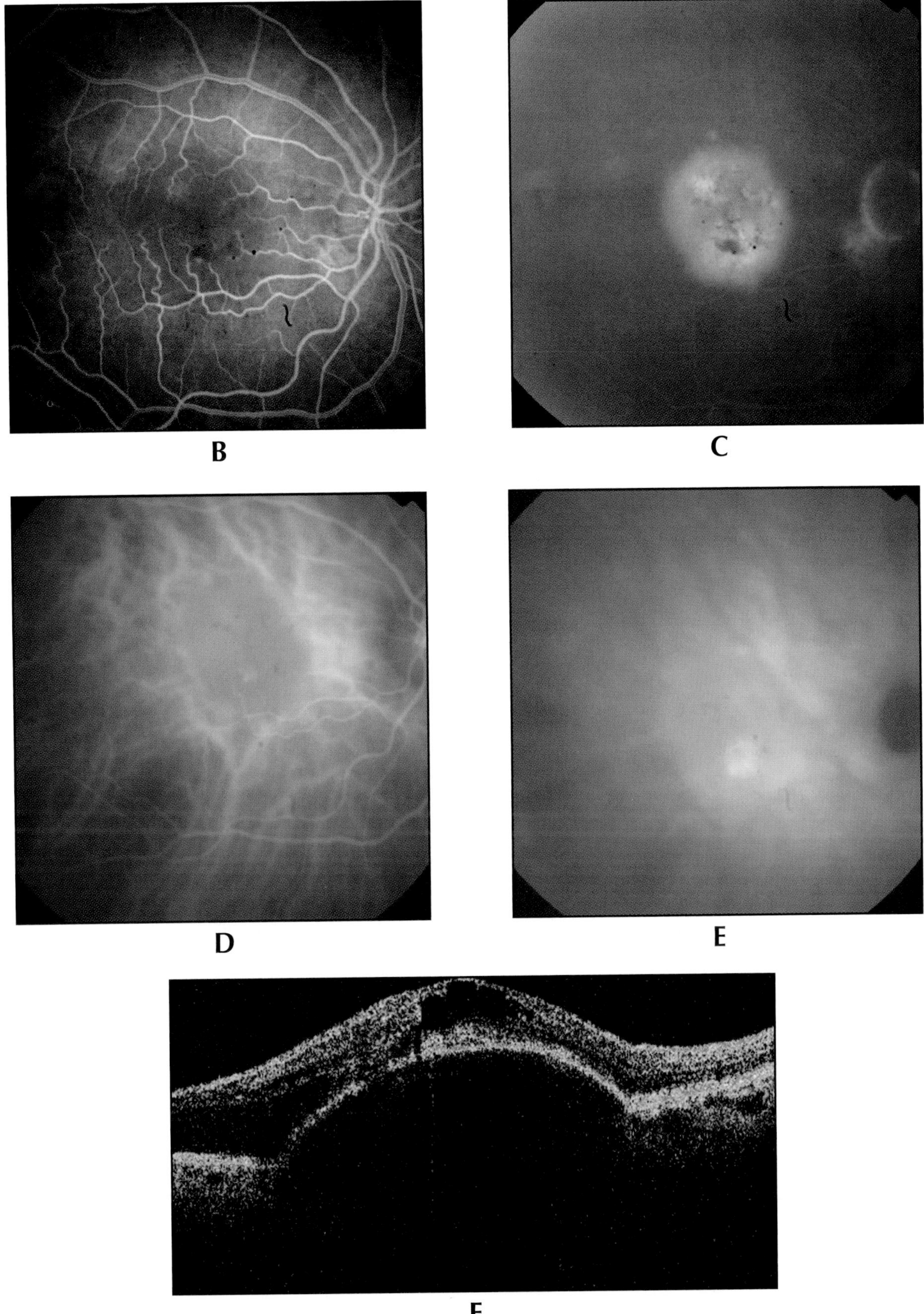
B
C
D
E
F

Case 7-22A. Retinal Angiomatous Proliferation

Clinical Summary

A 90-year-old woman complained of decreasing visual acuity in both eyes for 1 year. Visual acuity was 20/30 in the right eye. Fundus examination of the right eye (A) showed central macular thickening and a focal intraretinal hemorrhage inferior to the foveal center. FA (B) showed stippled hyperfluorescence early with late leakage and well-defined margins (C) diagnostic of occult CNV. ICGA (D and E) showed three well-defined hot spots corresponding to chorioretinal anastomoses, confirming the presence of a retinal angiomatous lesion.

Optical Coherence Tomography

Oblique scan through the foveal center of the right eye (F) showed loss of the foveal contour and increased thickness due to the presence of cystic intraretinal edema. There were juxtafoveal elevations of the highly reflective external band indicating serous detachment of the pigment epithelium.

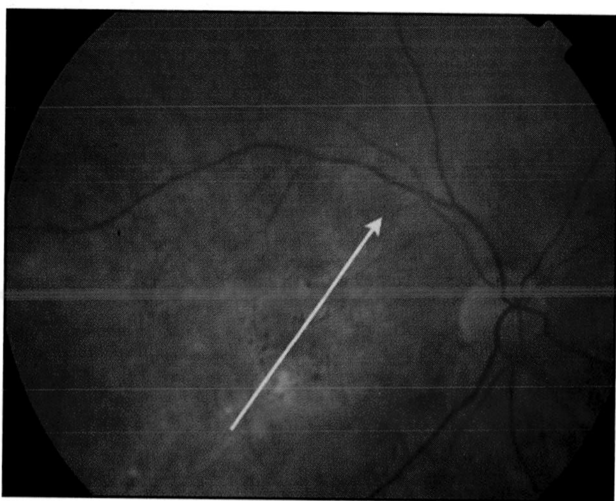

A

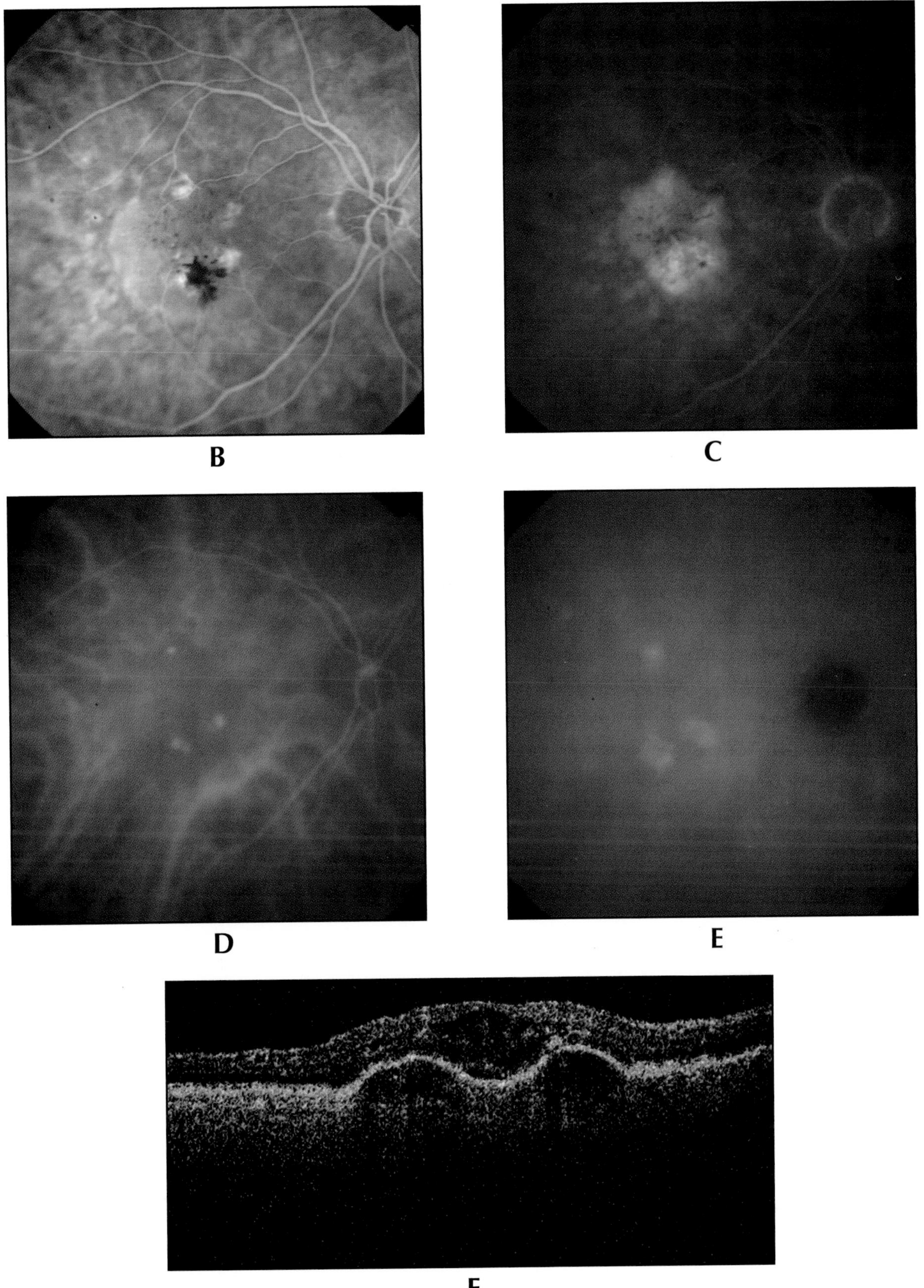
B
C
D
E
F

Case 7-22B. Retinal Angiomatous Proliferation Progression

Continuation of Clinical Summary

Four weeks later, vision in the right eye decreased to 20/100. The PED appeared larger on the fundus exam (G) with the presence of new intraretinal hemorrhages. The fluorescein angiogram (H and I) showed areas of localized hypofluorescence corresponding to the intraretinal hemorrhages in the early phases and diffuse late leakage of the dye in the area of the PED.

Follow-Up Optical Coherence Tomography

A repeat scan through the foveal center (J) showed a single, dome-shaped elevation corresponding to a serous PED. The PED showed significant enlargement from the previous study. The highly reflective external band appeared thin and discontinuous. Subretinal fluid was present adjacent to the PED. The intraretinal cystic edema was more pronounced.

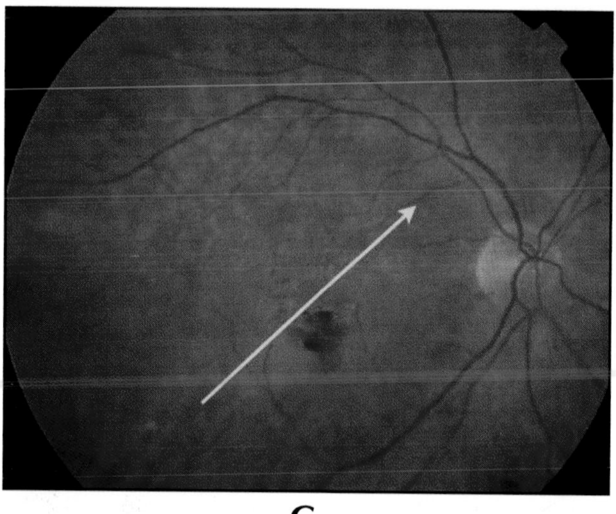

G

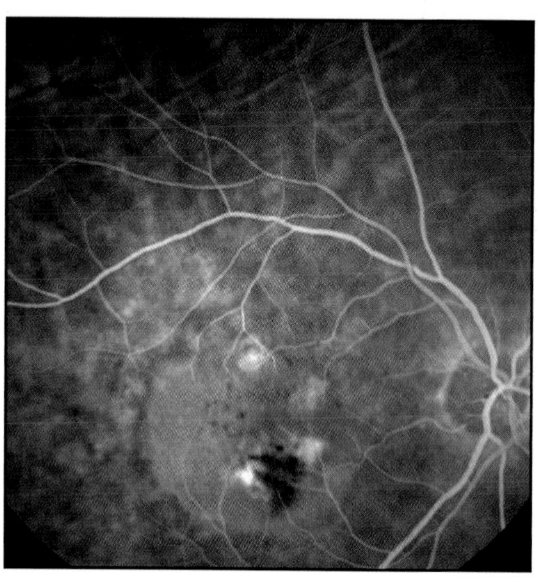

H

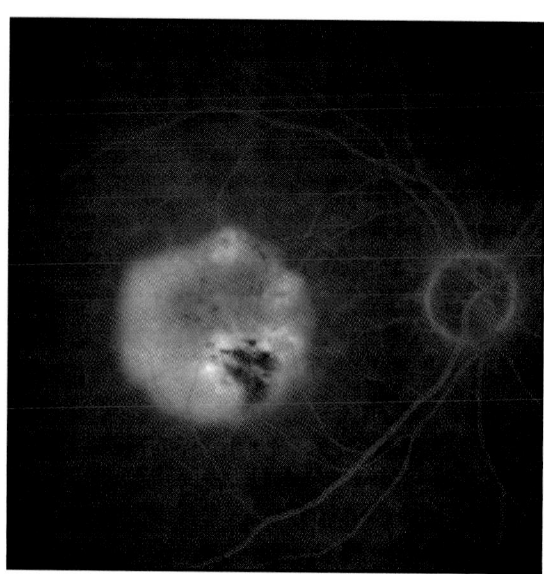

I

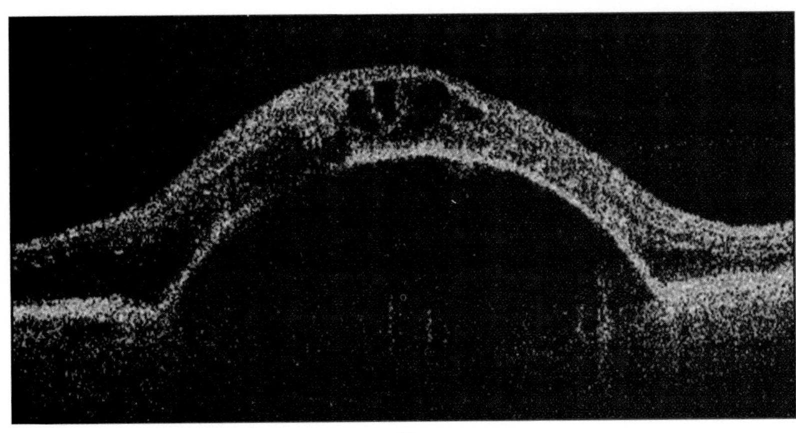

J

Case 7-23A. Retinal Angiomatous Proliferation

Clinical Summary

The left eye of the same patient in case 7-25 had a visual acuity of 20/70. Fundus examination (A) revealed drusen and pigment mottling. There was a central PED occupying an area of approximately two disc diameters. Small intraretinal hemorrhages were present within the superonasal quadrant of the PED. An early transit angiographic image of the left eye (B) revealed two focal fluorescent areas identified as early retinal angiomatous proliferations with overlying retinal anastomoses. A late phase angiogram (C) revealed leakage throughout the PED. ICGA (D and E) showed two well-defined hot spots corresponding to chorioretinal anastomoses, confirming the presence of a retinal angiomatous lesion.

Optical Coherence Tomography

An oblique scan through the foveal center of the left eye (F) showed a large, highly elevated, dome-shaped PED. The overlying retina was thickened with extensive intraretinal cystic edema. The highly reflective external band appeared attenuated and discontinuous, but this may have been an optical artifact due to its elevation. Subretinal fluid was present at the edges of the PED.

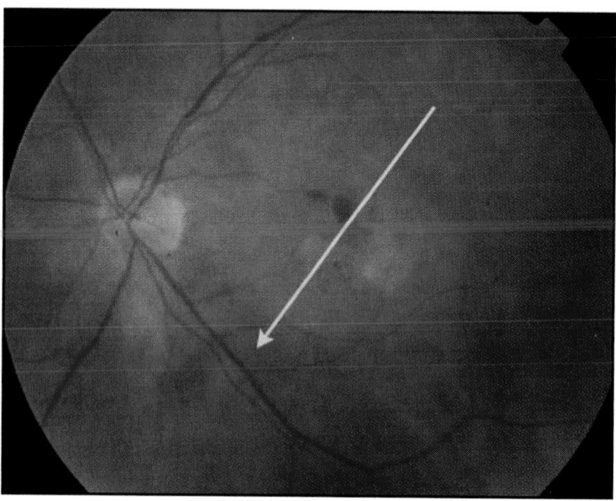

A

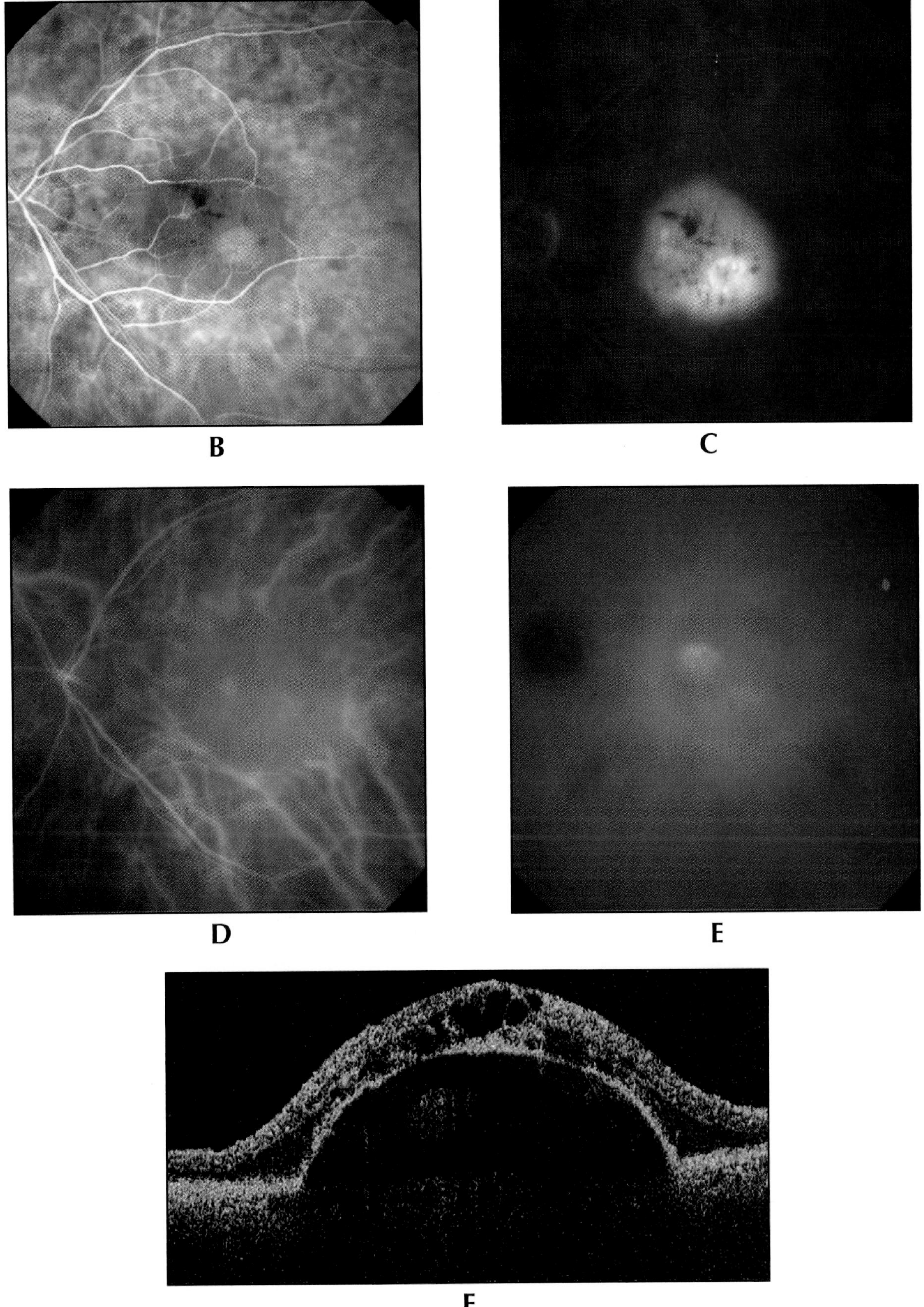
B
C
D
E
F

Case 7-23B. Four Weeks Later

Continuation of Clinical Summary

Four weeks later, vision in the left eye decreased to 20/400. Increased elevation of the PED was observed on the fundus exam (G) with presence of new intraretinal hemorrhages. FA showed the two focal areas of fluorescence and an outline of the PED (H). The late angiographic image showed increased fluorescence delineating the PED (I). An intravitreal triamcinolone injection was performed.

Follow-Up Optical Coherence Tomography

An OCT scan through the foveal center (J) continued to show the highly elevated PED with overlying CME. Once again, the highly reflective external band appeared focally attenuated and discontinuous. Subretinal fluid was still evident at the base of the PED.

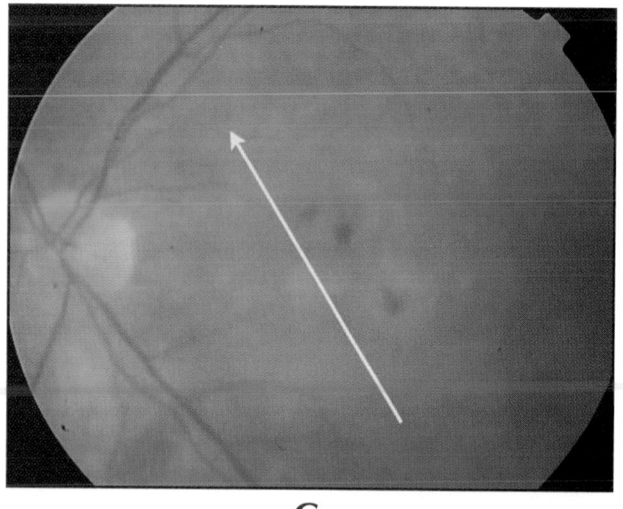

G

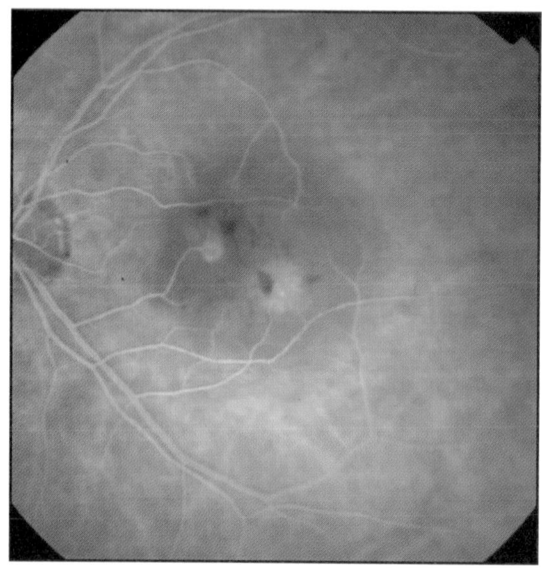

H

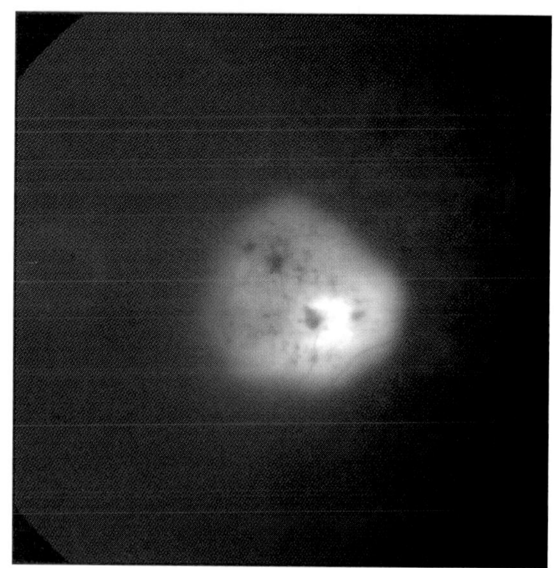

I

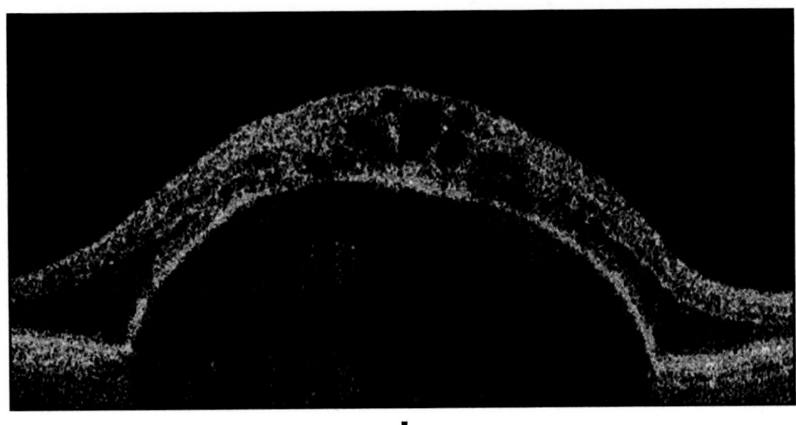

J

Case 7-23C. Three Months After Intravitreal Triamcinolone Injection

Continuation of Clinical Summary

Three months after the triamcinolone injection, vision in the left eye improved from 20/400 to 20/200. On examination (K), the retinal thickness, the intraretinal hemorrhages, and the elevation of the PED had diminished. FA revealed persistent leakage characteristic of a PED associated with RAP (L and M).

Follow-Up Optical Coherence Tomography

Repeat OCT scan through the foveal center (N) showed an increase in the macular edema and central retinal thickness but further decrease in the elevation of the PED. Increased reflectivity of the fluid within the PED probably represented changes in the composition due to differential absorption of its components. There was a decrease in the amount of subretinal fluid adjacent to the PED.

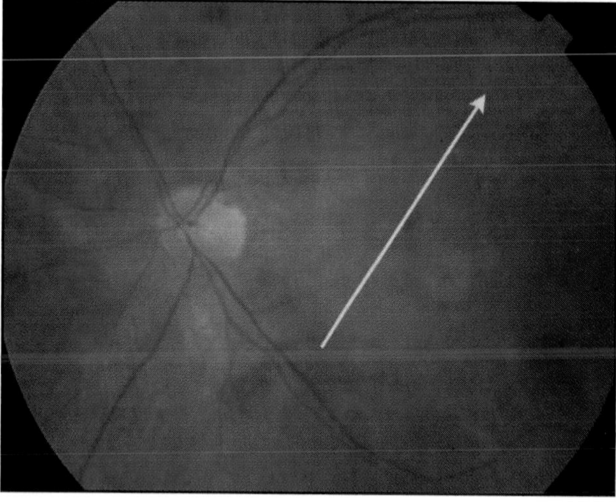

K

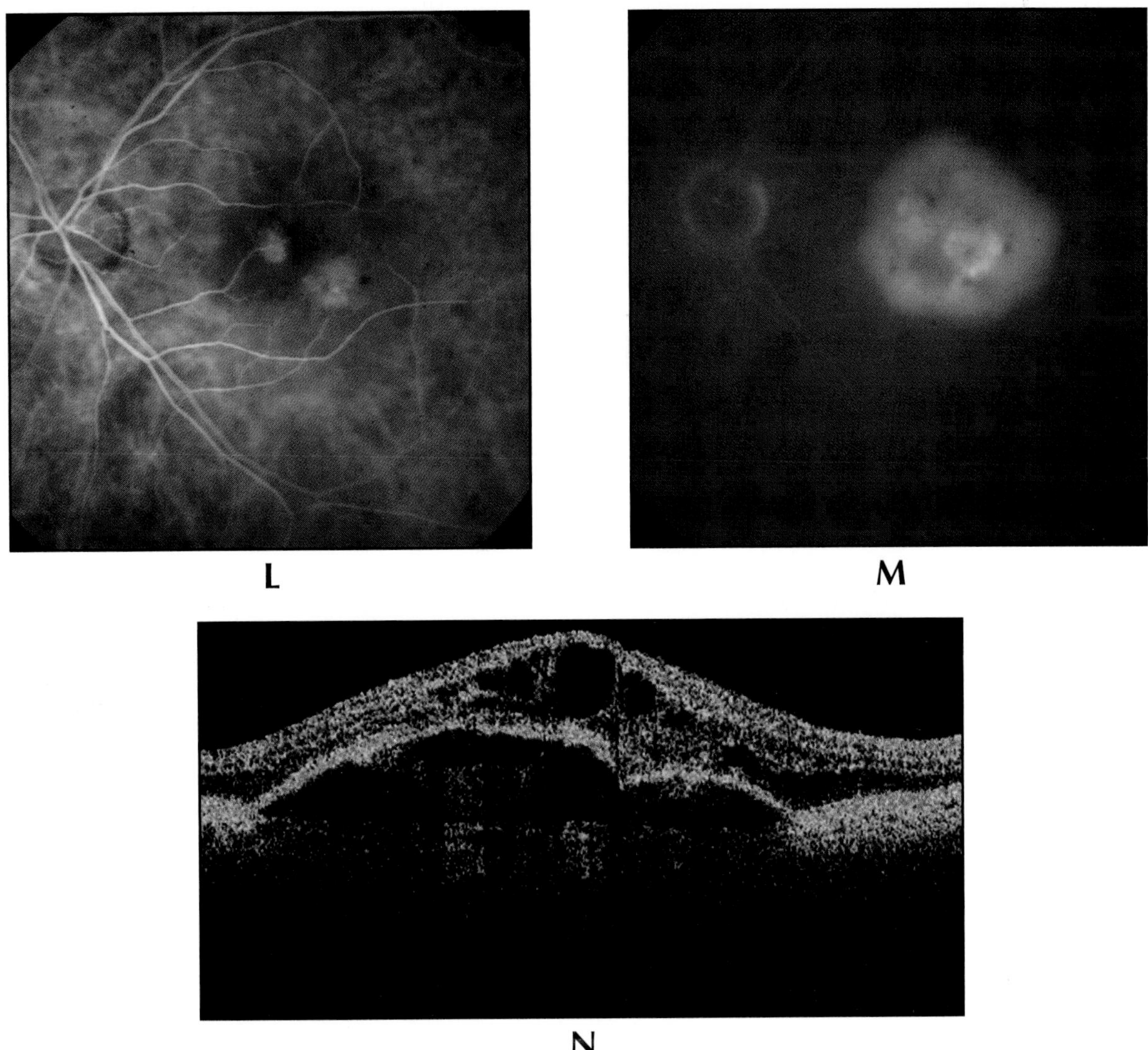
L
M
N

Case 7-23D. Seven Months After Intravitreal Triamcinolone Injection

Continuation of Clinical Summary

Seven months after the triamcinolone injection, vision in the left eye was decreased to 20/300. On examination (O), the PED was more elevated, the retinal thickness had increased, and there were new small intraretinal hemorrhages. FA revealed persistent leakage characteristic of a PED associated with RAP (P and Q). The patient received combined treatment of PDT and intravitreal triamcinolone.

Follow-Up Optical Coherence Tomography

A repeat OCT scan through the foveal center (R) showed increased cystoid retinal edema with central thickening. The PED was more elevated, and there was an increase in the subretinal surrounding the lesion. A central area of discontinuity in the highly reflective external band could also be seen.

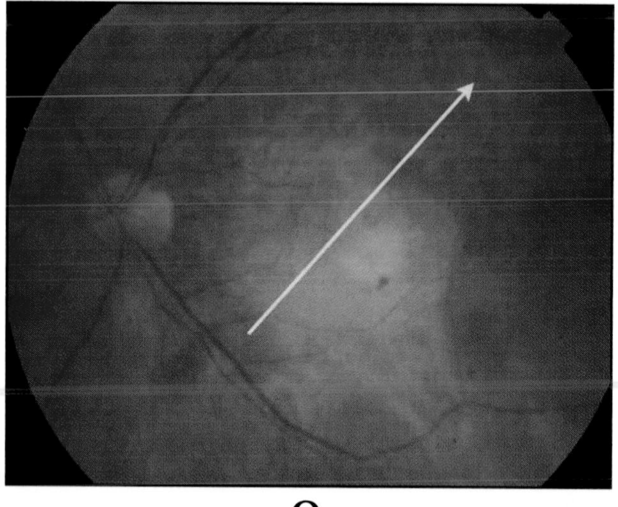

O

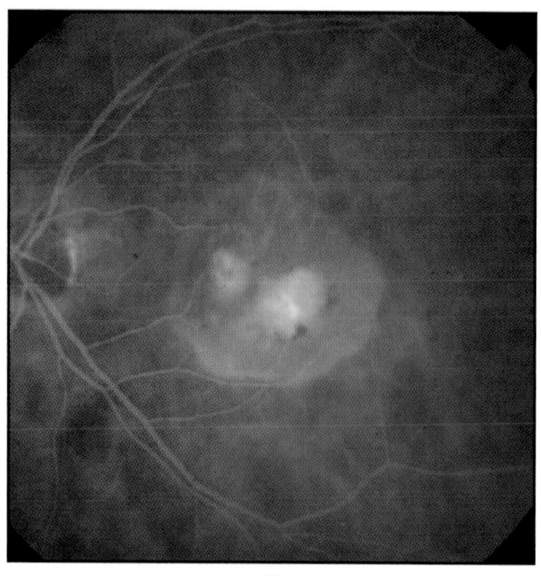

P

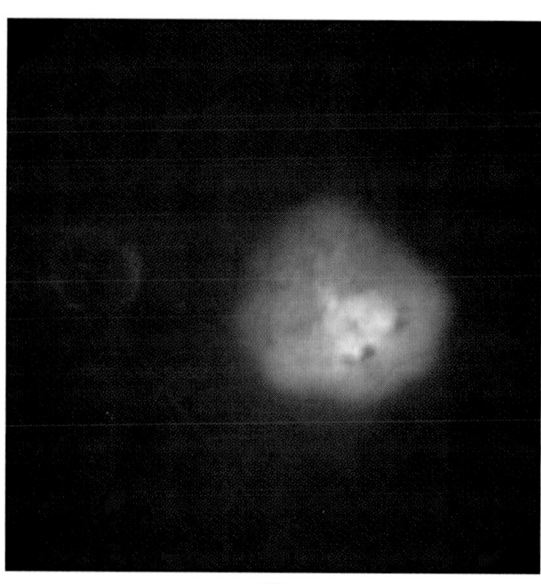

Q

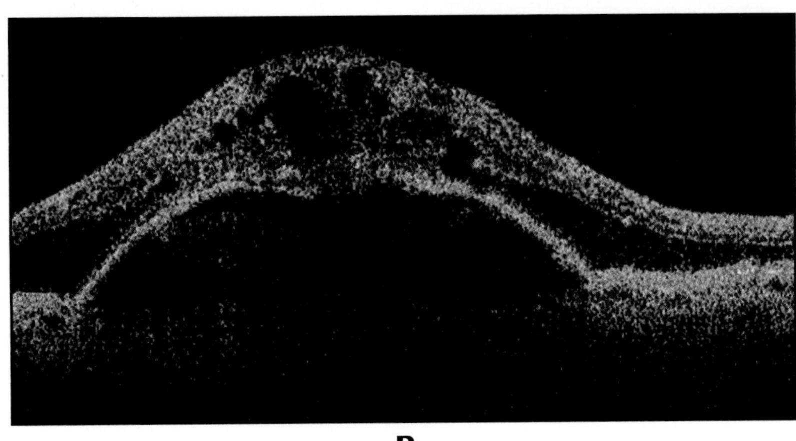

R

Case 7-23E. Four Weeks After Combined Photodynamic Therapy and Intravitreal Triamcinolone Injection

Continuation of Clinical Summary

Four weeks after PDT and triamcinolone injection, vision in the left eye improved to 20/200. On examination (S), the retinal thickness, intraretinal hemorrhages, and the elevation of the PED had diminished. FA (T and U) revealed only one well-defined fluorescent lesion temporal to the foveal center with decreased leakage throughout the PED compared with the previous visit.

Follow-Up Optical Coherence Tomography

An OCT scan through the foveal center (V) now showed improved foveal contour with a decrease in central retinal thickness and resolution of the intraretinal cytic edema. Some details of the layered appearance of the retina were visualized, but the photoreceptor layer appeared indistinct. There was a marked decrease in the elevation of the PED. The sub-PED space appeared highly reflective, probably due to a change in its composition and absorption of the fluid components. There was also a decrease in the amount of subretinal fluid adjacent to the PED.

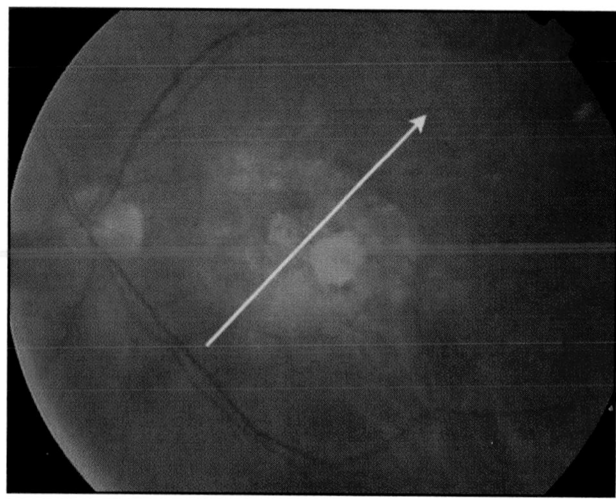

S

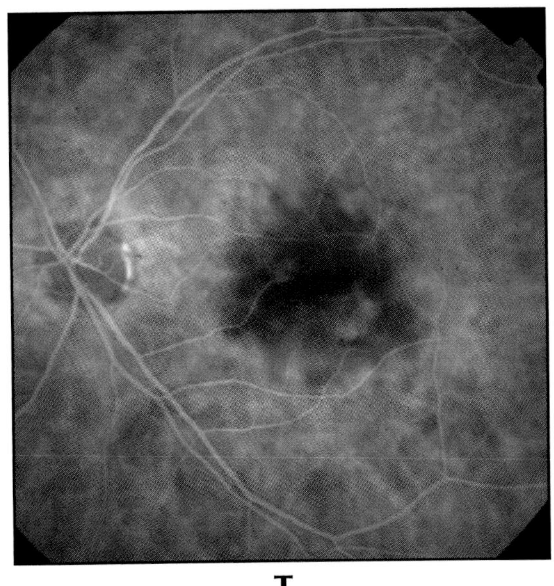

T

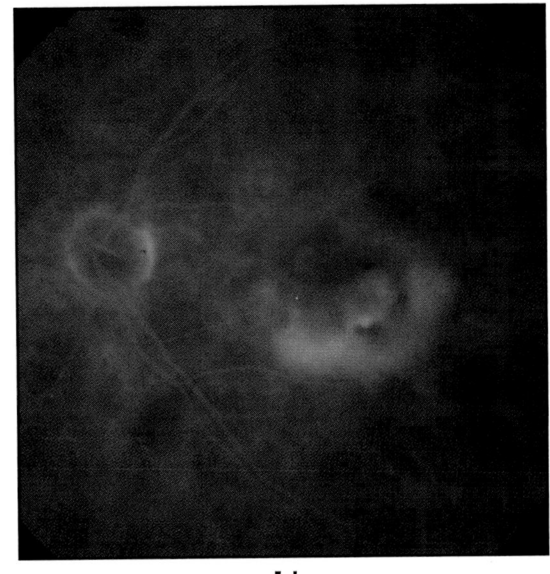

U

V

Case 7-23F. Three Months After Combined Photodynamic Therapy and Intravitreal Triamcinolone Injection

Continuation of Clinical Summary

Three months after PDT and triamcinolone injection, vision in the left eye was still 20/200. On examination (W), the central area appeared flat with RPE atrophy and mottling. Early subretinal fibrosis was present. FA (X and Y) revealed early hypofluorescence throughout the PED with late staining of the two angiomatous lesions.

Follow-Up Optical Coherence Tomography

An OCT scan through the foveal center (Z) showed a further decrease in the elevation of the PED. The highly reflective external band remained irregular, and areas of increased reflectivity from the central choroid probably represent fibrosis from the collapsed PED. There was no evidence of residual subretinal or intraretinal fluid.

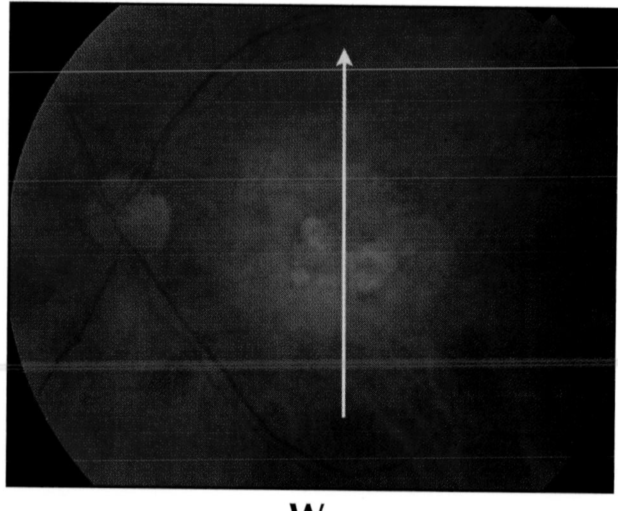

W

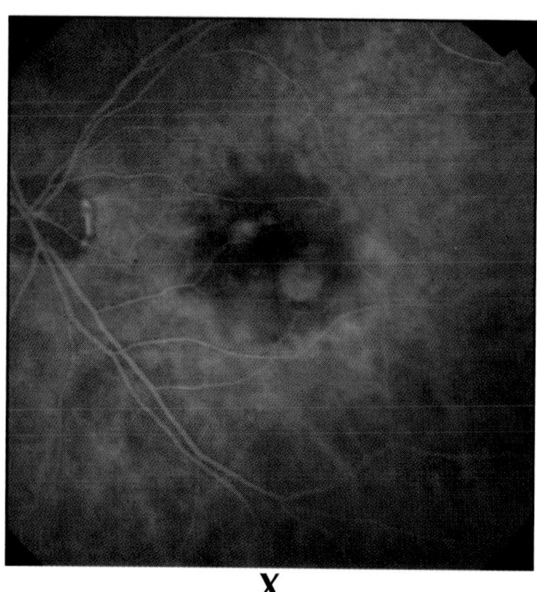

X

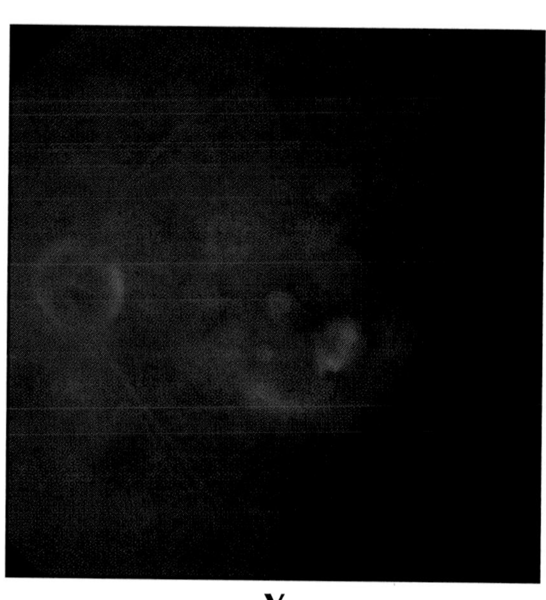

Y

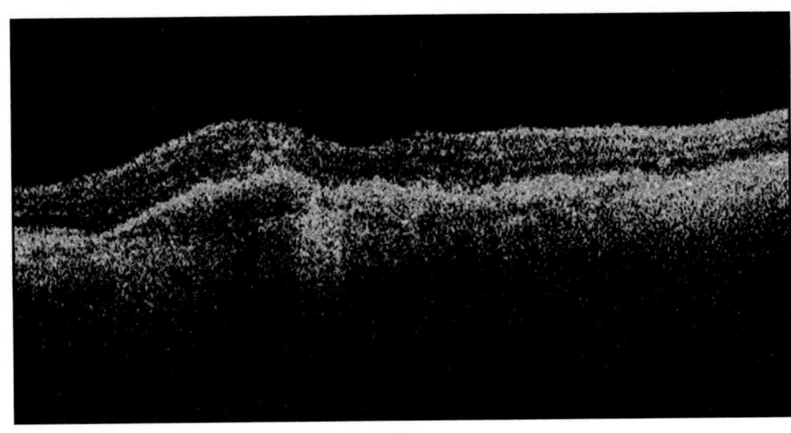

Z

Case 7-24. Retinal Pigment Epithelium Tear

Clinical Summary

A 76-year-old woman with a 1-year history of poor visual acuity in her left eye from exudative ARMD complained of decreased vision in the right eye for the past month. Her visual acuity was 20/40 in the right eye. Fundus examination (A) showed evidence of subretinal fluid in the central macula. Beneath this area, there was a sharply demarcated area of hypopigmentation adjacent to an area of hyperpigmentation. FA (B and C) confirmed the presence of an RPE tear.

Optical Coherence Tomography

A vertical OCT scan through the fovea (D) showed elevation of the neurosensory retina above a cavity of subretinal fluid. As the scan passed through the hyperpigmented area (central portion of the scan), the highly reflective external band appeared elevated and irregular. As the scan proceeded superiorly through the area of pigment loss (right side of the scan), the external band was no longer evident. The retina overlying this area showed only mild edema with preservation of the layered organization.

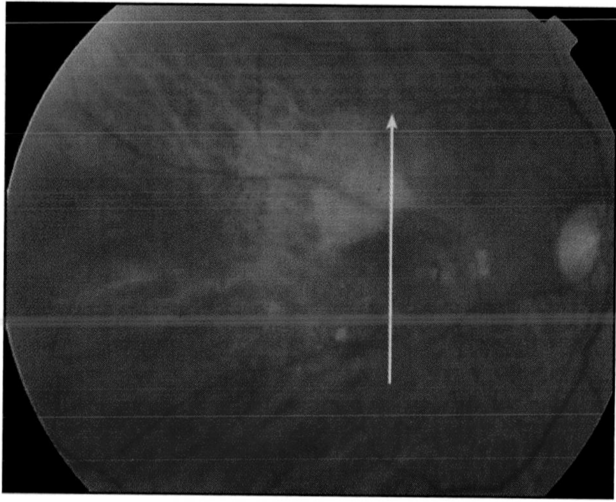

A

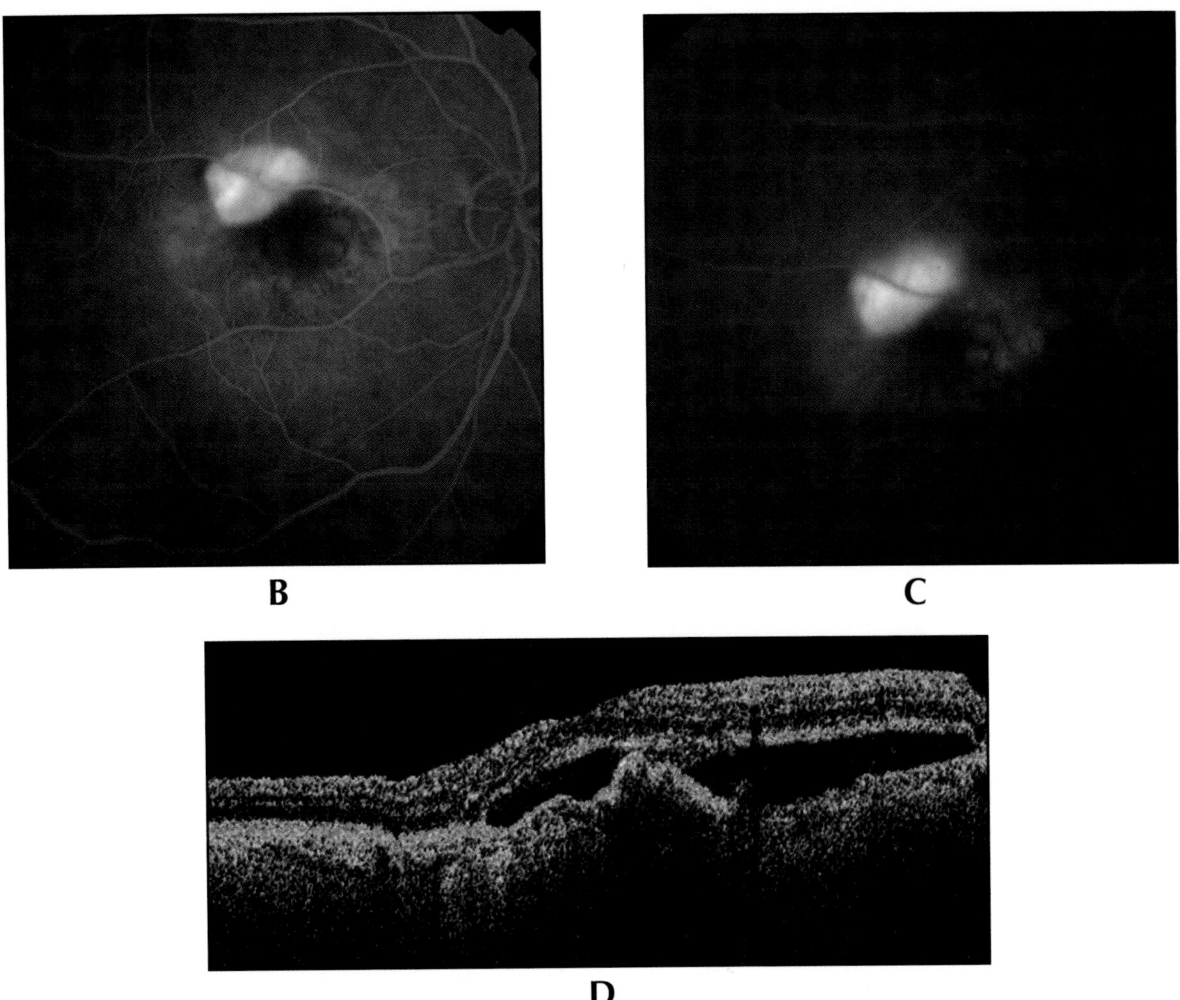
B
C
D

Case 7-25A. Occult Choroidal Neovascularization With Progression to a Retinal Pigment Epithelium Tear

Clinical Summary

An 86-year-old woman complained of decreased vision in her right eye over the past month. Her visual acuity was 20/50 in this eye. Fundus examination (A) showed irregular pigmentary mottling with a PED in the macula. FA (B and C) demonstrated occult CNV with early mottled fluorescence and late leakage. Observation of this lesion was recommended.

Optical Coherence Tomography

A vertical OCT scan through the fovea (D) confirmed the presence of a PED with dome-shaped elevation of the highly reflective external band. There was a small amount of subretinal fluid at the base of the PED. The overlying retina showed mild thickening with loss of the foveal contour.

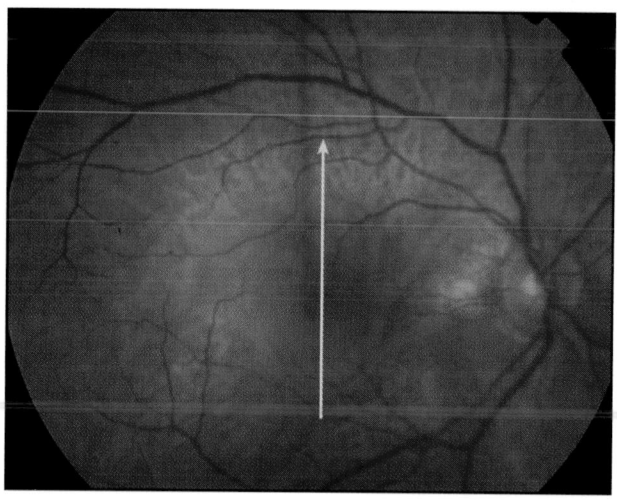

A

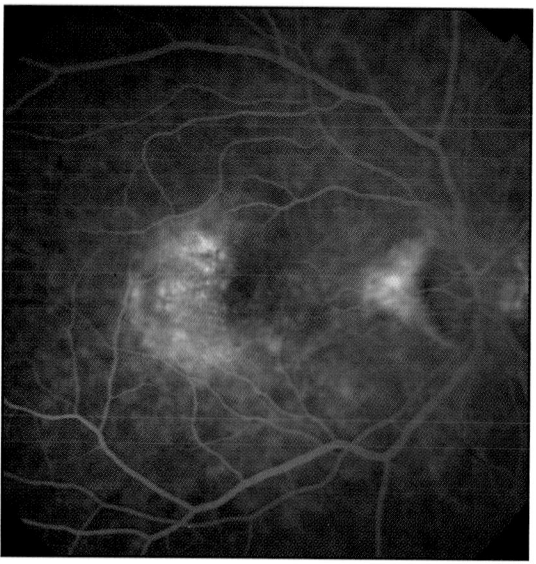

B

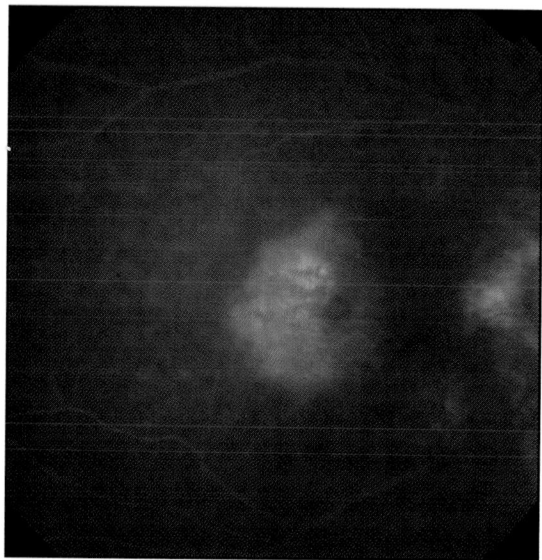

C

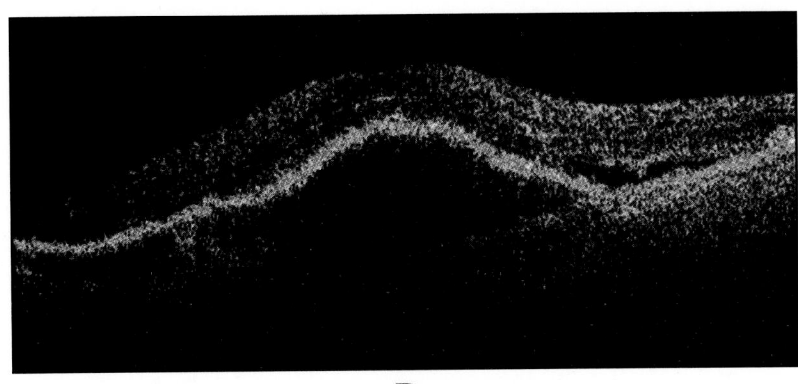

D

Case 7-25B. Retinal Pigment Epithelium Tear Formation

Continuation of Clinical Summary

The patient returned 4 months later and reported a mild decrease in her vision over the past 2 weeks. Her visual acuity in the right eye was now 20/60. Examination (E) showed a decrease in the height of the PED. There was an area of hypopigmentation temporally that was sharply demarcated from the dark fovea. FA (F and G) confirmed the presence of an RPE tear.

Follow-Up Optical Coherence Tomography

A horizontal OCT scan was taken through the fovea (H). As the scan passed through the area of RPE loss (left side of scan), there was enhanced penetration/reflectivity from the choroid. This appeared as thickening of the highly reflective external band in this area. Centrally, the PED was decreased in height, and the external band showed numerous corrugations indicating irregular folding of the torn RPE. The retina shows an irregular contour, but there is no evidence of subretinal or intraretinal fluid.

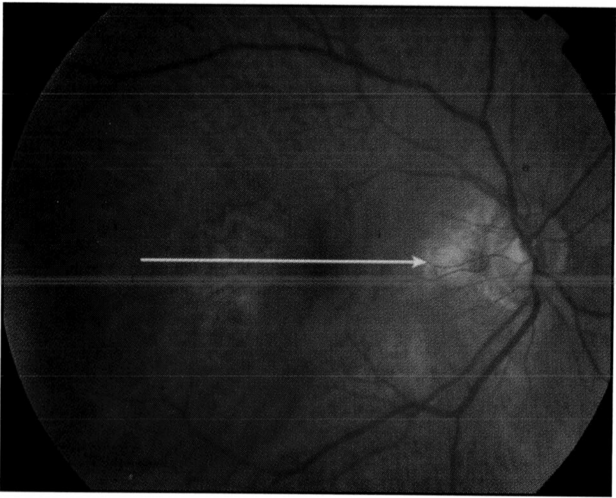

E

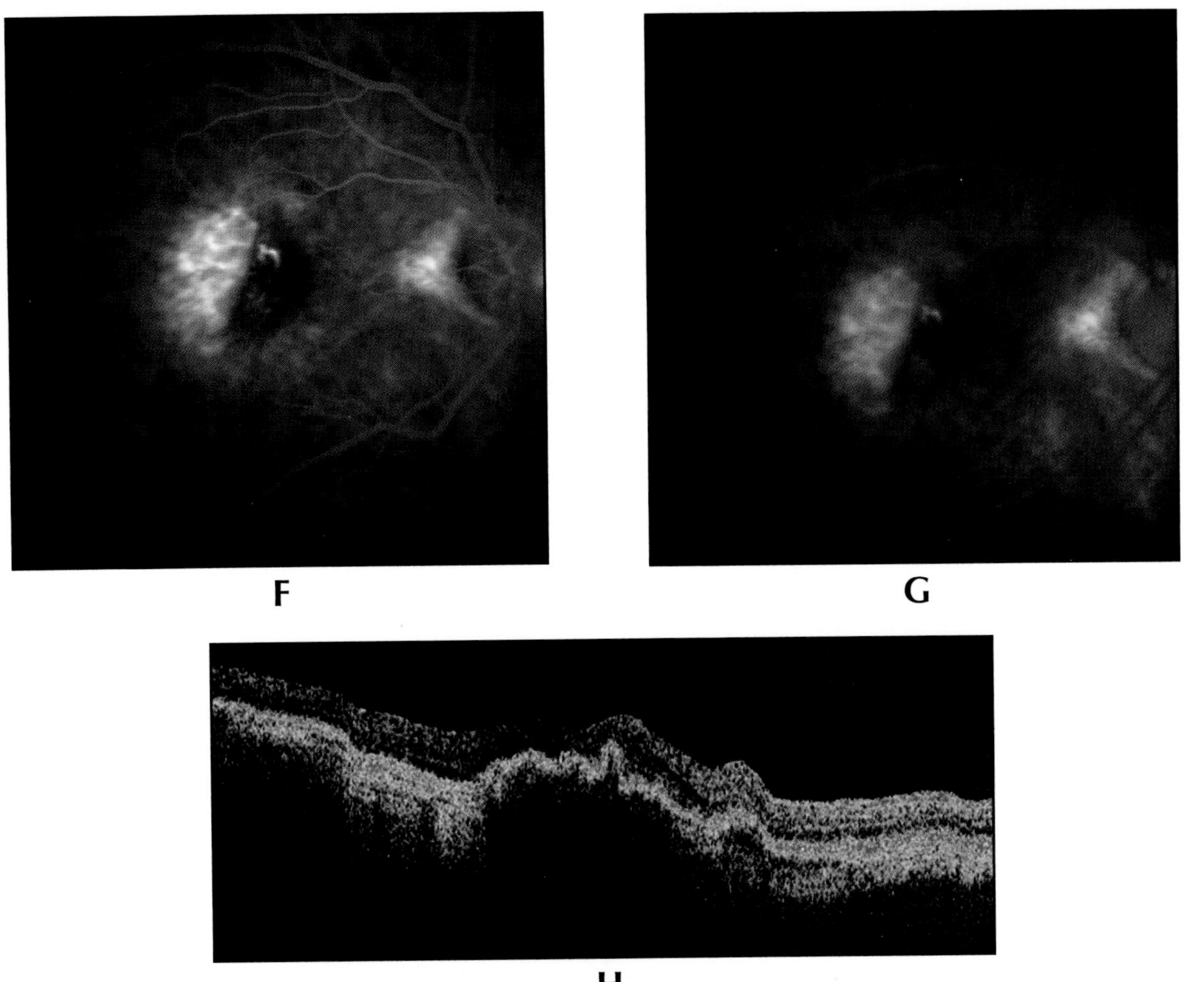
F
G
H

Case 7-26. Subretinal Hemorrhage

Clinical Summary

A 70-year-old man presented with sudden loss of vision in his left eye 2 weeks earlier. His visual acuity was 20/200 in this eye. Fundus examination (A) showed evidence of a subretinal hemorrhage involving the fovea. FA (B and C) demonstrated blockage of the normal fluorescence in the area of hemorrhage. ICGA (D and E) did not show evidence of a hot spot.

Optical Coherence Tomography

An oblique OCT scan through the fovea (F) showed a dome-shaped area of retinal elevation. Although there was distortion of the retinal contour, the intraretinal organization was relatively normal. Beneath the retina in this area, there was a thick and irregular band of high reflectivity that corresponds to the subretinal blood. Attenuation of the signal resulted in shadowing of the underlying layers, limiting visualization of these structures. However, a second, elevated band could be seen underneath this thicker initial band. This may represent elevation of the RPE due to a localized area of sub-RPE blood.

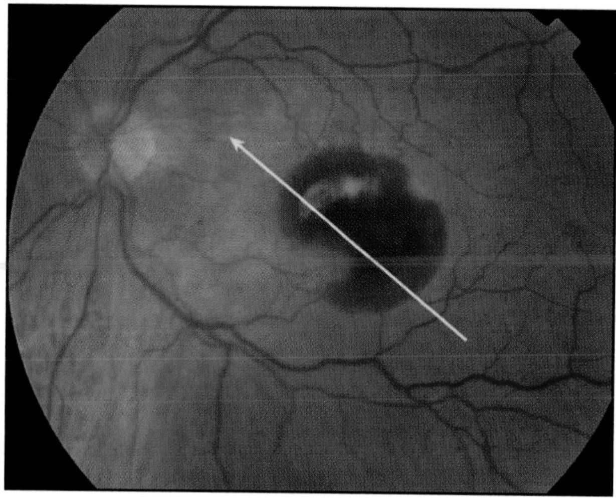

A

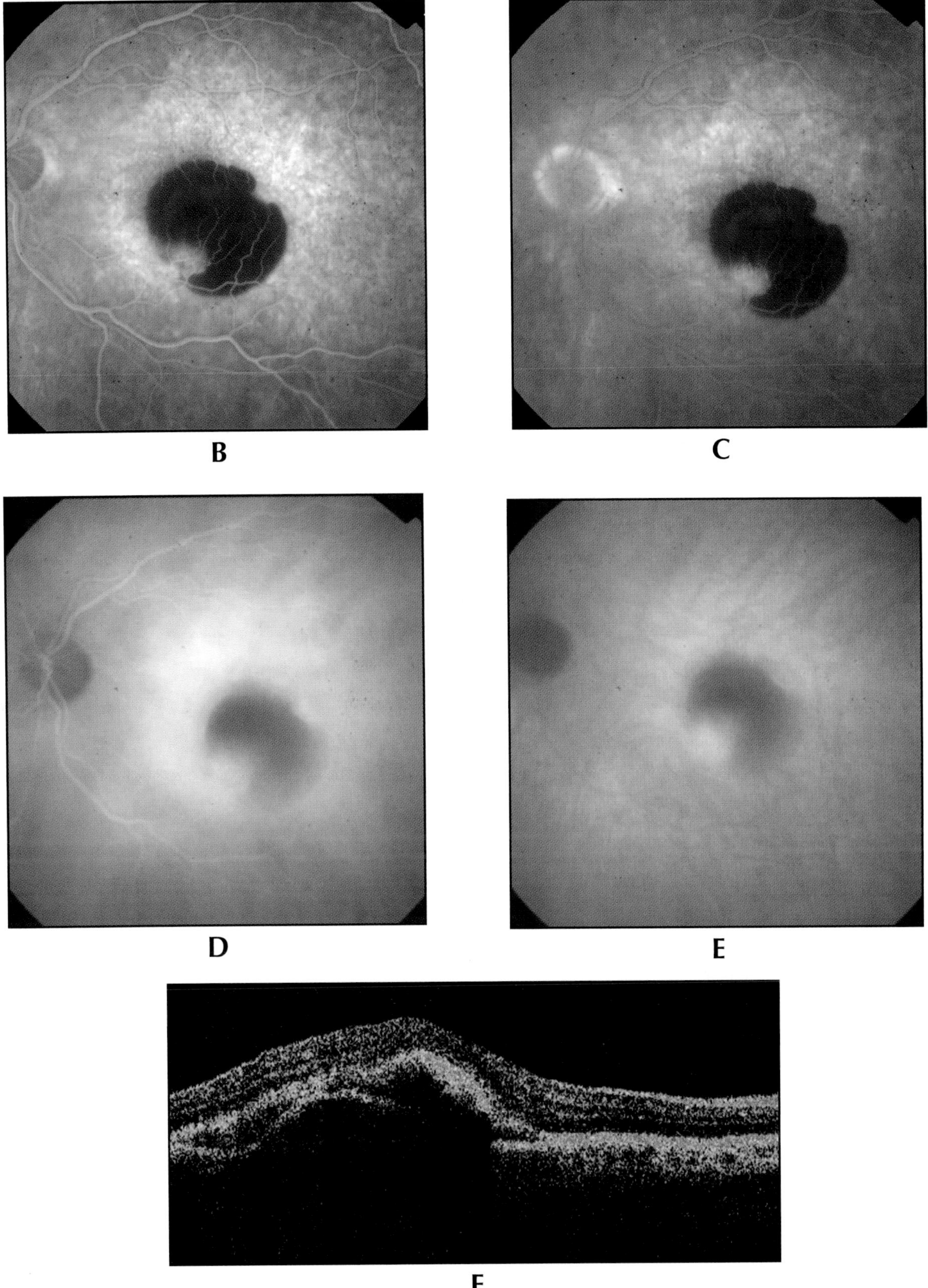
B
C
D
E
F

Case 7-27. Subretinal Hemorrhage

Clinical Summary

A 78-year-old woman with a history of ARMD complained of a sudden decrease in vision with her right eye to hand motions. Fundus examination (A) revealed a massive submacular hemorrhage. ICGA (B and C) showed blocked fluorescence in the area of the hemorrhage with some subfoveal fluorescence.

Optical Coherence Tomography

A horizontal scan through the macula (D) showed marked elevation of the central retina with a distortion of the retinal contour but preservation of the intraretinal organization. There was a thick and highly reflective band beneath the retina that represents the subretinal hemorrhage. This hemorrhage shadows the underlying choroidal reflections. Near the optic nerve, the choroidal reflectivity appeared enhanced due to the localized pigment atrophy seen on exam.

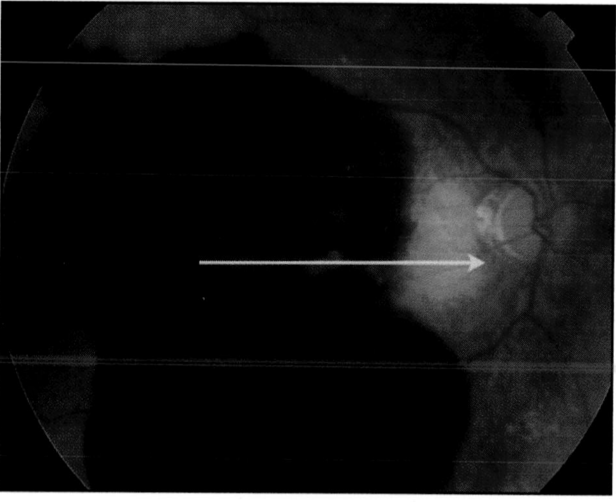

A

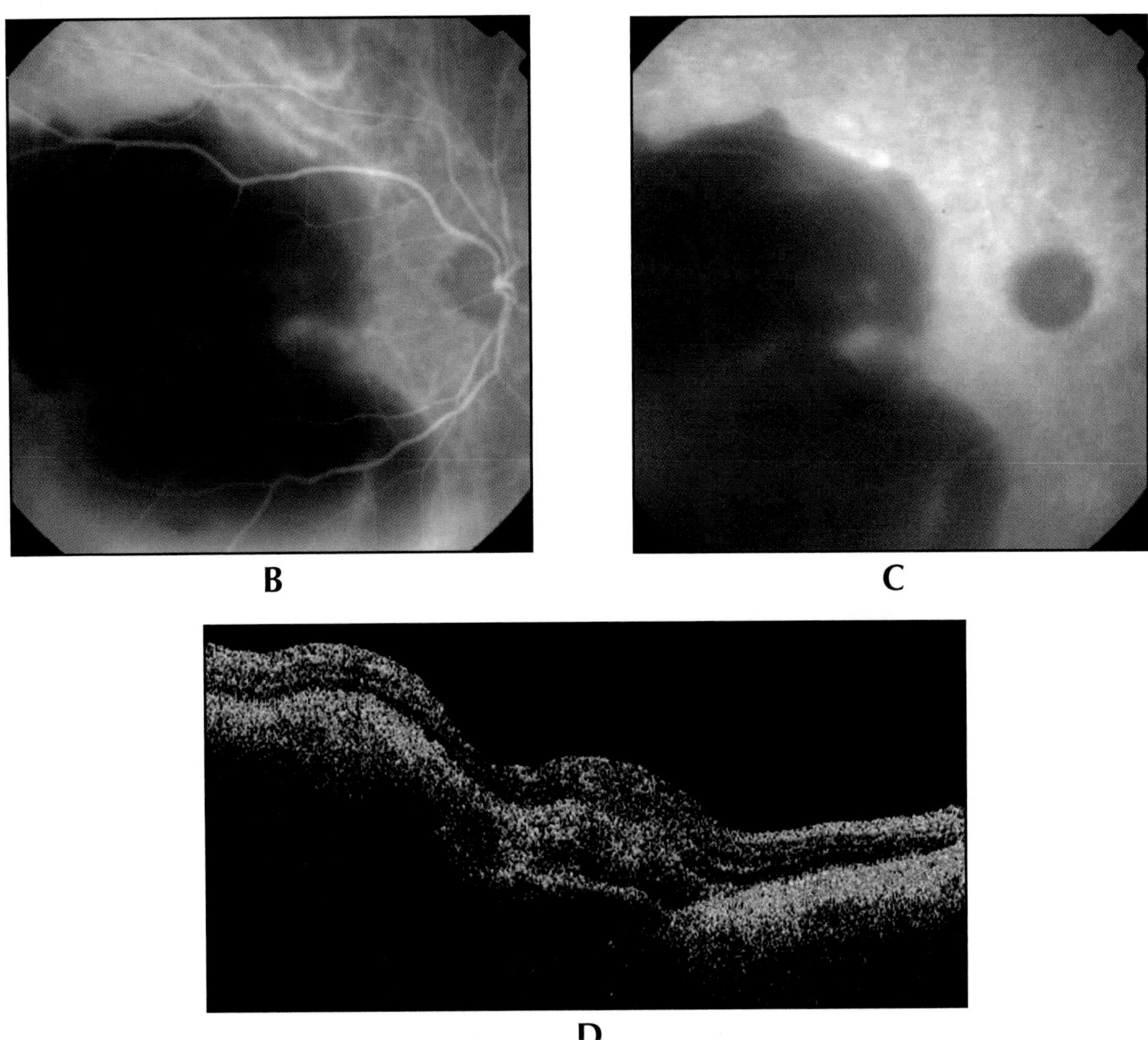

B

C

D

Case 7-28.
Disciform Scar With Macular Edema

Clinical Summary

A 79-year-old man with a history of exudative ARMD had a visual acuity of 20/400 after three PDT treatments. Fundus examination (A) revealed retinal edema with extensive disciform subfoveal fibrosis. FA showed an early well-defined fluorescent lesion (B) with late staining (C).

Optical Coherence Tomography

A horizontal scan through the macula (D) showed elevation and enlargement of the highly reflective band representing the fibrous scar with overlying cystoid retinal edema. There is shadowing of the choroid beneath the elevated scar. There is no evidence of subretinal fluid accumulation. Atrophy adjacent to the optic nerve results in increased reflectivity from the choroid (right side of the scan).

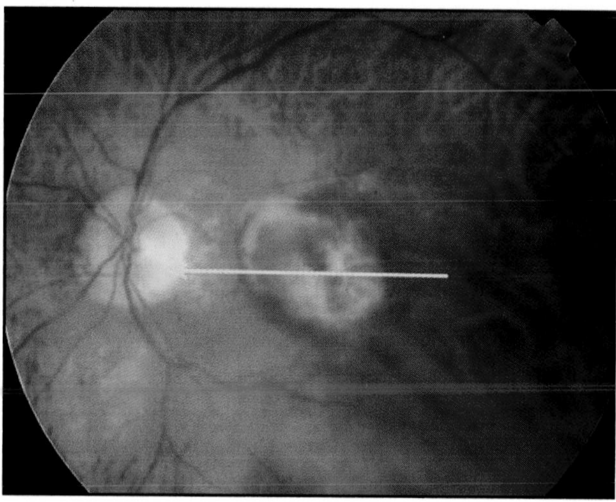

A

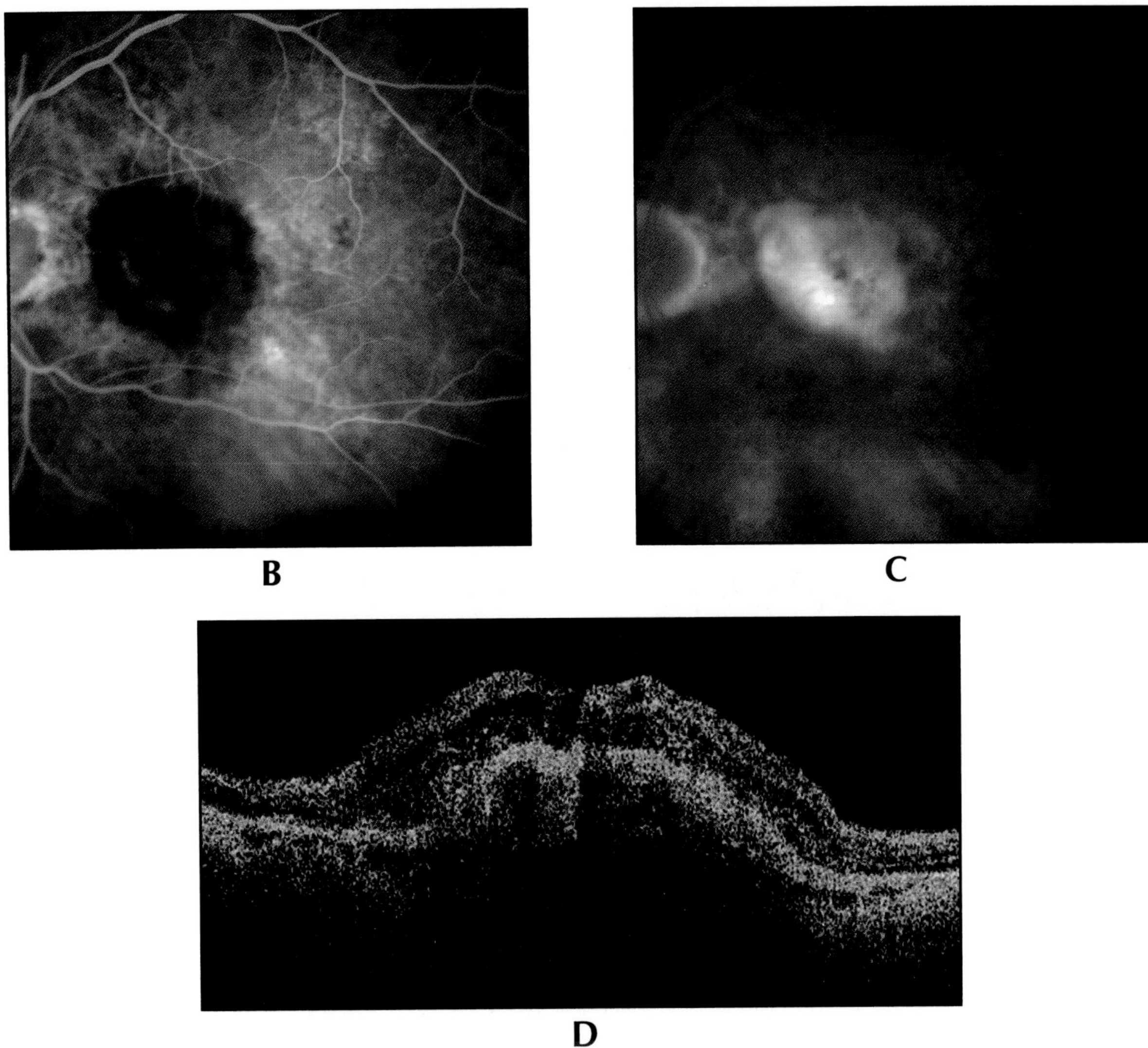
B
C
D

Case 7-29. Fibrotic Disciform Scar and Central Atrophy

Clinical Summary

A 79-year-old man with ARMD and right visual acuity of 20/400 for over a year presented for an evaluation. The right eye has not received any treatment. Fundus examination (A) revealed extensive subfoveal fibrosis, atrophy, and pigment mottling of the right macula extending to the peripapillary area. Early FA showed a window defect corresponding with the disciform area of atrophy (B) and late staining of the fibrotic component of the scar (C).

Optical Coherence Tomography

A horizontal scan through the macula (D) showed marked elevation of the area corresponding to the fibrosis (left side of the scan). Pigmentary atrophy allows enhanced penetration and reflectivity of the signal from the choroid, resulting in a thick area of intense reflectivity beneath the retina. The overlying retina is extremely thin and atrophic. There is no evidence of active subretinal or intraretinal fluid.

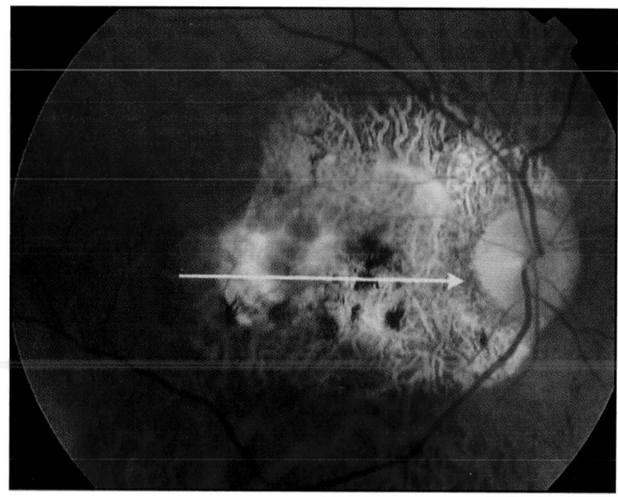

A

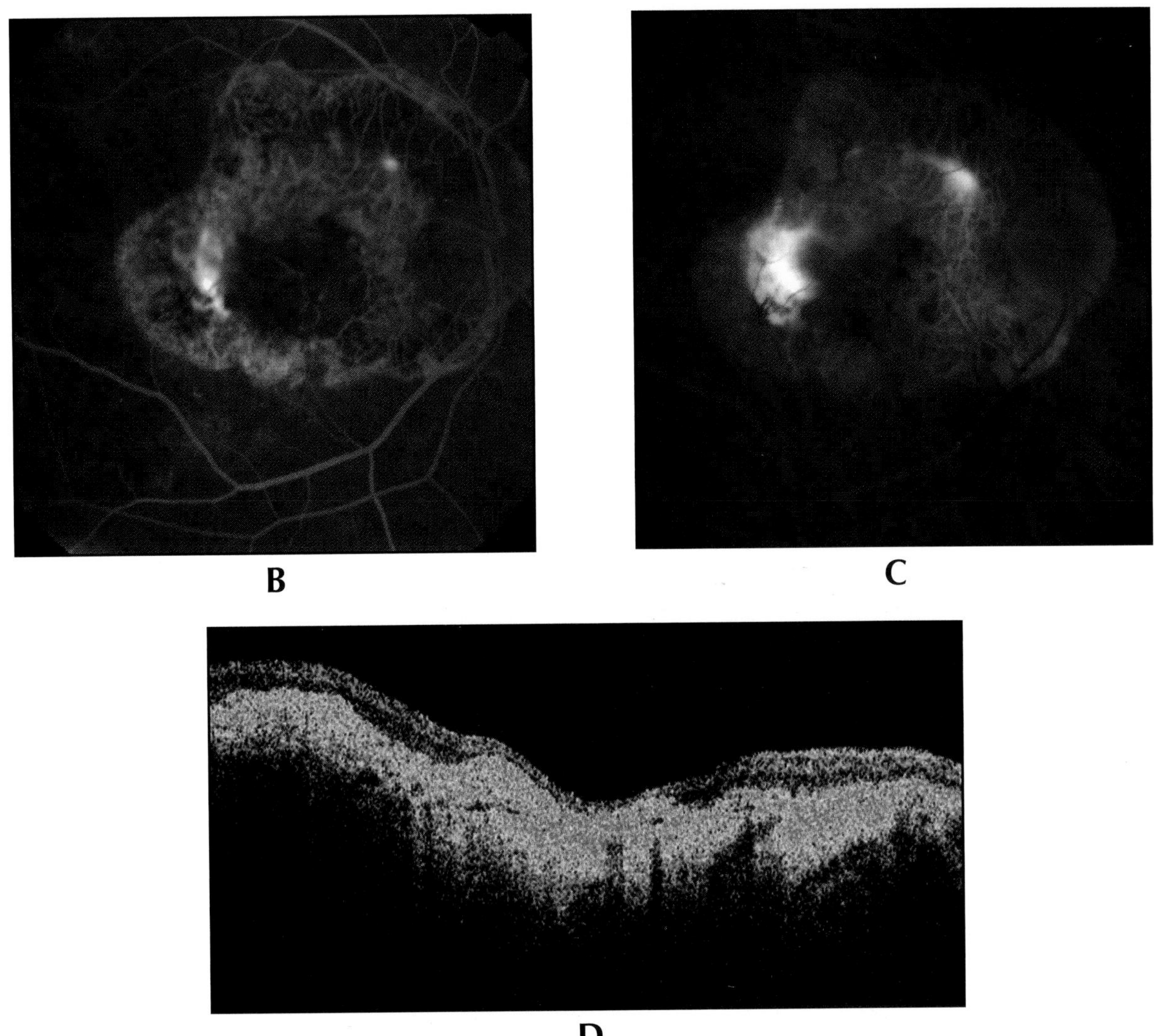
B
C
D

Chapter 8

Miscellaneous Macular Degenerations

Elias C. Mavrofrides, MD and Carmen A. Puliafito, MD

- Pathologic Myopia
- Angioid Streaks
- Idiopathic Choroidal Neovascularization
- Central Serous Chorioretinopathy With Choroidal Neovascularization
- Juxtafoveal Telangiectasis With Choroidal Neovascularization
- Presumed Ocular Histoplasmosis

In addition to age-related macular degeneration (ARMD), numerous conditions have been associated with the development of choroidal neovascularization (CNV). These conditions, which primarily affect younger patients, include pathologic myopia, angioid streaks, presumed ocular histoplasmosis, inflammatory chorioretinopathies, hereditary maculopathies, and trauma.[1] Abnormalities of the retinal pigment epithelium (RPE) and Bruch's membrane predispose to the development of CNV in these conditions. In some cases, an underlying cause for the CNV cannot be identified and these are termed *idiopathic*.

CNV in association with these conditions often differs from neovascularization due to ARMD. Gass described two patterns of neovascularization: type 1 growth of new vessels beneath the pigment epithelium and type 2 growth of vessels above the RPE in the subretinal space.[2] Type 2 neovascularization is more readily identified ophthalmoscopically and usually has a "classic" appearance on fluorescein angiography (FA). ARMD most commonly exhibits type 1 neovascularization, while these miscellaneous macular degenerations usually show type 2.[2] CNV in these miscellaneous macular degenerations is also typically smaller, more likely to regress spontaneously, and has a better prognosis than ARMD.

As with ARMD, optical coherence tomography (OCT) can be a valuable tool in the evaluation of patients with these conditions. The CNV in these cases usually appears as a highly reflective mass protruding above the RPE signal into the subretinal space. This appearance is consistent with the type 2 CNV as described by Gass.[2] The overlying retina is usually thickened with hyporeflective cystic spaces indicating intraretinal fluid accumulation.[3-6] In some cases of myopic CNV, intraretinal fluid accumulation does not occur, and the overlying retina may actually appear thinner than the adjacent tissue.[4] Subretinal fluid is also frequently identified around these lesions and appears on the OCT image as a nonreflective space beneath the neurosensory retina. Shadowing of the choroid beneath the CNV varies depending on the density/reflectivity of the lesion.

Several authors have described changes in the appearance of the CNV lesion on the OCT image as activity deceases and scarring develops.[4-6] Histopathologically, the regressing vessels are enveloped by RPE cells and become more fibrotic. As these changes occur, the CNV lesion often exhibits increased reflectivity on the OCT image and may become more fusiform in shape. These changes often make the lesion less distinct from the adjacent RPE signal. The most definitive sign of membrane regression, however, is resolution of the associated subretinal and intraretinal edema.

Less frequently, CNV in these conditions adopts a type 1 growth pattern. The OCT image shows changes similar to CNV associated with ARMD (see Chapter 7). These changes typically include disruption and elevation of the RPE with associated subretinal and intraretinal fluid accumulation. Because there is less penetration of the signal beneath the RPE, the neovascularization is usually not well defined on the OCT image in these instances.

Large subretinal hemorrhages can also occur in association with CNV in these conditions. Visualization of the neovascular lesion can initially be prevented by the hemorrhage. Because the reflectivity of the retina and blood can be similar, the separation between these two layers on OCT may be indistinct. Shadowing of the underlying RPE and choroid signal depends on the degree of elevation of the subretinal blood. Usually, penetration of the signal is adequate enough to define the position of the RPE and confirm the subretinal (versus sub-RPE) location of the blood. With subsequent resolution of the hemorrhage, the OCT can then help define the extent and activity of the associated neovascular complex.

The utility of OCT imaging in these conditions is not only characterization of the lesion, but also using this information to direct management and monitor response. As mentioned previously, these lesions may regress spontaneously without significant visual alteration. OCT can be useful in confirming and/or monitoring spontaneous regression of the lesion, thus obviating the need for intervention.

In many cases, however, intervention is beneficial for active lesions. The MPS study has shown the benefit of focal laser treatment for extrafoveal and juxtafoveal lesions in POHS and idiopathic CNV.[7] Photodynamic therapy (PDT) has subsequently been used for the treatment of subfoveal CNV in many of these conditions.[8-11] Identification of active or progressive CNV on OCT imaging can establish the need for these interventions.

OCT can then be used to monitor tissue response to these treatments and thus direct further management. Involution of the subretinal lesion with resolution of the associated edema indicates adequate treatment response and the need for observation. Increases in the size of the lesion or amount of surrounding edema can indicate persistent activity of the neovascularization and the need for additional intervention.

The role of OCT in the surgical removal of subfoveal CNV has also been evaluated.[12,13] Patients with type 2 CNV appear to have better outcomes after surgical removal than those with type 1 lesions. OCT can thus be used to define the anatomic location of the lesion to determine eligibility for surgical intervention.[12] Other lesion characteristics on the OCT image, such as well-defined edges, may also be important in predicting visual outcome after surgery.[13]

References

1. Cohen SY, Laroche A, Leguen Y, Soubrane G, Coscas GJ. Etiology of choroidal neovascularization in young patients. *Ophthalmology*. 1996;103:1241-1244.
2. Gass JDM. Biomicroscopic and histopathologic considerations regarding the feasibility of surgical excision of subfoveal neovascular membranes. *Am J Ophthalmol*. 1994;118:285-289.
3. Hee MR, Baumal CR, Puliafito CA, et al. Optical coherence tomography of age-related macular degeneration and choroidal neovascularization. *Ophthalmology*. 1996;103:1260-1270.
4. Baba T, Ohno-Matsui K, Yoshida T, et al. Optical coherence tomography of choroidal neovascularization in high myopia. *Acta Ophthalmol Scand*. 2002;80:82-87.
5. Fukuchi T, Takahasi K, Ida H, Sho K, Matsumura M. Staging of idiopathic choroidal neovascularization by optical coherence tomography. *Graefe's Arch Clin Exp Ophthalmol*. 2001;239:424-429.
6. Iida T, Hagimura N, Sato T, Kishi S. Optical coherence tomographic features of idiopathic submacular choroidal neovascularization. *Am J Ophthalmol*. 2000;130:763-768.
7. Ho AC. Miscellaneous macular degenerations. In: Regillo CD, Brown GC, Flynn HW JR, eds. *Vitreoretinal Diseases—The Essentials*. New York, NY: Thieme Medical Publishers Inc; 1999:241-253.
8. Verteporfin in Photodynamic Therapy Study Group. Photodynamic therapy of subfoveal choroidal neovascularization in pathologic myopia with verteporfin: 1 year results of a randomized clinical trial—VIP report no 1. *Ophthalmology*. 2001;108:841-852.
9. Sickenberg M, Schmidt-Erfurth U, Miller JW, et al. A preliminary study of photodynamic therapy using verteporfin for choroidal neovascularization in pathologic myopia, ocular histoplasmosis syndrome, angioid streaks, and idiopathic causes. *Arch Ophthalmol*. 2000;118:327-336.
10. Karacorlu M, Karacorlu S, Ozdemir H, Mat C. Photodynamic therapy with verteporfin for choroidal neovascularization in patients with angioid streaks. *Am J Ophthalmol*. 2002;134:360-366.
11. Spaide RF, Martin ML, Slakter J, et al. Treatment of idiopathic subfoveal choroidal neovascular lesions using photodynamic therapy with verteporfin. *Am J Ophthalmol*. 2002;134:62-68.
12. Giovannini A, Amato GP, Mariotti C, Scassellati-Sforzolini B. OCT imaging of choroidal neovascularization and its role in the determination of patients' eligibility for surgery. *Br J Ophthalmol*. 1999;83:438-442.
13. Brindaeu C, Glacet-Bernard A, Coscas F, Mimoun G, Coscas G, Soubrane G. Surgical removal of subfoveal choroidal neovascularization: visual outcome and prognostic value of fluorescein angiography and optical coherence tomography. *Eur J Ophthalmol*. 2001;11:287-295.

Case 8-1. Pathologic Myopia With Choroidal Neovascularization

Clinical Summary

A 40-year-old female has a history of high myopia (-22 diopters [D]) and poor visual acuity in her left eye from previous CNV. She complains of decreased central vision in her right eye over the past month. Her visual acuity has decreased from 20/30 to 20/200. Dilated fundus examination (A) of the right eye shows myopic pigmentary atrophy in the macular region and a pigmented lesion in the fovea. There is a small amount of edema surrounding this lesion. FA (B) shows early hyperfluorescence with late leakage consistent with subfoveal classic CNV.

Optical Coherence Tomography

The OCT image (C) shows a well-defined oval lesion extending above the RPE signal beneath the fovea. This lesion corresponds to the neovascularization identified on angiography. The overlying retina is mildly thickened, and there is a small pocket of adjacent subretinal fluid. There is shadowing of the choroidal signal beneath the neovascular lesion. The increased intensity of the choroid signal around this lesion results from enhanced penetration of the signal due to the myopic pigmentary atrophy.

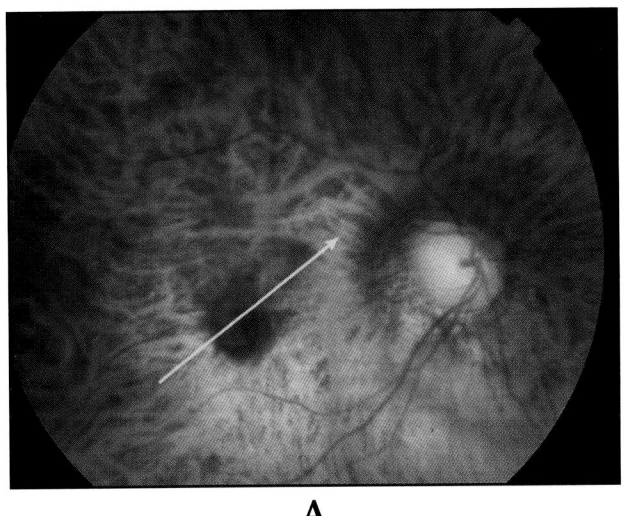

A

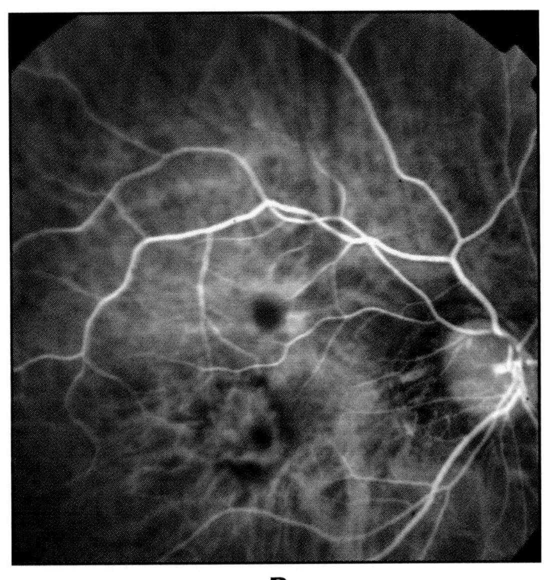

B

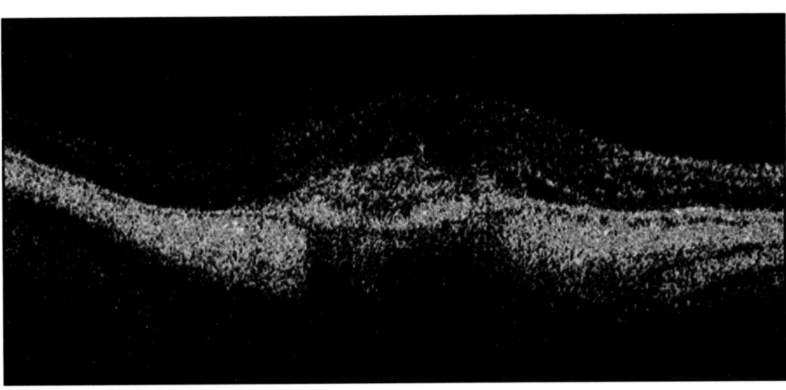

C

Case 8-2A. Pathologic Myopia With Choroidal Neovascularization

Clinical Summary

A 37-year-old male with a history of high myopia is referred for evaluation of a hemorrhage in his left eye. He has noticed mild distortion in this eye for the past month, and his visual acuity is 20/50. Retinal examination (A) shows myopic pigmentary changes in the macula and a Fuch's spot adjacent to the fovea. There is no evidence of associated retinal edema or hemorrhage on clinical exam. FA (B) shows an area of early hyperfluorescence with mild late leakage, indicating CNV.

Optical Coherence Tomography

The neovascular lesion is clearly identified on the OCT image (C) as a dome-shaped area extending above the RPE signal. There is mild distortion of the retinal contour, but no evidence of intraretinal or subretinal edema. The foveal pit can still be identified, and the lesion appears to be in a juxtafoveal position.

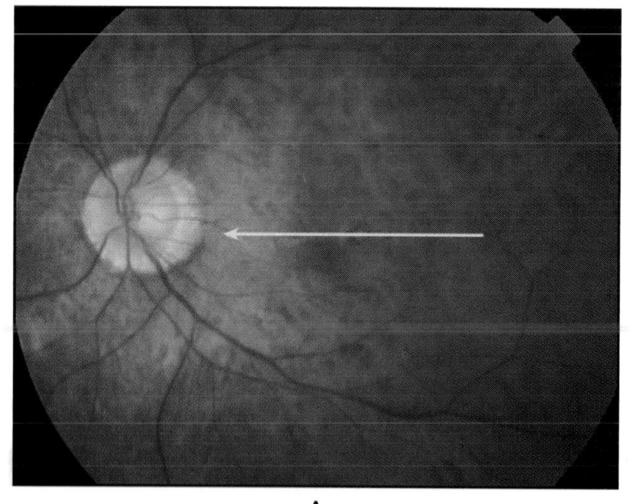

A

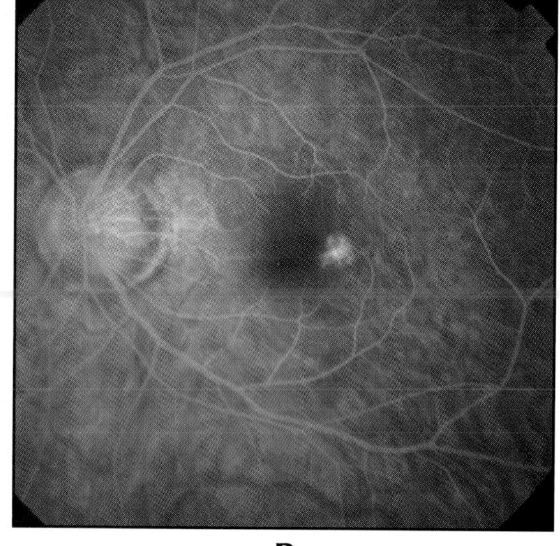

B

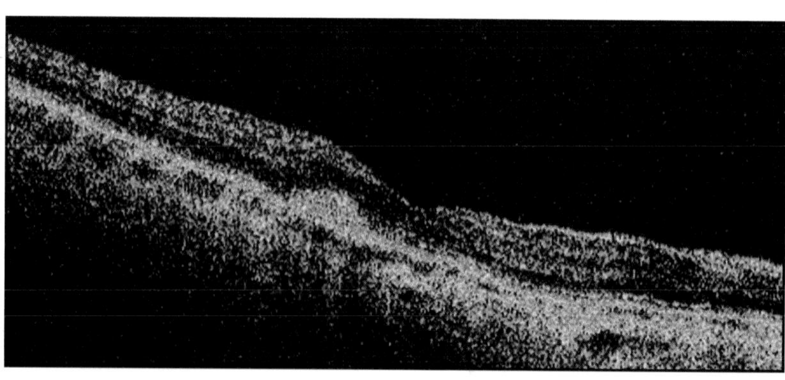

C

Case 8-2B. Enlargement of the Lesion

Continuation of Clinical Summary

The patient elects for observation and returns 3 months later for re-evaluation. He has noticed increased distortion in his left eye during the past 2 weeks. His visual acuity has now declined to 20/100. Retinal examination and FA (D and E) demonstrate enlargement of the neovascular lesion with subfoveal extension.

Follow-Up Optical Coherence Tomography

Progression of the lesion is confirmed on the OCT tomogram (F). The CNV, which is still well-visualized between the RPE and retina, appears much larger in size and definitely extends beneath the center of the fovea. Shadowing of the underlying choroid occurs because of the increased density of the lesion. Exudation from the lesion has resulted in retinal thickening and subretinal fluid accumulation.

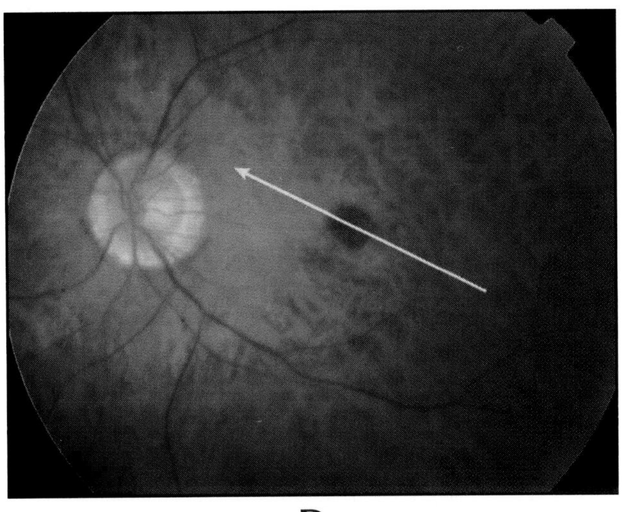

D

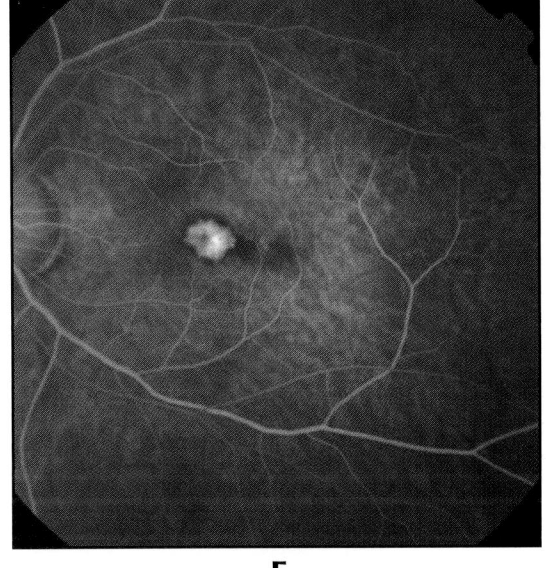

E

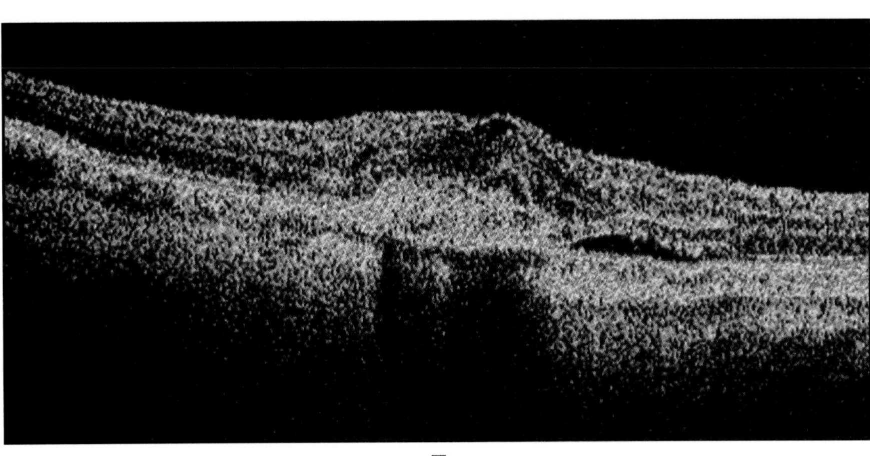

F

Case 8-3A. Myopic Degeneration With Choroidal Neovascularization

Clinical Summary

A 50-year-old female with a history of high myopia complains of central visual distortion in her right eye for 1 month. Her visual acuity has decreased in this eye from 20/30 to 20/70. Dilated fundus examination (A) shows peripapillary and macular pigmentary changes consistent with myopic degeneration. In the foveal region, there is a localized area of hyperpigmentation with overlying subretinal fluid. FA (B) shows a small area of hyperfluorescence in the fovea that leaks in the late phase consistent with classic CNV.

Optical Coherence Tomography

The OCT tomogram (C) shows an oval, hyperreflective lesion above the RPE signal that corresponds to the neovascular complex seen on the angiogram. There is a pocket of subretinal fluid adjacent to this lesion and mild overlying retinal edema. The RPE signal shows mild irregularity but no evidence of significant elevation or disruption.

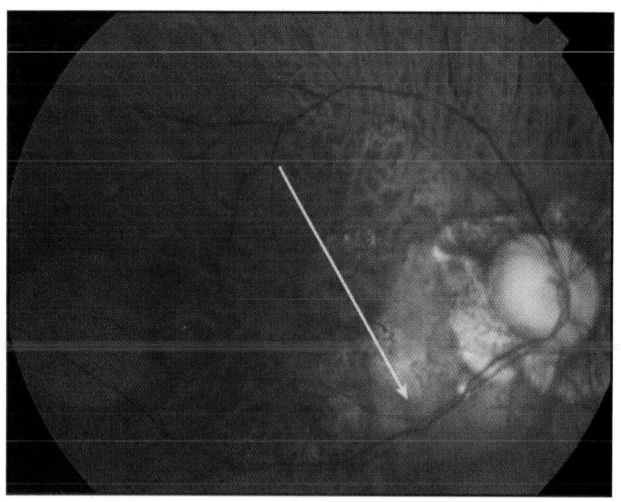

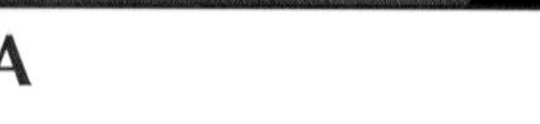

A

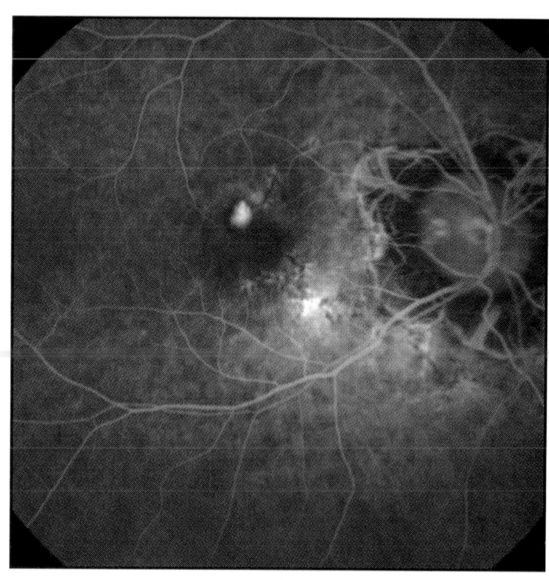

B

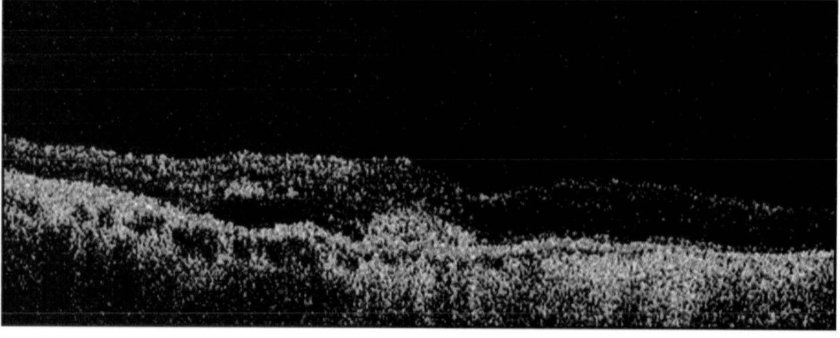

C

Case 8-3B.
Treatment With Photodynamic Therapy

Continuation of Clinical Summary

PDT is performed at the initial visit. The patient returns 6 weeks later and reports decreased distortion. Her visual acuity in this eye has improved to 20/50. Retinal examination (D) shows pigmentary degeneration but no evidence of persistent subretinal fluid. There is still an area of hyperfluorescence on angiography (E) but no evidence of active leakage.

Follow-Up
Optical Coherence Tomography

An OCT cut is obtained in the same location and direction as the pretreatment image shown. The hyperreflective lesion previously seen above the RPE signal is no longer identified (F), suggesting regression of the neovascular complex. There has also been resolution of the subretinal fluid. The underlying RPE signal remains irregular, consistent with the pigmentary changes identified on exam.

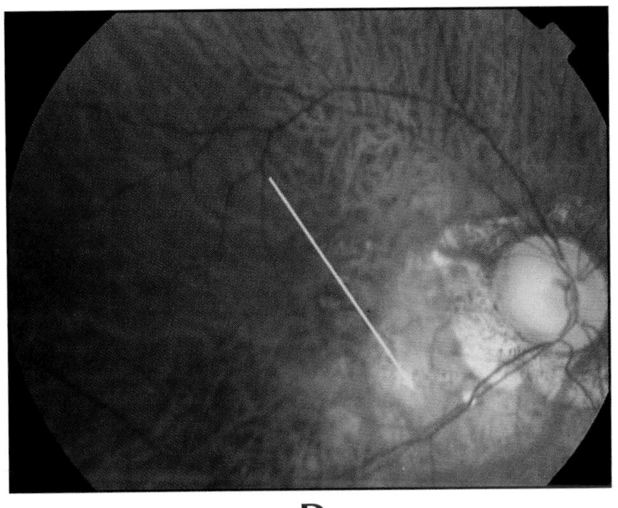

D

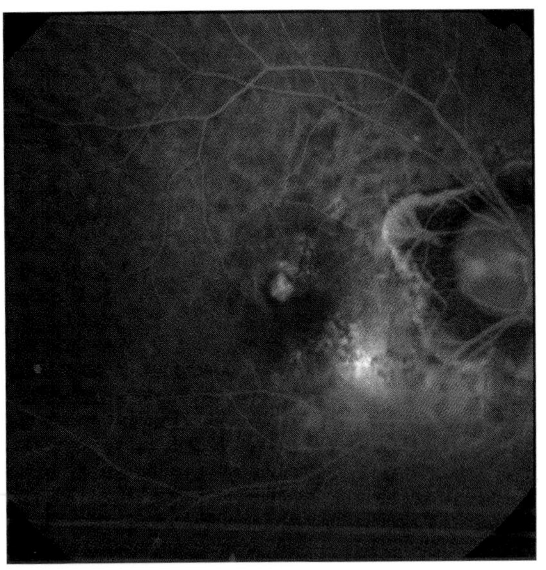

E

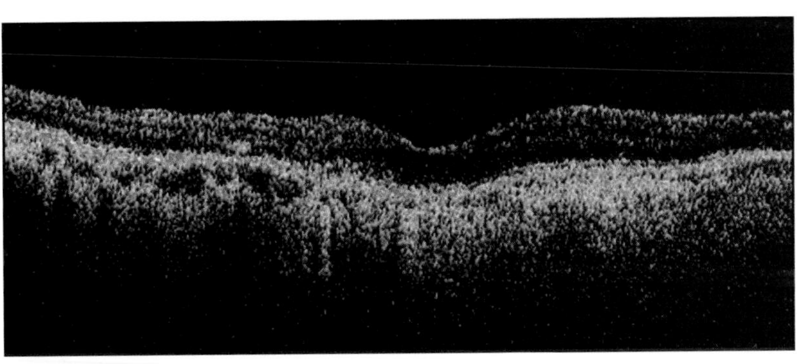

F

Case 8-4A. Pathologic Myopia With Choroidal Neovascularization

Clinical Summary

A 60-year-old female with a history of high myopia complains of a dark spot in the central visual acuity of her left eye for 4 months. Her visual acuity is 20/40 in this eye, and there is central metamorphopsia on Amsler grid testing. Dilated fundus examination (A) shows peripapillary and macular pigmentary atrophy consistent with pathologic myopia. There is a large neovascular complex in the macula with extensive overlying edema. FA (B) confirms a large classic neovascular lesion that extends under the fovea and leaks in the late phase of the study.

Optical Coherence Tomography

The OCT image (C) shows the neovascularization as a fusiform area of moderate reflectivity extending above the RPE signal into the subretinal space. This lesion shows slightly more intense reflectivity than the overlying retina but is slightly less intense than the adjacent RPE signal. The overlying retina is thickened with intraretinal cystic edema. The retina around the lesion does not show evidence of edema, and there is no associated subretinal fluid. The RPE signal does not show evidence of disruption, although there is mild shadowing beneath the CNV.

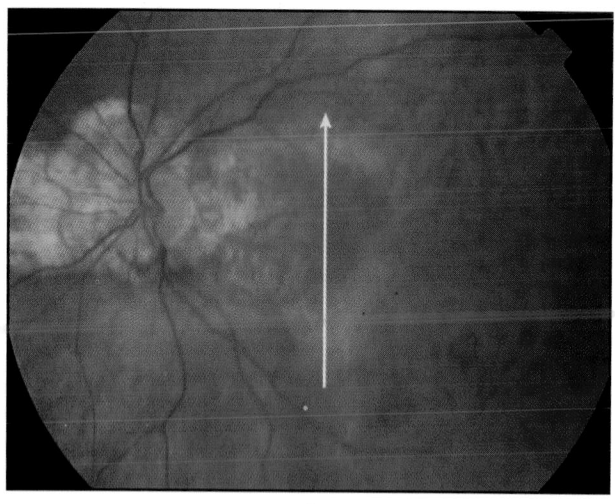

A

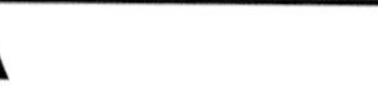

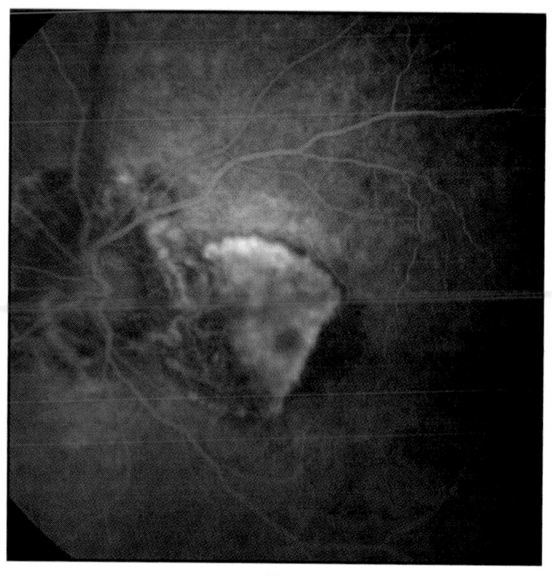

B

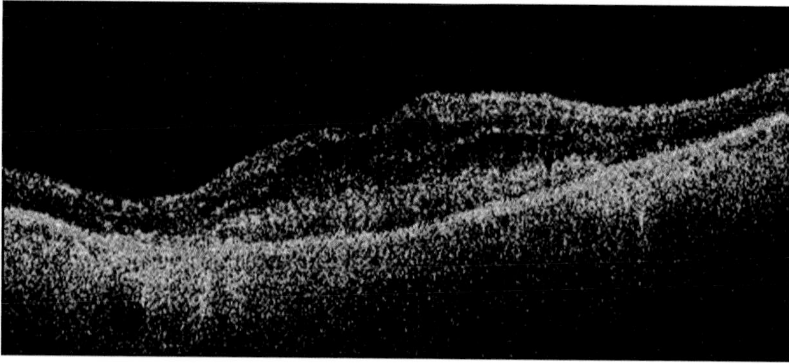

C

Case 8-4B. Treatment With Photodynamic Therapy

Continuation of Clinical Summary

Photodynamic therapy is performed at the initial visit. She returns 1 month later and reports improvement in her distortion. Her visual acuity in this eye is now 20/30. Dilated fundus examination (D) shows pigmentary mottling but no evidence of active neovascularization or edema. On FA (E), there is now a large area of hypofluorescence in the area of previous neovascularization.

Follow-Up Optical Coherence Tomography

The previously identified neovascular lesion is no longer evident on the post-treatment OCT image (F). There has also been resolution of the retinal edema with normalization of the retinal contour. These changes confirm involution of the CNV after the PDT treatment.

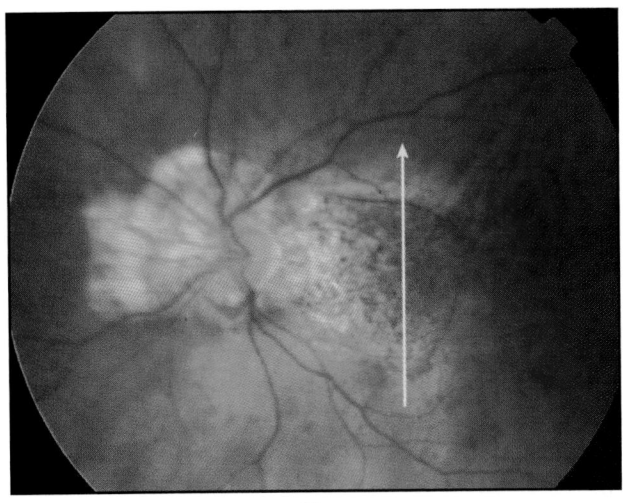

D

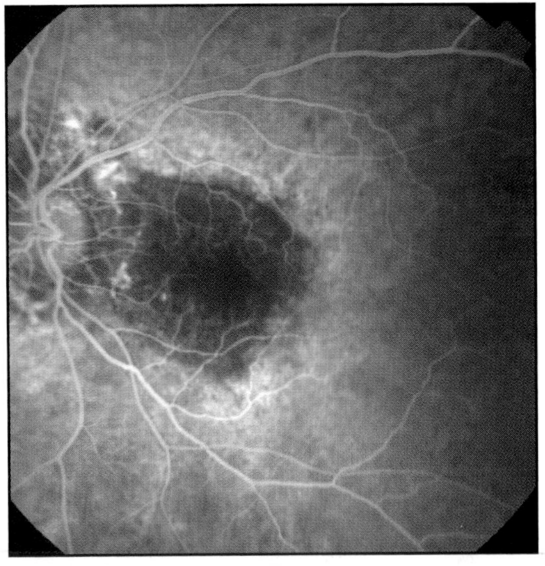

E

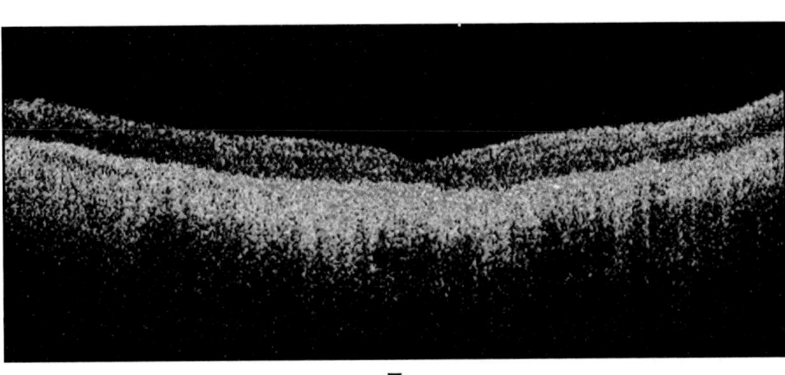

F

Case 8-5A. Pathologic Myopia With Choroidal Neovascularization

Clinical Summary

A 32-year-old female who is 5 months pregnant complains of decreased visual acuity in her left eye over the past 2 months. She has a history of high myopia (-14 D) with central macular scarring from previous CNV in her right eye. Her visual acuity in the left eye is 20/30. Dilated fundus examination (A) shows peripapillary atrophy and myopic pigmentary mottling in the macula. There appears to be a small amount of edema superior to the fovea. FA is deferred because the patient is pregnant.

Optical Coherence Tomography

There is a small dome-shaped area of increased reflectivity above the RPE signal on the OCT image (B). This represents early CNV with a type 2 growth pattern. The CNV extends to, but does not involve, the fovea. Adjacent to this lesion there is a clear cavity beneath the retina that represents subretinal fluid. The retina above this lesion is edematous, but the foveal pit contour is preserved. Macular pigmentary atrophy allows deeper penetration and increased reflectivity of the signal, resulting in a more intense choroidal band.

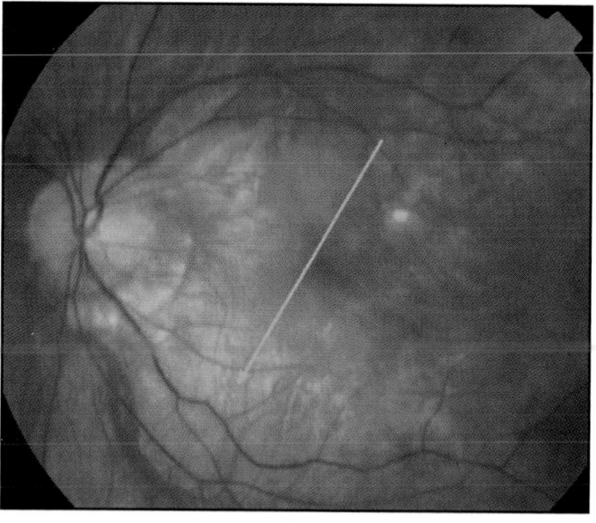

A

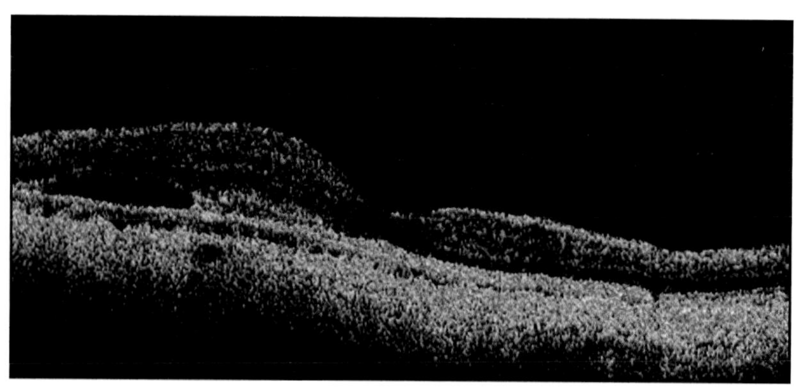

B

Case 8-5B. Pathologic Myopia With Choroidal Neovascularization

Continuation of Clinical Summary

Observation is recommended because the patient is pregnant. She is subsequently followed with serial clinical and OCT examinations. Over the next month, the patient notices slight worsening and her visual acuity decreases to 20/40. Fundus examination is unchanged from initial. Although intravitreal triamcinolone injection is considered, continued observation is recommended. Three months after her initial visit, her visual acuity declines further to 20/80. She delivers her child by uncomplicated C-section at 8 months gestation. Shortly after delivery, PDT is performed. Her visual acuity after PDT improves to 20/30 and remains stable 6 months after treatment.

Follow-Up Optical Coherence Tomography

The OCT image at her 1-month follow-up (C) confirms enlargement of the subretinal CNV lesion with extension toward the fovea. The foveal distortion has increased, but the intraretinal and subretinal edema are mostly unchanged. Three months after the initial exam, there has again been progression of the lesion. The OCT image (D) now shows growth of the lesion with increased intraretinal and subretinal edema. The OCT image (E) taken after PDT confirms a dramatic response to treatment. The neovascularization has regressed with only a thin band of increased reflectivity in the area of the previous lesion. The intraretinal and subretinal fluid has resolved, and the foveal pit contour has been restored.

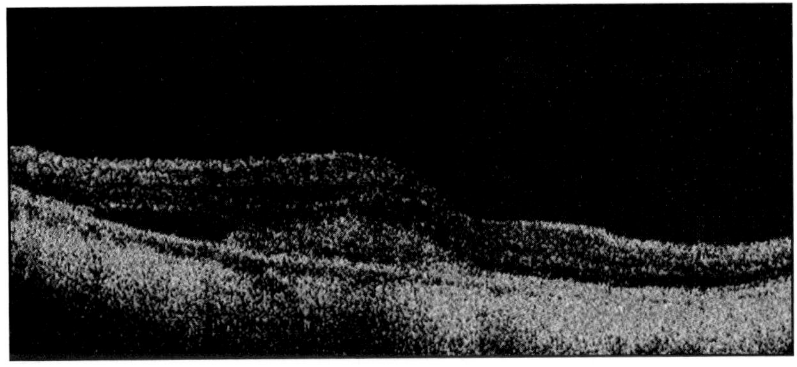

C

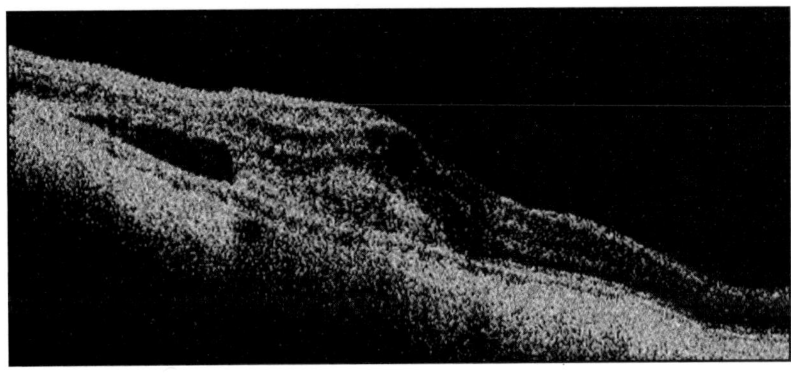

D

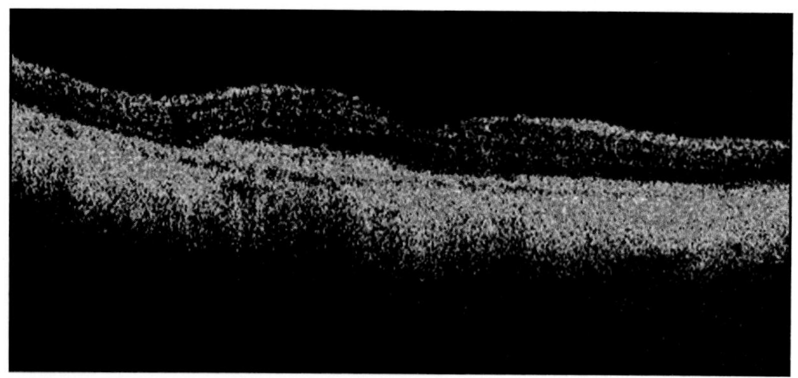

E

Case 8-6. Angioid Streaks

Clinical Summary

A 45-year-old female presents for evaluation of mild central visual distortion in her right eye for the past 6 months. Her visual acuity in this eye is 20/25. Dilated fundus examination (A) shows evidence of angioid streaks radiating from the disc. One of the streaks passes horizontally through the macula just above the fovea. In the temporal periphery, this is mild pigmentary mottling suggesting a "peau d' orange" appearance. FA (B) shows hyperfluorescence along the angioid streaks with late staining but no leakage.

Optical Coherence Tomography

A vertical OCT image (C) through the macula shows a normal appearing neurosensory retina with a normal foveal contour. The high-intensity RPE/choroid signal is normal in appearance in the inferior macula (left portion of the tomogram) but shows irregular undulations as the scan passes through the area of the angioid streak. There is no evidence of associated CNV since subretinal and/or intraretinal fluid are not present.

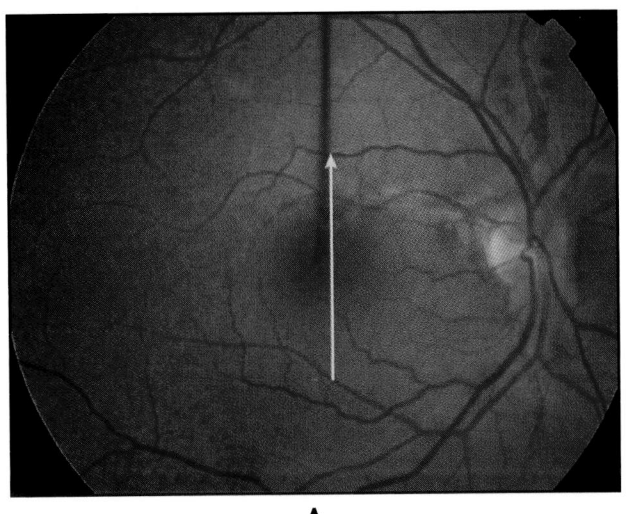

A

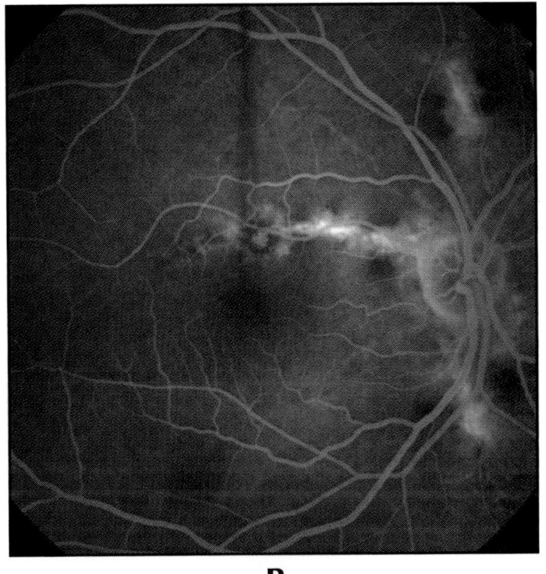

B

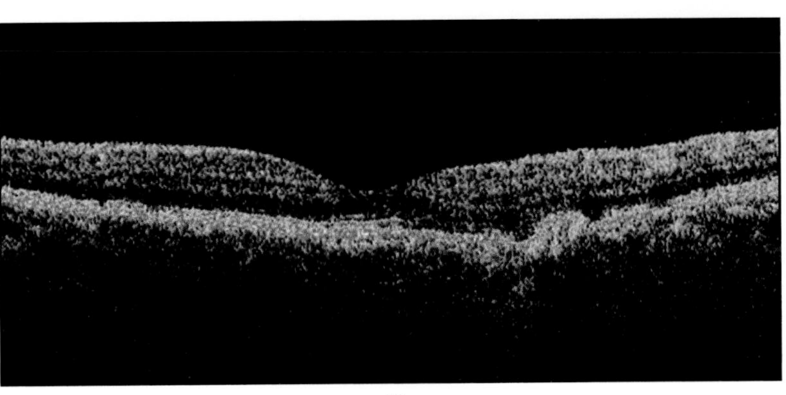

C

Case 8-7A.
Angioid Streaks With Choroidal Neovascularization

Clinical Summary

A 56-year-old male complains of progressive loss of the central vision in the left eye over that past 4 months. His visual acuity in this eye is 20/100. Dilated fundus examination (A) shows peripapillary pigmentary mottling with numerous angioid streaks radiating from the optic nerve. In the foveal region, there is a yellow-grey lesion with adjacent pigment clumping and surrounding subretinal fluid. FA (B) confirms the presence of classic CNV in the fovea.

Optical Coherence Tomography

The CNV can be seen on the OCT image (C) as a fusiform thickening along the high intensity RPE signal. The overlying retina is edematous with numerous intraretinal cysts. Along the edge of the lesion, there is a nonreflective space beneath the fovea, indicating a localized area of subretinal fluid.

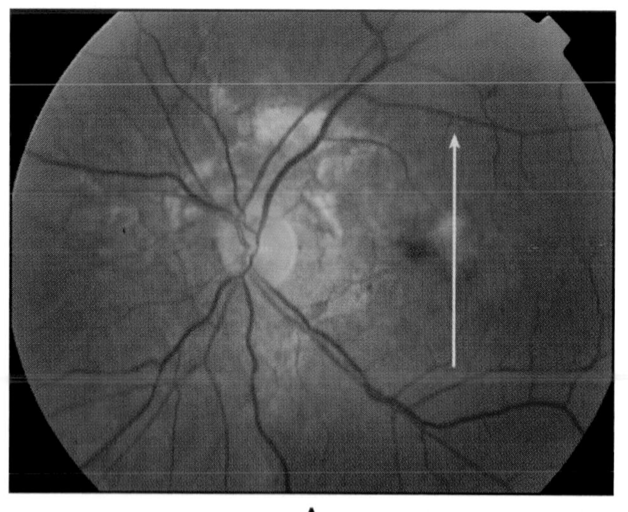

A

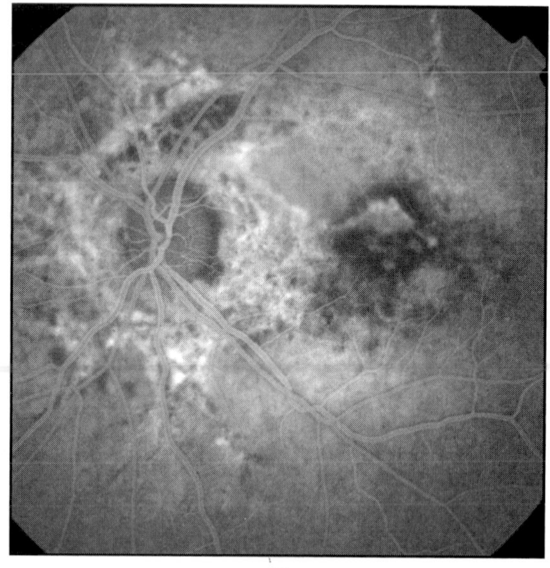

B

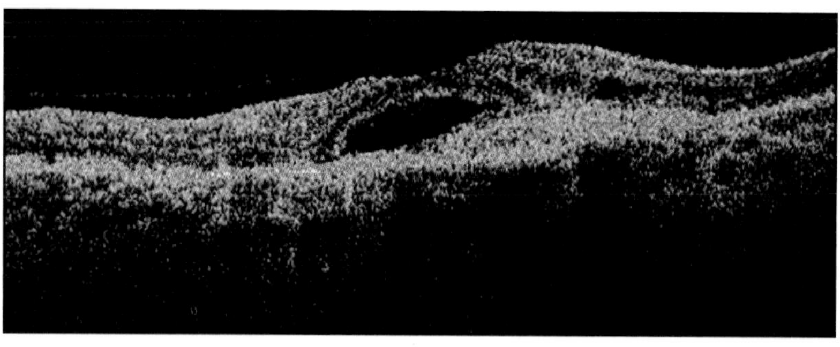

C

Case 8-7B.
Treatment With Photodynamic Therapy

Continuation of Clinical Summary

PDT is performed at the initial visit. Three months after treatment, his visual acuity remains 20/100. Although the lesion appears slightly more fibrotic on clinical exam (D), adjacent subretinal fluid is still present. On FA (E), the area of early hyperfluorescence is smaller than previous, but there still is active leakage in the late phase of the study.

Follow-Up Optical Coherence Tomography

The neovascularization appears smaller and more compact on the post-treatment OCT image (F). Cystoid edema is still present in the overlying retina, and the fovea remains elevated above a pocket of subretinal fluid. After confirming persistent exudation from the neovascularization, retreatment with PDT was recommended.

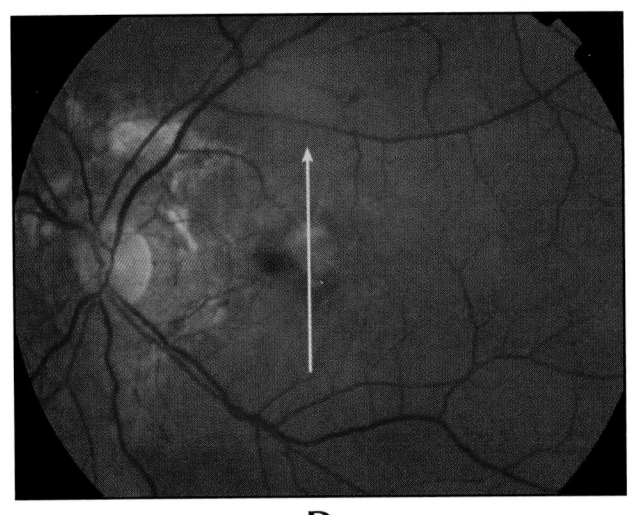

D

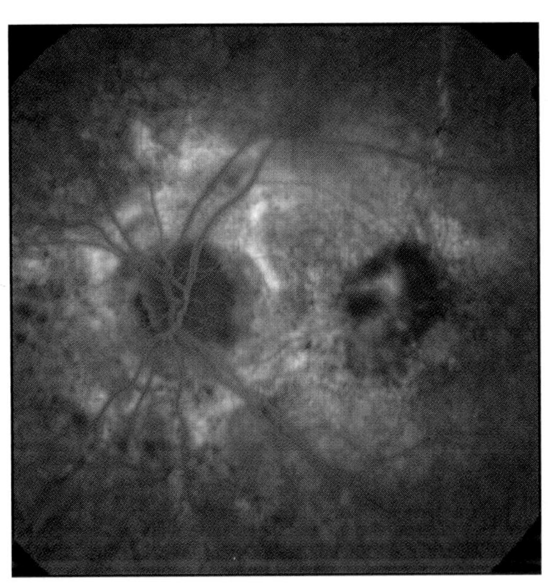

E

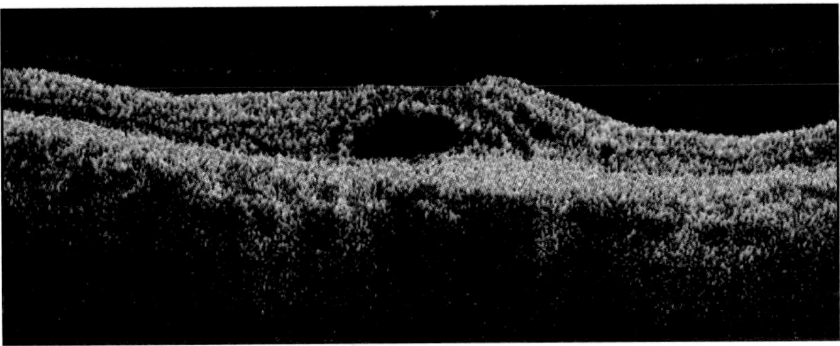

F

Case 8-8A. Idiopathic Choroidal Neovascularization With Subretinal Hemorrhage

Clinical Summary

A 50-year-old male complains of a sudden decrease in the visual acuity of his right eye 3 days earlier. He has no history of previous ocular problems. His visual acuity in this eye has decreased from 20/20 to 20/200. Dilated fundus examination (A) shows a large subretinal hemorrhage in the macula. There is extensive blockage from the blood on FA (B). Indocyanine angiography (ICGA) (C) reveals an irregular area of hyperfluorescence within the area of blockage.

Optical Coherence Tomography

OCT through the macula (D) shows elevation of the retina by the blood. The separation between the retina and subretinal blood is indistinct because these layers exhibit similar reflectivity. Although the retinal contour shows some distortion, the foveal pit can still be identified. Attenuation of the signal by the blood results in shadowing of the RPE and choroid. The RPE signal is faintly evident, confirming the subretinal location of the blood. A distinct neovascular complex cannot be identified.

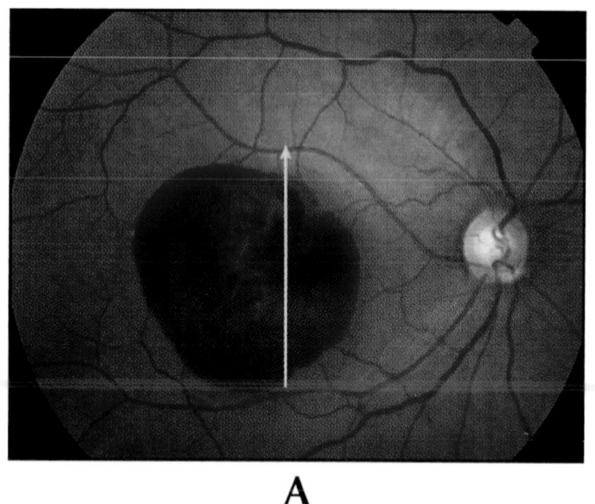

A

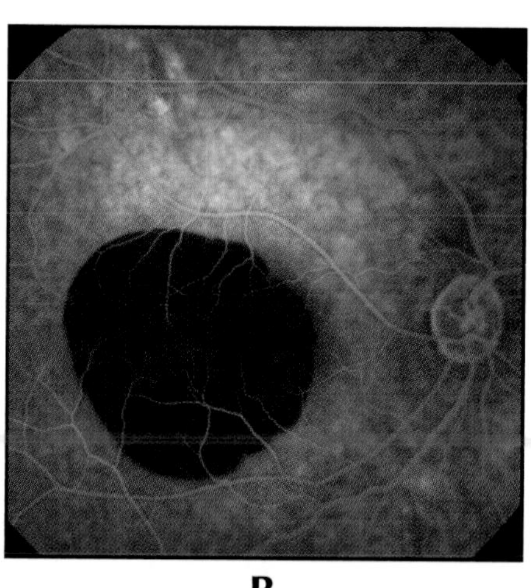

B

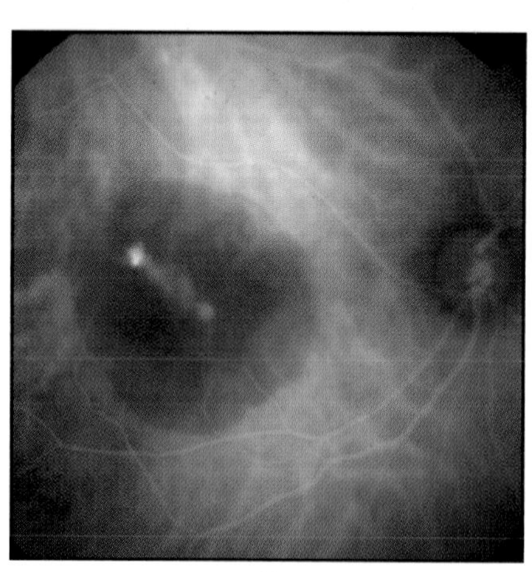

C

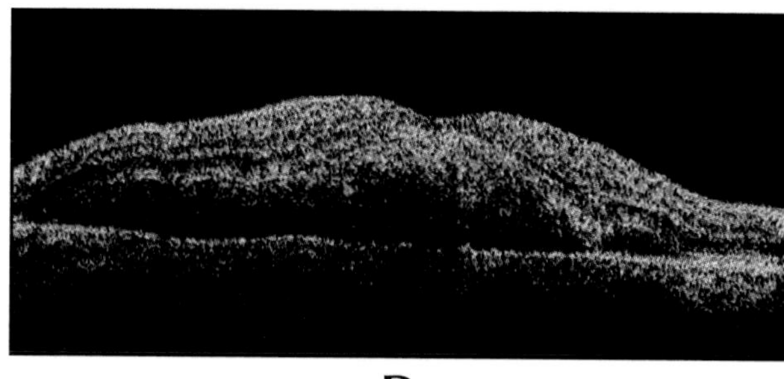

D

Case 8-8B.
Spontaneous Resolution of the Hemorrhage

Continuation of Clinical Summary

Observation is recommended. Six weeks later, the patient denies improvement and the visual acuity remains 20/200. On dilated fundus examination (E), there has been some resolution of the hemorrhage. An irregular area of subretinal fibrosis surrounded by a cuff of shallow subretinal blood is now evident. FA (F) now shows mottled hyperfluorescence in the midphase with late staining. After 6 more weeks of observation, the patient's visual acuity improves to 20/60. Retinal examination shows almost complete resolution of the subretinal hemorrhage.

Follow-Up Optical Coherence Tomography

The OCT image taken at the 6-week follow-up (G) shows dramatic resolution of the subretinal hemorrhage. There is irregular thickening of the high-intensity RPE/choroid signal in the area of the previous hemorrhage, but a distinct neovascular lesion is not identified. There is also no evidence of subretinal or intraretinal edema.

At the 3-month follow-up (H), the foveal retina and subfoveal RPE signal have become more normal in appearance. The RPE/choroid signal still shows some thickening, but this has become more localized temporal to the fovea. There is still no evidence of subretinal or intraretinal edema at this time.

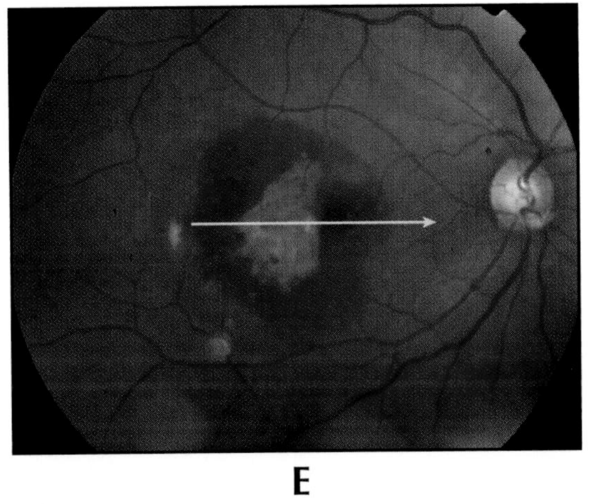

E

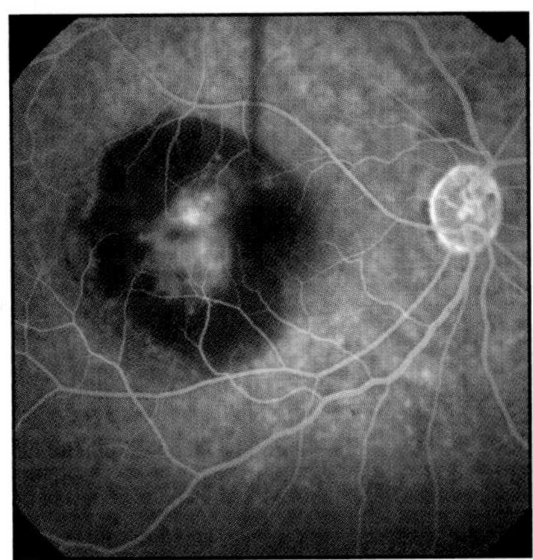

F

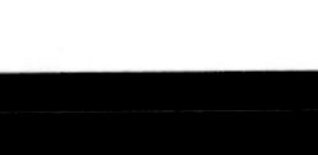

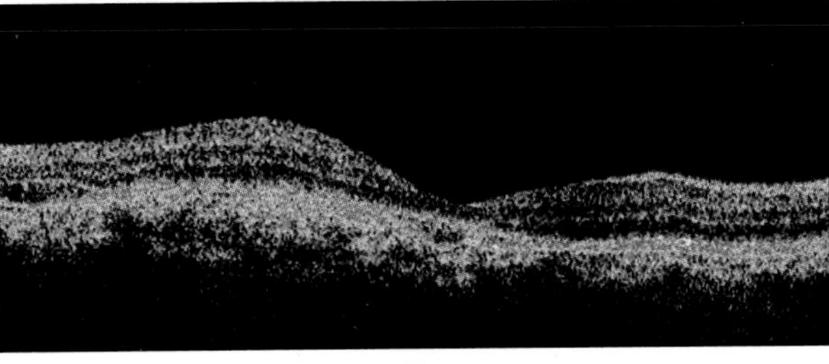

G

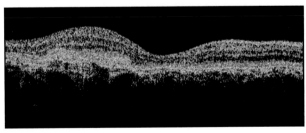

H

Case 8-9A. Idiopathic Choroidal Neovascularization

Clinical Summary

A 25-year-old female is referred for evaluation of decreased visual acuity in her left eye over the past 2 months. She has a history of idiopathic CNV in this eye that was treated with PDT 2 years earlier. Her visual acuity has now decreased from 20/50 to 20/100. Retinal examination (A) shows a localized area of subretinal fibrosis with associated pigmentary mottling and surrounding subretinal fluid. On FA (B), there is a central, circular area of early hyperfluorescence with surrounding mottled fluorescence. Leakage is evident along the inferior aspect of this lesion in the late frames.

Optical Coherence Tomography

The vertical OCT tomogram (C) shows a hyperreflective lesion sitting above the RPE signal in the subretinal space. A small nonreflective cavity between the lesion and the retina indicates a pocket of subretinal fluid. There is thickening of the retina over this lesion especially inferiorly. These findings indicate active exudation from the CNV.

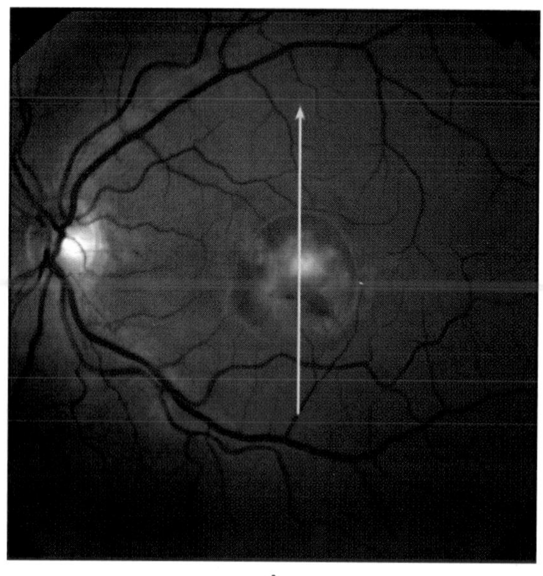

A

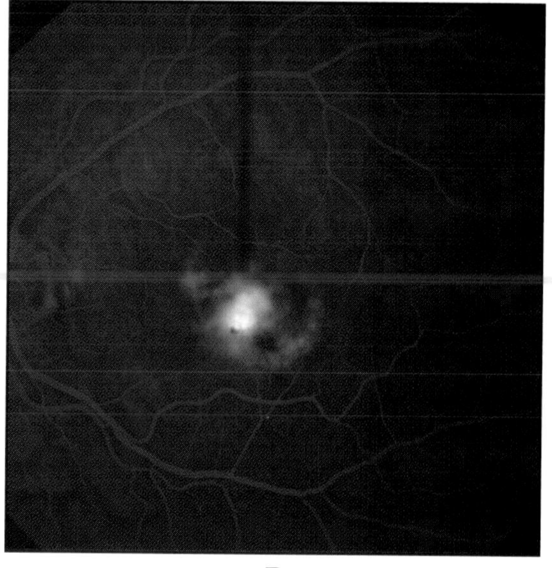

B

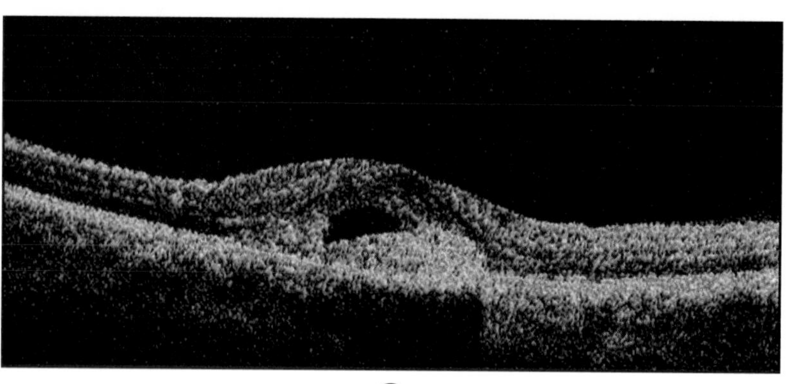

C

Case 8-9B. Treatment With Photodynamic Therapy

Continuation of Clinical Summary

The patient undergoes PDT. She returns 6 weeks later, and her visual acuity has improved to 20/50. Retinal evaluation (D) shows subretinal fibrosis and pigmentary mottling without definite edema. On the FA (E), there is mottled early hyperfluorescence with questionable staining versus mild leakage in the late frames. Three months after treatment, her visual acuity, retinal examination, and FA are stable. Further observation is recommended.

Follow-Up Optical Coherence Tomography

The vertical OCT tomogram (F) taken 6 weeks after the PDT continues to show a well-defined subretinal lesion that is mostly unchanged in appearance. The previously seen subretinal and intraretinal edema has almost completely resolved, indicating decreased exudation from the lesion. Three months after PDT (G), there is increased reflectivity from the lesion and shadowing of the underlying choroid. There is also no evidence of associated subretinal or intraretinal edema. These findings suggest fibrotic involution of the CNV.

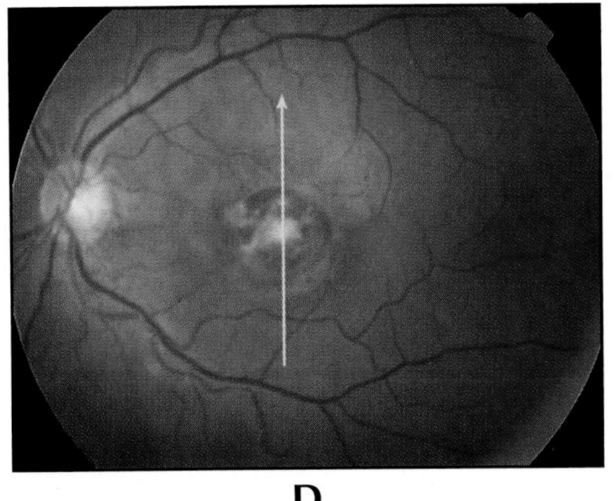

D

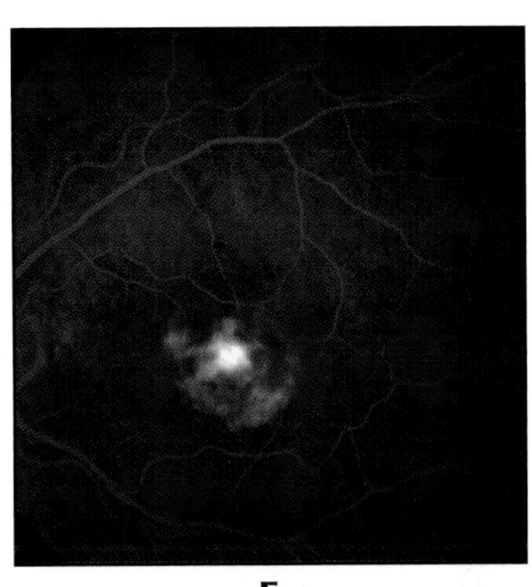

E

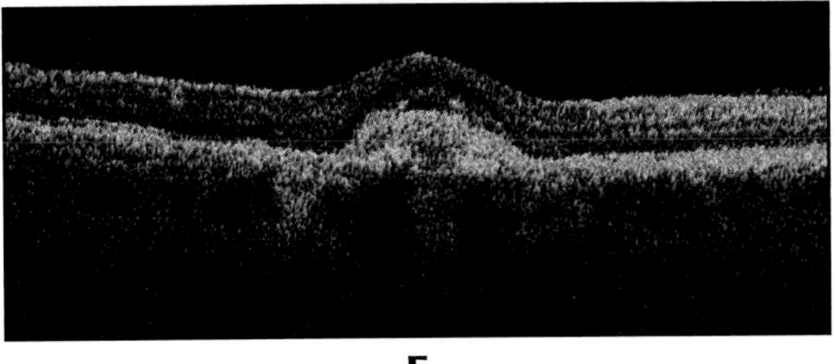

F

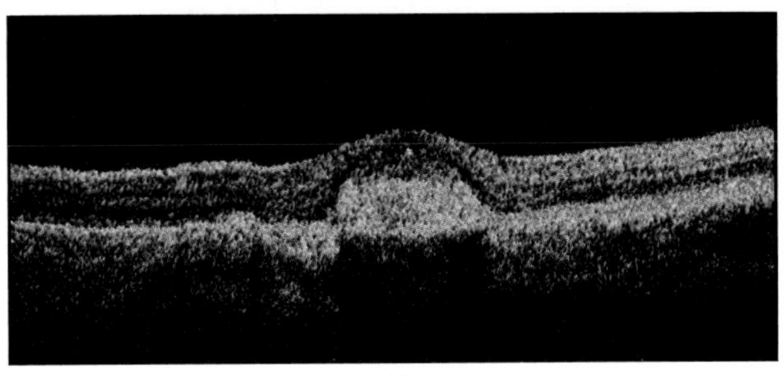

G

Case 8-10. Idiopathic Central Serous Chorioretinopathy With Choroidal Neovascularization

Clinical Summary

A 80-year-old male complains of decreased visual acuity in the right eye for 1 month. He has a history of idiopathic central serous chorioretinopathy and underwent laser treatment to the right eye 20 years earlier. He reports good visual acuity without recurrence after the laser treatment in this eye. His visual acuity is 20/200, and dilated fundus exam (A) reveals extensive pigmentary mottling in the macular region. There is a hyperpigmented lesion with surrounding edema beneath the fovea. FA (B) shows a well-defined area of hyperfluorescence that progressively leaks consistent with CNV.

Optical Coherence Tomography

The OCT image (C) shows the neovascularization as a dome-shaped lesion with high reflectivity that protrudes into the subretinal space. There is a large nonreflective space over the lesion corresponding to an intraretinal cystic cavity. Smaller intraretinal cysts are also present, and the retinal tissue in this area is thickened. There is no evidence of subretinal fluid on this tomogram.

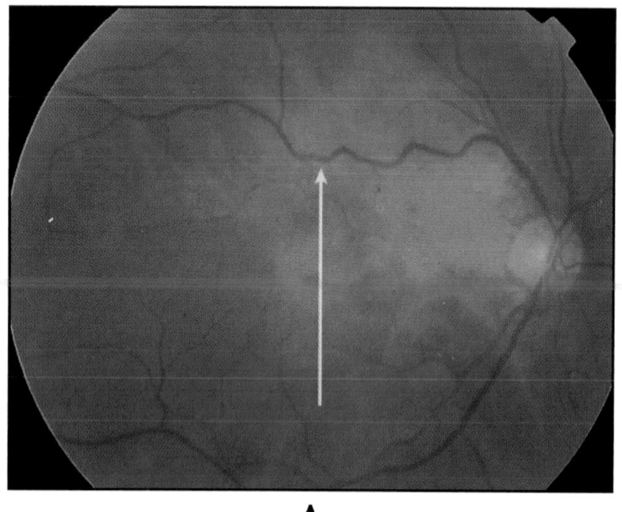

A

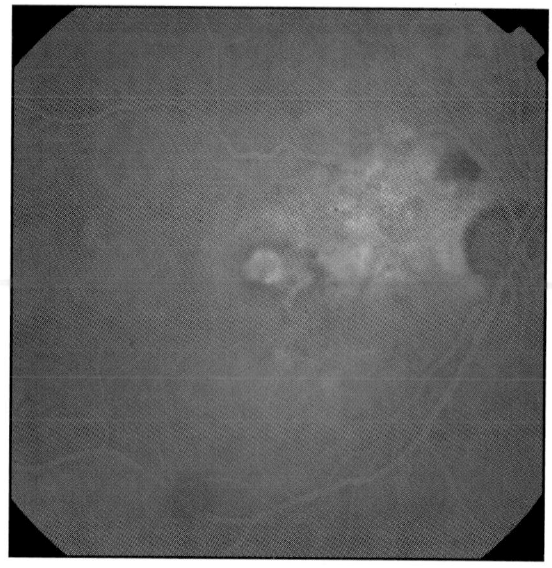

B

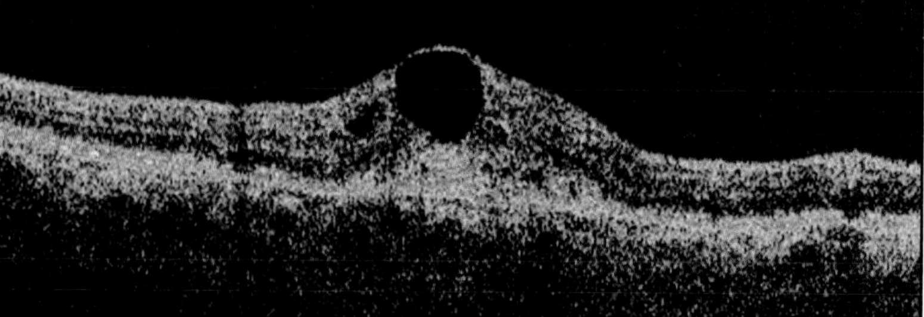

C

Case 8-11A. Juxtafoveal Retinal Telangiectasis With Choroidal Neovascularization

Clinical Summary

A 67-year-old male complains of worsening vision in both eyes over the past year. His visual acuity is 20/60 in the right eye. The dilated fundus examination (A) shows telangiectatic vessels temporal to the fovea in this eye. FA (B) demonstrates hyperfluorescence surrounding the fovea.

Optical Coherence Tomography

The OCT image (C) shows a clear, nonreflective space within the retina at the fovea. There is blunting of the foveal pit, but the retina is otherwise normal in thickness and contour. The high-intensity RPE signal is relatively uniform in appearance without evidence of disruption or thickening. This retinal configuration on OCT is consistent with juxtafoveal telangiectasis (JFT).

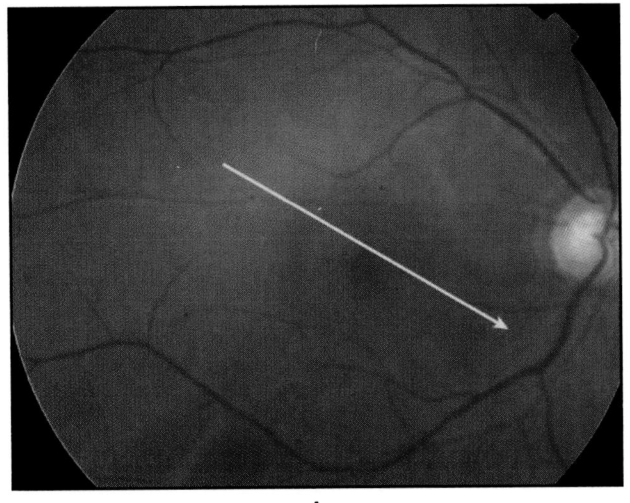

A

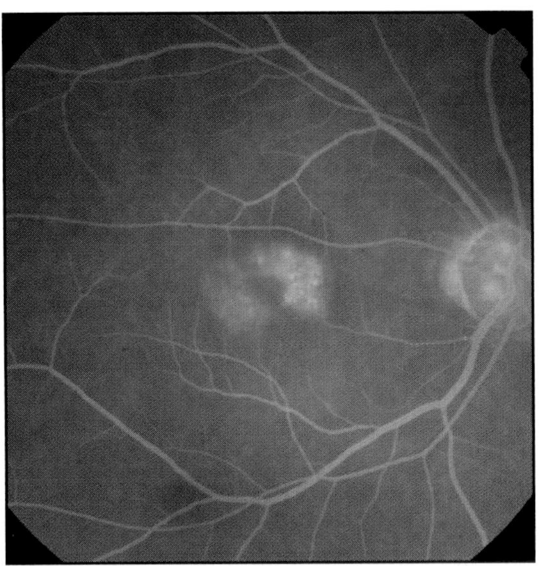

B

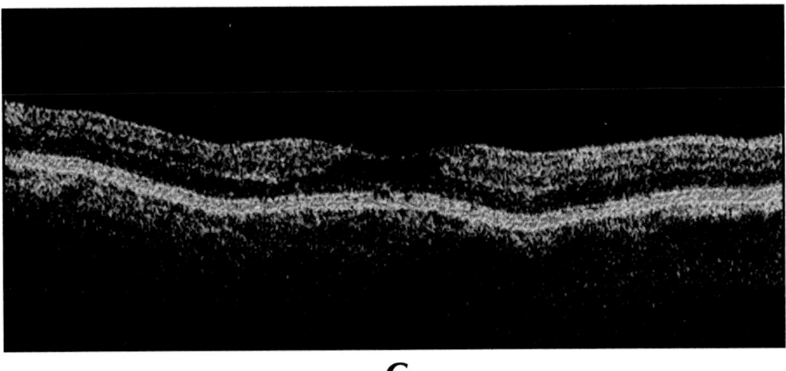

C

Case 8-11B. Juxtafoveal Retinal Telangiectasis With Choroidal Neovascularization

Clinical Summary

The visual acuity in his left eye is 20/70. The dilated fundus examination (D) shows a localized area of pigmentary mottling with associated edema adjacent to the fovea. Telangiectatic vessels, similar to those in the other eye, were also present in this area. FA (E) reveals a well-defined area of early hyperfluorescence with late leakage indicating CNV.

Optical Coherence Tomography

OCT images taken through this area (F and G) show a small oval area of thickening along the RPE signal that corresponds to the neovascularization. This lesion can be seen better on the processed image (G) than the scanned image (F). There is mild thickening of the retina but no evidence of subretinal fluid around this lesion. Intraretinal cystic spaces consistent with JFT are also identified in this eye.

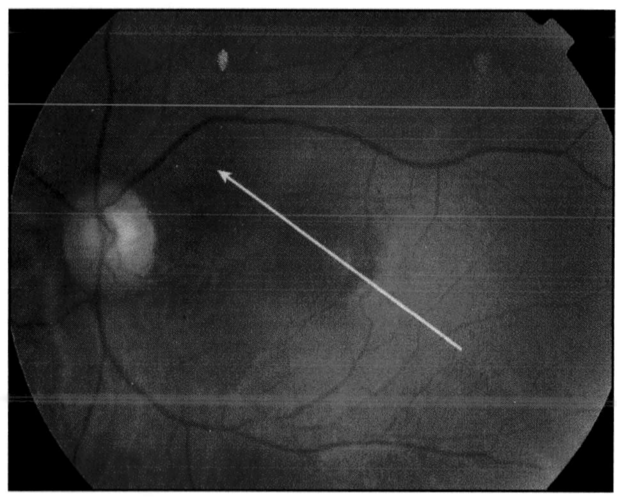

D

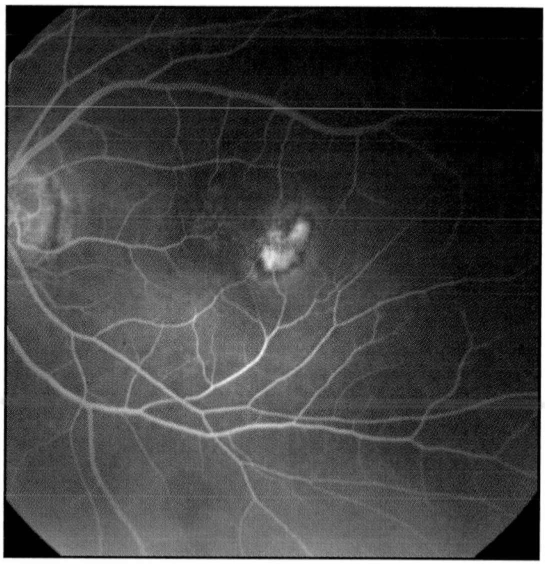

E

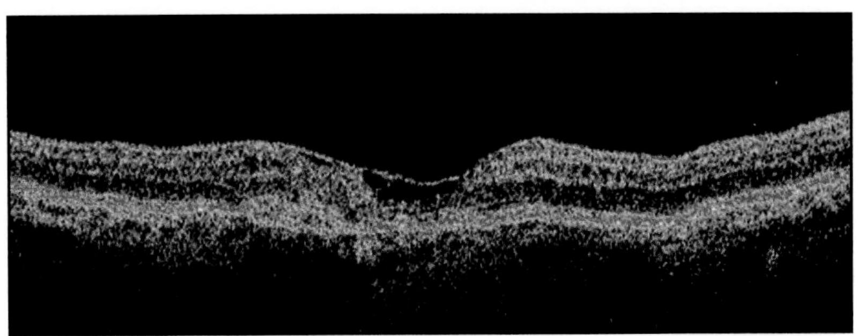

F

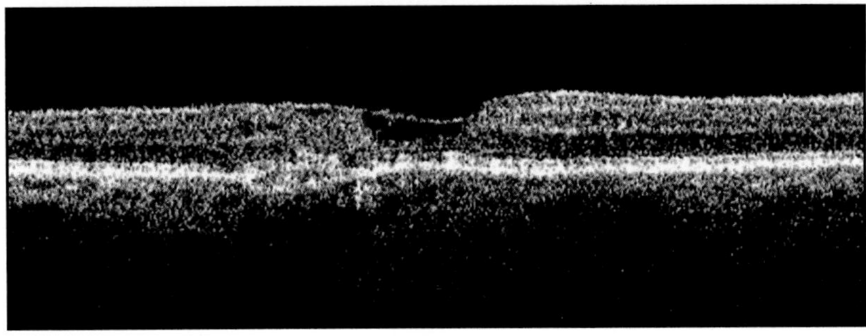

G

Case 8-12A. Presumed Ocular Histoplasmosis

Clinical Summary

A 39-year-old woman has a diagnosis of ocular histoplasmosis. She has undergone two laser treatments in her right eye for CNV in the past. She has been stable for the past 5 years, until 1 month ago when she started noticing decreased vision in her right eye. Her visual acuity in this eye was 20/30 at her last exam 4 months ago but has now declined to 4/200. Retinal examination shows a hypopigmented scar with focal RPE hyperplasia inferior to fixation (A). The foveal edge of the scar appears blurry, indicating the presence of subretinal fluid. FA reveals a mottled hyperfluorescence in the early phases (B) with late leakage (C) consistent with CNV.

Optical Coherence Tomography

An oblique scan is taken through the scar and fovea (D). As the scan passes through the atrophic scar (left side of the image), the OCT image shows increased intensity of the choroidal signal. This results from the enhanced penetration and reflectivity of the signal through the area of atrophy. The overlying retina appears thinned and irregular. Adjacent to the scar in the fovea (center of the image), there is a small reflective lesion extending above the RPE signal into the subretinal space. This corresponds to the neovascularization. The retina overlying this lesion is edematous with small intraretinal cysts.

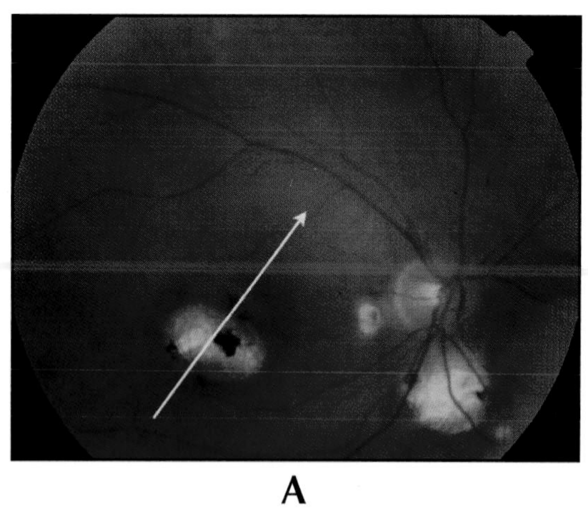

A

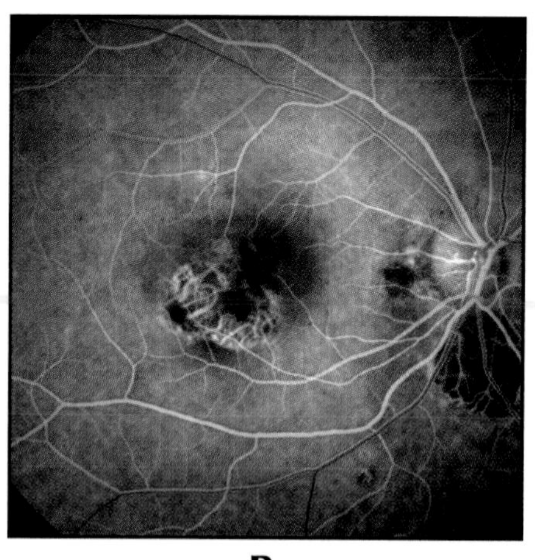

B

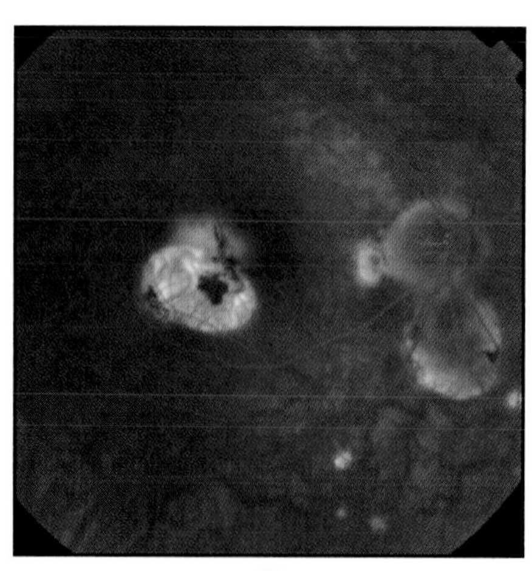

C

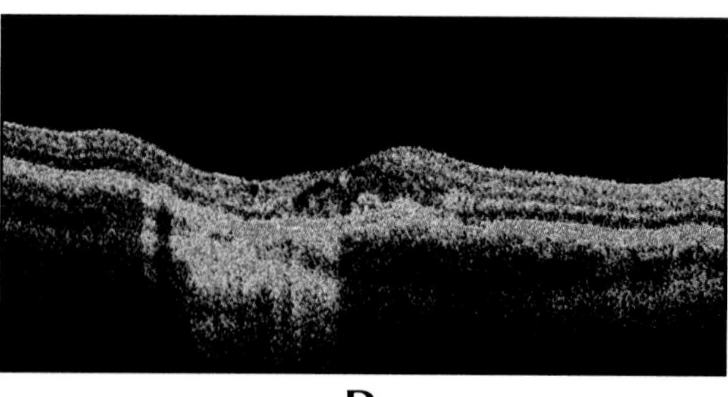

D

Case 8-12B. Treatment With Photodynamic Therapy

Continuation of Clinical Summary

She is treated with PDT at her initial visit. Six weeks after treatment, the visual acuity in the right eye has improved to 20/200. The foveal edge of the scar now appears flat (E). FA reveals mottled hyperfluorescence (F) with late staining (G) but no evidence of persistent leakage.

Follow-Up Optical Coherence Tomography

Repeat scan in the same location and direction as before (H) shows stable changes associated with the atrophic scar. The previously seen subretinal CNV lesion is no longer identified, and the intraretinal edema has also resolved. These changes indicate good response to the PDT.

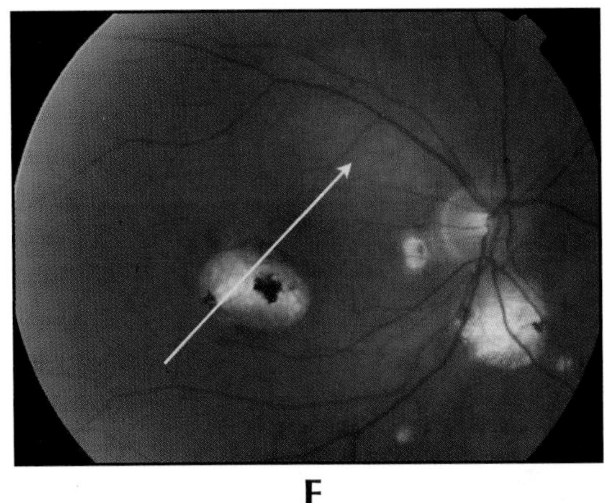

E

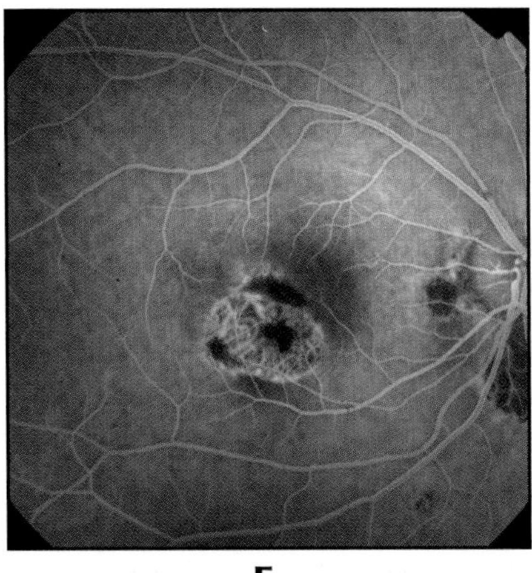

F

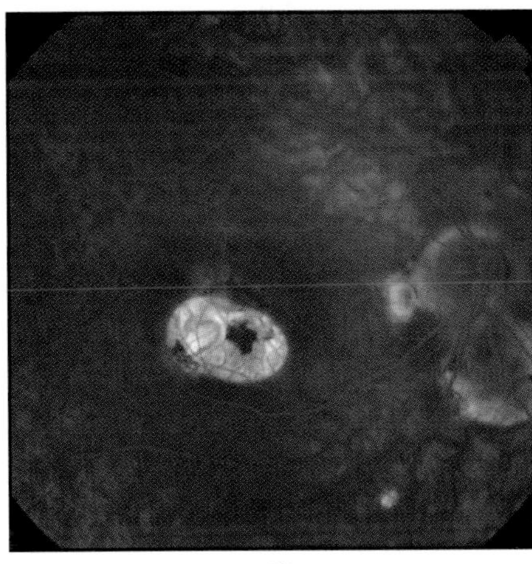

G

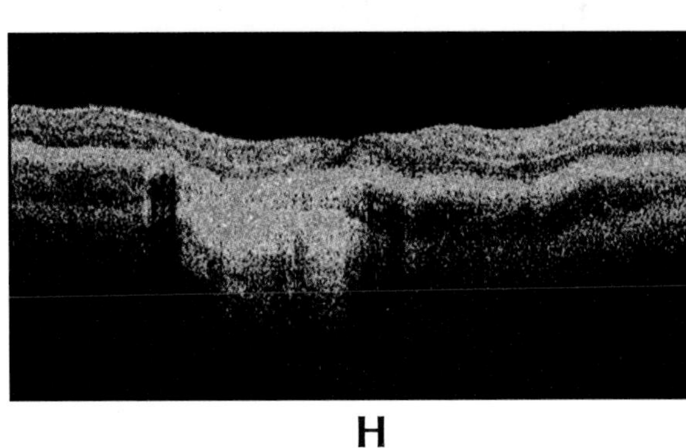

H

Chapter 9

Chorioretinal Inflammatory Diseases

Natalia Villate, MD; Elias C. Mavrofrides, MD; and Janet Davis, MD

- Intermediate Uveitis
- Idiopathic Retina Vasculitis and Neuroretinitis
- Multifocal Choroiditis
- Sarcoidosis
- Vogt-Koyanagi-Harada Disease
- Sympathetic Ophthalmia
- Birdshot Chorioretinopathy
- Toxoplasmosis
- Syphilitic Uveitis
- Cytomegalovirus Retinitis With Immune Recovery Uveitis

Uveitis is classified according to anatomic location and secondarily to the underlying cause. Location, etiology, duration, and severity determine the extent of damage to intraocular tissues. Complications secondary to uveitis are similar to those observed in other retinal diseases: cystoid macular edema (CME), choroidal neovascularization (CNV), and chorioretinal scarring. Optical coherence tomography (OCT) provides an effective means of quantifying reflectivity, location, and extent of these secondary complications of uveitis.[1] It may also have relevance in imaging inflammatory lesions that are specific to particular types of uveitis that affect the posterior segment.[2]

OCT produces high-resolution cross-sectional imaging of the retina that directly measures the z-plane, with a theoretical axial resolution of 10 to 14 microns (μm). A high degree of reproducibility in measuring macular thickness in normal individuals and diabetic patients has been described.[3] Therefore, it is well-suited to repeated measurements of macular status in uveitis patients in whom management decisions are required longitudinally.

The use of OCT in the precise depiction of CME is perhaps its most practical use in the management of ocular inflammatory diseases. CME is the most common sight-threatening complication of uveitis and has the potential for long-term visual morbidity. When compared to fluorescein angiography (FA),[4] OCT is effective in detecting CME. It has the advantage of being noninvasive and without risk for the patient. Furthermore, OCT can provide reliable information in patients with moderate vitreous opacities or small pupils resulting from posterior synechiae, both common findings in uveitis patients that can prevent acceptable stereoscopic FA.

In chronic CME, retinal thickness, size and location of cysts, and subretinal fluid accumulation can be monitored by OCT in order to determine results of, or need for, therapy.[5] Sequential OCT scans of CME can demonstrate anatomic changes from persistence of CME. In the late stages, CME may be associated with lamellar or full-thickness macular hole formation. OCT may help distinguish between holes and large central cysts. Detection of vitreomacular traction or an epiretinal membrane by OCT may lead to consideration of membrane peeling to release traction on the macula.[1] In contrast, retinal thinning in the aftermath of CME may lead the clinician to conclude that vision loss is irreversible and further therapy is not indicated.

CNV is an uncommon complication of uveitis, but one that is uniquely suited to imaging with OCT. OCT has the potential to help distinguish between inflammatory lesions and adjacent CNV in some cases, such as neovascularization arising from toxoplasmic chorioretinitis. In eyes with subfoveal neovascular membranes secondary to multifocal choroiditis, a hyperreflective band anterior to the RPE and an optically clear separation zone underneath the RPE have been associated with a good postoperative outcome after subretinal surgery to remove the CNV.[6]

The use of OCT for the examination of posterior inflammatory lesions is largely untested. Hypothetically, inflammation would increase optical reflectivity because infiltrates of inflammatory cells would increase the optical scattering. However, tissue swelling from inflammation may decrease optical reflectivity and inflammatory infiltrates may cause shadowing of posterior structures. Careful interpretation of OCT images is therefore required along with clinical and angiographic correlation.[2] It seems likely that OCT will help localize inflammatory infiltrates to specific retinal and inner choroidal layers and thereby provide information regarding the pathophysiology of posterior uveitis.

We have selected cases that demonstrate the OCT appearance of either ocular complications of uveitis or posterior inflammatory lesions. OCT data on both topics will likely accrue rapidly in the future.

Reference

1. Hassenstein A, Bialasiewicz AA, Richard G. Optical coherence tomography in uveitis patients. *Am J Ophthalmol*. 2000;130(5):669-670.
2. Wang RC, Zamir E, Dugel PU, et al. Progressive subretinal fibrosis and blindness associated with multifocal granulomatous chorioretinitis: a variant of sympathetic ophthalmia. *Ophthalmology*. 2002;109(8):1527-1531.
3. Hee MR, Puliafito CA, Wong C, et al. Quantitative assessment of macular edema with optical coherence tomography. *Arch Ophthalmol*. 1995;113(8):1019-1029.
4. Antcliff RJ, Stanford MR, Chauhan DS, et al. Comparison between optical coherence tomography and fundus fluorescein angiography for the detection of cystoid macular edema in patients with uveitis. *Ophthalmology*. 2000; 107(3):593-599.
5. Antcliff RJ, Spalton DJ, Stanford MR, Graham EM, Ffytche TJ, Marshall J. Intravitreal triamcinolone for uveitic cystoid macular edema: an optical coherence tomography study. *Ophthalmology*. 2001;108(4):765-772.
6. Zolf R, Glacet-Bernard A, Benhamou N, Mimoun G, Coscas G, Soubrane G. Imaging analysis with optical coherence tomography: relevance for submacular surgery in high myopia and in multifocal choroiditis. *Retina*. 2002; 22(2):192-201.

Case 9-1A.
Intermediate Uveitis With Cystoid Macular Edema

Clinical Summary

A 50-year-old African-American woman had a 3-year history of chronic bilateral intermediate uveitis. Systemic work-up was negative. She had received focal laser treatment for macular edema in both eyes by her previous physician. Best-corrected visual acuity (BCVA) was 20/50 in both eyes. On examination, she had persistent low-grade inflammation. Fundus exam of the right eye (A) revealed pigment mottling and macular thickening. FA showed early mottled hyperfluorescence in the posterior pole (B) with late diffuse leakage in a cystoid pattern (C). Of note is the presence of a nonfilling central cyst.

Optical Coherence Tomography

An oblique scan through the macula (D) reveals partial loss of the foveal contour with large cystic cavities within the retina. A neurosensory detachment is observed directly beneath the fovea. Tissue bands separate the fluid-filled cavities, probably representing stretched Müller cells. The central retinal elevation is 514 µm, including both the thickened retina and the subretinal fluid. The retinal map (E) depicts a 3-mm area of marked elevation centered on the fovea with moderate elevation in the 6-mm area of the map. The "nonfilling cyst" seen on FA may correspond to lack of pooling in the neurosensory detachment.

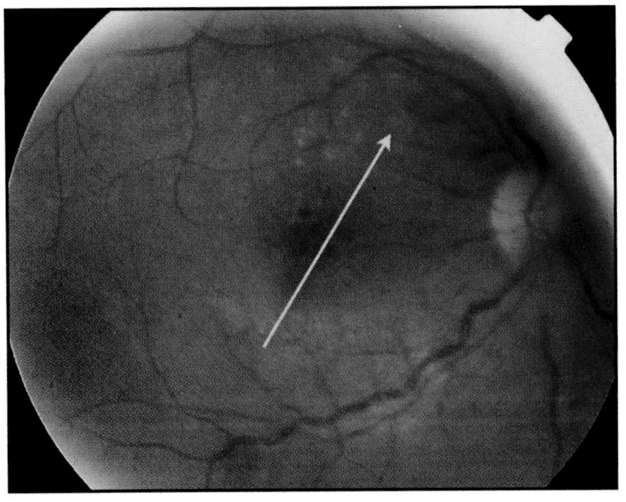

A

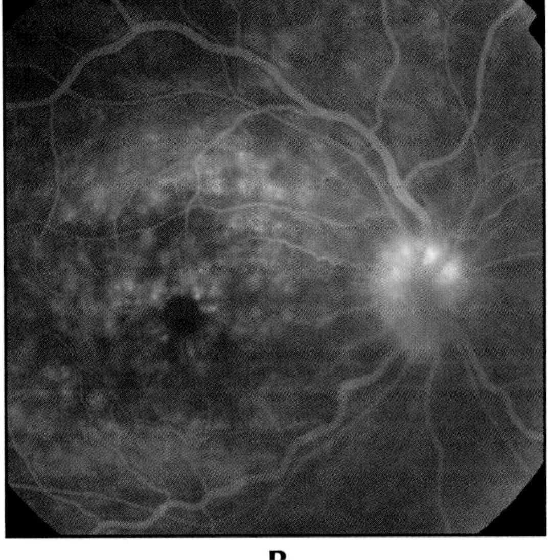

B

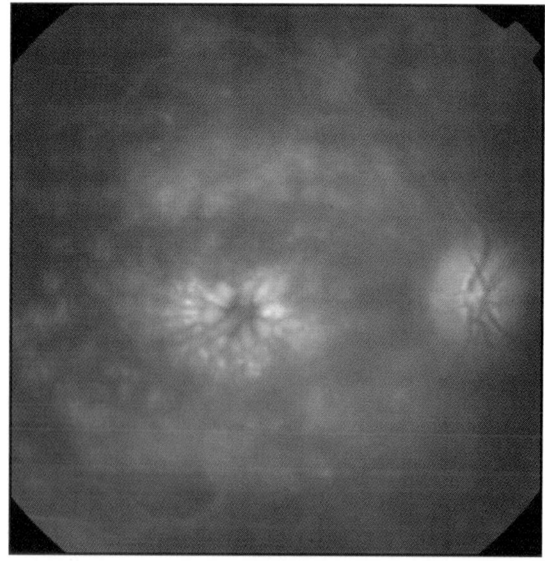

C

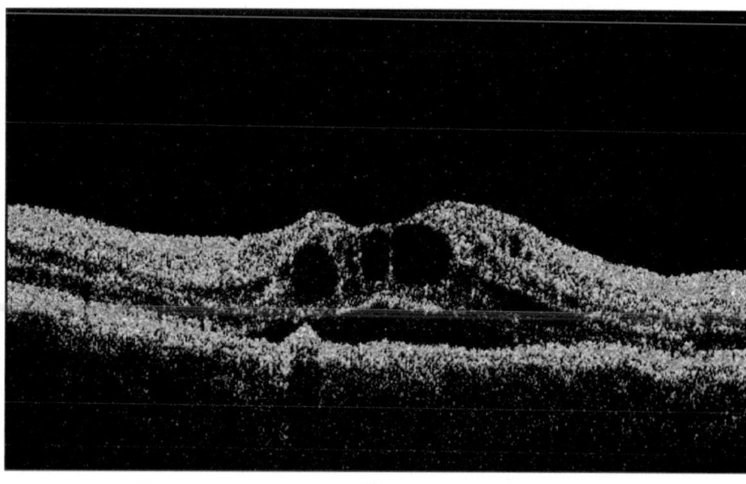

D

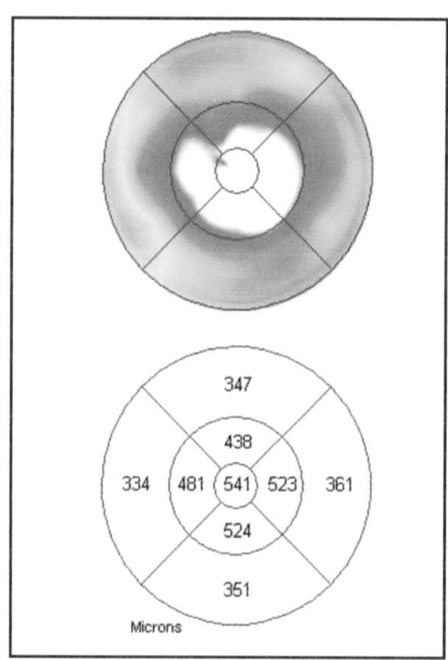

E

Case 9-1B. Intermediate Uveitis With Cystoid Macular Edema

Clinical Summary

The left eye showed similar findings (F). A late petalloid pattern of CME with a filled center and diffuse macular leakage were evident on the FA (G).

Optical Coherence Tomography

A vertical scan through the center of the fovea (H) shows loss of foveal contour with flattening and irregularity of the inner retinal surface. The central elevation is increased to 547 µm (I) and there are cystic cavities occupying the center of the fovea. No subretinal fluid is detected in the central macula, corresponding to the filled center on the FA.

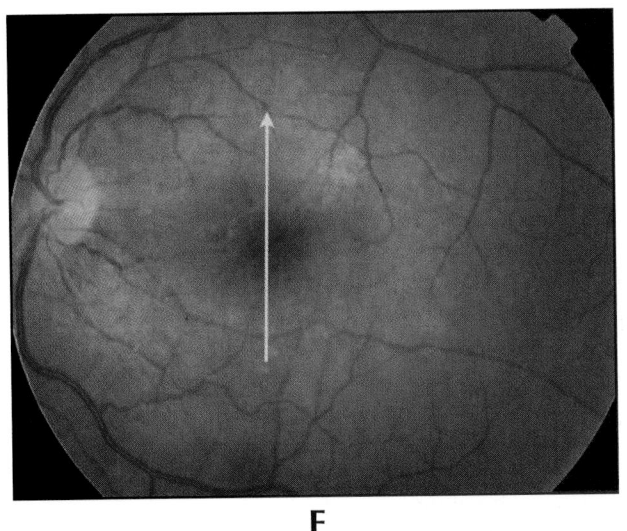

F

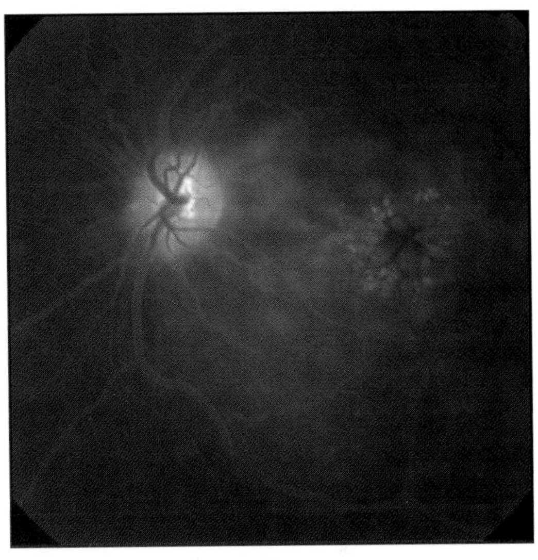

G

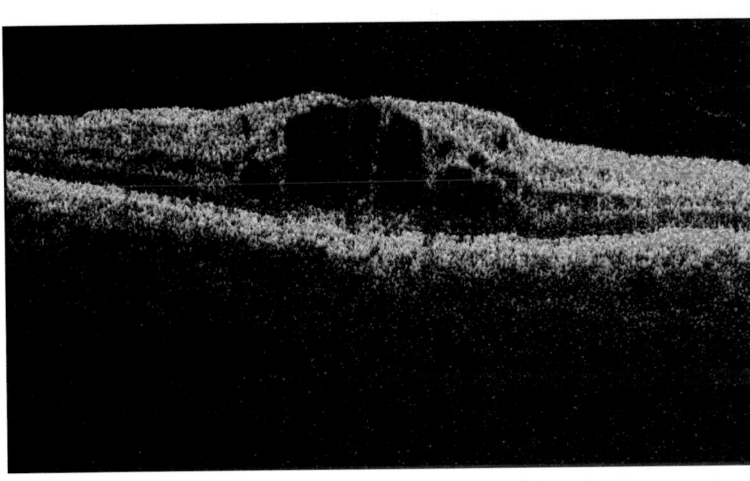

H

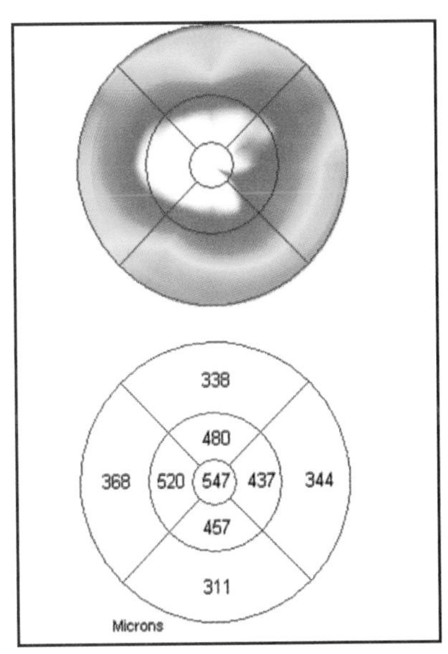

I

Case 9-2A. Idiopathic Retinal Vasculitis and Neuroretinitis With Exudative Maculopathy

Clinical Summary

A 21-year-old woman had a history of bilateral retinal vasculitis for 2 years with poor vision for 1 year. Visual acuity was 20/300 in both eyes. Examination of the fundus (A) revealed lipid exudates around the nerve and macula in the right eye. The disc appeared congested with engorgement and distortion of the vessels. The angiogram (B) shows the characteristic aneurysmal dilations of the retinal arteries. Peripheral vascular occlusion with neovascularization at the border zone between perfused and nonperfused retina were also observed. There was late leakage from the optic nerve and from the major vessels (C). The late phases of the angiogram do not support the diagnosis of CNV.

Optical Coherence Tomography

An oblique scan through the foveal center (D) shows preserved foveal contour. Beneath the fovea, there is a thick band of increased reflectivity that elevates the retina. The appearance is similar to that seen with CNV, but the location of the exudates suggests that this "red line" most likely represents reflections from the dense subretinal material rather than anterior protrusion of the RPE. This is more clearly seen in the vertical scan through the lesion (E). Small highly reflective round and irregular opacities corresponding to lipid exudates are observed in the outer retina along with optically clear subretinal fluid adjacent to the optic nerve.

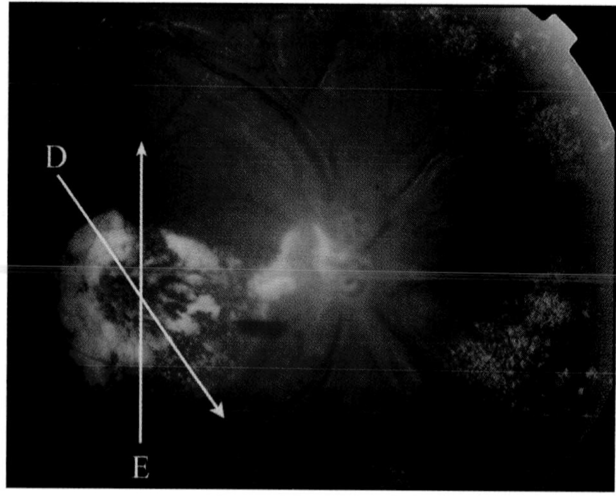

A

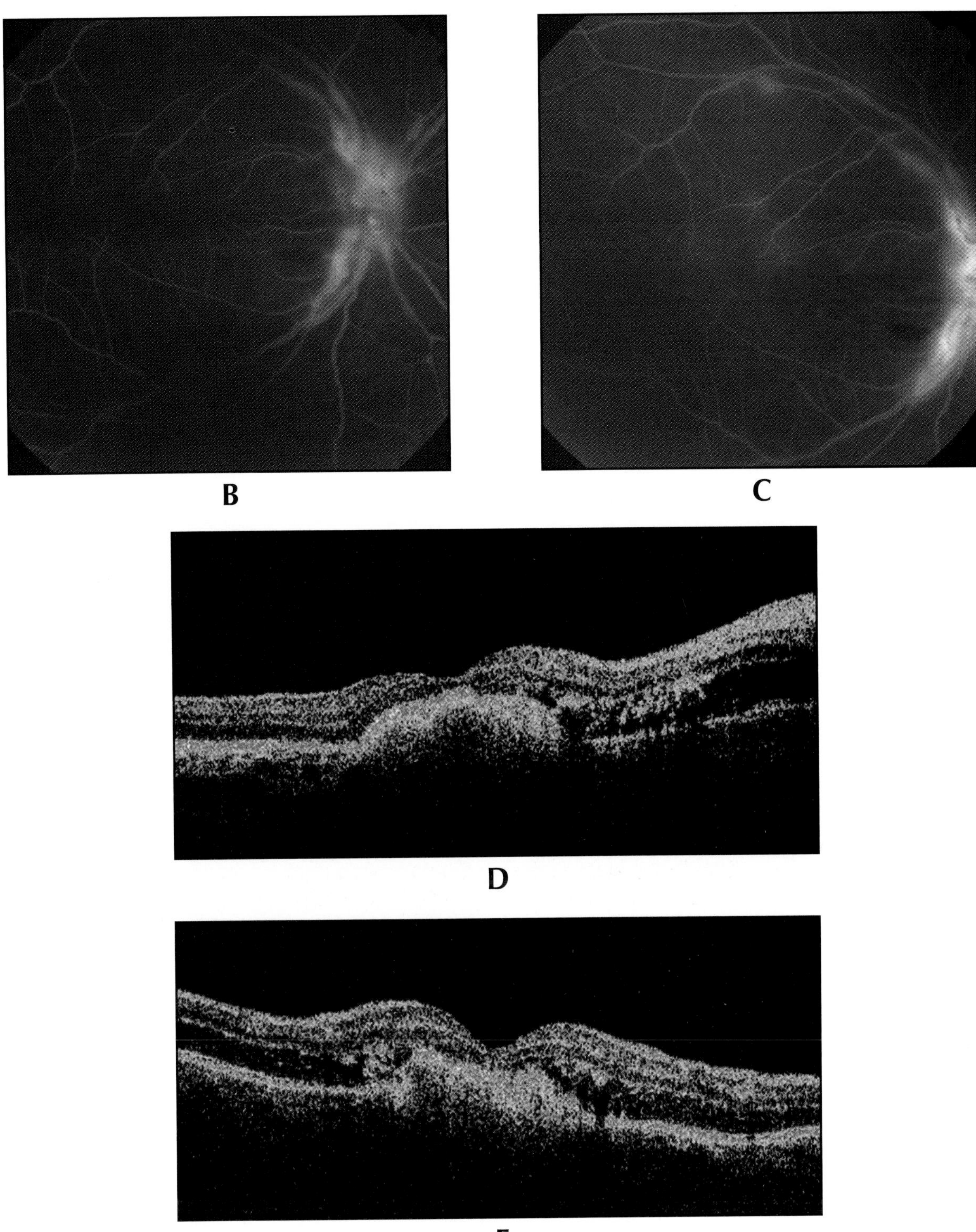
B
C
D
E

Case 9-2B. Idiopathic Retinal Vasculitis and Neuroretinitis With Exudative Maculopathy

Clinical Summary

Examination of the left eye (F) revealed more extensive exudation around the nerve and an elevated lipid nodule centered in the macula. The retinal vessels terminated within the substance of the nodule. There was condensation of the posterior hyaloid over the optic nerve with distortion of the vessels. On FA (G), the characteristic retinal arteriolar macroaneurysms were visible close to the optic nerve along the superior and inferior vascular arcades. The lipid nodule stained with fluorescein dye without evidence of leakage (H).

Optical Coherence Tomography

A vertical scan through the fovea (I) shows a marked elevation of the foveal center. There is an elevated, highly reflective lesion occupying the subretinal space that corresponds to the lipid nodule. This dense material causes extensive shadowing of the underlying signal. Focal, highly reflective exudates are seen in the inferior portion of the scan line. A thick, highly reflective membrane appears fused to the inner retinal surface in the center of the fovea and extends to the sides in a plateau configuration, consistent with a taut, adherent posterior hyaloid.

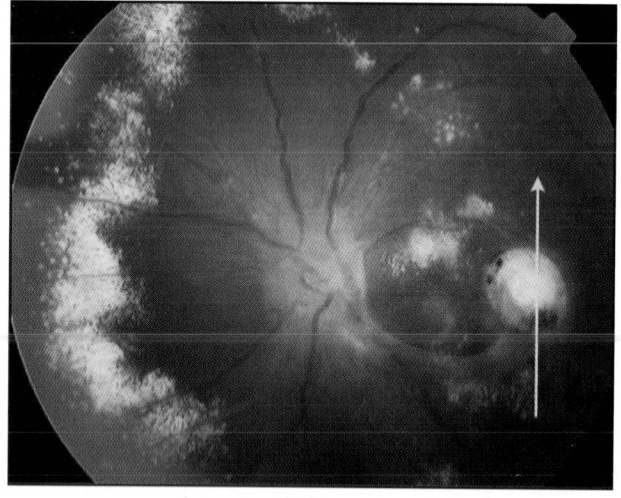

F

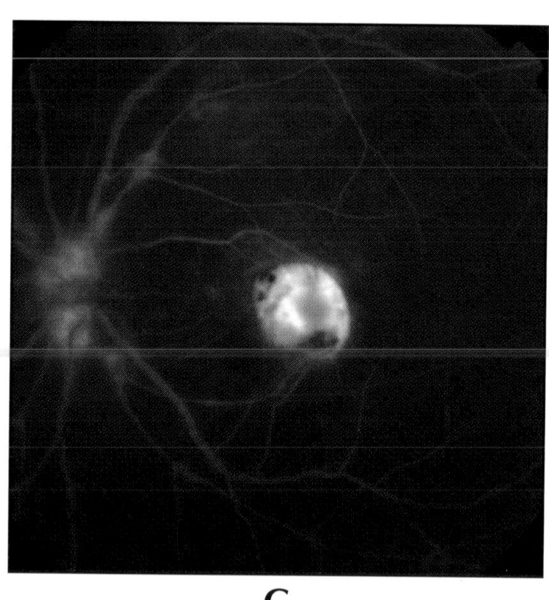

G

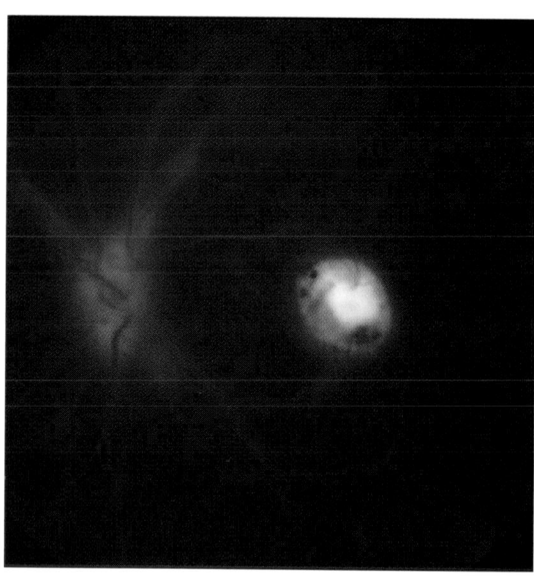

H

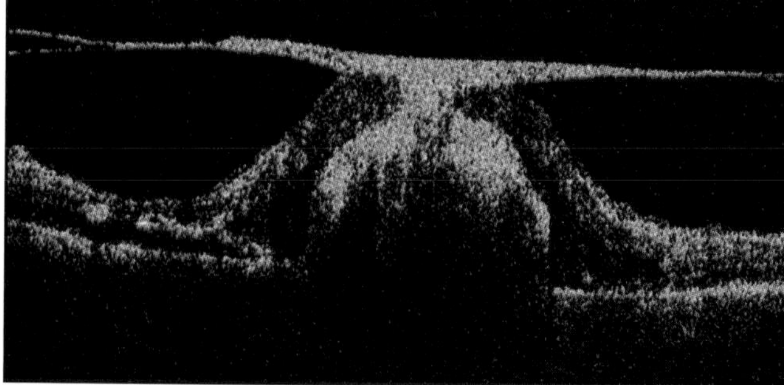

I

Case 9-3A.
Multifocal Choroiditis With Panuveitis

Clinical Summary

A 36-year-old man had chronic inflammation of unknown etiology in his right eye for 4 years. Visual acuity was 20/400 in the right eye and 20/20 in the left eye. Anterior chamber cellular reaction and posterior synechiae were noted on slit-lamp exam. Retinal examination (A) showed hazy media limiting the view of the posterior fundus. FA (B) showed profuse leakage in the macula in the late phases.

Optical Coherence Tomography

A vertical scan through the foveal center (C) before treatment shows loss of the normal foveal contour with increased central thickness of 487 µm. Large cystic cavities are observed within the retinal layers. The signal is decreased in intensity due to the vitreous opacity. The retinal map (D) shows thickening of the perifoveal area with irregularity and artifact.

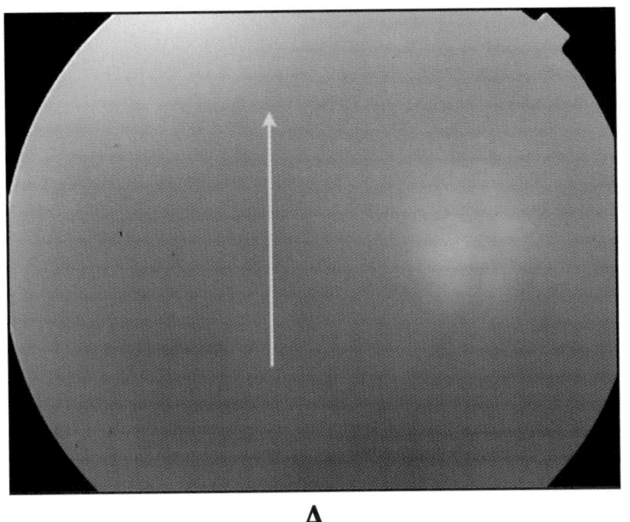

A

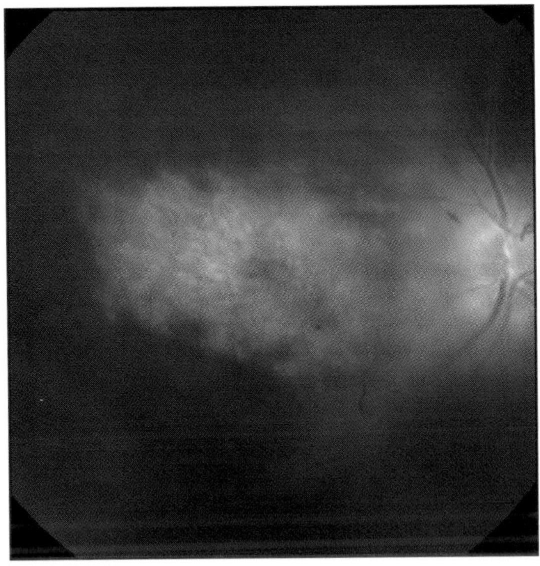

B

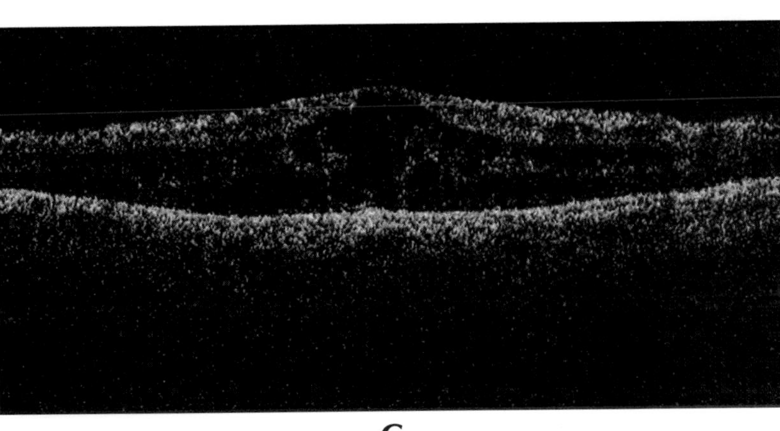

C

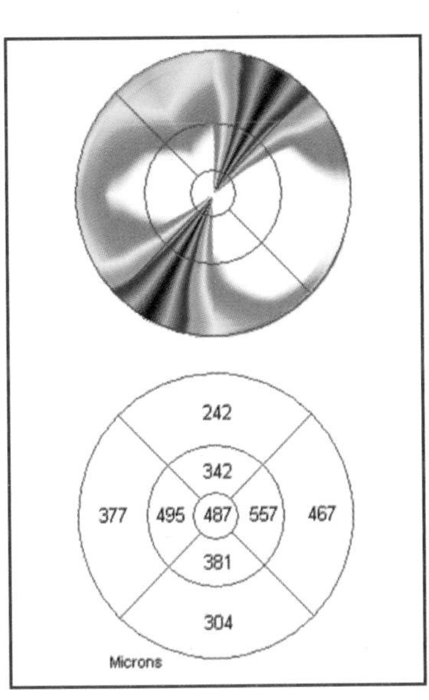

D

Case 9-3B. Response to Treatment

Continuation of Clinical Summary

The patient received two periocular steroid injections within a 3-month interval. Four months after the last injection, visual acuity improved to 20/100 and the media were clearer (E). Multiple chorioretinal inflammatory lesions were now visible outside the vascular arcades, suggesting a diagnosis of multifocal choroiditis with panuveitis.

Follow-Up Optical Coherence Tomography

OCT after treatment (F) shows a restored foveal contour with normal retinal architecture. The retinal map (G) shows remodeling of the central surface with persistent mild thickening of the perifoveal retina. The peripheral choroidal lesions could not be imaged by OCT.

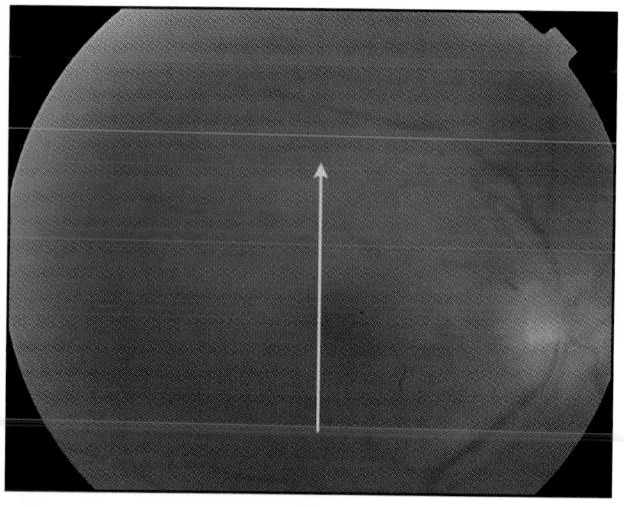

E

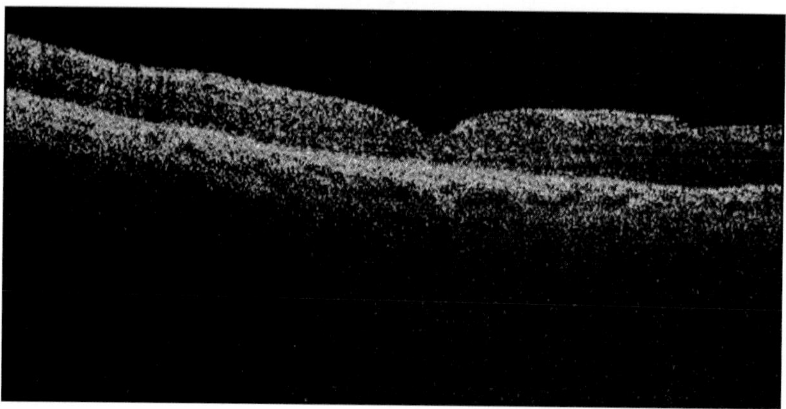

F

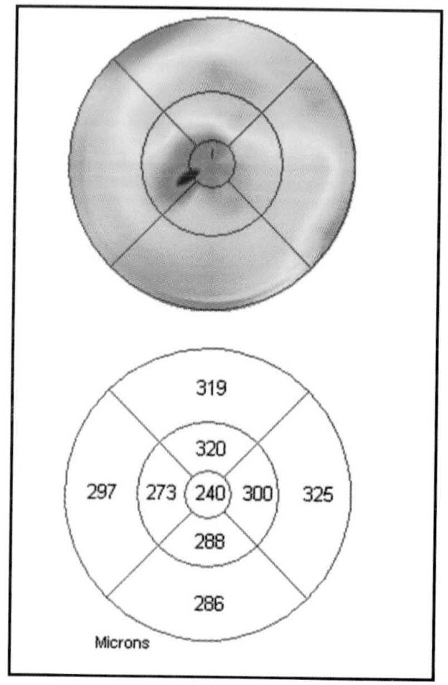

G

Case 9-4A. *Multifocal Choroiditis With Subretinal Fibrosis*

Clinical Summary

A 10-year-old girl had a recent change in the vision of the left eye. Exam showed trace anterior segment and vitreous inflammation. There were multiple choroidal lesions with various degrees of scarring in the posterior poles and periphery of both eyes. A diagnosis of multifocal choroiditis was made. The visual acuity was 20/20 in the right eye and 20/30 in the left. Fundus examination of the right eye (A) showed pigmented scars near the fovea, and stellate to round multifocal chorioretinal scars throughout the posterior fundus (B). FA (C) showed late staining of the lesions.

Optical Coherence Tomography

An oblique scan through the perifoveal scar (D) shows marked anterior protrusion of the RPE/choriocapillaris band with posterior shadowing due to the heavy pigmentation. The foveal contour is preserved, and the retinal thickness is within normal limits.

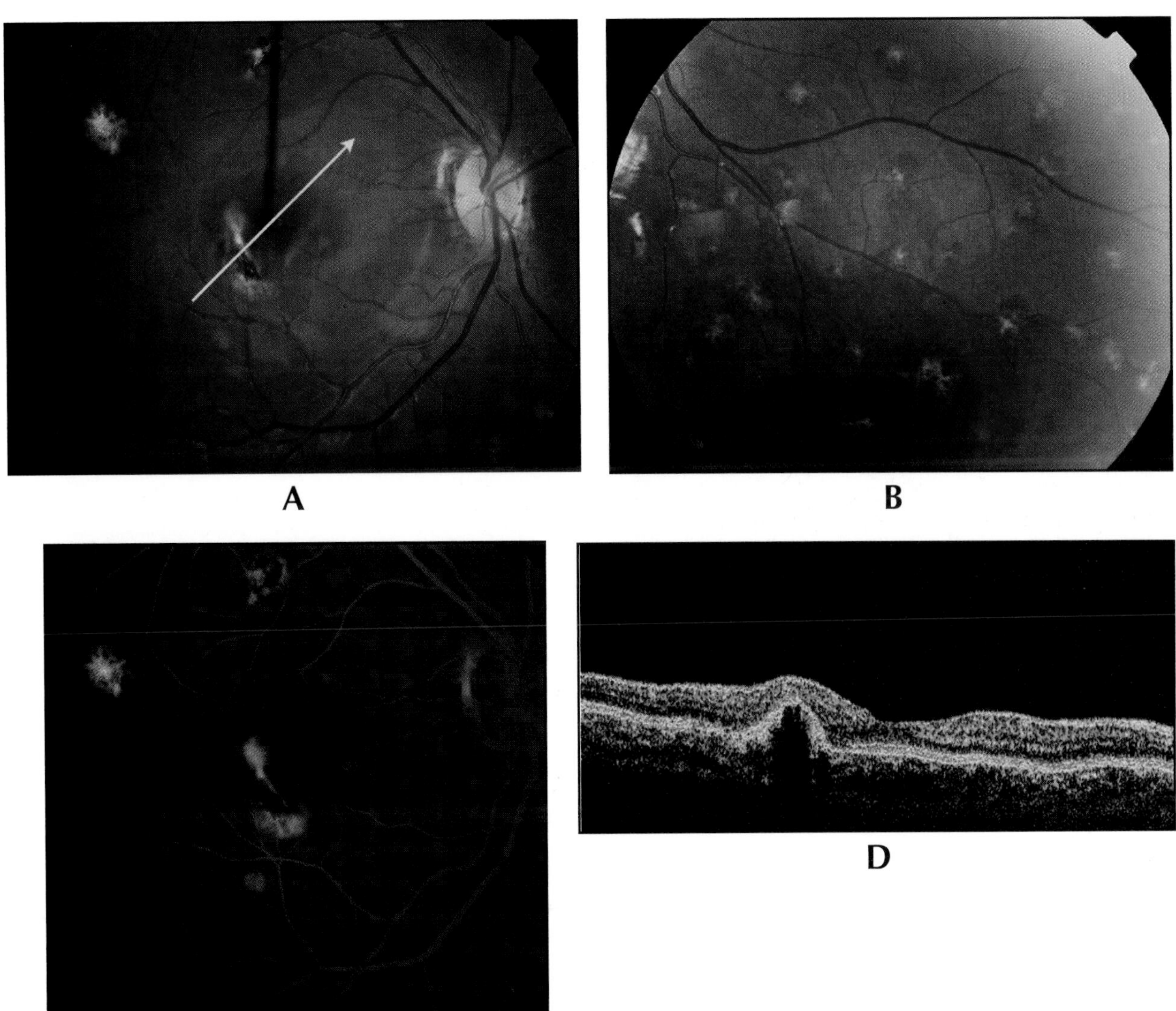

A B C D

Case 9-4B. Multifocal Choroiditis With Subretinal Fibrosis

Clinical Summary

Examination of the left eye (E) revealed the presence of fresh choroidal lesions in the posterior pole. Hemorrhage was present surrounding a large lesion superonasal to the fovea. The angiogram (F) showed two early well-defined hyperfluorescent lesions superonasal and inferotemporal to the fovea. These lesions were surrounded by a rim of blockage and were suspicious for CNV.

Optical Coherence Tomography

An oblique scan through the macula (G) passes through both suspicious lesions. They appear as localized thickenings of the external high reflective band. The superonasal lesion shows anterior protrusion of the RPE layer with highly backscattering material beneath. The overlying retina appears layered and well organized. No subretinal fluid accumulation is detected.

Comment

Laser treatment was not applied because of the lack of subretinal fluid. The patient did well on medical treatment (oral corticosteroids and methotrexate) with resolution of the macular lesions to stable scars.

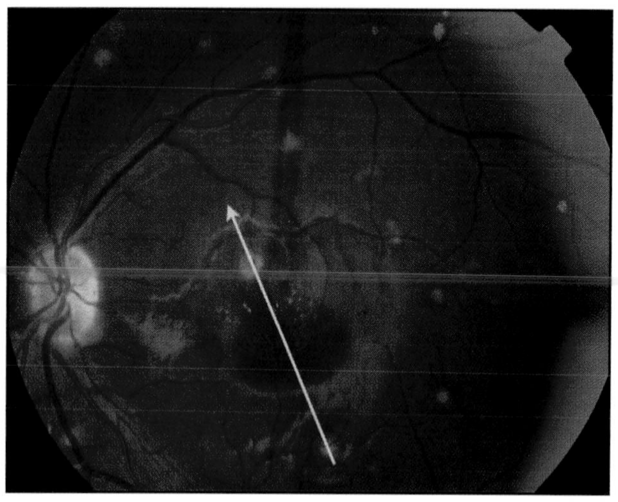

E

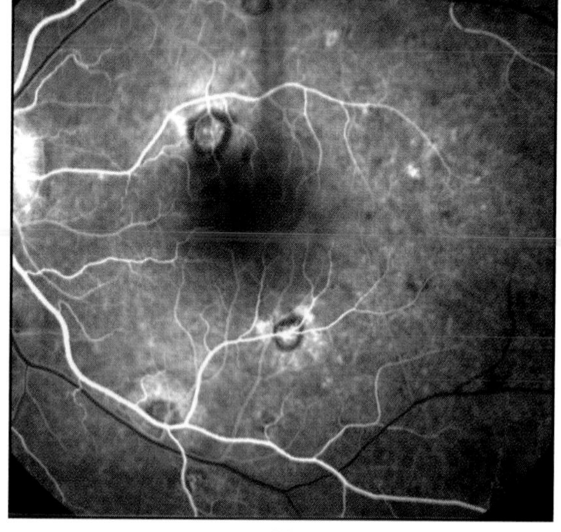

F

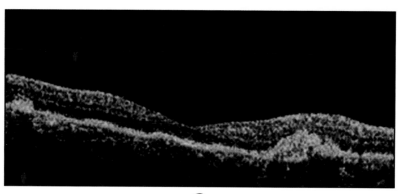

G

Case 9-5A. Sarcoidosis With Choroidal Granulomas

Clinical Summary

A 51-year-old Caucasian woman presented with acute anterior granulomatous uveitis in her right eye and vision of 20/60. Systemic work up revealed a positive ACE and hilar adenopathy. A diagnosis of sarcoidosis was made. The anterior segment inflammation resolved on topical corticosteroids. Subsequently, slightly elevated, pale choroidal lesions were noted in the macular area as shown in the color fundus photograph (A). Similar lesions were also visible in the midperiphery of the right eye. These indistinct, slightly elevated choroidal lesions appeared hypofluorescent in the early phases of the angiogram (B) and stained faintly in the late phases (C).

Optical Coherence Tomography

A vertical scan through the macula (D) shows a preserved foveal contour and normal central thickness. There are two oval-shaped, well-demarcated low reflective areas localized in the choroid, causing mild elevation of the overlying high reflective band. Since the retinal map measures thickness from the inner retinal surface to the outer high reflective band, the elevation caused by the choroidal change is not evident on the map (E).

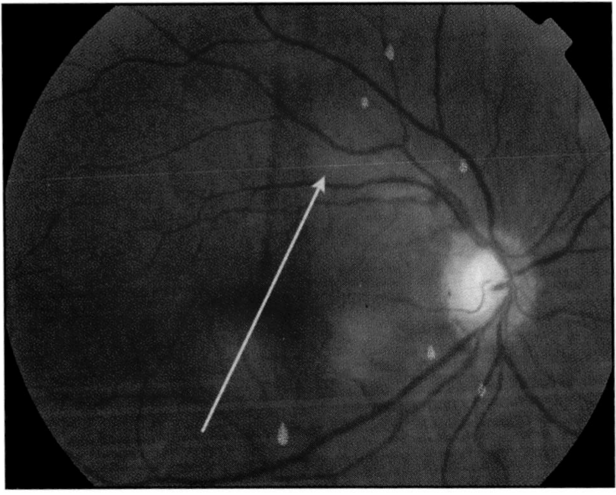

A

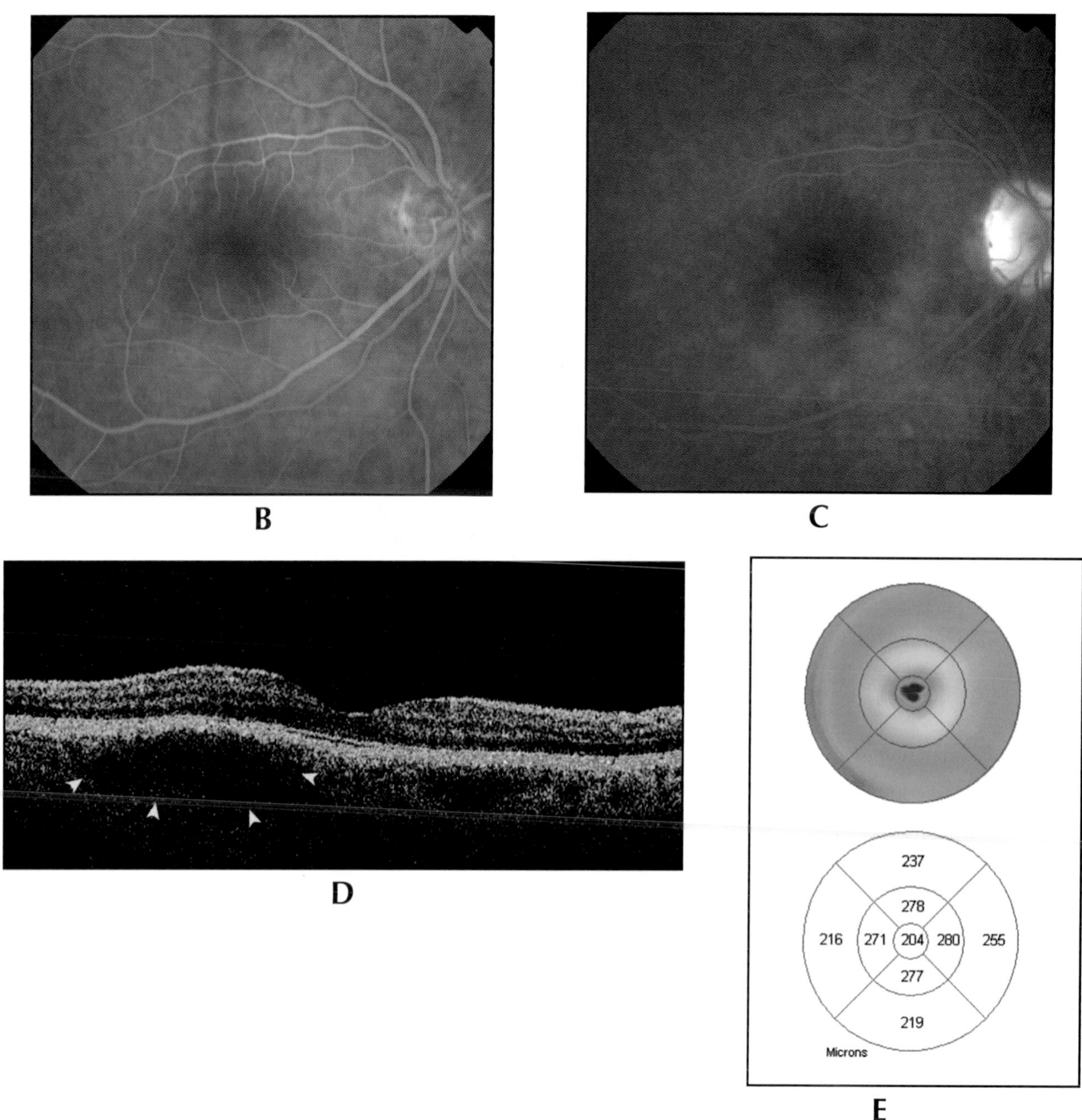
B
C
D
237
278
216
271
204
280
255
277
219
Microns
E

Case 9-5B.
Response to Treatment With Systemic Corticosteroids

Continuation of Clinical Summary

The patient was treated with oral prednisone for 3 weeks. Vision in the right eye returned to 20/40. Retinal examination (F) revealed flattening of the lesions with a persistent discoloration of the area inferior to the foveal center.

Follow-Up Optical Coherence Tomography

Repeat scan through the macula (G) shows resolution of the hyporeflective lesions beneath the retinal pigment epithelium (RPE) and flattening of the red band. The choroidal backscattering signal has returned to normal with visualization of the lumen of choroidal vessels.

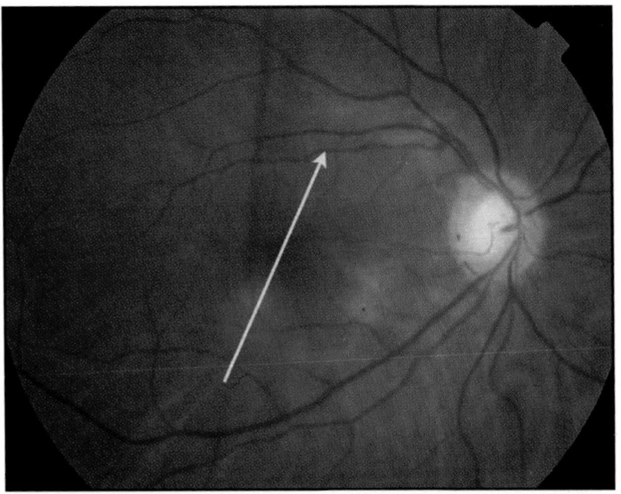

F

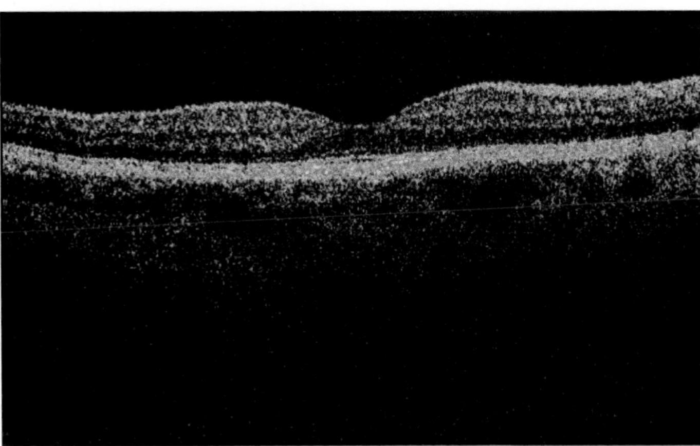

G

Case 9-6A. Vogt-Koyanagi-Harada Disease

Clinical Summary

A 31-year-old woman presented with loss of vision in both eyes to the 20/400 level for 3 days. Fundus evaluation (A) of the right eye revealed serous retinal detachment involving the macula. FA (B) showed multiple punctate hyperfluorescent lesions at the level of the RPE. Pooling of the dye under the areas of serous detachment was observed in the late frames of the angiogram (C).

Optical Coherence Tomography

A horizontal scan through the macula (D) showed extensive elevation of the neurosensory retina. The inner retinal layers were relatively well-preserved, and the foveal contour could still be identified. There appeared to be complex infolding of the outer retinal layers, creating variably sized cystic cavities. Although some of the fluid was clearly subretinal, in other areas it was difficult to differentiate subretinal from intraretinal location of the fluid. The fluid in these spaces showed a moderate amount of backscattering signal, probably indicating higher protein content. The retinal map (E) confirms elevation of the central macula to a peak of 727 μm.

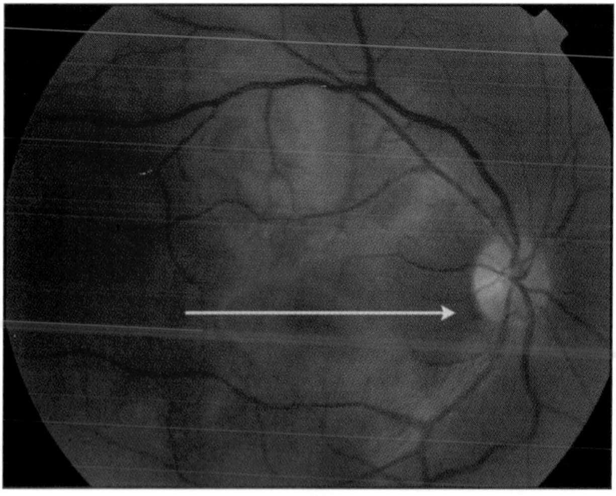

A

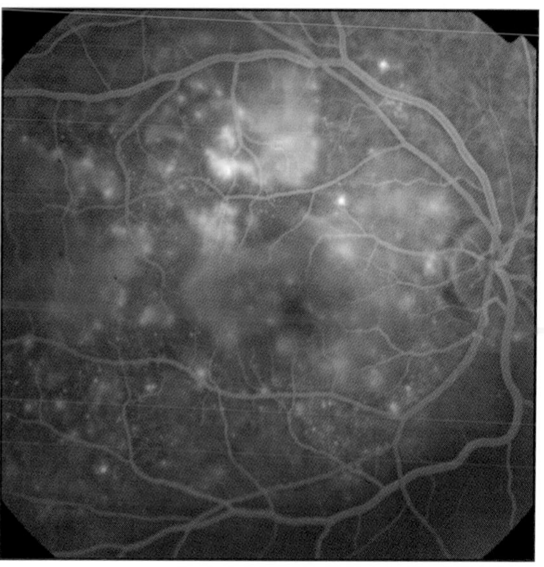

B

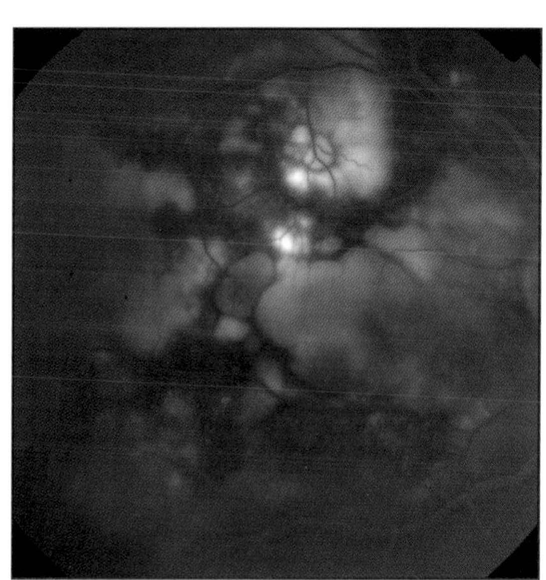

C

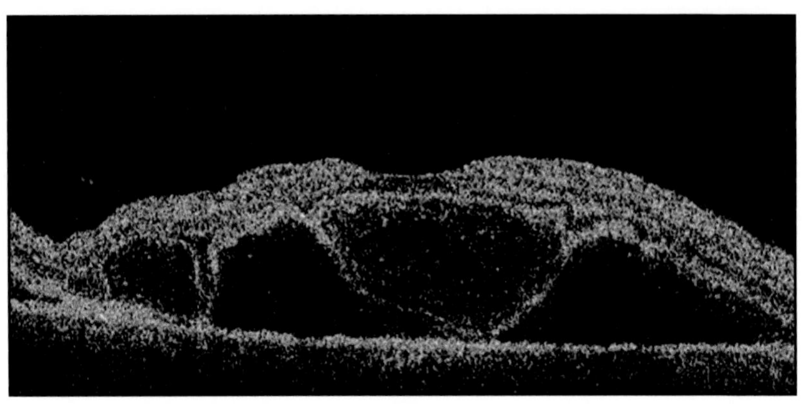

D

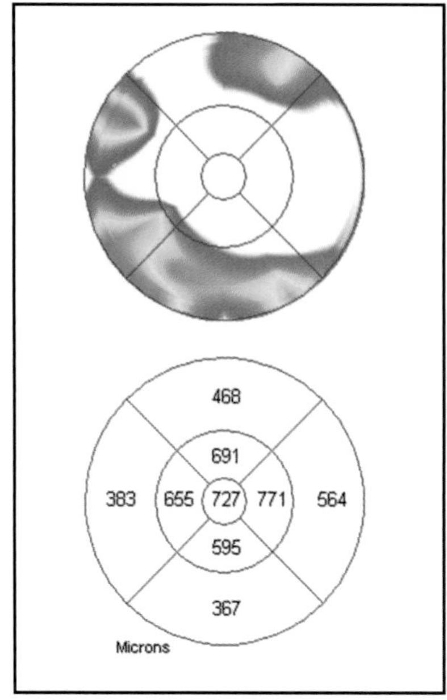

E

Case 9-6B. Vogt-Koyanagi-Harada Disease

Clinical Summary

Fundus evaluation (F) of the left eye also showed serous retinal detachments involving the posterior pole. FA (G) showed punctate peripapillary and macular hyperfluorescent lesions in the early phase of the study. Many of these hyperfluorescent areas became confluent with pooling of the dye in the late phase (H).

Optical Coherence Tomography

A horizontal scan through the foveal center (I) showed similar changes with significant elevation of the retina. The inner retina was again relatively normal, while the outer retina showed areas of irregular infolding. The thick subretinal fluid showed a moderate amount of reflectivity. The map (J) revealed marked elevation and irregularity of the retinal surface.

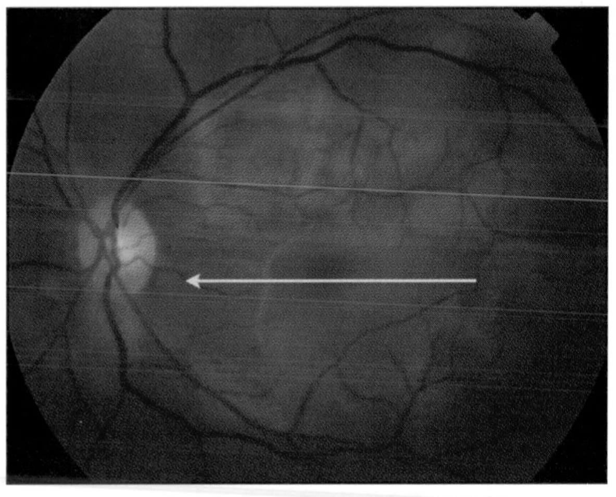

F

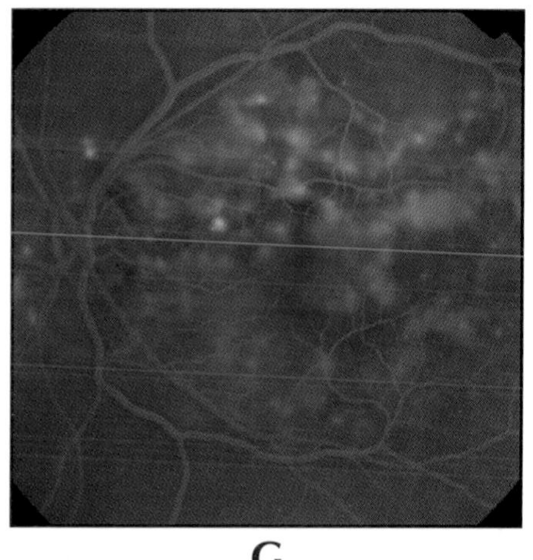

G

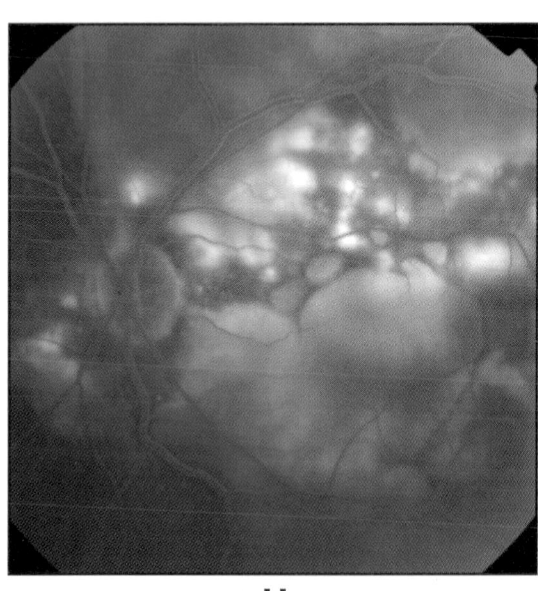

H

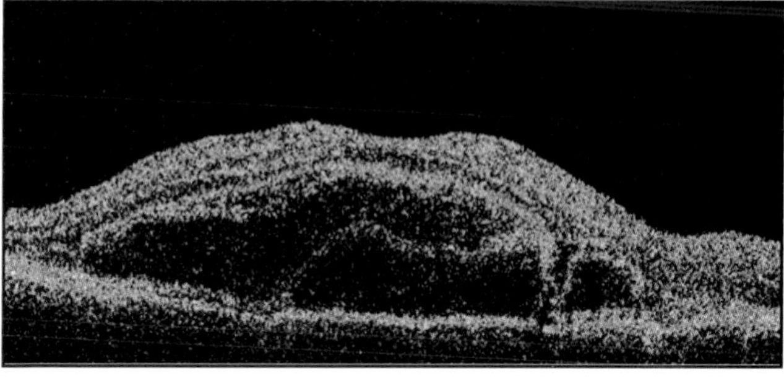

I

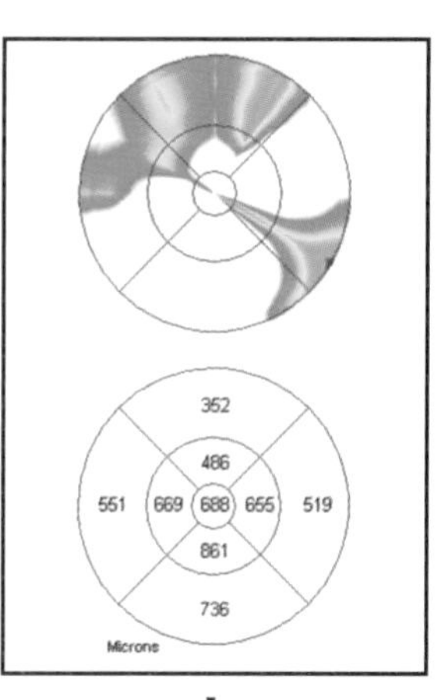

J

Case 9-6C. Response to Treatment With Corticosteroids

Continuation of Clinical Summary

High-dose oral corticosteroids were started. Two weeks later, vision returned to 20/20 in both eyes. Fundus examination (K and L) revealed complete resolution of the subretinal fluid. Mild residual pigment mottling was noted in both foveas.

Follow-Up Optical Coherence Tomography

Post-treatment tomograms (M and N) through the fovea show restored foveal contour in both eyes. The central thickness and anatomic configuration of the fovea returned to normal. The retinal maps (O and P) confirmed normalization of the retinal thickness.

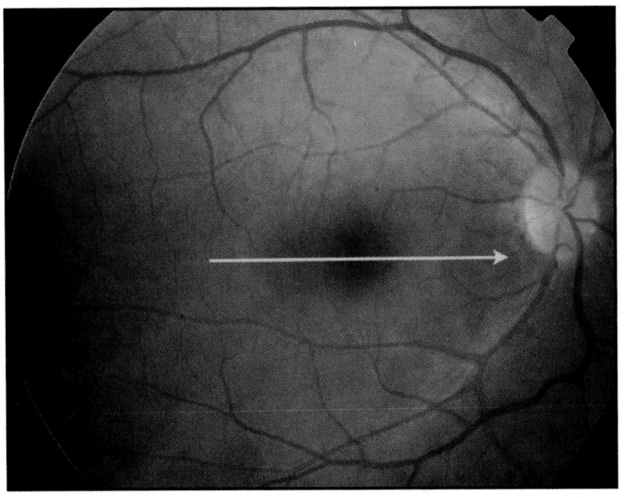

K

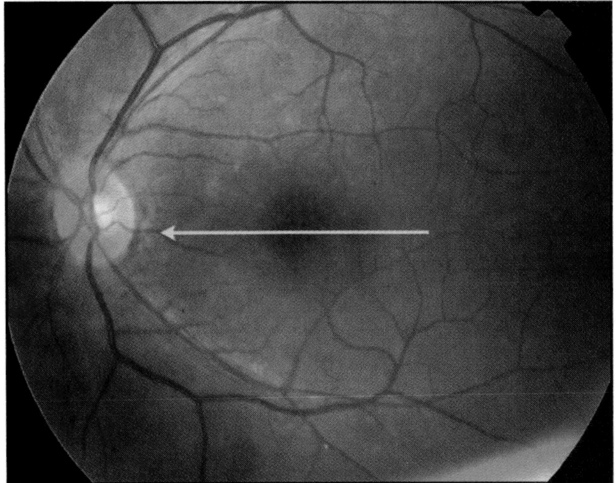

L

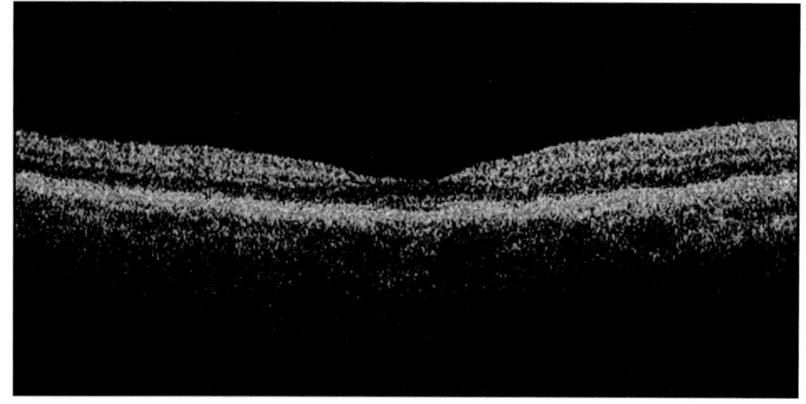

M

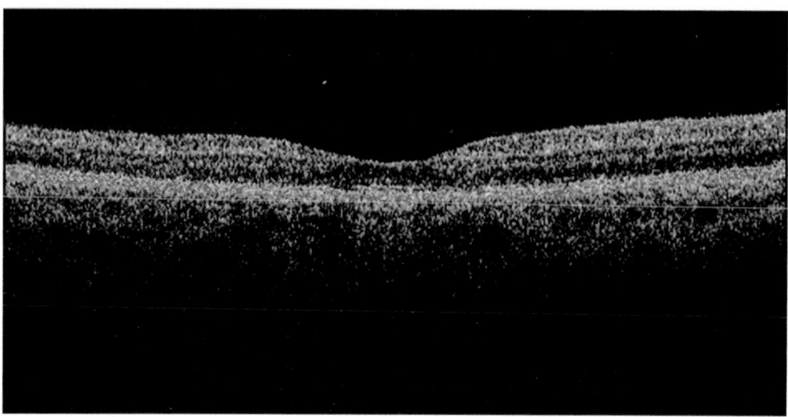

N

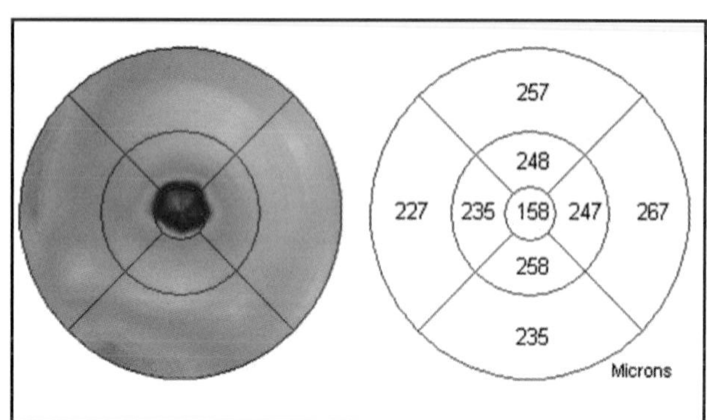
257
248
227
235
158
247
267
258
235
Microns

O

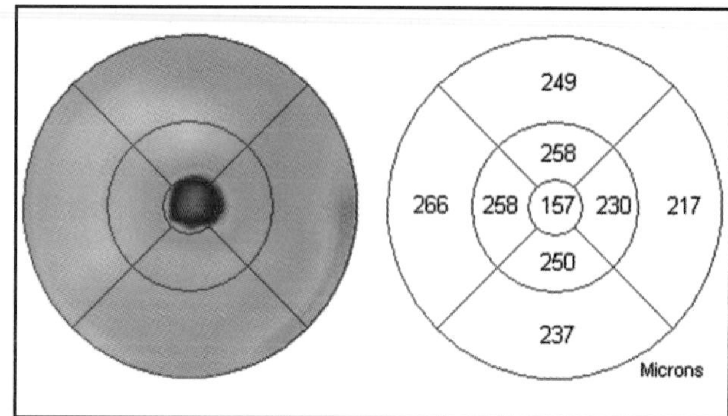
249
258
266
258
157
230
217
250
237
Microns

P

Case 9-7. *Acute Sympathetic Ophthalmia*

Clinical Summary

A 20-year-old man with a history of penetrating trauma in the left eye presented with decreased vision in the right eye for 10 days. Visual acuity in the right eye was 20/100 with anterior segment and vitreous inflammation. Retina examination (A) showed subretinal fluid in the macular area and around the optic nerve. FA (B) showed early punctate hyperfluorescent lesions around the fovea with late diffuse leakage involving the foveal center and the optic nerve (C). The left eye was not suitable for scanning. Vision returned to 20/15 in the right eye after pulse treatment with high dose oral corticosteroids, followed by a combination of low dose oral corticosteroids and methotrexate.

Optical Coherence Tomography

A horizontal scan through the fovea (D) showed central elevation of the retina over a cavity of subretinal fluid. As the scan passes nasally (right side of the image), the exact location of the fluid cavity (subretinal versus intraretinal) was difficult to determine. The thick, proteinaceous nature of this fluid was indicated by the moderate amount of reflectivity. The structure of the inner retina appeared preserved except for flattening of the foveal contour. The retinal map (E) highlights the extensive macular thickening. This OCT pattern is similar to that seen in Vogt-Koyanagi-Harada disease (VKH) (as demonstrated in case 9-6).

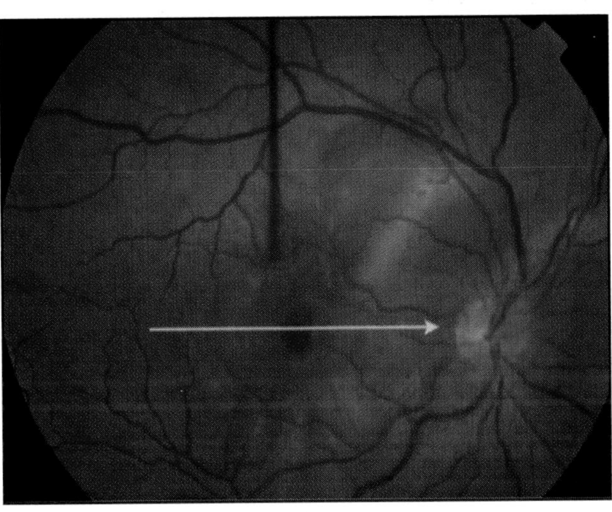

A

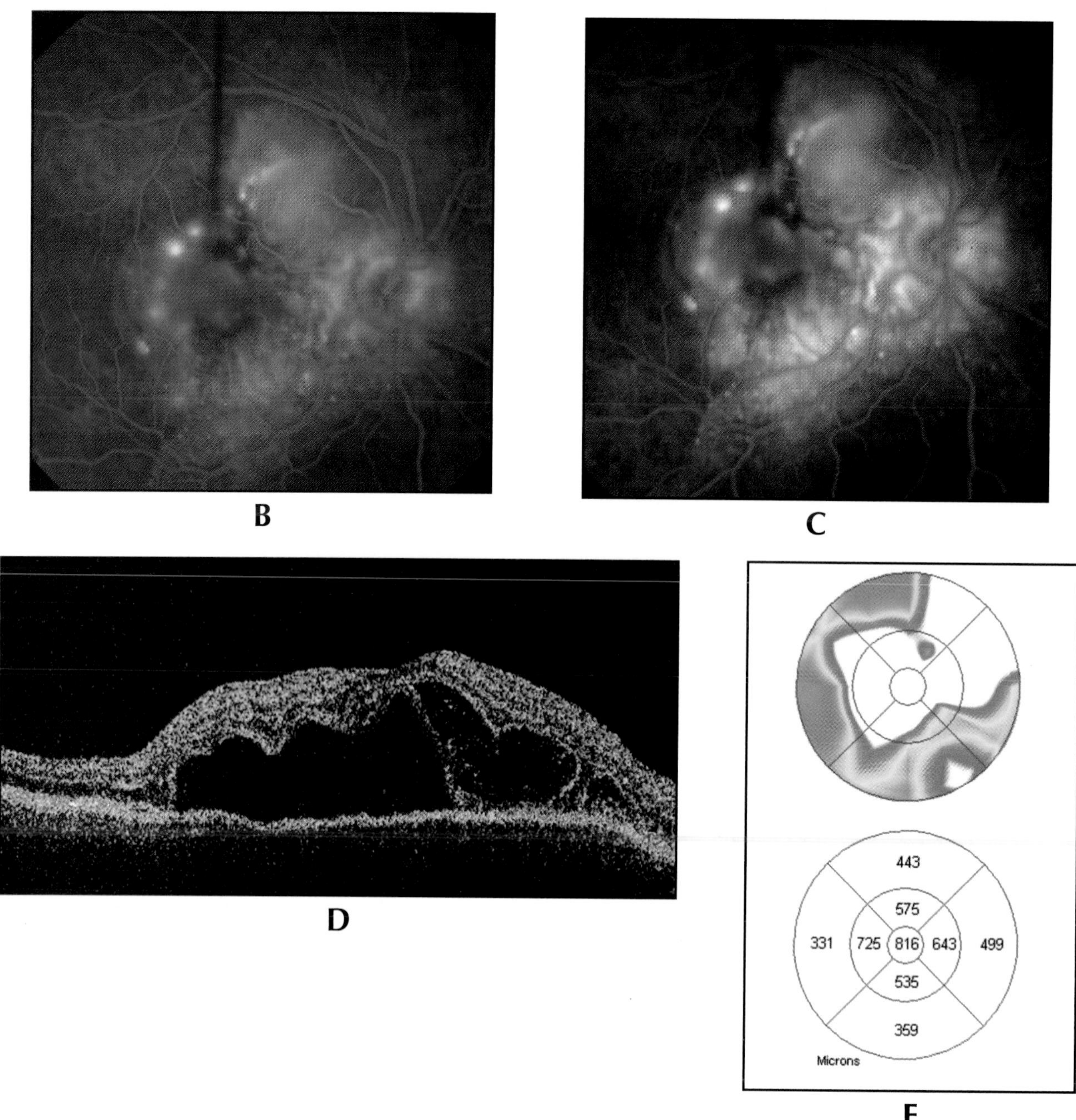
B
C
D
443
575
331
725
816
643
499
535
359
Microns
E

Case 9-8. Chronic Sympathetic Ophthalmia

Clinical Summary

A 76-year-old woman had a history of complicated retinal detachment surgery in the left eye, followed by inflammatory changes in both eyes. The left eye was enucleated and the pathology was consistent with sympathetic ophthalmia. During tapering of corticosteroid therapy, a severe exacerbation of inflammation occurred. Her visual acuity was 20/400. Examination of the retina (A) through hazy media revealed 360-degree peripapillary subretinal inflammation. Discoloration and mottling of the macula was noted. FA (B) showed extensive peripapillary leakage and perifoveal CME. Treatment with intravitreal triamcinolone acetonide, high doses of oral prednisone, azathioprine, and ultimately cyclophosphamide did not result in visual improvement.

Optical Coherence Tomography

A horizontal scan through the foveal center (C) reveals loss of the foveal contour and of the layered organization of the retina. There is extensive cystoid edema in the retina. The external band has nodular irregularities with high backscattering signal from the sub-RPE space. Toward the nasal end of the scan line, the outer retina is hyporeflective with posterior shadowing. This corresponds to the region of the peripapillary subretinal deposits.

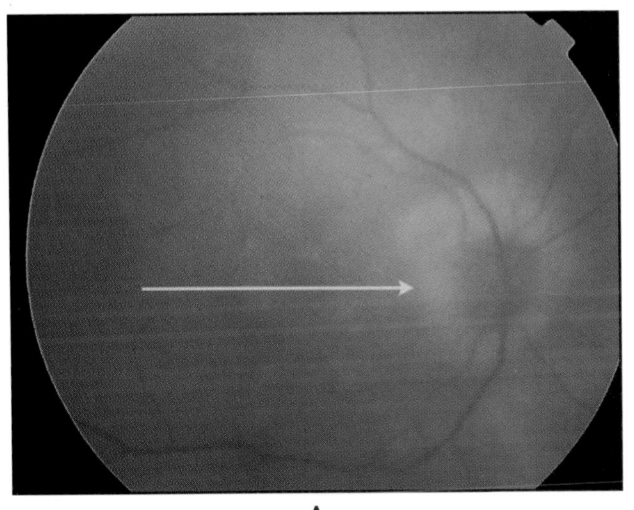

A

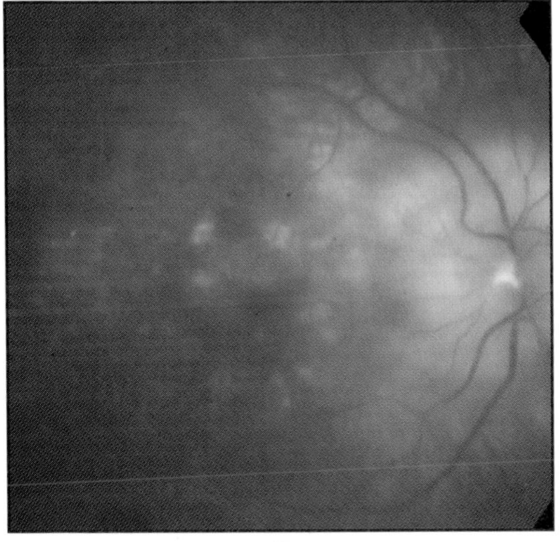

B

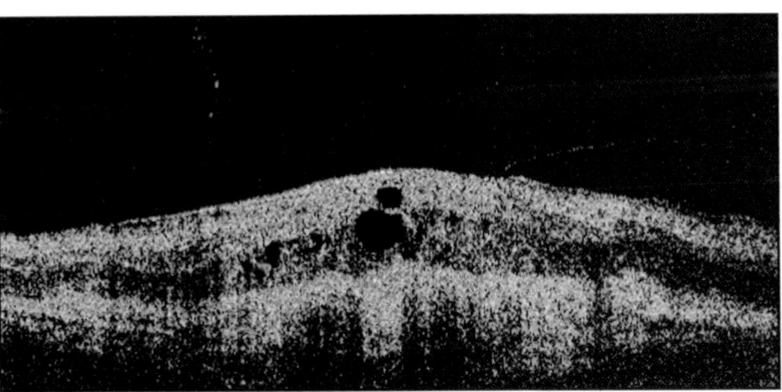

C

Case 9-9A. Birdshot Chorioretinopathy

Clinical Summary

A 54-year-old woman complained of decreased vision in both eyes for 5 years. She was HLA-A29 positive. Periocular steroid injections resolved the vitreous inflammation. BCVA was 20/20 in each eye. Retinal examination of the right eye (A) showed a hypopigmented fundus. Large choroidal vessels were visible throughout the posterior pole. Indocyanine green angiography (ICGA) (B) showed large well-defined hyperfluorescent lesions in the choroid.

Optical Coherence Tomography

An oblique scan through the foveal center (C) showed marked thinning of the retina. Despite this thinning, there was some preservation of the foveal contour and retinal architecture. The highly reflective external band was slightly thickened and irregular. A zone of reduced signal intensity was seen in the choroid. The retinal map (D) confirms diffuse thinning of the retina throughout the macula.

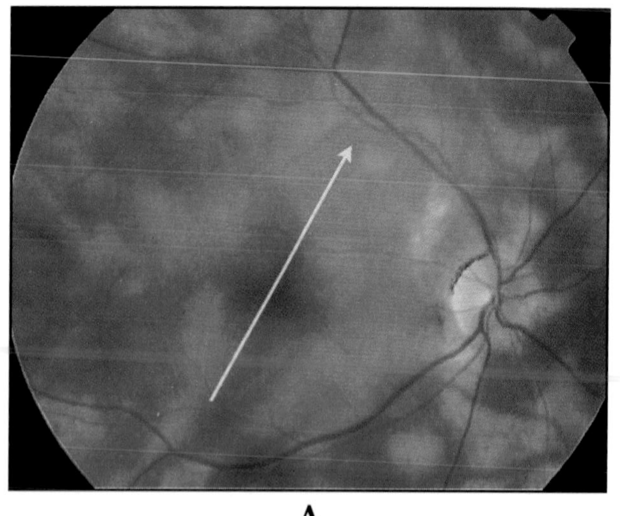

A

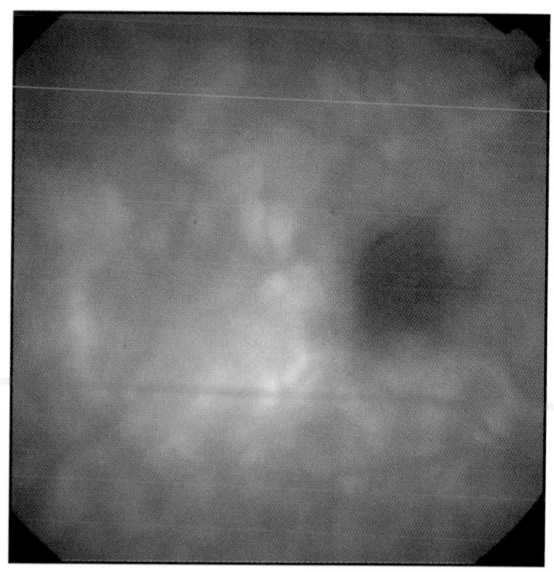

B

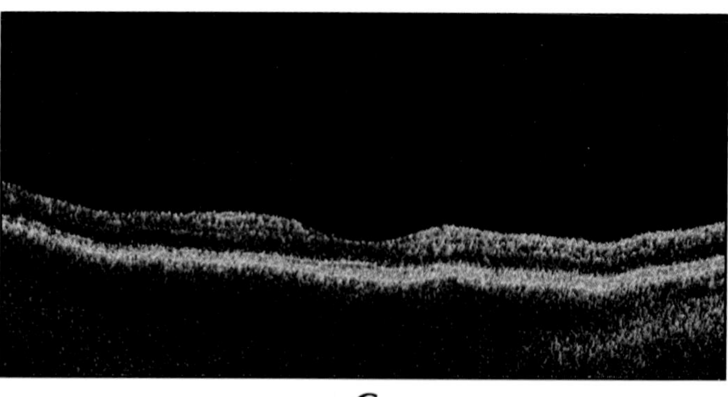

C

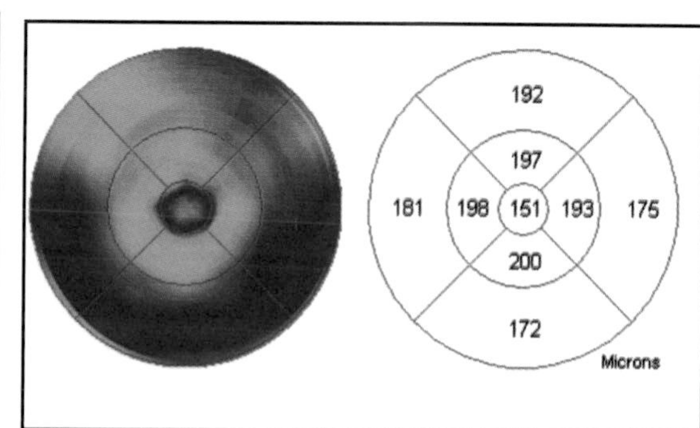

D

Case 9-9B. Birdshot Chorioretinopathy

Clinical Summary

Retinal examination of the left eye (E) showed a pale optic nerve, attenuated retinal vessels, and large choroidal vessels visible through a depigmented RPE. ICGA (F) showed large hypofluorescent areas during the early phase.

Optical Coherence Tomography

An oblique scan through the foveal center (G) again showed thinning of the retina with preservation of the foveal contour and retinal architecture. The highly reflective external band showed mild changes similar to those seen in the other eye. A horizontal area of hyporeflective choroidal tissue was also observed under the external band in this eye. The retinal map (H) further highlighted the extensive retinal thinning.

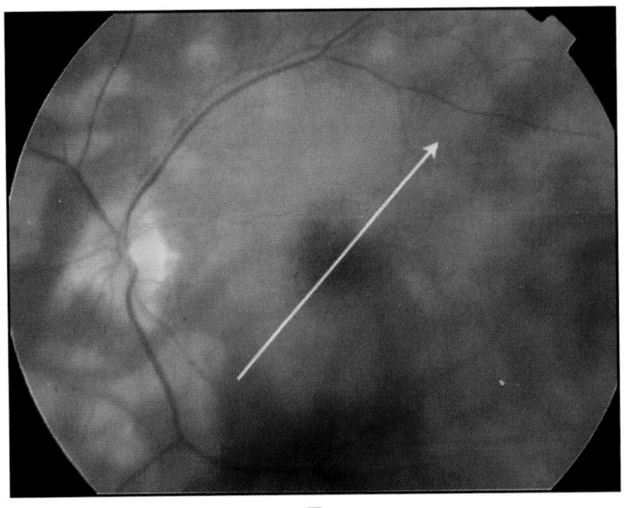

E

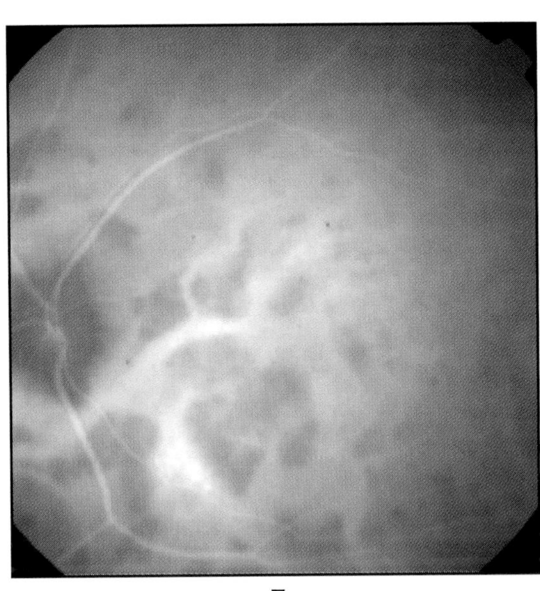

F

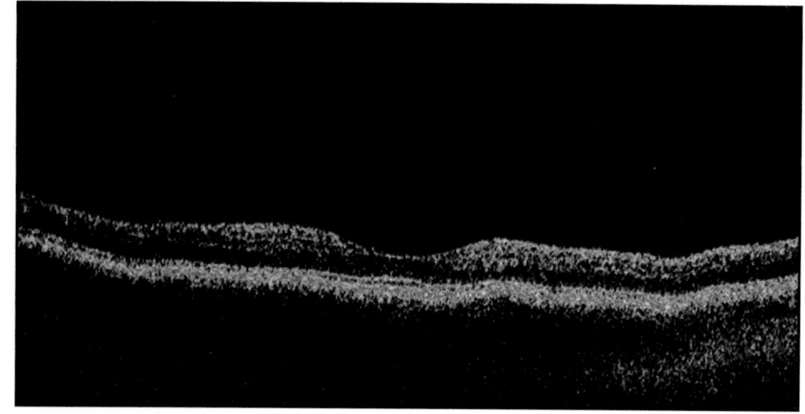

G

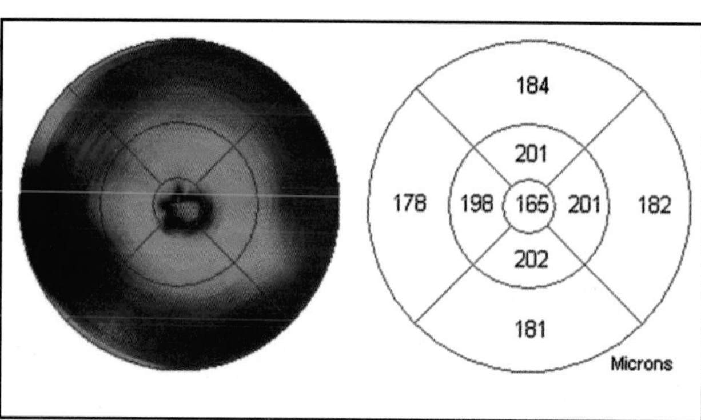

H

Case 9-10A.
Toxoplasmic Chorioretinitis

Clinical Summary

A 15-year-old female presented with decreased vision in the right eye for 4 days. Visual acuity was 1/200 in the right eye and 20/20 in the left eye. IgG toxoplasmosis titers were positive. Retinal examination (A) revealed vitreous haze and a well-circumscribed white area of retinitis with a surrounding hypopigmented halo and distortion of the foveal architecture secondary to the presence of subretinal fluid. FA (B) showed early blocked fluorescence in the area of focal inflammation with profuse late leakage extending to the foveal center (C). She received treatment with daraprim, sulfadiazine, and oral prednisone. Anterior segment examination showed no cell or flare reaction.

Optical Coherence Tomography

A vertical scan through the center of the lesion (D) shows increased intraretinal reflectivity corresponding with the area of retinitis, with shadowing of the underlying choroidal tissue. Subretinal fluid accumulation elevating the fovea is observed inferiorly. The retinal map (E) shows diffuse thickening of the central area.

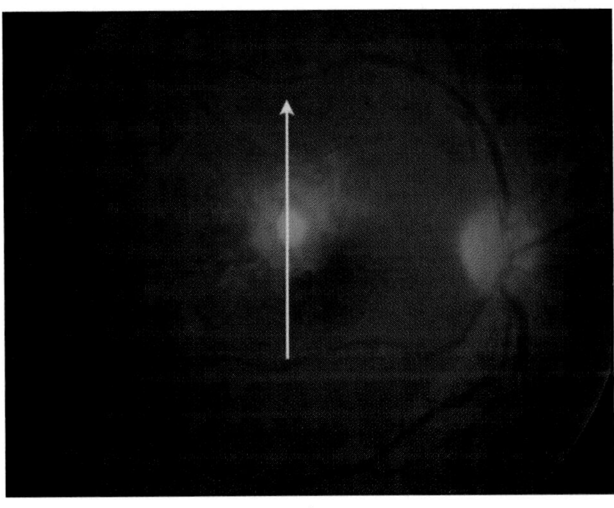

A

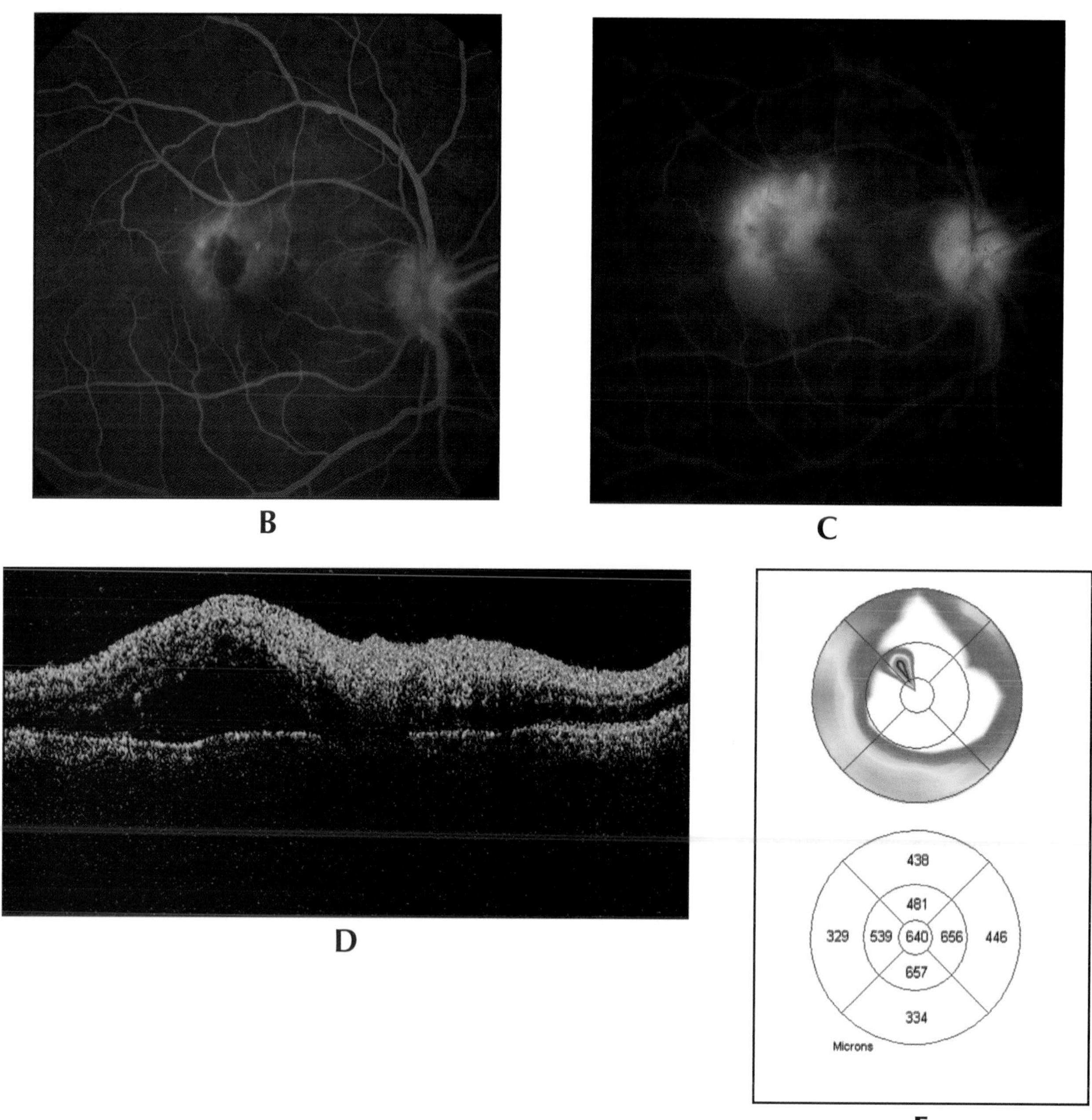
B
C
D
438
481
329
539
640
656
446
657
334
Microns
E

Case 9-10B. Response to Treatment

Continuation of Clinical Summary

Two weeks after starting treatment, vision in the right eye improved to 20/400. The lesion appeared to be more sharply demarcated, and there was partial flattening of the subretinal fluid in the area inferior to the foveal center (F). Four weeks after the initial visit (I), there was further improvement of the vision to 20/200 and a decrease in the size of the active lesion.

Follow-Up Optical Coherence Tomography

A repeat scan through the exact same location was obtained at every follow-up visit. The retinal tissue at the site of the lesion appears more compact and highly reflective (G) after 2 weeks of treatment. It still causes localized shadowing of the underlying choroid. The subfoveal fluid has decreased, and retinal anatomy appears more normal. High reflective vitreous opacities are visible overlying the retina. The map (H) shows persistent thickening, especially superior and nasal to the fovea. A repeat scan at 4 weeks (J) shows partial restoration of the foveal contour. The intraretinal lesion appears highly reflective shadowing the underlying choroid. Retinal thickness (K) has returned to normal except for some thinning in the perifoveal region.

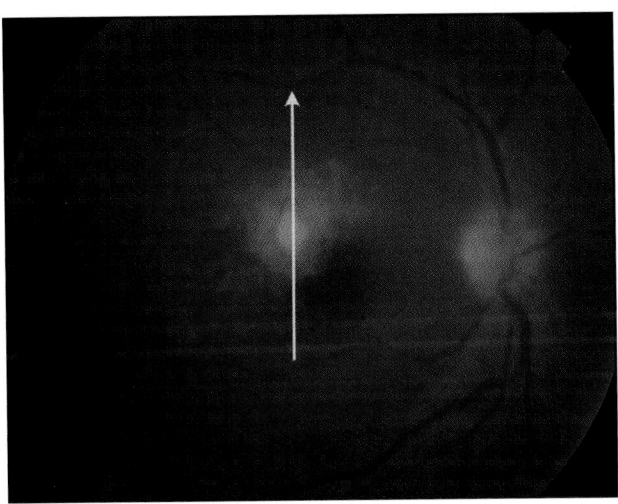

F

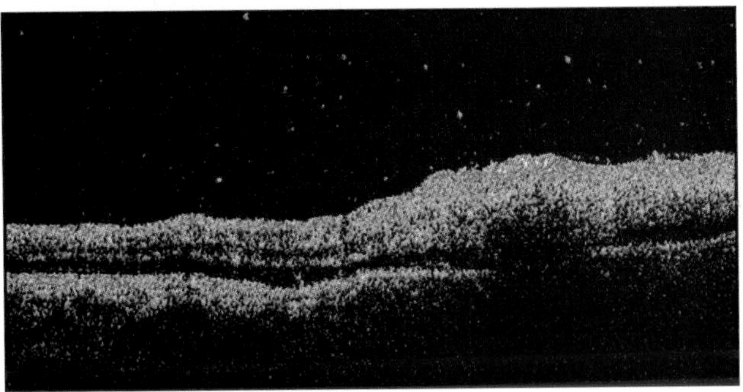

G

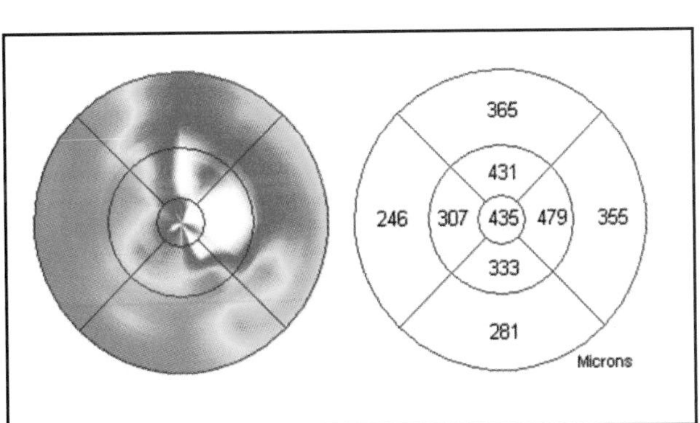

H

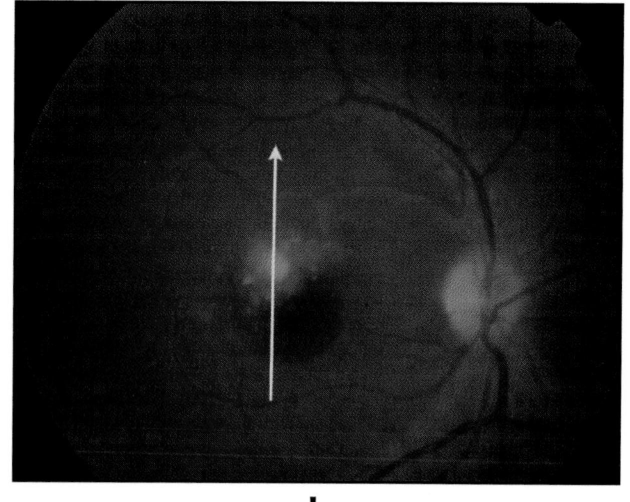

I

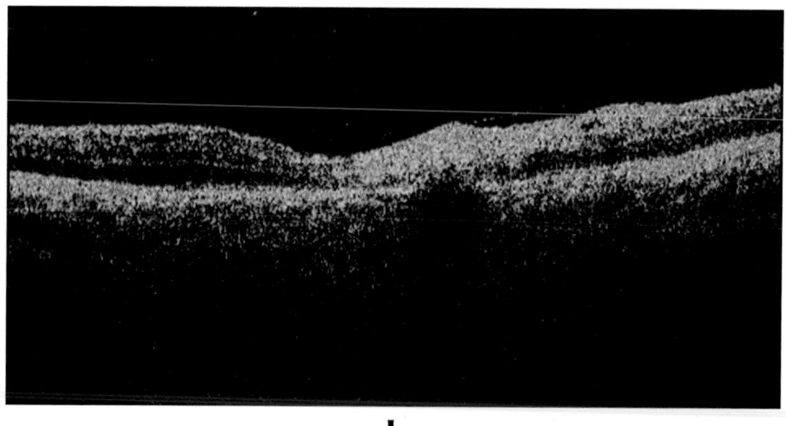

J

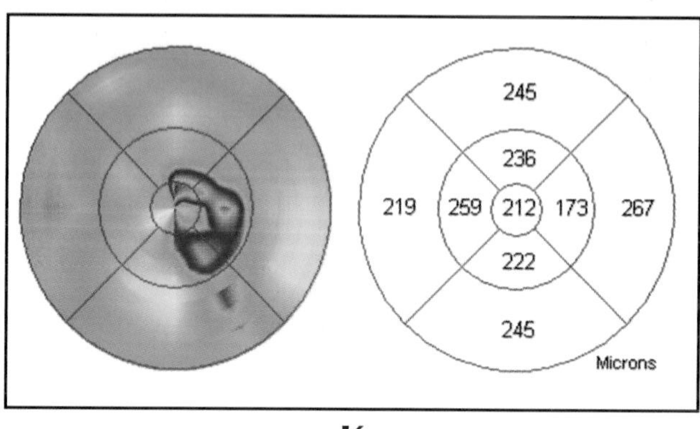

K

Case 9-11A. Toxoplasmosis With Subretinal Neovascularization

Clinical Summary

A 19-year-old male had a macular scar from ocular toxoplasmosis in his right eye from early childhood. CNV developed and he was treated with TTT. Two months later there was reduction in vision to 20/200 with fresh subretinal hemorrhage and fluid accumulation. Examination of the macula (A) revealed a pigmented chorioretinal scar temporal to fixation, but the boundaries between it and the CNV at the nasal edge were not clear. FA (B) showed minimal early leakage with late leakage from the nasal edge of the lesion on late frames (C).

Optical Coherence Tomography

A horizontal scan is taken through the toxoplasmosis scar and foveal center (D). In the area of the scar, there is increased density of the retinal layers and fusion to the RPE/choroid. A subretinal neovascular membrane is adjacent to the scar and poorly defined. The RPE is shadowed directly beneath this lesion but appears flat rather than anteriorly protruded. Areas of low reflectivity beneath the retina indicate subretinal fluid accumulation. The retinal map (E) highlights the extensive thickening in the foveal region.

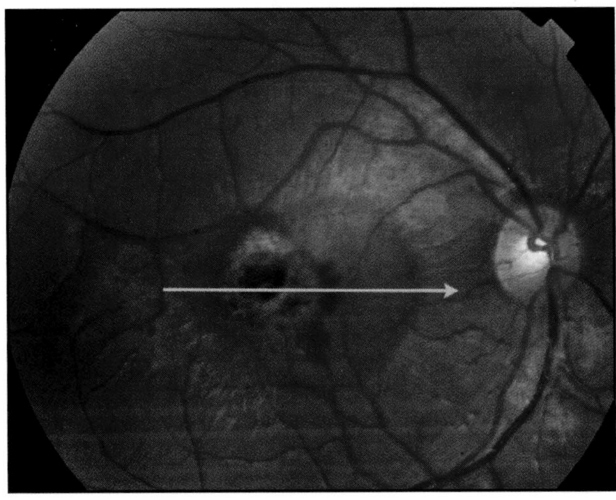

A

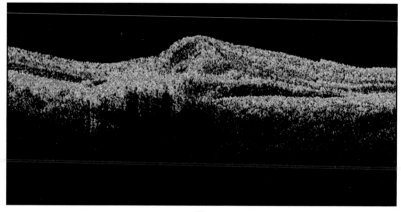

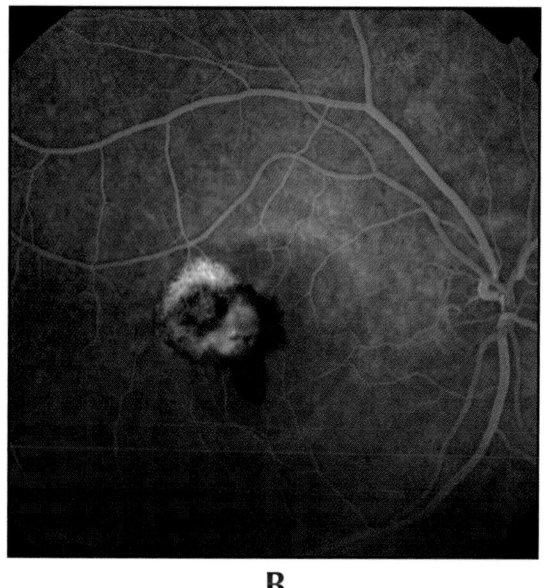

B

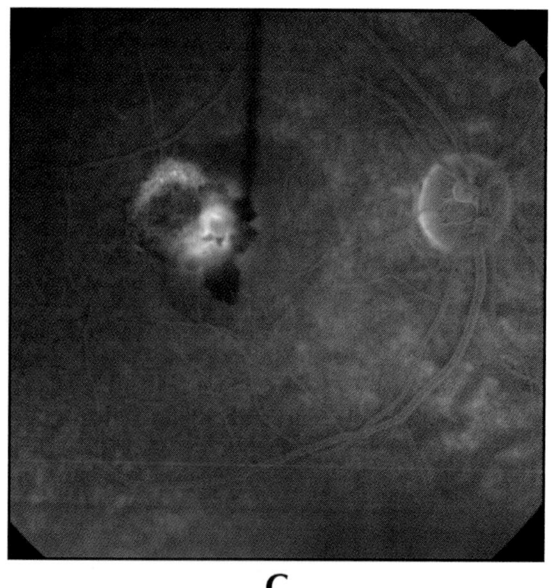

C

D

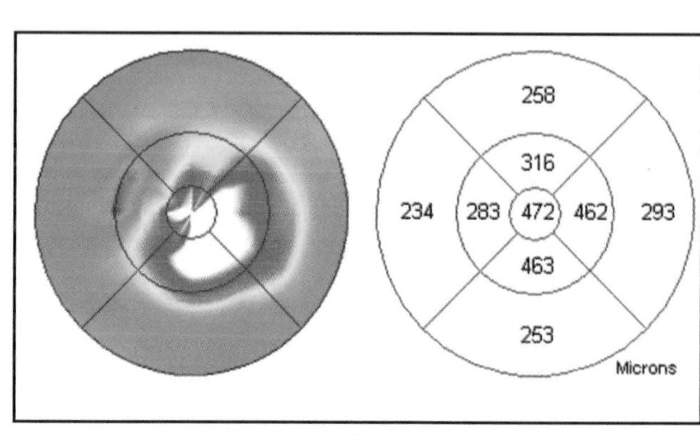

E

Case 9-11B.
Treatment With Photodynamic Therapy

Continuation of Clinical Summary

The patient is treated with photodynamic therapy at this initial visit. Six weeks after treatment, vision in the right eye improved to 20/50. The nasal edge of the scar appeared healed, and the subfoveal fluid resolved (F). There was a small amount of hemorrhage still present. No leakage is observed on FA (G).

Follow-Up Optical Coherence Tomography

A repeat OCT scan (H) shows irregular elevation of the RPE band with shadowing of the underlying choroid in the area of the toxoplasmosis scar. There has been resolution of the adjacent subretinal and intraretinal fluid, indicating inactivation of the neovascularization. The retinal map (I) shows thinning of the retina over the scar with normalization of the adjacent foveal thickness.

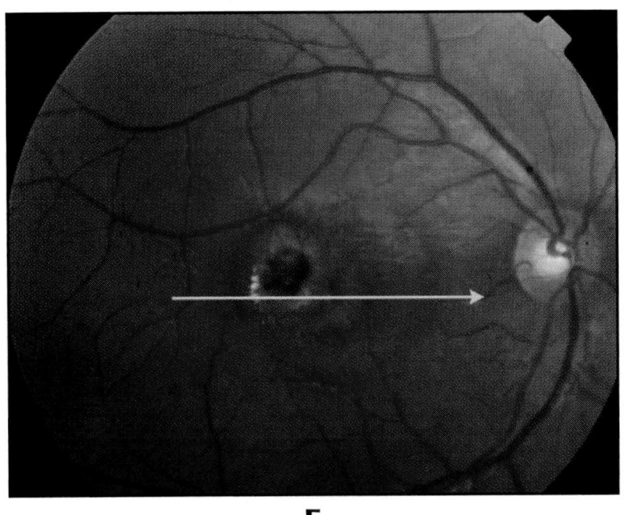

F

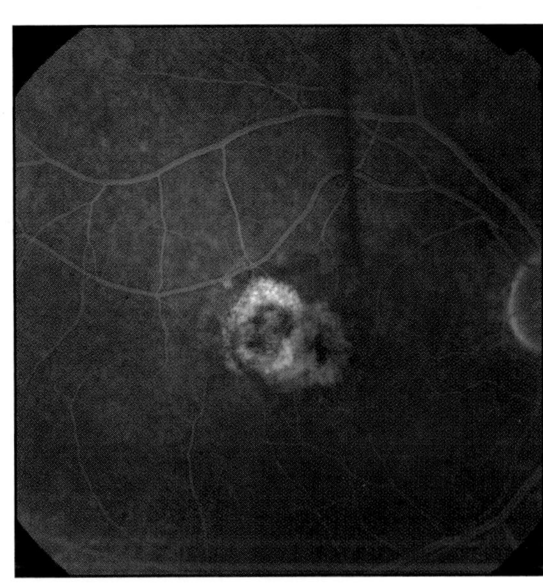

G

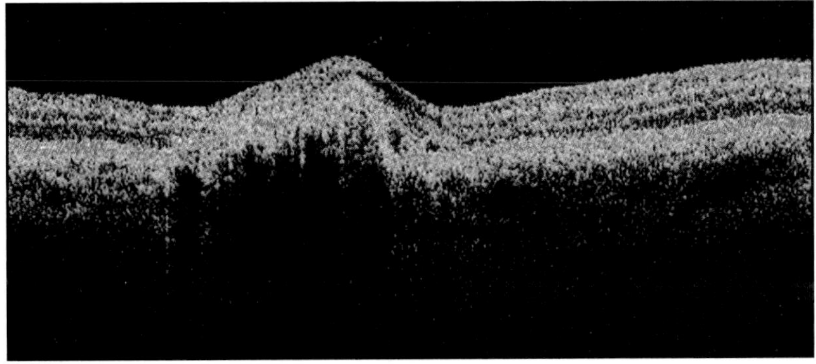

H

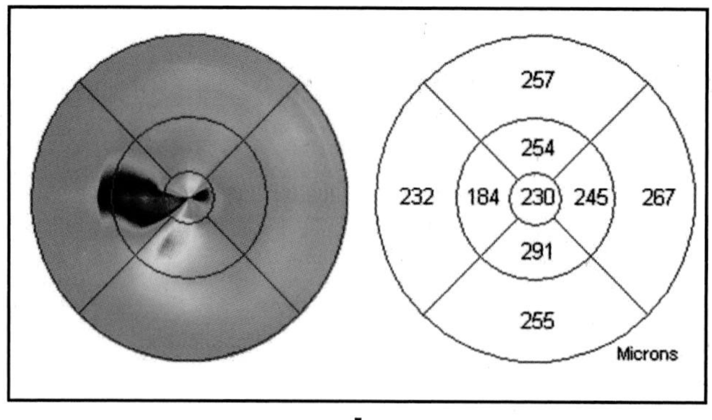

I

Case 9-12A. Syphillitic Uveitis

Clinical Summary

A 43-year-old man presented with symptoms of severe, progressive bilateral decrease in vision for 6 days. Visual acuity was 20/400 in the right eye and 20/300 in the left eye at presentation. Systemic work up revealed positive RPR and FTA-Abs. A diagnosis of bilateral syphilitic chorioretinitis was made. Examination of the left eye (A) revealed hazy media. The disc appeared inflamed and with blurry margins, and there were diffuse, patchy areas of retinal whitening involving the posterior pole. FA (B) demonstrated early peripapillary leakage with localized areas of choroidal hypofluorescence. Late diffuse leakage was observed (C). The patient received treatment with penicillin at neurosyphilis doses.

Optical Coherence Tomography

A vertical scan through the fovea (D) shows altered foveal contour with preserved inner retinal architecture. The generalized tissue hyporeflectivity is probably secondary to the diffuse vitreous opacity. There is thick subretinal fluid with a low to moderate reflective signal, causing shadowing of the underlying structures. The retinal map (E) shows marked thickening and irregularity throughout the center.

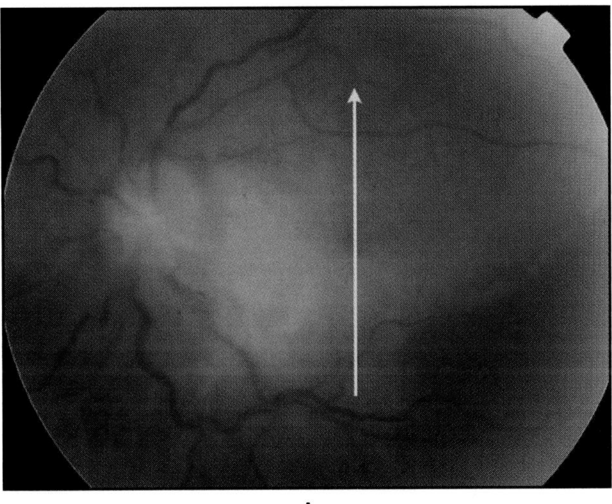

A

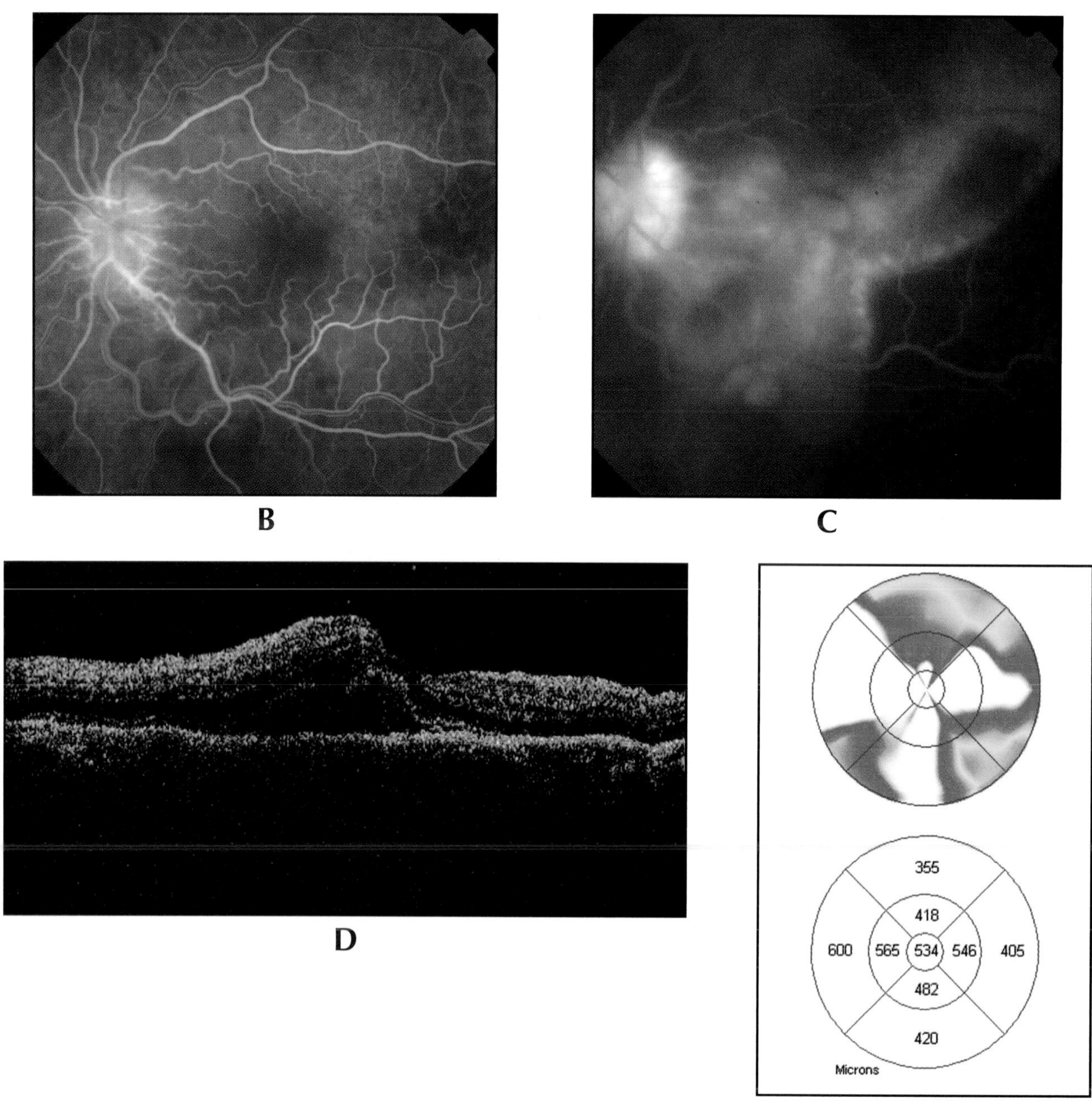
B
C
D
355
418
600
565
534
546
405
482
420
Microns
E

Case 9-12B. Response to Treatment

Continuation of Clinical Summary

Ten weeks after starting the treatment, visual acuity had returned to 20/30 in the right eye and 20/20 in the left eye. Examination of the left eye (F) showed persistent vitreous opacities and peripapillary inflammation. FA (G) revealed resolution of the exudative detachment involving the macula of the left eye. There was early mottled hyperfluorescence in the macula without leakage in the late phase (H). The optic nerve showed mild leakage.

Follow-Up Optical Coherence Tomography

A repeat scan through the macula (I) reveals restored foveal contour with a normal appearing retinal architecture. There has been complete resolution of the subretinal fluid. The signal coming from the underlying choroid is within normal limits, and the choroidal vasculature appears well delineated. The retinal map (J) shows remodeling of the perifoveal retina with normal central thickness but mild residual optic nerve swelling.

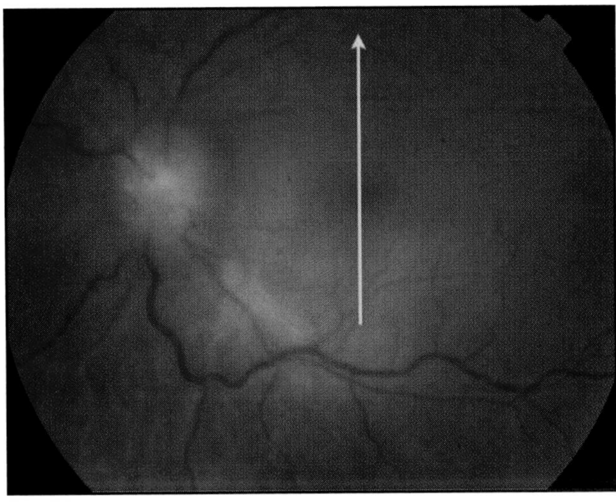

F

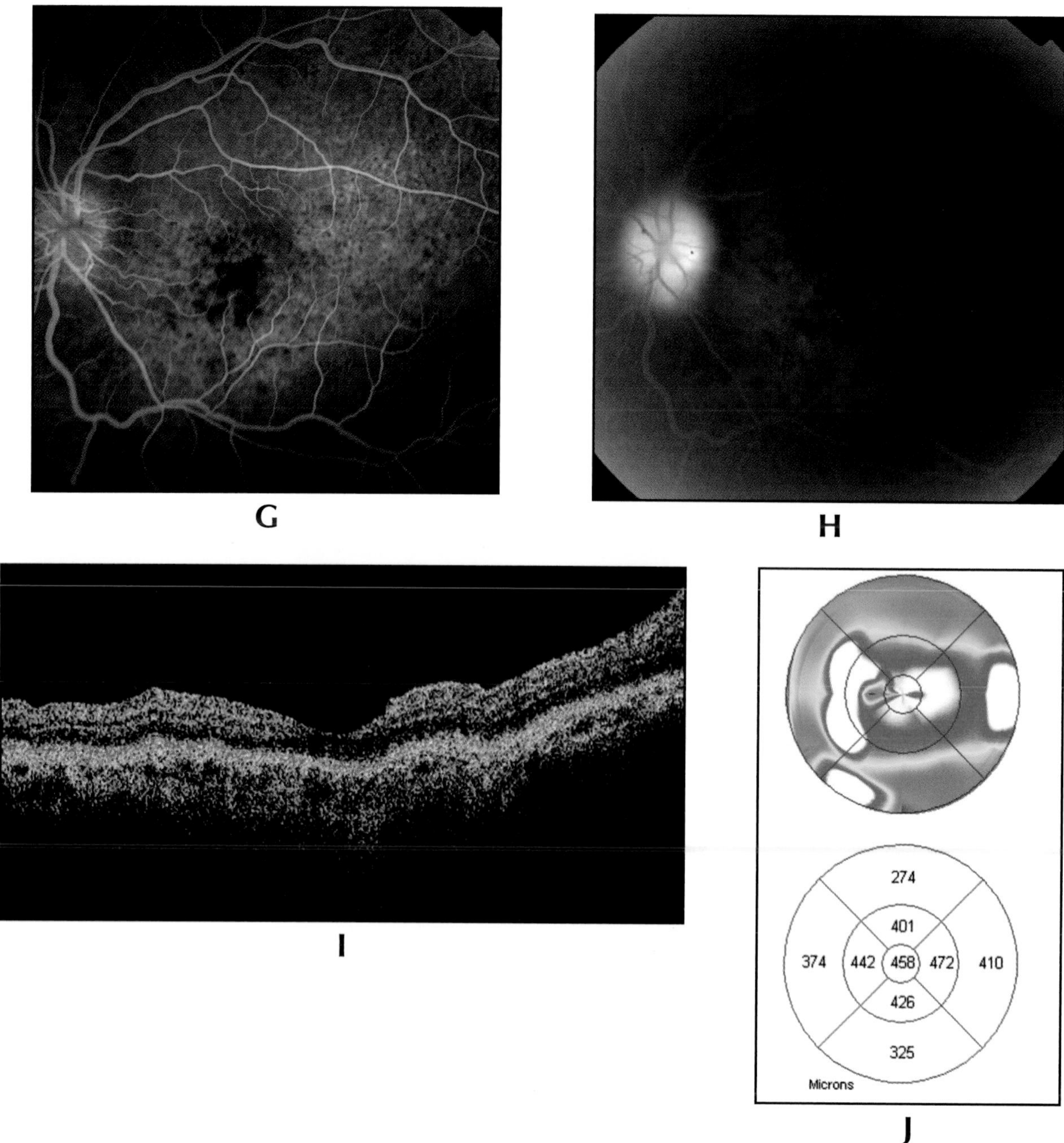
G
H
274
401
374
442
458
472
410
426
325
Microns
I
J

Case 9-13A. Cytomegalovirus Retinitis With Immune Recovery Vitreitis and Cystoid Macular Edema

Clinical Summary

A 31-year-old male had CMV retinitis successfully treated 5 years before. After starting on highly active antiretroviral therapy, he had no further reactivations but developed chronic anterior uveitis. He complained of persistent decrease in vision and floaters in both eyes. BCVA was 20/60 in the right eye. Anterior segment examination revealed trace cellular reaction. There was mild vitreous inflammation with vitreous strand formation. Retinal examination of the right eye (depicted in the OCT video image—A) showed extensive areas of healed retinitis extending into the macula. Pigment abnormalities and focal thickening were noted in the foveal region. He was diagnosed with immune recovery uveitis.

Optical Coherence Tomography

A vertical scan through the foveal center of the right eye (B) shows vitreous opacities parallel to the inner retina. These may represent focal cellular infiltrates on the posterior hyaloid surface. There is a mild increase in central thickness with CME. The superior aspect of the scan cuts through an area of healed retinitis, where the retinal tissue is compacted and highly reflective.

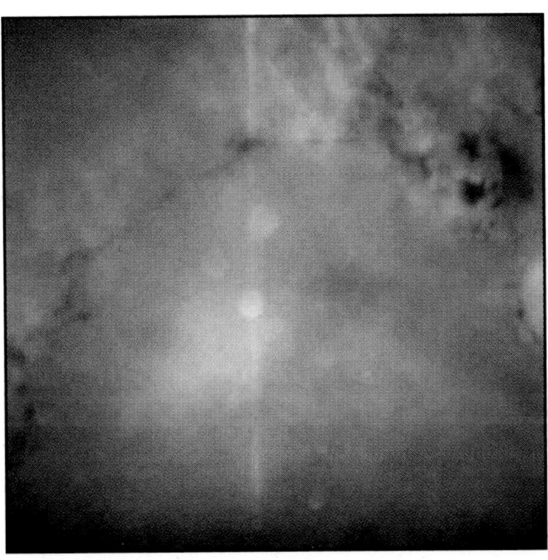

A

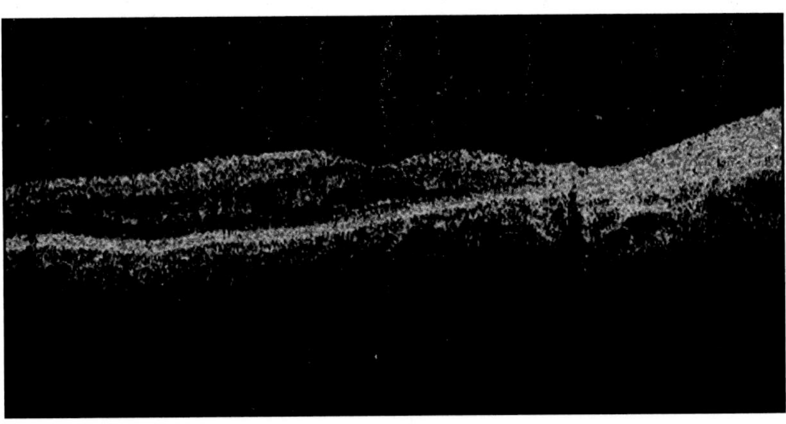

B

Case 9-13B. Cytomegalovirus Retinitis With Immune Recovery Vitreitis and Cystoid Macular Edema

Clinical Summary

BCVA was 20/50 in the left eye. There was mild cellular reaction in the anterior chamber and vitreous cavity of this eye. Retinal examination (depicted in the OCT video image—C) shows peripheral scarring from the previous retinitis. There is extensive CME in this eye.

Optical Coherence Tomography

A vertical scan through the fovea of the left eye (D) also shows vitreous opacities lying above the retinal surface. There is a suggestion of focal attachment to the foveal center with possible traction. There is loss of the foveal contour with intraretinal thickening. CME is seen as nonreflective cavities within the retina.

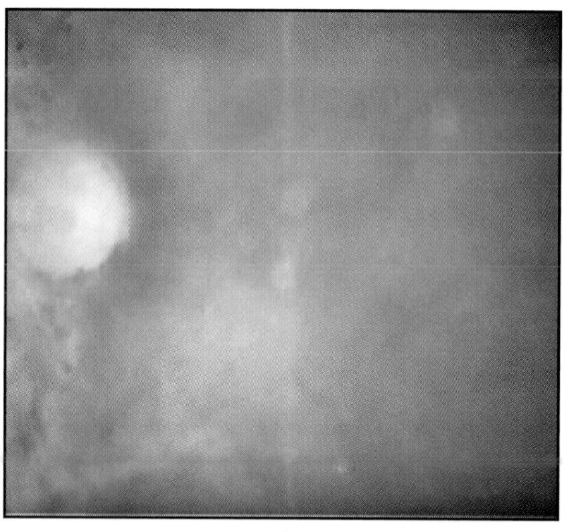

C

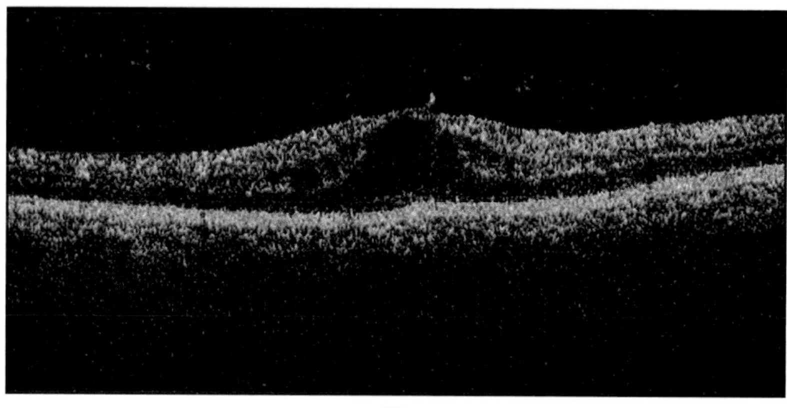

D

Chapter 10

Retinal Dystrophies

Vanessa Cruz-Villegas, MD; Philip J. Rosenfeld, MD; and Carmen A. Puliafito, MD

- Retinitis Pigmentosa
- Cone-Rod Dystrophy
- Stargardt's Disease
- Best's Disease
- Pattern Dystrophy
- X-Linked Juvenile Retinoschisis

Optical coherence tomography (OCT) plays a pivotal role in diagnosing, monitoring, and assessing treatment benefit in different macular conditions such as diabetic and cystoid macular edema (CME), epiretinal membranes, macular holes, vitreomacular traction syndrome, and macular edema secondary to retinal vein occlusions. This noninvasive diagnostic tool can also help in the clinical evaluation and management of hereditary retinal disorders.[1] OCT contributes to our understanding of the histopathology of these disorders by providing high-resolution cross-sectional imaging of the retina and retinal pigment epithelium (RPE)/choriocapillaris.

Retinitis Pigmentosa

Retinitis pigmentosa is one of the most common hereditary retinal disorders seen in clinical practice. Patients with retinitis pigmentosa typically experience nyctalopia and peripheral vision loss. Clinical findings include pale optic nerve heads; attenuated retinal vessels; peripheral pigmentary changes; or bone-spicule formation and peripheral atrophy of the retina, RPE, and choriocapillaris. CME is a common, potentially treatable cause of central visual loss in retinitis pigmentosa. OCT can detect the presence of CME in a noninvasive way and quantify the response to treatment to acetalozamide.[1,2] CME is visualized in OCT as cystic intraretinal spaces of reduced optical reflectivity. In retinitis pigmentosa or rod-cone dystrophies, thinning of the affected neurosensory retina and RPE/choriocapillaris complex may be observed by OCT.[3,4] This atrophy or thinning of the neurosensory retina allows better penetration of light and hence, enhanced reflectivity from the choroid is evident in these cases.[3] The pigmented lesions are seen as hyperreflective areas.[3]

Cone-Rod Dystrophy

Cone-rod dystrophies comprise a heterogeneous group of diseases characterized by cone and rod involvement. The cone involvement is more predominant. Patients with this condition may experience progressive central vision loss, photoaversion, and poor color vision. As the condition progresses, rod dysfunction becomes evident and patients may share symptoms and signs of retinitis pigmentosa, such as nyctalopia, peripheral visual loss, peripheral atrophic changes, and bone-spicule formation. The macular appearance of cone-rod dystrophies may range from central RPE mottling to a bull's eye pattern or more diffuse atrophy. OCT may show central thinning of the neurosensory retina.[5] In 1986, a histopathologic study confirmed the loss of photoreceptor cells in the macular area and the peripheral retina. However, the equatorial retina had a relative preservation of photoreceptors.[6] OCT images of cone-rod dystrophy correlate with these histopathologic findings, revealing disorganization of the outer retinal layers and reduced reflectivity at the level of the outer nuclear layer consistent with the disappearance of photoreceptors.

Stargardt's Disease

Stargardt's disease is also a common hereditary condition that usually affects individuals in their first or second decade of life. Individuals with this disease may present with bilateral yellowish flecks at the level of the RPE and macular atrophic changes. Histopathologic studies reveal accumulation of lipofuscin-like material at the RPE level and loss of RPE and photoreceptor cells.[7] OCT findings correlate with these descriptions and provide an in vivo evaluation of the histopathology of this condition. Patients with Stargardt's disease may show thinning of the affected retina and disorganization and loss of the outer nuclear layer in OCT. Atrophy of the neurosensory retina and RPE lets better light penetration, resulting in increased choroidal reflectivity.

Best's Disease

Best's disease is an inherited macular dystrophy characterized by the presence of bilateral subretinal vitelliform lesions. These vitelliform lesions may progress and evolve over time to an atrophic end-stage. It is not unusual to observe choroidal neovascularization (CNV) in patients with this disorder. Histopathologic reports reveal degeneration of photoreceptors, accumulation of lipofuscin at the level of the RPE, and sub-RPE fibrillar material deposition.[8] Unfortunately, there are no histopathology reports describing the vitelliform stage. OCT contributes to our knowledge of this macular dystrophy by providing high-resolution in vivo imaging of the retina and RPE/choriocapillaris complex. OCT findings seen in Best's disease vary depending of the stage of the condition. The findings described in the literature include elevation and/or splitting of the RPE/choriocapillaris complex. A hyporeflective space is sometimes visualized between the split layers of this complex.[9] Also, central neurosensory retinal detachments like the ones observed in idiopathic central serous chorioretinopathy may be observed.[9,10] Since Best's disease is a dynamic macular dystrophy that evolves into different stages, OCT findings disclose the changing and variegate nature of the disorder. In addition, OCT not only provides an insight into the nature of the disease, it also helps to follow the evolution of the condition. This is particularly important in cases of CNV in which OCT may assist in the assessment of treatment response.[11]

Pattern Dystrophy

Pattern dystrophy is a dominantly inherited macular condition characterized by yellowish deposits at the level of the RPE in the macular region. The configuration of the foveal lesions may present in different patterns, including vitelliform round or oval lesions, reticular, and triradiate or butterfly lesions.[12] OCT findings seen in this condition correlate with the diversity of the clinical presentation. Thickening at the level of the RPE[10] as well as hyperreflective deposits under the neurosensory retina overlying the RPE have been described in the literature.[13] Also, thinning of the neurosensory retina and photoreceptor loss may be observed in the macular area.

X-Linked Juvenile Retinoschisis

X-linked juvenile retinoschisis is a vitreoretinal dystrophy characterized by the presence of foveal schisis in almost all cases and peripheral retinoschisis in approximately 50% of cases.[12] Later in the course of the condition, the cystic macular changes may evolve into atrophic macular changes. Histopathologic reports reveal that the splitting occurs at the nerve fiber layer level, suggesting an abnormality of the Müller cells.[14-16] An intraretinal periodic acid Schiff positive material has been described in areas next to the schitic regions.[16] Cystic changes at the outer retinal layers have been reported not only in the macular region but also in the peripheral schitic area.[17] OCT images of hereditary retinoschisis correlate well with the histopathologic findings. Splitting in the neural retina with bridging retinal elements may be observed.[18] Cystic alterations and schisis cavities may be subtle and difficult to visualize clinically. OCT may depict these subtle changes not apparent on clinical exam.[18] This modality determines the extent of macular involvement and provides precise and objective information that is valuable for surgical intervention. With OCT, monitoring the response to surgery is feasible. Resolution of foveal schisis by OCT after surgery correlates with visual outcome.[19]

References

1. Stanga PE, Downes SM, Ahuja RM, et al. Comparison of optical coherence tomography and fluorescein angiography in assessing macular edema in retinal dystrophies: preliminary results. *Int Ophthalmol*. 2001;23(4-6):321-325.
2. Rumen F, Souied E, Oubraham H, Coscas G, Soubrane G. Optical coherence tomography in the follow up of macular edema treatment in retinitis pigmentosa. *J Fr Ophthalmol*. 2001;24(8):854-859.
3. Hamada S, Yoshida K, Chihara E. Optical coherence tomography images of retinitis pigmentosa. *Ophthalmic Surg Lasers*. 2000;31(3):253-256.

4. Jacobson SG, Buraczynska M, Milam AH, et al. Disease expression in X-linked retinitis pigmentosa caused by a putative null mutation in the RPGR gene. *Invest Ophthalmol Vis Sci*. 1997;38(10):1983-1997.
5. Jacobson SG, Cideciyan AV, Huang Y, et al. Retinal degenerations with truncation mutations in the cone-rod homeobox (CRX) gene. *Invest Ophthalmol Vis Sci*. 1998;39(12): 2417-2426.
6. Rabb MF, Tso MO, Fishman GA. Cone-rod dystrophy. A clinical and histopathologic report. *Ophthalmology*. 1986; 93(11):1443-1451.
7. Birnbach CD, Jarvelainen M, Possin DE, Milam AH. Histopathology and immunocytochemistry of the neurosensory retina in fundus flavimaculatus. *Ophthalmology*. 1994;101(7):1211-1219.
8. Frangieh GT, Green WR, Fine SL. A histopathologic study of Best's macular dystrophy. *Arch Ophthalmol*. 1982;100(7): 1115-1121.
9. Pianta MJ, Aleman TS, Cideciyan AV, et al. In vivo micropathology of Best macular dystrophy with optical coherence tomography. *Exp Eye Res*. 2003;76(2):203-211.
10. Pierro L, Tremolada G, Introini U, Calori G, Brancato R. Optical coherence tomography findings in adult-onset foveomacular vitelliform dystrophy. *Am J Ophthalmol*. 2002;134(5):675-680.
11. Andrade RE, Farah ME, Cardillo JA, Hofling-Lima AL, Uno F, Costa RA. Optical coherence tomography in choroidal neovascular membrane associated with Best's vitelliform dystrophy. *Acta Ophthalmol Scand*. 2002;80(2): 216-218.
12. Gass JDM. *Stereoscopic Atlas of Macular Diseases*. 4th ed. St. Louis, Mo: CV Mosby; 1997:314-325, 374-376.
13. Benhamou N, Souied EH, Zolf R, Coscas F, Coscas G, Soubrane G. Adult-onset foveomacular vitelliform dystrophy: a study by optical coherence tomography. *Am J Ophthalmol*. 2003;135(3):362-367.
14. Manschot WA. Pathology of hereditary juvenile retinoschisis. *Arch Ophthalmol*. 1972;88:131-138.
15. Yanoff M, Rahn EK, Zimmerman LE. Histopathology of juvenile retinoschisis. *Arch Ophthalmol*. 1968;79:49-53.
16. Condon GP, Brownstein S, Wang NS, Kearns JA, Ewing CC. Congenital hereditary (juvenile X-linked) retinoschisis. Histopathologic and ultrastructural findings in three eyes. *Arch Ophthalmol*. 1986;104(4):576-583.
17. Ando A, Takahashi K, Sho K, Matsushima M, Okamura A, Uyama M. Histopathological findings of X-linked retinoschisis with neovascular glaucoma. *Graefes Arch Clin Exp Ophthalmol*. 2000;238(1):1-7.
18. Stanga PE, Chong VNH, Reck AC, Hardcastle AJ, Holder GE. Optical coherence tomography and electrophysiology in X-linked juvenile retinoschisis associated with a novel mutation in the XLRS1 gene. *Retina*. 2001;21:78-80.
19. Azzolini C, Pierro L, Codenotti M, Brancato R. OCT images and surgery of juvenile macular retinoschisis. *Eur J Ophthalmol*. 1997;7(2):196-200.

Case 10-1A. Retinitis Pigmentosa

Clinical Summary

A 17-year-old man with a history of retinitis pigmentosa (RP) was examined. His visual acuity was 20/40 in the right eye. Dilated fundus examination of this eye revealed slightly attenuated retinal vessels and mottling with patches of atrophic RPE throughout the midperiphery and periphery. In addition to the "moth-eaten" appearance, relative preservation of the RPE adjacent to the retinal vessels was observed consistent with the preserved para-arteriolar RPE variety of RP. The macula revealed cystic intraretinal changes (A). Fluorescein angiography (FA) (B) showed faint areas of perifoveal hyperfluorescence associated with late leakage as the angiogram progressed into late frames.

Optical Coherence Tomography

OCT (C) illustrated cystic areas of low reflectivity in the outer plexiform layer consistent with CME. Retinal map analysis showed a foveal thickness of 635 microns (μm) in this eye (D).

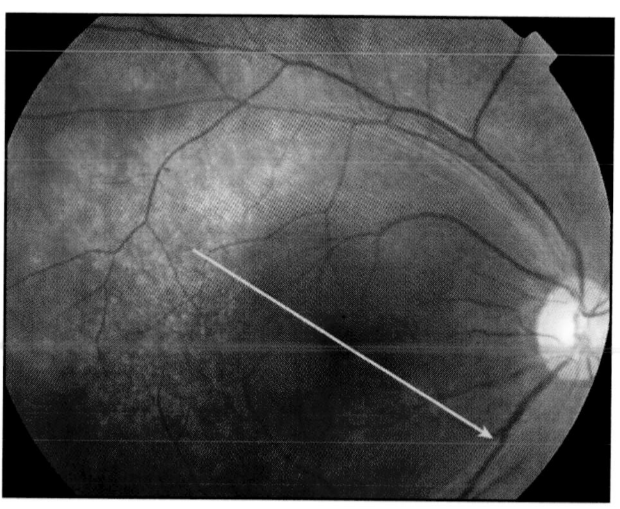

A

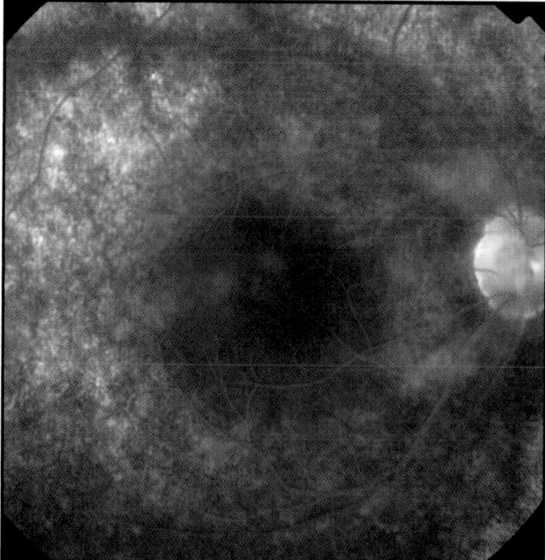

B—Early

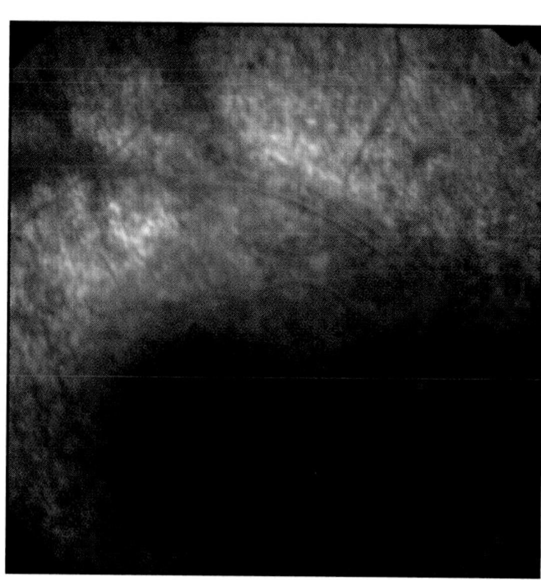

B—Late

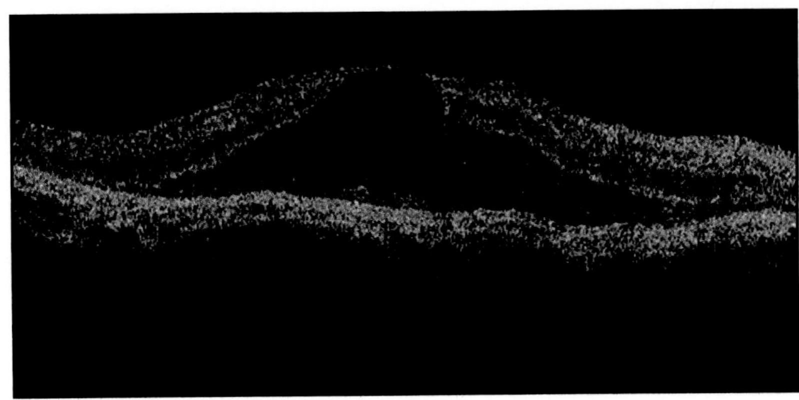

C

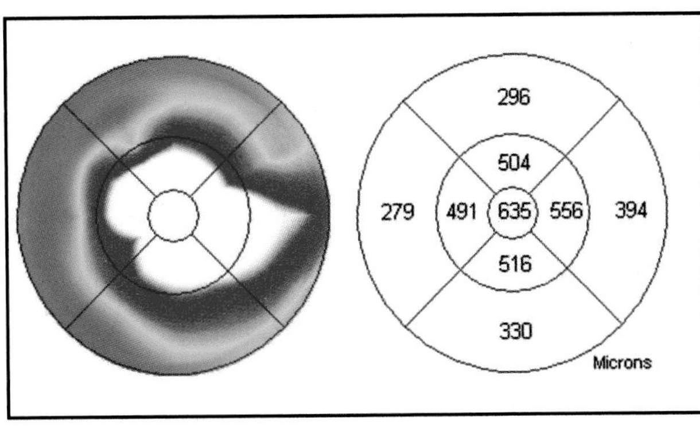

D

Case 10-1B. Retinitis Pigmentosa

Clinical Summary

Evaluation of the patient's left eye revealed the same findings (E). Visual acuity was 20/50 in this eye. Again, FA (F) showed late leakage consistent with macular edema.

Optical Coherence Tomography

An OCT scan obtained through the fovea (G) also showed big spaces of reduced reflectivity at the level of the outer plexiform layer representing CME. The foveal thickness measured 546 µm (H).

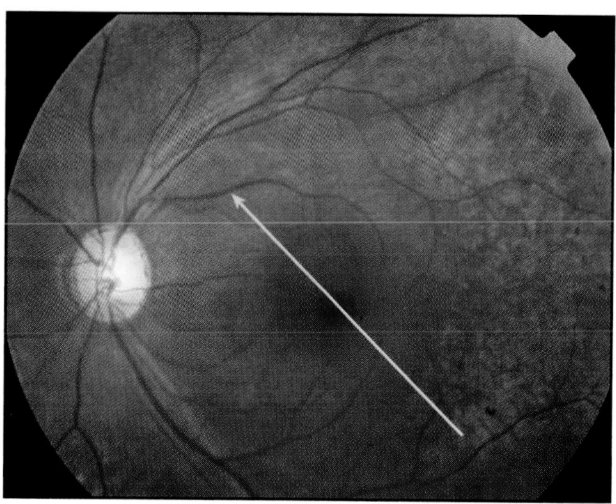

E

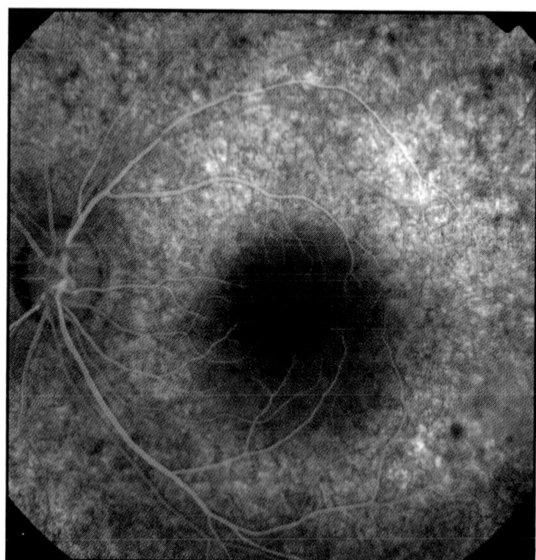

F—Early

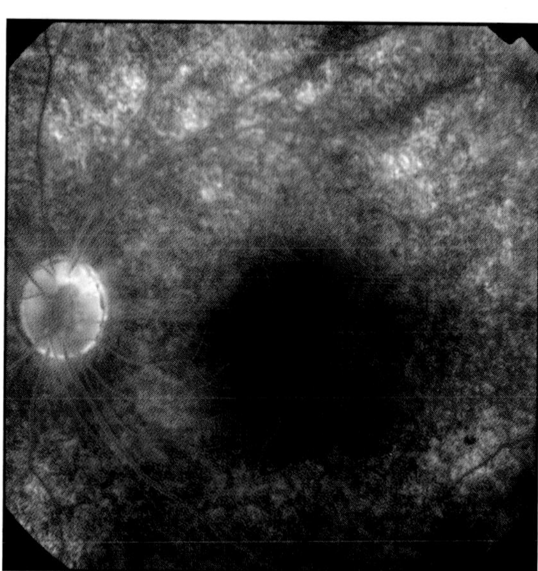

F—Late

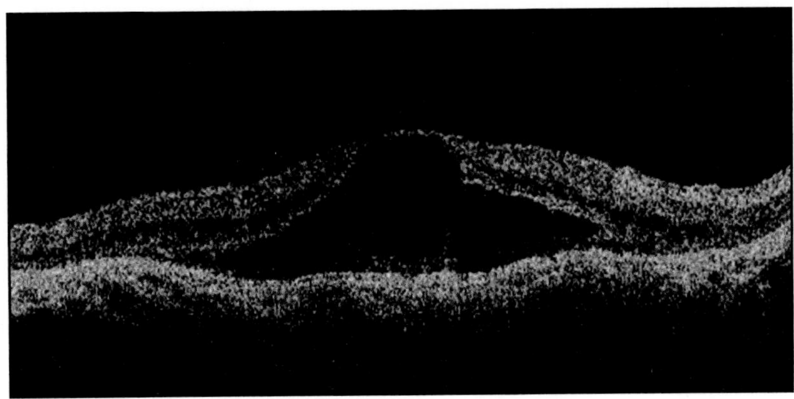

G

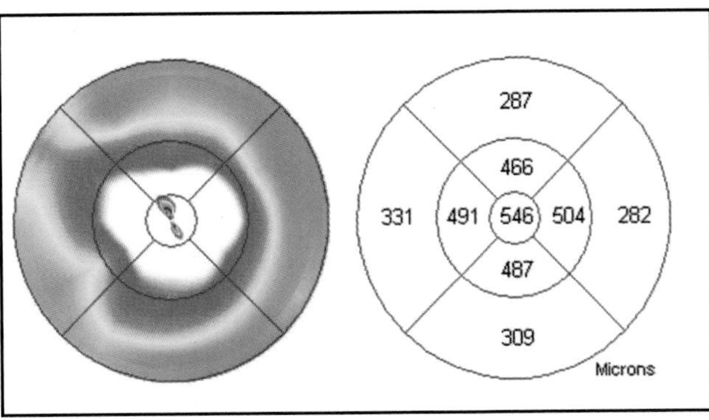

H

Case 10-2A. Retinitis Pigmentosa

Clinical Summary

A 43-year-old man complained of bilateral peripheral visual loss and central distortion. His visual acuity was 20/50 in the right eye. Examination revealed attenuated retinal vessels, cystic macular changes, and peripheral retinal and RPE atrophy (A). Bone-spicule formation was observed beyond the equator (B). Full-field ERG revealed markedly reduced and prolonged photopic and scotopic responses consistent with RP.

Optical Coherence Tomography

An OCT scan obtained through the fovea (C) showed optically clear cystic spaces representing CME. The central macular thickness measured 411 μm (D). A scan obtained through an atrophic area inferotemporal to the fovea (E) revealed decreased thickness of the neurosensory retina. This retinal tissue loss allowed increased light penetration into the choroid. The choroidal vessels were seen as dark hyporeflective circles beneath the highly reflective band (choriocapillaris/choroid complex). A scan obtained superiorly to the fovea in the midperiphery (F) again confirmed the presence of retinal thinning and increased reflectivity from the choroid.

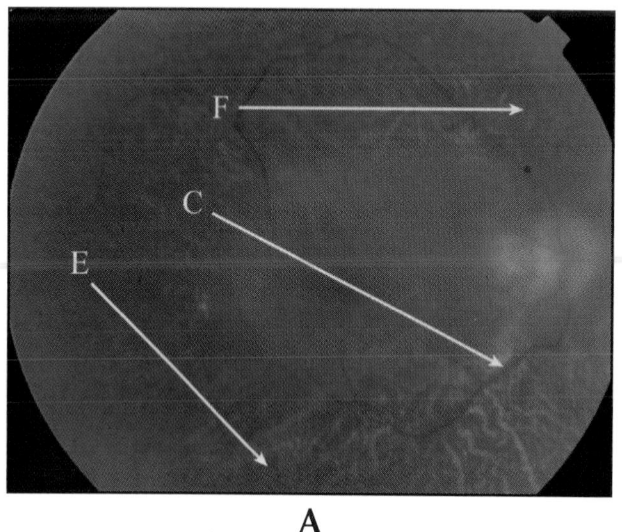

A

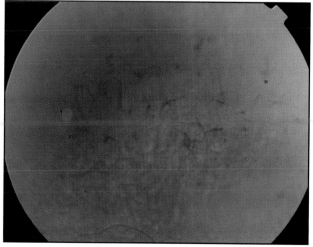

B

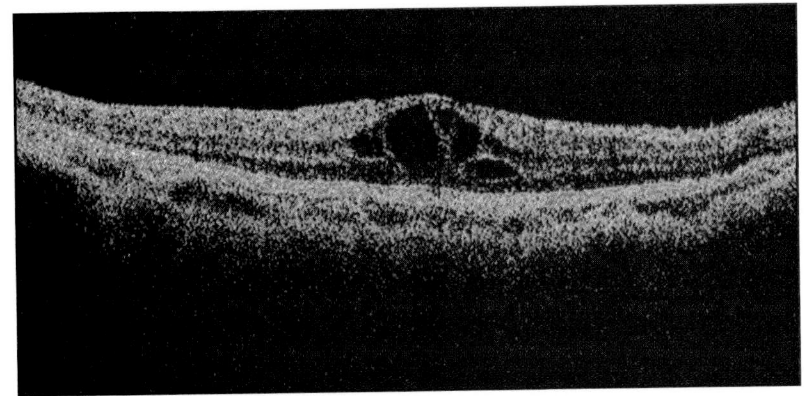

C

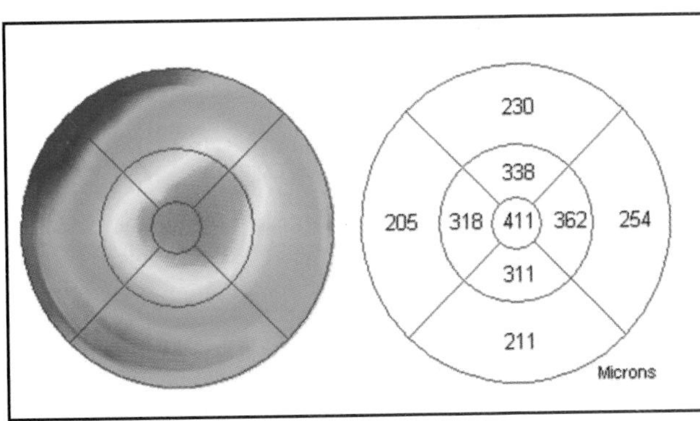

D

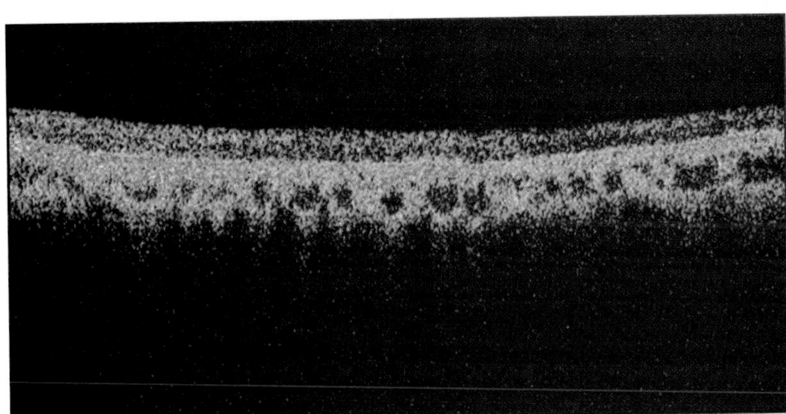

E

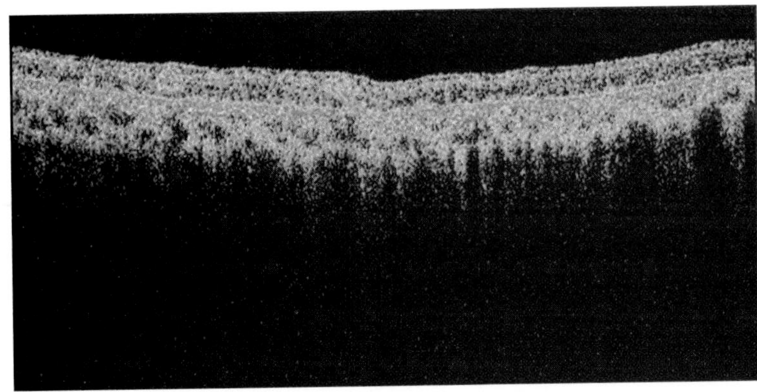

F

Case 10-2B. Retinitis Pigmentosa

Clinical Summary

Evaluation of the patient's left eye revealed the same clinical findings (G and H). Visual acuity measured 20/25 in this eye.

Optical Coherence Tomography

An OCT scan obtained through the fovea (I) revealed central thickening and spaces of low optical reflectivity consistent with CME. However, the degree of macular edema is less prominent in this eye than in the right eye as evidenced by the retinal map analysis, which showed a foveal thickness of 328 μm (J). OCT scans obtained in atrophic regions inferior (K) and temporal the fovea (L) showed a remarkable reduced retinal thickness with enhanced reflections from the choroid. Again, the choroidal vessels were visualized as dark round spaces. The reduced reflectance from the neurosensory retina corresponded to the degree of cellular loss principally in the outer layers. Loss of the RPE layer was also noted.

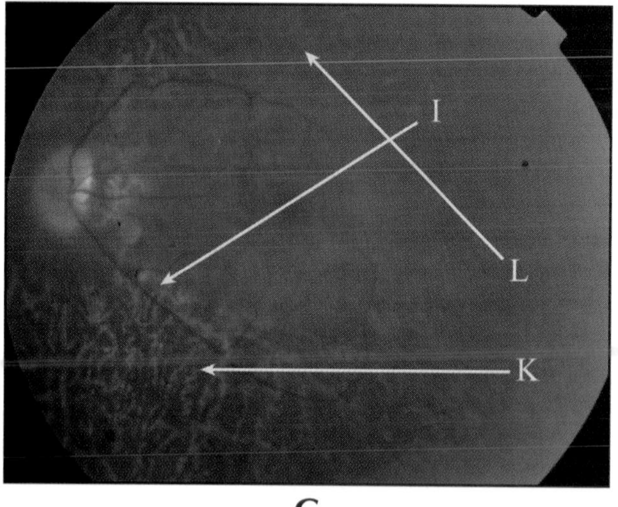

G

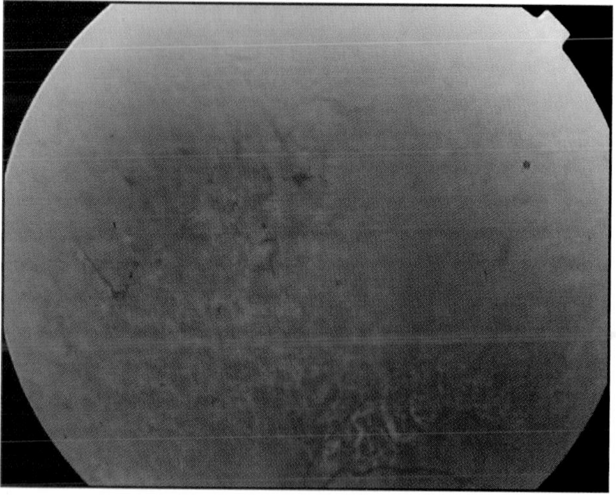

H

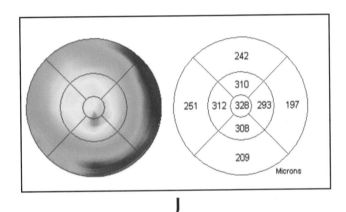

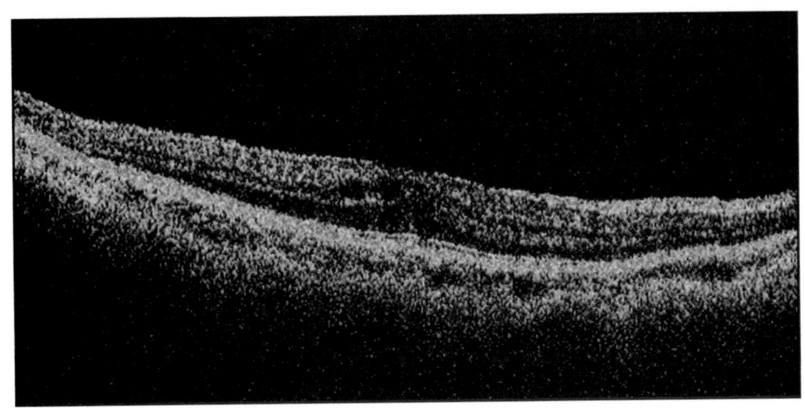

I

242
310
251 312 328 293 197
308
209
Microns

J

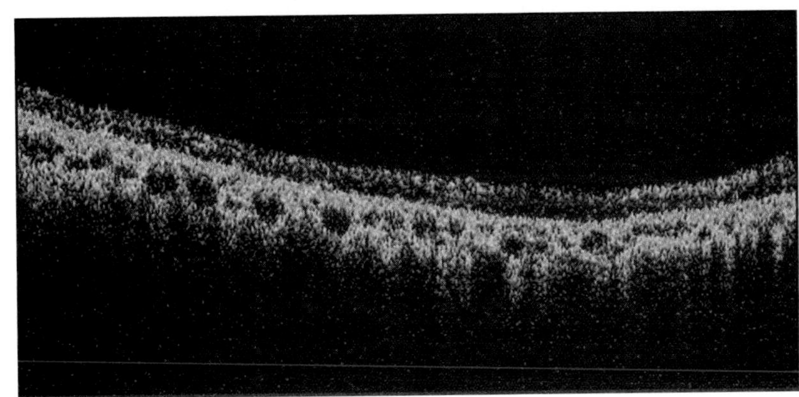

K

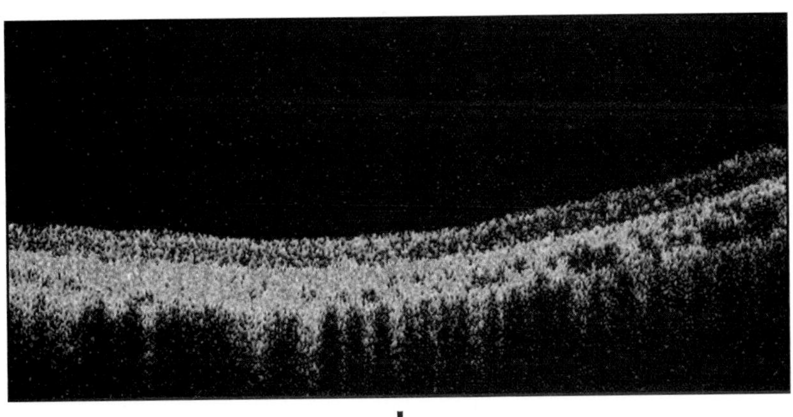

L

Case 10-3A. Retinitis Punctata Albescens

Clinical Summary

A 10-year-old girl with a history of retinitis punctata albescens was examined. Her visual acuity was 20/25 in the right eye. Retinal examination of the right eye revealed wrinkling of the internal limiting membrane in the posterior pole and cystoid macular changes (A). Mottling and patchy atrophic alterations were visualized throughout the midperiphery and periphery. White dots were observed scattered throughout the fundus (B, C, and D).

Optical Coherence Tomography

OCT (E) depicted loss of the normal foveal contour and cystic areas of reduced reflectivity at the level of the outer plexiform layer consistent with CME. The central macular thickness measured 362 μm in this eye (F).

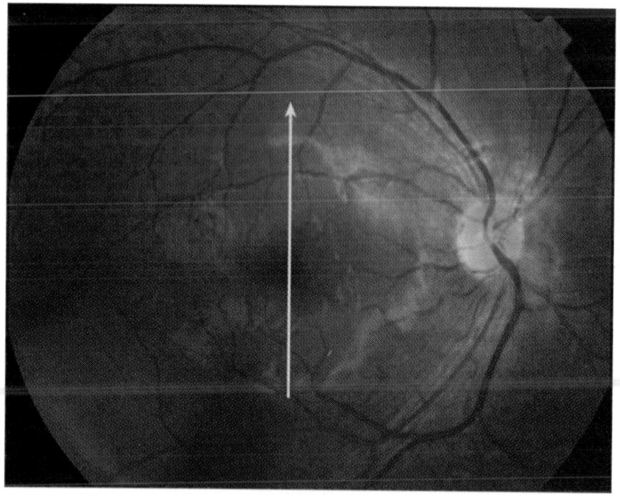

A

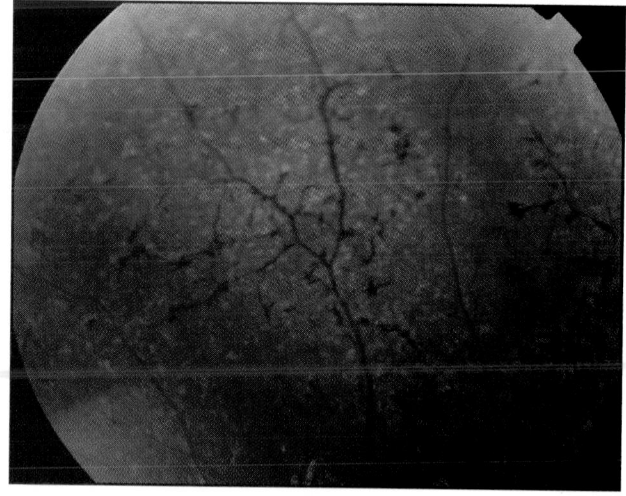

B

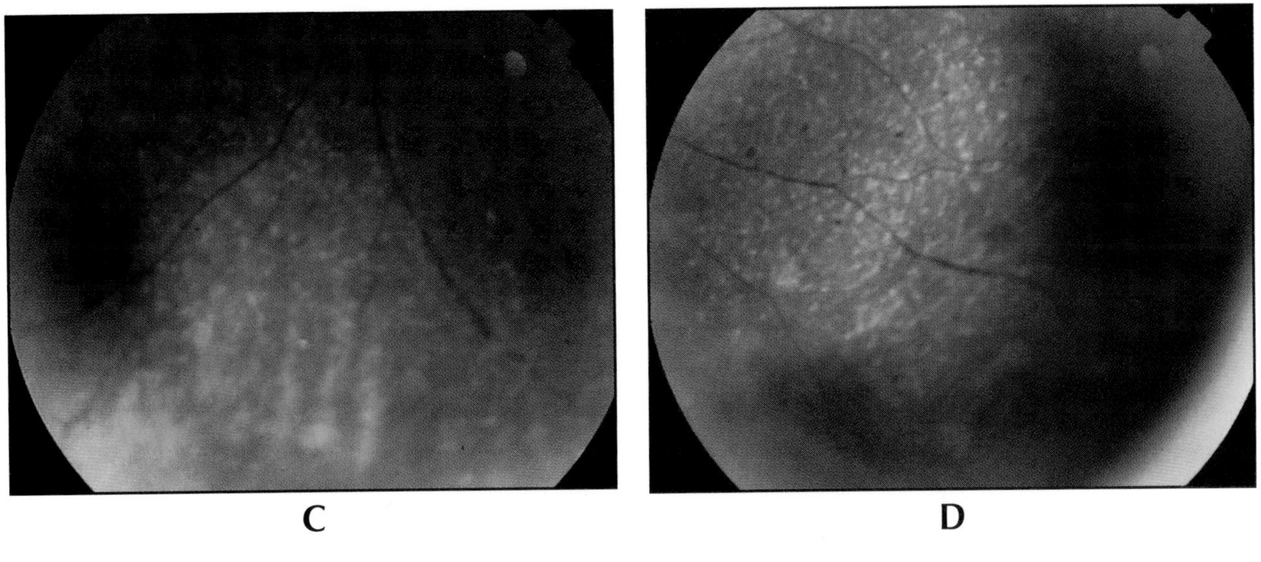

C D

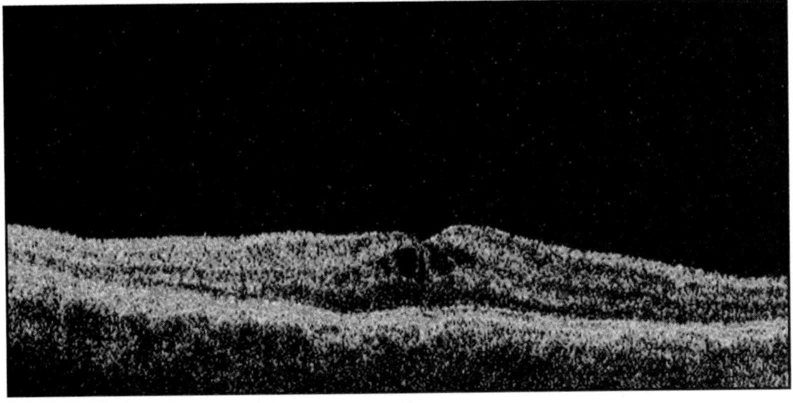

E

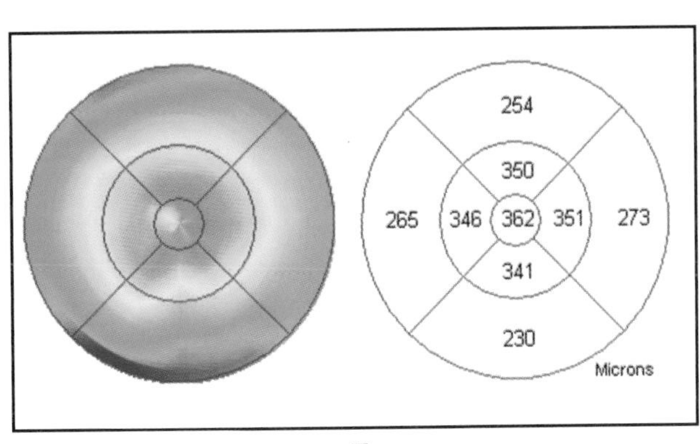

F

Case 10-3B. Retinitis Punctata Albescens

Clinical Summary

Evaluation of the patient's left eye revealed the same clinical findings (G to J). Visual acuity measured 20/20 in this eye.

Optical Coherence Tomography

An OCT scan obtained through the fovea (K) showed tiny low reflective cystic spaces representing CME. The foveal thickness measured 322 μm (L).

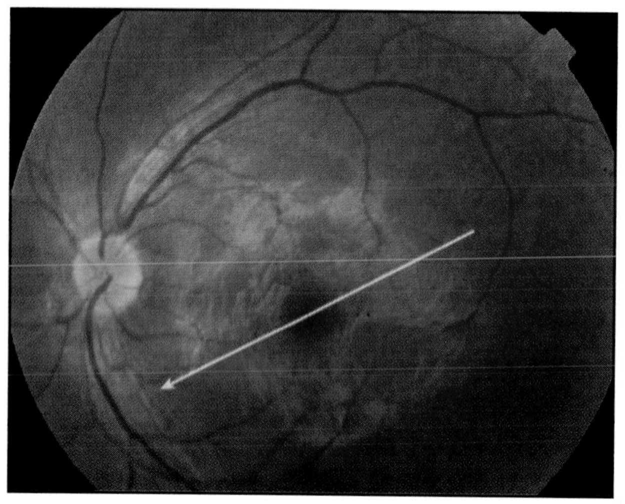

G

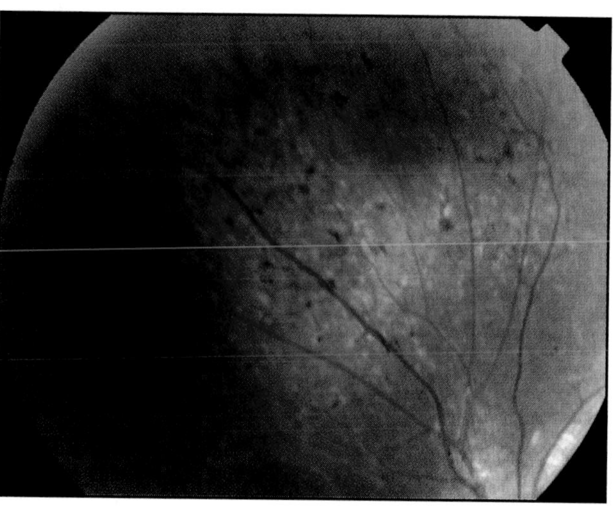

H

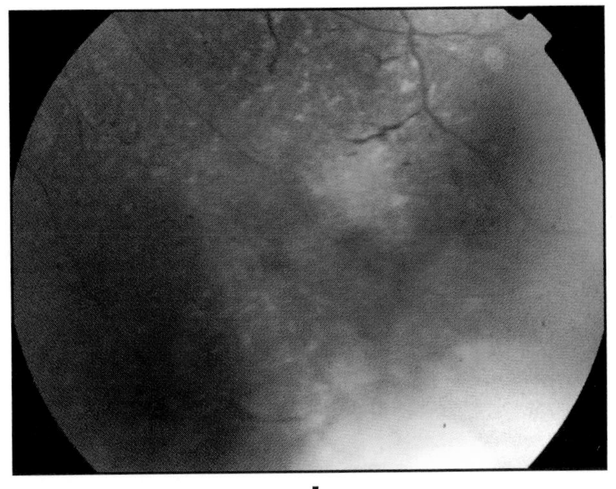

I

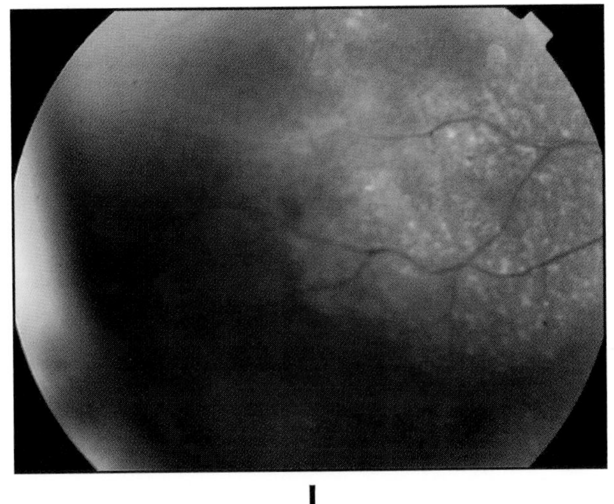

J

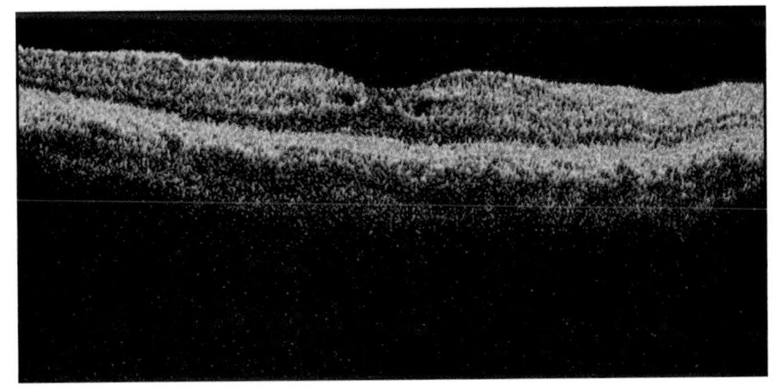

K

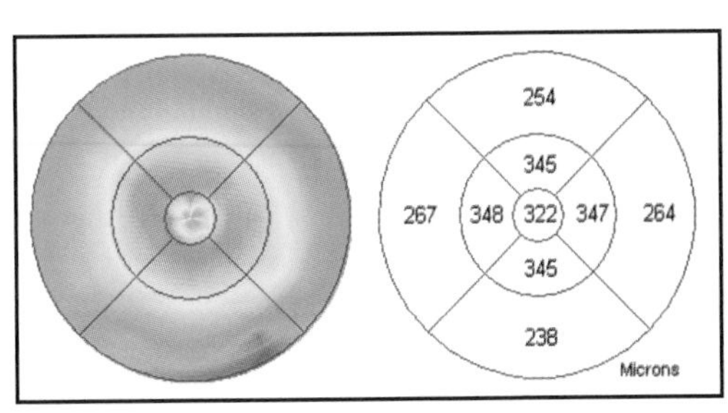

L

Case 10-4A.
Rod-Cone Dystrophy

Clinical Summary

A 47-year-old man was diagnosed with rod-cone dystrophy. His visual acuity was 20/50 in the right eye. Retinal examination of this eye revealed a slight optic nerve pallor, attenuation of retinal vessels, and RPE atrophy more prominently seen in the macular area. The macula also showed some cystic alterations (A). FA (B) showed staining and window defects corresponding to the areas of RPE atrophy.

Optical Coherence Tomography

Despite the fact that no obvious dye leakage was appreciated in FA, a horizontal OCT scan (C) showed cystic spaces of reduced reflectivity in the outer retinal layers consistent with CME. The perifoveal area surrounding the central cystic fovea showed enhanced reflectivity of the choroid due to increased optical penetration in this atrophic area. The central macular thickness was 409 μm. The perifoveal area was thin, with a thickness ranging from 188 μm to 232 μm (D).

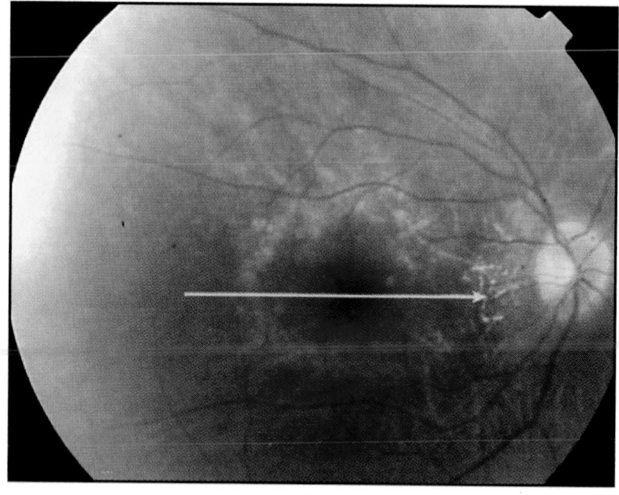

A

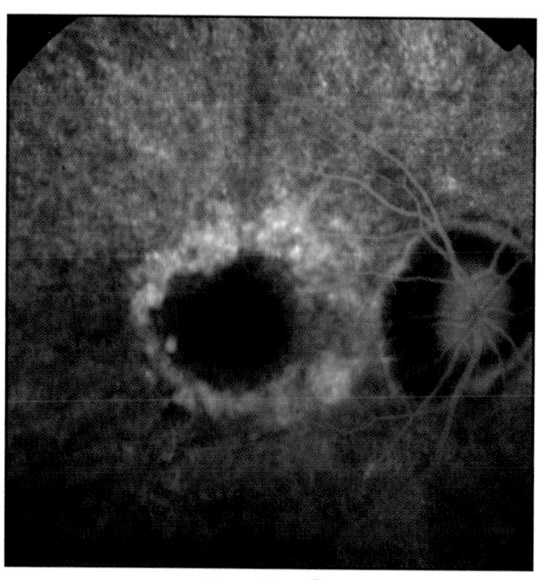

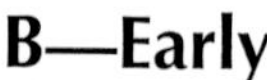

B—Early

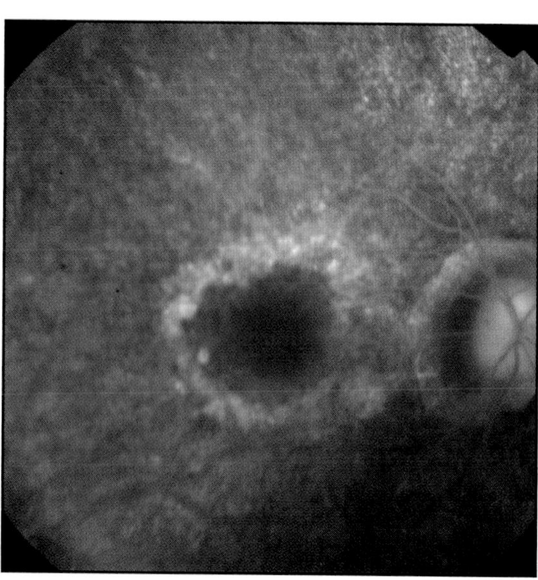

B—Late

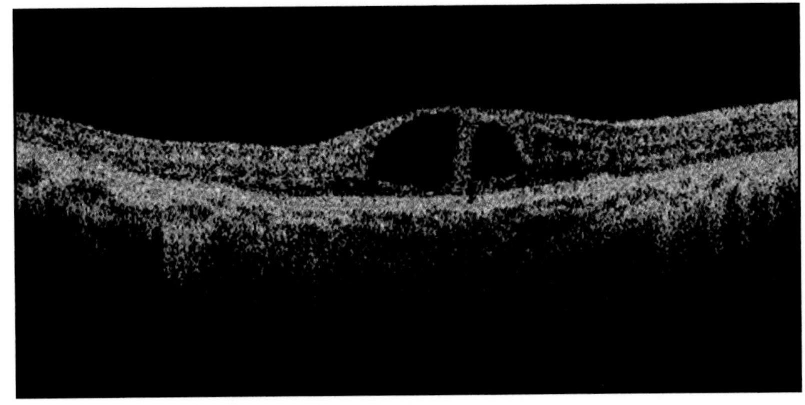

C

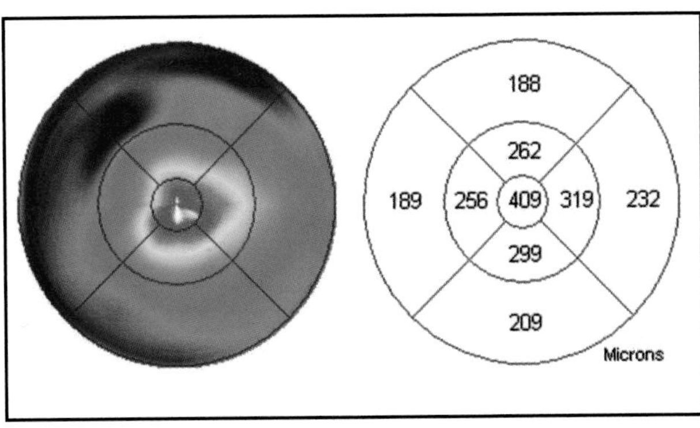

D

Case 10-4B. Rod-Cone Dystrophy

Clinical Summary

The left eye showed similar findings (E). The vision was 20/40 in this eye. FA (F) revealed window defects consistent with RPE atrophy in the macular area but no apparent leakage.

Optical Coherence Tomography

A horizontal OCT scan (G) obtained through the fovea revealed intraretinal fluid accumulation represented by cystic spaces of reduced reflectivity. Enhanced choroidal reflectivity secondary to increased light penetration was appreciated in the perimacular area, which correlates with the aforementioned atrophic alterations. The retinal map analysis showed a central foveal thickness of 351 μm. The perimacular ring measured from 196 μm to 241 μm in thickness (H).

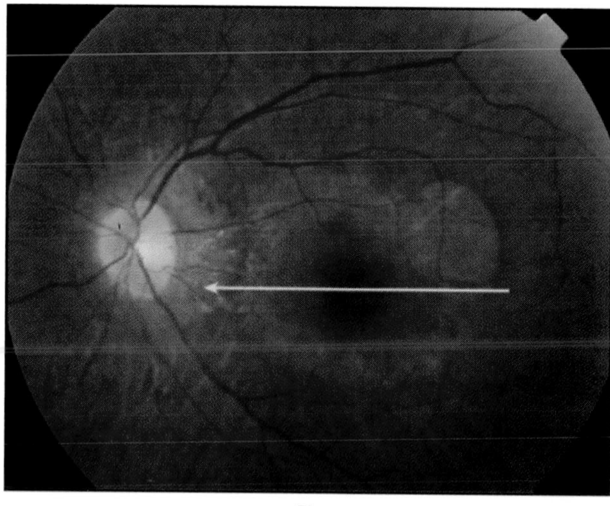

E

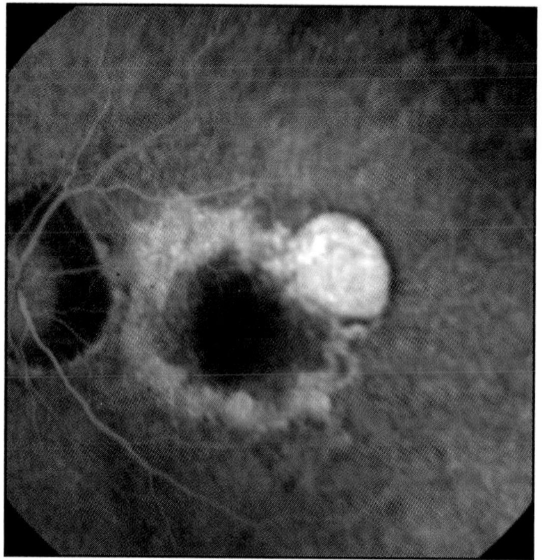

F—Early

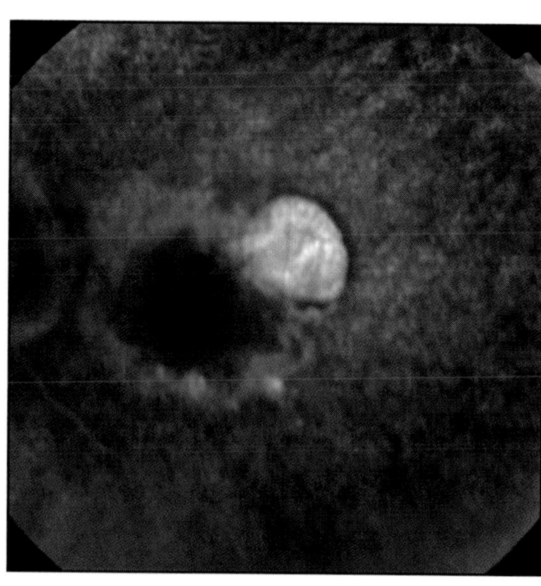

F—Late

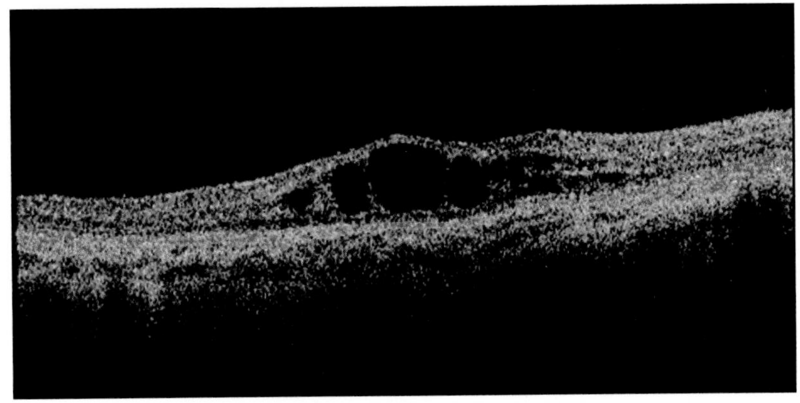

G

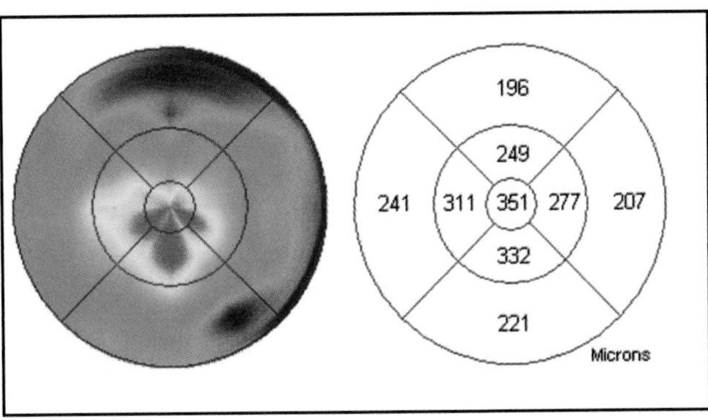

H

Case 10-5A. Cone-Rod Dystrophy

Clinical Summary

A 51-year-old woman was referred for retinal evaluation of pigmentary macular changes. She was asymptomatic, and her best-corrected visual acuity (BCVA) measured 20/30 in the right eye. Dilated fundus examination showed an annular area of hypopigmentation surrounding the fovea consistent with a bull's eye appearance. A darkly pigmented flat lesion was noticed inferotemporal to the fovea consistent with a choroidal nevus (A). FA (B) revealed an oval area of hyperfluorescence corresponding to the hypopigmented ring surrounding the central region of hypofluorescence. Full-field electroretinogram showed rod-cone dysfunction, and multifocal ERG responses were decreased especially centrally. A diagnosis of cone-rod dystrophy was established.

Optical Coherence Tomography

OCT (C) showed blunting of the foveal contour with thinning of the retinal tissue. Decreased reflectivity and loss or disorganization of the normal retinal architecture was visualized in the outer retinal layers of the foveal center, probably representing partial loss of the photoreceptor layer. The inferotemporal choroidal nevus (left side of the scan) showed increased choroidal reflectivity. The retinal map analysis showed a central thickness of 216 μm (D).

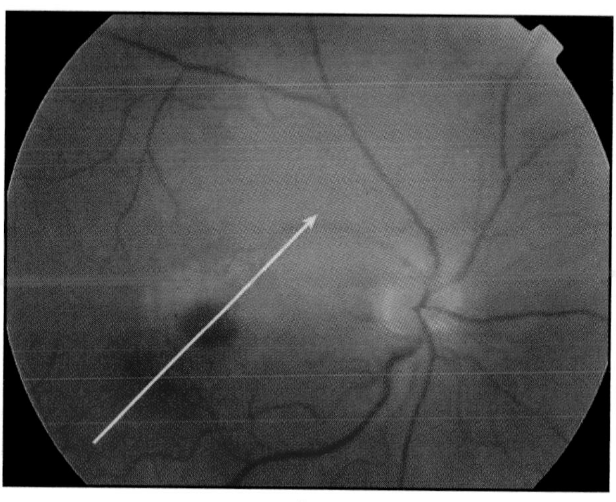

A

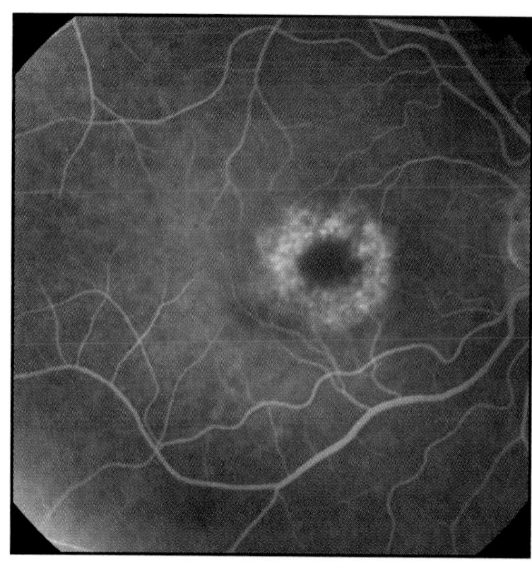

B—Early

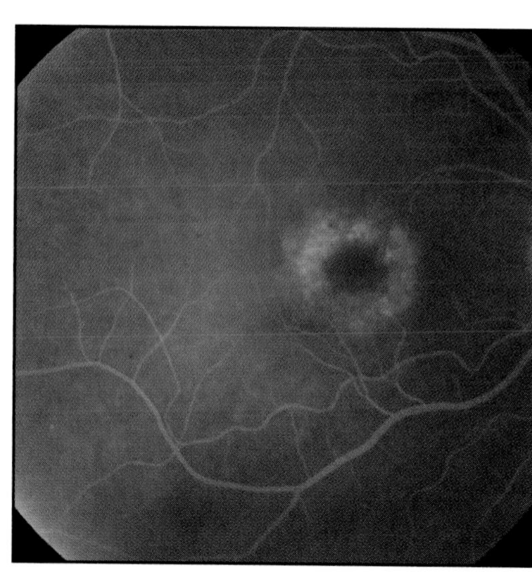

B—Late

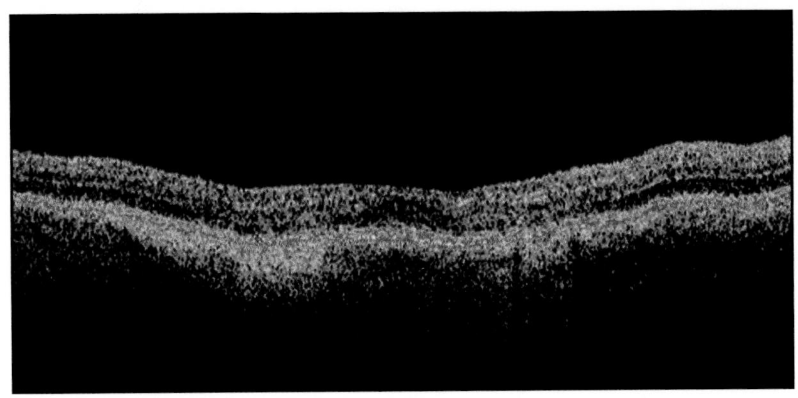

C

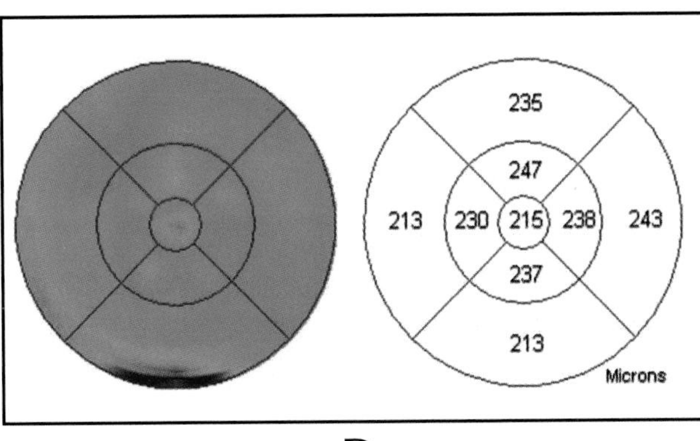

D

Case 10-5B. Cone-Rod Dystrophy

Clinical Summary

Vision in the left eye measured 20/25. A bull's eye maculopathy was observed on examination (E). FA of the left eye (F) revealed the same pattern of hypofluorescence surrounded by hyperfluorescence. Electrophysiologic studies were compatible with cone-rod dystrophy.

Optical Coherence Tomography

OCT scan (G) showed retinal thinning, blunting of the foveal pit, and disappearance of the outer nuclear layer. The foveal center measured 215 μm (H).

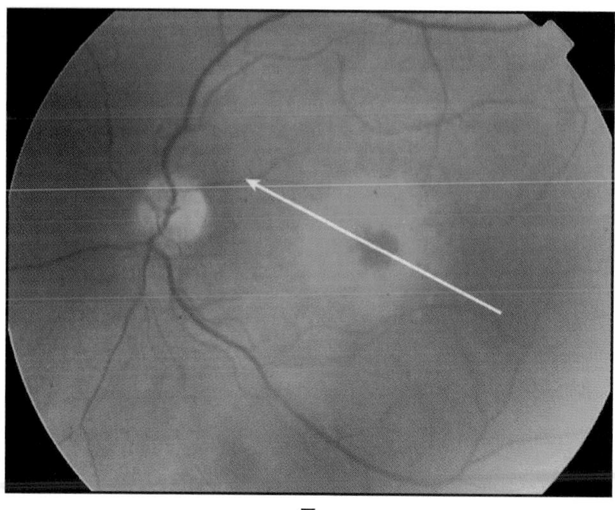

E

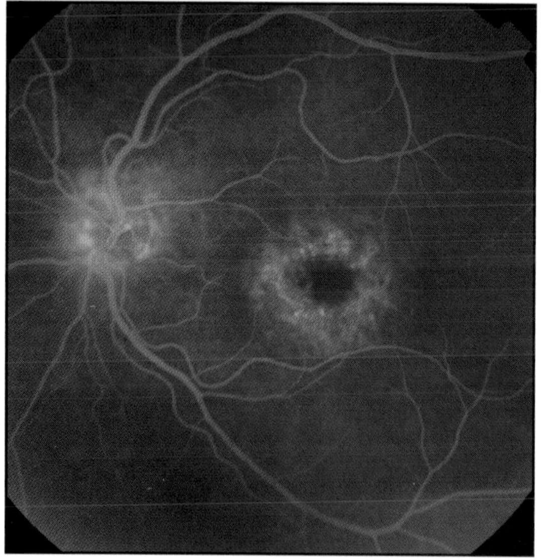

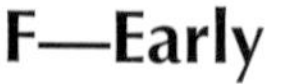

F—Early

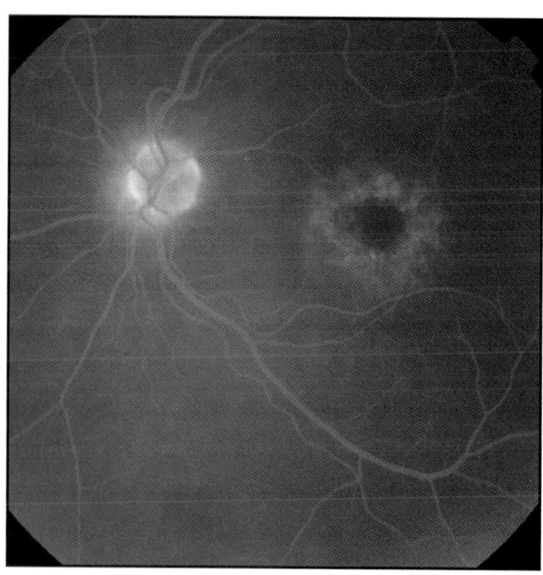

F—Late

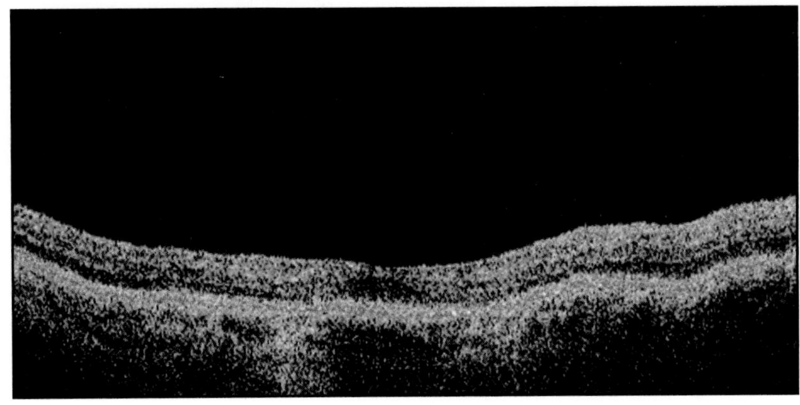

G

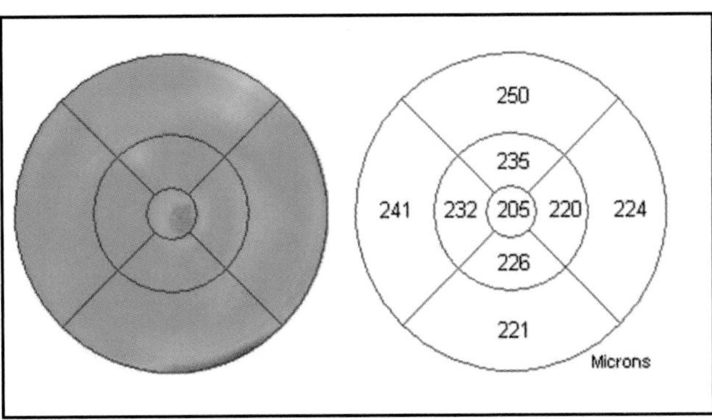

H

Case 10-6A. Stargardt's Disease

Clinical Summary

A 61-year-old man with a history of Stargardt's disease was examined. His visual acuity was 4/200 in the right eye. Fundus examination showed disciform yellowish flecks encircling the arcades and patches of RPE atrophy. The macula was notable for central geographic atrophy with pigment clumping (A).

Optical Coherence Tomography

A horizontal OCT scan obtained through the fovea (B) showed marked thinning of the neurosensory retina. Enhanced reflectivity from the choroid was evident especially centrally as atrophic areas allowed better penetration of light. Partial loss of the outer nuclear layer (nuclei of photoreceptors) was observed. An intraretinal hyperreflective central dot was observed corresponding to pigment metaplasia. The foveal thickness measured 178 μm (C).

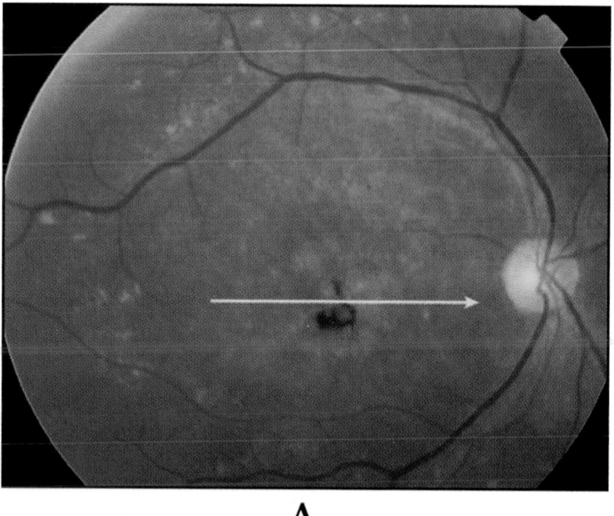

A

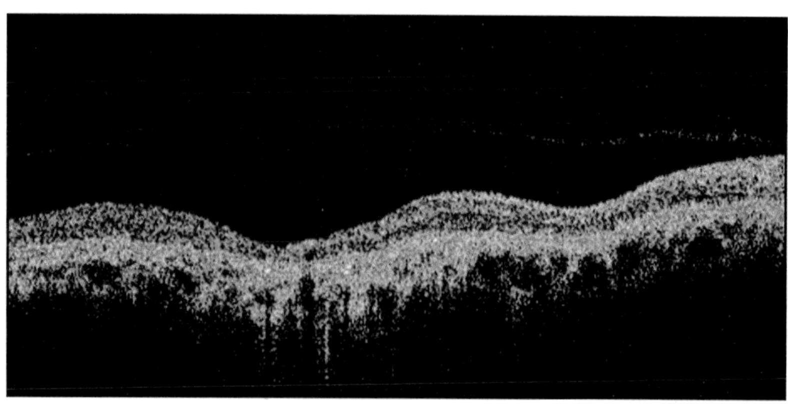

B

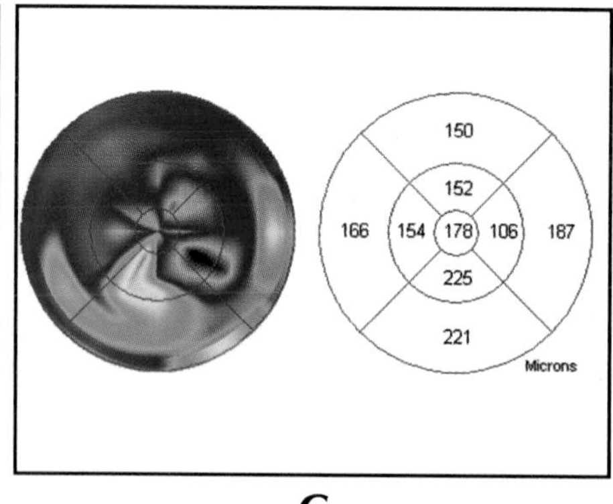

C

Case 10-6B. Stargardt's Disease

Clinical Summary

The patient's left eye had a visual acuity of 20/400. Retinal examination also showed scattered triradiate flecks and a "beaten metal" atrophic macular appearance (D).

Optical Coherence Tomography

An OCT scan (E) was obtained slightly off set to include the area superonasal to the fovea. Thinned neurosensory retina was observed. Increased choroidal reflectivity was evident under the macula correlating with the atrophic central region previously described. The choroidal reflectivity was not enhanced in the area superonasal to the fovea because this region, although thin, is not markedly atrophic. Partial disorganization of the photoreceptor nuclear layer was observed. The foveal center measured 199 μm (F).

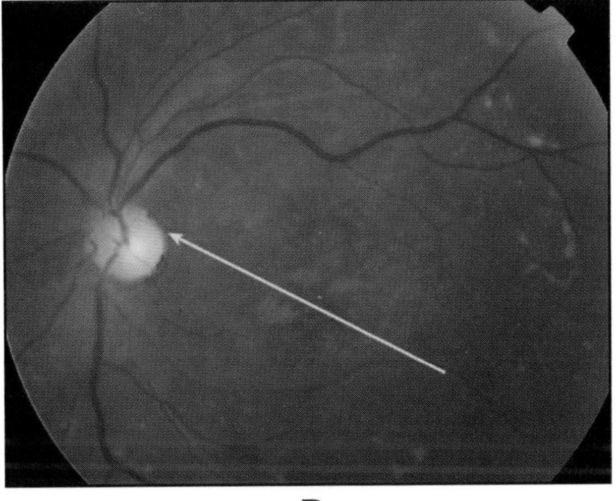

D

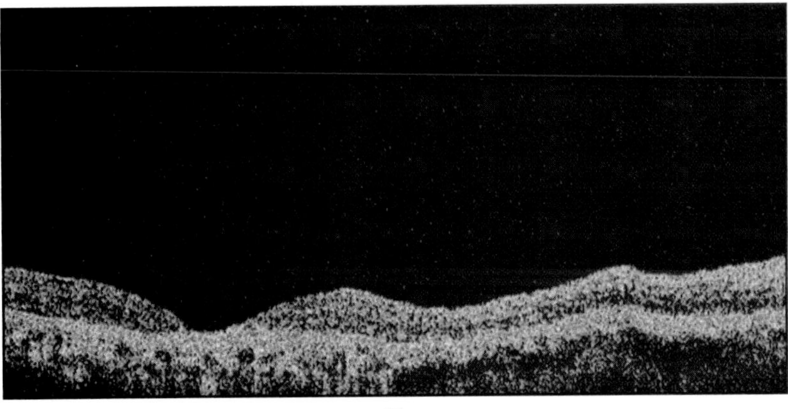

E

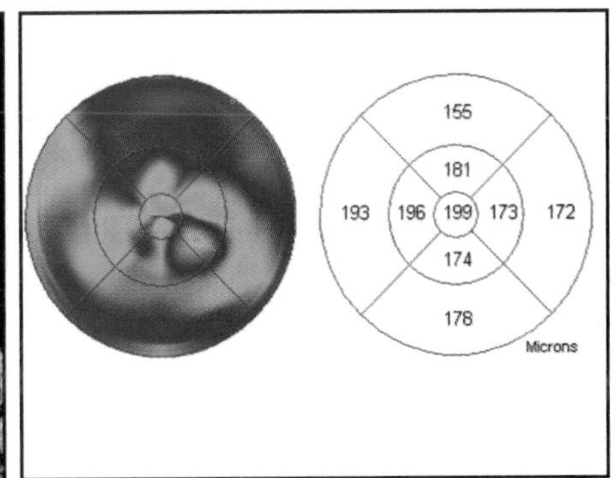

F

Case 10-7A. Stargardt's Disease

Clinical Summary

A 35-year-old man was diagnosed with Stargardt's disease. His visual acuity was 20/400 in the right eye. Retinal examination showed striking hyperplasia of the RPE surrounded by a border of RPE atrophy (A). FA (B) revealed a central area of blocked fluorescence corresponding to the pigment accumulation surrounded by staining and window defects from the atrophic RPE.

Optical Coherence Tomography

OCT obtained through the fovea (C) showed remarkable thinning of the neurosensory retina. Retinal hyporeflectivity was evident especially at the level of the photoreceptor nuclear layer, which correlates with the degree of cellular loss and the histopathology reports in the literature. Atrophy of the outer retinal layers, as well as of the RPE, enhanced light penetration, resulting in increased optical reflectivity from the choroid. The foveal thickness measured 105 μm (D).

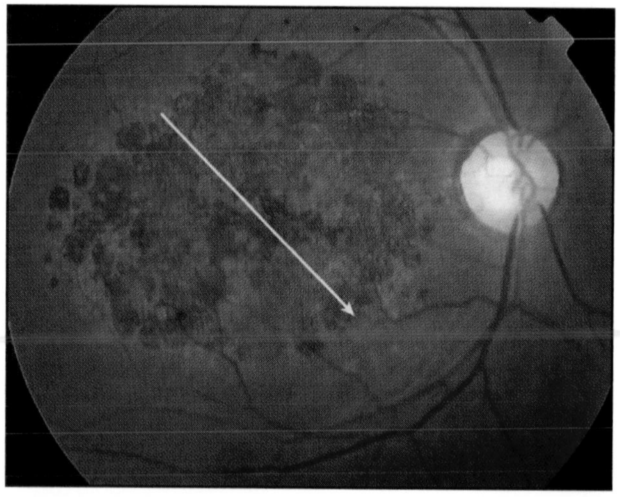

A

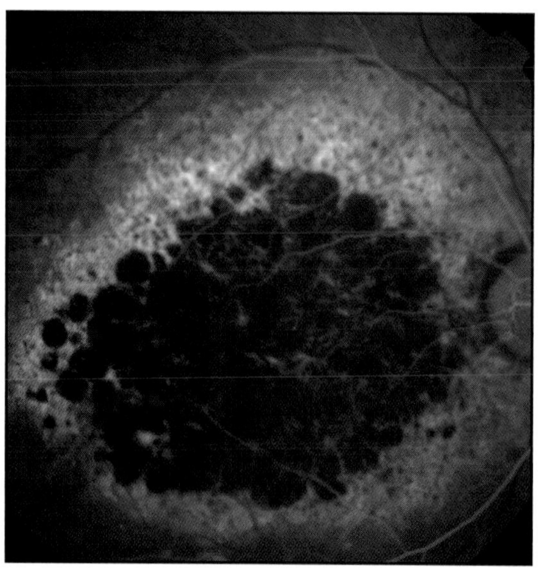

B—Early

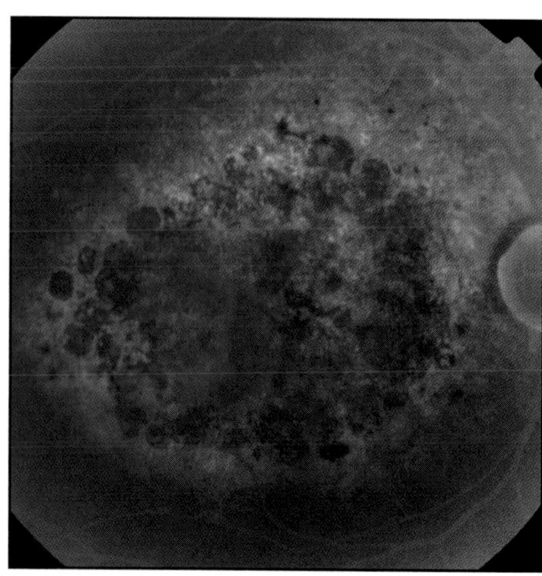

B—Late

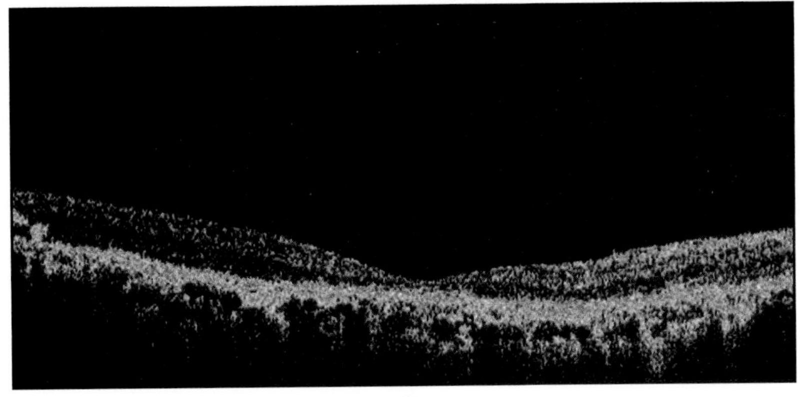

C

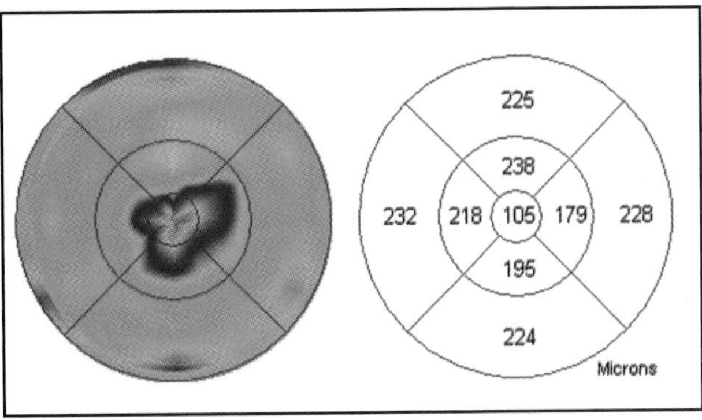

D

Case 10-7B. Stargardt's Disease

Clinical Summary

Examination of the left eye again revealed end-stage maculopathy characterized by hyperpigmented and hypopigmented areas (E). The visual acuity was 20/400 in this eye. FA (F) was alike in this eye.

Optical Coherence Tomography

OCT scan (G) illustrated a very atrophic neurosensory retina and enhanced optical reflectivity from the choroid. The outer nuclear layer was hyporeflective probably due to loss of photoreceptors. The retinal map analysis showed a central thickness of 96 μm (H).

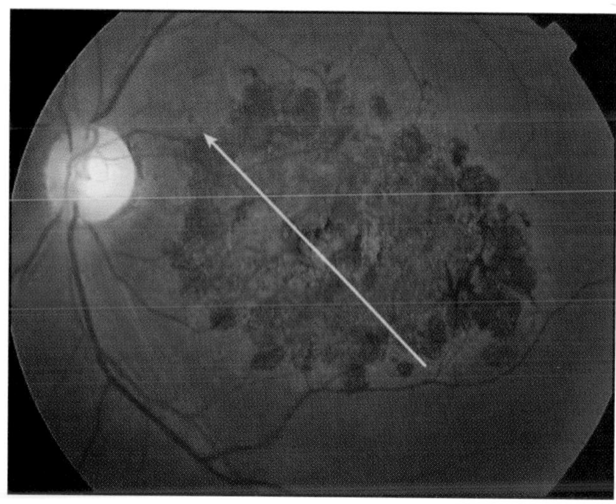

E

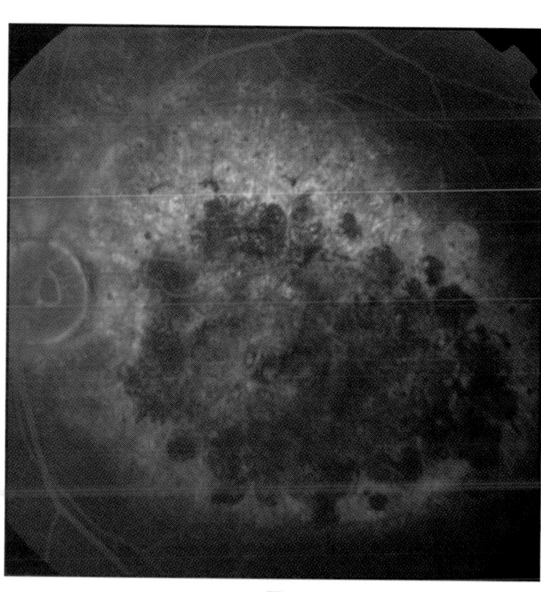

F

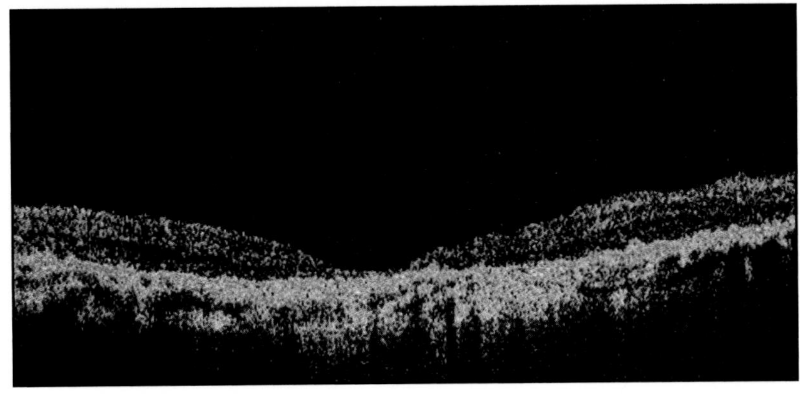

G

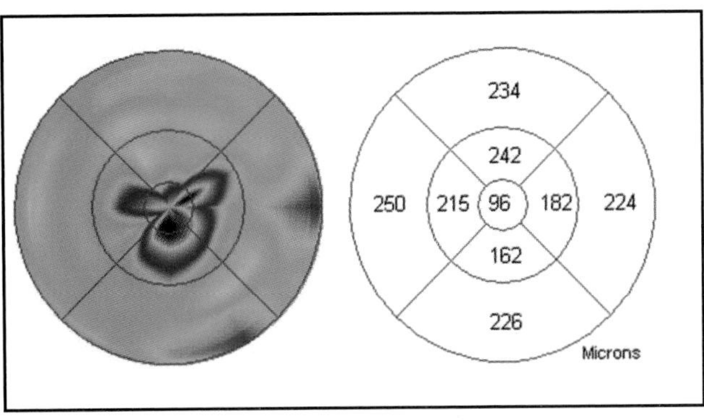

H

Case 10-8A. Stargardt's Disease

Clinical Summary

A 67-year-old woman complained of a gradual and bilateral decrease in vision. Her visual acuity was 20/200 in the right eye. Dilated fundus examination showed a central macular area of RPE atrophy with a beaten-bronze appearance. Scattered yellowish flecks were seen throughout the posterior pole (A). FA (B) revealed a central window RPE defect associated with late staining. A silent choroid was evident. A diagnosis of Stargardt's disease was made.

Optical Coherence Tomography

OCT obtained through the fovea (C) showed striking thinning and atrophy of the neurosensory retina. This marked retinal thinning allowed better light penetration, resulting in increased reflectivity from the choroidal tissue. The central macular thickness measured 113 µm (D).

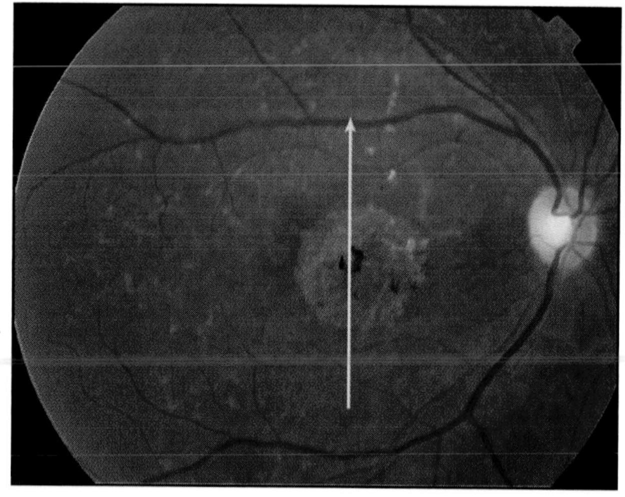

A

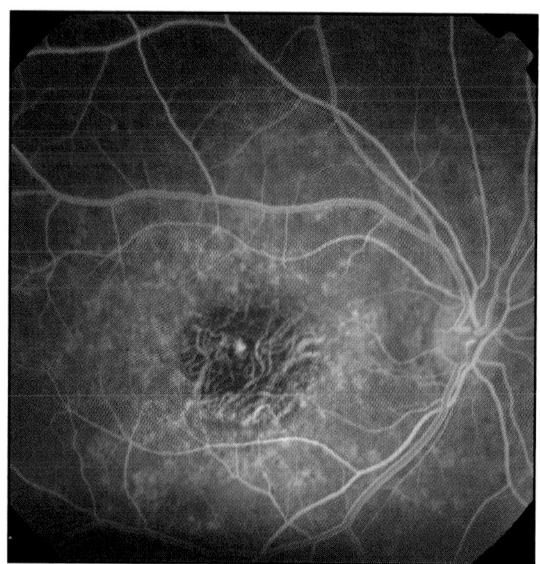

B—Early

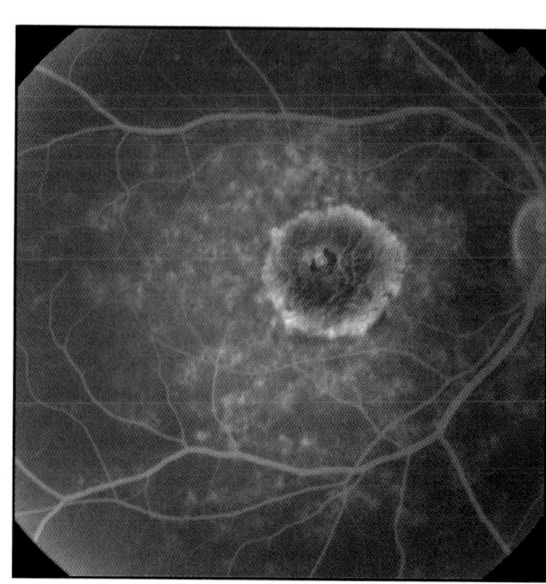

B—Late

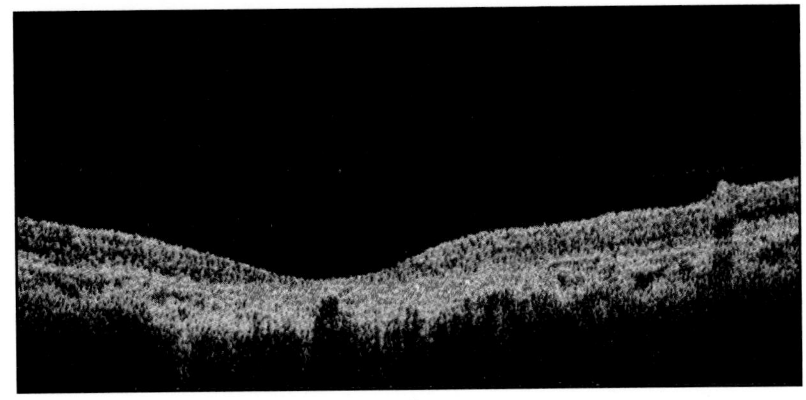

C

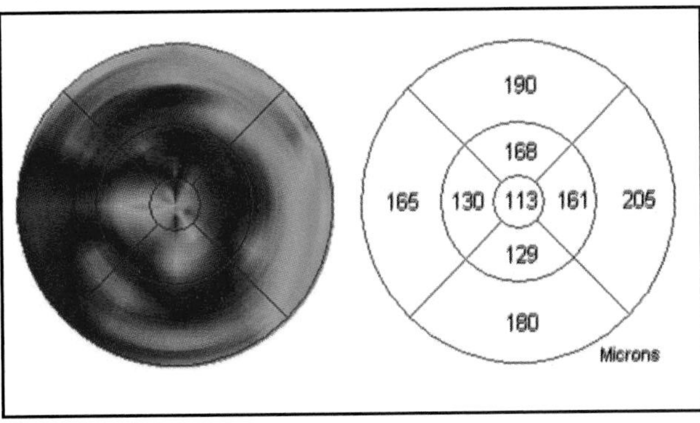

D

Case 10-8B. Stargardt's Disease

Clinical Summary

Examination of the left eye revealed the same central beaten-bronze appearance with few perimacular disciform yellowish lesions (E). The visual acuity was also 20/200 in the left eye. Findings in FA (F) were the same.

Optical Coherence Tomography

OCT scan (G) revealed a thin neurosensory retina. Some of the choroidal vessels were adequately visualized since the optical choroidal signal was enhanced due to the fact that light penetrates better through an atrophic retina. The retinal map analysis showed a central thickness of 102 μm (H).

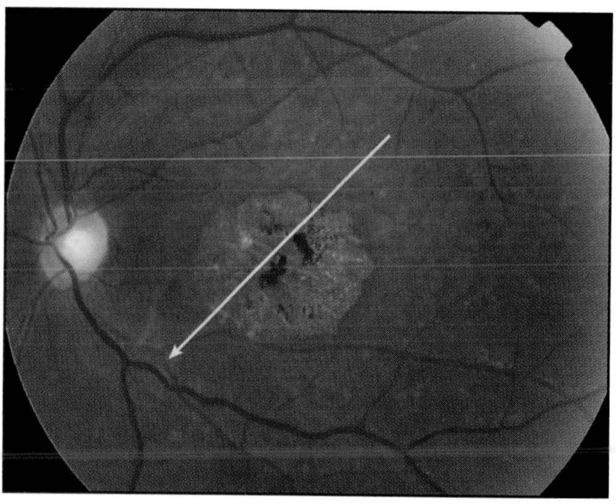

E

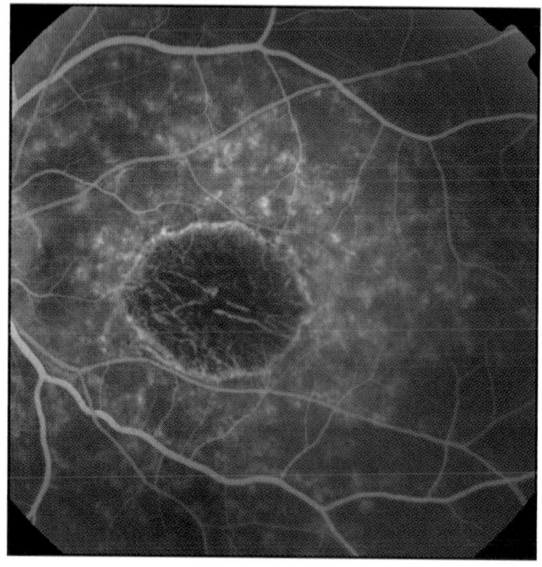

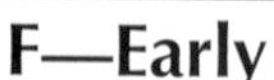

F—Early

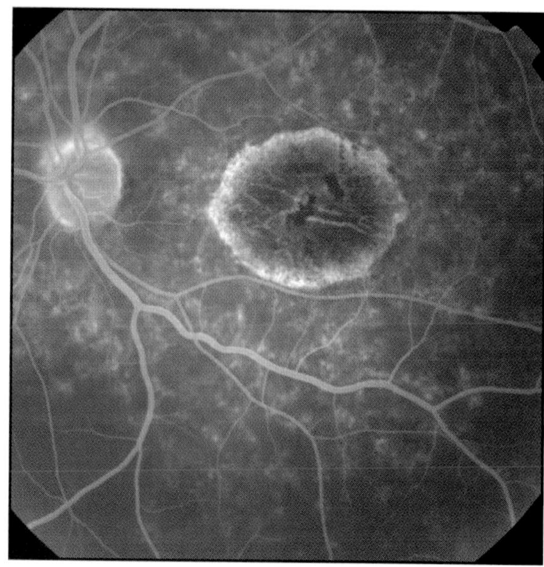

F—Late

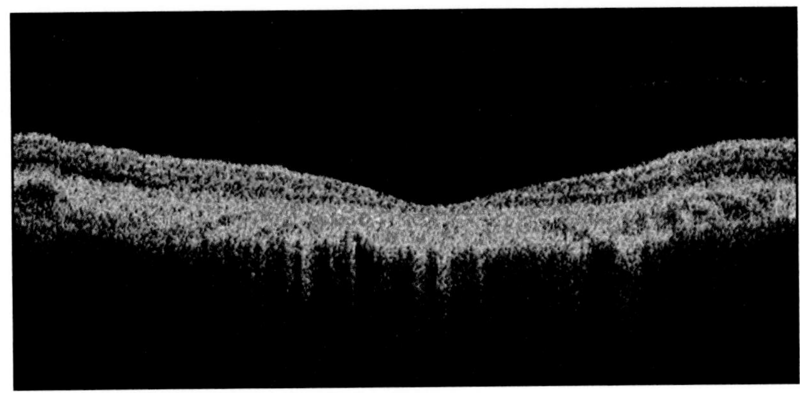

G

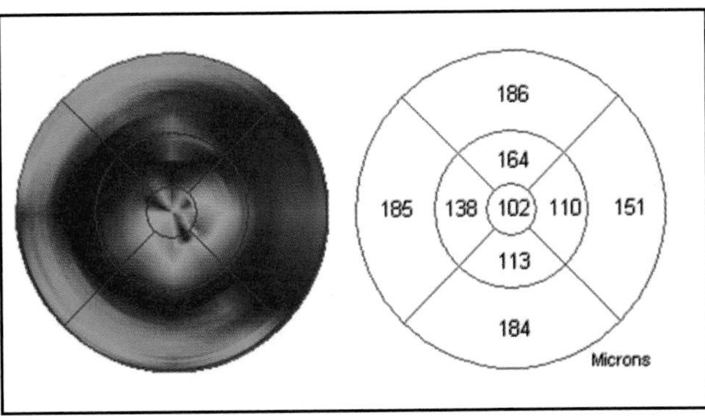

H

Case 10-9A. Best's Disease

Clinical Summary

A 7-year-old girl was referred for retinal evaluation. She has been experiencing increasing difficulty seeing the blackboard at school. The visual acuity was 20/80 in the right eye. On examination, a yellowish material was evident inferior to the foveal center. Subretinal fluid accumulation was appreciated involving the foveal center. Drusen-like deposits were encircling the macular region (A). A presumptive diagnosis of Best's disease was made.

Optical Coherence Tomography

OCT (B) revealed an elevated highly reflective nodular lesion at the level of the RPE protruding into the subretinal space. The apex of this nodular subretinal lesion looked in apposition with the neurosensory retina. This may represent subretinal neovascularization. The neurosensory retina was elevated but without evidence of intraretinal fluid accumulation. The low reflective space underneath the retina corresponded to subretinal fluid accumulation. The optical reflections from choriocapillaris/choroid complex were shadowed by the presence of the neurosensory detachment. An OCT scan (C) was obtained through the yellowish subretinal material inferotemporal to the fovea. It showed a highly reflective and irregular nodular thickening at the level of the RPE.

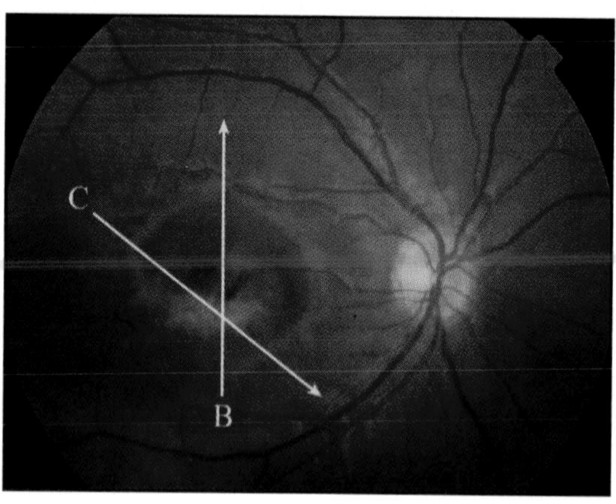

A

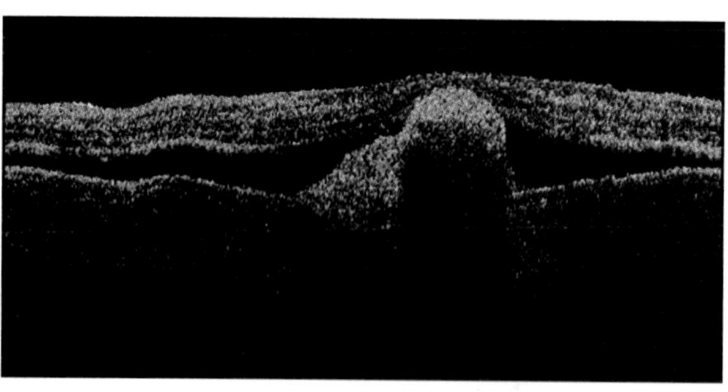

B

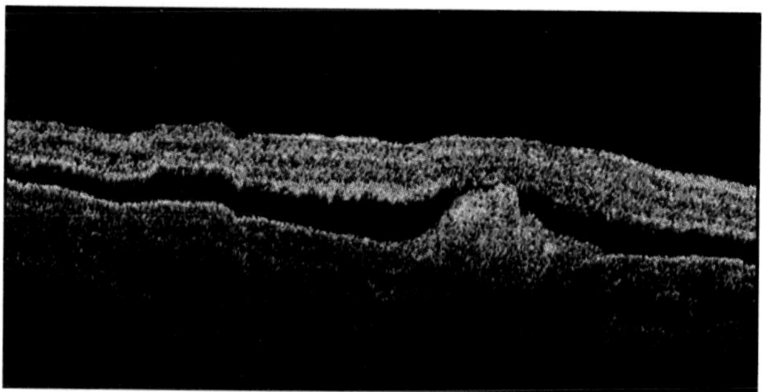

C

Case 10-9B.
Best's Disease

Clinical Summary

Evaluation of the patient's left eye revealed the subretinal yellowish material more granular in appearance. Subretinal fluid and a streak of intraretinal blood were also evident. Drusen-like subretinal deposits or flecks were more conspicuous temporal to the macular area (D). Visual acuity was 20/60 in this eye.

Optical Coherence Tomography

An OCT scan (E) obtained through fixation illustrated highly reflective and irregular nodular deposits or lesions at the RPE level protruding toward and merging with the neurosensory retina. This could be consistent with subretinal neovascularization and fibrosis. A neurosensory detachment was also observed corresponding to the low reflective subretinal fluid accumulation. Shadowing of the choroidal optical reflections was visualized.

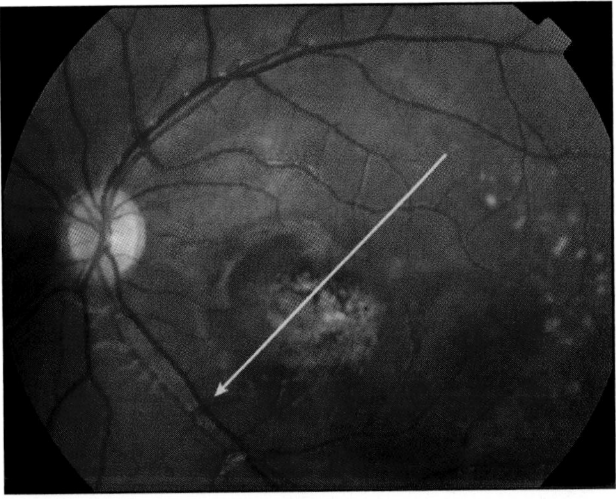

D

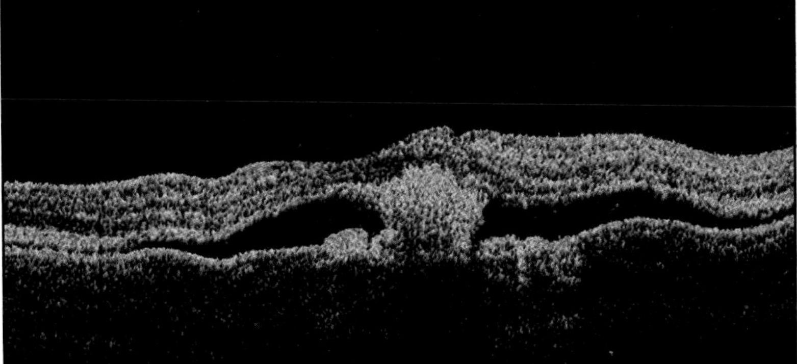

E

Case 10-10A. Best's Disease

Clinical Summary

An 18-year-old young woman with a history of Best's disease was examined. Her brother and mother also have the condition. The visual acuity was 20/50 in the right eye. Upon examination, a yellowish vitelliform lesion of approximately 1500 μm was evident in the foveal center. A subretinal elevated slightly pigmented lesion was notable adjacent to the inferonasal margin of the vitelliform lesion (A).

Optical Coherence Tomography

OCT (B) showed a low reflective space that appeared to split the RPE. An OCT scan (C) obtained through the pigmented lesion revealed an elevated highly reflective sub-RPE excrescence that shadowed the optical signals from the choroid underneath. This lesion probably represented a choroidal neovascular complex in the process of involution. The retina looked elevated in that area but no intraretinal edema was present. A low reflective space was appreciated below the neurosensory retina.

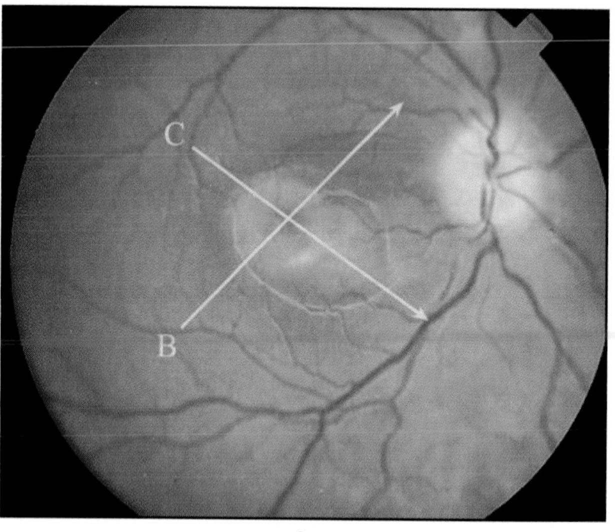

A

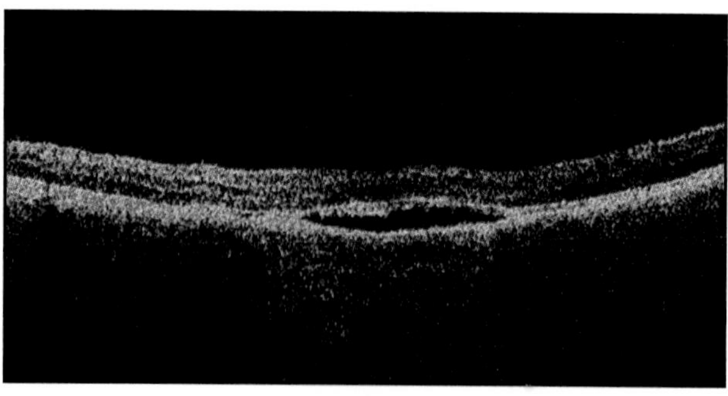

B

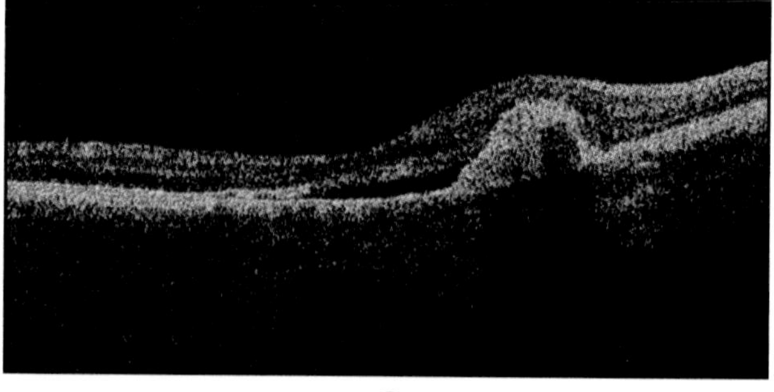

C

Case 10-10B. Best's Disease

Clinical Summary

The left eye also revealed a subretinal yellowish vitelliform lesion of approximately one disc in diameter (D). Visual acuity was 20/20 in this eye.

Optical Coherence Tomography

A horizontal OCT scan (E) obtained through the vitelliform lesion showed an irregularly thickened RPE. The RPE showed a split configuration with a low reflective space between the anterior and posterior layers. Shadowing of the optical reflections from the choroid was noticeable.

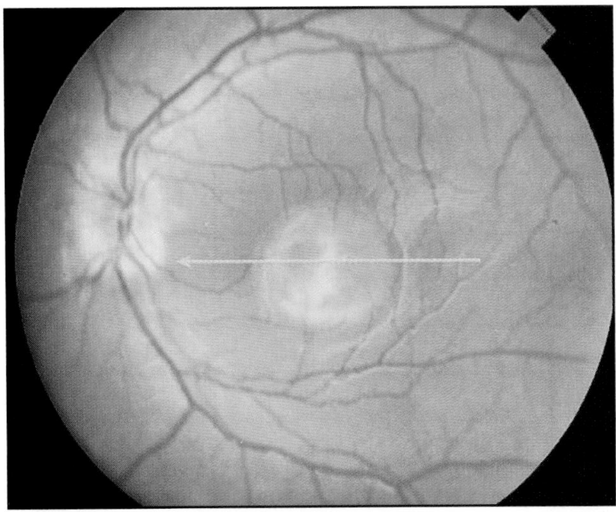

D

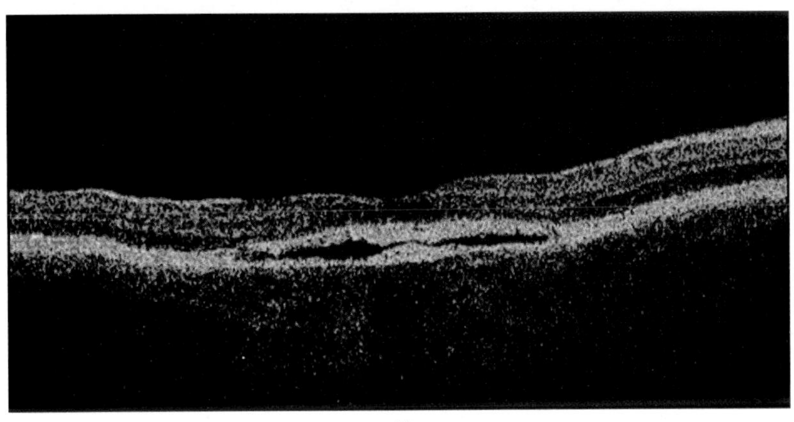

E

Case 10-11A. Best's Disease

Clinical Summary

A 69-year-old man with a history of long-standing central metamorphopsia was examined. His visual acuity was 20/25 in the right eye. Slit-lamp biomicroscopy showed a macular yellowish vitelliform lesion of approximately half a disc diameter in size (A). An electro-oculogram was abnormal with an Arden ratio of 1:3 in both eyes. A diagnosis of Best's disease was established.

Optical Coherence Tomography

OCT (B) revealed a small low reflective space that appeared to be underneath the photoreceptor layer and above the RPE corresponding to the vitelliform lesion. Disruption or discontinuity of the photoreceptor layer was observed. Thinning of the neurosensory retina above this lesion was visualized. Central retinal thickness measured 191 μm (C).

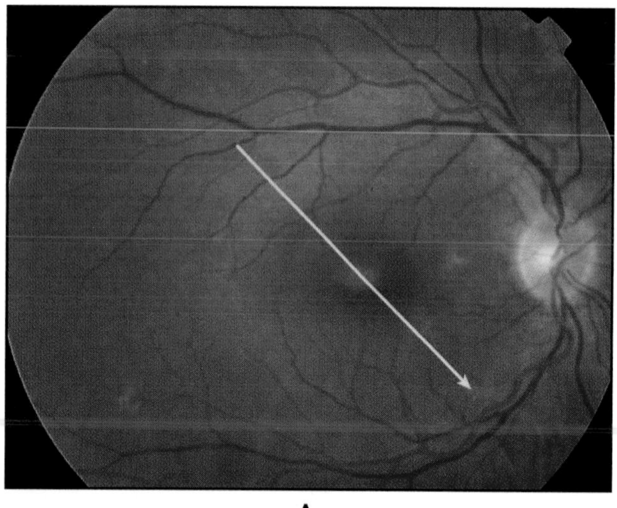

A

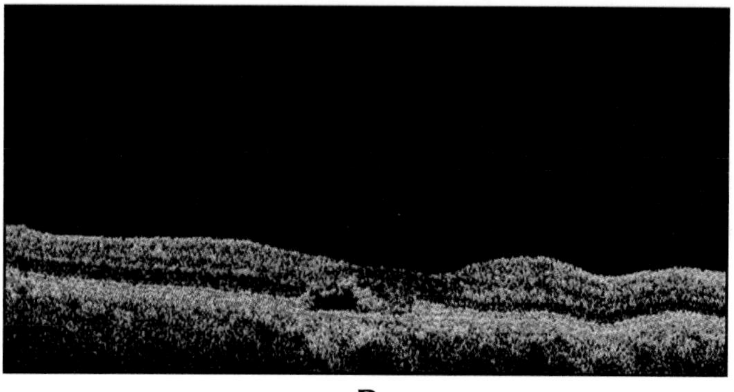

B

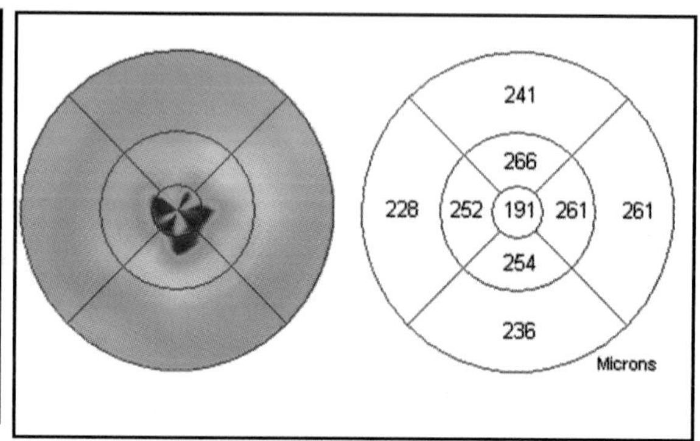

C

Case 10-11B. Best's Disease

Clinical Summary

Examination of the left eye showed a vitelliform lesion in the pseudohypopyon stage of approximately one disc diameter in size (D). Visual acuity was 20/100 in this eye.

Optical Coherence Tomography

A vertical OCT scan (E) obtained through this vitelliform lesion revealed a low reflective cavity that appeared to be underneath the photoreceptor layer and above the RPE. The photoreceptor layer appeared to be irregular and disrupted. The yellowish material seen inferiorly in the pseudohypopyon lesion was visualized as a hyperreflective material on the OCT (left side of the scan). The normal foveal contour was lost. Central macular thickness measured 304 μm (F).

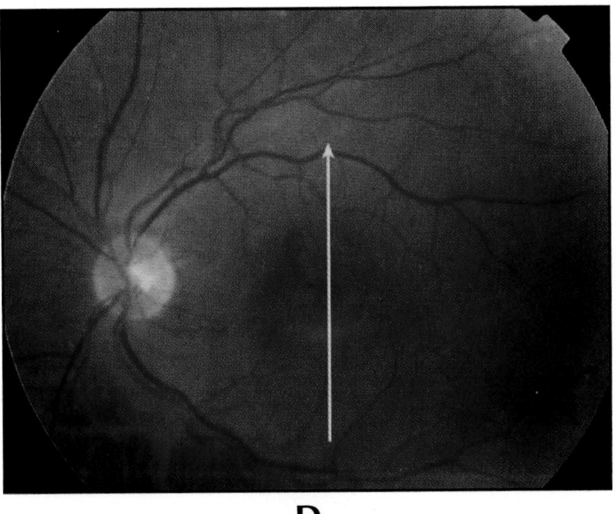

D

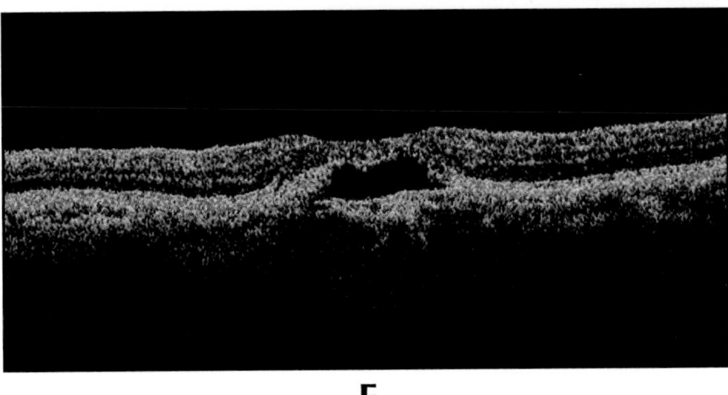

E

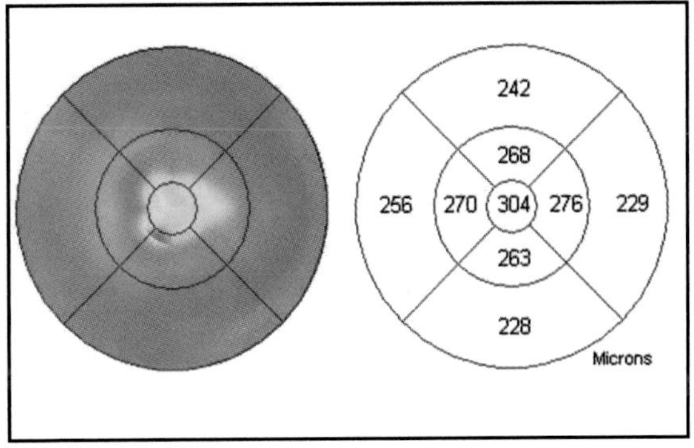

F

Case 10-12A. Pattern Dystrophy

Clinical Summary

A 55-year-old man with pattern dystrophy was examined. His visual acuity was 20/70 in the right eye. Fundus examination showed a butterfly or triradiate yellow lesion at the level of the RPE in the macular area (A).

Optical Coherence Tomography

An OCT scan obtained through the fovea (B) revealed an irregularly elevated configuration of the RPE corresponding to the yellow lesion. Central macular thinning was observed. The foveal thickness measured 174 μm (C).

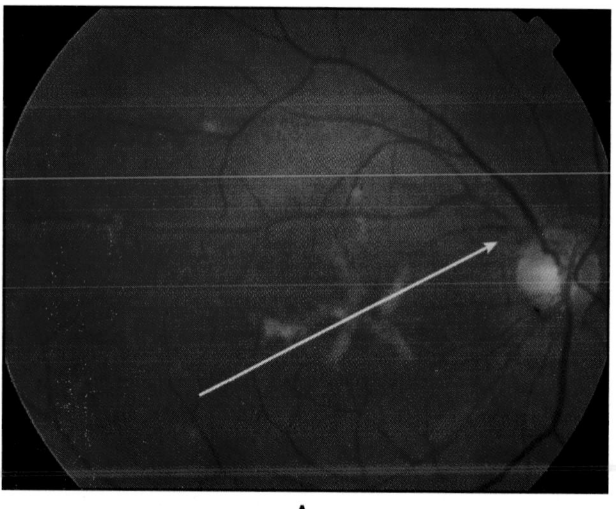

A

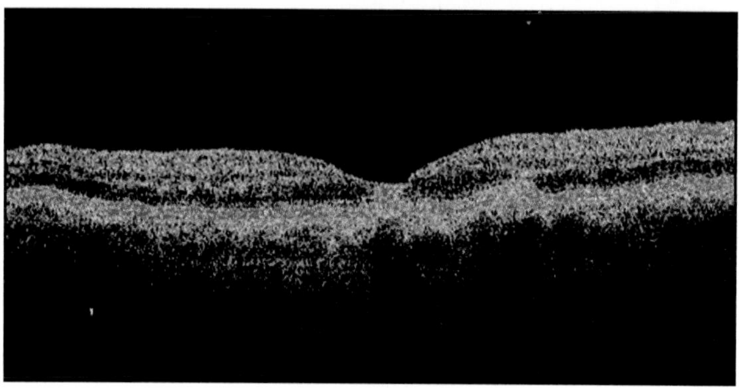

B

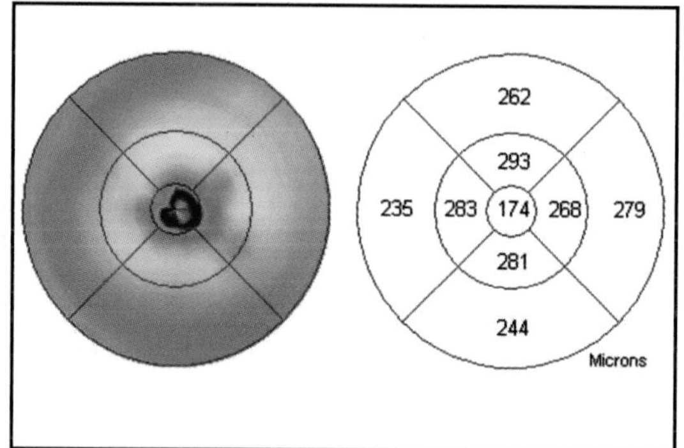

C

Case 10-12B. Pattern Dystrophy

Clinical Summary

Examination of the patient's left eye showed a central area of RPE atrophy surrounded by yellow lesions (D). The visual acuity of this eye was 20/200.

Optical Coherence Tomography

An OCT scan (E) was obtained through the fovea. Thinning of the neurosensory retina and photoreceptor loss was observed centrally. Increased choroidal reflectivity was evident under the fovea due to enhanced light penetration through the atrophic central region previously described. Small irregular elevations of the highly reflective RPE band were observed corresponding to the yellow lesions around the central atrophic area. The foveal thickness measured 156 μm (F).

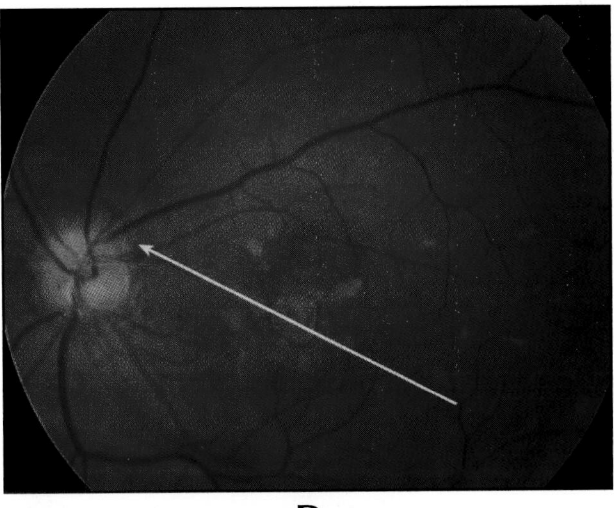

D

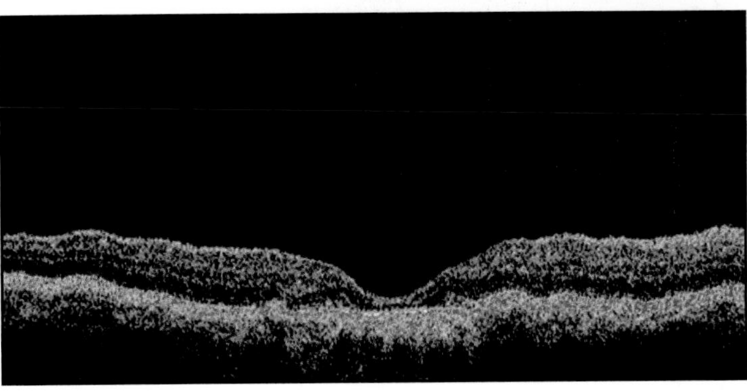

E

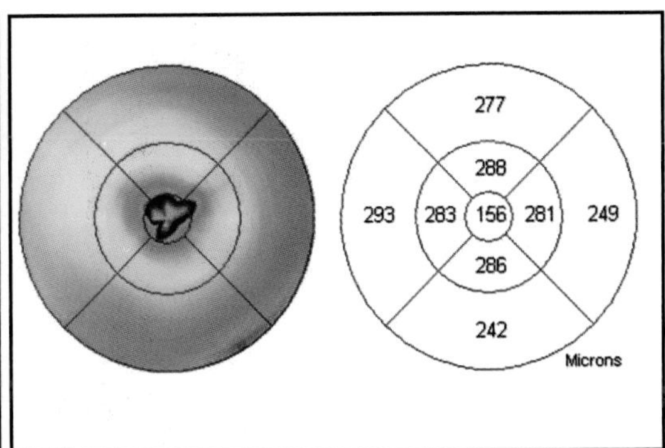

F

Case 10-13. X-Linked Juvenile Retinoschisis

Clinical Summary

An 8-year-old boy with a history of X-linked juvenile retinoschisis was examined. His visual acuity was 20/60 in the right eye. Retinal examination showed a stellate maculopathy and a peripheral schisis extending from the inferotemporal quadrant toward the inferotemporal arcade in the posterior pole. Retinal pigment alterations were also noticed (A).

Optical Coherence Tomography

A vertical OCT scan obtained through the fovea (B) confirmed the presence of the foveal cystic alterations predominantly in the outer layers. Cleavage or splitting in the retinal tissue at the level of the nerve fiber layer and bridging retinal elements were noticeable inferior to the fovea where the peripheral schisis cavity was observed.

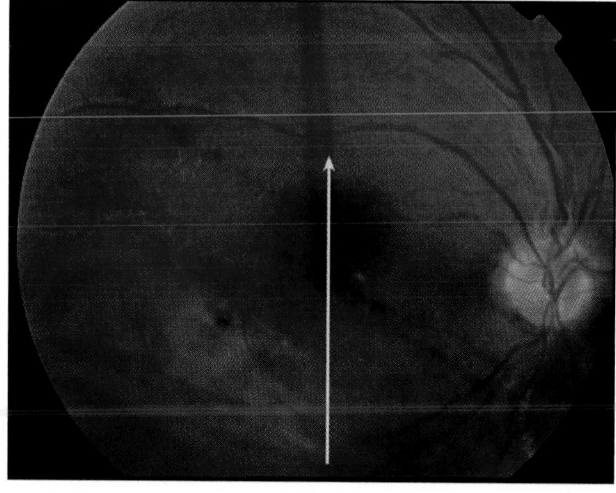

A

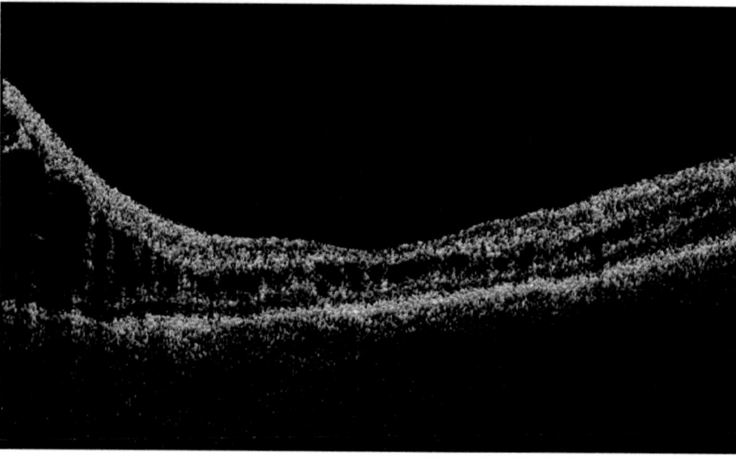

B

Chapter 11

Miscellaneous Retinal Diseases

Elias C. Mavrofrides, MD; Vanessa Cruz-Villegas, MD; and Carmen A. Puliafito, MD

- Pseudophakic Cystoid Macular Edema
- Cystoid Macular Edema Associated With Glaucoma Therapy
- Rhegmatogenous Retinal Detachment
- Posterior Segment Trauma
- Congenital Pit of the Optic Disc
- Myelinated Nerve Fiber Layer
- Cancer-Associated Retinopathy

Optical coherence tomography (OCT) can be useful in the evaluation of a broad range of retinal conditions. This chapter provides additional examples of the application of OCT in various clinical situations.

Cystoid Macular Edema

One of the most powerful applications of OCT is in the evaluation and management of patients with cystoid macular edema (CME) regardless of the underlying etiology. CME appears as retinal thickening with intraretinal cavities of reduced reflectivity on OCT.[1] The use of OCT for CME caused by diabetic retinopathy, retinal vein occlusion, choroidal neovascularization (CNV), inflammatory conditions, and retinal dystrophies has been detailed in other chapters.

CME can also occur in many other clinical settings, most notably following intraocular surgery. Clinically significant CME is estimated to occur in 1% to 2% of patients undergoing cataract extraction and is likely more common after other types of intraocular surgery.[2] Establishing the diagnosis by fundus examination alone can be difficult, and fluorescein angiography (FA) is often needed for confirmation. OCT appears to be equally effective as angiography in establishing the diagnosis but is far less invasive and significantly quicker. OCT also has the advantage of providing a quantitative assessment of macular thickness, which can be used to monitor the clinical course. Repeated quantitative evaluations with OCT can be invaluable in therapeutic decision making. Resolution of the edema without improvement of visual acuity can prompt evaluation for other factors contributing to vision loss. Persistent edema unresponsive to initial therapy (ie, topical medications) can establish the need for more invasive intervention (ie, steroid injection or vitrectomy).

Rhegmatogenous Retinal Detachment

As with other types of retinal detachment, OCT can be useful in the evaluation of patients with rhegmatogenous retinal detachments. OCT is extremely sensitive in identifying elevation of the neurosensory retina because of the distinct difference in optical reflectivity between the retina and underlying retinal pigment epithelium (RPE)/choroid. Detachment of the neurosensory retina can be seen as nonreflective space between the elevated retinal signal and the underlying high-intensity RPE/choroidal band.

In patients with rhegmatogenous retinal detachment, OCT can confirm the presence of shallow subretinal fluid that may be difficult to identify on ophthalmoscopy. OCT can also help distinguish true retinal detachment from other entities in the differential, such as retinoschisis.

Following retinal detachment repair, there is a great deal of variability in the degree and time course of visual recovery. OCT has been used to identify the presence of shallow subretinal fluid beneath the fovea in patients with delayed visual recovery after successful detachment surgery.[3,4] This shallow fluid could not be identified on clinical exam or FA. As a result, OCT can provide important information about visual outcomes and prognosis after retinal detachment repair.

Posterior Segment Trauma

Several characteristics make OCT an effective tool in the management of patients with posterior segment trauma. OCT is usually more comfortable for the traumatized patient than other examination techniques since it is noninvasive and uses infrared illumination.[5] OCT images can often be obtained even when the view to the retina is limited since only a small aperture is need for effective imaging. OCT is also highly sensitive in identifying small anatomic changes, such as a traumatic macular hole, that may be difficult to confirm clinically.

Post-traumatic retinal alterations, such as edema or inflammation, manifest as changes in the contour and reflectivity of neurosensory retina on OCT. Retinal atrophy can be seen as thinning of the retinal signal, while scarring usually results in increased reflectivity.

Hemorrhage, a common finding in trauma, results in relatively high reflectivity with shadowing of the underlying layers on the OCT image. The degree of shadowing depends on the thickness and density of the hemorrhage. In some cases, the reflectivity of the hemorrhage may be similar to the retina, making distinction of these two layers slightly difficult.

Changes in the RPE and choroid following trauma can also be seen on the OCT image. Detachment of the RPE can be seen as elevation of the high intensity outer band with shadowing of the underlying choroidal signal. RPE defects or choroidal rupture allow deeper penetration and increased reflectivity of the signal resulting in a thick, intense outer band.

Optic Nerve Head Pits

OCT imaging has also helped our understanding of the retinal changes associated with optic nerve pits. In many cases, OCT shows severe outer retinal edema causing a schisis-like configuration in the macula. This is often associated with the accumulation of subretinal fluid creating bilaminar structure. Fluid appears to pass directly from the optic nerve pit into the retinal stroma and then secondarily into the subretinal space.[6,7] Several authors have subsequently demonstrated the usefulness of OCT in the monitoring of patients that have undergone surgical intervention for this condition.[7-10]

References

1. Hee MR, Puliafito CA, Wong C, et al. Quantitative assessment of macular edema with optical coherence tomography. *Arch Ophthalmol*. 1995;113(8):1019-1029.
2. Nelson ML, Martidis A. Managing cystoid macular edema after cataract surgery. *Curr Opin Ophthalmol*. 2003;14(1): 39-43.
3. Hagimura N, Iida T, Suto K, Kishi S. Persistent foveal detachment after successful rhegmatogenous retinal detachment surgery. *Am J Ophthalmol*. 2002;133(4):516-520.
4. Wolfensberg TJ, Gonvers M. Optical coherence tomography in the evaluation of incomplete visual acuity recovery after macula-off retinal detachments. *Graefes Arch Clin Exp Ophthalmol*. 2002;240(2):85-89.
5. Hee MP, Izatt JA, Huang D, et al. Optical coherence tomography of the human retina. *Arch Ophthalmol*. 1995;113:325-332.
6. Rutledge BK, Puliafito CA, Duker JS, Hee MR, Cox MS. Optical coherence tomography of macular lesions associated with optic nerve head pits. *Ophthalmology*. 1996;103(7): 1047-1053.
7. Lincoff H, Schiff W, Krivoy D, Ritch R. Optical coherence tomography of pneumatic displacement of optic disc pit maculopathy. *Br J Ophthalmol*. 1998;82(4):367-372.
8. Theodossiadis GP, Theodossiadis PG. Optical coherence tomography in optic disk pit maculopathy treated by the macular buckling procedure. *Am J Ophthalmol*. 2001; 132(2):184-190.
9. Konno S, Akiba J, Sato E, Kuriyama S, Yoshida A. OCT in successful surgery of retinal detachment associated with optic nerve head pit. *Ophthalmic Surg Lasers*. 2000;31(3): 236-239.
10. Todokoro D, Kishi S. Reattachment of retina and retinoschisis in pit-macular syndrome by surgically-induced vitreous detachment and gas tamponade. *Ophthalmic Surg Lasers*. 2000;31(3):233-235.

Case 11-1. Pseudophakic Cystoid Macular Edema

Clinical Summary

A 72-year-old woman who underwent cataract extraction with an intraocular lens (IOL) implant in her right eye 6 months earlier had been experiencing poor vision for 4 months. Her visual acuity was 20/400 in this eye. Slit-lamp biomicroscopy showed retinal thickening and cystic macular changes (A). FA (B) revealed perifoveal areas of early hyperfluorescence associated with late leakage in a petalloid fashion consistent with CME. Staining of the optic nerve head was also observed. A diagnosis of Irvine-Gass syndrome was done.

Optical Coherence Tomography

A horizontal OCT scan (C) showed marked retinal thickening with cystic areas of reduced reflectivity, especially in the outer plexiform layer consistent with CME. In addition, a low reflective space was noted beneath the retina indicative of a neurosensory retinal detachment. The central foveal thickness measured 768 µm (D).

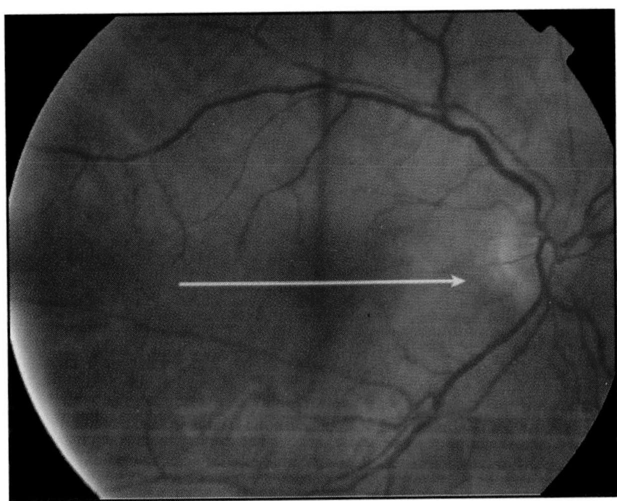

A

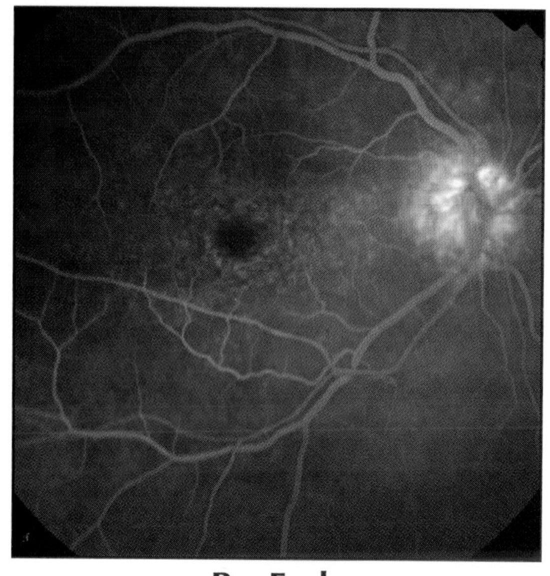

B—Early

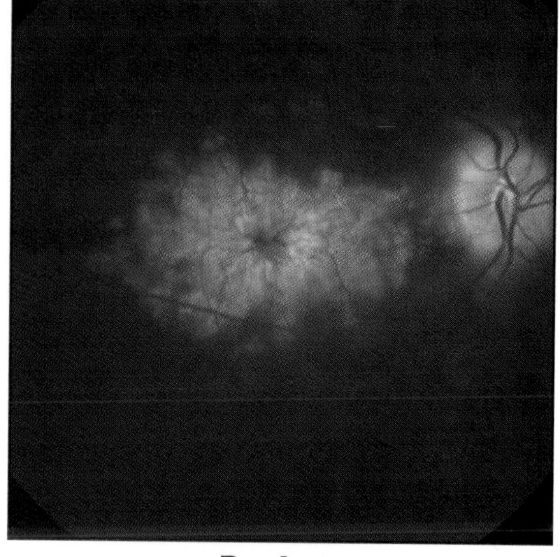

B—Late

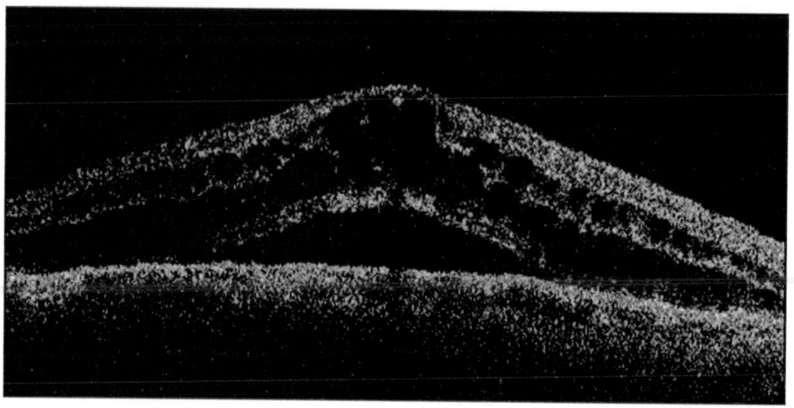

C

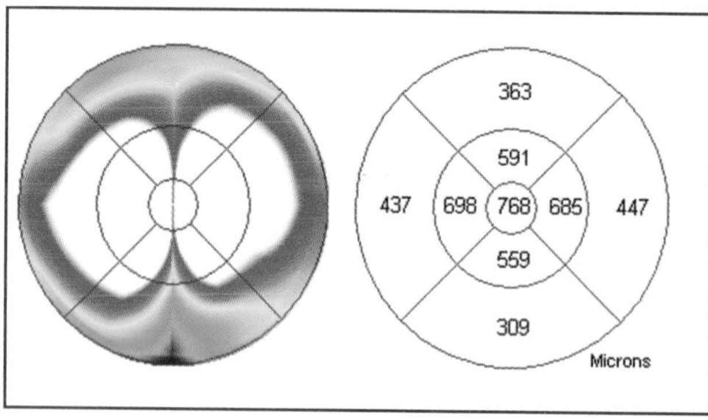

D

Case 11-2A. Postoperative Cystoid Macular Edema Treated With Intravitreal Triamcinolone

Clinical Summary

A 60-year-old female complains of decreased visual acuity in the right eye starting 1 month after uncomplicated phacoemulsification cataract extraction with IOL placement. Her visual acuity in this eye is 20/100, and dilated fundus examination (A) shows CME with a large central cyst. Late frames of the FA (B) reveal petalloid hyperfluorescence in the fovea.

Optical Coherence Tomography

On the OCT image (C), there is extensive retinal thickening with numerous large optically clear cavities within the retina corresponding to the macular cysts. Fluid accumulation and cyst formation are most extensive in the outer retina. A small pocket of subretinal fluid is also present. The retinal thickness map (D) delineates the circular area of thickening centered on the fovea. The retinal thickness reaches a peak of 723 µm at the fovea.

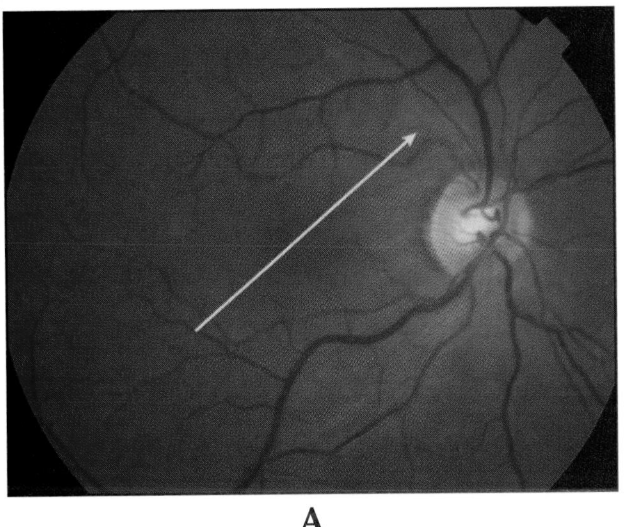

A

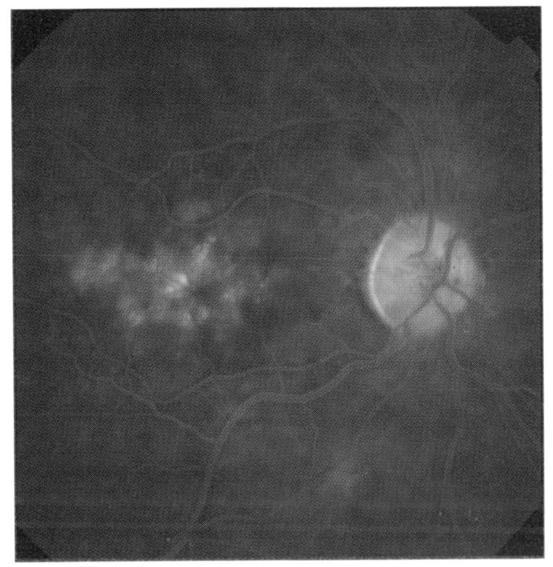

B

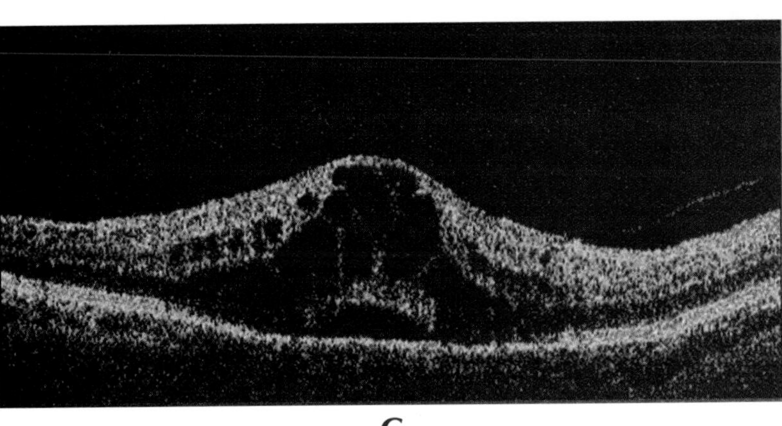

C

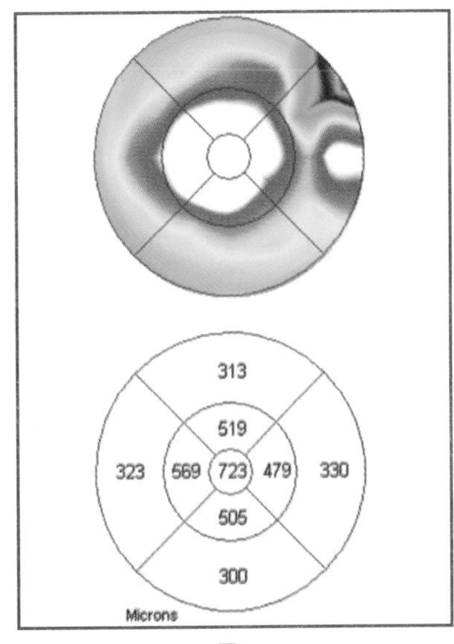

D

Case 11-2B. Treatment With Intravitreal Triamcinolone

Continuation of Clinical Summary

An intravitreal injection of triamcinolone was performed at this initial visit. The patient returns 1 month later and reports significant improvement of her vision. Her visual acuity is 20/20, and there is no evidence of macular edema on clinical exam (E).

Follow-Up Optical Coherence Tomography

Postinjection OCT imaging (F) confirms resolution of the macular edema. The intraretinal cystic cavities are no longer present, and the retinal contour has normalized. The retinal map (G) confirms a significant reduction in retinal thickness throughout the macular region, and central foveal thickness has returned to a normal level of 269 µm.

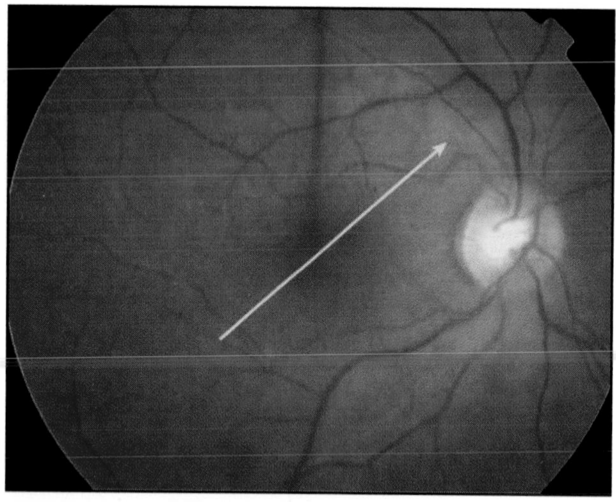

E

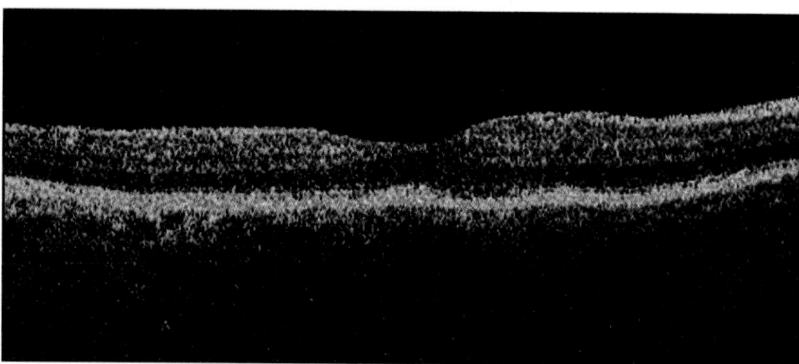

F

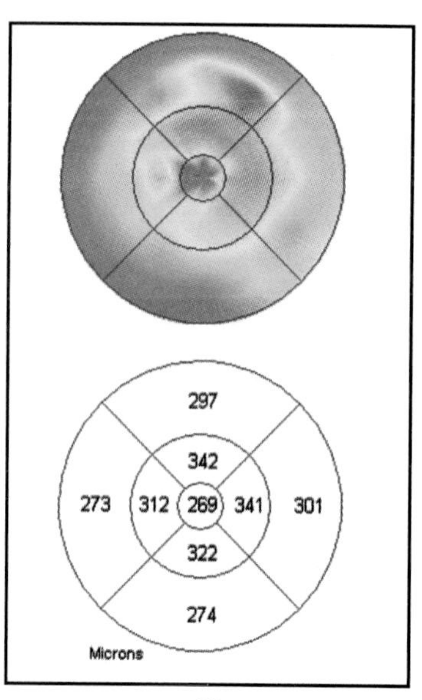

G

Case 11-3A. Cystoid Macular Edema Associated With Glaucoma Drops

Clinical Summary

A 58-year-old female was referred for evaluation of macular edema in the left eye. She has a history of glaucoma and underwent tube shunt placement in the left eye 6 months earlier. She currently uses multiple glaucoma drops, including a prostaglandin analog in both eyes, for persistent elevation of the intraocular pressure. Her visual acuity is 20/60 in the left eye, and dilated fundus exam (A) reveals macular edema.

Optical Coherence Tomography

The initial OCT image (B and C) shows extensive thickening of the foveal retina. There are a few small cystic cavities in the inner retinal layers. A larger area of decreased reflectivity in the outer retina indicates extensive cystoid edema. Bridging retinal elements can be seen passing through this area, and a thin layer of retinal tissue is seen at the base of this cavity, confirming the anatomic location as intraretinal. The central foveal thickness measures 479 µm and reaches a peak of 536 µm superior to the fovea.

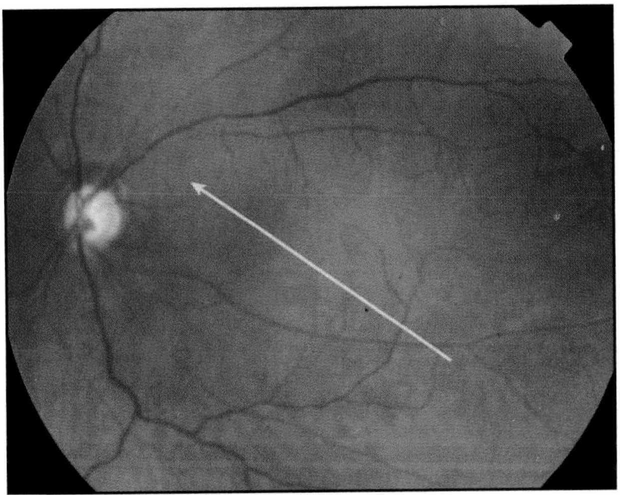

A

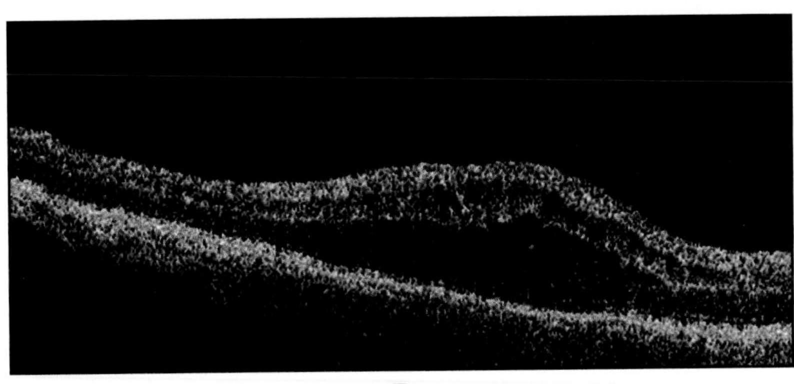

B

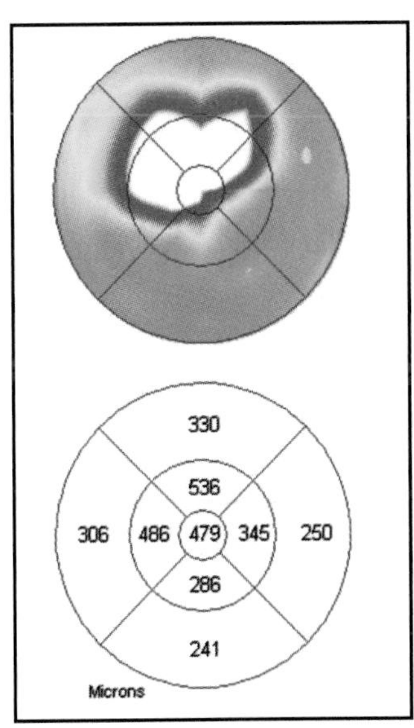

C

Case 11-3B. Improvement With Topical Medication Change

Continuation of Clinical Summary

Her prostaglandin analog was discontinued, and she was started on a topical nonsteroidal anti-inflammatory drug (NSAID). Six weeks later, her visual acuity had improved to 20/40, and there was minimal edema evident on exam.

Follow-Up Optical Coherence Tomography

Six weeks after changing her medications, there is a significant decrease in retinal thickness on the OCT image (D and E). A cyst is still present in the fovea, but the large outer retinal cystic cavity has resolved. Central foveal thickness has decreased to 367 μm, and there has been a reduction of retinal thickness throughout the macula.

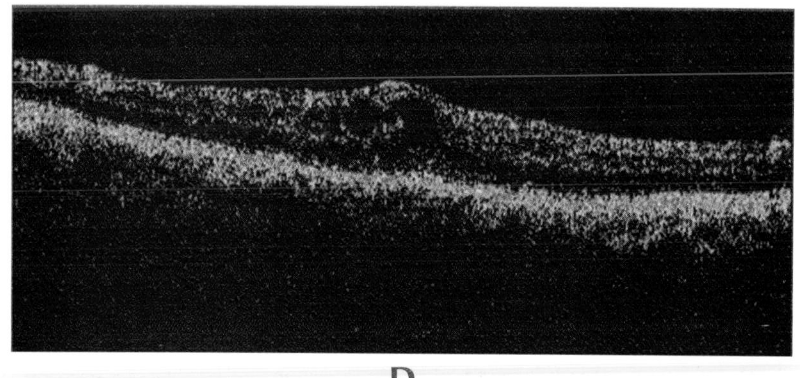

D

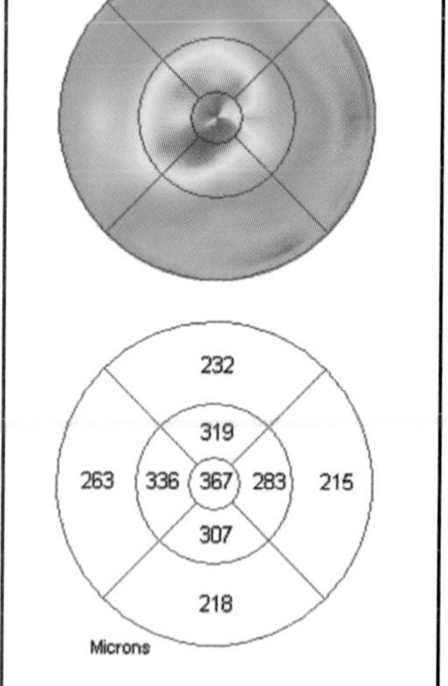

E

Case 11-4. Rhegmatogenous Retinal Detachment

Clinical Summary

A 30-year-old man with a history of high intraocular pressure (IOP) and iridocyclitis in the right eye was referred for evaluation. The patient had a 6-month history of decreased vision in this eye. His visual acuity was 20/50. Slit-lamp examination revealed pigmented cells in the anterior chamber. He was currently using timolol maleate 0.5% and dorzolamide hydrochloride 2%. His IOP was 18 mmHg in this eye. Dilated fundus examination revealed a chronic shallow superior rhegmatogenous retinal detachment involving the upper half of the macula (A). FA (B) revealed late staining of the optic nerve and pooling of fluorescein dye in the superior portion of the retina. No CME was present.

Optical Coherence Tomography

A vertical OCT scan (C) confirmed the presence of an optically clear space beneath the neurosensory retina consistent with subretinal fluid superior to the fovea (right side of the scan). The foveola was not involved. Cystic spaces of reduced reflectivity were visualized in the detached portion of the retina corresponding to chronic intraretinal fluid accumulation. A horizontal OCT scan (D) was obtained through the detached retina superiorly. It showed a shallow retinal detachment with subretinal fluid accumulation. Again, cystic intraretinal changes denoted the chronic nature of the detachment.

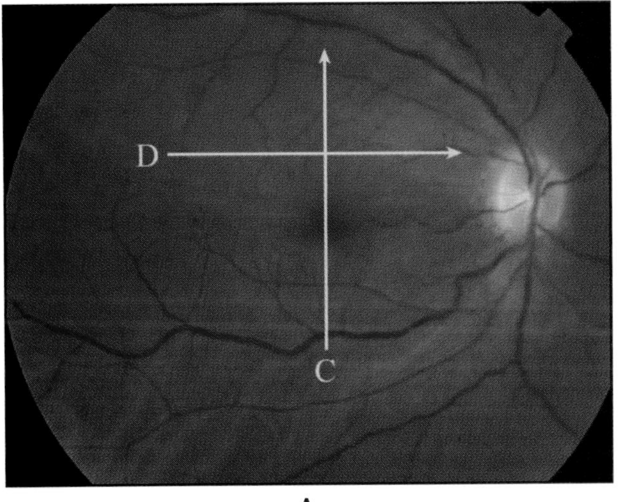

A

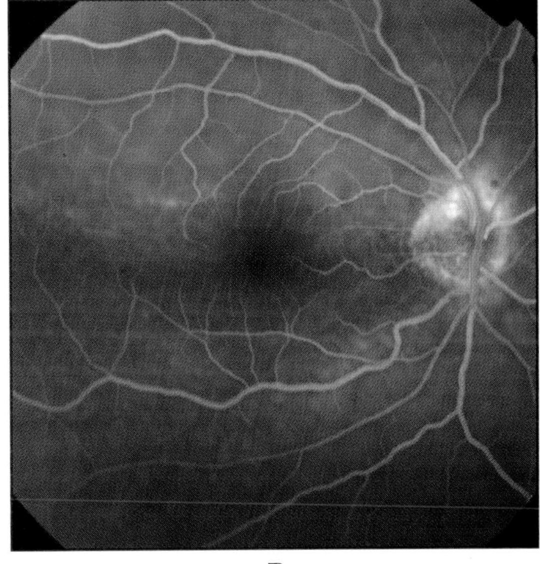
B

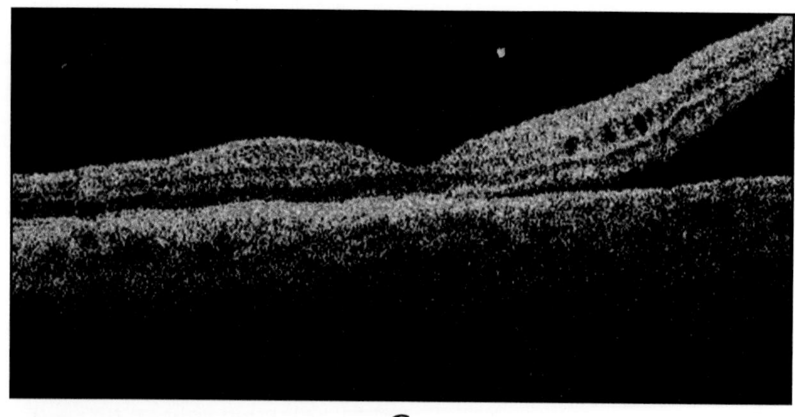

C

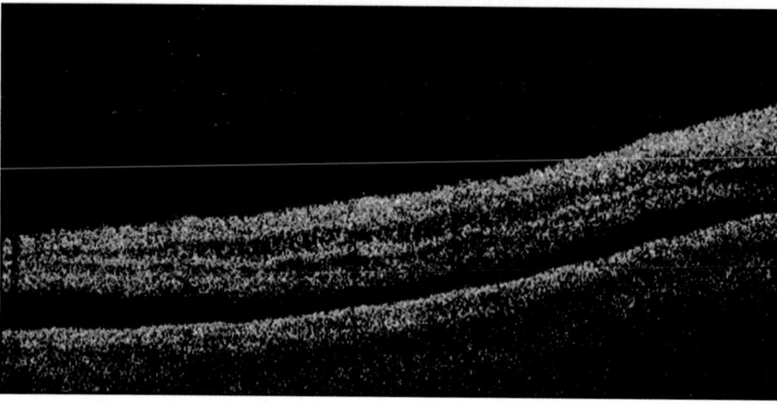

D

Case 11-5A. Persistent Subfoveal Fluid After Retinal Detachment Repair

Clinical Summary

A 70-year-old male is referred for evaluation of persistently decreased central visual acuity after retinal detachment repair. The patient underwent a pars plana vitrectomy with drainage retinotomy and fluid-gas exchange 3 months earlier. Although the retina appeared attached clinically (A), the visual acuity remained 20/200.

Optical Coherence Tomography

OCT (B) reveals shallow elevation of the neurosensory retina above an optically clear cavity of subretinal fluid. The subretinal fluid cavity reaches a maximum height of only 190 μm and is therefore difficult to identify ophthalmoscopically. There is a high-intensity reflection off of the outer surface of the neurosensory retina. This can be differentiated from an RPE detachment by the presence of a second high-intensity signal beneath the clear cavity (which is the actual RPE signal) and the lack of significant choroidal shadowing.

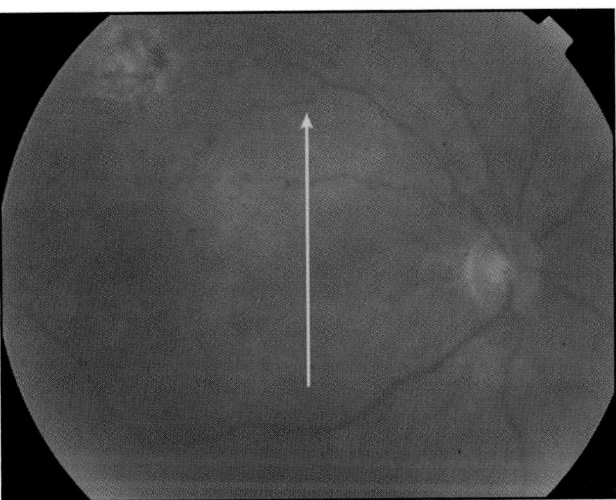

A

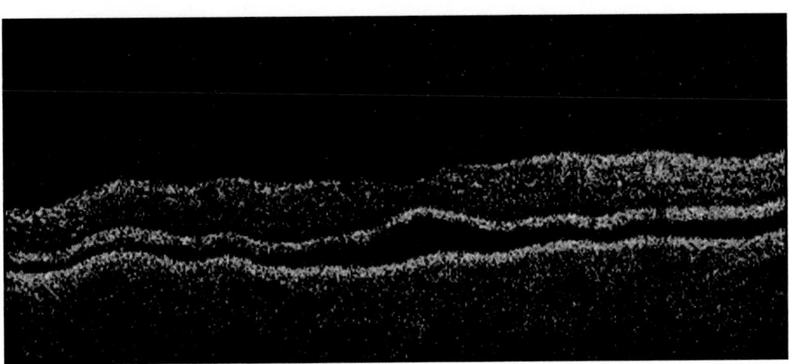

B

Case 11-5B. Persistent Subfoveal Fluid After Retinal Detachment Repair

Continuation of Clinical Summary

Two months later, the patient has not noticed any improvement and his visual acuity remains 20/200. Although there is blunting of the foveal reflex, definite subretinal fluid is not seen on exam. Four months later, the patient notes improvement and his visual acuity increases to 20/60.

Follow-Up Optical Coherence Tomography

At the 2-month follow-up, the OCT tomogram (C) continues to show a small amount of persistent subretinal fluid. Although the subretinal fluid has decreased in height to 90 μm, the fovea remains completely detached. Four months later, there is almost complete resolution of the subretinal fluid on the OCT tomogram (D).

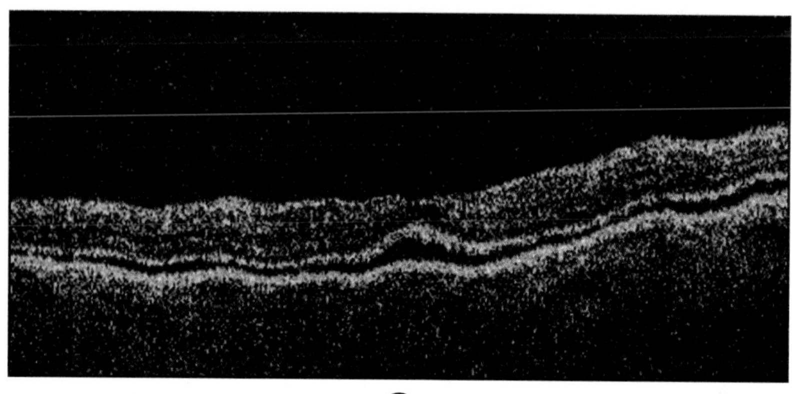

C

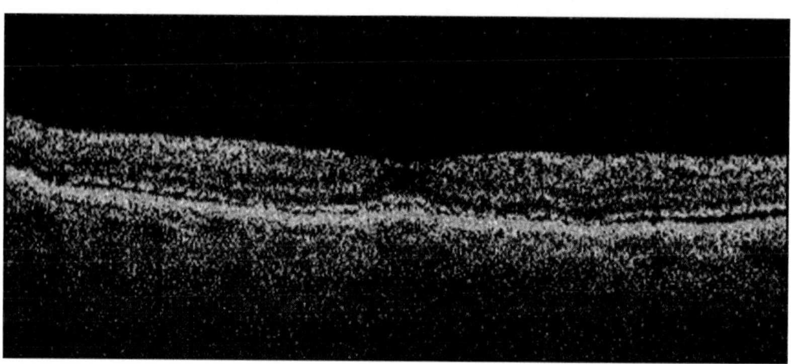

D

Case 11-6. *Post-Traumatic Choroidal Rupture*

Clinical Summary

A 23-year-old female complains of decreased vision in her left eye after being punched in this eye earlier that evening. Her visual acuity is 20/200. There is extensive periorbital edema and bruising. Dilated fundus examination (A) shows evidence of a choroidal rupture through the macula with associated submacular hemorrhage. The choroidal ruptures are seen as hyperfluorescent window defects on the angiogram (B). Three parallel areas of choroidal rupture can be seen inferotemporal to the fovea.

Optical Coherence Tomography

OCT (C) shows elevation of the fovea from the subretinal hemorrhage. Because the retina and blood have similar reflectivity, it is difficult to precisely differentiate these layers. As the scan passes through the inferotemporal macula (left side of the tomogram), there are three areas of increased choroidal reflectivity. These areas result from increased penetration and reflectivity of the signal as it passes through the choroidal ruptures.

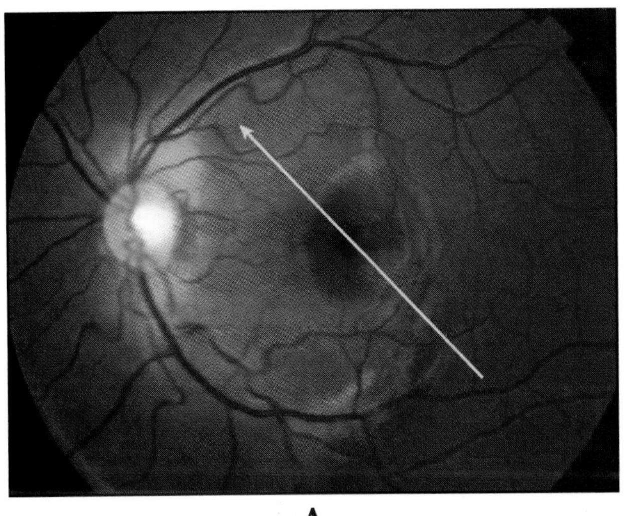

A

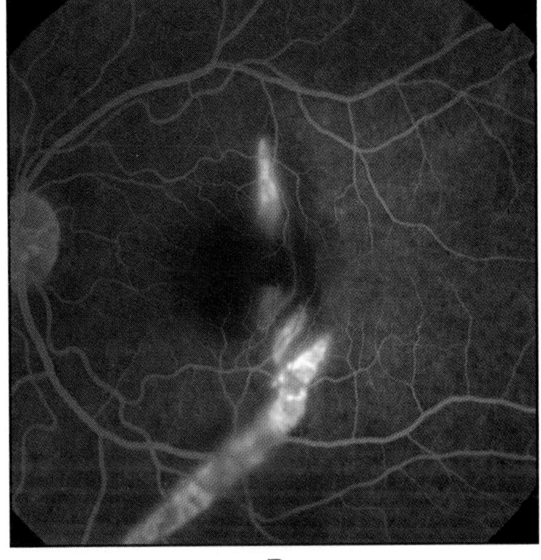

B

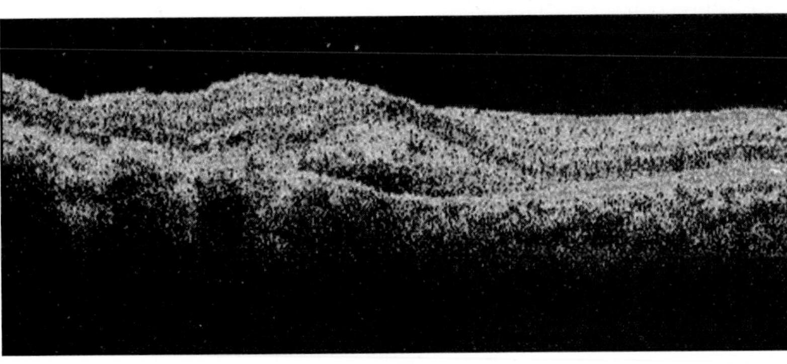

C

Case 11-7. Valsalva Retinopathy

Clinical Summary

A 19-year-old woman experienced vision decrease after several episodes of vomiting during her third trimester of pregnancy. Her vision was 20/80 in this eye. Dilated fundus examination showed a subhyaloid hemorrhage involving the foveal center (A).

Optical Coherence Tomography

An OCT scan through the fovea (B) revealed a dome-shaped reflective area consistent with subhyaloid blood beneath a reflective band corresponding to the posterior hyaloid. The neurosensory retina was visualized underneath the blood. The hemorrhage blocked to some degree the optical reflections returning from the retina and RPE/choriocapillaris layers. Scan C showed a region inferonasal to the fovea (right side of the scan) where the subhyaloid hemorrhage is less dense, allowing better light propagation and resulting in adequate visualization of the neurosensory retina as well as the RPE/choriocapillaris.

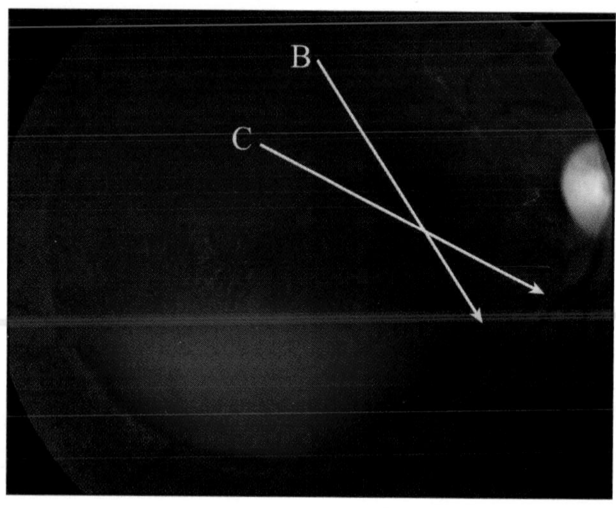

A

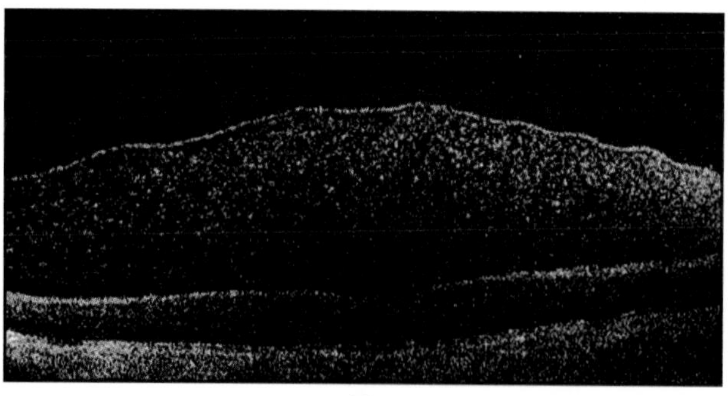

B

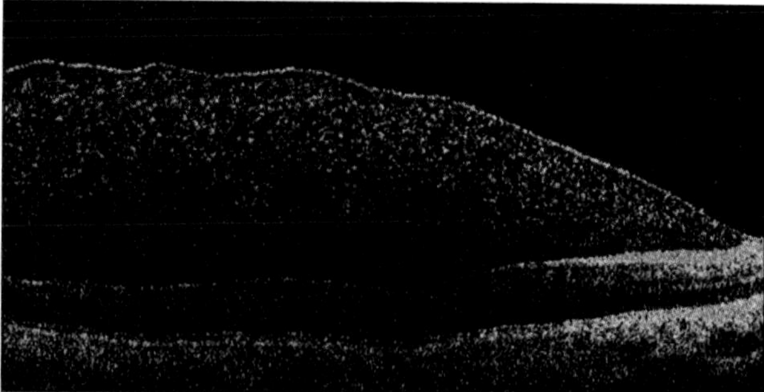

C

Case 11-8.
Chorioretinitis Sclopetaria

Clinical Summary

A 24-year-old man suffered a gunshot wound to the left periorbital region 8 months earlier. The bullet entered through the left inferior orbital rim. The patient underwent facial bone reconstruction and complained of poor vision in his left eye. Visual acuity measured 20/200 in this eye. Dilated fundus examination showed extensive chorioretinal scarring and fibrosis involving the macular region (A) and inferior retina (B).

Optical Coherence Tomography

A horizontal OCT scan (C) obtained through the fovea showed thinning of the overlying neurosensory retina in association with irregular thickening of the RPE/choroid layer. A reflective band was visible anterior to the retinal tissue consistent with a posterior vitreous detachment. Another OCT scan (D) showed marked retinal atrophy. The underneath RPE layer showed a highly reflective irregular configuration. Shadowing of the choroidal optical reflections was observed below this highly reflective area. Scan E depicted a region of high backscattering consistent with fibrosis fusing the neurosensory retina and RPE/choroid. A horizontal scan obtained inferior to the optic nerve (F) revealed preretinal fibrosis, seen as a region of increased reflectivity (right side of the scan) in association with a highly reflective and thickened RPE/choroid underneath. The atrophic retina lost its normal architecture. The central macular area measured 177 µm (G).

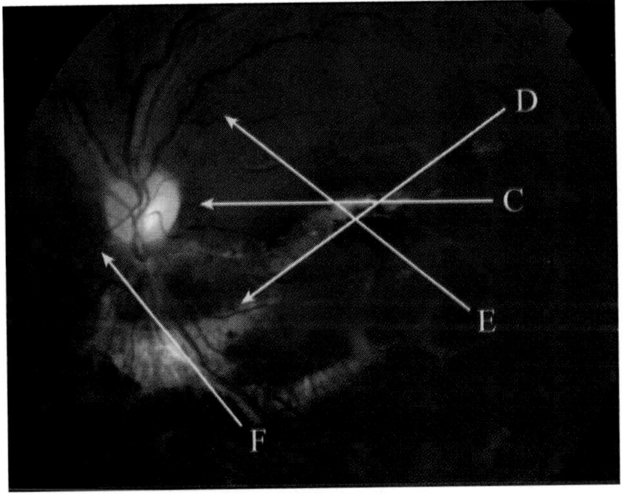

A

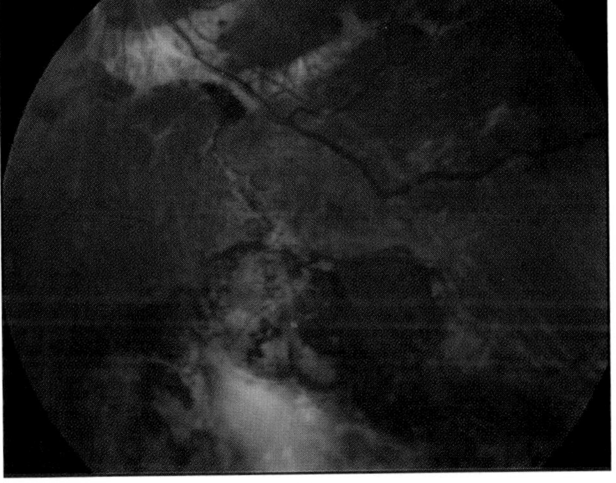

B

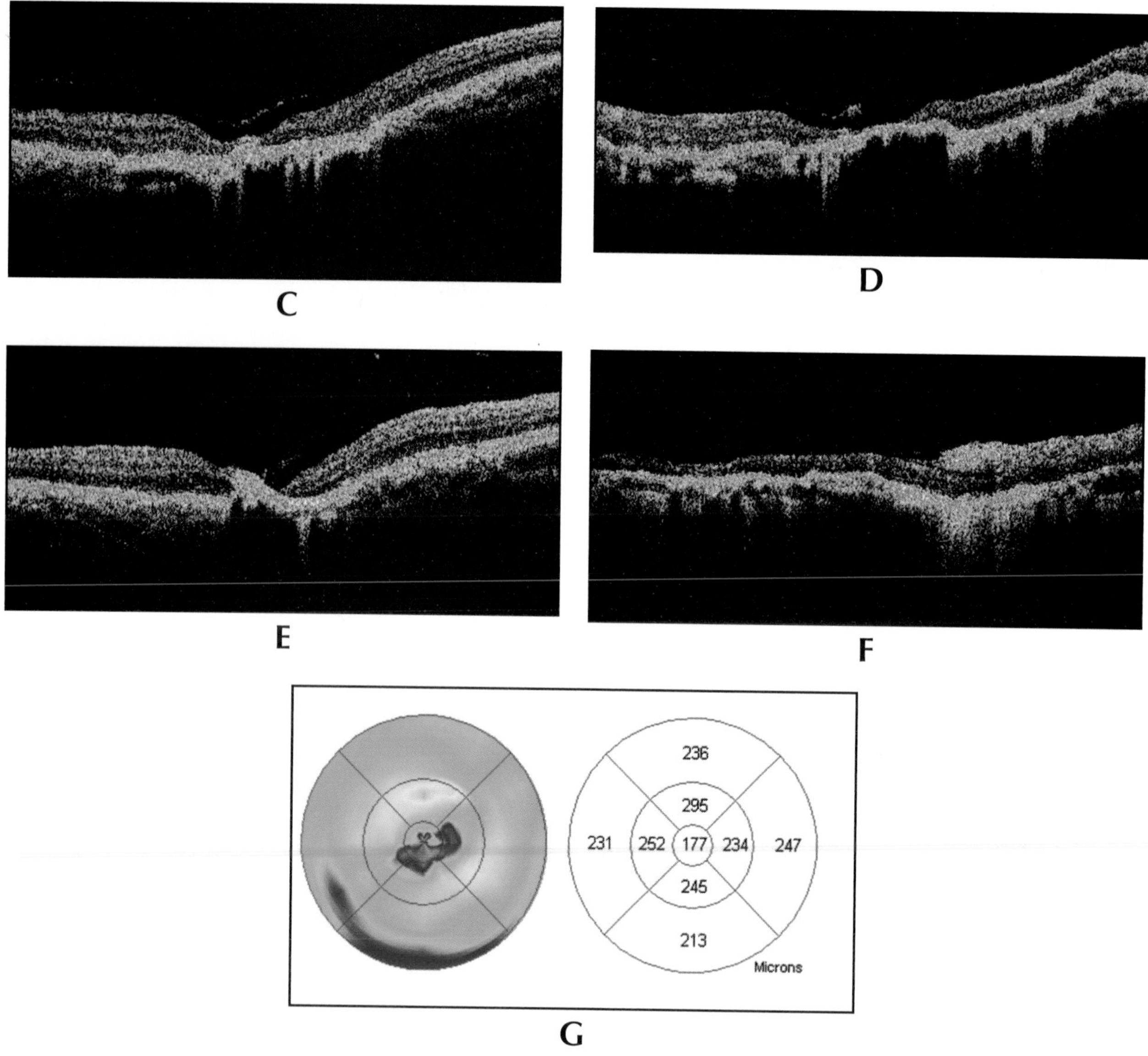
C
D
E
F
236
295
231
252
177
234
247
245
213
Microns
G

Case 11-9. Congenital Pit of the Optic Disc

Clinical Summary

A 45-year-old woman was referred for evaluation of macular elevation in the right eye. She was asymptomatic, and her vision was 20/20 in that eye. Slit-lamp biomicroscopy showed a temporal congenital optic disc pit and cystic retinal alterations in the papillomacular bundle area (A and B). FA (C) showed no obvious leakage.

Optical Coherence Tomography

A horizontal OCT scan (D) showed optically clear cystic spaces in the inner and outer retinal layers involving the center of the fovea as well as the nasal retina (right side of the scan). This schisis configuration revealed vertical structures corresponding to Müller cells bridging the outer and inner retina.

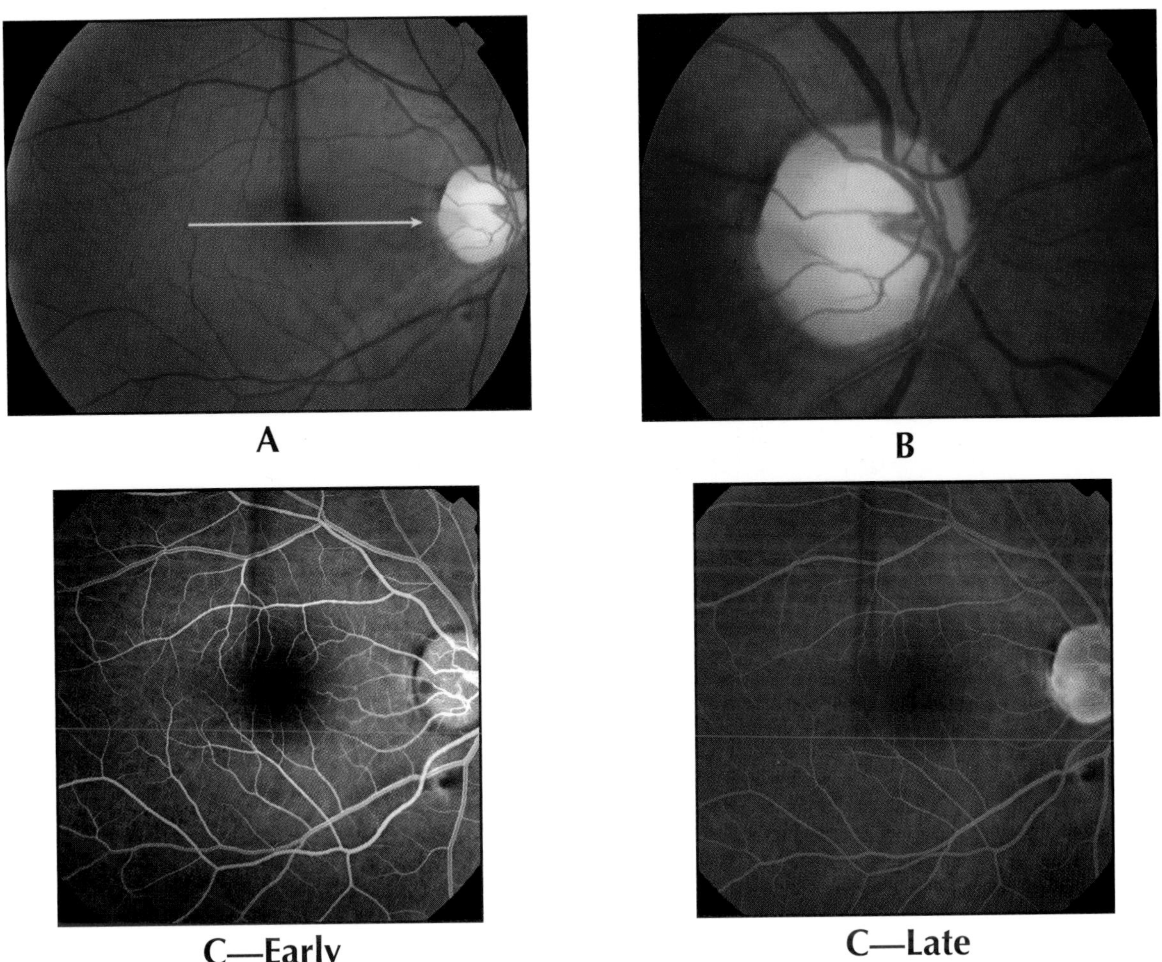

A

B

C—Early

C—Late

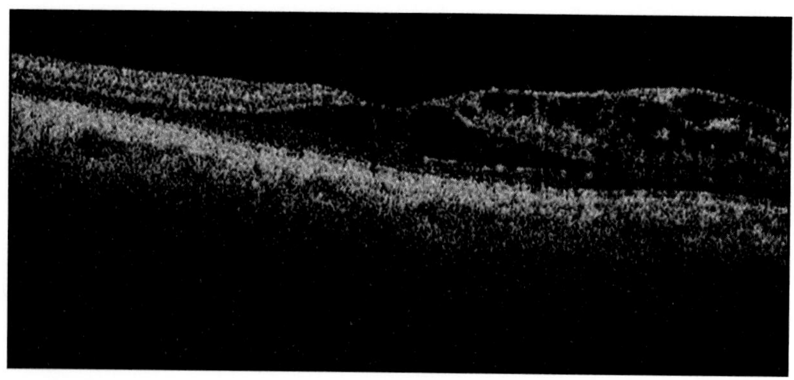

D

Case 11-10. Congenital Pit of the Optic Disc and Chorioretinal Colobomatous Defect

Clinical Summary

A 33-year-old woman was evaluated for a macular serous elevation associated with a congenital pit of the optic nerve head in her right eye. Her vision was 20/40 in this eye. Slit-lamp biomicroscopy showed an inferotemporal congenital optic disc pit and serous elevation of the macular area associated with pigmentary changes. A chorioretinal colobomatous defect was noticed just inferior to the optic nerve head (A).

Optical Coherence Tomography

OCT (B) confirmed the presence of a neurosensory retinal detachment, visualized as an elevation of the neurosensory retina over an optically clear space, adjacent to the edge of the optic disc pit. A reflective protrusion was noticed at the level of the RPE probably consistent with hyperplasia of this tissue. This finding suggests chronicity of the condition. An OCT scan (C) obtained through the fovea again showed the low reflective space under the neurosensory retina representing the neurosensory retinal detachment and mild intraretinal cystic changes in the fovea. An OCT scan (D) was obtained through the colobomatous area and nasal macular region. An area of thinning with lack of the normal retinal and RPE architecture was observed consistent with the colobomatous defect. The optical reflections from the scleral tissue underneath were enhanced due to the increased light penetration through the overlying thin tissue. The neurosensory retinal elevation was again observed.

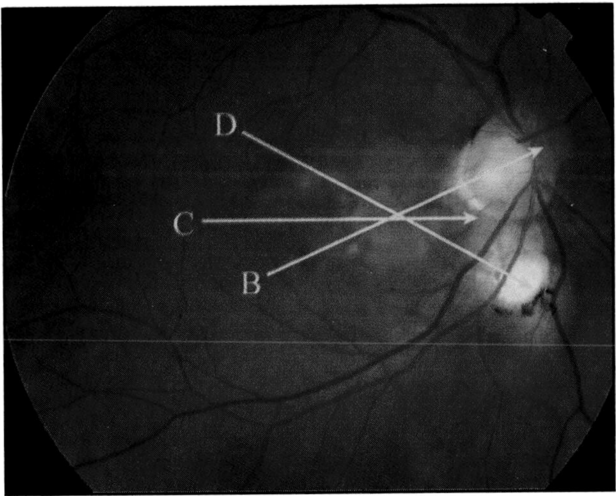

A

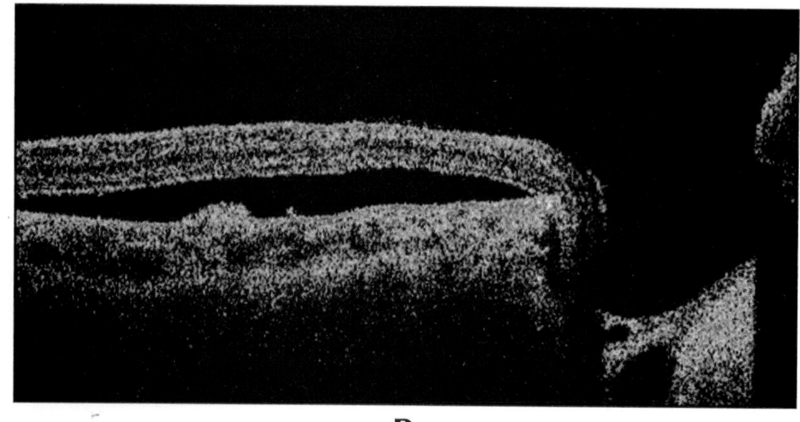

B

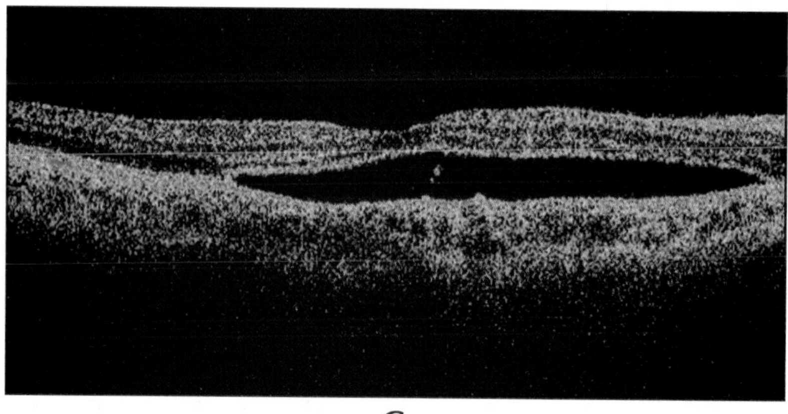

C

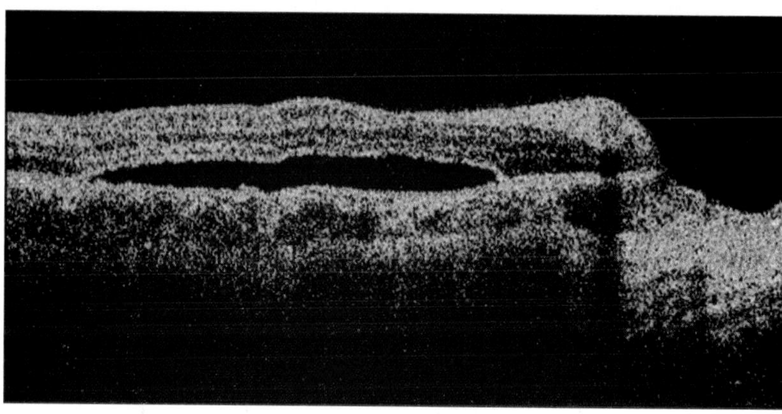

D

Case 11-11. Myelinated Fibers

Clinical Summary

A 70-year-old man recently diagnosed with type II diabetes mellitus was examined. The visual acuity in the left eye was 20/20. Dilated fundus examination of the left eye revealed myelinated nerve fibers inferior to the optic nerve head (A and B).

Optical Coherence Tomography

A vertical OCT scan (C) obtained inferior to the optic disc showed an area of increased reflectivity at the level of the nerve fiber layer correlating with the myelinated fibers. Shadowing of the optic signal from the tissues below this highly reflective area was appreciated.

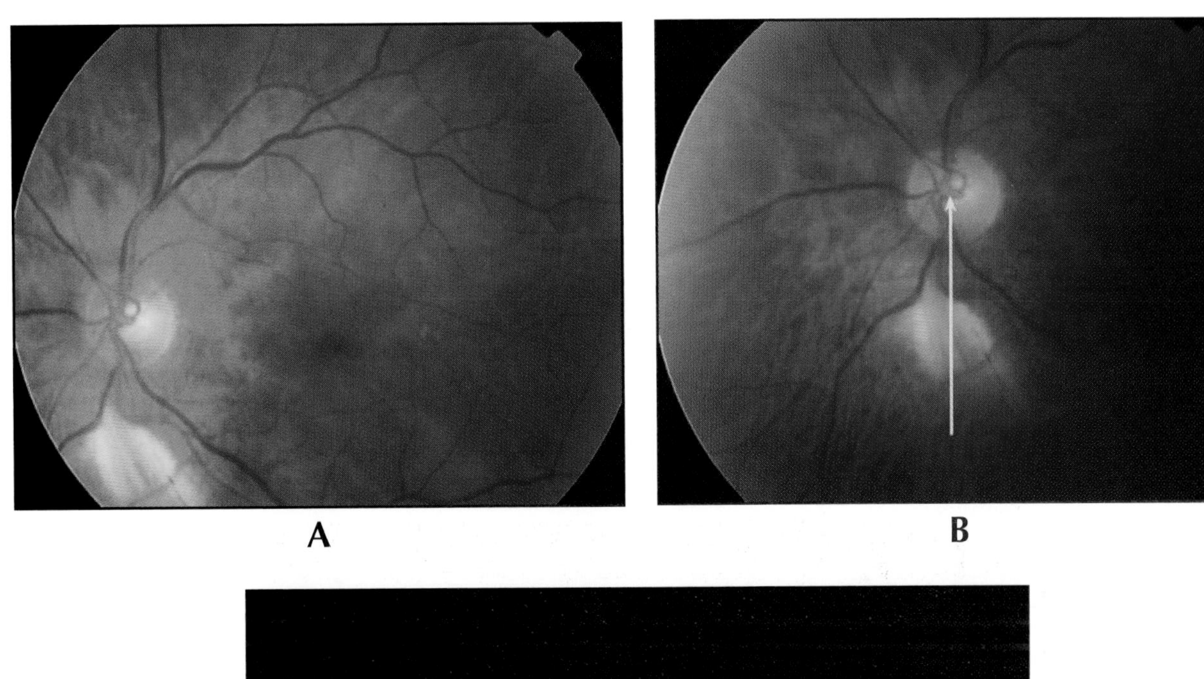

A B

C

Case 11-12. Cancer-Associated Retinopathy

Clinical Summary

A 65-year-old female is referred for evaluation of unexplained vision loss. She complains of progressive dimming of her vision in both eyes over the past 3 months. Her visual acuity is 20/25, and formal visual field testing shows extensive constriction of the peripheral field in both eyes. Dilated fundus exam (A and B) shows mild narrowing of the retinal arterioles but is otherwise unremarkable. FA shows a mild delay in A-V transit time but is otherwise normal. Full-field ERG demonstrates bilateral photoreceptor degeneration. A computer tomography (CT) scan of the chest shows a pulmonary mass with hilar lymphadenopathy, and subsequent biopsy confirms small cell lung cancer.

Optical Coherence Tomography

The OCT (C and D) shows thinning of the neurosensory retina in the peripheral macula. The foveal thickness and contour are relatively normal, but the neurosensory retina thins dramatically as the scan passes away from the fovea. This is best demonstrated on the retinal thickness map (E) where the peripheral macular thickness is approximately half normal. This pattern of retinal thinning appears similar to other conditions that result in photoreceptor degeneration (see Chapter 10).

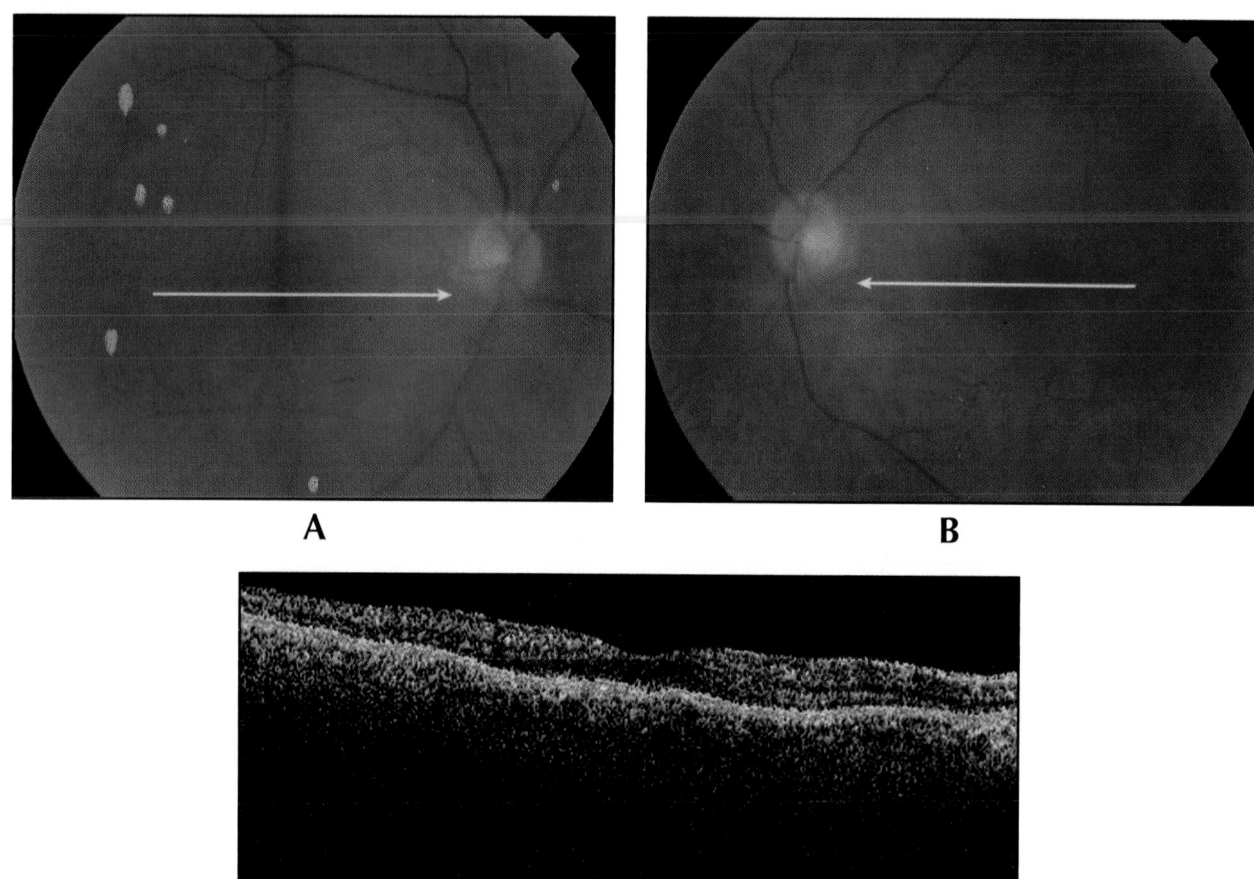

A B

C

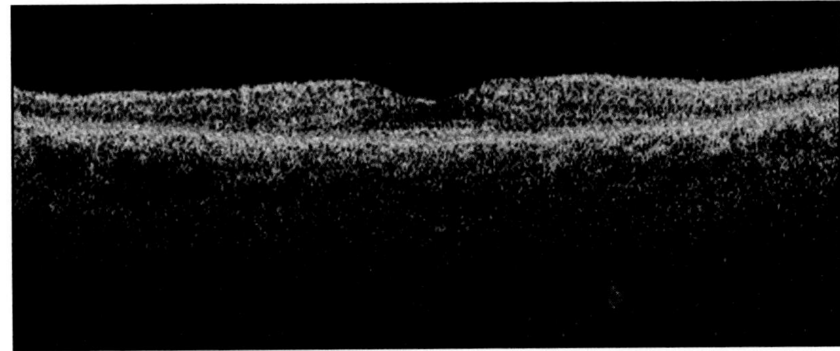

D

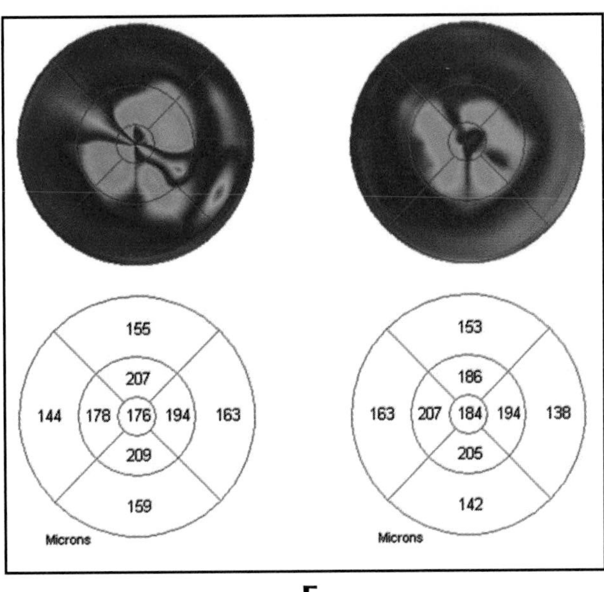
155
207
144
178
176
194
163
209
159
Microns
153
186
163
207
184
194
138
205
142
Microns

E

Section III

Optical Coherence Tomography in Glaucoma, Neuro-Ophthalmology, and the Anterior Segment

Chapter 12

Optical Coherence Tomography in Glaucoma

Gadi Wollstein, MD; Siobahn Beaton; Adelina Paunescu, PhD; Hiroshi Ishikawa, MD; James G. Fujimoto, PhD; and Joel S. Schuman, MD

Interpretation of the Optical Coherence Tomography Image

Glaucoma is characterized by irreversible loss of the retinal nerve fiber layer (NFL) and ganglion cell layer with corresponding typical visual field (VF) changes. The morphological changes are evaluated clinically by optic nerve head (ONH) and NFL assessment. However, qualitative assessment is highly observer-dependent and therefore prone to large interobserver variation.[1-4] In addition, detection of tissue changes during follow-up is crucial for determining the need for treatment, although this imposes a great clinical challenge.

VF testing is used to estimate the functional glaucomatous damage. The test is a subjective assessment that requires patient cooperation and can suffer large intervisit variation. Due to the large variation, detection of VF changes requires repetition of the test, thus deferring diagnosis.

Several studies have suggested that glaucomatous field abnormalities may be preceded by structural changes of the ONH[5-7] and NFL (Figure 12-1).[8-10] Histological evaluation of the NFL estimated that up to 50% of the retinal NFL may be lost prior to the appearance of initial VF damage.[11] This damage may be detected in 60% of NFL photographs up to 6 years prior to the appearance of a detectable VF defect.[10] Detection of early structural damage may help identify patients who require preventive therapy because they are at a high risk for visual loss and may spare patients without damage the cost and morbidity of treatment.

Several imaging devices are currently available, all aimed to provide objective quantitative measures of posterior segment ocular structures:

1. Confocal scanning laser ophthalmoscopy (CSLO)—This device acquires sequential scans of the ONH to provide a three-dimensional reconstruction of the imaged area. The CSLO is capable of scanning only the ONH and due to the large normal anatomical variability and the structural complexity of this region, the capability of this device to detect glaucomatous damage is limited. Moreover, in order to obtain the stereometric measures, the operator is required to trace the ONH margin, thus inducing an operator-dependent variability. An additional limitation of this technology is the necessity of using an intraocular reference plane in order to establish the height measurements. This plane might be different between subjects and may change over time in certain pathological circumstances. The transverse resolution of the commercially available device is 10 microns (μm) and the axial resolution is 300 μm
2. Scanning laser polarimetry (SLP)—This device uses the birefringence properties of the retinal NFL to estimate the thickness of this layer in the peripapillary region. Since other ocular structures—mainly the cornea—influence the birefringence properties of the eye, the capability of the device to detect glaucomatous changes is reduced. A newer version of this device, with a dynamic compensation modality, shows promise in reducing confounding due to anterior segment birefringence. Since SLP evaluates the peripapillary region, pathologic processes in this location, such as peripapillary atrophy, also confound analysis. The resolution of this device is reportedly 13 μm
3. Scanning laser biomicroscopy—This device utilizes a method similar to biomicroscopy in which light is projected at an angle on the scanned area and the backscattered light is detected. The device is capable of scanning the ONH, macula, and peripapillary region. Since the incoming and the outgoing lights

pass through different locations, this device requires pupil dilation. Furthermore, corneal opacities as well as cataractous changes can make image acquisition difficult. The resolution of this device is 50 μm

Optical coherence tomography (OCT) is a quantitative, objective high resolution device capable of scanning the ONH, macula, and peripapillary region. The capability to scan all these regions improves the ability to detect and confirm the ocular structure. The resolution of the OCT (StratusOCT, Carl Zeiss Meditec, Dublin, Calif) is 8 μm to 10 μm, better than any other available glaucoma imaging device.

OCT offers the ability to perform structural imaging in glaucoma patients and glaucoma suspects and allows structure-function correlation. Early in the disease, patients the OCT disclosed structural abnormalities without any detectable VF loss. If VF loss is present, a structural abnormality should be detectable. One excellent use of OCT is in identifying corresponding structural and functional abnormalities, eliminating the need for repeated VF tests to confirm the presence of a new or subtle defect.

OCT has become a valuable tool in glaucoma management for identifying the presence of disease or confirming its absence and is useful for the detection of disease progression over time.

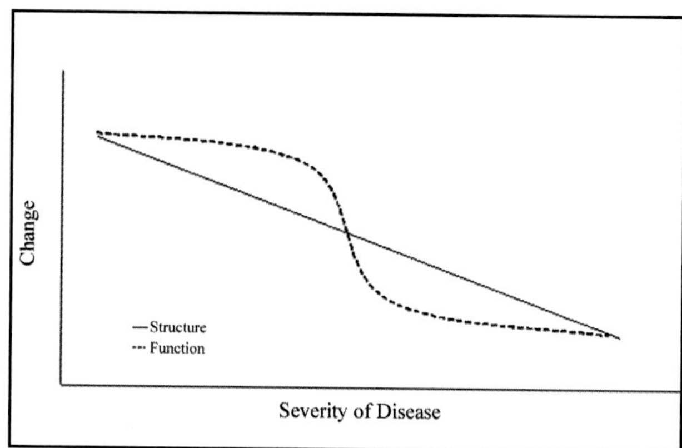

Figure 12-1. A disconnect exists between structure and function in the visual system. Approximately 40% to 50% of retinal ganglion cells (RGCs) may be lost prior to the development of a detectable functional abnormality, whereas structural abnormalities are detectable in a more linear fashion. This graph illustrates that early in the disease, structural imaging is a more sensitive indicator of glaucomatous damage, while once functional disease is detectable, it is a very sensitive parameter to follow. Late in the disease, functional measures again fail, as the disease moves beyond perimetry's dynamic range, and structural imaging may still be able to measure ongoing change.

References

1. Sturmer J, Poinoosawmy D, Broadway DC, Hitchings RA. Intra- and interobserver variation of optic nerve head measurements in glaucoma suspects using disc-data. *Int Ophthalmol*. 1992;16(4-5):227-233.
2. Abrams LS, Scott IU, Spaeth GL, et al. Agreement among optometrists, ophthalmologists, and residents in evaluating the optic disc for glaucoma. *Ophthalmology*. 1994;101(10): 1662-1667.
3. Gaasterland DE, Blackwell B, Dally LG, et al. The Advanced Glaucoma Intervention Study (AGIS): 10. Variability among academic glaucoma subspecialists in assessing optic disc notching. *Trans Am Ophthalmol Soc*. 2001;99:177-84; discussion 84-85.
4. Tielsch JM, Katz J, Quigley HA, et al. Intraobserver and interobserver agreement in measurement of optic disc characteristics. *Ophthalmology*. 1988;95(3):350-356.
5. Sommer A, Pollack I, Maumenee AE. Optic disc parameters and onset of glaucomatous field loss. I. Methods and progressive changes in disc morphology. *Arch Ophthalmol*. 1979;97(8):1444-1448.
6. Pederson J, Anderson D. The mode of progressive disc cupping in ocular hypertension and glaucoma. *Arch Ophthalmol*. 1980;98:490-495.
7. Quigley HA, Katz J, Derick RJ, et al. An evaluation of optic disc and nerve fiber layer examinations in monitoring progression of early glaucoma damage. *Ophthalmology*. 1992;99(1):19-28.
8. Sommer A, Miller NR, Pollack I, et al. The nerve fiber layer in the diagnosis of glaucoma. *Arch Ophthalmol*. 1977;95(12):2149-2156.
9. Sommer A, Quigley H, Robin A. Evaluation of nerve fiber layer assessment. *Arch Ophthalmol*. 1984;102:1766-1771.
10. Sommer A, Katz J, Quigley HA, et al. Clinically detectable nerve fiber atrophy precedes the onset of glaucomatous field loss. *Arch Ophthalmol*. 1991;109(1):77-83.
11. Quigley HA, Addicks EM, Green WR. Optic nerve damage in human glaucoma. III. Quantitative correlation of nerve fiber loss and visual field defect in glaucoma, ischemic neuropathy, papilledema, and toxic neuropathy. *Arch Ophthalmol*. 1982;100(1):135-146.

Index to Cases

Normal Eyes

Case 12-1 Normal Nerve Fiber Layer, Macula, and Optic Nerve Head Imaging and a Full Visual Field Characterized This Healthy Eye 488

Case 12-2 Improper Alignment Made a Normal Eye Appear to Have a Thin Nerve Fiber Layer 490

Structure-Function Correspondence

Case 12-3 Excellent Correspondence Was Seen Between All Structural and Functional Analyses 492

Case 12-4 All Structural Measures Were Consistent With Each Other and With Functional Findings in Location and Severity. 496

Case 12-5 Structure-Function Correlation Allowed Diagnosis and Treatment of Glaucoma 500

Case 12-6 Nerve Fiber Layer, Optic Nerve Head, and Macula Showed Excellent Correspondence With Visual Fields in Advanced Glaucoma 504

Case 12-7 Nerve Fiber Layer and Macular Analysis Corresponded to Visual Field Abnormality in Advanced Glaucoma 508

Case 12-8 Advanced Glaucoma Was Demonstrated by Loss of the Majority of the Nerve Fiber Layer, Severe Macular Thinning, and Only a Central Island Remaining on the Visual Field . . . 510

The Utility of Imaging in Early Glaucoma

Case 12-9 Structure and Function Combined to Disclose Glaucoma in the Right Eye and Preperimetric Glaucoma on the Left. 514

Case 12-10 Optical Coherence Tomography, Heidelberg Retina Tomograph, and Visual Field Correlation Supported Authenticity of Early Visual Field Abnormalities 517

Glaucoma is Global

Case 12-11 Even With Field Loss on One Side of the Horizontal Meridian, Structural Imaging Revealed That Glaucoma Damage Was Global. 521

Imaging Supports Early, Questionable Visual Field Findings

Case 12-12 Structural and Functional Imaging Corresponded to Both Eyes, Reinforced Significance of Early Superior Visual Field Defect OD 523

Case 12-13 Structural Imaging Corresponded With Visual Field, Reinforced Significance of Early Superior Visual Field Defect 527

Case 12-14 Nerve Fiber Layer and Neuroretinal Rim Loss Corresponded With Visual Field, Reinforced Significance of Early Visual Field Defect; Macula Did Not Equal Visual Field 529

Case 12-15 Nerve Fiber Layer, Macular, and Optic Nerve Head Scanning All Corresponded With Visual Field Loss. Structural Correspondence With Questionable Visual Field Loss Corroborated Findings 531

Imaging Discloses Functional Artifact

Case 12-16 Corresponding Optical Coherence Tomography, Heidelberg Retinal Tomograph, and Visual Field Findings Supported Glaucomatous Damage in the Right Eye; Lack of Structural Correlation Suggested Visual Field Defect Was Artifact on the Left. 535

Case 12-17 Structural Testing Corresponded With Superior Functional Loss, Suggested Inferior Loss Was Either Mild or Artifact 539

Case 12-18 Structural Imaging Suggested That Visual Field Abnormalities Were Erroneous in One Eye and Valid in the Other . . . 541

Case 12-19 Structural Measures Supported Superior But Not Inferior Visual Field Defects . . . 545

Imaging Suggests Actual Glaucoma Damage Exceeds Visual Fields

Case 12-20 Correspondence Between Structural and Functional Measures Was Good, But There Was Less Functional Loss Than Might Be Expected Based on Retinal Nerve Fiber Layer, Macular, and Optic Nerve Head Abnormalities, Particularly. This Suggested That This Patient Should Be Watched Closely For Future Functional Loss . . . 547

Case 12-21 Structure and Function Corresponded, But Structural Loss Exceeded Detectable Functional Damage. Macular Imaging Helped to Explain Why Functional Loss May Have Been Missed . . . 551

Case 12-22 The Amount of Structural Loss Appeared to Exceed the Functional Loss Present . . . 553

Beware Artifact

Case 12-23 Nerve Fiber Layer and Macular Thinning Corresponded to a Disc Hemorrhage and Visual Field Loss. A Poor Quality Image Demonstrated That Data From Poor Scans Should Be Disregarded . . . 557

Nerv Fiber Layer is Superior to Optic Nerve Head and Macula in Sensitivity to Glaucomatous Damage

Case 12-24 Optical Coherence Tomography and Heidelberg Retinal Tomograph Showed Good Correspondence With Each Other and With Visual Fields. Nerve Fiber Layer and Macular Measurements Gave Better Indications of Functional Loss Than Optic Nerve Head Assessments . . . 559

Case 12-25 Good Correspondence Among Visual Field Damage and Retinal Nerve Fiber Layer, Macular, and Optic Nerve Head Measurements . . . 562

Case 12-26 Retinal Nerve Fiber Layer Assessment Corresponded to Visual Field Findings, but the Optic Nerve Head and Macular Measures Missed the Superior Temporal Loss of Tissue . . . 566

Case 12-27 Retinal Nerve Fiber Layer Measurements Corresponded to Functional Loss. A Small Disc on the Right Confounded Optic Nerve Head Analysis. Macular Thickness Was Reduced in Accordance With Functional Loss . . . 568

Case 12-28 A Focal Nerve Fiber Layer Defect Was Demonstrated on Optical Coherence Tomography, Nerve Fiber Layer, Macular Imaging, and Perimetry, But Not by Optic Nerve Head Analysis . . . 572

Case 12-29 Nerve Fiber Layer and Macular Scans Showed Excellent Correspondence With Visual Fields, But Small Optic Nerves Confounded Optic Nerve Head Analysis . . . 575

Case 12-30 Nerve Fiber Layer Proved to Correspond Better to Visual Field Abnormalities Than Optic Nerve Head or Macular Imaging . . . 579

Case 12-31 Structure and Function Corresponded, With Retinal Nerve Fiber Layer Having the Closest Relationship to Visual Field Loss . . . 583

Case 12-32 Nerve Fiber Layer Thinning Corresponded to Severe Visual Field Loss in Advanced Glaucoma. Macular Thickness Was Normal, Which Suggested Confounding by Another Macular Disease . . . 587

Abnormal Structure With Normal Function May Suggest Future Functional Loss

Case 12-33 Good Structure-Function Correspondence of Glaucomatous Damage on the Right With Borderline Abnormal Structure on the Left Suggested That Functional Loss May Develop on the Left . . . 589

Case 12-34 Structural Damage on Optical Coherence Tomography May Be Harbinger of Future Further Visual Field Loss 592

Case 12-35 Nerve Fiber Layer, Optic Nerve Head, and Macula Corresponded With Visual Field; Superior Structural Abnormalities May Presage Inferior Visual Field Loss 596

Longitudinal Analysis

Case 12-36 A Patient With Narrow Angles But No Glaucoma Was Stable by Nerve Fiber Layer and Visual Field Throughout Follow-Up 598

Case 12-37 A Normal and Stable Circumpapillary Nerve Fiber Layer Suggested the Absence of Glaucoma in the Presence of Pseudoexfoliation and Fluctuating Visual Field Defects 600

Case 12-38 Longitudinal Evaluation of Optical Coherence Tomography and Visual Fields Demonstrated Loss of Nerve Fiber Layer Prior to Development of Visual Field Defect 602

Case 12-39 Progressive Nerve Fiber Layer and Visual Field Loss Went Hand-in-Hand 605

Case 12-40 Loss of Nerve Fiber Layer Paralleled Visual Field Loss 608

Case 12-1. Normal Nerve Fiber Layer, Macula, and Optic Nerve Head Imaging and a Full Visual Field Characterized This Healthy Eye

A 51-year-old Caucasian man had presbyopia. Visual acuity was 20/20 and the intraocular pressure (IOP) was 16 millimeters of mercury (mmHg) in the left eye. The anterior chamber was normal. Dilated fundus examination revealed a normal appearing ONH (A) with no other abnormalities noted. Humphrey VFs were full in the left eye (B). Heidelberg retina tomograph (HRT) showed a normal size ONH with a small cup (C).

Optical Coherence Tomography

The circumpapillary scan showed a retinal NFL with normal thickness, with the typical pattern of thickest NFL in the superior and inferior regions (the "double hump" pattern) (D). This pattern actually contains two peaks superiorly and a peak and a shoulder inferiorly, but by convention continues to be referred to as the "double hump" pattern in this book. The macular retinal thickness was normal and was thinner in the outer inferior and temporal regions than elsewhere (E). Note the normally thicker retina nasally compared to temporally, corresponding to the papillomacular bundle. A normal sized optic disc with a small cup was noted in the ONH scan (F).

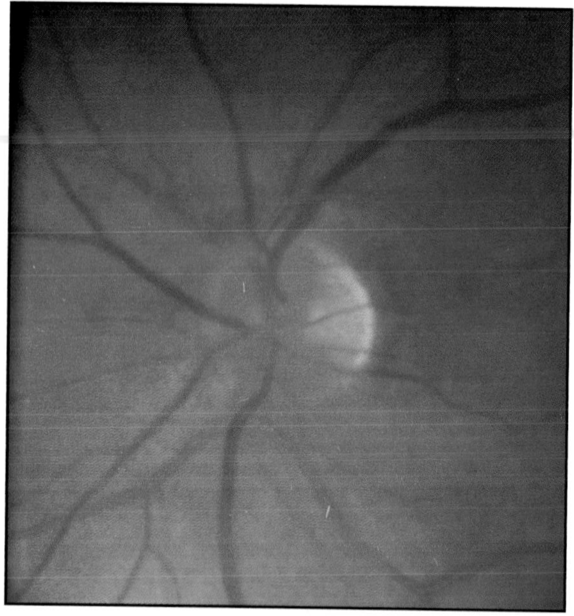

A

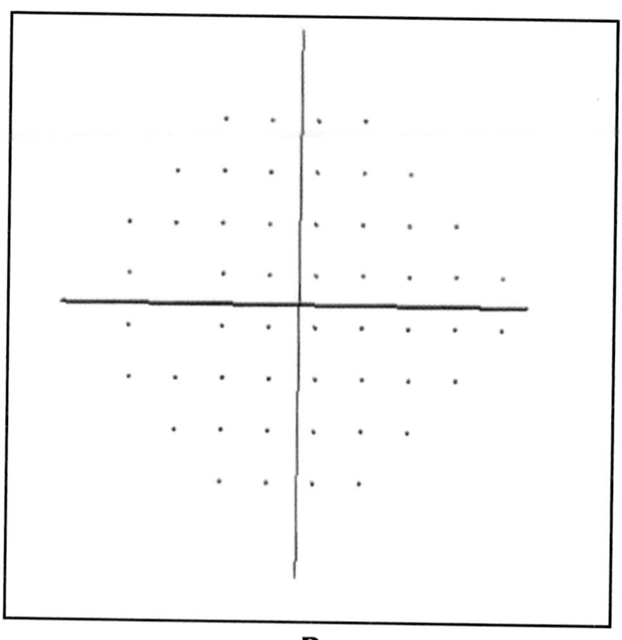

B

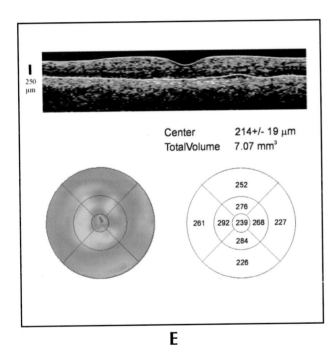

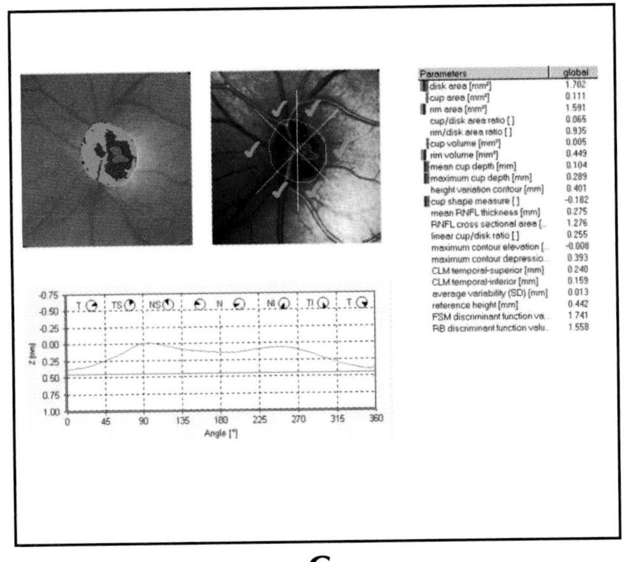

Parameters | global
disk area [mm²] 1.702
cup area [mm²] 0.111
rim area [mm²] 1.591
cup/disk area ratio [] 0.065
rim/disk area ratio [] 0.935
cup volume [mm³] 0.005
rim volume [mm³] 0.449
mean cup depth [mm] 0.104
maximum cup depth [mm] 0.289
height variation contour [mm] 0.401
cup shape measure [] -0.182
mean RNFL thickness [mm] 0.275
RNFL cross sectional area [... 1.276
linear cup/disk ratio [] 0.255
maximum contour elevation [... -0.008
maximum contour depressio... 0.393
CLM temporal-superior [mm] 0.240
CLM temporal-inferior [mm] 0.159
average variability (SD) [mm] 0.013
reference height [mm] 0.442
FSM discriminant function va... 1.741
RB discriminant function valu... 1.558
Angle [°]

C

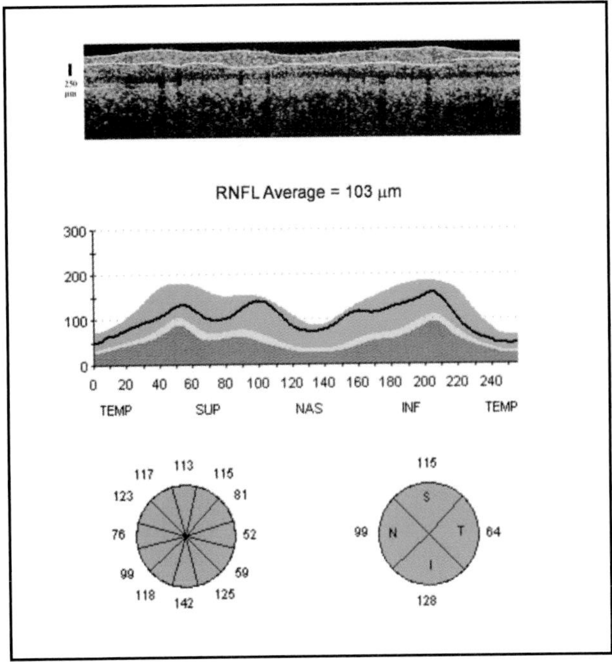

D

250 µm

Center 214+/- 19 µm
TotalVolume 7.07 mm³

252
261 292 239 268 227
276
284
226

E

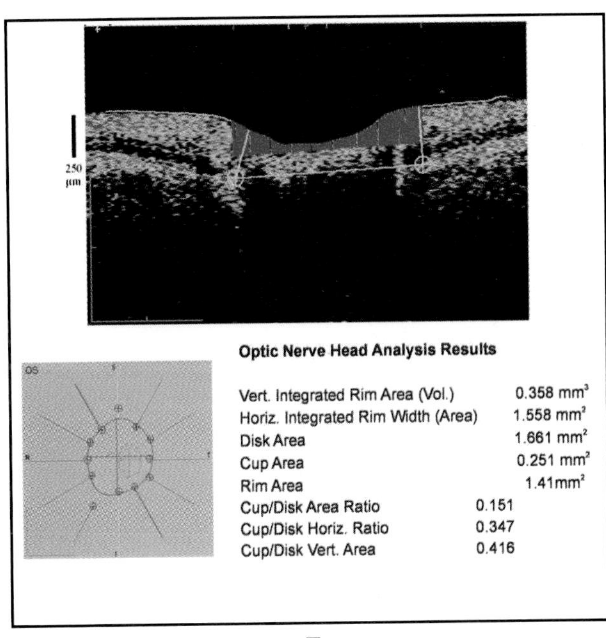

250 µm
Optic Nerve Head Analysis Results
Vert. Integrated Rim Area (Vol.) 0.358 mm³
Horiz. Integrated Rim Width (Area) 1.558 mm²
Disk Area 1.661 mm²
Cup Area 0.251 mm²
Rim Area 1.41mm²
Cup/Disk Area Ratio 0.151
Cup/Disk Horiz. Ratio 0.347
Cup/Disk Vert. Area 0.416

F

Case 12-2. Improper Alignment Made a Normal Eye Appear to Have a Thin Nerve Fiber Layer

A 43-year-old healthy Caucasian man had no ocular disease. Visual acuity was 20/20 in the left eye and IOP was 15 mmHg. The anterior chamber examination was unremarkable and no ocular abnormality was found on examination of the posterior segment. VF test was full (A). HRT showed small optic disc size with a small cup and normal neuroretinal rim (B).

Optical Coherence Tomography

The circumpapillary retinal NFL thickness was in the low range of normal with thinning nasally (C). A repeat NFL scan showed normal NFL thickness. Normal and symmetrical macular retinal thickness was noted (D). The ONH scan showed a small cup in a normal size disc (E).

Comment

Low normal NFL thickness was noted in the nasal region of the initial peripapillary scan. Careful evaluation of the scan revealed slight asymmetry in the alignment of the eye. This could be appreciated by evaluating the signal intensity of the retinal pigment epithelium (RPE) layer (the red inferior band). In a properly aligned scan, the intensity of this band would be homogenous along the entire scan. The left side of the scan had a wider band, while the right side had a thinner band, reflecting inappropriate alignment. The NFL scan was normal once the patient was properly aligned.

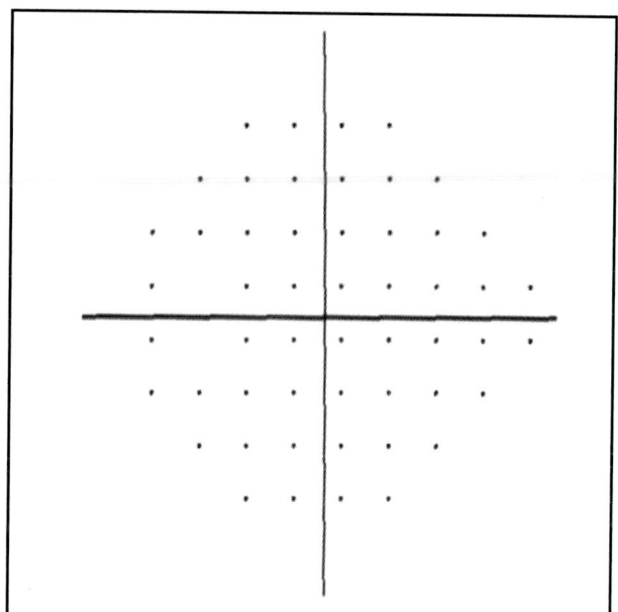

A

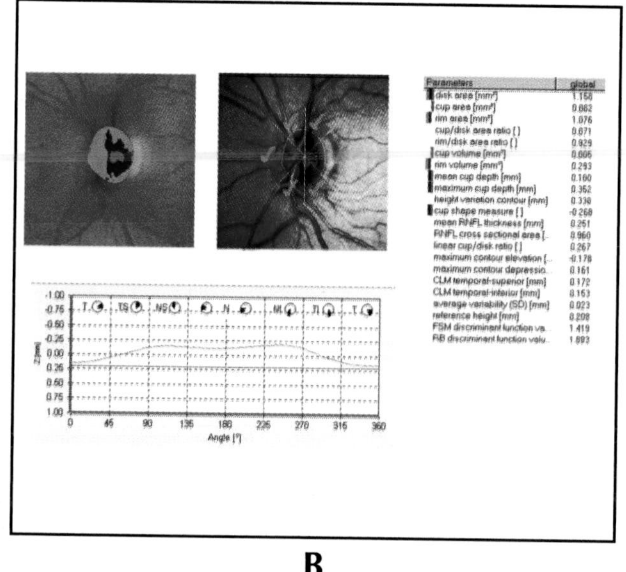

Parameters global
disk area [mm²] 1.158
cup area [mm²] 0.082
rim area [mm²] 1.076
cup/disk area ratio [ ] 0.071
rim/disk area ratio [ ] 0.929
cup volume [mm³] 0.006
rim volume [mm³] 0.293
mean cup depth [mm] 0.100
maximum cup depth [mm] 0.352
height variation contour [mm] 0.338
cup shape measure [ ] -0.268
mean RNFL thickness [mm] 0.251
RNFL cross sectional area [... 0.960
linear cup/disk ratio [ ] 0.267
maximum contour elevation [... -0.178
maximum contour depressio... 0.161
CLM temporal-superior [mm] 0.172
CLM temporal-inferior [mm] 0.163
average variability (SD) [mm] 0.023
reference height [mm] 0.208
FSM discriminant function va... 1.419
RB discriminant function valu... 1.893

B

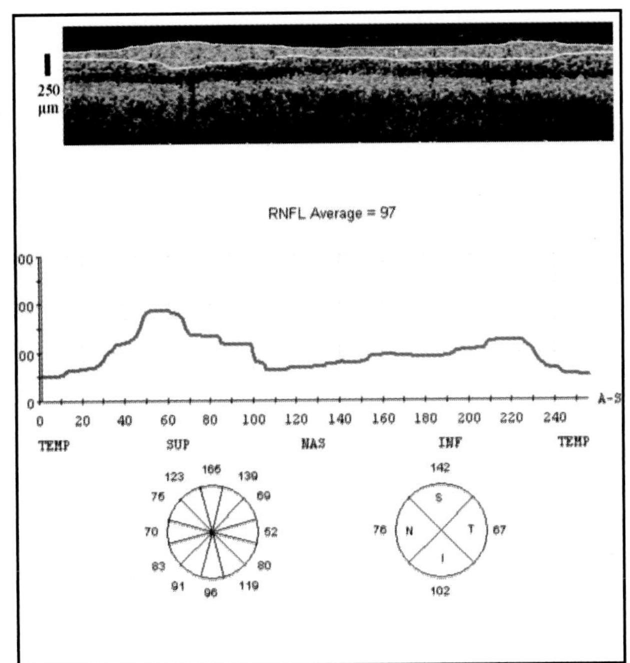

C

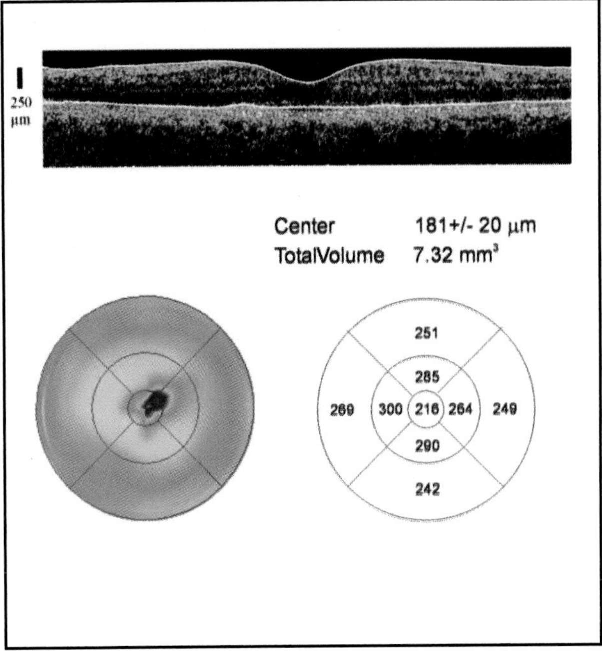

D

Optic Nerve Head Analysis Results

Vert. Integrated Rim Area (Vol.)	0.562 mm³
Horiz. Integrated Rim Width (Area)	1.71 mm²
Disk Area	1.771 mm²
Cup Area	0.171 mm²
Rim Area	1.6 mm²
Cup/Disk Area Ratio	0.097
Cup/Disk Horiz. Ratio	0.334
Cup/Disk Vert. Area	0.309

E

Case 12-3. Excellent Correspondence Was Seen Between All Structural and Functional Analyses

A 68-year-old Caucasian man with primary open-angle glaucoma was treated with bimatoprost 0.03% and brimonidine 0.2%. The visual acuity was 20/16 in the right eye and 20/25 in the left eye and the IOP was 16 mmHg in both eyes. The anterior segment examination was normal with wide open angles and the funduscopy revealed asymmetric cupping with a larger cup in the left eye (A and B). The VF test showed early inferior paracentral and nasal defects in the right eye (C) and paracentral and nasal defects in the left eye (D) more pronounced in the inferior hemifield. Asymmetric cupping was shown with the HRT with larger cupping on the left (E and F) and abnormal thinning of the neuroretinal rim superior and inferior temporally.

Optical Coherence Tomography

The retinal NFL was markedly thinner in the left than the right eye (G and H). The abnormal thinning in the right eye was located at the 9:00 through 11:00 positions, with borderline thinning elsewhere, and in the left eye in the entire temporal half of the disc. The macular volume was markedly reduced in the left eye (J) compared to the right eye (I) with reduced thickness in the superior and temporal outer segments in the right eye and the entire outer region and the inferior and temporal inner regions in the left eye. Asymmetric cupping was evident by ONH analysis; cup/disc area ratio was larger in the left eye (K and L). A rim notch was noted superior temporally in the right eye with elimination of the neuroretinal rim in most of the temporal half of the disc in the left eye.

Comment

Excellent correspondence was seen between all structural and functional analyses.

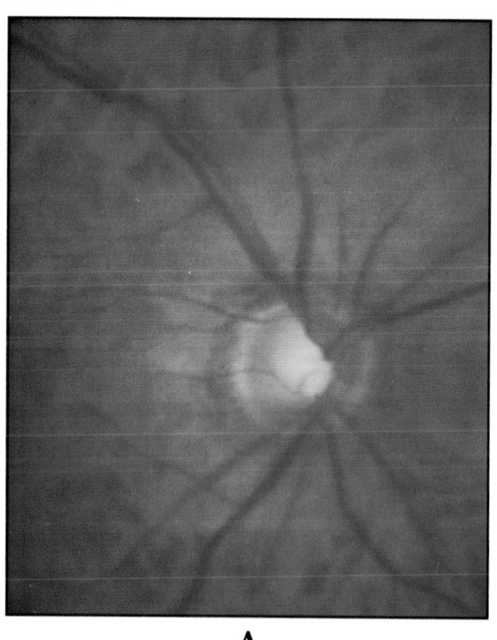

A

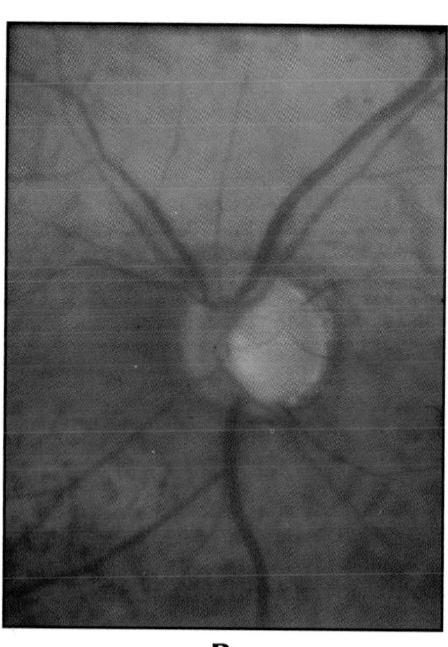

B

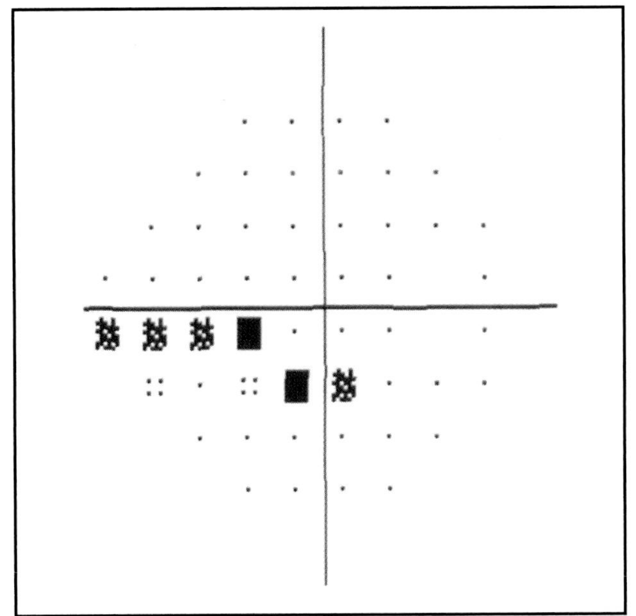

C

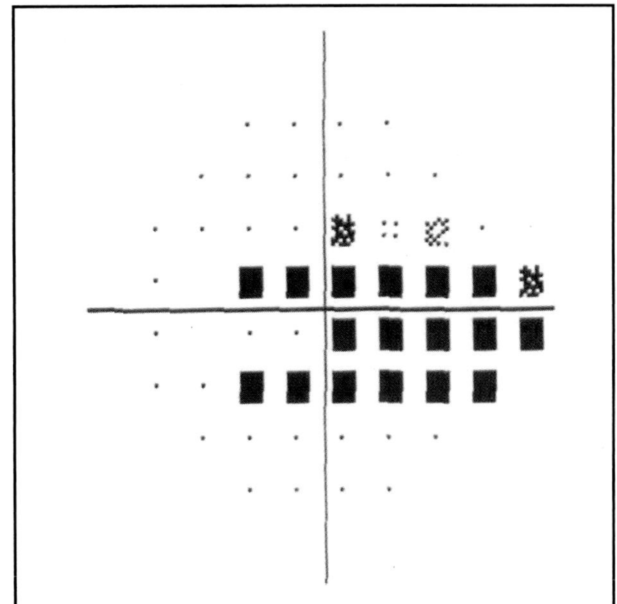

D

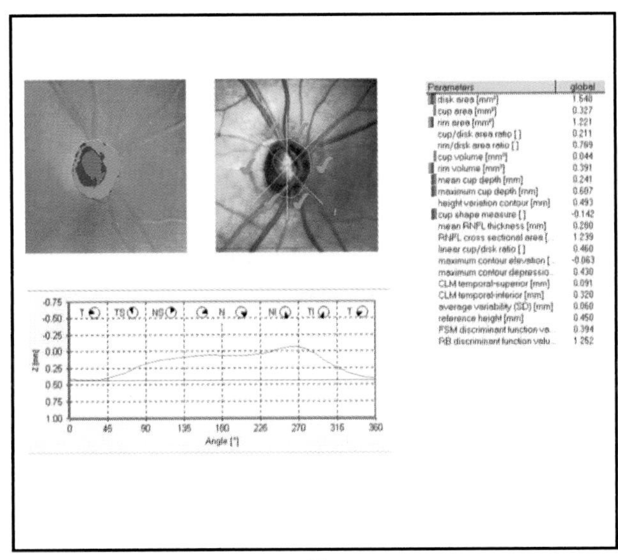

Parameters	global
disk area [mm²]	1.540
cup area [mm²]	0.327
rim area [mm²]	1.221
cup/disk area ratio [ ]	0.211
rim/disk area ratio [ ]	0.789
cup volume [mm³]	0.044
rim volume [mm³]	0.391
mean cup depth [mm]	0.241
maximum cup depth [mm]	0.607
height variation contour [mm]	0.493
cup shape measure [ ]	-0.142
mean RNFL thickness [mm]	0.280
RNFL cross sectional area [	1.239
linear cup/disk ratio [ ]	0.460
maximum contour elevation [	-0.063
maximum contour depressio	0.430
CLM temporal-superior [mm]	0.091
CLM temporal-inferior [mm]	0.320
average variability (SD) [mm]	0.060
reference height [mm]	0.450
FSM discriminant function va	0.394
RB discriminant function valu	1.252

E

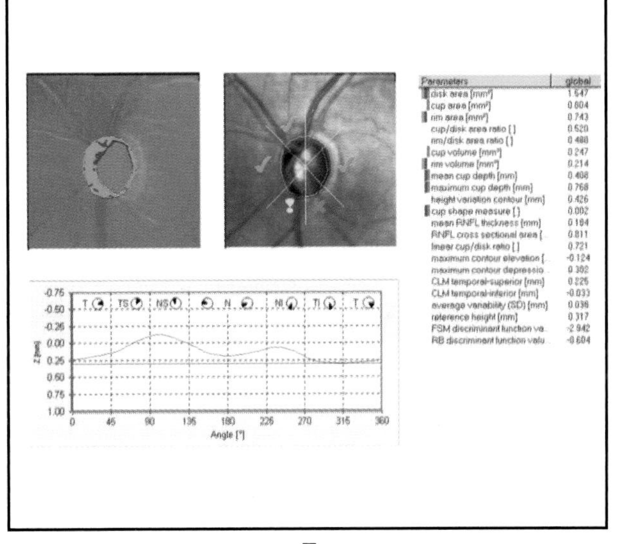

Parameters	global
disk area [mm²]	1.547
cup area [mm²]	0.804
rim area [mm²]	0.743
cup/disk area ratio [ ]	0.520
rim/disk area ratio [ ]	0.480
cup volume [mm³]	0.247
rim volume [mm³]	0.214
mean cup depth [mm]	0.408
maximum cup depth [mm]	0.768
height variation contour [mm]	0.426
cup shape measure [ ]	0.002
mean RNFL thickness [mm]	0.184
RNFL cross sectional area [	0.811
linear cup/disk ratio [ ]	0.721
maximum contour elevation [	-0.124
maximum contour depressio	0.302
CLM temporal-superior [mm]	0.225
CLM temporal-inferior [mm]	-0.033
average variability (SD) [mm]	0.038
reference height [mm]	0.317
FSM discriminant function va	-2.942
RB discriminant function valu	-0.604

F

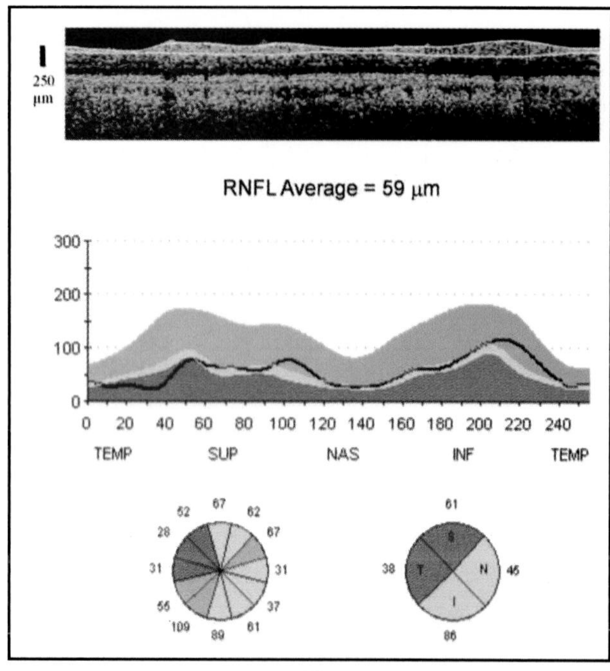
250 µm
RNFL Average = 59 µm
300
200
100
0
0 20 40 60 80 100 120 140 160 180 200 220 240
TEMP SUP NAS INF TEMP
S
T
N
I

G

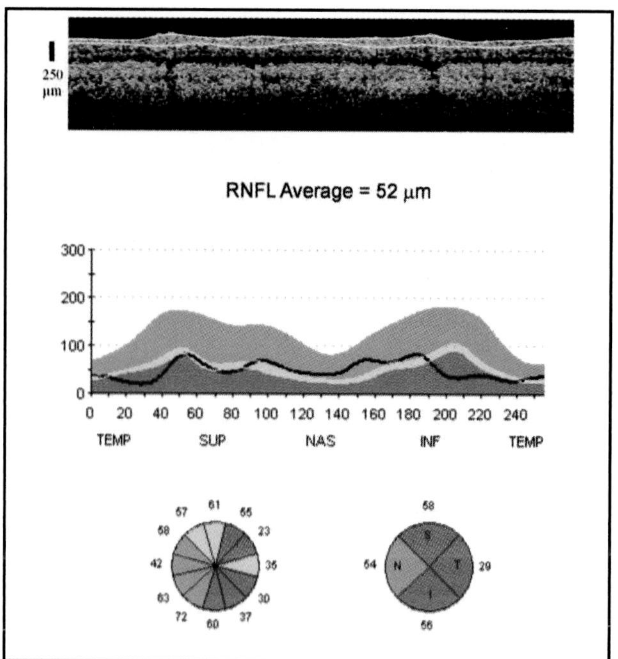
250 µm
RNFL Average = 52 µm
300
200
100
0
0 20 40 60 80 100 120 140 160 180 200 220 240
TEMP SUP NAS INF TEMP
S
N
T
I

H

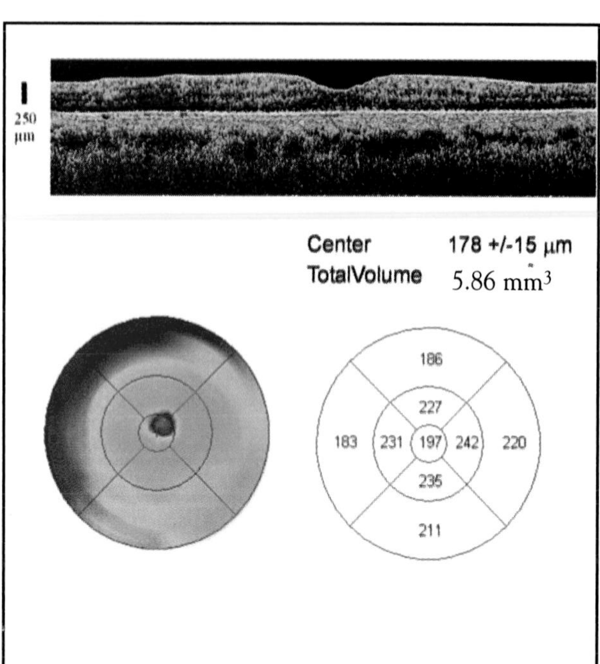
250 µm
Center 178 +/-15 µm
TotalVolume 5.86 mm³
186
227
183 231 197 242 220
235
211

I

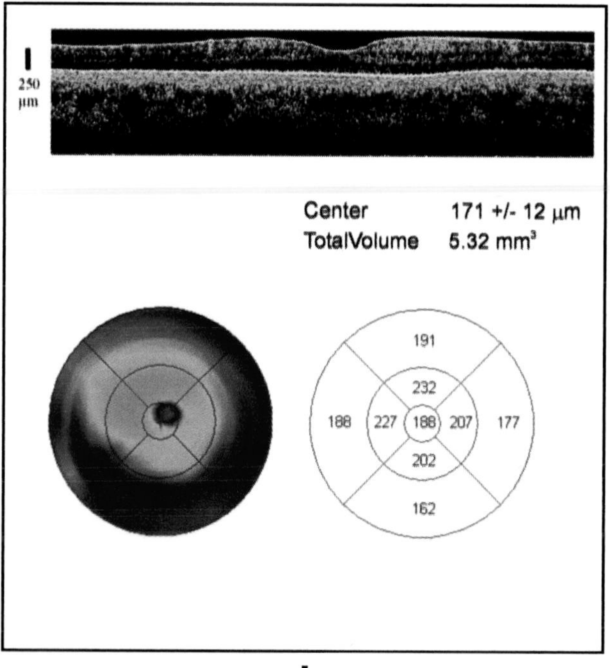
250 µm
Center 171 +/- 12 µm
TotalVolume 5.32 mm³
191
232
188 227 188 207 177
202
162

J

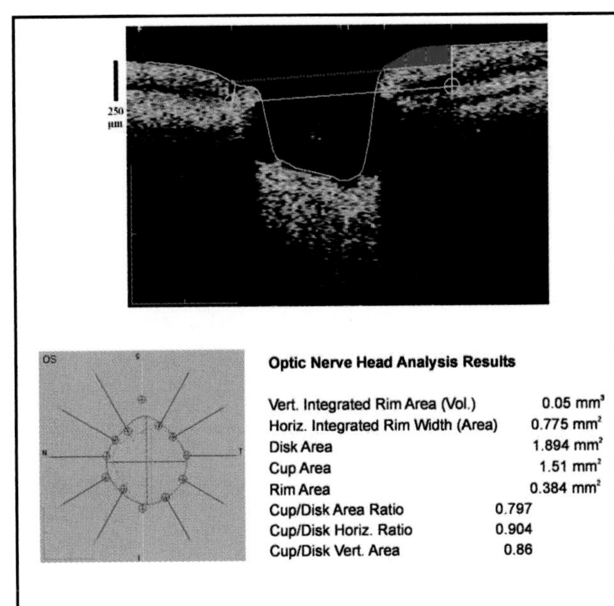
250 µm
OS
S
N
T
I
Optic Nerve Head Analysis Results
Vert. Integrated Rim Area (Vol.) 0.05 mm³
Horiz. Integrated Rim Width (Area) 0.775 mm²
Disk Area 1.894 mm²
Cup Area 1.51 mm²
Rim Area 0.384 mm²
Cup/Disk Area Ratio 0.797
Cup/Disk Horiz. Ratio 0.904
Cup/Disk Vert. Area 0.86

K

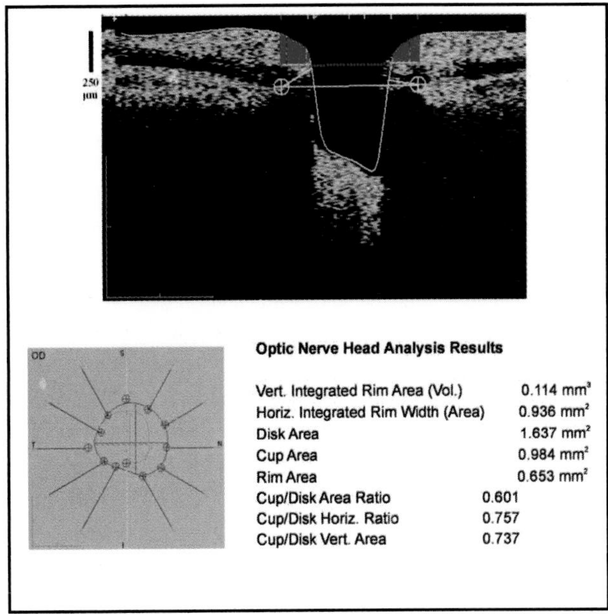
250 µm
OD
S
T
N
I
Optic Nerve Head Analysis Results
Vert. Integrated Rim Area (Vol.) 0.114 mm³
Horiz. Integrated Rim Width (Area) 0.936 mm²
Disk Area 1.637 mm²
Cup Area 0.984 mm²
Rim Area 0.653 mm²
Cup/Disk Area Ratio 0.601
Cup/Disk Horiz. Ratio 0.757
Cup/Disk Vert. Area 0.737

L

Case 12-4. All Structural Measures Were Consistent With Each Other and With Functional Findings in Location and Severity

A 64-year-old African-American woman with normal tension glaucoma in both eyes was treated with selective laser trabeculoplasty and medically with brinzolamide 1% and bimatoprost 0.03%. The visual acuity was 20/25 and the IOP was 13 mmHg in both eyes. The examination of the anterior and posterior segments was unremarkable except for large ONH cups in both eyes (A and B) with peripapillary atrophy in the left eye. Red-free photography showed a NFL defect in the right eye (C) from 6:00 to 7:30 and in the left eye (D), a smaller defect from 4:00 to 5:00. The Humphrey VF showed superior paracentral defects in both eyes (E and F). HRT showed larger disc and cup areas in the right eye (G) compared to the left (H) and thinning of the neuroretinal rim in the temporal and inferior segments in the right eye. The left disc showed a thinner neuroretinal rim inferiorly.

Optical Coherence Tomography

Abnormal thinning of the retinal NFL was noted at 6:00 and 7:00 in the right eye, with borderline thinning at 8:00, 12:00, 1:00, and 3:00 (I), and thickness was abnormal at 5:00 and 6:00 and slightly reduced at 10:00 in the left (J). Macular scanning showed a reduction in inferior and temporal retinal thickness in both eyes (K and L). A larger disc area was noted in the left eye (M) than the right eye (N) with a larger cup in the right eye.

Comment

All structural measures were consistent with each other and with functional findings. The depth of the defects in the right and left eyes was mirrored by structural and functional testing.

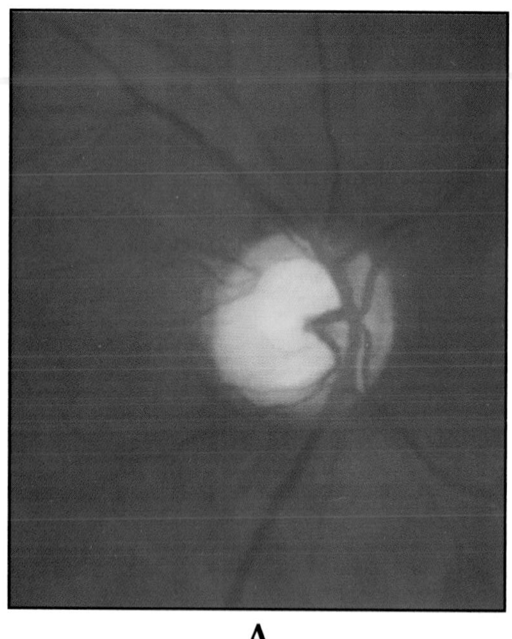

A

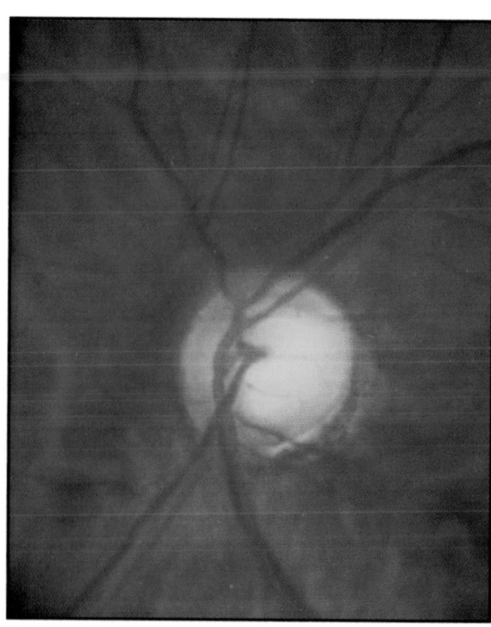

B

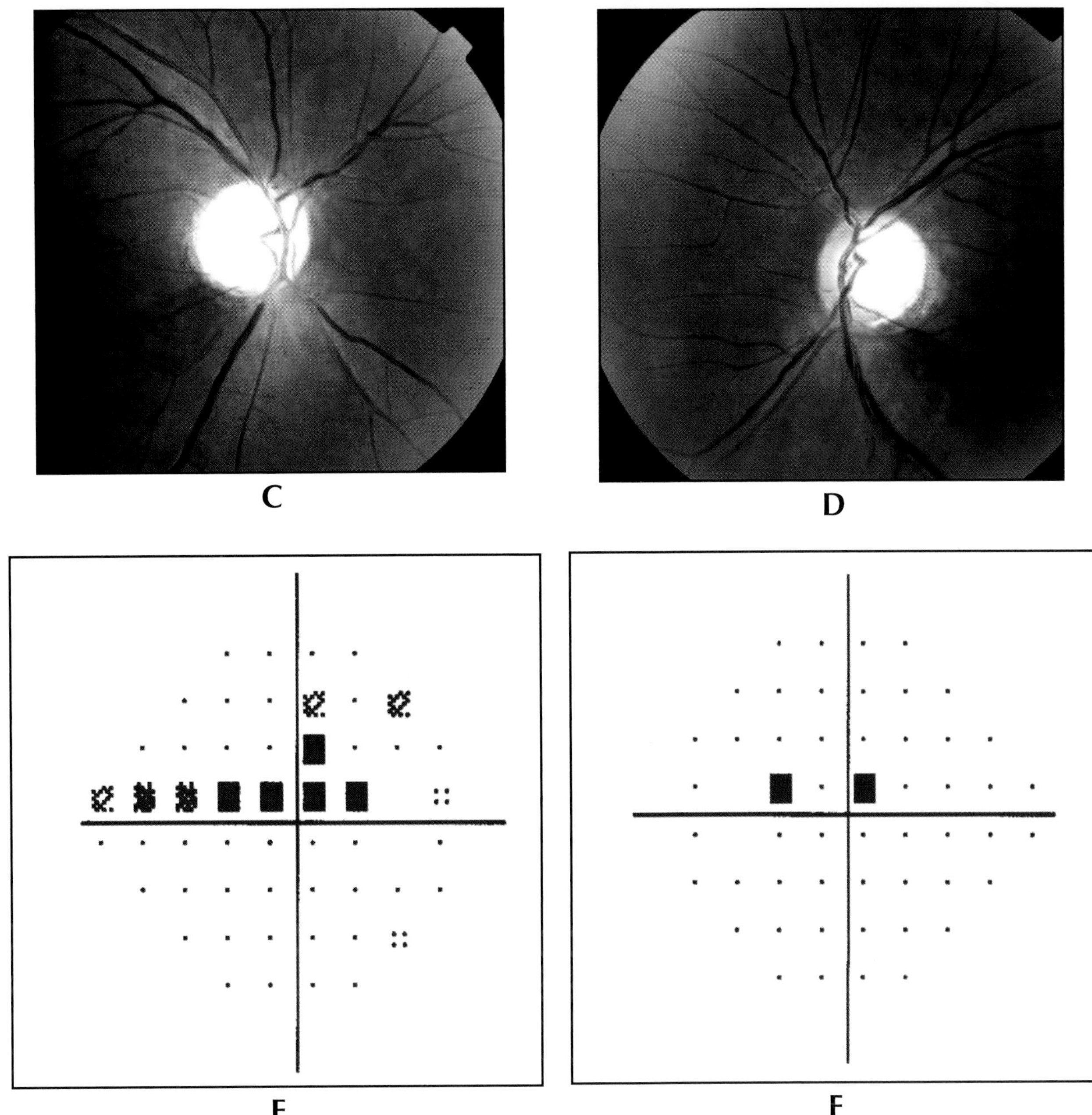
C
D
E
F

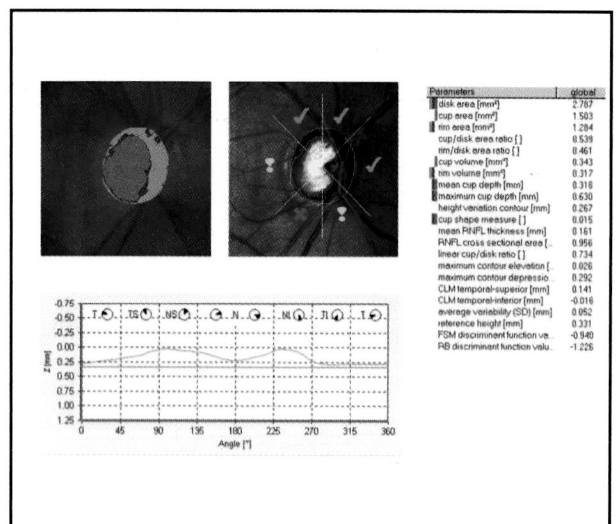
Parameters
global
Angle [°]

G

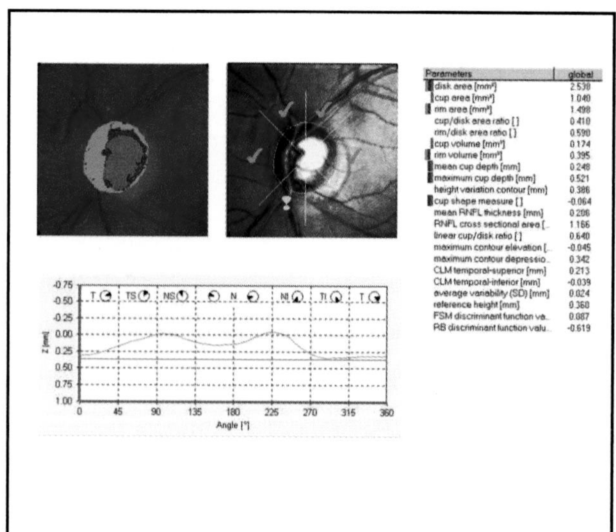
Parameters
global
Angle [°]

H

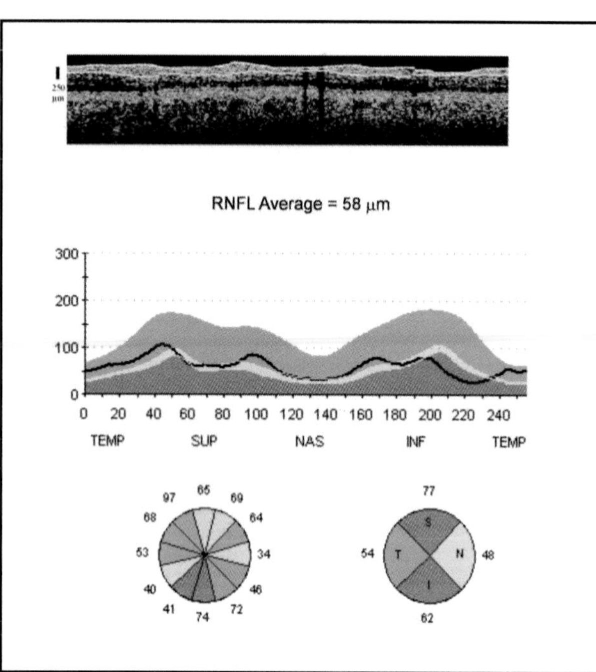
RNFL Average = 58 µm
TEMP
SUP
NAS
INF
TEMP

I

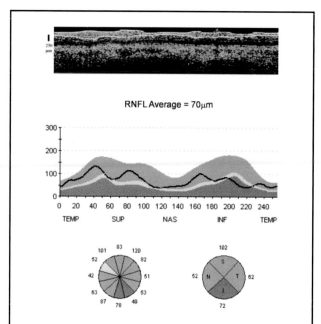

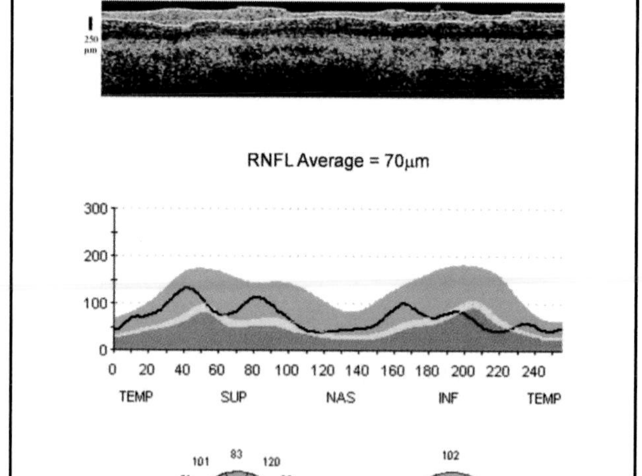
RNFL Average = 70µm
TEMP
SUP
NAS
INF
TEMP

J

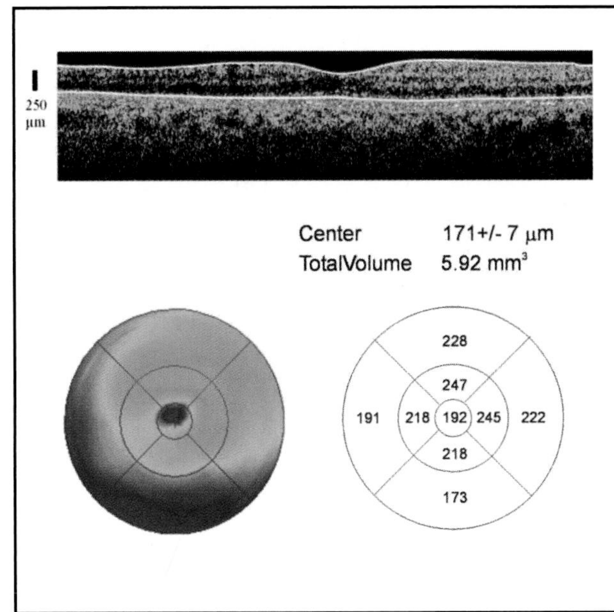
250 µm
Center 171+/- 7 µm
TotalVolume 5.92 mm³
228
247
191 218 192 245 222
218
173

K

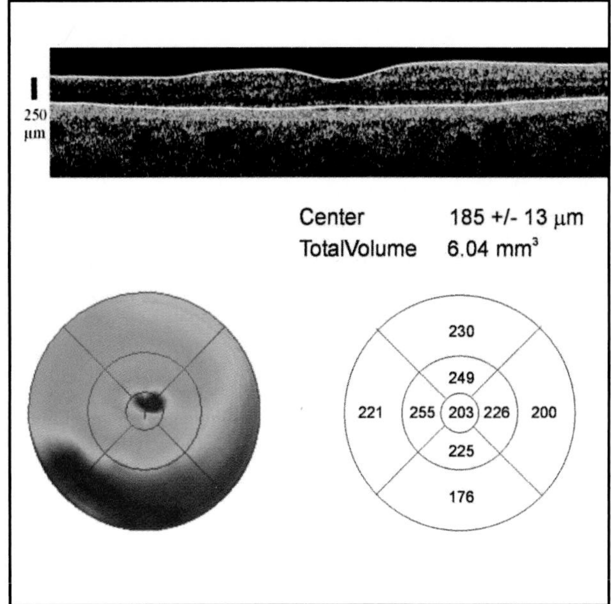
250 µm
Center 185 +/- 13 µm
TotalVolume 6.04 mm³
230
249
221 255 203 226 200
225
176

L

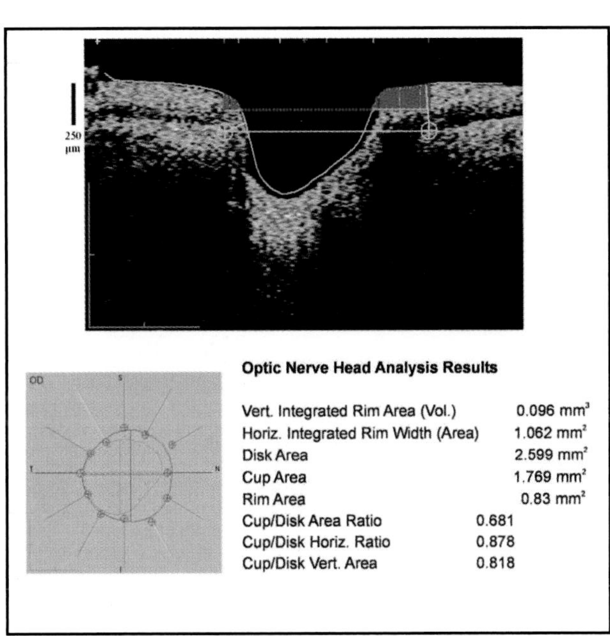
250 µm
OD
Optic Nerve Head Analysis Results
Vert. Integrated Rim Area (Vol.) 0.096 mm³
Horiz. Integrated Rim Width (Area) 1.062 mm²
Disk Area 2.599 mm²
Cup Area 1.769 mm²
Rim Area 0.83 mm²
Cup/Disk Area Ratio 0.681
Cup/Disk Horiz. Ratio 0.878
Cup/Disk Vert. Area 0.818

M

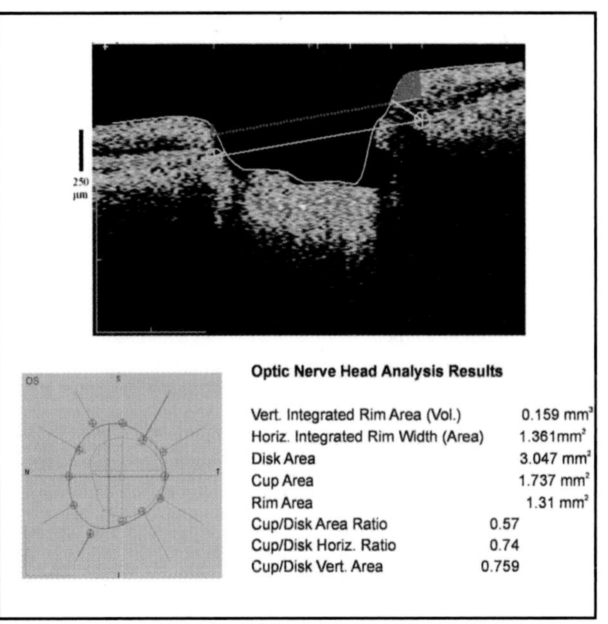
250 µm
OS
Optic Nerve Head Analysis Results
Vert. Integrated Rim Area (Vol.) 0.159 mm³
Horiz. Integrated Rim Width (Area) 1.361mm²
Disk Area 3.047 mm²
Cup Area 1.737 mm²
Rim Area 1.31 mm²
Cup/Disk Area Ratio 0.57
Cup/Disk Horiz. Ratio 0.74
Cup/Disk Vert. Area 0.759

N

Case 12-5. Structure-Function Correlation Allowed Diagnosis and Treatment of Glaucoma

A 41-year-old Asian man had primary open-angle glaucoma in both eyes. Visual acuity was 20/20 in the right eye and 20/60 in the left eye. The IOPs were 14 mmHg bilaterally. A normal anterior segment was noted with wide open anterior chamber angles and a normal appearing posterior segment, except for asymmetric cupping with a larger optic disc cup in the left eye (A and B). Frequency doubling technology showed superior paracentral and inferior nasal defects in the right eye (C) and both superior and inferior paracentral defects in the left eye (D), more pronounced inferiorly. Normal ONH with equal cup sizes was noted with the HRT analysis (E and F).

Optical Coherence Tomography

There was a slight reduction in the average retinal NFL thickness noted in both eyes, with localized thinning at 10:00 in the right eye (G) and at 3:00 in the left eye (H). Macular scanning showed a general reduction in total volume of the left eye (J) compared to the right eye (I). The optic disc analysis showed a slightly larger disc size in the left eye with equal cup size in both eyes (K and L).

Comment

In this patient with early glaucoma, there were normal Swedish interactive thresholding algorithm (SITA) VFs and the frequency doubling technology (FDT) showed early abnormalities. Structural testing was mildly abnormal, but the correspondence of the structure and function allowed the diagnosis and treatment of the patient's glaucoma.

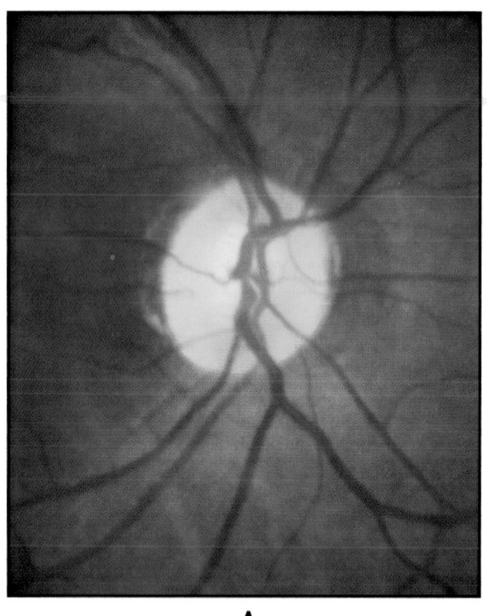

A

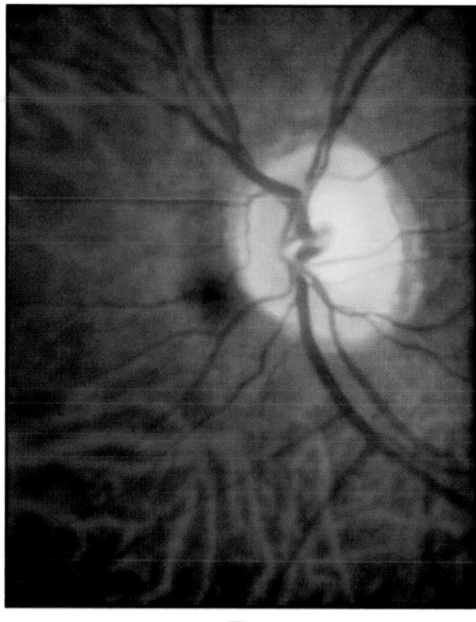

B

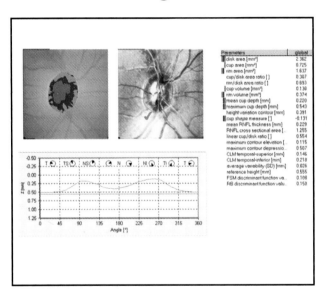

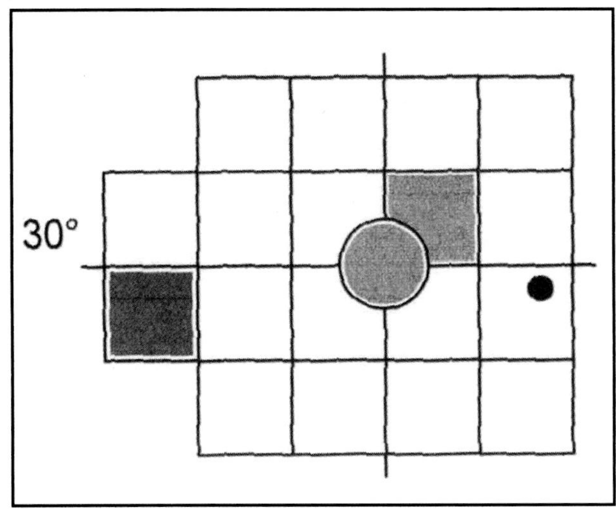

C

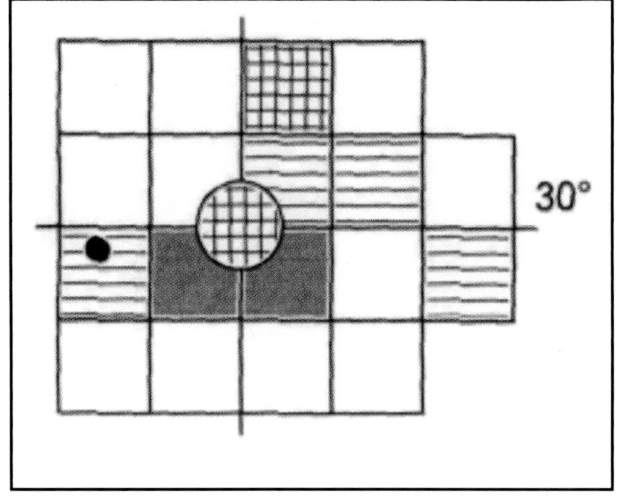

D

Parameters	global
disk area [mm²]	2.362
cup area [mm²]	0.725
rim area [mm²]	1.637
cup/disk area ratio [ ]	0.307
rim/disk area ratio [ ]	0.693
cup volume [mm³]	0.138
rim volume [mm³]	0.374
mean cup depth [mm]	0.220
maximum cup depth [mm]	0.543
height variation contour [mm]	0.391
cup shape measure [ ]	-0.131
mean RNFL thickness [mm]	0.229
RNFL cross sectional area [...	1.255
linear cup/disk ratio [ ]	0.554
maximum contour elevation [...	0.115
maximum contour depressio...	0.507
CLM temporal-superior [mm]	0.146
CLM temporal-inferior [mm]	0.218
average variability (SD) [mm]	0.026
reference height [mm]	0.555
FSM discriminant function va...	0.108
RB discriminant function valu...	0.150

E

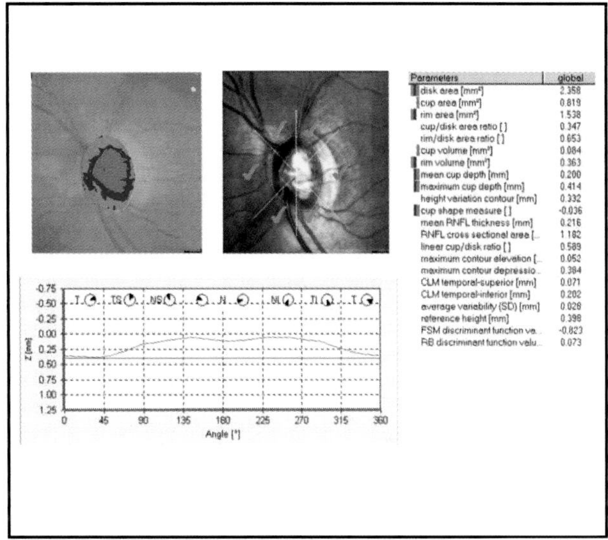

Parameters	global
disk area [mm²]	2.358
cup area [mm²]	0.819
rim area [mm²]	1.538
cup/disk area ratio [ ]	0.347
rim/disk area ratio [ ]	0.653
cup volume [mm³]	0.084
rim volume [mm³]	0.363
mean cup depth [mm]	0.200
maximum cup depth [mm]	0.414
height variation contour [mm]	0.332
cup shape measure [ ]	-0.036
mean RNFL thickness [mm]	0.216
RNFL cross sectional area [...	1.182
linear cup/disk ratio [ ]	0.589
maximum contour elevation [...	0.052
maximum contour depressio...	0.384
CLM temporal-superior [mm]	0.071
CLM temporal-inferior [mm]	0.202
average variability (SD) [mm]	0.028
reference height [mm]	0.398
FSM discriminant function va...	-0.823
RB discriminant function valu...	0.073

F

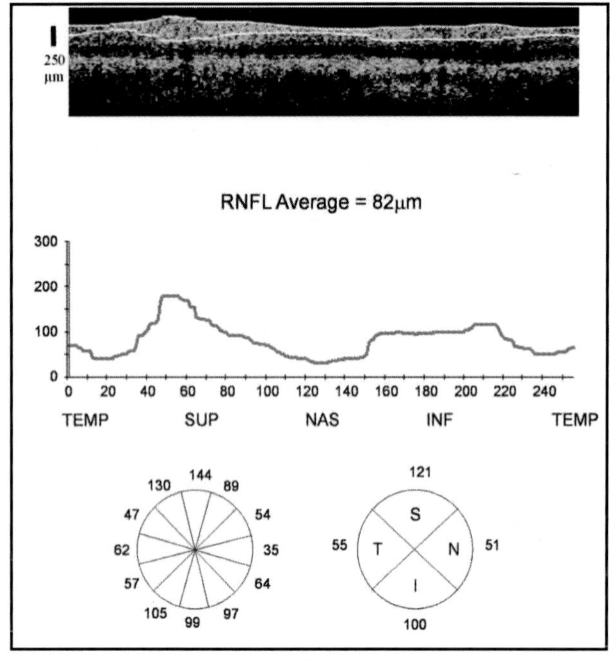
250 µm
RNFL Average = 82µm
300
200
100
0
0 20 40 60 80 100 120 140 160 180 200 220 240
TEMP SUP NAS INF TEMP
144 89 54 35 64 97 99 105 57 62 47 130
121
S
T N
I
55 51
100

G

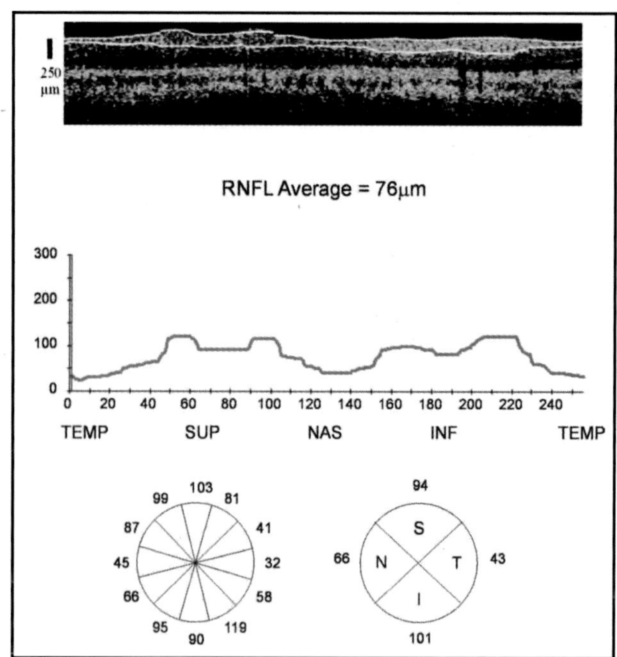
250 µm
RNFL Average = 76µm
300
200
100
0
0 20 40 60 80 100 120 140 160 180 200 220 240
TEMP SUP NAS INF TEMP
103 81 41 32 58 119 90 95 66 45 87 99
94
S
N T
I
66 43
101

H

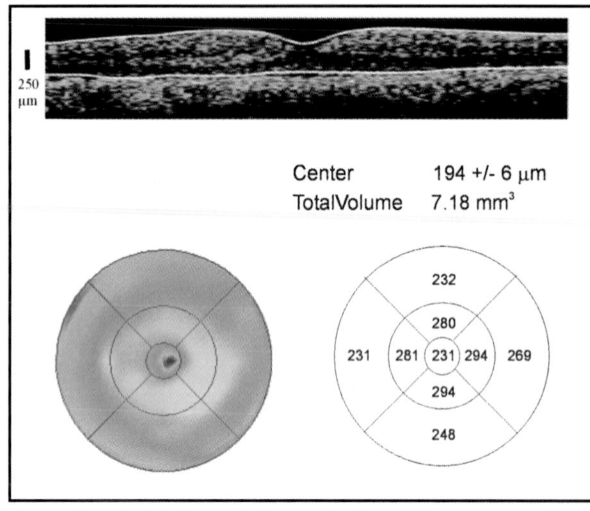
250 µm
Center 194 +/- 6 µm
TotalVolume 7.18 mm³
232
280
231 281 231 294 269
294
248

I

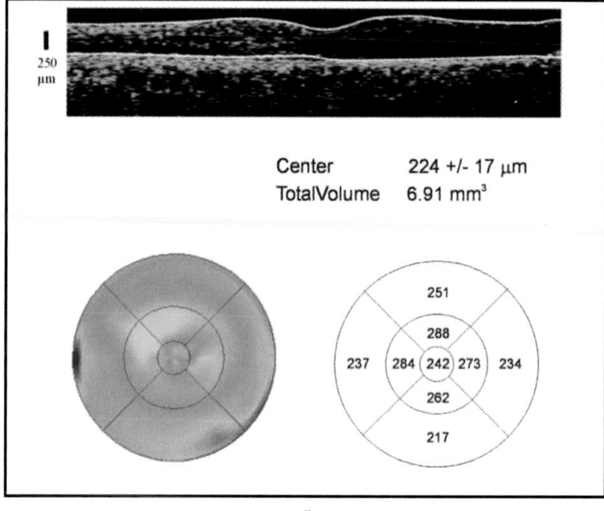
250 µm
Center 224 +/- 17 µm
TotalVolume 6.91 mm³
251
288
237 284 242 273 234
262
217

J

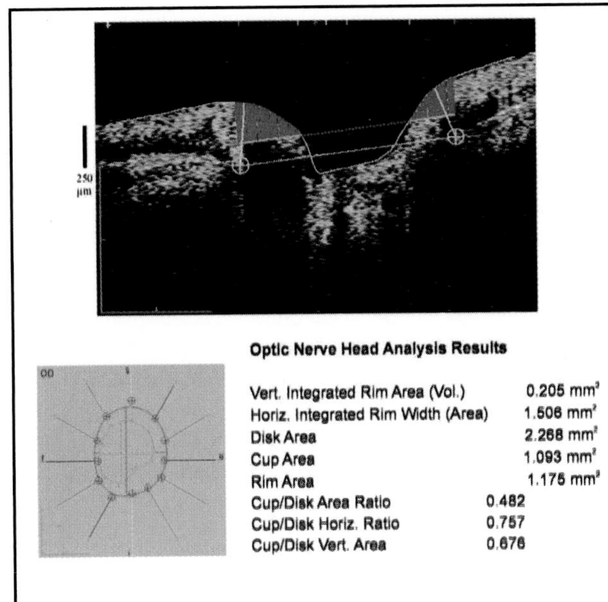
250 µm
OD
Optic Nerve Head Analysis Results
Vert. Integrated Rim Area (Vol.) 0.205 mm³
Horiz. Integrated Rim Width (Area) 1.506 mm²
Disk Area 2.268 mm²
Cup Area 1.093 mm²
Rim Area 1.175 mm²
Cup/Disk Area Ratio 0.482
Cup/Disk Horiz. Ratio 0.757
Cup/Disk Vert. Area 0.676

K

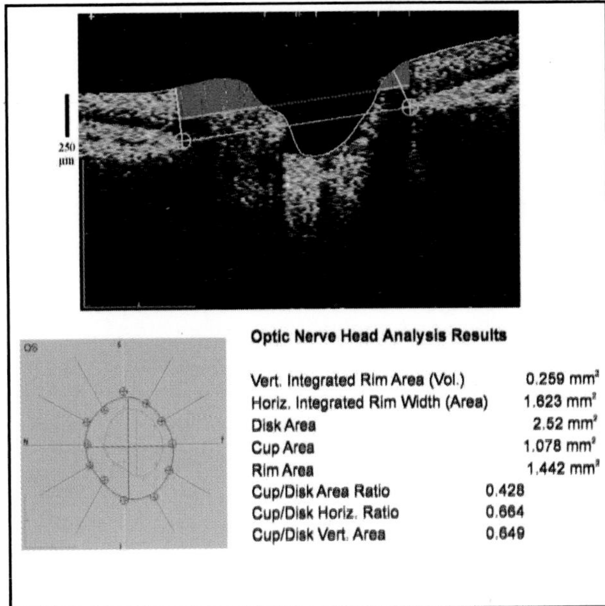
250 µm
OS
Optic Nerve Head Analysis Results
Vert. Integrated Rim Area (Vol.) 0.259 mm³
Horiz. Integrated Rim Width (Area) 1.623 mm²
Disk Area 2.52 mm²
Cup Area 1.078 mm²
Rim Area 1.442 mm²
Cup/Disk Area Ratio 0.428
Cup/Disk Horiz. Ratio 0.664
Cup/Disk Vert. Area 0.649

L

Case 12-6. Nerve Fiber Layer, Optic Nerve Head, and Macula Showed Excellent Correspondence With Visual Fields in Advanced Glaucoma

A 76-year-old Caucasian woman had advanced primary open-angle glaucoma well controlled with treatment, including timolol gel 0.5% and latanoprost 0.005% in both eyes. On examination, visual acuity was 20/15 and intraocular pressures were 11 mmHg bilaterally. The anterior and posterior segment examinations were unremarkable except for posterior vitreous detachments in both eyes. A tilted ONH was noted in the left eye, and there was peripapillary atrophy in both eyes (A and B). The VF tests demonstrated superior hemifield and inferior nasal defects in both eyes with more pronounced superior damage in the right eye (C) and inferior damage in the left eye (D). HRT showed a small disc in the right eye (E) with abnormally thin neuroretinal rim in all but the temporal sector and a tilted small sized disc with abnormal neuroretinal rim in the superior and inferior sectors of the left eye (F).

Optical Coherence Tomography

Retinal NFL thickness as measured in the circumpapillary scan was markedly reduced in the right eye (G) (average retinal NFL of 42 μm) and to a lesser degree in the left eye (H) (60 μm). In both eyes, the retinal NFL loss was noted mainly inferiorly and temporally. Significant thinning was also noted at 1:00 and 2:00 in the right eye. The macular scans showed reduction in the retinal thickness in the outer ring of the superior, temporal, and inferior regions in both eyes (I and J) and the inferior inner ring in the right eye. The ONH analysis (K and L) was an inadequate study in the left eye (L).

Comments

Macular volume was similar for both eyes; however, the right eye had thinner measurements in the inferior compared to the superior region, compatible with the VF defect. In the left eye, the macular thickness was similar in the outer superior and inferior regions, again corresponding to the superior and inferior VF defects. Circumpapillary OCT and HRT ONH analysis showed good correspondence with VFs as well.

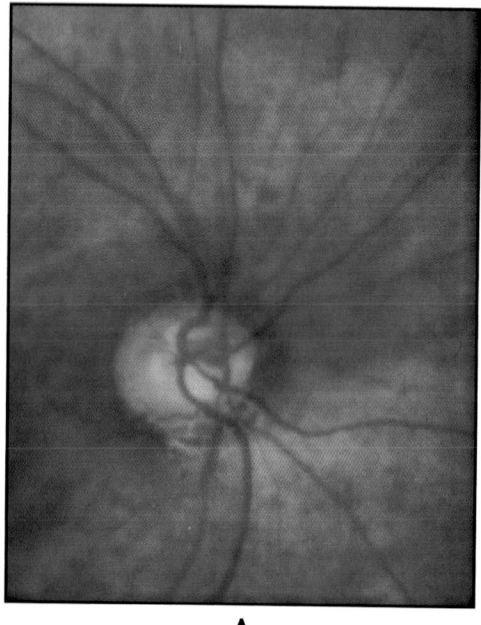

A

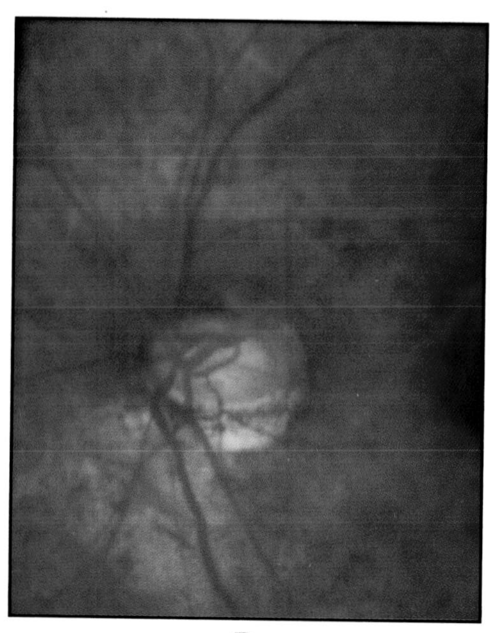

B

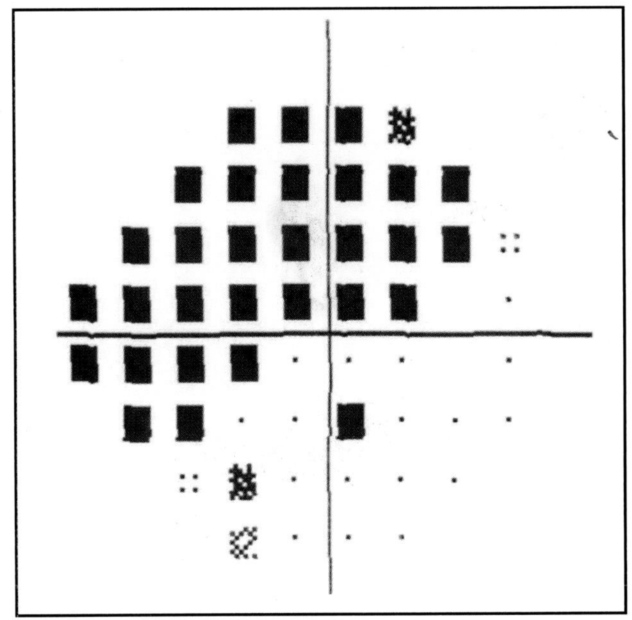

C

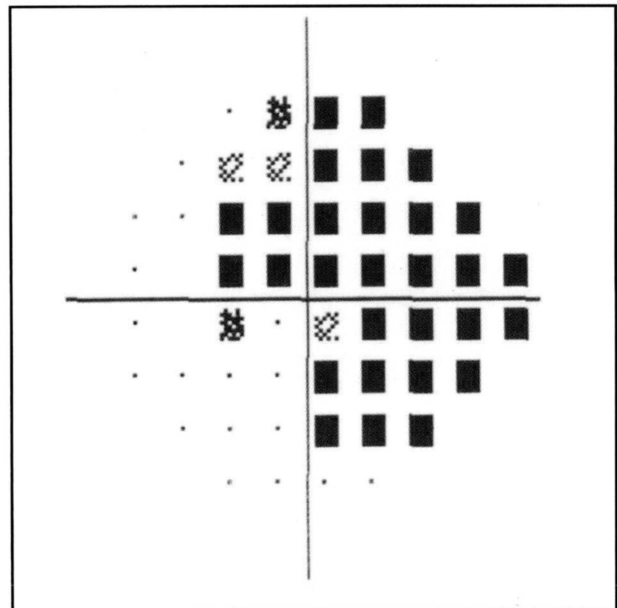

D

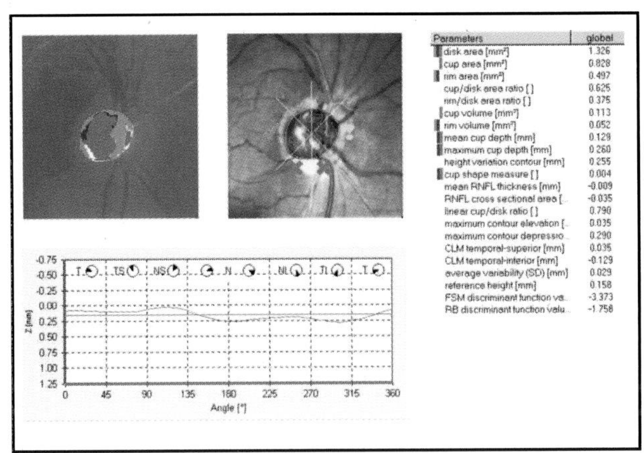
Parameters global
disk area [mm²] 1.326
cup area [mm²] 0.828
rim area [mm²] 0.497
cup/disk area ratio [ ] 0.625
rim/disk area ratio [ ] 0.375
cup volume [mm³] 0.113
rim volume [mm³] 0.052
mean cup depth [mm] 0.129
maximum cup depth [mm] 0.260
height variation contour [mm] 0.255
cup shape measure [ ] 0.004
mean RNFL thickness [mm] -0.009
RNFL cross sectional area [... -0.035
linear cup/disk ratio [ ] 0.790
maximum contour elevation [... 0.035
maximum contour depressio... 0.290
CLM temporal-superior [mm] 0.035
CLM temporal-inferior [mm] -0.129
average variability (SD) [mm] 0.029
reference height [mm] 0.158
FSM discriminant function va... -3.373
RB discriminant function valu... -1.758
T TS NS N NI TI T
Z [mm]
Angle [°]

E

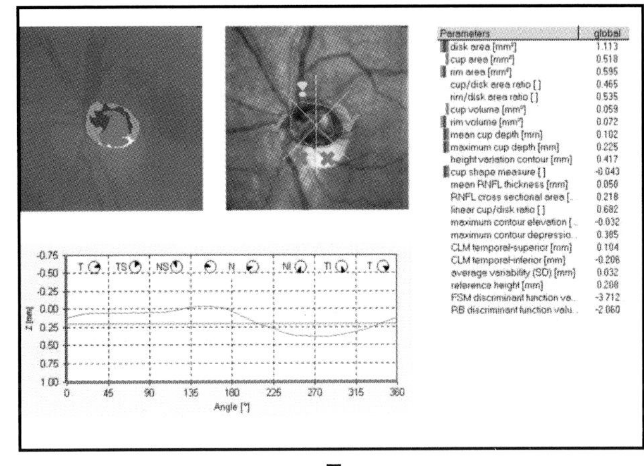
Parameters global
disk area [mm²] 1.113
cup area [mm²] 0.518
rim area [mm²] 0.595
cup/disk area ratio [ ] 0.465
rim/disk area ratio [ ] 0.535
cup volume [mm³] 0.059
rim volume [mm³] 0.072
mean cup depth [mm] 0.102
maximum cup depth [mm] 0.225
height variation contour [mm] 0.417
cup shape measure [ ] -0.043
mean RNFL thickness [mm] 0.058
RNFL cross sectional area [... 0.218
linear cup/disk ratio [ ] 0.682
maximum contour elevation [... -0.032
maximum contour depressio... 0.385
CLM temporal-superior [mm] 0.104
CLM temporal-inferior [mm] -0.206
average variability (SD) [mm] 0.032
reference height [mm] 0.208
FSM discriminant function va... -3.712
RB discriminant function valu... -2.060
T TS NS N NI TI T
Z [mm]
Angle [°]

F

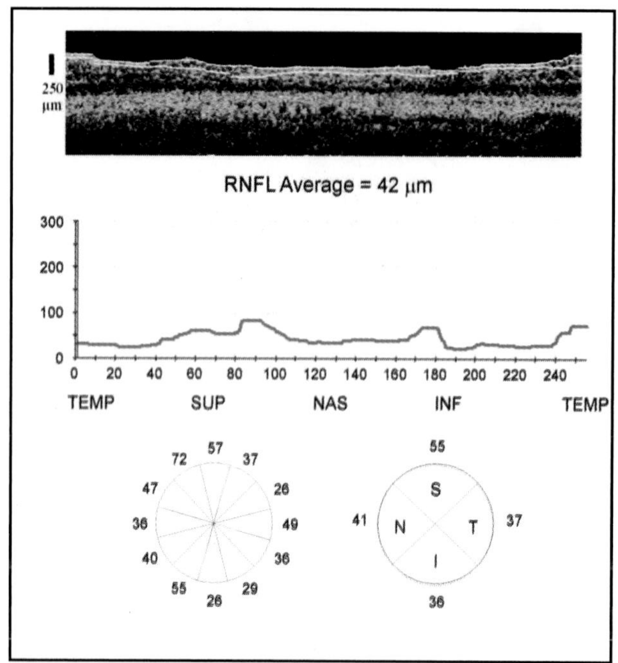
250 µm
RNFL Average = 42 µm
TEMP
SUP
NAS
INF
TEMP
S
N
T
I

G

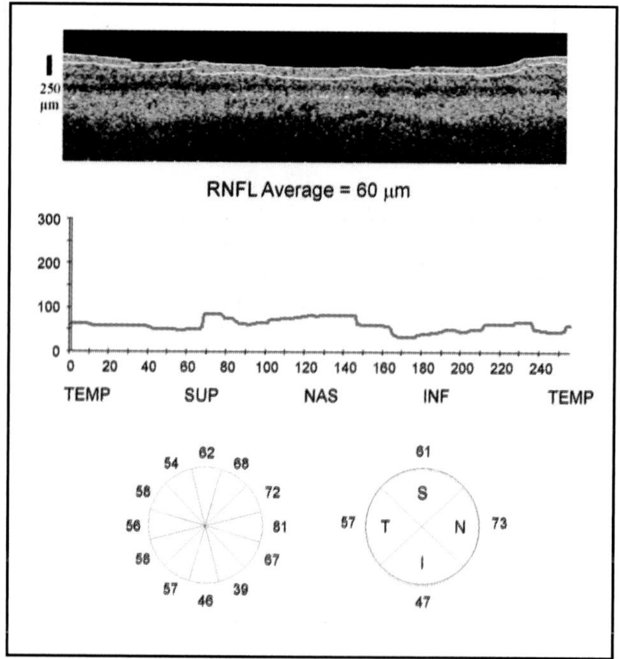
250 µm
RNFL Average = 60 µm
TEMP
SUP
NAS
INF
TEMP
S
T
N
I

H

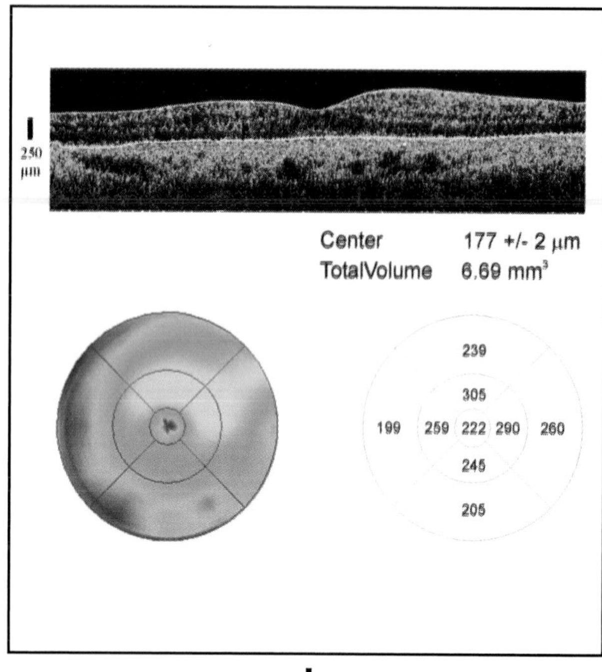
250 µm
Center 177 +/- 2 µm
TotalVolume 6.69 mm³

I

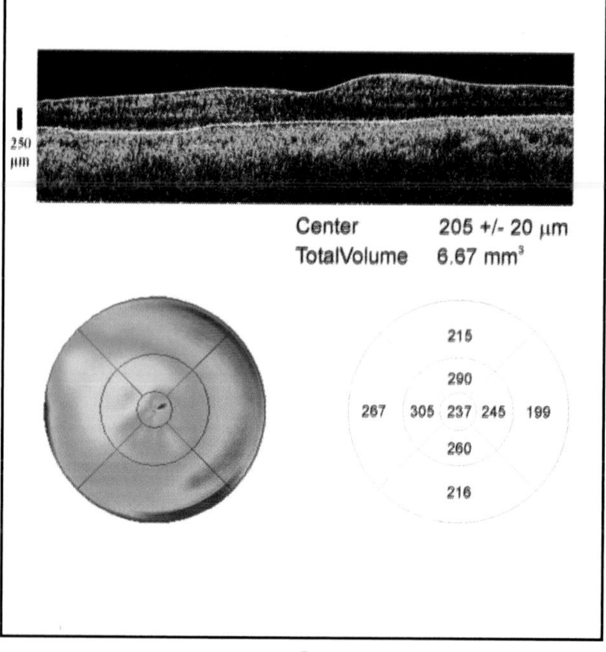
250 µm
Center 205 +/- 20 µm
TotalVolume 6.67 mm³

J

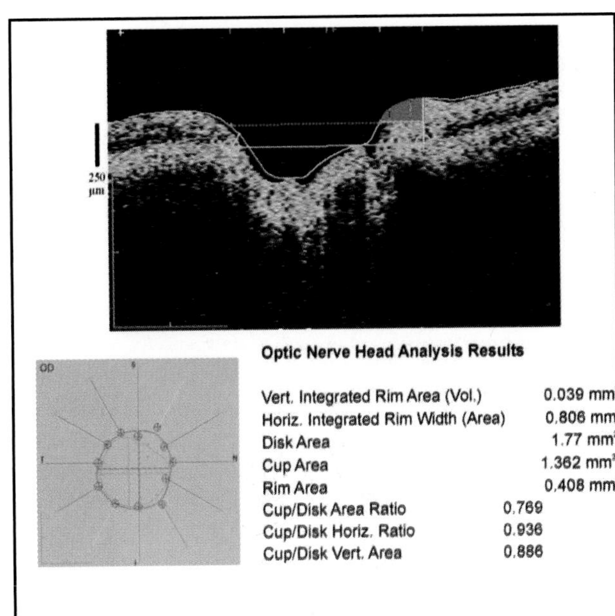
250 µm
OD
Optic Nerve Head Analysis Results
Vert. Integrated Rim Area (Vol.) 0.039 mm³
Horiz. Integrated Rim Width (Area) 0.806 mm²
Disk Area 1.77 mm²
Cup Area 1.362 mm²
Rim Area 0.408 mm²
Cup/Disk Area Ratio 0.769
Cup/Disk Horiz. Ratio 0.936
Cup/Disk Vert. Area 0.886

K

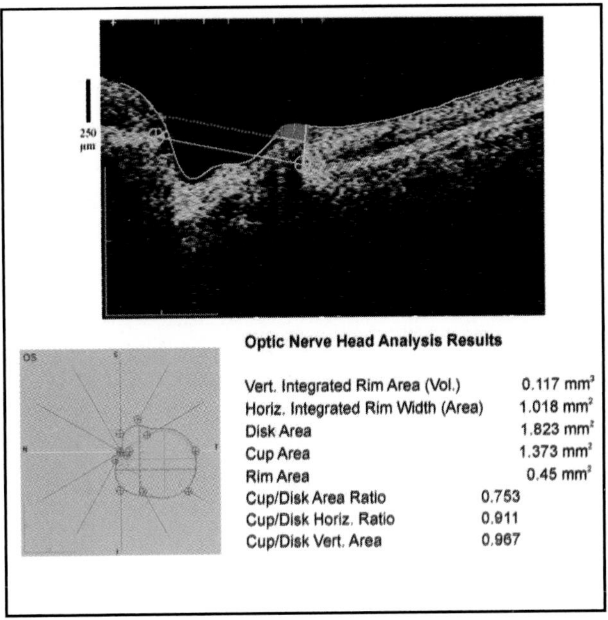
250 µm
OS
Optic Nerve Head Analysis Results
Vert. Integrated Rim Area (Vol.) 0.117 mm³
Horiz. Integrated Rim Width (Area) 1.018 mm²
Disk Area 1.823 mm²
Cup Area 1.373 mm²
Rim Area 0.45 mm²
Cup/Disk Area Ratio 0.753
Cup/Disk Horiz. Ratio 0.911
Cup/Disk Vert. Area 0.967

L

Case 12-7. Nerve Fiber Layer and Macular Analysis Corresponded to Visual Field Abnormality in Advanced Glaucoma

A 63-year-old Caucasian man with normal tension glaucoma in the left eye was treated with bimatoprost 0.03% and brimonidine 0.2%. On examination, the visual acuity was 20/60 and the IOP was 13 mmHg. The anterior segment was unremarkable, and the posterior segment examination revealed large optic disc cups with loss of the temporal neuroretinal rim and peripapillary atrophy (A). VF showed advanced superior and inferior defects (B). HRT showed a large cup with abnormal thinning of the neuroretinal rim in all segments except the temporal (C).

Optical Coherence Tomography

The circumpapillary NFL scan showed marked thinning superiorly inferiorly and temporally (D). The macula scan showed marked inferior outer thinning and milder thinning temporally and nasally in the outer regions and in the inner inferior sector (E). The ONH disclosed a large cup (F).

Comment

Circumpapillary NFL thickness corresponds with the VF abnormality, as does macular thickness. HRT ONH assessment correlates with the superior but not the inferior VF abnormality.

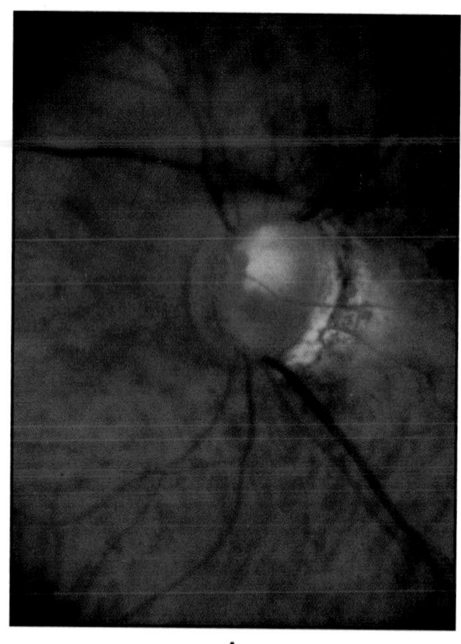

A

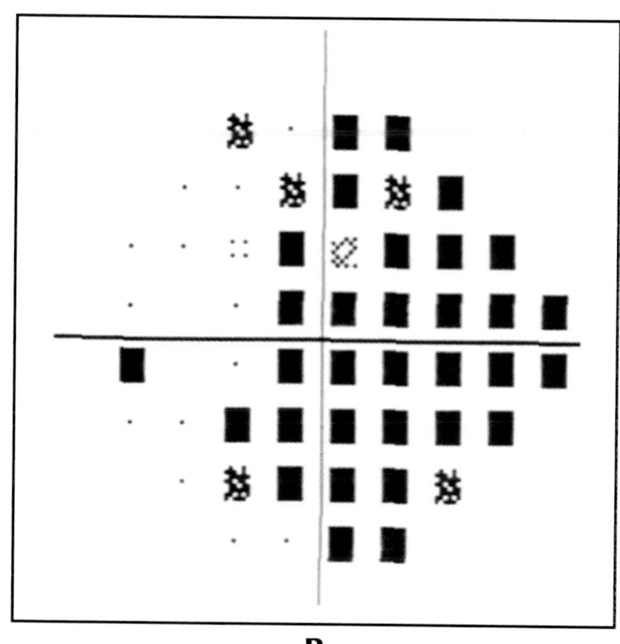

B

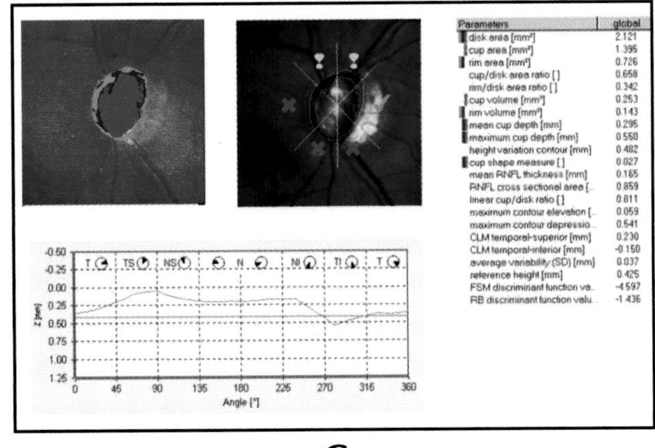
Parameters global
disk area [mm²] 2.121
cup area [mm²] 1.395
rim area [mm²] 0.726
cup/disk area ratio [ ] 0.658
rim/disk area ratio [ ] 0.342
cup volume [mm³] 0.253
rim volume [mm³] 0.143
mean cup depth [mm] 0.295
maximum cup depth [mm] 0.550
height variation contour [mm] 0.482
cup shape measure [ ] 0.027
mean RNFL thickness [mm] 0.165
RNFL cross sectional area [... 0.859
linear cup/disk ratio [ ] 0.811
maximum contour elevation [... 0.059
maximum contour depressio... 0.541
CLM temporal-superior [mm] 0.230
CLM temporal-inferior [mm] -0.150
average variability (SD) [mm] 0.037
reference height [mm] 0.425
FSM discriminant function va... -4.597
RB discriminant function valu... -1.436
T TS NS N NI TI T
Angle [°]

C

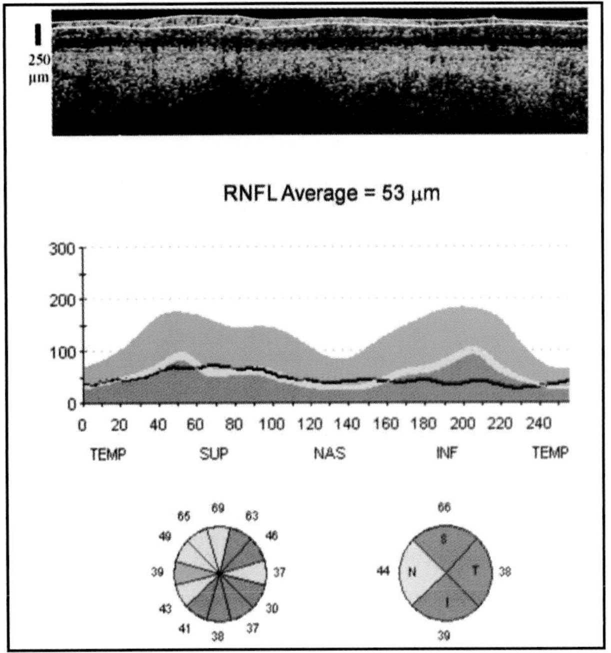
250 µm
RNFL Average = 53 µm
300
200
100
0
0 20 40 60 80 100 120 140 160 180 200 220 240
TEMP SUP NAS INF TEMP
69 63 46 37 30 37 38 41 43 39 49 65
66 S
44 N
T 38
I
39

D

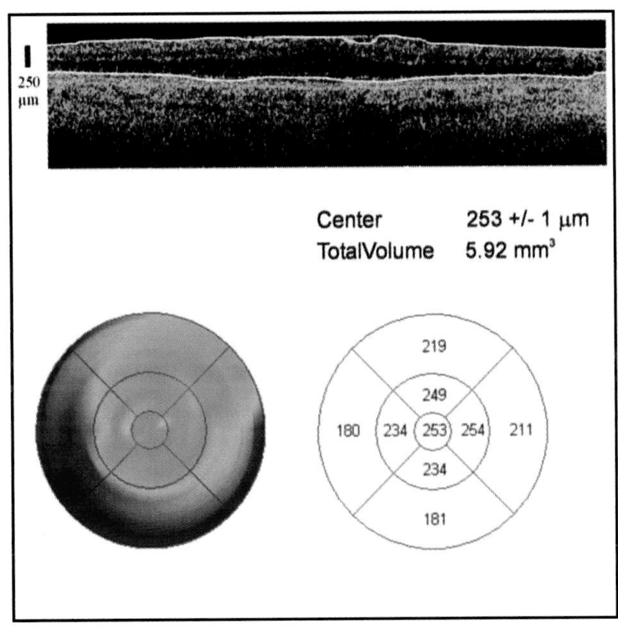
250 µm
Center 253 +/- 1 µm
TotalVolume 5.92 mm³
219
249
180 234 253 254 211
234
181

E

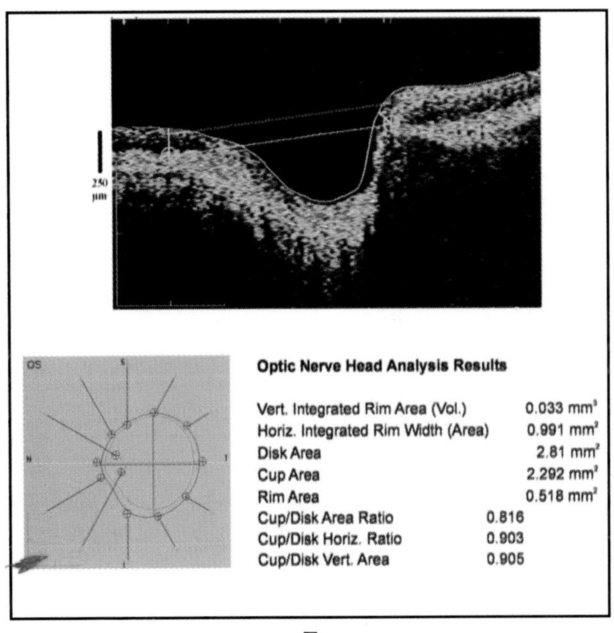
250 µm
OS
Optic Nerve Head Analysis Results
Vert. Integrated Rim Area (Vol.) 0.033 mm³
Horiz. Integrated Rim Width (Area) 0.991 mm²
Disk Area 2.81 mm²
Cup Area 2.292 mm²
Rim Area 0.518 mm²
Cup/Disk Area Ratio 0.816
Cup/Disk Horiz. Ratio 0.903
Cup/Disk Vert. Area 0.905

F

Case 12-8. Advanced Glaucoma Was Demonstrated by Loss of the Majority of the Nerve Fiber Layer, Severe Macular Thinning, and Only a Central Island Remaining on the Visual Field

An 88-year-old Asian woman had primary open-angle glaucoma in both eyes treated with bimatoprost 0.03% and a combination of timolol 0.5% and dorzolamide 2%. The visual acuity was 20/100 in the right eye and 20/50 in the left, and the IOPs were 16 mmHg and 14 mmHg, respectively. The anterior and posterior segments were unremarkable, except for loss of the temporal neuroretinal rim in the right eye (A) and thinning of the inferior temporal neuroretinal rim in the left eye (B). Humphrey VF testing of the central 10 degrees disclosed a remnant of an inferior temporal central island in the right eye (C) and a slightly wider field in the left eye (D). HRT of the right eye showed a normal sized disc with thinning of the neuroretinal rim in all sectors except for the superior segments (E) and all segments in the left eye (F).

Optical Coherence Tomography

The retinal NFL thickness in the circumpapillary scan was remarkably attenuated, with an average measurement of 36 μm in the right eye (G) and 40 μm in the left (H). The severe retinal damage was noted also in the macular scan of the right eye (I) with diminished retinal thickness and volume. The macular scan was of very poor quality on the left (J). The ONH disclosed near complete cupping in both eyes (K and L).

Comment

This patient with advanced glaucoma had lost the majority of her NFL, as shown by the circumpapillary OCT and macular scans, and had only a central island of vision remaining as seen on VF. The ONH imaging reflected these abnormalities less well than the other structural parameters.

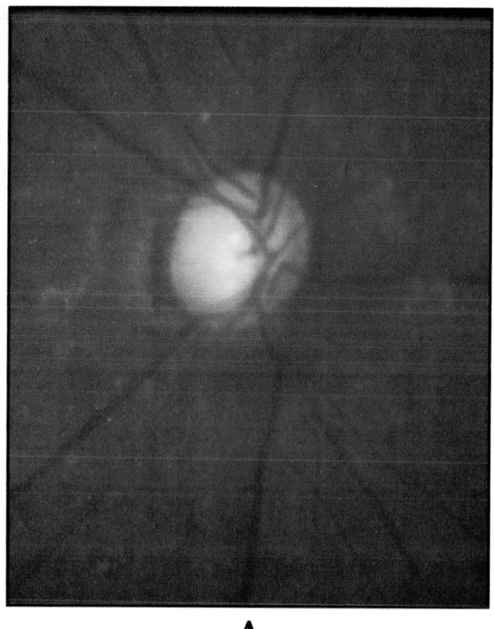

A

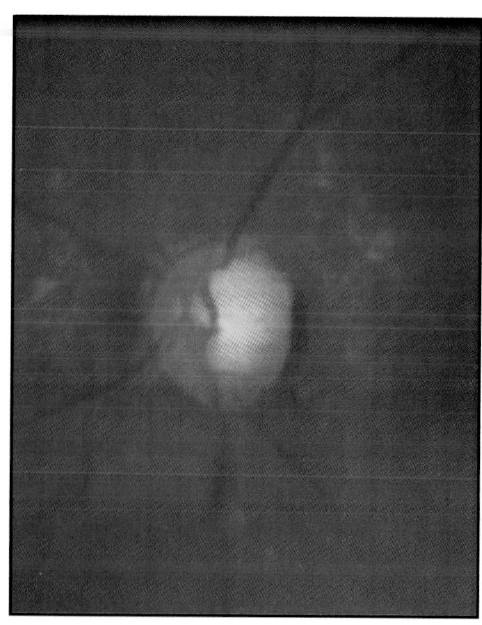

B

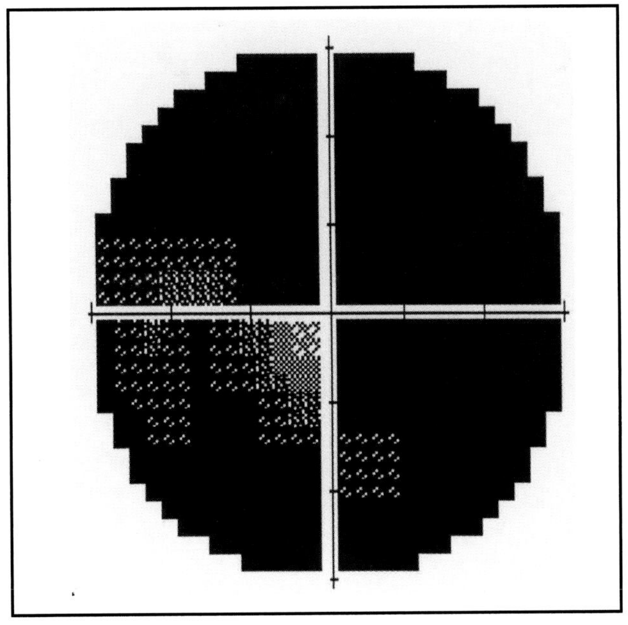

C

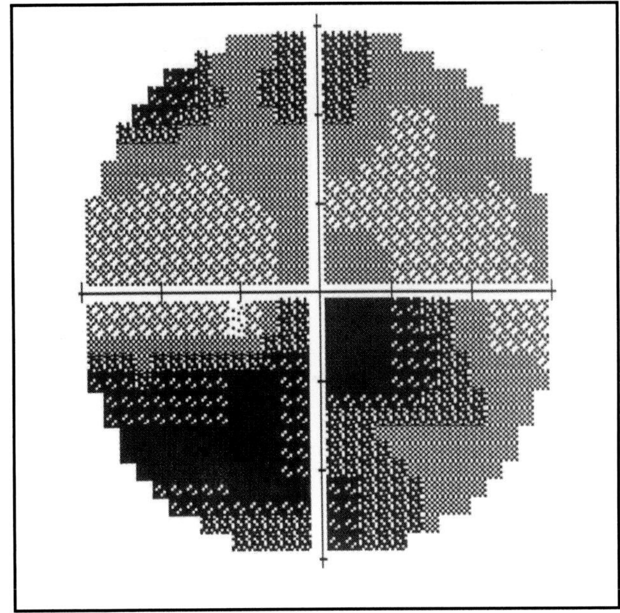

D

Parameters	global
disk area [mm²]	1.889
cup area [mm²]	0.924
rim area [mm²]	0.965
cup/disk area ratio [ ]	0.489
rim/disk area ratio [ ]	0.511
cup volume [mm³]	0.384
rim volume [mm³]	0.206
mean cup depth [mm]	0.406
maximum cup depth [mm]	0.971
height variation contour [mm]	0.431
cup shape measure [ ]	-0.125
mean RNFL thickness [mm]	0.091
RNFL cross sectional area [...	0.446
linear cup/disk ratio [ ]	0.699
maximum contour elevation [...	0.005
maximum contour depressio...	0.437
CLM temporal-superior [mm]	0.092
CLM temporal-inferior [mm]	0.063
average variability (SD) [mm]	0.116
reference height [mm]	0.377
FSM discriminant function va...	-0.905
RB discriminant function valu...	-0.046

E

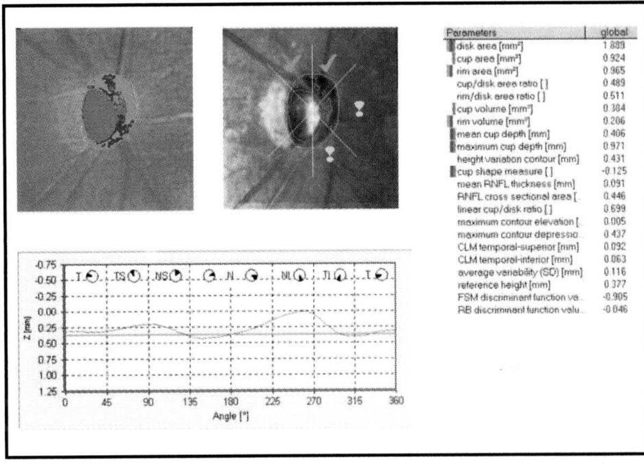

F

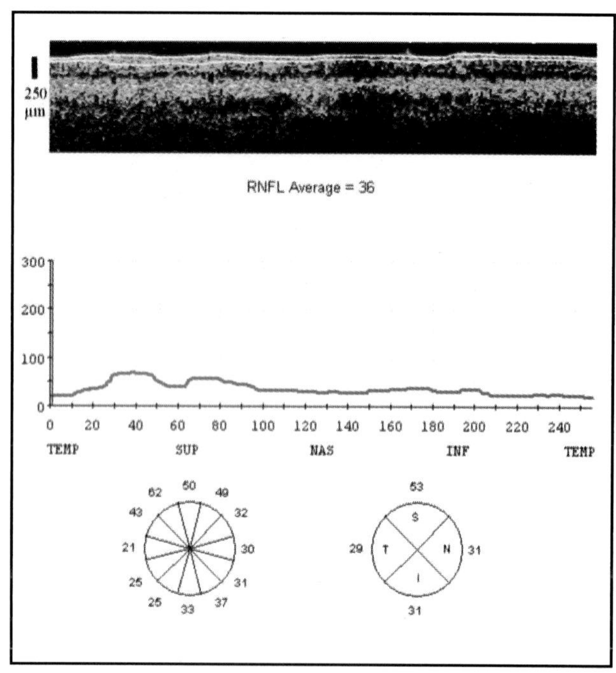
250 µm
RNFL Average = 36
300
200
100
0
0 20 40 60 80 100 120 140 160 180 200 220 240
TEMP SUP NAS INF TEMP
50 49 32 30 31 37 33 25 25 21 43 62
53 S T N I 29 31 31

G

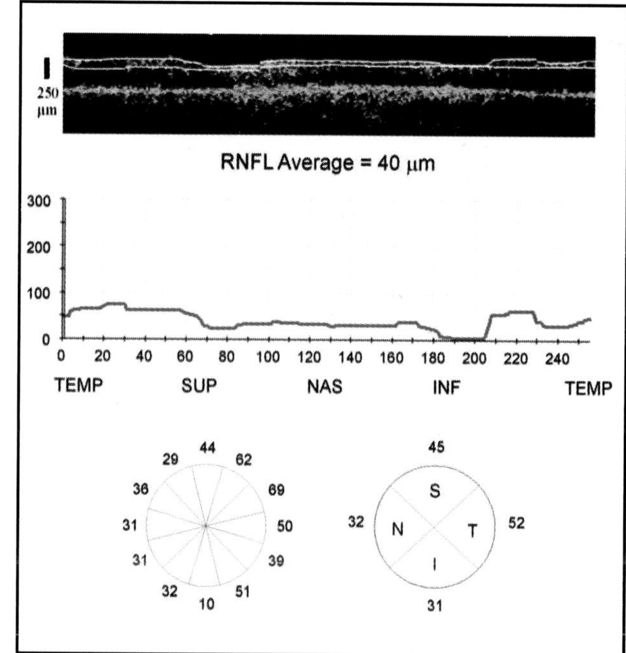
250 µm
RNFL Average = 40 µm
300
200
100
0
0 20 40 60 80 100 120 140 160 180 200 220 240
TEMP SUP NAS INF TEMP
44 62 69 50 39 51 10 32 31 31 36 29
45 S N T I 32 52 31

H

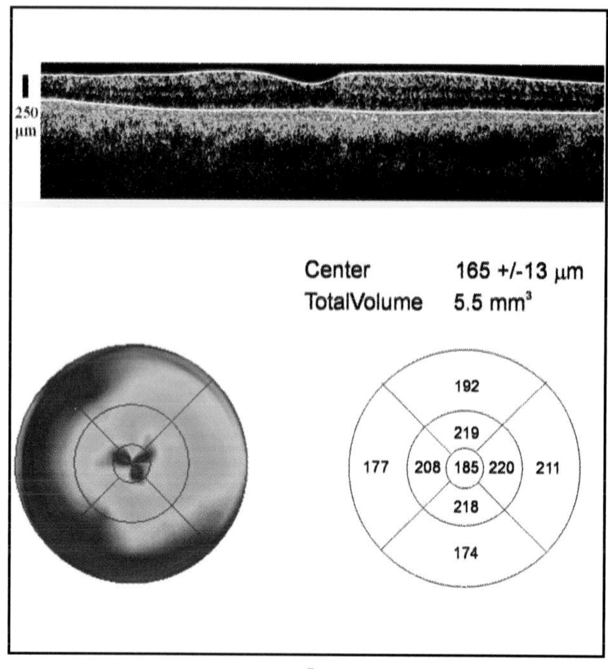
250 µm
Center 165 +/-13 µm
TotalVolume 5.5 mm³
192
219
177 208 185 220 211
218
174

I

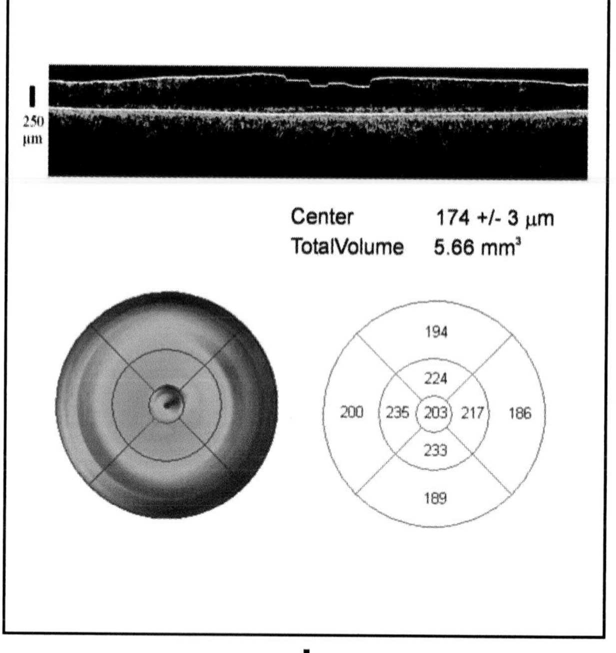
250 µm
Center 174 +/- 3 µm
TotalVolume 5.66 mm³
194
224
200 235 203 217 186
233
189

J

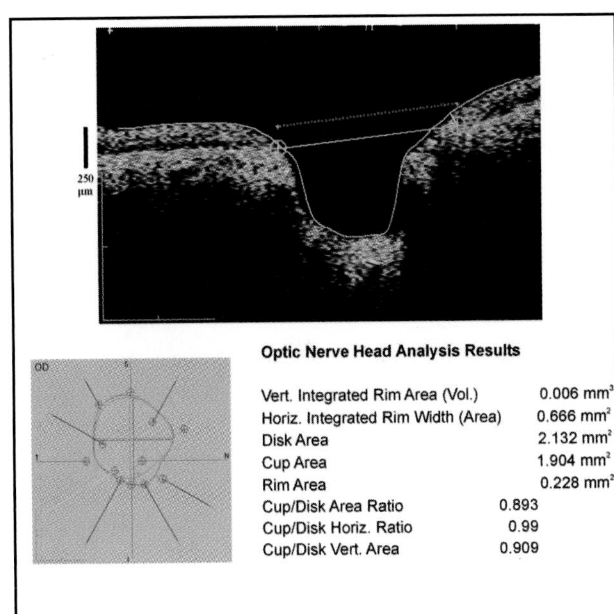
250 μm
OD
S
T
N
I
Optic Nerve Head Analysis Results
Vert. Integrated Rim Area (Vol.) 0.006 mm³
Horiz. Integrated Rim Width (Area) 0.666 mm²
Disk Area 2.132 mm²
Cup Area 1.904 mm²
Rim Area 0.228 mm²
Cup/Disk Area Ratio 0.893
Cup/Disk Horiz. Ratio 0.99
Cup/Disk Vert. Area 0.909

K

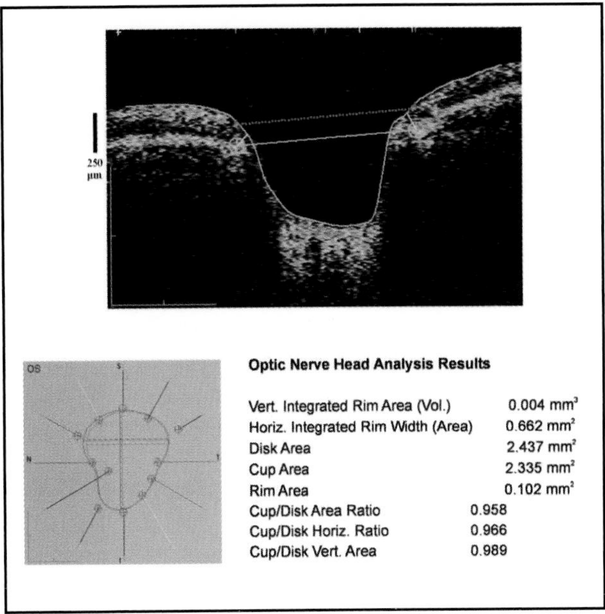
250 μm
OS
S
N
T
I
Optic Nerve Head Analysis Results
Vert. Integrated Rim Area (Vol.) 0.004 mm³
Horiz. Integrated Rim Width (Area) 0.662 mm²
Disk Area 2.437 mm²
Cup Area 2.335 mm²
Rim Area 0.102 mm²
Cup/Disk Area Ratio 0.958
Cup/Disk Horiz. Ratio 0.966
Cup/Disk Vert. Area 0.989

L

Case 12-9. Structure and Function Combined to Disclose Glaucoma in the Right Eye and Preperimetric Glaucoma on the Left

A 62-year-old Caucasian man had normal tension glaucoma treated with brinzolamide twice a day OU. On examination, visual acuity was 20/20 and IOPs were 16 mmHg in each eye. Pachymetry showed that the corneas were slightly thin in each eye, at 486 μm OD and 497 μm OS centrally. The anterior chamber angles were open to ciliary body band bilaterally. The ONH examination disclosed asymmetric cupping with a larger cup on the right, and thinning of the superior temporal and inferior neuroretinal rim (A and B). Frequency-doubling technology demonstrated an early inferior arcuate scotoma OD (C) and a full field OS (D). HRT highlighted the larger disc and cup in the right (E) compared to the left eye (F), with abnormal sectors identified in all segments except for temporally on the right.

Optical Coherence Tomography

Peripapillary NFL thinning was noted in the right eye primarily in the superior, temporal, and inferior sectors and could be seen as attenuation of the normal "double hump" pattern (G). Abnormal NFL thinning was present superior temporally and inferior temporally in the left eye as well (H), although there was no VF loss detectable. Similar macular maps were seen for both eyes with retinal thinning in the outer ring sectors (I and J). ONH analysis showed large cupping in both eyes (K and L).

Comment

This patient was just at the threshold of VF loss, but structural testing, particularly peripapillary NFL thickness but also HRT ONH evaluation and macular thickness, showed that this patient was abnormal and had glaucoma. The patient had an FDT VF defect in the right eye, but not in the left, where he had preperimetric glaucoma.

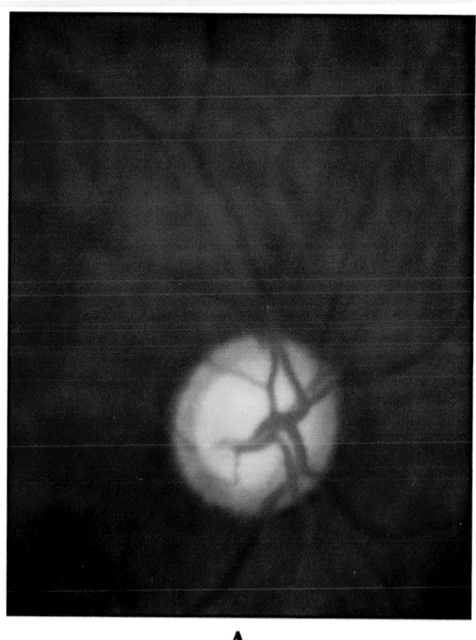

A

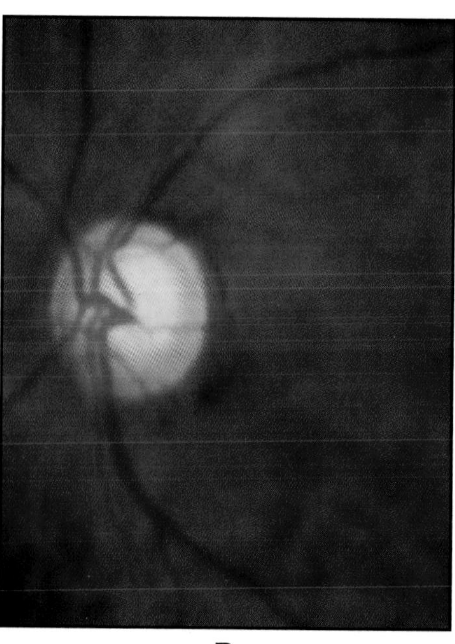

B

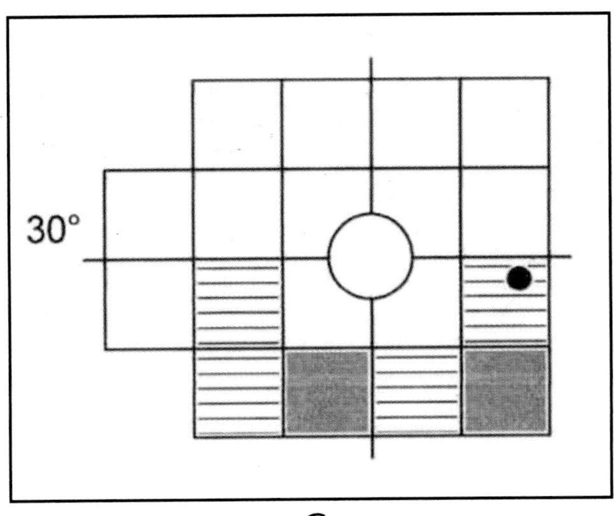

C

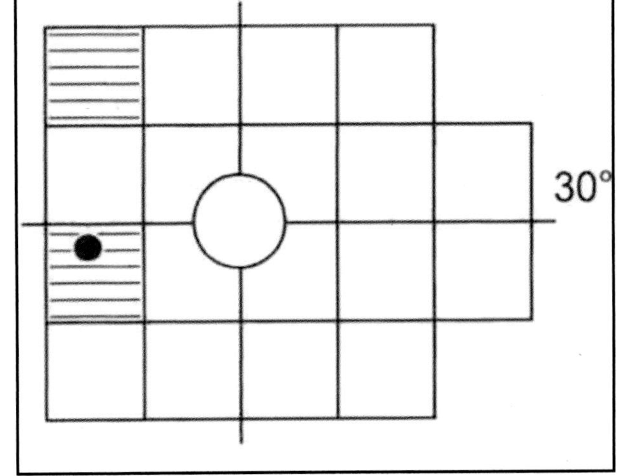

D

Parameters	global
disk area [mm²]	2.298
cup area [mm²]	1.571
rim area [mm²]	0.727
cup/disk area ratio []	0.684
rim/disk area ratio []	0.316
cup volume [mm³]	0.716
rim volume [mm³]	0.101
mean cup depth [mm]	0.487
maximum cup depth [mm]	0.850
height variation contour [mm]	0.128
cup shape measure []	0.087
mean RNFL thickness [mm]	0.076
RNFL cross sectional area [...	0.408
linear cup/disk ratio []	0.827
maximum contour elevation [...	0.111
maximum contour depressio...	0.238
CLM temporal-superior [mm]	0.029
CLM temporal-inferior [mm]	0.001
average variability (SD) [mm]	0.040
reference height [mm]	0.247
FSM discriminant function va...	-3.298
RB discriminant function valu...	-2.014

E

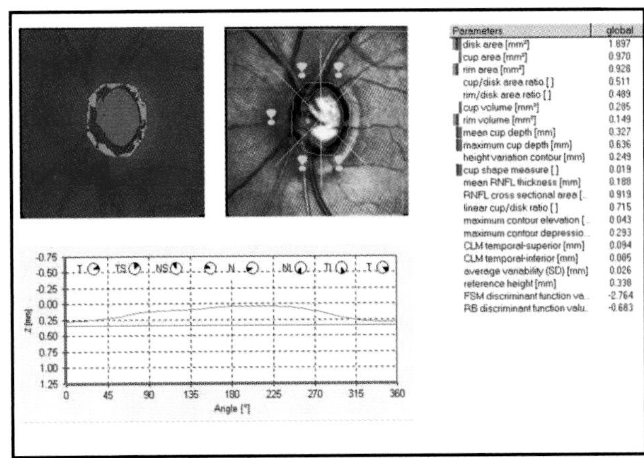

F

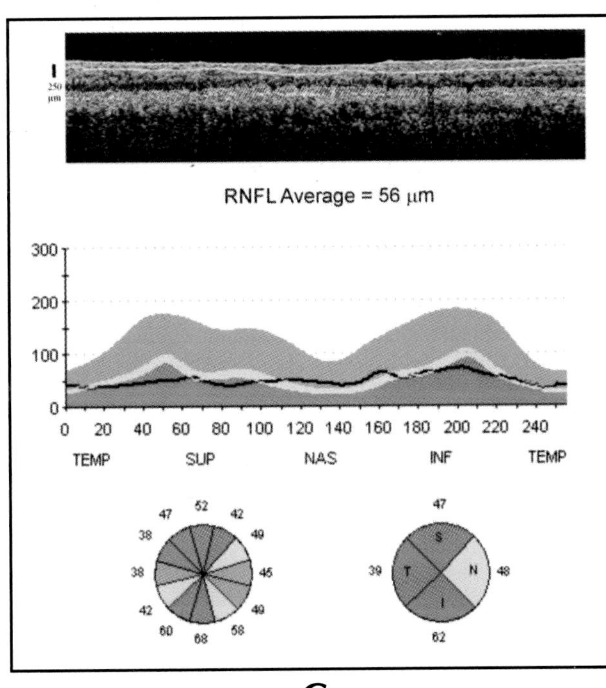

G

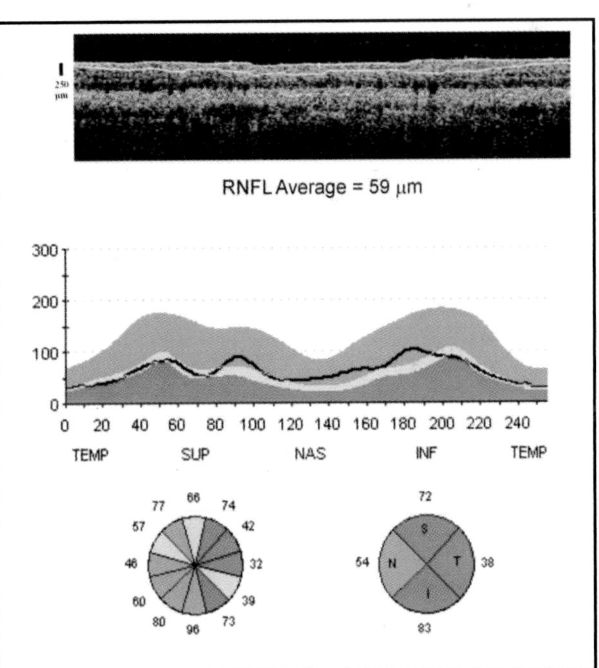

H

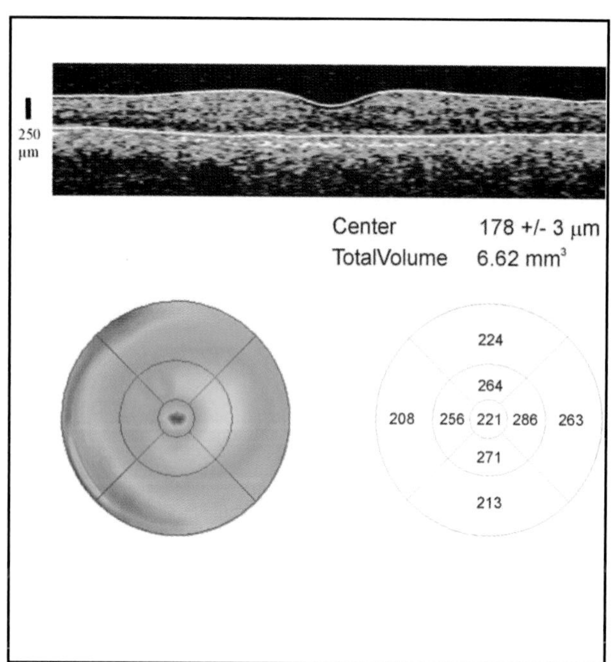

I

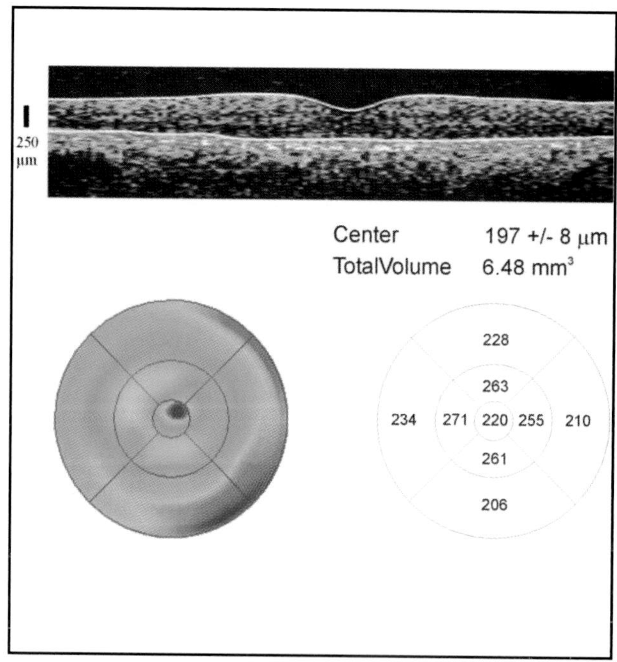

J

250 µm

OD

Optic Nerve Head Analysis Results

Vert. Integrated Rim Area (Vol.)	0.048 mm³
Horiz. Integrated Rim Width (Area)	1.016 mm²
Disk Area	2.726 mm²
Cup Area	2.238 mm²
Rim Area	0.488 mm²
Cup/Disk Area Ratio	0.821
Cup/Disk Horiz. Ratio	0.97
Cup/Disk Vert. Area	0.842

K

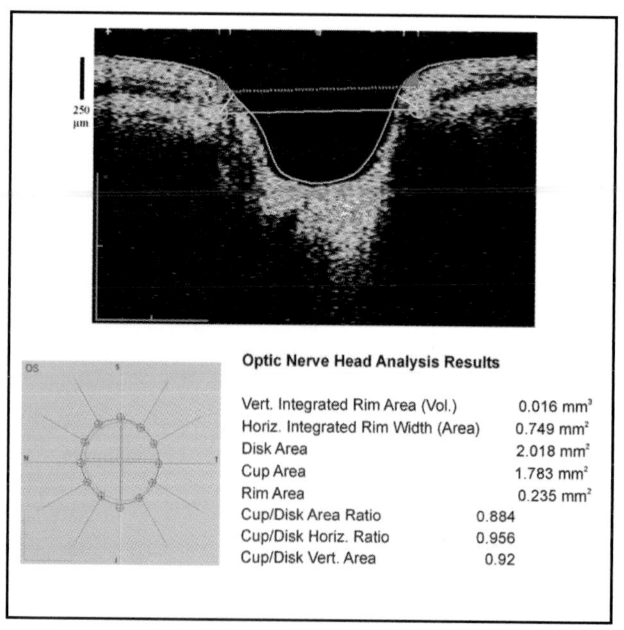

250 µm
OS
Optic Nerve Head Analysis Results
Vert. Integrated Rim Area (Vol.) 0.016 mm³
Horiz. Integrated Rim Width (Area) 0.749 mm²
Disk Area 2.018 mm²
Cup Area 1.783 mm²
Rim Area 0.235 mm²
Cup/Disk Area Ratio 0.884
Cup/Disk Horiz. Ratio 0.956
Cup/Disk Vert. Area 0.92

L

Case 12-10. Optical Coherence Tomography, Heidelberg Retina Tomograph, and Visual Field Correlation Supported Authenticity of Early Visual Field Abnormalities

A 75-year-old African-American man with primary open-angle glaucoma in both eyes was treated with latanoprost 0.005% and a combination of timolol 0.5% and dorzolamide 2%. Visual acuity was 20/32 and the IOP was 15 mmHg in both eyes. Slit-lamp examination revealed normal anterior chambers. Dilated fundus examination showed a larger optic disc cup in the right (A) eye compared to the left (B), with peripapillary atrophy in both eyes. Humphrey VF showed superior paracentral defects in both eyes, worse on the right than the left (C and D). HRT analysis showed greater cupping in the right eye (E) than the left eye (F) with overall thinning of the neuroretinal rim, excluding the temporal superior segment. A complete obliteration of the inferior NFL peak was noted in NFL analysis. In the left eye, there was a lesser reduction of the inferior NFL peak with abnormal thinning of the rim in the temporal inferior segment.

Optical Coherence Tomography

The circumpapillary NFL analysis showed thinning in the nasal quadrant and at 6:00 to 8:00 in the right eye (G). The left eye analysis showed a localized defect confined to 8:00 (H). Macular scans showed retinal thinning inferiorly, more on the right (I) than on the left (J). Optic disc analysis revealed equal disc sizes with a larger cup inferiorly on the right (K and L).

Comment

This patient with early-to-moderate glaucoma—worse on the right than the left—had corresponding OCT, HRT, and VF findings. The findings were consistent both in location and severity. The presence of structural abnormalities, especially in the left eye, supported the mild VF abnormalities.

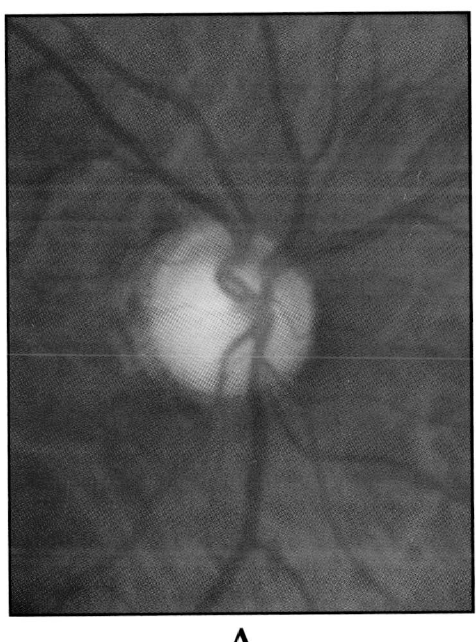

A

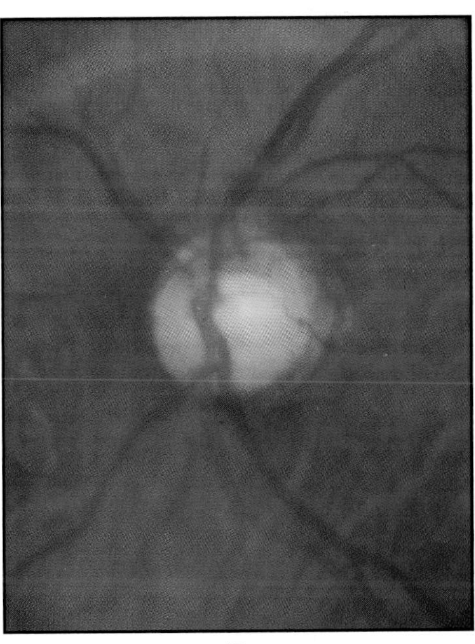

B

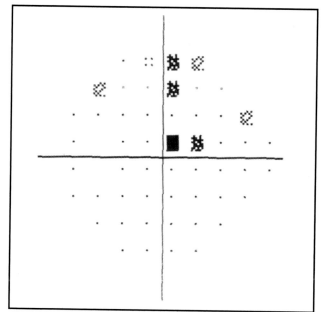

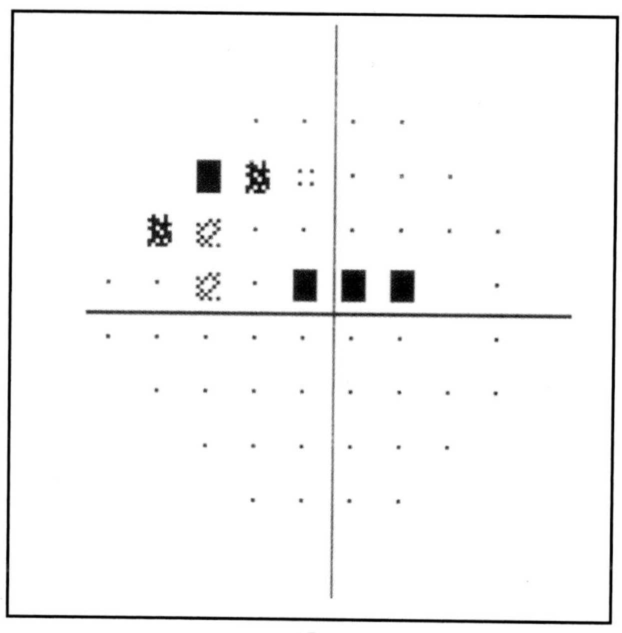

C

D

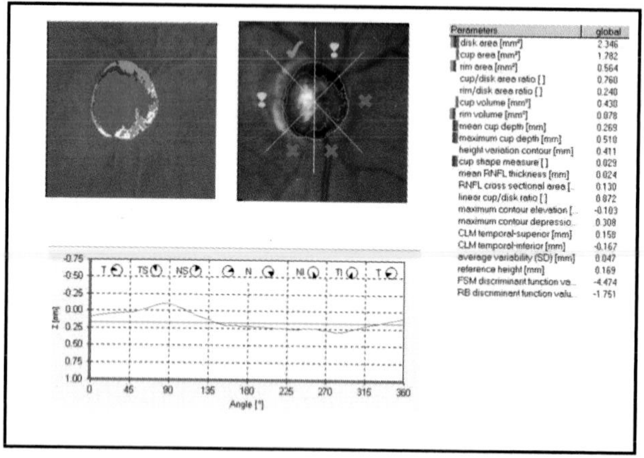
Parameters global
disk area [mm²] 2.346
cup area [mm²] 1.782
rim area [mm²] 0.564
cup/disk area ratio [] 0.760
rim/disk area ratio [] 0.240
cup volume [mm³] 0.430
rim volume [mm³] 0.078
mean cup depth [mm] 0.269
maximum cup depth [mm] 0.510
height variation contour [mm] 0.411
cup shape measure [] 0.029
mean RNFL thickness [mm] 0.024
RNFL cross sectional area [... 0.130
linear cup/disk ratio [] 0.872
maximum contour elevation [... -0.103
maximum contour depressio... 0.308
CLM temporal-superior [mm] 0.158
CLM temporal-inferior [mm] -0.167
average variability (SD) [mm] 0.047
reference height [mm] 0.169
FSM discriminant function va... -4.474
RB discriminant function valu... -1.751
Angle [°]

E

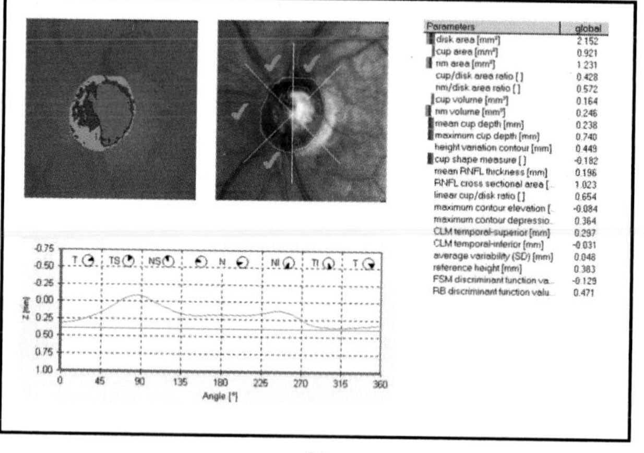
Parameters global
disk area [mm²] 2.152
cup area [mm²] 0.921
rim area [mm²] 1.231
cup/disk area ratio [] 0.428
rim/disk area ratio [] 0.572
cup volume [mm³] 0.164
rim volume [mm³] 0.246
mean cup depth [mm] 0.238
maximum cup depth [mm] 0.740
height variation contour [mm] 0.449
cup shape measure [] -0.182
mean RNFL thickness [mm] 0.196
RNFL cross sectional area [... 1.023
linear cup/disk ratio [] 0.654
maximum contour elevation [... -0.084
maximum contour depressio... 0.364
CLM temporal-superior [mm] 0.297
CLM temporal-inferior [mm] -0.031
average variability (SD) [mm] 0.048
reference height [mm] 0.383
FSM discriminant function va... -0.129
RB discriminant function valu... 0.471
Angle [°]

F

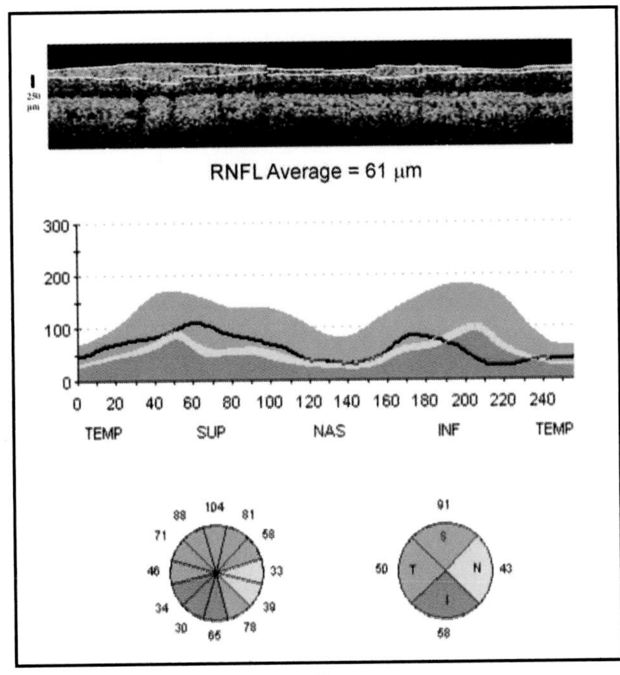
RNFL Average = 61 µm
300
200
100
0
0 20 40 60 80 100 120 140 160 180 200 220 240
TEMP SUP NAS INF TEMP
104 81 58 33 39 78 65 30 34 46 71 88
91
50 T S N I 43
58

G

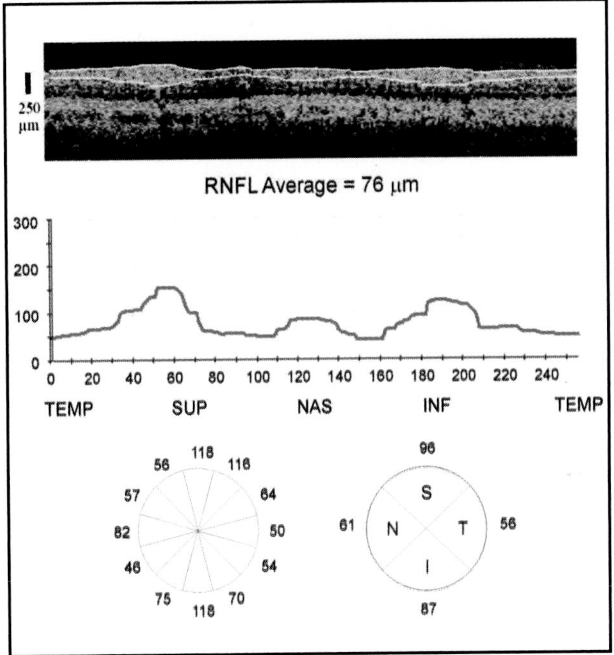
250 µm
RNFL Average = 76 µm
300
200
100
0
0 20 40 60 80 100 120 140 160 180 200 220 240
TEMP SUP NAS INF TEMP
118 116 64 50 54 70 118 75 46 82 57 56
96
S
61 N T 56
I
87

H

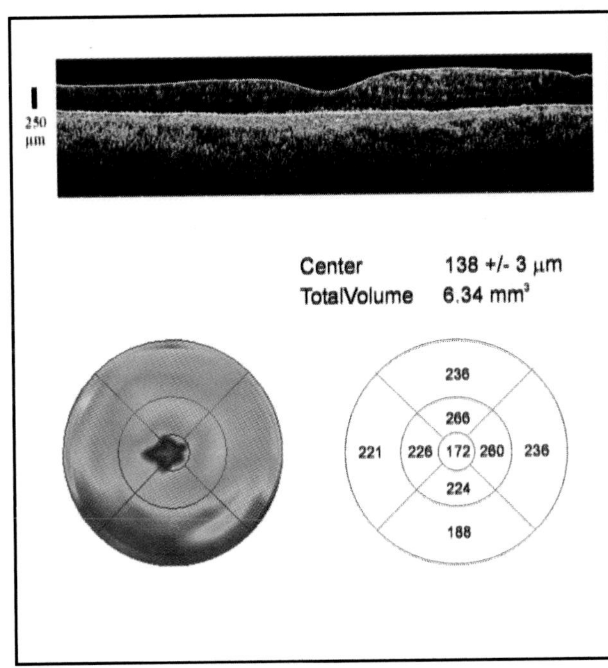
250 µm
Center 138 +/- 3 µm
TotalVolume 6.34 mm³
236
266
221 226 172 260 236
224
188

I

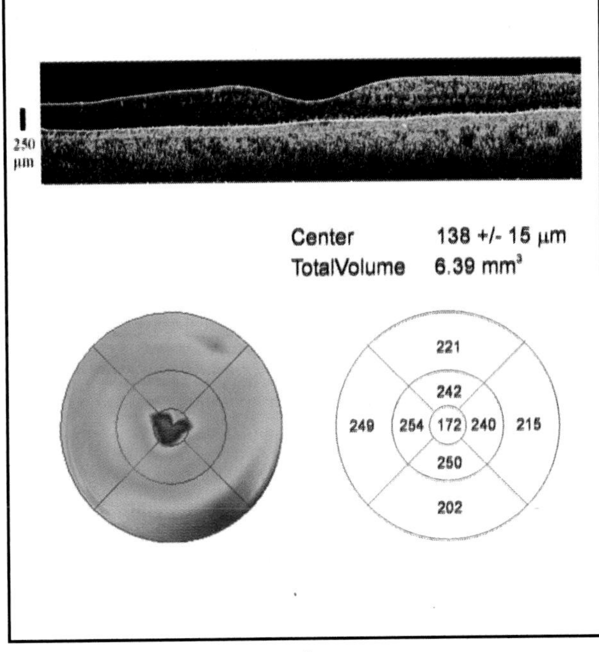
250 µm
Center 138 +/- 15 µm
TotalVolume 6.39 mm³
221
242
249 254 172 240 215
250
202

J

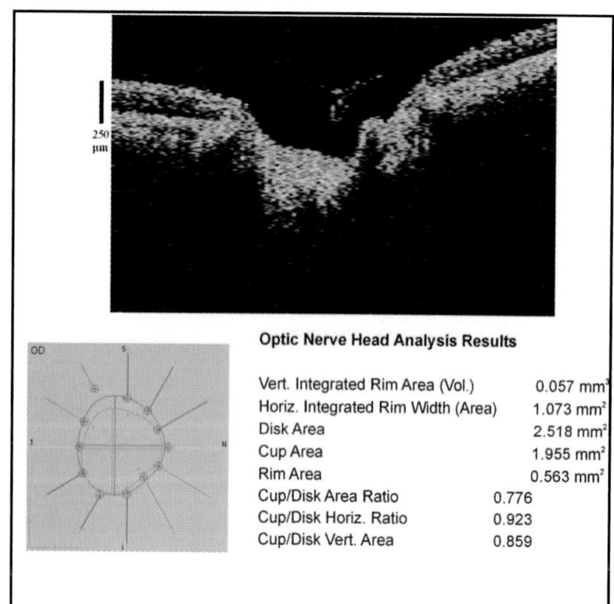
250 µm
OD
Optic Nerve Head Analysis Results
Vert. Integrated Rim Area (Vol.) 0.057 mm³
Horiz. Integrated Rim Width (Area) 1.073 mm²
Disk Area 2.518 mm²
Cup Area 1.955 mm²
Rim Area 0.563 mm²
Cup/Disk Area Ratio 0.776
Cup/Disk Horiz. Ratio 0.923
Cup/Disk Vert. Area 0.859

K

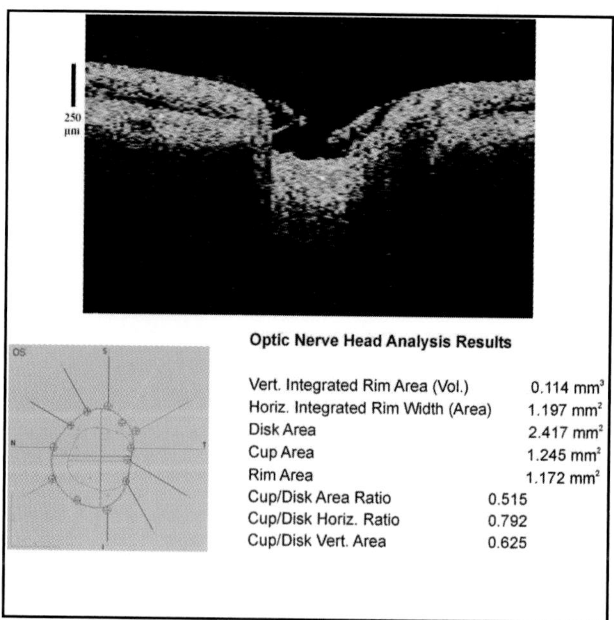
250 µm
OS
Optic Nerve Head Analysis Results
Vert. Integrated Rim Area (Vol.) 0.114 mm³
Horiz. Integrated Rim Width (Area) 1.197 mm²
Disk Area 2.417 mm²
Cup Area 1.245 mm²
Rim Area 1.172 mm²
Cup/Disk Area Ratio 0.515
Cup/Disk Horiz. Ratio 0.792
Cup/Disk Vert. Area 0.625

L

Case 12-11. Even With Field Loss on One Side of the Horizontal Meridian, Structural Imaging Revealed That Glaucoma Damage Was Global

A 70-year-old Caucasian man with a branch retinal vein occlusion in the left eye and primary open-angle glaucoma in both eyes was treated with latanoprost 0.005% once daily and brimonidine 0.2% twice daily in both eyes. Visual acuity was 20/20 and IOP was 13 mmHg in the right eye. The anterior segment of the right eye (A) was unremarkable, and the posterior segment was notable for peripapillary atrophy marked cupping of the ONH to the disc margin superior temporally. Humphrey VF showed a dense inferior hemifield defect (B). HRT showed neuroretinal rim thinning over the entire temporal half of the right eye (C).

Optical Coherence Tomography

Retinal NFL was distinctly diminished superiorly in the right eye but was clearly thinned throughout the entire scan (D). Macular scanning demonstrated retinal thinning in the outer rings as well as in the superior inner ring corresponding to the VF defect (E). The ONH scan showed dramatic cupping with diminution of the temporal and superior temporal neuroretinal rim (F).

Comments

This case again demonstrated the global nature of glaucomatous damage. While only the inferior hemifield showed glaucomatous VF loss, there was clear structural damage throughout the eye disclosed by OCT NFL, macular, and ONH analysis, as well as HRT ONH topography. There was a hint of a superior VF defect, but this would plainly have been disregarded without the corresponding structural abnormalities.

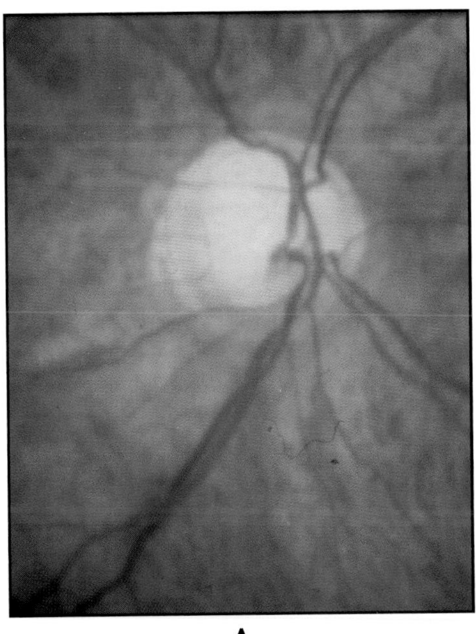

A

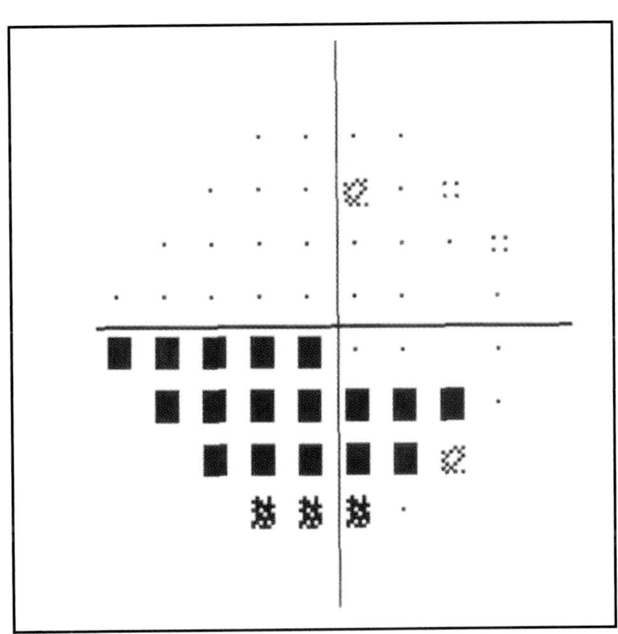

B

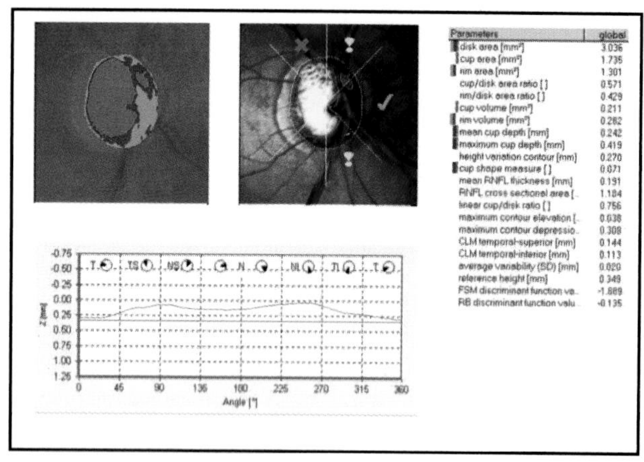
Parameters global
disk area [mm²] 3.036
cup area [mm²] 1.735
rim area [mm²] 1.301
cup/disk area ratio [ ] 0.571
rim/disk area ratio [ ] 0.429
cup volume [mm³] 0.211
rim volume [mm³] 0.282
mean cup depth [mm] 0.242
maximum cup depth [mm] 0.419
height variation contour [mm] 0.270
cup shape measure [ ] 0.071
mean RNFL thickness [mm] 0.191
RNFL cross sectional area [... 1.184
linear cup/disk ratio [ ] 0.756
maximum contour elevation [... 0.038
maximum contour depressio... 0.308
CLM temporal-superior [mm] 0.144
CLM temporal-inferior [mm] 0.113
average variability (SD) [mm] 0.020
reference height [mm] 0.349
FSM discriminant function va... -1.889
RB discriminant function valu... -0.135
T TS NS N NI TI T
Angle [°]

C

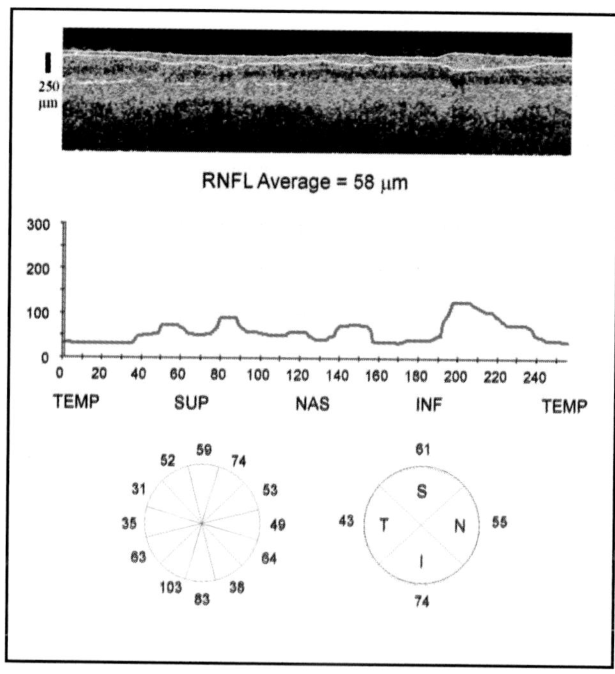
250 µm
RNFL Average = 58 µm
300
200
100
0
0 20 40 60 80 100 120 140 160 180 200 220 240
TEMP SUP NAS INF TEMP
59 74 53 49 64 38 83 103 63 35 31 52
61
S
T N
I
43 55
74

D

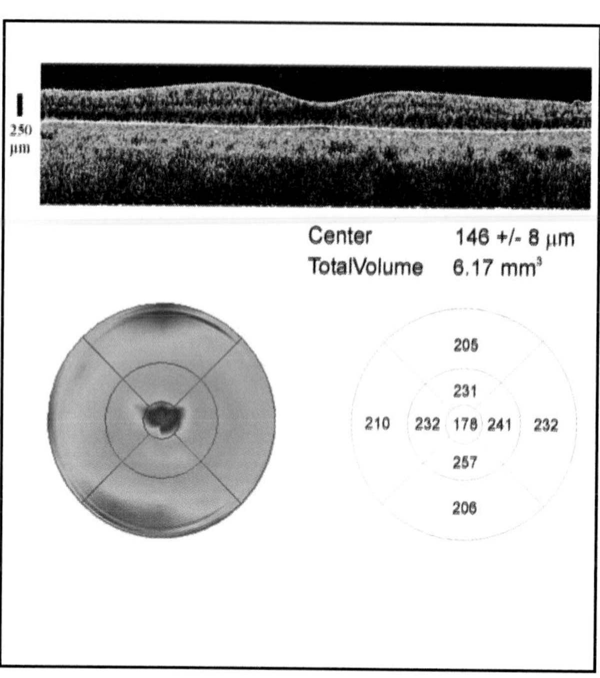
250 µm
Center 146 +/- 8 µm
TotalVolume 6.17 mm³
205
231
210 232 178 241 232
257
206

E

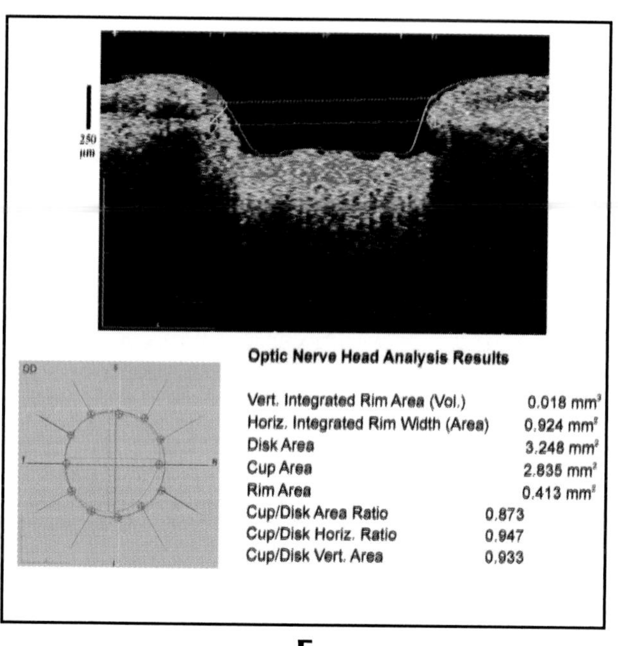
250 µm
Optic Nerve Head Analysis Results
Vert. Integrated Rim Area (Vol.) 0.018 mm³
Horiz. Integrated Rim Width (Area) 0.924 mm²
Disk Area 3.248 mm²
Cup Area 2.835 mm²
Rim Area 0.413 mm²
Cup/Disk Area Ratio 0.873
Cup/Disk Horiz. Ratio 0.947
Cup/Disk Vert. Area 0.933

F

Case 12-12. Structural and Functional Imaging Corresponded to Both Eyes, Reinforced Significance of Early Superior Visual Field Defect OD

A 52-year-old Caucasian woman with bilateral primary open-angle glaucoma underwent selective laser trabeculoplasty and was being treated with bimatoprost 0.03% and brinzolamide 1% bilaterally. The visual acuity was 20/20 and the IOP was 16 mmHg in both eyes. The anterior segments were normal with open angles observed in gonioscopy. The ONHs were cupped, and a minute disc hemorrhage was visible at 5:00 in the left eye (A and B). Humphrey VFs showed inferior nasal and paracentral defects in the right eye (C) and an inferior nasal and paracentral defect in the left eye (D). HRT disclosed neuroretinal thinning in the temporal superior segment in both eyes (E and F).

Optical Coherence Tomography

The circumpapillary scan showed normal scan in the right eye (E) and NFL thinning at 1:00 and 5:00 in the left eye (F). The right macular thickness was reduced in the inferior and temporal outer and inner sectors (I) and a slight retinal thickness reduction in the left eye in the superior, temporal, and inferior segments (J). Optic nerve cupping was noted mainly in the temporal superior sector in both eyes (K and L).

Comments

The OCT thickness measurements in the outer ring of the left macula were only slightly reduced; however, evaluating the thickness map highlighted retinal thinning mainly in the superior part of the macula. The macular, ONH, and NFL findings corresponded with the VF defects in both eyes.

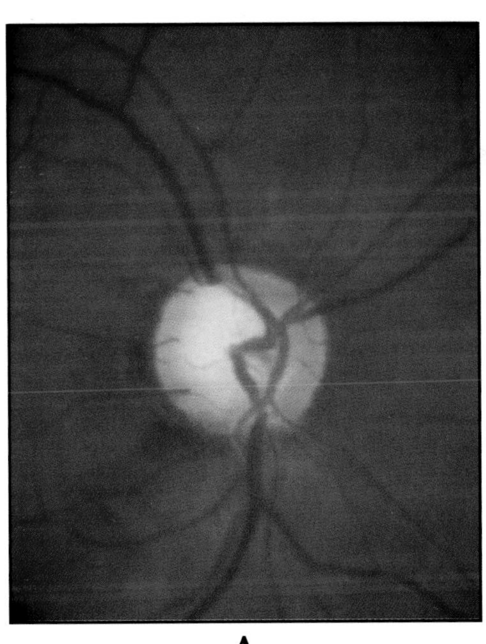

A

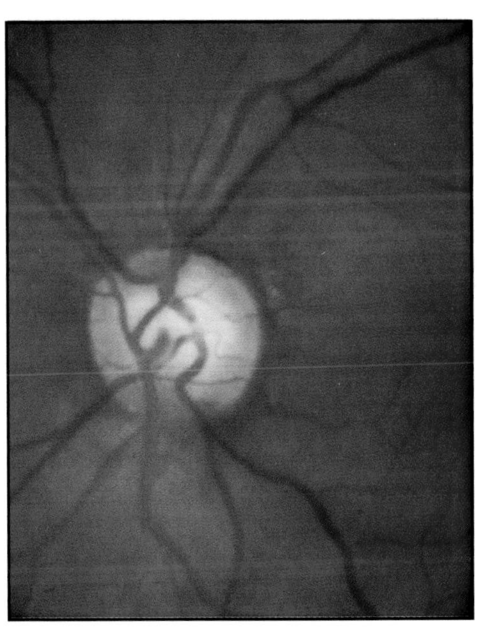

B

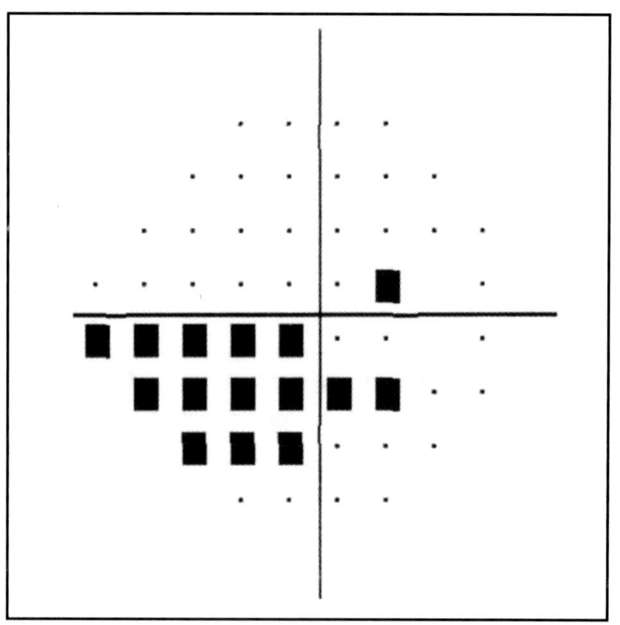

C

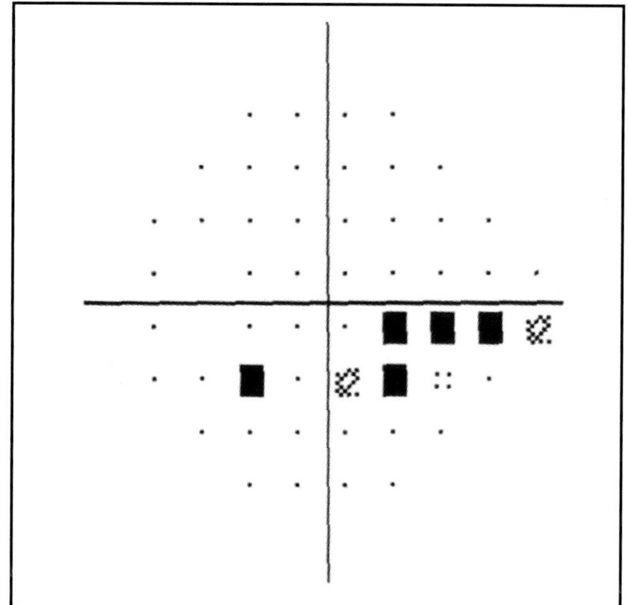

D

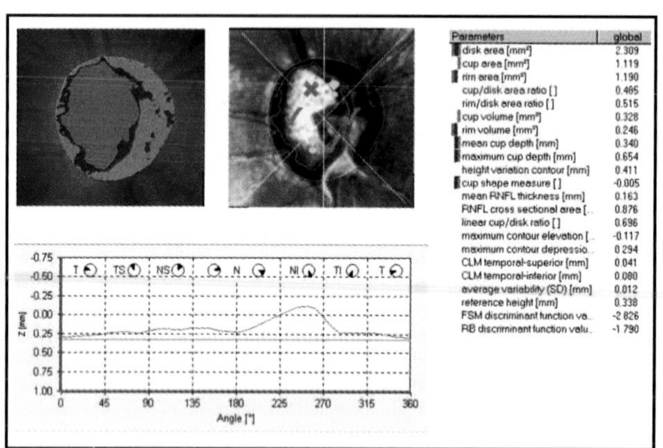

Parameters	global
disk area [mm²]	2.309
cup area [mm²]	1.119
rim area [mm²]	1.190
cup/disk area ratio [ ]	0.485
rim/disk area ratio [ ]	0.515
cup volume [mm³]	0.328
rim volume [mm³]	0.246
mean cup depth [mm]	0.340
maximum cup depth [mm]	0.654
height variation contour [mm]	0.411
cup shape measure [ ]	-0.005
mean RNFL thickness [mm]	0.163
RNFL cross sectional area [...	0.876
linear cup/disk ratio [ ]	0.696
maximum contour elevation [...	-0.117
maximum contour depressio...	0.294
CLM temporal-superior [mm]	0.041
CLM temporal-inferior [mm]	0.080
average variability (SD) [mm]	0.012
reference height [mm]	0.338
FSM discriminant function va...	-2.826
RB discriminant function valu...	-1.790

E

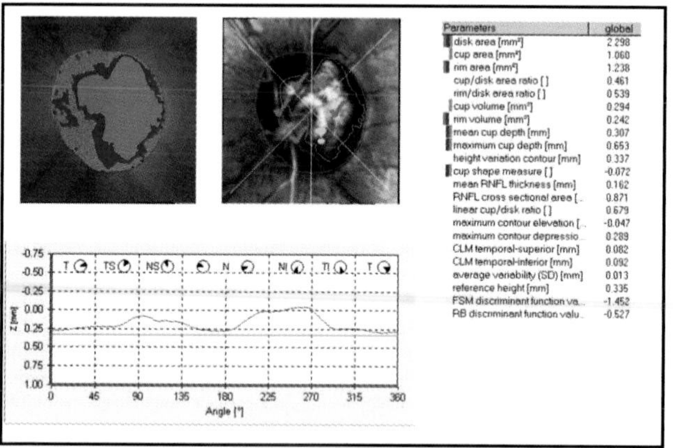

Parameters	global
disk area [mm²]	2.298
cup area [mm²]	1.060
rim area [mm²]	1.238
cup/disk area ratio [ ]	0.461
rim/disk area ratio [ ]	0.539
cup volume [mm³]	0.294
rim volume [mm³]	0.242
mean cup depth [mm]	0.307
maximum cup depth [mm]	0.653
height variation contour [mm]	0.337
cup shape measure [ ]	-0.072
mean RNFL thickness [mm]	0.162
RNFL cross sectional area [...	0.871
linear cup/disk ratio [ ]	0.679
maximum contour elevation [...	-0.047
maximum contour depressio...	0.289
CLM temporal-superior [mm]	0.082
CLM temporal-inferior [mm]	0.092
average variability (SD) [mm]	0.013
reference height [mm]	0.335
FSM discriminant function va...	-1.452
RB discriminant function valu...	-0.527

F

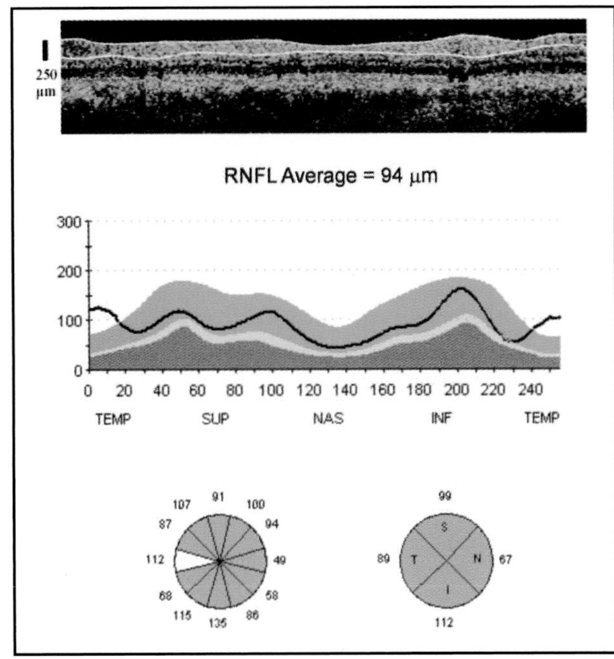

250 µm
RNFL Average = 94 µm
300
200
100
0
0 20 40 60 80 100 120 140 160 180 200 220 240
TEMP SUP NAS INF TEMP
107 91 100
87 94
112 49
68 58
115 135 86
99
S
89 T N 67
I
112

G

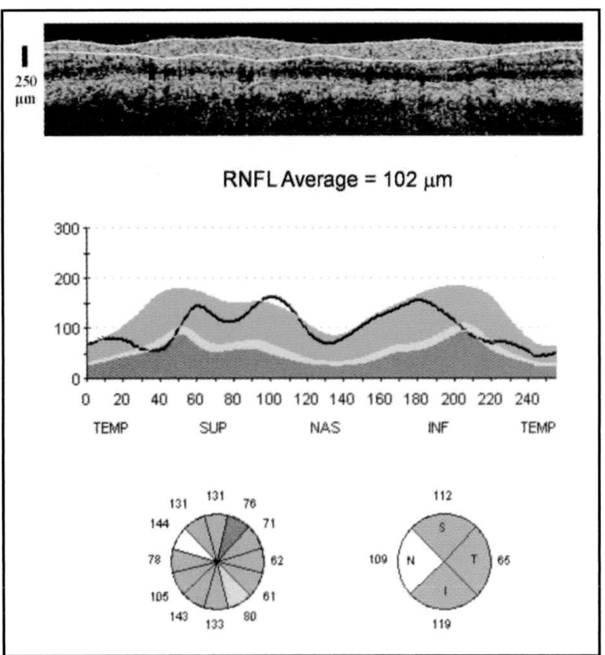

250 µm
RNFL Average = 102 µm
300
200
100
0
0 20 40 60 80 100 120 140 160 180 200 220 240
TEMP SUP NAS INF TEMP
131 131 76
144 71
78 62
105 61
143 133 80
112
S
109 N T 65
I
119

H

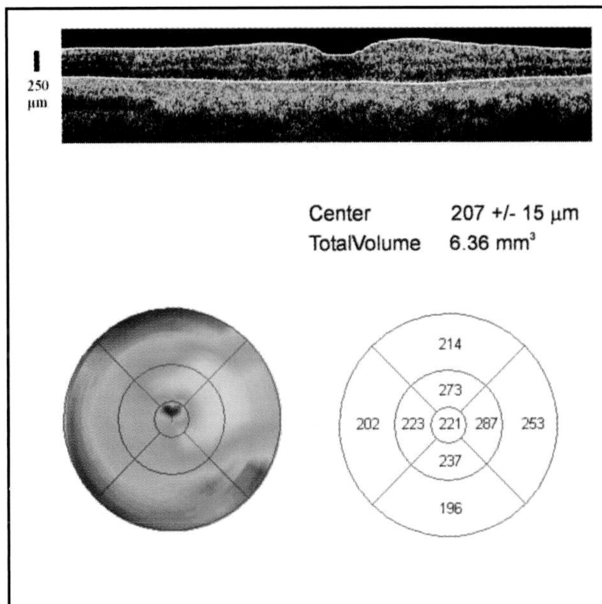

250 µm
Center 207 +/- 15 µm
TotalVolume 6.36 mm³
214
273
202 223 221 287 253
237
196

I

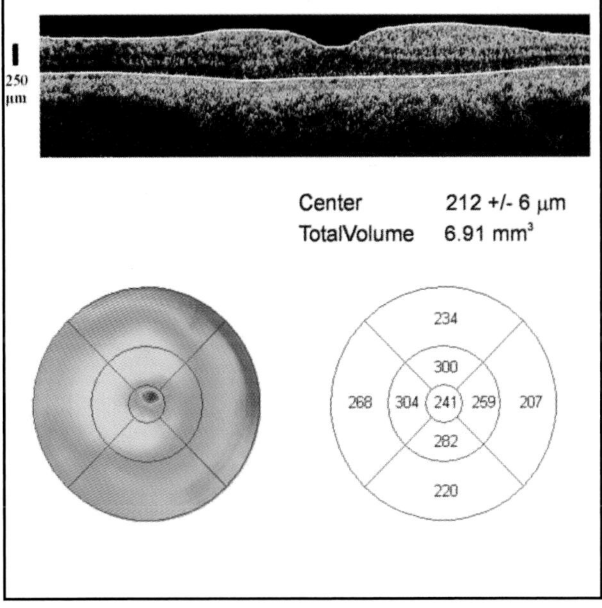

250 µm
Center 212 +/- 6 µm
TotalVolume 6.91 mm³
234
300
268 304 241 259 207
282
220

J

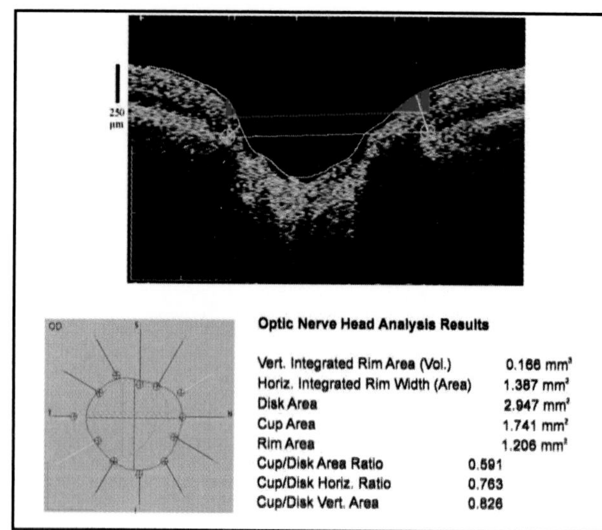
250 µm
OD
S
T
N
I
Optic Nerve Head Analysis Results
Vert. Integrated Rim Area (Vol.) 0.166 mm³
Horiz. Integrated Rim Width (Area) 1.387 mm²
Disk Area 2.947 mm²
Cup Area 1.741 mm²
Rim Area 1.206 mm²
Cup/Disk Area Ratio 0.591
Cup/Disk Horiz. Ratio 0.763
Cup/Disk Vert. Area 0.826

K

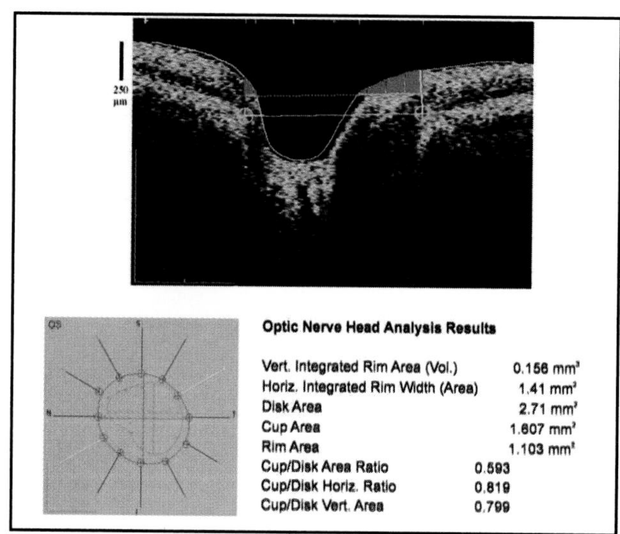
250 µm
OS
S
N
T
I
Optic Nerve Head Analysis Results
Vert. Integrated Rim Area (Vol.) 0.156 mm³
Horiz. Integrated Rim Width (Area) 1.41 mm²
Disk Area 2.71 mm²
Cup Area 1.607 mm²
Rim Area 1.103 mm²
Cup/Disk Area Ratio 0.593
Cup/Disk Horiz. Ratio 0.819
Cup/Disk Vert. Area 0.799

L

Case 12-13. Structural Imaging Corresponded With Visual Field, Reinforced Significance of Early Superior Visual Field Defect

A 49-year-old Caucasian woman with primary open-angle glaucoma in the right eye was treated with brinzolamide 1% and bimatoprost 0.03%. On examination, visual acuity was 20/16 and the IOP was 16 mmHg. No abnormal finding was noted in the anterior segment, and indirect ophthalmoscopy showed marked excavation of the ONH (A). Perimetry demonstrated an inferior nasal defect (B). HRT scanning revealed borderline thinning of the neuroretinal rim in the nasal sectors as well as the superior temporal and the inferior temporal regions (C).

Optical Coherence Tomography

The circumpapillary scan demonstrated generalized thinning of the retinal NFL, with extensive loss in the superior, inferior, and temporal quadrants (D). The outer temporal sector was thinner than expected in the macular scan (E). The ONH had thinning of the neuroretinal rim temporally (F).

Comment

Structure and function showed good correspondence in this case. Careful evaluation of the macular map disclosed the predominantly superior thinning of the outer temporal sector corresponding to the inferior nasal VF defect.

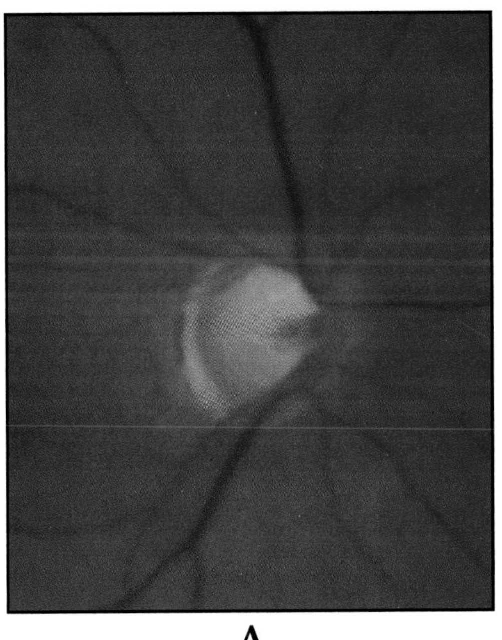

A

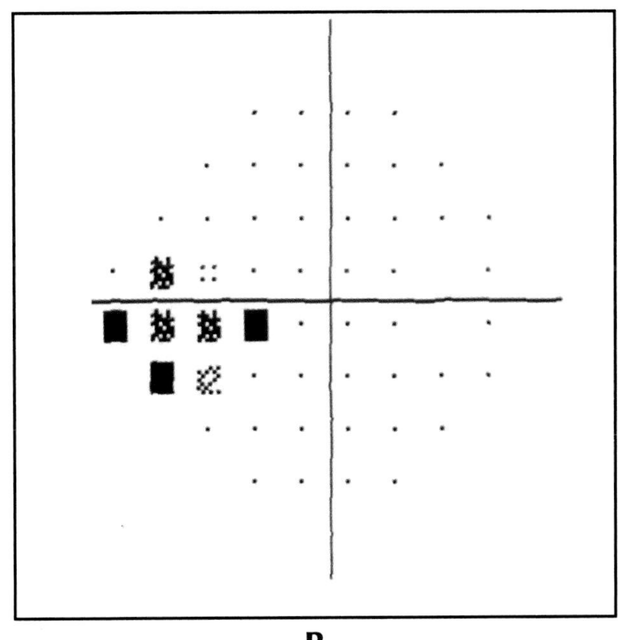

B

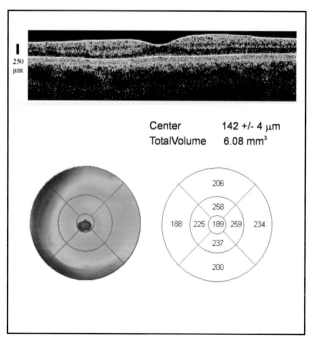

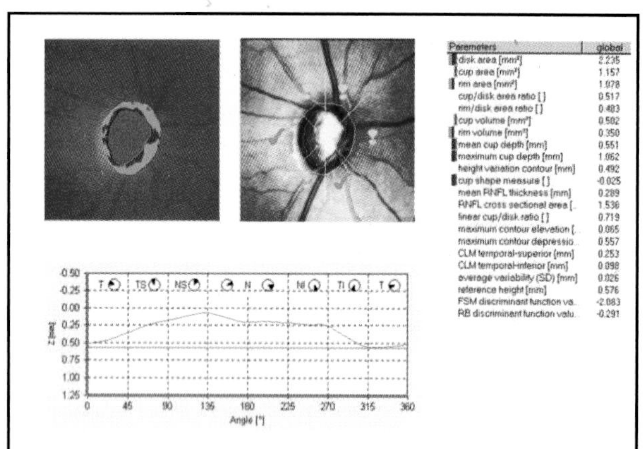

Parameters	global
disk area [mm²]	2.235
cup area [mm²]	1.157
rim area [mm²]	1.078
cup/disk area ratio [ ]	0.517
rim/disk area ratio [ ]	0.483
cup volume [mm³]	0.502
rim volume [mm³]	0.350
mean cup depth [mm]	0.551
maximum cup depth [mm]	1.062
height variation contour [mm]	0.492
cup shape measure [ ]	-0.025
mean RNFL thickness [mm]	0.289
RNFL cross sectional area [...	1.536
linear cup/disk ratio [ ]	0.719
maximum contour elevation [...	0.065
maximum contour depressio...	0.557
CLM temporal-superior [mm]	0.253
CLM temporal-inferior [mm]	0.098
average variability (SD) [mm]	0.026
reference height [mm]	0.576
FSM discriminant function va...	-2.083
RB discriminant function valu...	-0.291

C

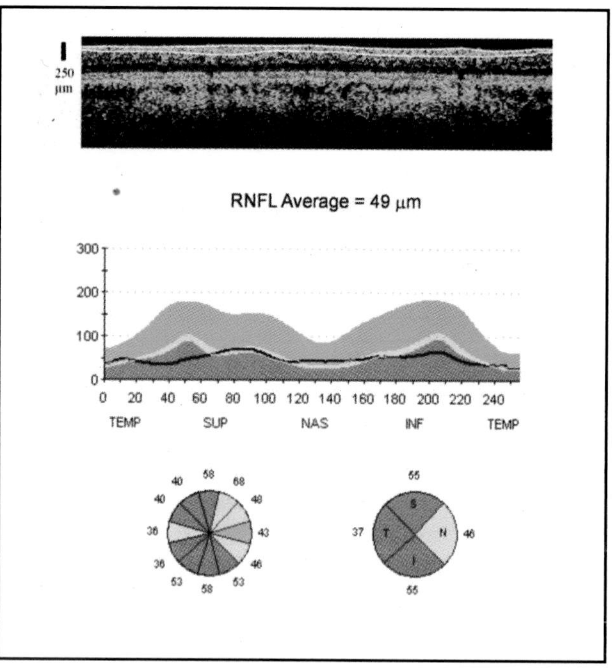

D

250 µm

Center 142 +/- 4 µm
TotalVolume 6.08 mm³

206
258
188 225 189 259 234
237
200

E

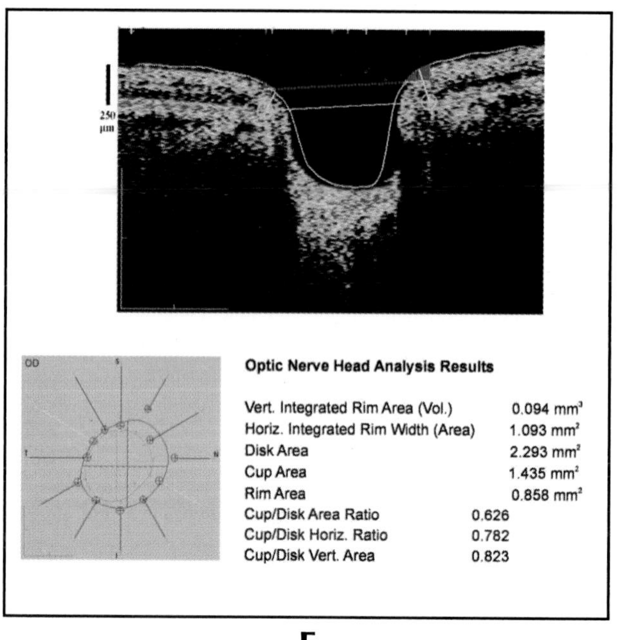

Optic Nerve Head Analysis Results

Vert. Integrated Rim Area (Vol.)	0.094 mm³
Horiz. Integrated Rim Width (Area)	1.093 mm²
Disk Area	2.293 mm²
Cup Area	1.435 mm²
Rim Area	0.858 mm²
Cup/Disk Area Ratio	0.626
Cup/Disk Horiz. Ratio	0.782
Cup/Disk Vert. Area	0.823

F

Case 12-14. Nerve Fiber Layer and Neuroretinal Rim Loss Corresponded With Visual Field, Reinforced Significance of Early Visual Field Defect; Macula Did Not Equal Visual Field

A 76-year-old Caucasian woman with primary open-angle glaucoma in the left eye was treated with bimatoprost 0.03% and brinzolamide 1%. Visual acuity was 20/32 and the IOP was 13 mmHg. Slit-lamp examination of the anterior segment did not reveal any abnormal finding, and the dilated fundus examination revealed symmetrical marked ONH cupping (A). Humphrey VF testing showed inferior nasal and paracentral defects (B). HRT scanning showed abnormal temporal thinning of the neuroretinal rim (C).

Optical Coherence Tomography

Circumpapillary scanning revealed significant retinal NFL thinning at the 4:00 and 5:00 positions as well as between 1:00 and 2:00 (D). There was borderline thinning in the adjacent, more nasal tissue. The macular scan showed inferior and temporal retinal thinning (E). The ONH scan showed obliteration of the temporal aspect of the neuroretinal rim (F).

Comments

Retinal NFL and ONH analysis demonstrated not only the established inferior VF loss but also confirmed the reality of the superior defect. While relatively mild by Humphrey VF, there was significant retinal NFL thinning and loss of neuroretinal rim. Macular imaging did not correspond with this patient's functional loss. Even though the macula was thin throughout, the inferior macula was thinner than the superior. It was unknown if this would be a harbinger of future superior functional loss or reflected a relative lack of sensitivity of macular imaging in glaucoma diagnosis.

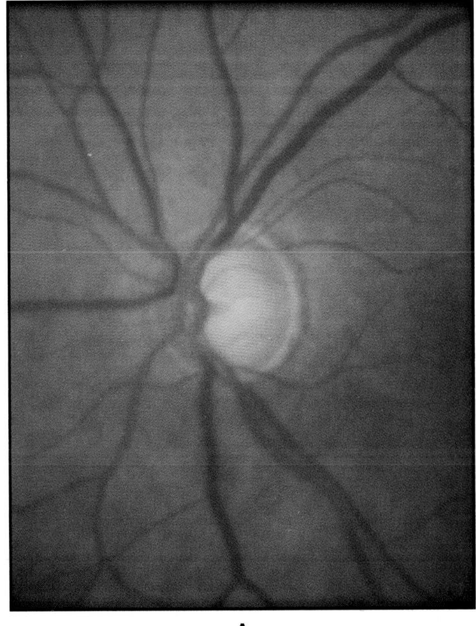

A

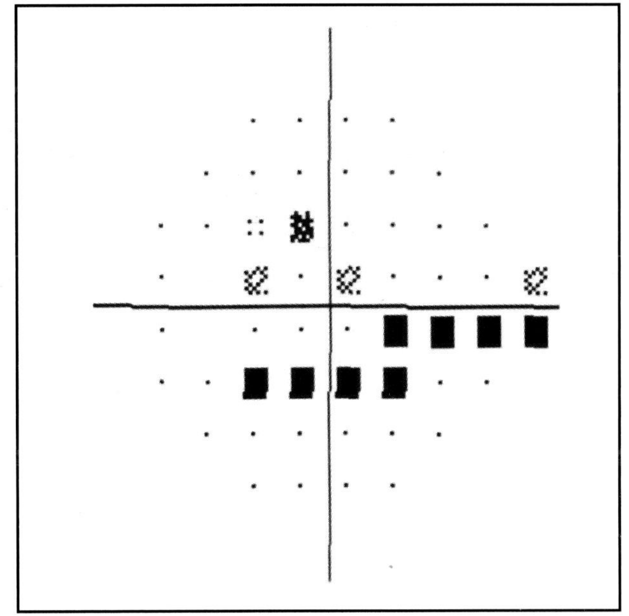

B

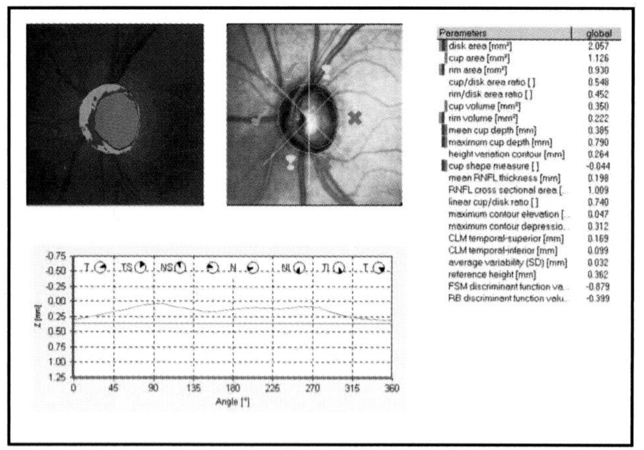
Parameters global
disk area [mm²] 2.057
cup area [mm²] 1.126
rim area [mm²] 0.930
cup/disk area ratio [ ] 0.548
rim/disk area ratio [ ] 0.452
cup volume [mm³] 0.350
rim volume [mm³] 0.222
mean cup depth [mm] 0.385
maximum cup depth [mm] 0.790
height variation contour [mm] 0.264
cup shape measure [ ] -0.044
mean RNFL thickness [mm] 0.198
RNFL cross sectional area [... 1.009
linear cup/disk ratio [ ] 0.740
maximum contour elevation [... 0.047
maximum contour depressio... 0.312
CLM temporal-superior [mm] 0.169
CLM temporal-inferior [mm] 0.099
average variability (SD) [mm] 0.032
reference height [mm] 0.362
FSM discriminant function va... -0.879
RB discriminant function valu... -0.399
Angle [°]

C

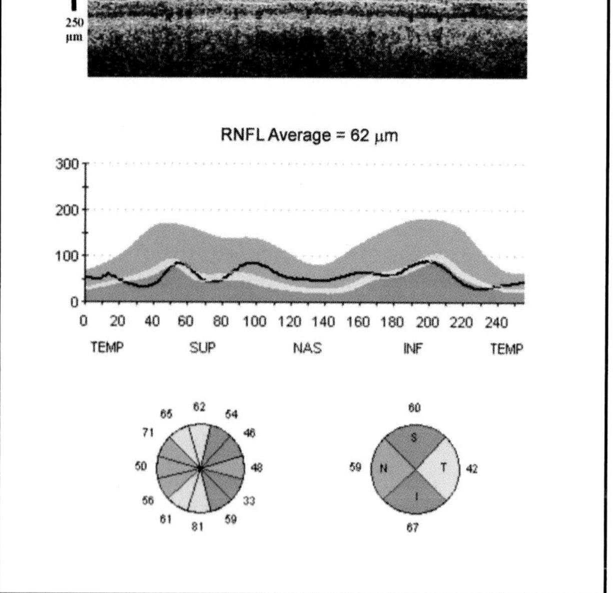
250 μm
RNFL Average = 62 μm
TEMP
SUP
NAS
INF
TEMP

D

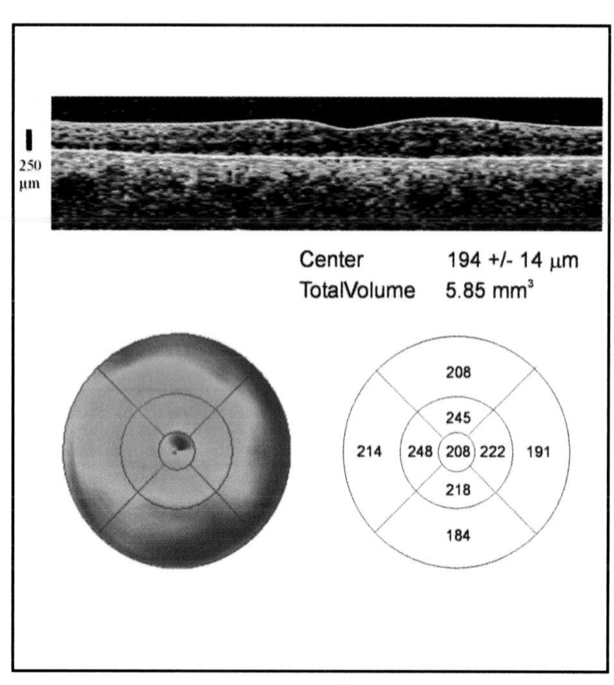
250 μm
Center 194 +/- 14 μm
TotalVolume 5.85 mm³
208
245
214
248
208
222
191
218
184

E

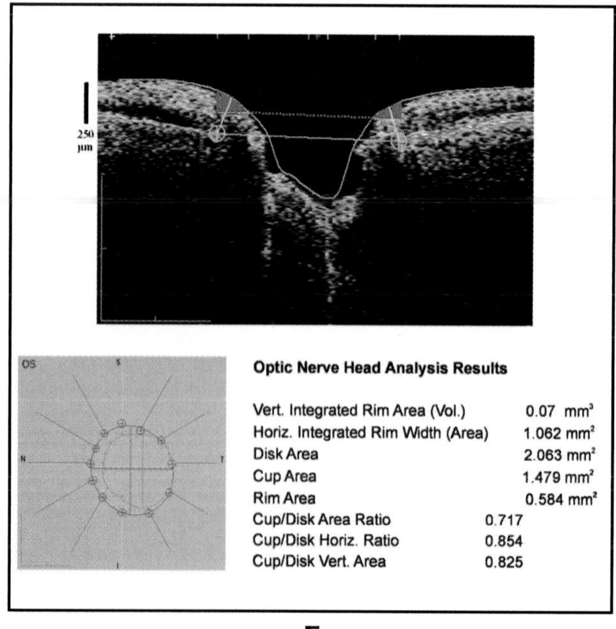
250 μm
OS
Optic Nerve Head Analysis Results
Vert. Integrated Rim Area (Vol.) 0.07 mm³
Horiz. Integrated Rim Width (Area) 1.062 mm²
Disk Area 2.063 mm²
Cup Area 1.479 mm²
Rim Area 0.584 mm²
Cup/Disk Area Ratio 0.717
Cup/Disk Horiz. Ratio 0.854
Cup/Disk Vert. Area 0.825

F

Case 12-15. Nerve Fiber Layer, Macular, and Optic Nerve Head Scanning All Corresponded With Visual Field Loss. Structural Correspondence With Questionable Visual Field Loss Corroborated Findings

A 70-year-old Caucasian woman with bilateral pseudoexfoliation glaucoma was treated with selective laser trabeculoplasty as well as latanoprost 0.005% and a combination of timolol 0.5% and dorzolamide 2%. Visual acuities were 20/20 and the IOPs were 20 mmHg in both eyes. On examination, pseudoexfoliation material was noted on the anterior lens capsule and in the anterior chamber angles bilaterally. Marked optic disc cupping was noted in both eyes, along with peripapillary atrophy (A and B). Humphrey VF testing showed an inferior nasal defect in the right eye (C) and an early inferior nasal defect in the left eye (D). HRT analysis showed similar disc sizes and cupping bilaterally, with thinning of the neuroretinal rim in the superior temporal segment in the right eye (E) and borderline thinning in the nasal superior and temporal inferior segments (F).

Optical Coherence Tomography

The circumpapillary scan disclosed similar average retinal NFL thickness in both eyes, with marked thinning superiorly more than inferiorly in the right eye (G) and superiorly in the left eye (H). The macular volume was lower in the right (I) than the left eye (J), mostly in the outer inferior and temporal sectors. ONH scans showed marked cupping on the right (K) more than the left (L).

Comment

NFL, macular, and ONH scanning all corresponded with VF loss. The structural measures emphasized the reality of what appeared to be mild VF loss superiorly in the right eye and inferiorly on the left, pointing out the importance of evaluating correspondence between structural and functional measures.

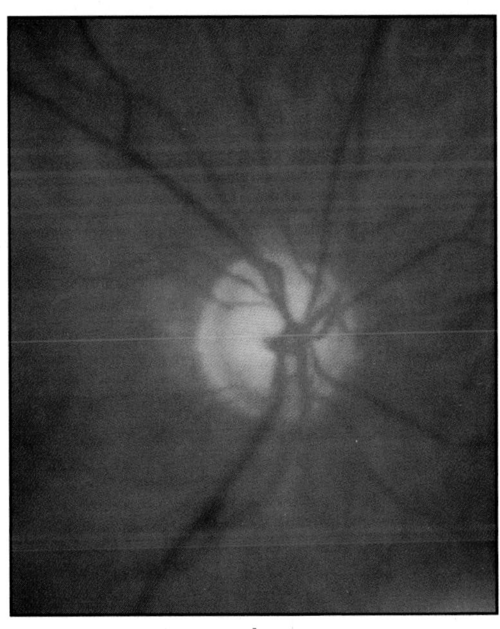

A

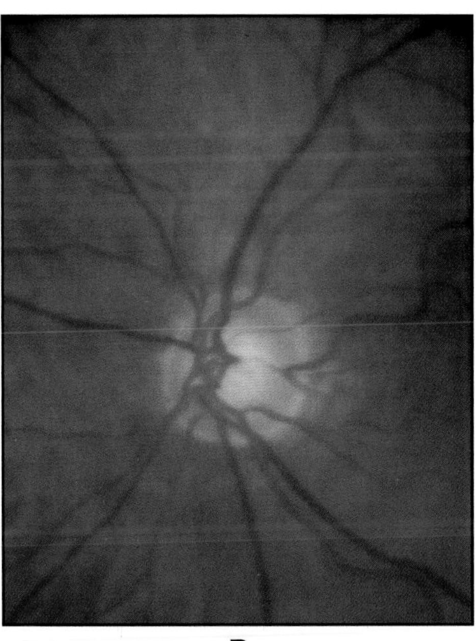

B

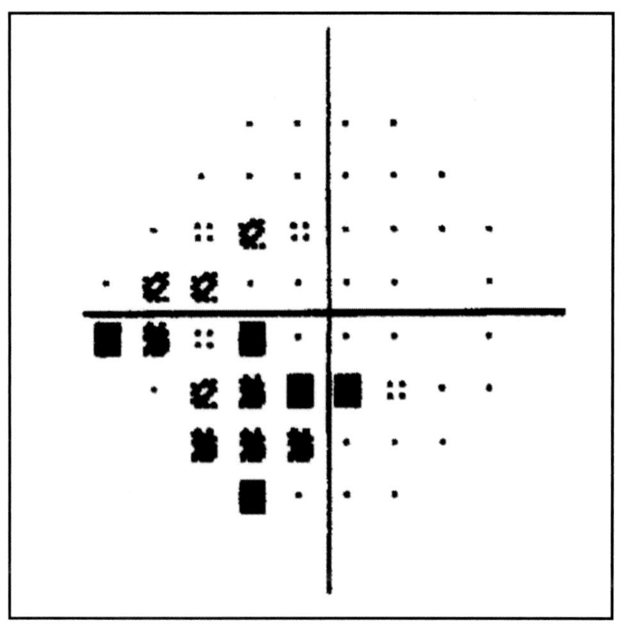

C

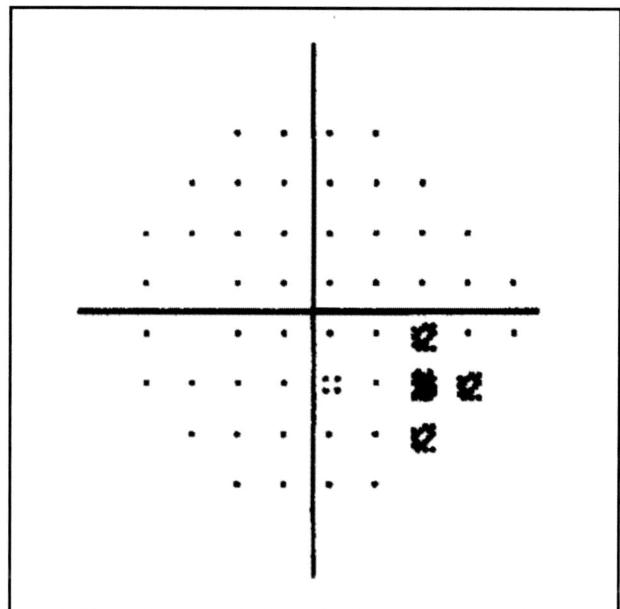

D

Parameters	global
disk area [mm²]	1.601
cup area [mm²]	0.723
rim area [mm²]	0.878
cup/disk area ratio [ ]	0.451
rim/disk area ratio [ ]	0.549
cup volume [mm³]	0.109
rim volume [mm³]	0.136
mean cup depth [mm]	0.206
maximum cup depth [mm]	0.445
height variation contour [mm]	0.163
cup shape measure [ ]	-0.062
mean RNFL thickness [mm]	0.143
RNFL cross sectional area [...	0.643
linear cup/disk ratio [ ]	0.672
maximum contour elevation [...	0.053
maximum contour depressio...	0.216
CLM temporal-superior [mm]	0.086
CLM temporal-inferior [mm]	0.065
average variability (SD) [mm]	0.018
reference height [mm]	0.259
FSM discriminant function va...	-1.000
RB discriminant function valu...	-0.321

E

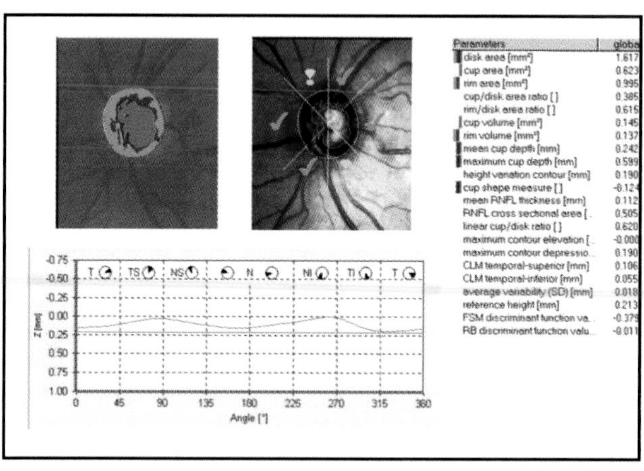

Parameters	globa
disk area [mm²]	1.617
cup area [mm²]	0.623
rim area [mm²]	0.995
cup/disk area ratio [ ]	0.385
rim/disk area ratio [ ]	0.615
cup volume [mm³]	0.145
rim volume [mm³]	0.137
mean cup depth [mm]	0.242
maximum cup depth [mm]	0.599
height variation contour [mm]	0.190
cup shape measure [ ]	-0.124
mean RNFL thickness [mm]	0.112
RNFL cross sectional area [...	0.505
linear cup/disk ratio [ ]	0.620
maximum contour elevation [...	-0.000
maximum contour depressio...	0.190
CLM temporal-superior [mm]	0.106
CLM temporal-inferior [mm]	0.055
average variability (SD) [mm]	0.018
reference height [mm]	0.213
FSM discriminant function va...	-0.379
RB discriminant function valu...	-0.011

F

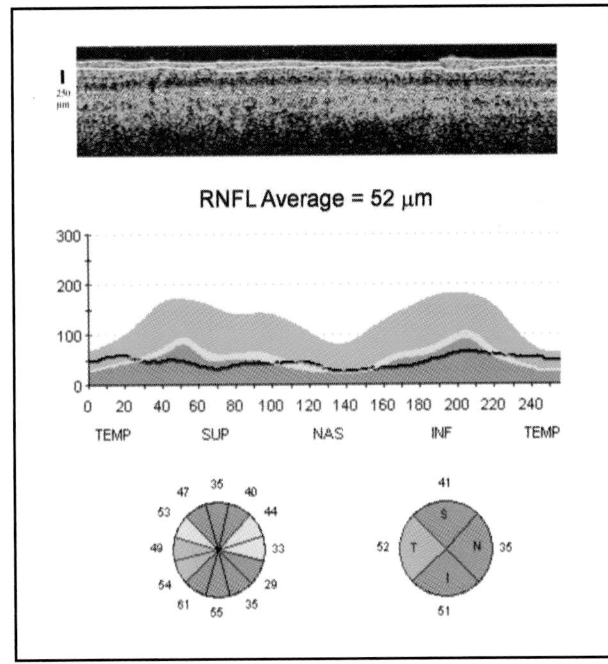
RNFL Average = 52 µm
300
200
100
0
0 20 40 60 80 100 120 140 160 180 200 220 240
TEMP SUP NAS INF TEMP
47 35 40
53 44
49 33
54 29
61 55 35
41
S
52 T N 35
I
51

G

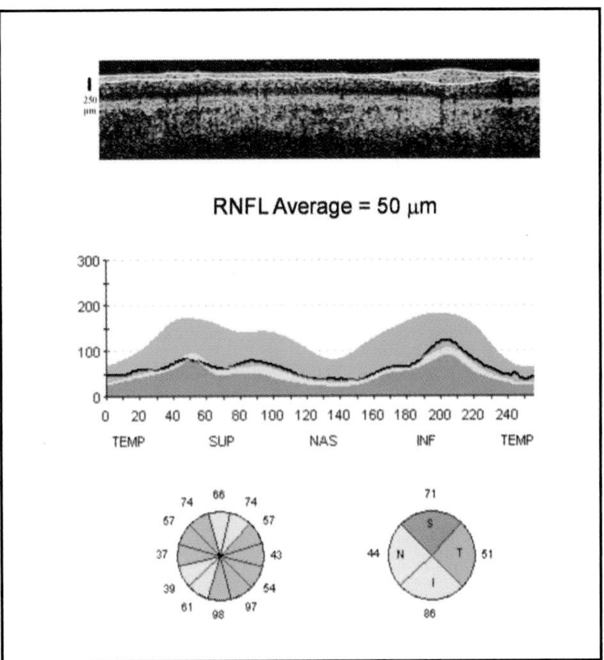
RNFL Average = 50 µm
300
200
100
0
0 20 40 60 80 100 120 140 160 180 200 220 240
TEMP SUP NAS INF TEMP
74 66 74
67 57
37 43
39 54
61 98 97
71
S
44 N T 51
I
86

H

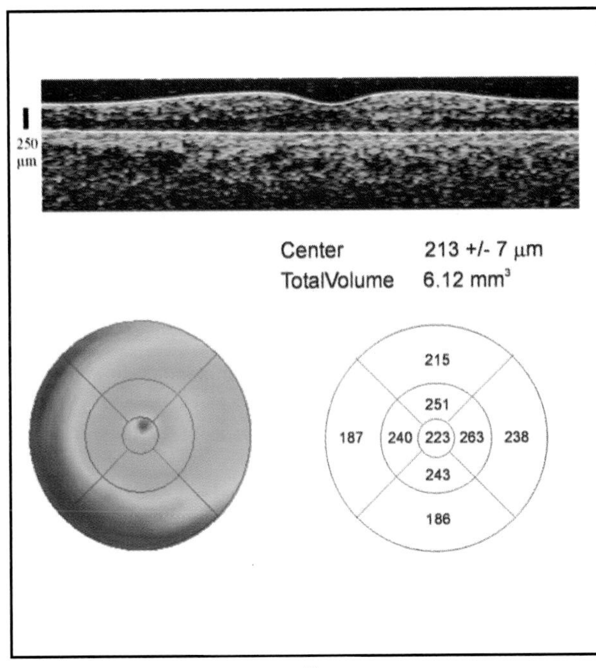
250 µm
Center 213 +/- 7 µm
TotalVolume 6.12 mm³
215
251
187 240 223 263 238
243
186

I

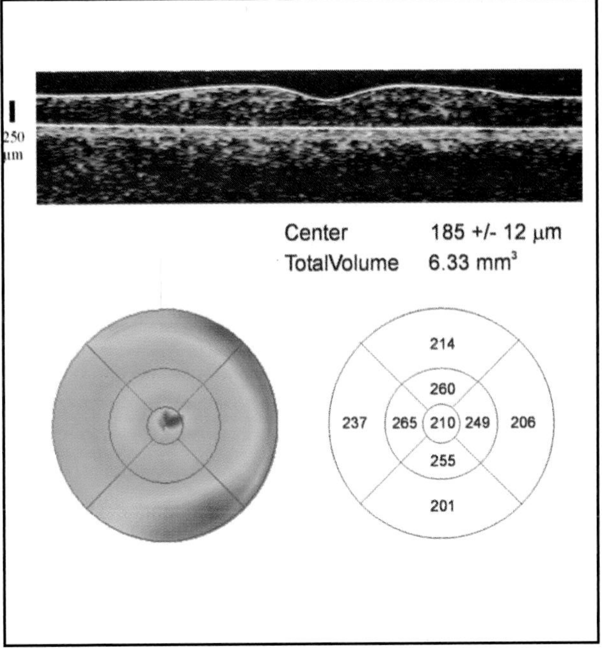
250 µm
Center 185 +/- 12 µm
TotalVolume 6.33 mm³
214
260
237 265 210 249 206
255
201

J

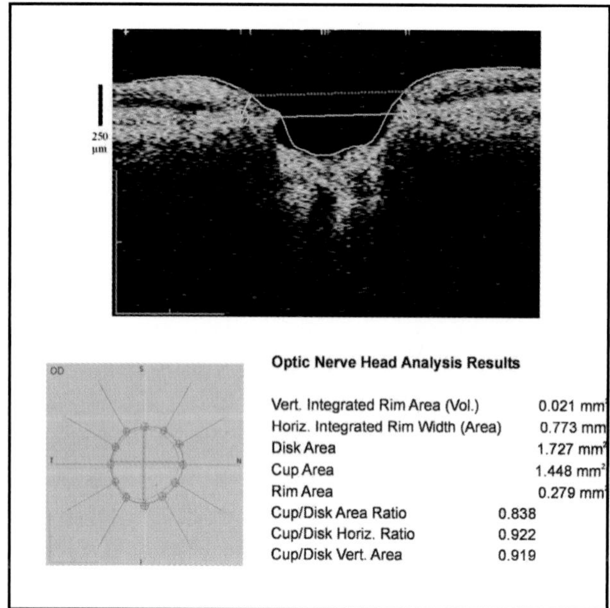
250 µm
OD
S
T
N
I
Optic Nerve Head Analysis Results
Vert. Integrated Rim Area (Vol.) 0.021 mm
Horiz. Integrated Rim Width (Area) 0.773 mm
Disk Area 1.727 mm²
Cup Area 1.448 mm²
Rim Area 0.279 mm
Cup/Disk Area Ratio 0.838
Cup/Disk Horiz. Ratio 0.922
Cup/Disk Vert. Area 0.919

K

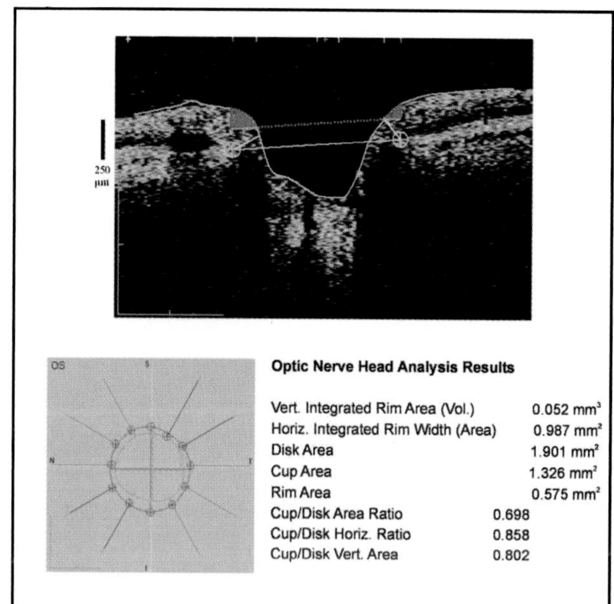
250 µm
OS
S
N
T
I
Optic Nerve Head Analysis Results
Vert. Integrated Rim Area (Vol.) 0.052 mm³
Horiz. Integrated Rim Width (Area) 0.987 mm²
Disk Area 1.901 mm²
Cup Area 1.326 mm²
Rim Area 0.575 mm²
Cup/Disk Area Ratio 0.698
Cup/Disk Horiz. Ratio 0.858
Cup/Disk Vert. Area 0.802

L

Case 12-16. Corresponding Optical Coherence Tomography, Heidelberg Retina Tomograph, and Visual Field Findings Supported Glaucomatous Damage in the Right Eye; Lack of Structural Correlation Suggested Visual Field Defect Was Artifact on the Left

A 58-year-old woman with bilateral pigmentary glaucoma and gradually progressing VF loss in the right eye was referred for a second opinion. On examination, visual acuity was 20/20 and IOPs were 17 mmHg OU. Krukenberg spindles were noted on the posterior surface of the corneas with midperipheral iris transillumination defects and a heavily pigmented trabecular meshwork. The anterior chamber angle was open 360 degrees to the ciliary body band. Posterior segment examination revealed marked ONH cupping in both eyes (A and B) with a NFL defect visible from 6:00 to 7:00 in the right eye (C and D). Humphrey VF testing demonstrated a superior arcuate scotoma in the right eye (E) and a possible inferior nasal step on the left (F). HRT scanning OD showed inferior temporal neuroretinal rim thinning and a NFL defect at the 6:30 position (G and H).

Optical Coherence Tomography

The retinal NFL (I and J) in the circumpapillary scan was substantially thinner on the right than the left, with diminished thickness at 7:00, corresponding to the superior arcuate VF defect. The macular scan showed reduced retinal thickness in the inferior outer ring in the right eye (K) and a normal scan on the left (L). ONH analysis showed a larger cup on the right (M) than the left (N).

Comments

A NFL defect was detected clinically in the inferior temporal aspect of the ONH. This defect corresponded to the superior VF defect and was seen in the peripapillary OCT as a marked thinning of the retinal NFL on the right side of the scanned image. There was good correspondence between the OCT, HRT, and VF. The normal scan of the left eye suggested that the possible VF defect in that eye was artifact.

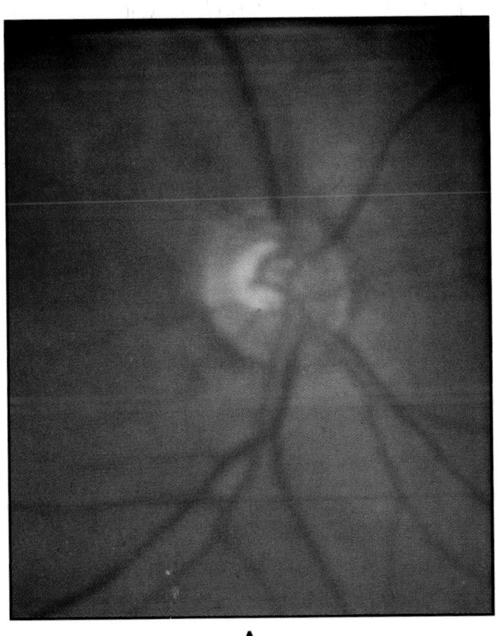

A

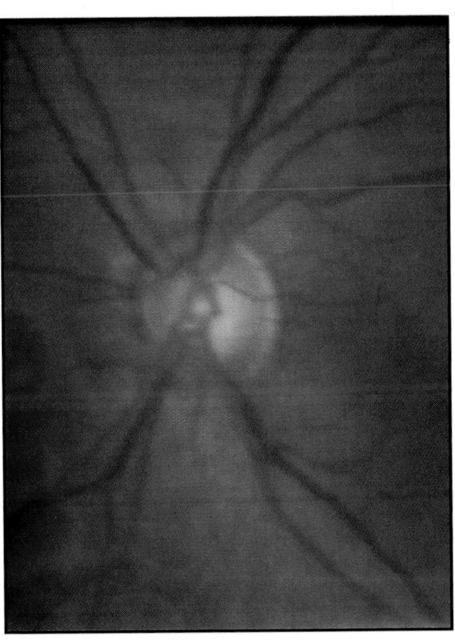

B

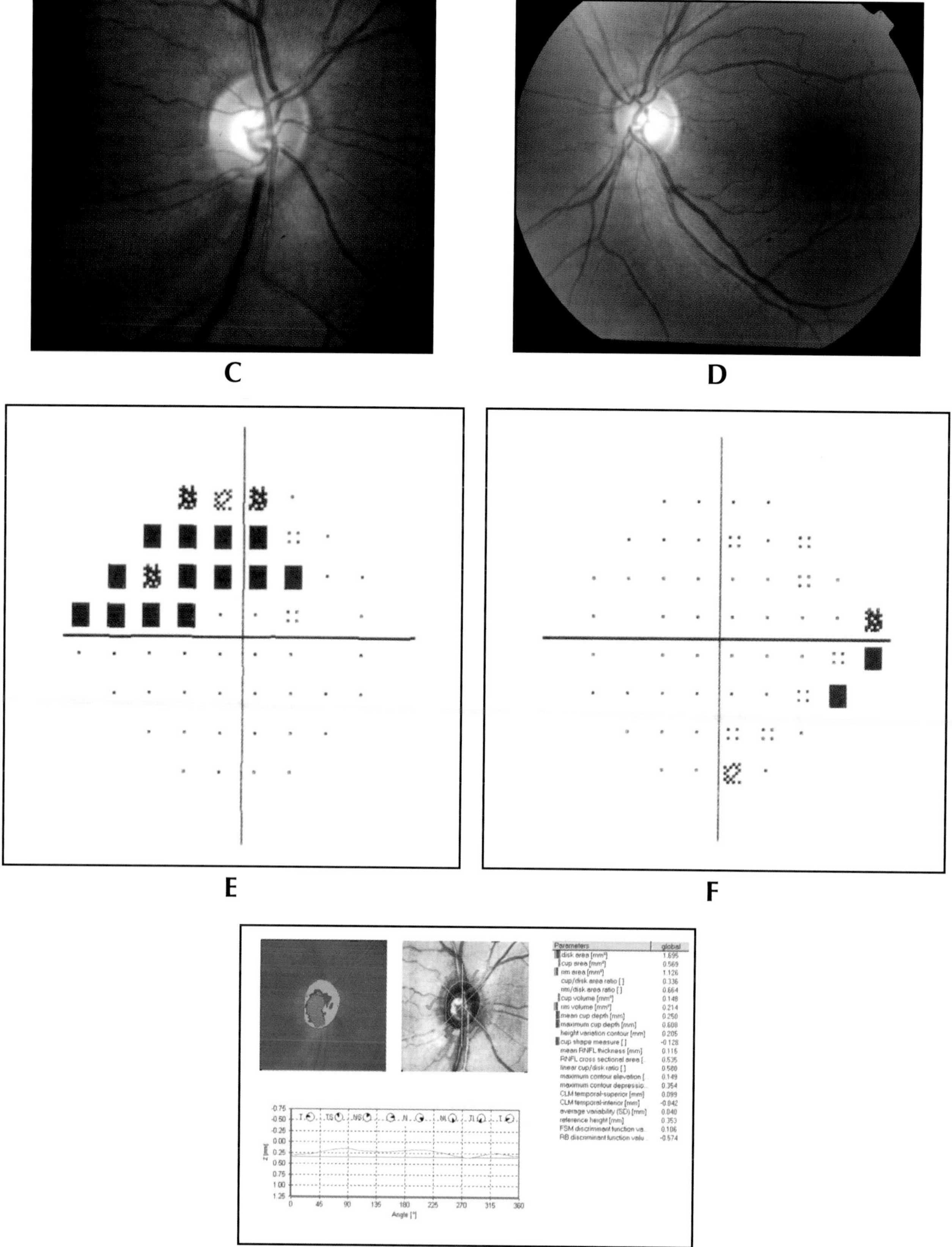
C
D
E
F
Parameters global
disk area [mm²] 1.695
cup area [mm²] 0.569
rim area [mm²] 1.126
cup/disk area ratio [ ] 0.336
rim/disk area ratio [ ] 0.664
cup volume [mm³] 0.148
rim volume [mm³] 0.214
mean cup depth [mm] 0.250
maximum cup depth [mm] 0.608
height variation contour [mm] 0.205
cup shape measure [ ] -0.128
mean RNFL thickness [mm] 0.116
RNFL cross sectional area [... 0.535
linear cup/disk ratio [ ] 0.580
maximum contour elevation [... 0.149
maximum contour depressio... 0.354
CLM temporal-superior [mm] 0.099
CLM temporal-inferior [mm] -0.042
average variability (SD) [mm] 0.040
reference height [mm] 0.353
FSM discriminant function va... 0.106
RB discriminant function valu... -0.574
z [mm]
Angle [°]
G

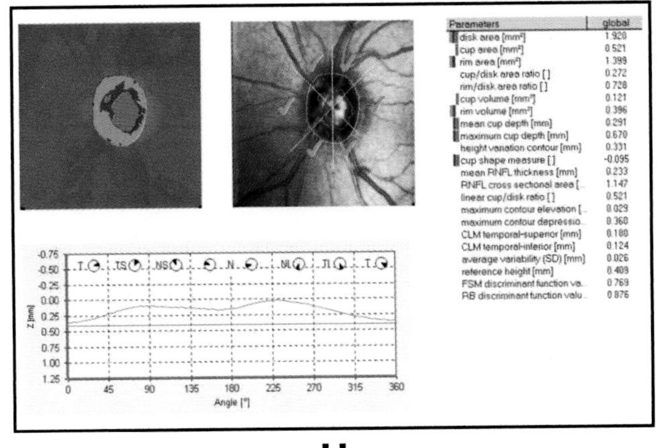
Parameters global
disk area [mm²] 1.920
cup area [mm²] 0.521
rim area [mm²] 1.399
cup/disk area ratio [] 0.272
rim/disk area ratio [] 0.728
cup volume [mm³] 0.121
rim volume [mm³] 0.396
mean cup depth [mm] 0.291
maximum cup depth [mm] 0.670
height variation contour [mm] 0.331
cup shape measure [] -0.095
mean RNFL thickness [mm] 0.233
RNFL cross sectional area [... 1.147
linear cup/disk ratio [] 0.521
maximum contour elevation [... 0.029
maximum contour depressio... 0.360
CLM temporal-superior [mm] 0.180
CLM temporal-inferior [mm] 0.124
average variability (SD) [mm] 0.026
reference height [mm] 0.409
FSM discriminant function va... 0.769
RB discriminant function valu... 0.876
Angle [°]

H

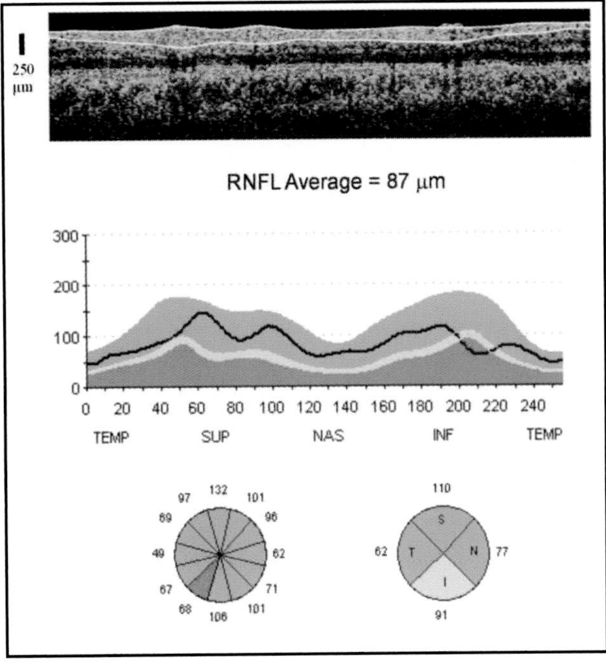
250 µm
RNFL Average = 87 µm
TEMP SUP NAS INF TEMP

I

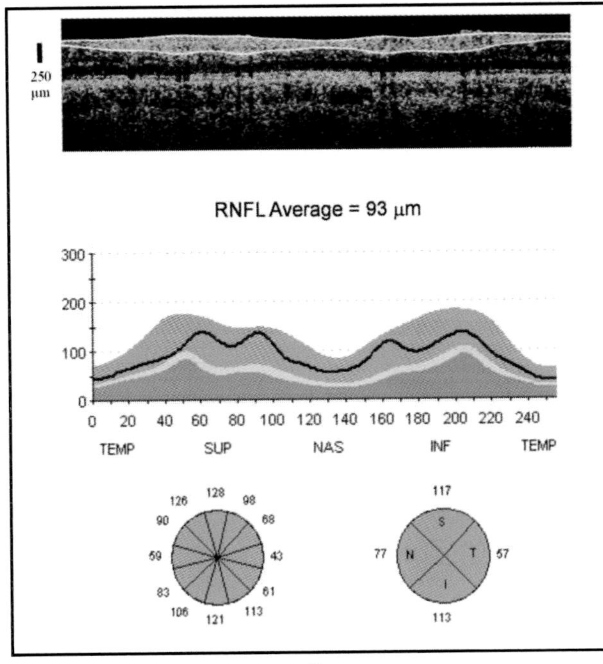
250 µm
RNFL Average = 93 µm
TEMP SUP NAS INF TEMP

J

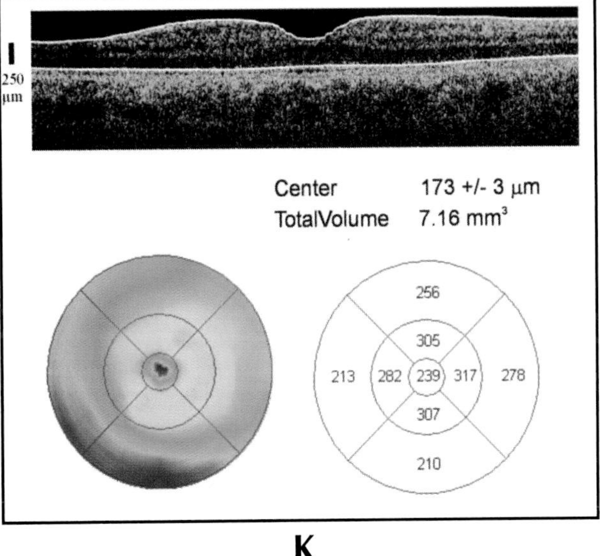
250 µm
Center 173 +/- 3 µm
TotalVolume 7.16 mm³

K

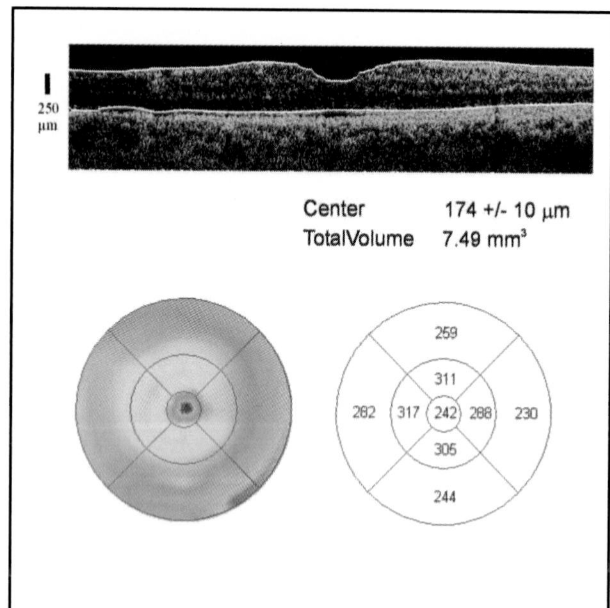

L

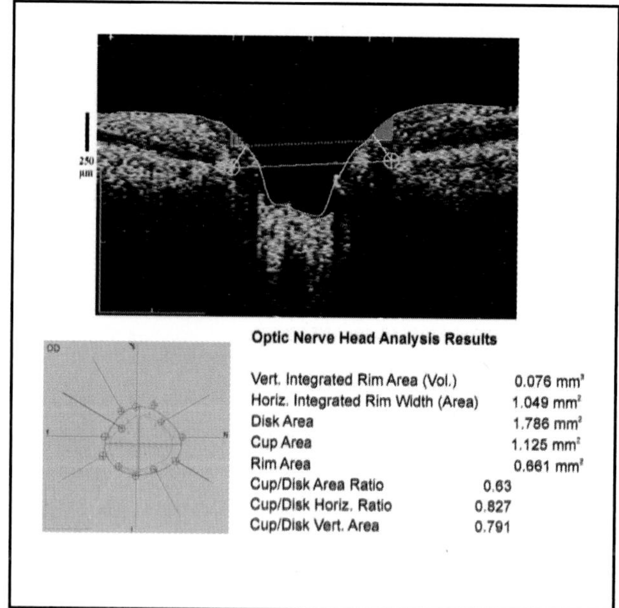

250 µm
OD
Optic Nerve Head Analysis Results
Vert. Integrated Rim Area (Vol.) 0.076 mm³
Horiz. Integrated Rim Width (Area) 1.049 mm²
Disk Area 1.786 mm²
Cup Area 1.125 mm²
Rim Area 0.661 mm²
Cup/Disk Area Ratio 0.63
Cup/Disk Horiz. Ratio 0.827
Cup/Disk Vert. Area 0.791

M

250 µm

OS

Optic Nerve Head Analysis Results

Vert. Integrated Rim Area (Vol.) 0.172 mm³
Horiz. Integrated Rim Width (Area) 1.309 mm²
Disk Area 1.734 mm²
Cup Area 0.803 mm²
Rim Area 0.931 mm²
Cup/Disk Area Ratio 0.463
Cup/Disk Horiz. Ratio 0.729
Cup/Disk Vert. Area 0.65

N

Case 12-17. Structural Testing Corresponded With Superior Functional Loss, Suggested Inferior Loss Was Either Mild or Artifact

A 55-year-old Caucasian woman with primary open-angle glaucoma was treated with brimonidine 0.2% and latanoprost 0.005% in her left eye. Visual acuity was 20/16 and the IOP was 20 mmHg. Slit-lamp examination revealed a deep and quiet anterior segment with a wide open angle. The ONH was cupped with the thinnest rim at the temporal inferior quadrant (A). VF testing showed an advanced superior nasal defect and earlier inferior nasal and superior temporal paracentral defects (B). The ONH was found to have abnormal rim thinning in the temporal and the inferior temporal segments with the HRT (C).

Optical Coherence Tomography

Retinal NFL thinning was present from 2:00 to 5:00 in the circumpapillary circular scan (D). Retinal thinning was noticed in the inferior and temporal segments in the macular scan (E). The optic nerve scan was notable for cupping in the inferior temporal quadrant (F).

Comments

Retinal NFL damage could be appreciated inferiorly in the circumpapillary scan. Inferior temporal neuroretinal rim loss was seen on ONH scans, and there was inferior temporal macular thinning. The structural tests corresponded strongly with the VF; however, they suggested that the inferior nasal VF loss was either mild or artifact.

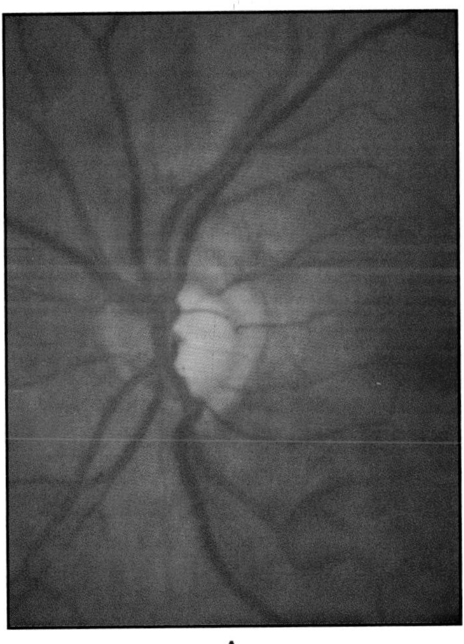

A

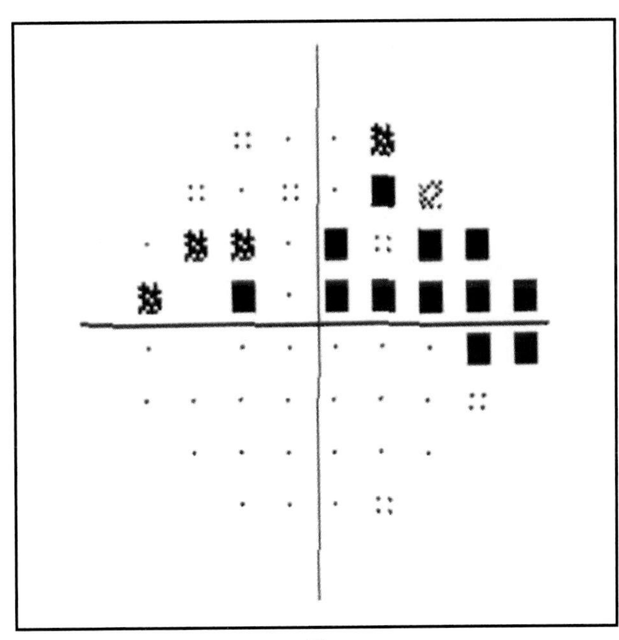

B

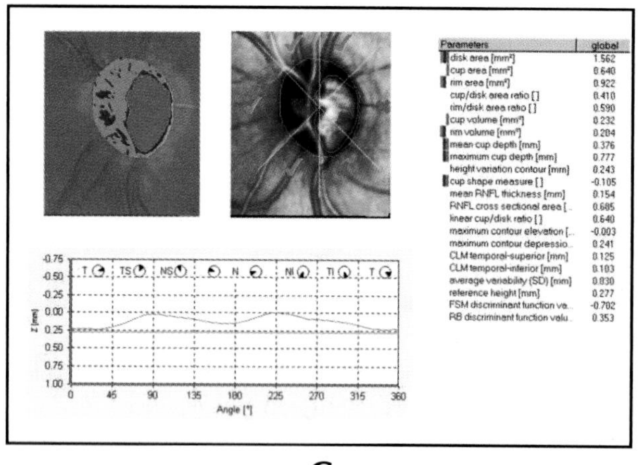

C

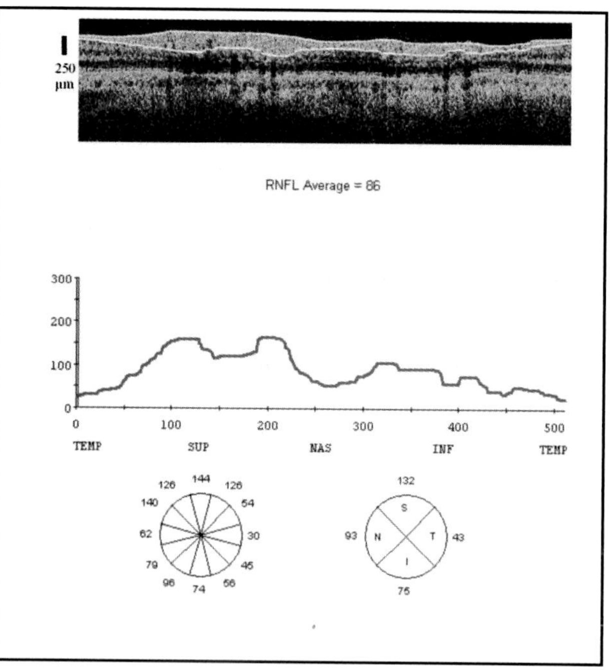

D

250 µm

Center 180 +/- 8 µm
TotalVolume 6.88 mm³

259
295
256 290 226 259 219
265
202

E

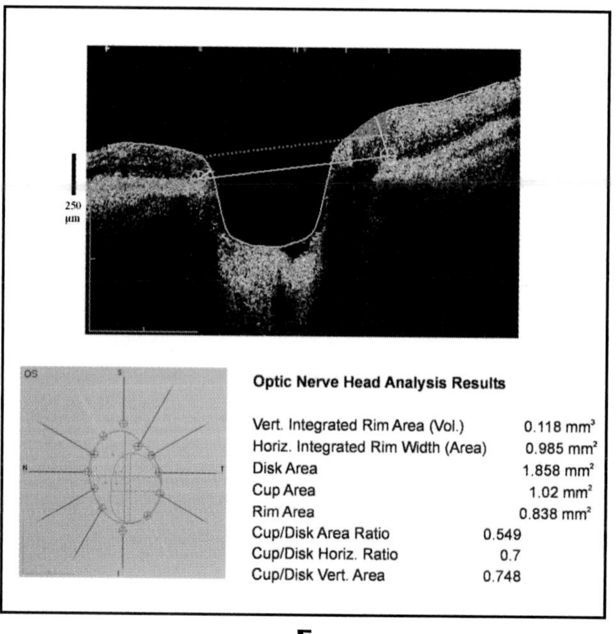

F

Case 12-18. Structural Imaging Suggested That Visual Field Abnormalities Were Erroneous in One Eye and Valid in the Other

A 13-year-old Hispanic boy with juvenile open-angle glaucoma in the left eye was treated with selective laser trabeculoplasty and trabeculectomy with mitomycin C. On examination, the visual acuity was 20/20 and the IOP was 12 mmHg. Slit-lamp examination revealed a functioning bleb, a deep and quiet anterior chamber, and a patent peripheral iridectomy in the left eye. A posterior subcapsular cataract was noted in the left eye, and there was marked ONH cupping (A and B). VFs showed superior and inferior arcuate defects in the right eye (C) and inferior nasal and paracentral defects as well as shallower superior nasal and paracentral defects in the left eye (D). HRT showed a normal ONH in the right side (E) and a small optic disc with normal cup (F).

Optical Coherence Tomography

The average circumpapillary retinal NFL thickness in the left eye (G) was 38 μm and in the healthy right eye (H) it was 116 μm. Reduced thickness was seen in all quadrants in the left eye with the least reduction in the inferior segment. The macular scan showed thinning in the temporal and inferior regions in the left eye and a healthy macular scan in the right eye (I and J). Marked optic nerve cup was noted with a small disc size in the left eye and normal size and shape in the right eye (K and L).

Comments

Reduced retinal thickness can be seen in the macular image. Note the loss of NFL in the left eye. Because of the small ONH size, the cup is small and confounds assessment. The VF is abnormal OD (more than OS), but structural assessment suggests that this represents artifact.

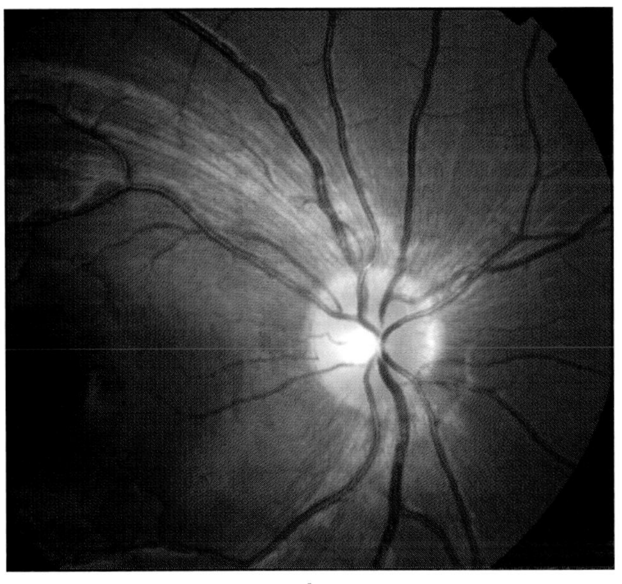

A

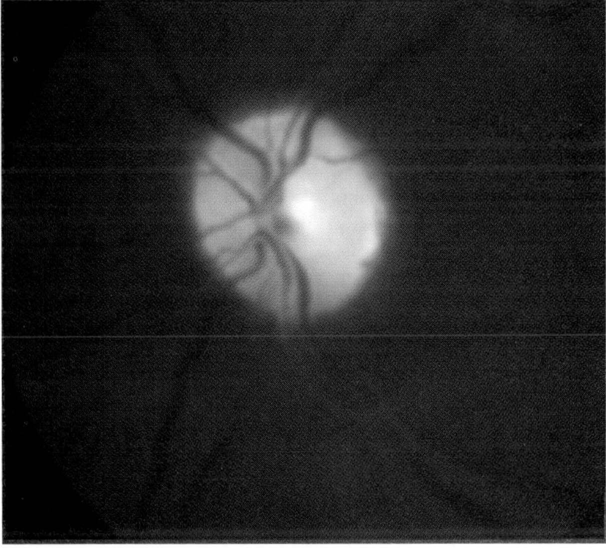

B

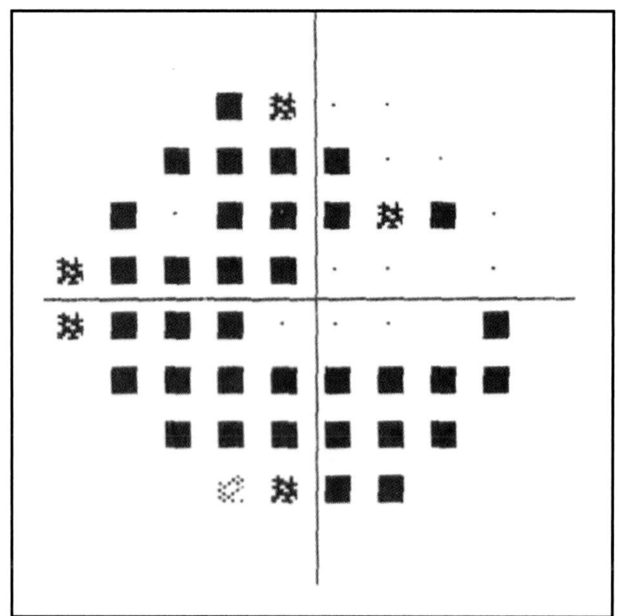

C

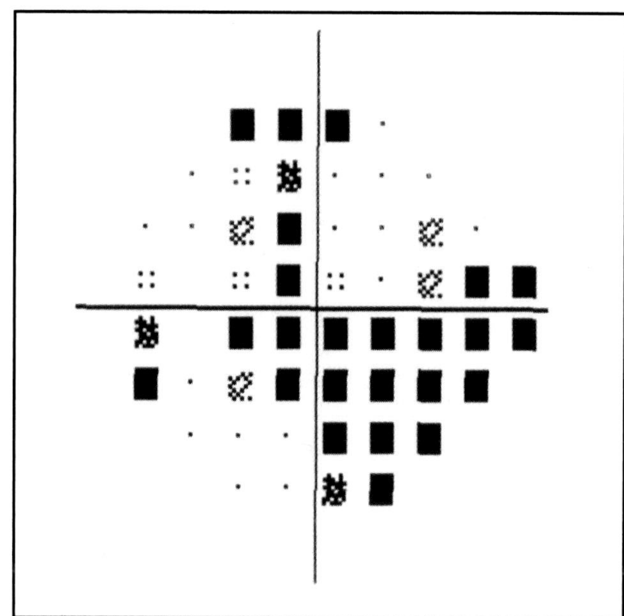

D

Parameters	global
disk area [mm²]	1.667
cup area [mm²]	0.330
rim area [mm²]	1.338
cup/disk area ratio [ ]	0.198
rim/disk area ratio [ ]	0.802
cup volume [mm³]	0.069
rim volume [mm³]	0.281
mean cup depth [mm]	0.168
maximum cup depth [mm]	0.764
height variation contour [mm]	0.356
cup shape measure [ ]	-0.368
mean RNFL thickness [mm]	0.248
RNFL cross sectional area [...	1.139
linear cup/disk ratio [ ]	0.446
maximum contour elevation [...	-0.163
maximum contour depressio...	0.192
CLM temporal-superior [mm]	0.172
CLM temporal-inferior [mm]	0.098
average variability (SD) [mm]	0.016
reference height [mm]	0.235
FSM discriminant function va...	1.705
RB discriminant function valu...	1.683

E

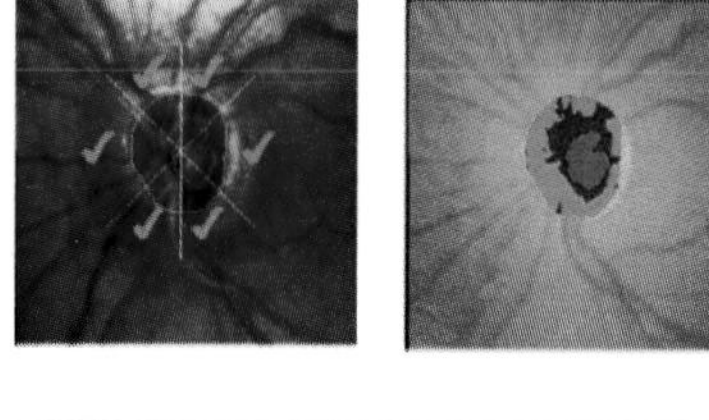

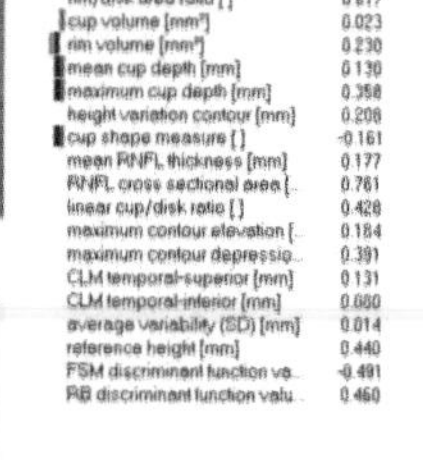

Parameters	global
disk area [mm²]	1.473
cup area [mm²]	0.270
rim area [mm²]	1.203
cup/disk area ratio [ ]	0.183
rim/disk area ratio [ ]	0.817
cup volume [mm³]	0.023
rim volume [mm³]	0.230
mean cup depth [mm]	0.130
maximum cup depth [mm]	0.358
height variation contour [mm]	0.208
cup shape measure [ ]	-0.161
mean RNFL thickness [mm]	0.177
RNFL cross sectional area [...	0.761
linear cup/disk ratio [ ]	0.428
maximum contour elevation [...	0.184
maximum contour depressio...	0.391
CLM temporal-superior [mm]	0.131
CLM temporal-inferior [mm]	0.080
average variability (SD) [mm]	0.014
reference height [mm]	0.440
FSM discriminant function va...	-0.491
RB discriminant function valu...	0.460

F

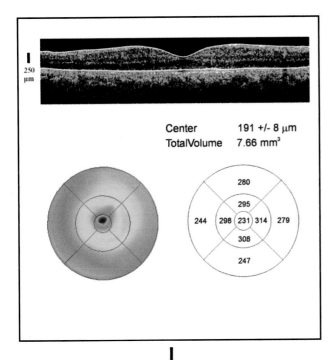

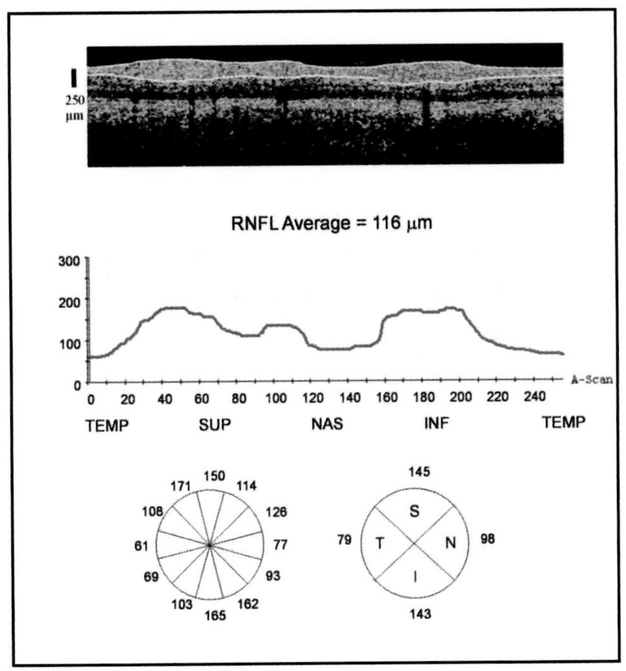

G

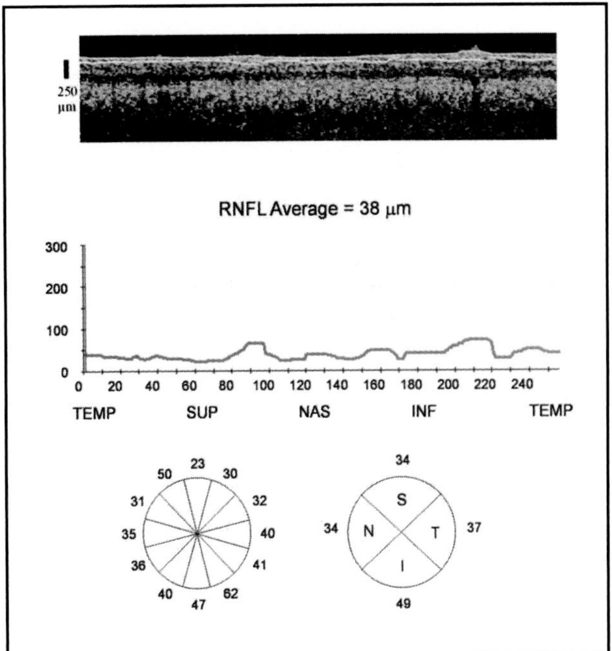

250
μm
Center 191 +/- 8 μm
TotalVolume 7.66 mm³
280
295
244 298 231 314 279
308
247

I

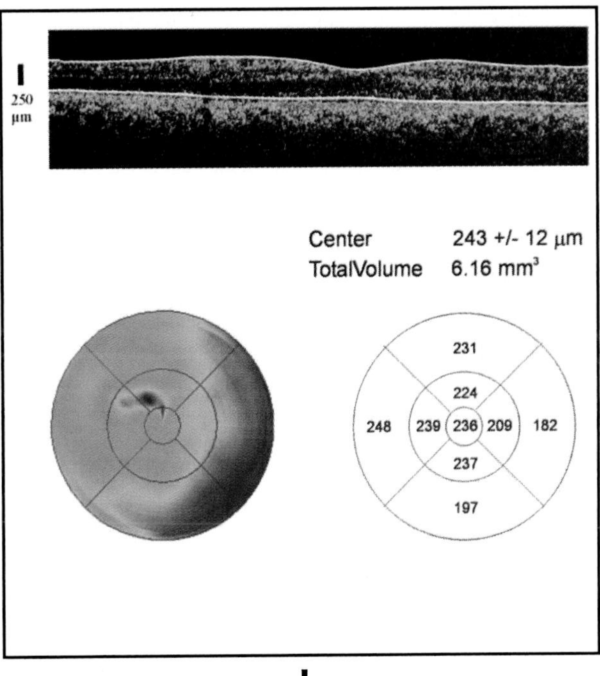

J

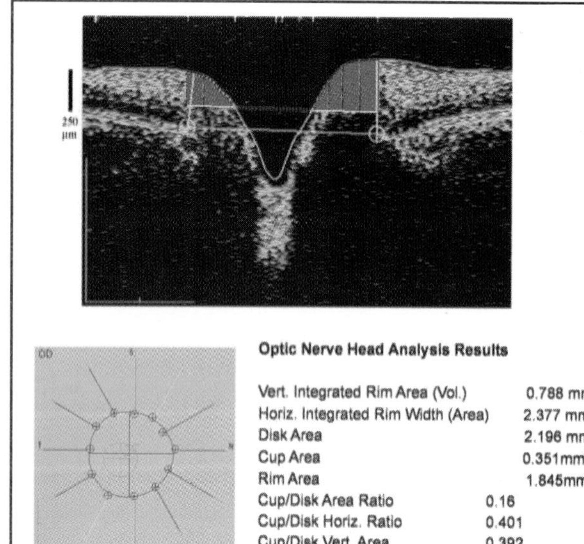
250 µm
OD
Optic Nerve Head Analysis Results
Vert. Integrated Rim Area (Vol.) 0.788 mm³
Horiz. Integrated Rim Width (Area) 2.377 mm²
Disk Area 2.196 mm²
Cup Area 0.351mm²
Rim Area 1.845mm²
Cup/Disk Area Ratio 0.16
Cup/Disk Horiz. Ratio 0.401
Cup/Disk Vert. Area 0.392

K

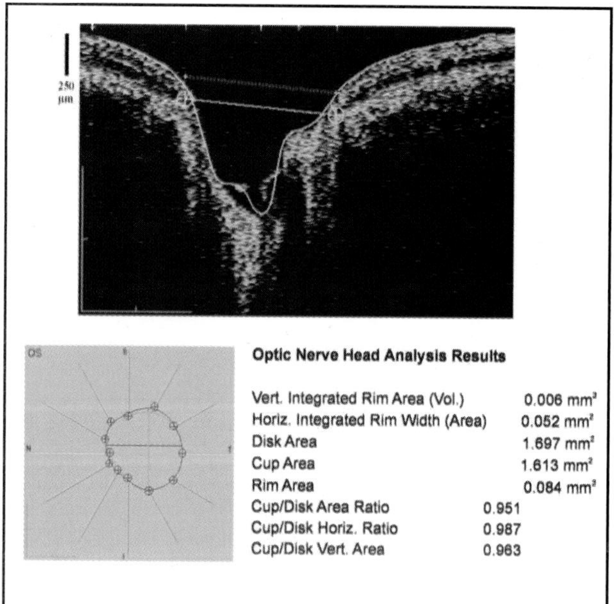
250 µm
OS
Optic Nerve Head Analysis Results
Vert. Integrated Rim Area (Vol.) 0.006 mm³
Horiz. Integrated Rim Width (Area) 0.052 mm²
Disk Area 1.697 mm²
Cup Area 1.613 mm²
Rim Area 0.084 mm²
Cup/Disk Area Ratio 0.951
Cup/Disk Horiz. Ratio 0.987
Cup/Disk Vert. Area 0.963

L

Case 12-19. Structural Measures Supported Superior But Not Inferior Visual Field Defects

A 78-year-old Caucasian man had normal tension glaucoma in the left eye. The visual acuity was 20/30 and IOP was 17 mmHg. The anterior segment examination revealed a deep anterior chamber with open angles. A large ONH cup was noted on fundus examination, with a myelinated NFL adjacent to the disc margin at 8:00 and a NFL defect at 5:00 (A). Humphrey VFs showed superior and inferior paracentral defects (B). HRT analysis revealed a rim notch inferior temporally compatible with the NFL defect noted on clinical examination (C).

Optical Coherence Tomography

Marked NFL thinning was noted at 4:00 and 5:00 and borderline thinning was present inferiorly and nasally (D). Thinning of the retina was noted in the macular scan inferiorly and in the outer temporal region (E). Optic nerve analysis showed near total excavation (F).

Comments

There was marked NFL thinning inferior temporally as shown in the peripapillary OCT scan, and this was consistent with the HRT ONH and macular analyses, as well as with the NFL defect noted clinically. The superior VF defects were explained by these findings, but the inferior VF abnormalities did not correlate with any structural measures. This supported the reality of the superior defects but put the veracity of the inferior VF findings into question.

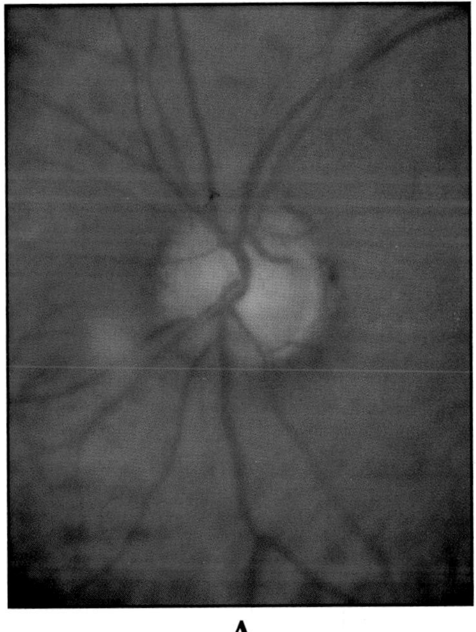

A

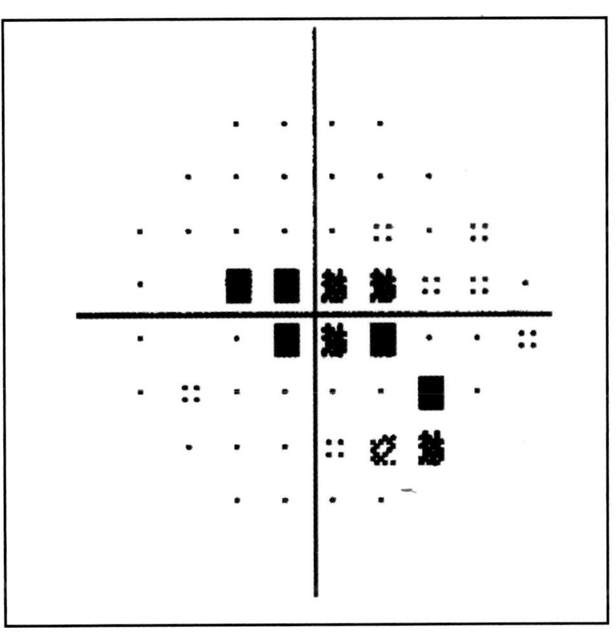

B

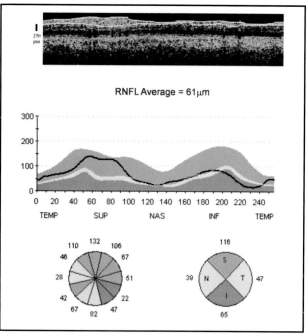

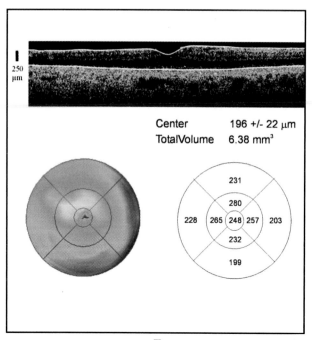

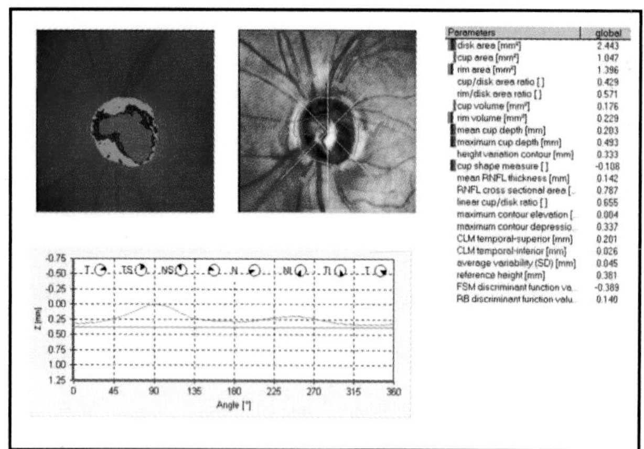

Parameters	global
disk area [mm²]	2.443
cup area [mm²]	1.047
rim area [mm²]	1.396
cup/disk area ratio []	0.429
rim/disk area ratio []	0.571
cup volume [mm³]	0.176
rim volume [mm³]	0.229
mean cup depth [mm]	0.203
maximum cup depth [mm]	0.493
height variation contour [mm]	0.333
cup shape measure []	-0.108
mean RNFL thickness [mm]	0.142
RNFL cross sectional area [...	0.787
linear cup/disk ratio []	0.655
maximum contour elevation [...	0.004
maximum contour depressio...	0.337
CLM temporal-superior [mm]	0.201
CLM temporal-inferior [mm]	0.026
average variability (SD) [mm]	0.045
reference height [mm]	0.381
FSM discriminant function va...	-0.389
RB discriminant function valu...	0.140

C

250 μm

RNFL Average = 61μm

0 20 40 60 80 100 120 140 160 180 200 220 240
TEMP SUP NAS INF TEMP

132 106 67 51 22 47 82 67 42 28 46 110

116 S
39 N T 47
I 65

D

250 μm

Center 196 +/- 22 μm
TotalVolume 6.38 mm³

231
280
228 265 248 257 203
232
199

E

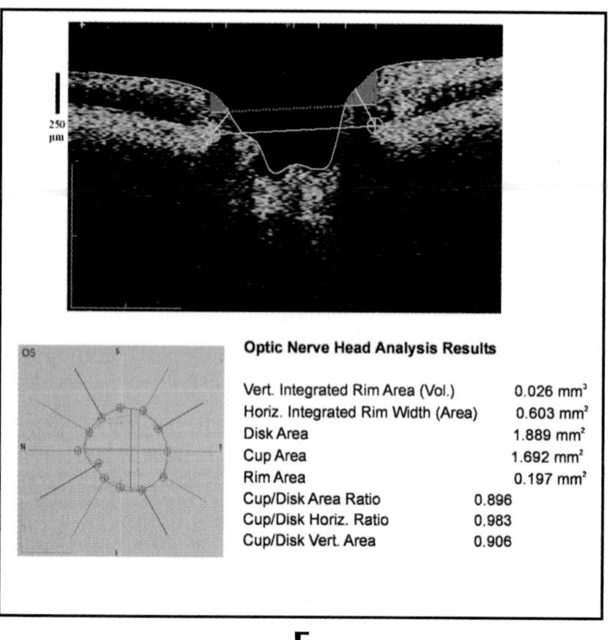

Optic Nerve Head Analysis Results

Vert. Integrated Rim Area (Vol.)	0.026 mm³
Horiz. Integrated Rim Width (Area)	0.603 mm²
Disk Area	1.889 mm²
Cup Area	1.692 mm²
Rim Area	0.197 mm²
Cup/Disk Area Ratio	0.896
Cup/Disk Horiz. Ratio	0.983
Cup/Disk Vert. Area	0.906

F

Case 12-20. Correspondence Between Structural and Functional Measures Was Good, But There Was Less Functional Loss Than Might Be Expected Based on Retinal Nerve Fiber Layer, Macular, and Optic Nerve Head Abnormalities, Particularly. This Suggested That This Patient Should Be Watched Closely For Future Functional Loss

A 79-year-old Caucasian woman had mild age-related macular degeneration (ARMD) and normal tension glaucoma treated with latanoprost 0.005% in both eyes. The visual acuity was 20/25 and the IOPs were 11 mmHg in both eyes. The anterior segment was normal and the posterior segment showed scattered hard drusen in the macula, large ONH cups, and peripapillary atrophy in both eyes (A and B). 24-2 SITA VFs showed dense inferior arcuate and superior nasal defects in the right eye (C) and were full on the left (D). Marked thinning of the neuroretinal rim was disclosed by the HRT in all segments except for nasal inferior in the right eye and temporal in the left eye (E and F).

Optical Coherence Tomography

Retinal NFL thinning was noted on the circumpapillary scan bilaterally, with an average retinal NFL thickness of 60 µm in the right eye (G) and 64 µm on the left (H). The thinning in the right eye was mainly superior and superior temporally, corresponding to the VF defect. The retinal thickness was reduced in the macula of the right eye in the outer ring in the superior, temporal, and inferior regions with a total retinal volume of 5.68 mm^3 (I). In the left eye, macular thinning was noted in the outer temporal ring with total volume of 6.35 mm^3 (J). ONH scanning demonstrated the absence of neuroretinal rim superior temporally in small sized discs in both eyes (K and L).

Comments

The OCT macular scan of the right eye showed thinning of the retina corresponding with the visual field defect; however, the scan illustrated that the macular damage was more pronounced than what was detected on the VF. The left eye showed overt signs of retinal damage that were not identified on the functional testing.

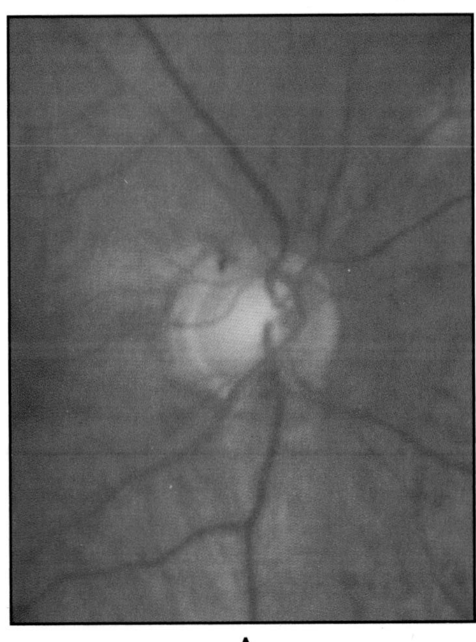

A

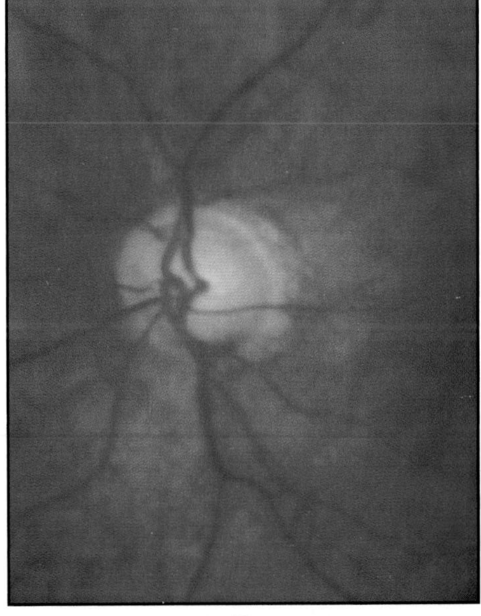

B

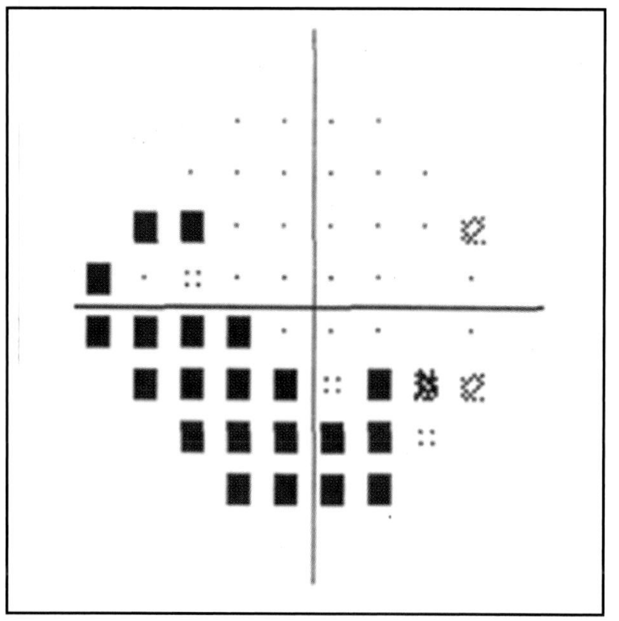

C

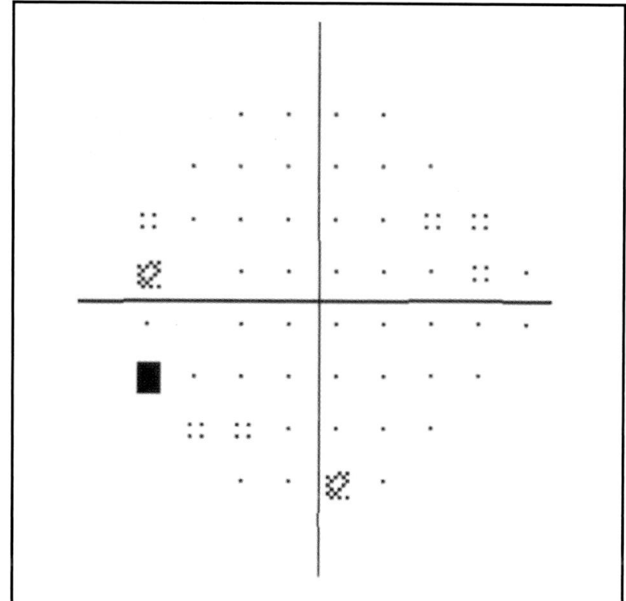

D

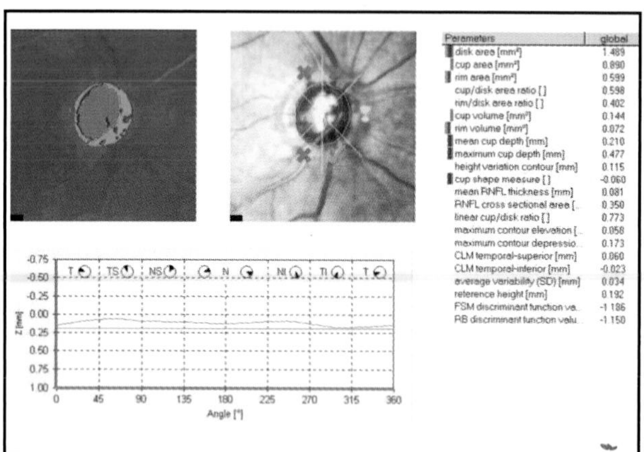
Parameters global
disk area [mm²] 1.489
cup area [mm²] 0.890
rim area [mm²] 0.599
cup/disk area ratio [] 0.598
rim/disk area ratio [] 0.402
cup volume [mm³] 0.144
rim volume [mm³] 0.072
mean cup depth [mm] 0.210
maximum cup depth [mm] 0.477
height variation contour [mm] 0.115
cup shape measure [] -0.060
mean RNFL thickness [mm] 0.081
RNFL cross sectional area [... 0.350
linear cup/disk ratio [] 0.773
maximum contour elevation [... 0.058
maximum contour depressio... 0.173
CLM temporal-superior [mm] 0.060
CLM temporal-inferior [mm] -0.023
average variability (SD) [mm] 0.034
reference height [mm] 0.192
FSM discriminant function va... -1.186
RB discriminant function valu... -1.150
T TS NS N NI TI T
Z [mm]
Angle [°]

E

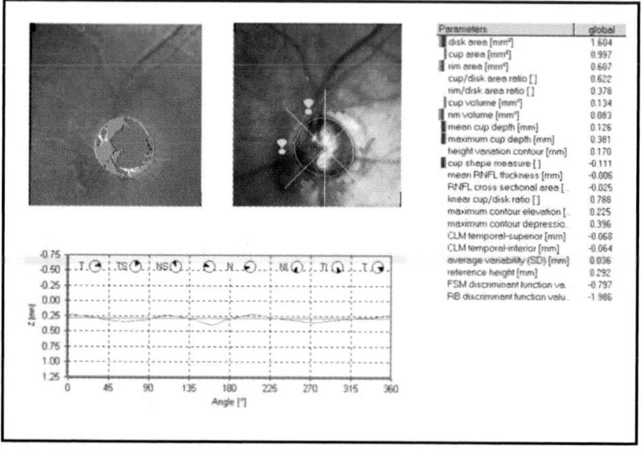
Parameters global
disk area [mm²] 1.604
cup area [mm²] 0.997
rim area [mm²] 0.607
cup/disk area ratio [] 0.622
rim/disk area ratio [] 0.378
cup volume [mm³] 0.134
rim volume [mm³] 0.083
mean cup depth [mm] 0.126
maximum cup depth [mm] 0.381
height variation contour [mm] 0.170
cup shape measure [] -0.111
mean RNFL thickness [mm] -0.006
RNFL cross sectional area [... -0.025
linear cup/disk ratio [] 0.788
maximum contour elevation [... 0.225
maximum contour depressio... 0.396
CLM temporal-superior [mm] -0.068
CLM temporal-inferior [mm] -0.064
average variability (SD) [mm] 0.036
reference height [mm] 0.292
FSM discriminant function va... -0.797
RB discriminant function valu... -1.986
T TS NS N NI TI T
Z [mm]
Angle [°]

F

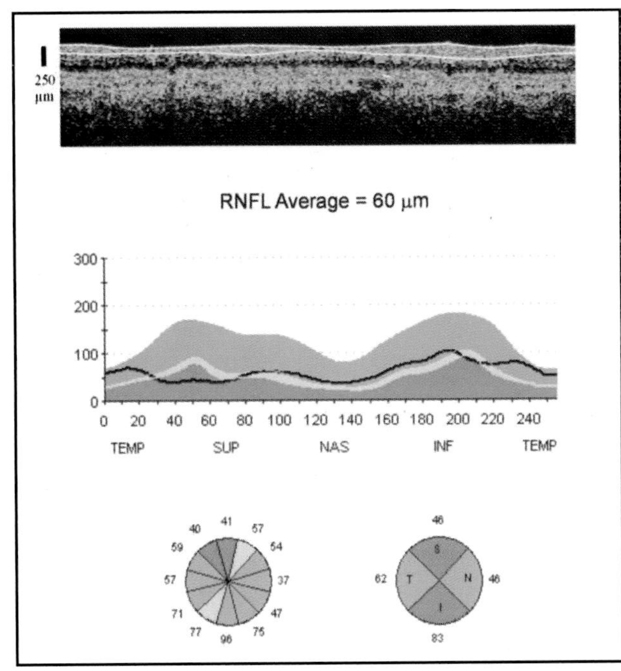

250 µm
RNFL Average = 60 µm
300
200
100
0
0 20 40 60 80 100 120 140 160 180 200 220 240
TEMP SUP NAS INF TEMP
40 41 57
59 54
57 37
71 47
77 96 75
46
S
62 T N 46
I
83

G

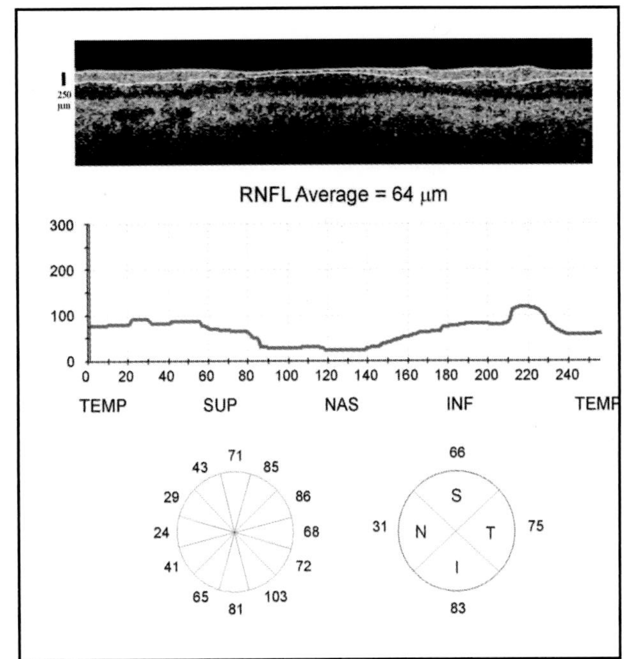

250 µm
RNFL Average = 64 µm
300
200
100
0
0 20 40 60 80 100 120 140 160 180 200 220 240
TEMP SUP NAS INF TEMP
43 71 85
29 86
24 68
41 72
65 81 103
66
S
31 N T 75
I
83

H

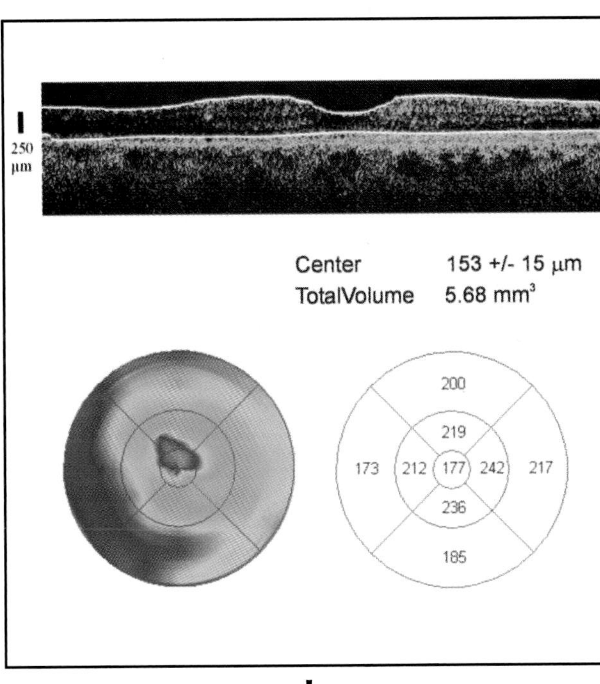

250 µm
Center 153 +/- 15 µm
TotalVolume 5.68 mm³
200
219
173 212 177 242 217
236
185

I

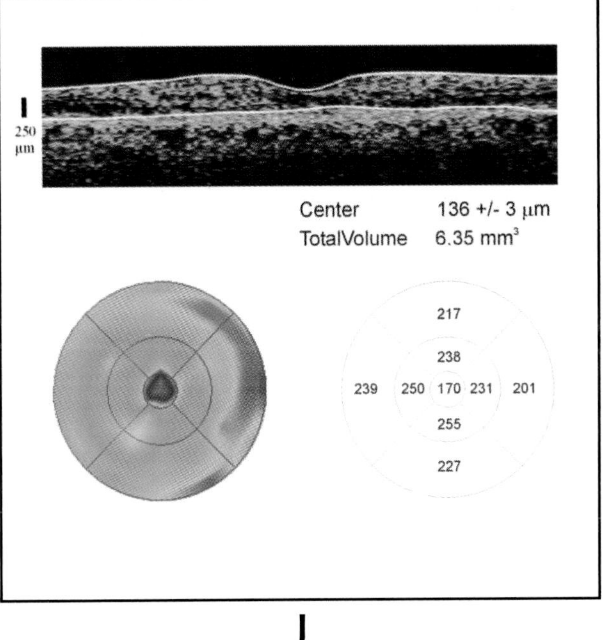

250 µm
Center 136 +/- 3 µm
TotalVolume 6.35 mm³
217
238
239 250 170 231 201
255
227

J

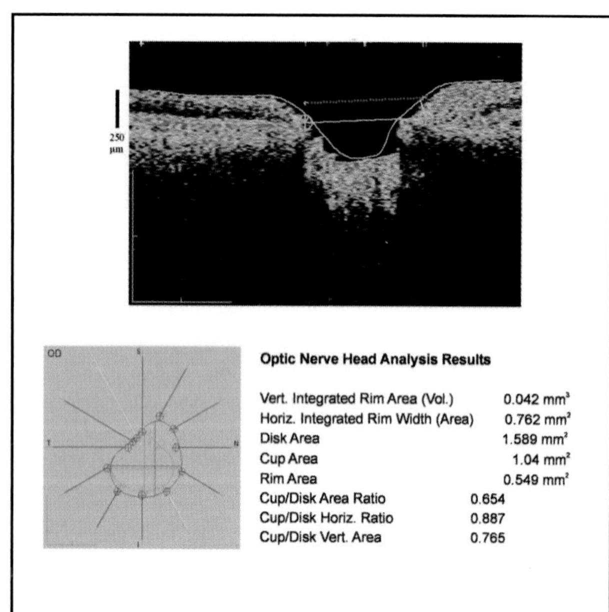
250
µm
OD
Optic Nerve Head Analysis Results
Vert. Integrated Rim Area (Vol.) 0.042 mm³
Horiz. Integrated Rim Width (Area) 0.762 mm²
Disk Area 1.589 mm²
Cup Area 1.04 mm²
Rim Area 0.549 mm²
Cup/Disk Area Ratio 0.654
Cup/Disk Horiz. Ratio 0.887
Cup/Disk Vert. Area 0.765

K

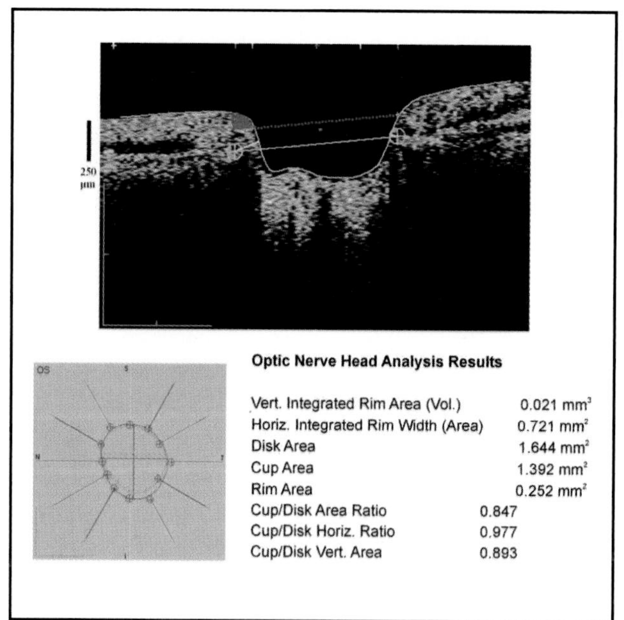
250
µm
OS
Optic Nerve Head Analysis Results
Vert. Integrated Rim Area (Vol.) 0.021 mm³
Horiz. Integrated Rim Width (Area) 0.721 mm²
Disk Area 1.644 mm²
Cup Area 1.392 mm²
Rim Area 0.252 mm²
Cup/Disk Area Ratio 0.847
Cup/Disk Horiz. Ratio 0.977
Cup/Disk Vert. Area 0.893

L

Case 12-21. Structure and Function Corresponded, But Structural Loss Exceeded Detectable Functional Damage. Macular Imaging Helped to Explain Why Functional Loss May Have Been Missed

A 22-year-old Caucasian man with advanced pseudoexfoliation glaucoma was treated in the left eye only with brimonidine 0.2% twice daily, bimatoprost 0.03% once daily, and a combination of timolol 0.5% with dorzolamide 2% twice daily. On examination, visual acuity was 20/20 OD and 20/200 OS, and IOPs were 14 mmHg in both eyes. Pseudoexfoliation material was seen on the anterior lens capsule of the left eye. Marked ONH asymmetry was noted, with advanced disc cupping in the left eye (A). 24-2 SITA VF testing was normal in the right eye and showed a severe inferior hemifield defect on the left (B). HRT scanning demonstrated marked cupping in the left eye, with more abnormalities shown inferiorly than superiorly (C). The HRT was normal on the right.

Optical Coherence Tomography

Dramatic overall NFL thinning was detected in the left eye; surprisingly, this was seen most significantly in the inferior sector (D). Macular scanning showed overall retinal thinning in the left eye with striking thinning superiorly more than inferiorly in the inner ring, and inferiorly more than superiorly in the outer ring (E). Circumpapillary and macular scans of the right eye were normal. The ONH scan was normal in the right and showed near total cupping in the left eye (F).

Comment

This case was interesting in that there was good structure-function correspondence, with global NFL, ONH, and macular damage present correlating with VF loss, but there was more inferior than superior structural damage by all measures, with the opposite true for function assessed by SITA 24-2 testing. This may have been related to the limited area tested by the 24-2 strategy, as the macular scan suggested that the outer ring revealed the inferior retinal defect, while the inner ring showed more superior retinal thinning. Since each millimeter of retina scanned corresponded to approximately 6 degrees, for a total of 36 degrees represented by the macular circular scan, this could have explained why the far peripheral damage shown by the 6 mm diameter macular scan might have been missed by 24-degree VF testing. The difference in macular location would have been difficult to determine based on the NFL or ONH testing alone.

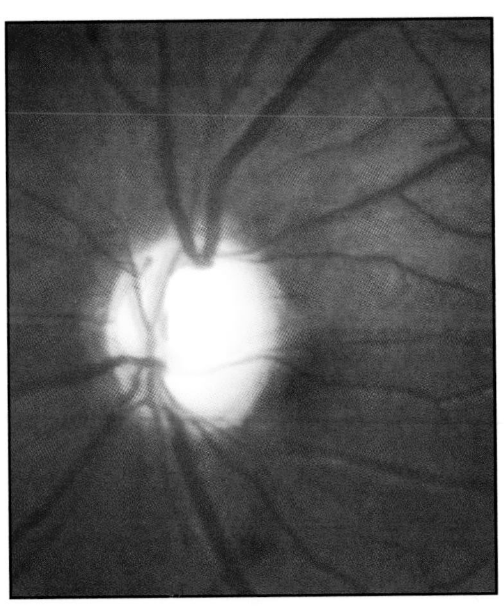

A

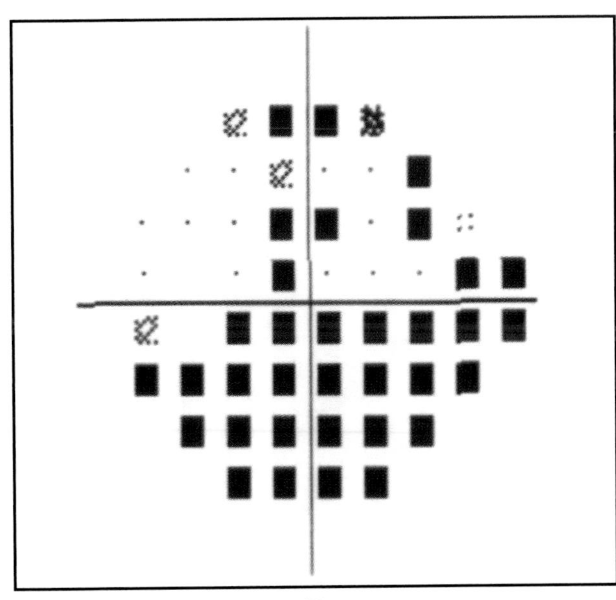

B

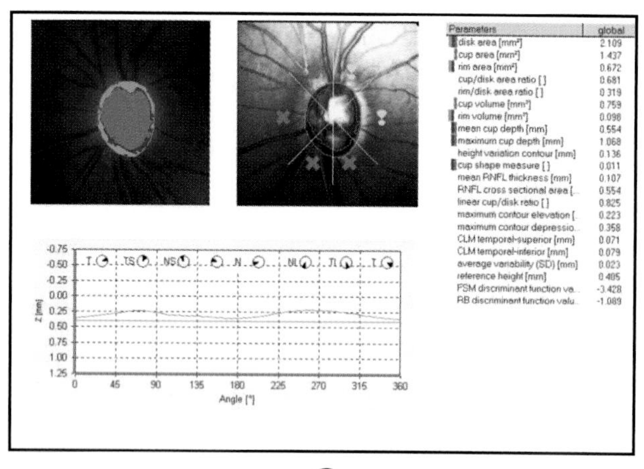
Parameters global
disk area [mm²] 2.109
cup area [mm²] 1.437
rim area [mm²] 0.672
cup/disk area ratio [] 0.681
rim/disk area ratio [] 0.319
cup volume [mm³] 0.759
rim volume [mm³] 0.098
mean cup depth [mm] 0.554
maximum cup depth [mm] 1.068
height variation contour [mm] 0.136
cup shape measure [] 0.011
mean RNFL thickness [mm] 0.107
RNFL cross sectional area [... 0.554
linear cup/disk ratio [] 0.825
maximum contour elevation [... 0.223
maximum contour depressio... 0.358
CLM temporal-superior [mm] 0.071
CLM temporal-inferior [mm] 0.079
average variability (SD) [mm] 0.023
reference height [mm] 0.405
FSM discriminant function va... -3.428
RB discriminant function valu... -1.089
Angle [°]

C

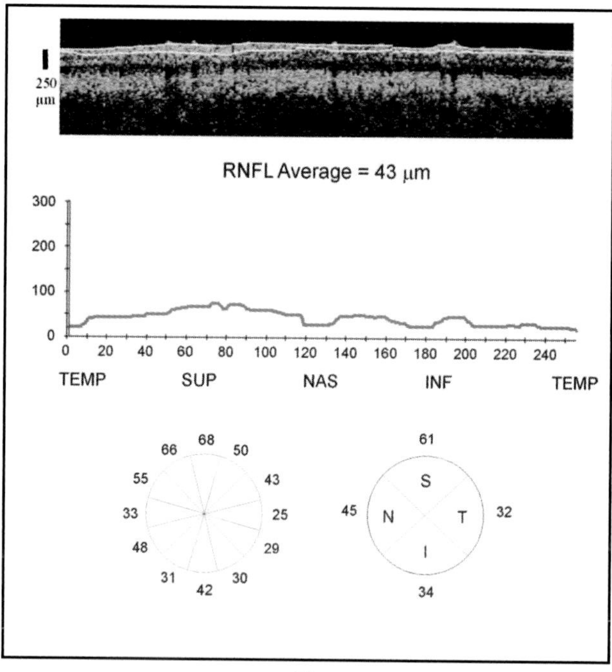
250 μm
RNFL Average = 43 μm
TEMP
SUP
NAS
INF
TEMP
S
N
T
I

D

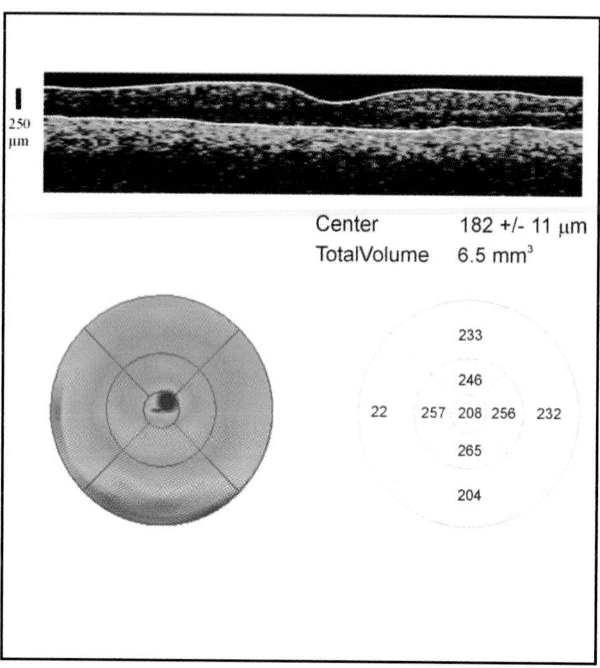
250 μm
Center 182 +/- 11 μm
TotalVolume 6.5 mm³
233
246
22 257 208 256 232
265
204

E

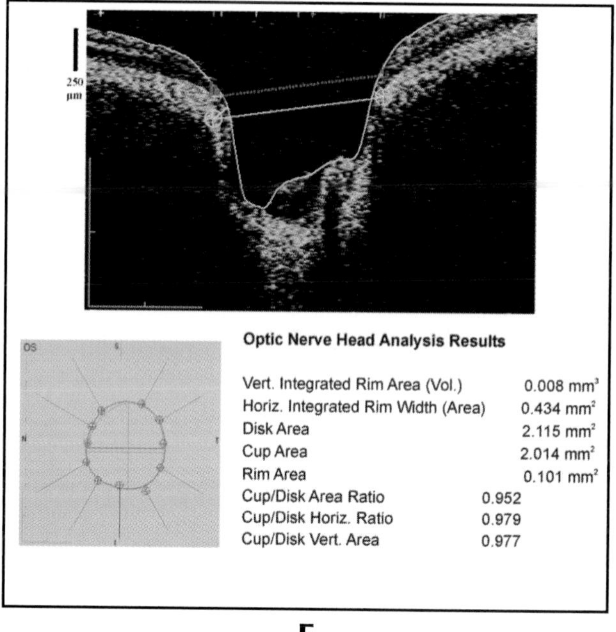
250 μm
Optic Nerve Head Analysis Results
Vert. Integrated Rim Area (Vol.) 0.008 mm³
Horiz. Integrated Rim Width (Area) 0.434 mm²
Disk Area 2.115 mm²
Cup Area 2.014 mm²
Rim Area 0.101 mm²
Cup/Disk Area Ratio 0.952
Cup/Disk Horiz. Ratio 0.979
Cup/Disk Vert. Area 0.977

F

Case 12-22. The Amount of Structural Loss Appeared to Exceed the Functional Loss Present

A 40-year-old Caucasian woman with bilateral primary open-angle glaucoma was treated with brimonidine 0.2%, latanoprost 0.005%, and a combination of timolol 0.5% and dorzolamide 2%. On examination, the visual acuity was 20/25 in both eyes and IOPs were 22 mmHg in the right eye and 18 mmHg on the left. The anterior segment was normal, and the ONH in the right eye had a thin neuroretinal rim in the temporal superior sector (A). In the left eye, a small disc hemorrhage was noted at 12:00 (B). Humphrey VFs showed dense inferior arcuate and early superior arcuate defects OD (C) and early superior and inferior arcuate and nasal defects OS (D). NFL photography disclosed a wedge defect spreading from 9:00 to 11:30 in the right eye (E) and normal NFL in the left eye (F). HRT of the right eye showed thinning of the neuroretinal rim throughout the temporal aspect of the ONH most pronounced superior temporally (G and H).

Optical Coherence Tomography

NFL thickness was reduced (average thickness of 57 µm) with flattening of the "double hump" pattern in the right eye mostly noted in the superior quadrant with an NFL thickness of 54 µm (I). The left eye showed overall retinal NFL thinning, most obvious superiorly and inferiorly (J). The retinal volume of the right macula was 6.25 mm^3 with thinning seen in the inferior, temporal, and superior outer ring regions (K). The volume of the left macula was 6.65 mm^3 with thinning detected in the inferior and temporal outer rings (L). The ONH scan showed marked asymmetry of cupping with obliteration of the neuroretinal rim superior temporally in the right eye (M and N).

Comments

Although the VF findings were substantially different between the eyes, the OCT scan showed somewhat similar tissue loss. This emphasizes the discrepancy between structural changes as detected by OCT and functional changes as determined by VF testing. On the other hand, there was more tissue loss by NFL, ONH, and macular measures in the right than the left eye, mirroring the VF loss in the two eyes.

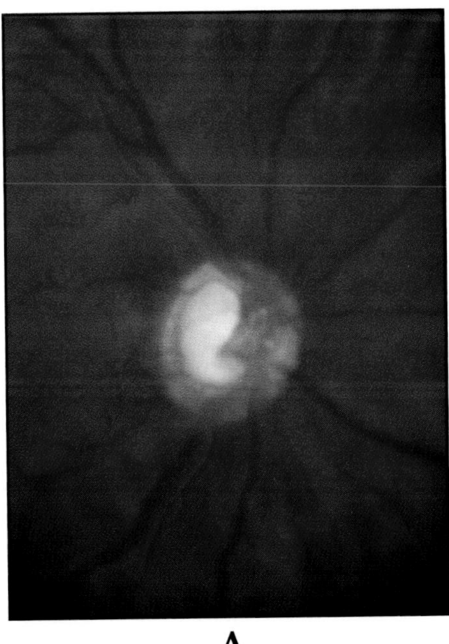

A

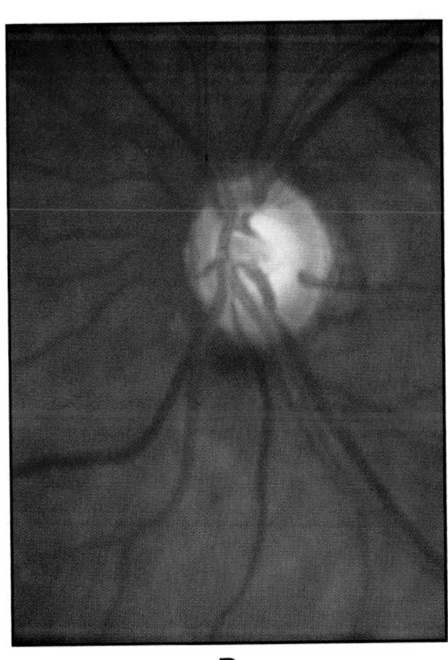

B

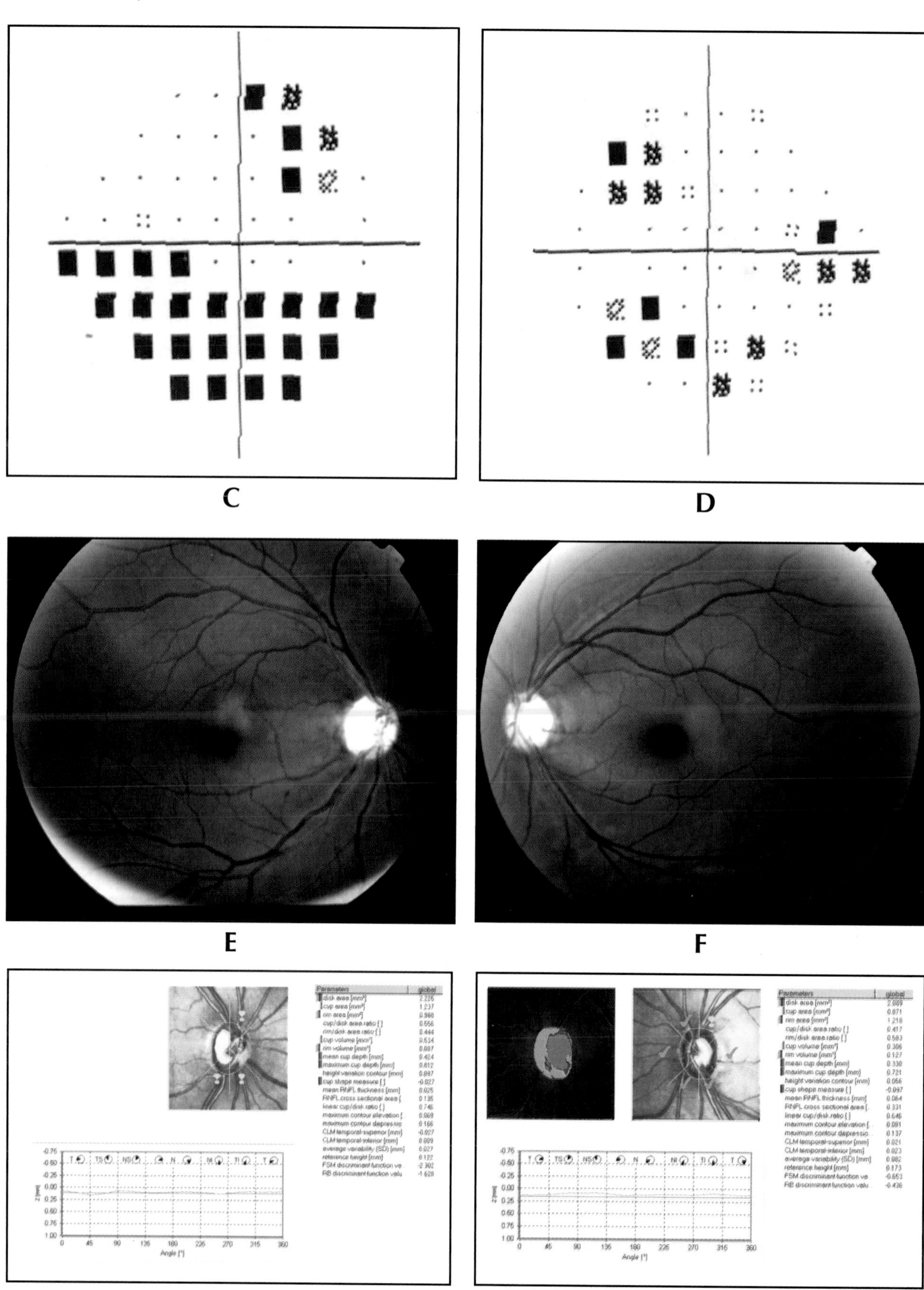
C
D
E
F
G
H

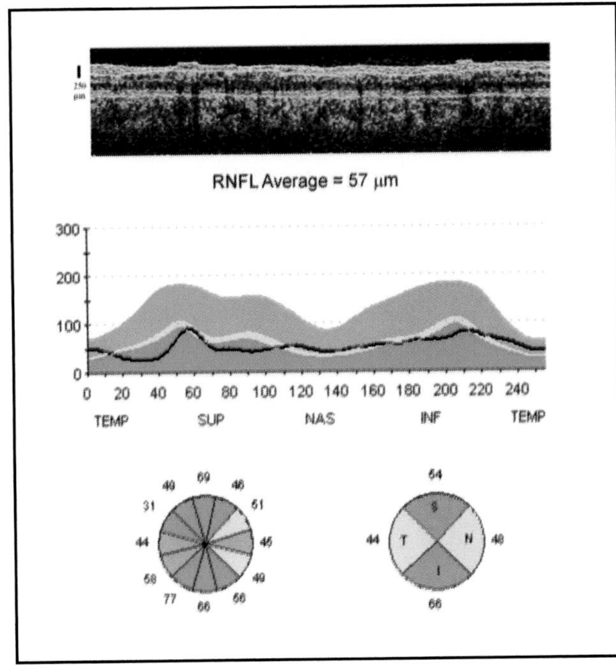

I

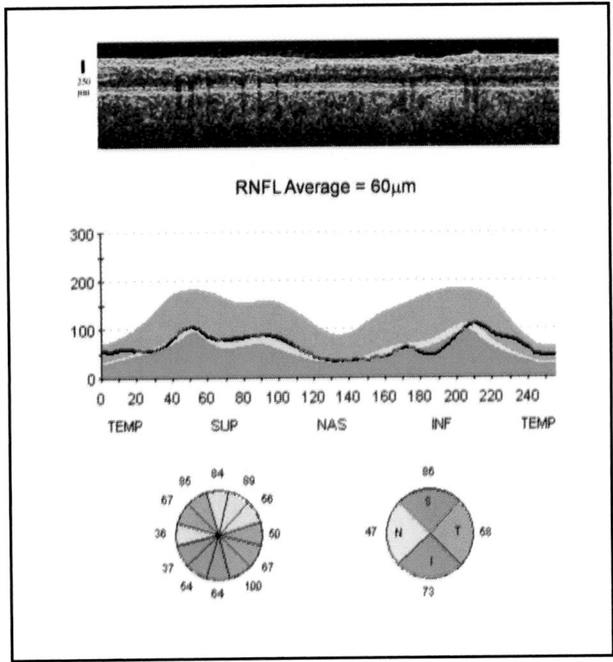

J

Center 169 +/- 3 µm
TotalVolume 6.25 mm³

208
249
200 249 209 272 234
267
199

K

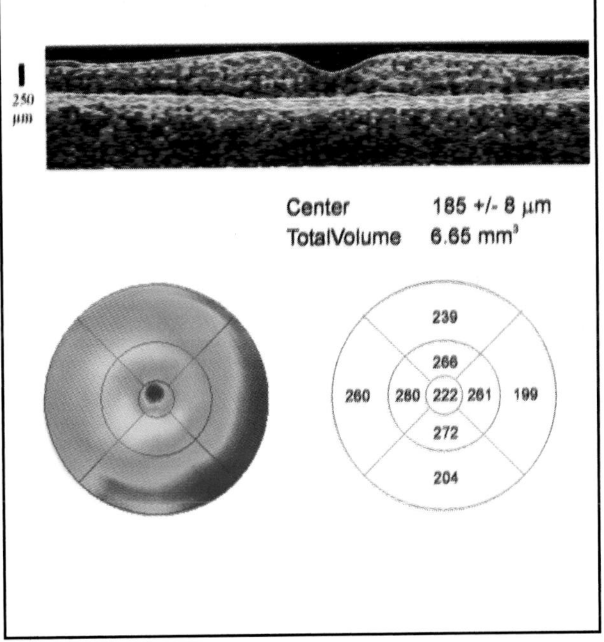

L

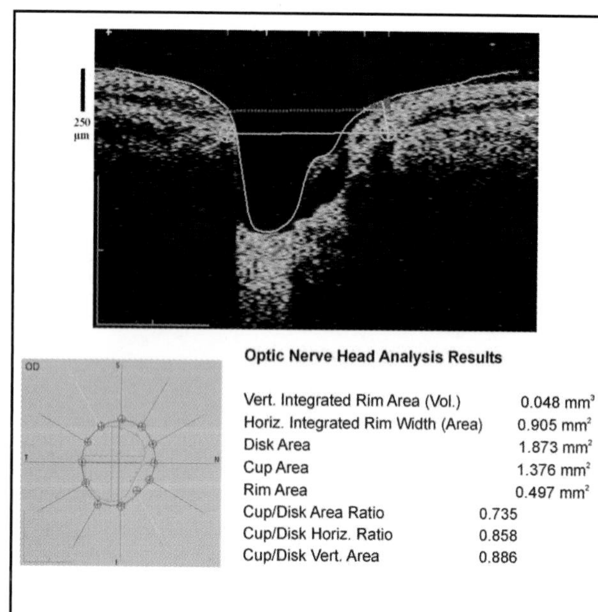
250 µm
OD
Optic Nerve Head Analysis Results
Vert. Integrated Rim Area (Vol.) 0.048 mm^3
Horiz. Integrated Rim Width (Area) 0.905 mm^2
Disk Area 1.873 mm^2
Cup Area 1.376 mm^2
Rim Area 0.497 mm^2
Cup/Disk Area Ratio 0.735
Cup/Disk Horiz. Ratio 0.858
Cup/Disk Vert. Area 0.886

M

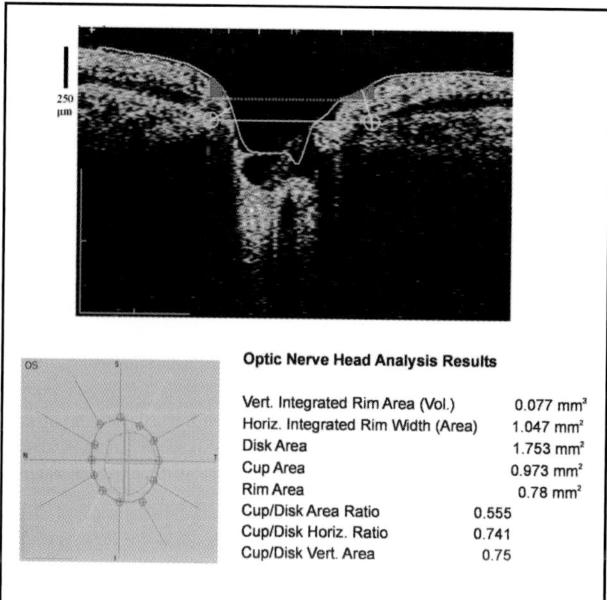
250 µm
OS
Optic Nerve Head Analysis Results
Vert. Integrated Rim Area (Vol.) 0.077 mm^3
Horiz. Integrated Rim Width (Area) 1.047 mm^2
Disk Area 1.753 mm^2
Cup Area 0.973 mm^2
Rim Area 0.78 mm^2
Cup/Disk Area Ratio 0.555
Cup/Disk Horiz. Ratio 0.741
Cup/Disk Vert. Area 0.75

N

Case 12-23. Nerve Fiber Layer and Macular Thinning Corresponded to a Disc Hemorrhage and Visual Field Loss. A Poor Quality Image Demonstrated That Data From Poor Scans Should Be Disregarded

A 77-year-old Caucasian man with normal tension glaucoma was treated with brimonidine and timolol in the left eye. On examination, the visual acuity was 20/20 and the IOP was 19 mmHg. The anterior chamber was deep with an open angle. Fundus examination revealed a larger cup in the left eye with thinning of the neuroretinal rim superior temporally, with adjacent peripapillary atrophy (A). A minute disc hemorrhage was noted at the 5:30 position at the disc margin. A Humphrey VF showed a superior paracentral defect (B). A poor quality HRT scan showed abnormal rim thinning at the nasal half and the temporal superior segments of the optic disc (C).

Optical Coherence Tomography

A thinned inferior retinal NFL was noted with flattening of the inferior component of the "double hump" configuration (D). The outer inferior macula was thinned (E). The ONH scan showed thinning of the neuroretinal rim (F).

Comments

Localized NFL thinning was seen in the circumpapillary OCT scan thickness chart between measuring points 198 to 210 corresponding to the location of the disc hemorrhage. Note that this localized defect was occupying part of two adjacent clock hours and when averaged with the remaining NFL, the measured value underestimated the tissue damage. The macular scan showed outer inferior thinning corresponding to the VF abnormality. The HRT was of poor quality and could not be read; this points out the sensitivity of both HRT and OCT to signal quality. Values created by such scans should be disregarded.

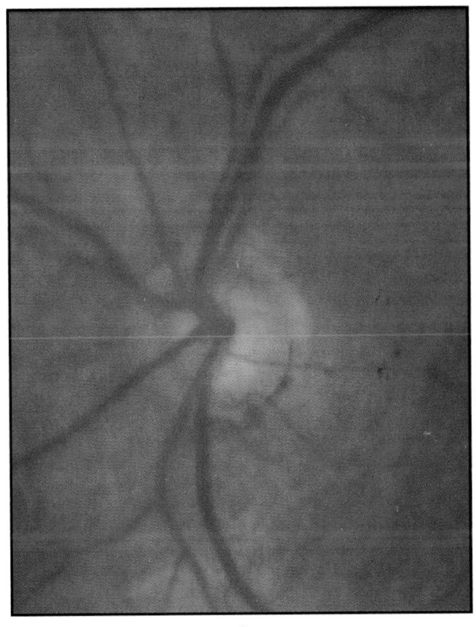

A

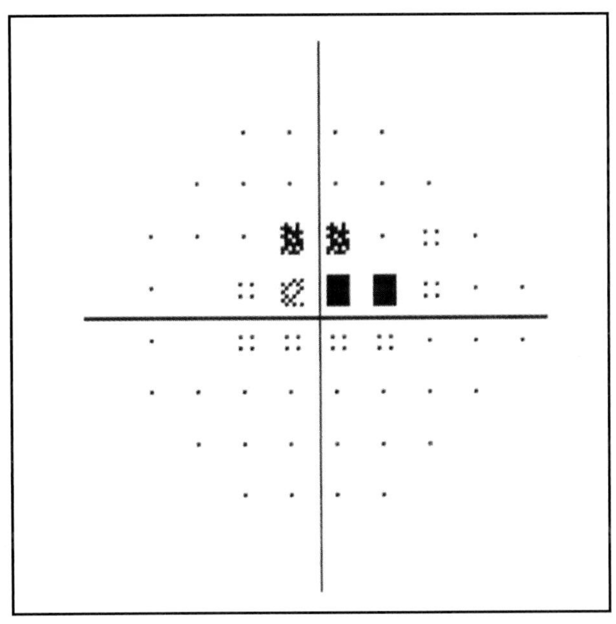

B

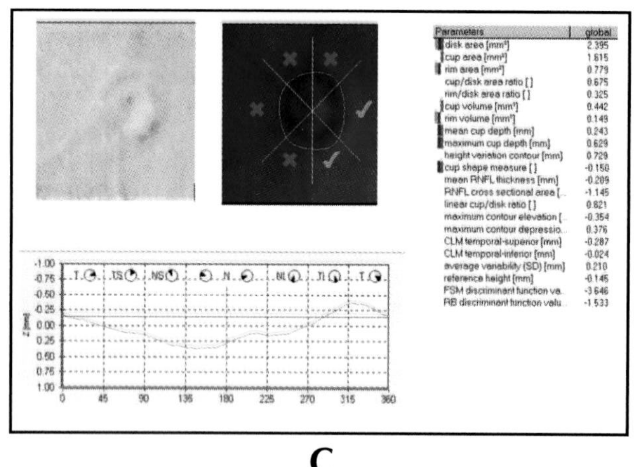

C

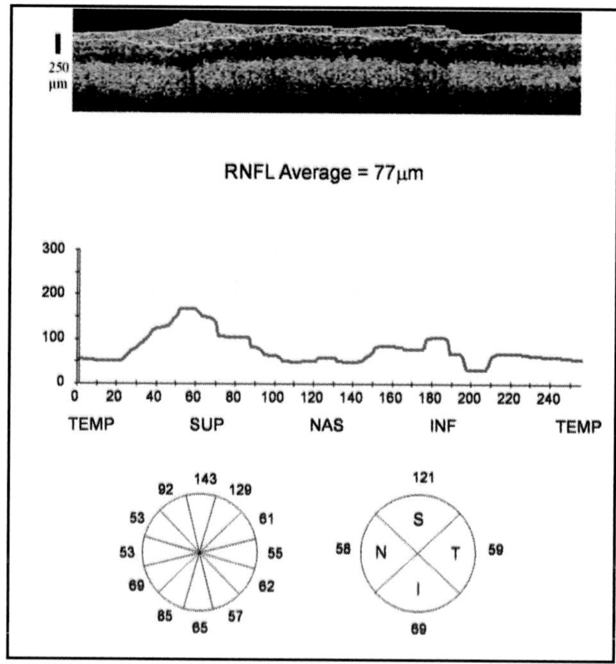

D

250 μm

Center 193 +/- 10 μm
TotalVolume 6.42 mm³

	228	
	243	
241	259 219 258	213
	255	
	196	

E

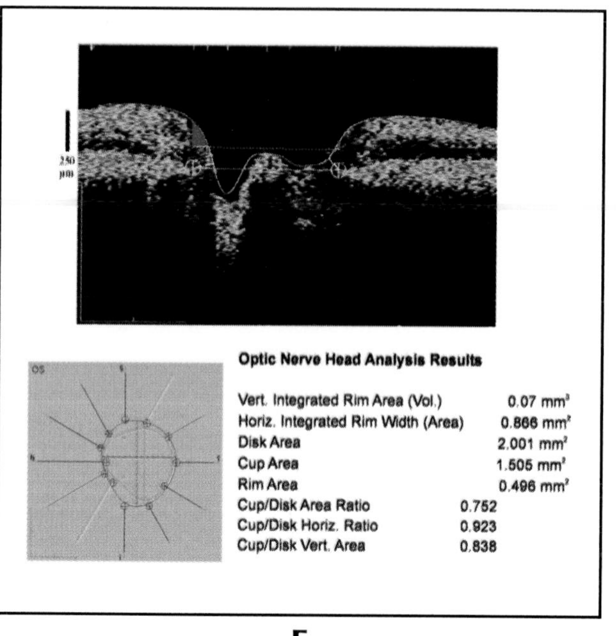

250 μm
OS
Optic Nerve Head Analysis Results
Vert. Integrated Rim Area (Vol.) 0.07 mm³
Horiz. Integrated Rim Width (Area) 0.866 mm²
Disk Area 2.001 mm²
Cup Area 1.505 mm²
Rim Area 0.496 mm²
Cup/Disk Area Ratio 0.752
Cup/Disk Horiz. Ratio 0.923
Cup/Disk Vert. Area 0.838

F

Case 12-24. Optical Coherence Tomography and Heidelberg Retina Tomograph Showed Good Correspondence With Each Other and With Visual Fields. Nerve Fiber Layer and Macular Measurements Gave Better Indications of Functional Loss Than Optic Nerve Head Assessments

A 30-year-old African-American woman was treated with travoprost 0.004% for normal tension glaucoma. The visual acuity was 20/20, and the IOPs were 12 mmHg in both eyes. The anterior segments were normal with widely open angles. Marked symmetrical ONH cupping was noted in both eyes. Frequency doubling technology demonstrated bilateral inferior arcuate defects more pronounced in the left eye (A and B). HRT scanning showed slightly greater cupping in the right eye than the left, with borderline thinning of the neuroretinal rim temporally in the right eye and superior temporally in both eyes (C and D).

Optical Coherence Tomography

Circumpapillary scanning demonstrated significant thinning of the retinal NFL at 9:00 to 12:00 in the right eye, with borderline thinning from 1:00 to 3:00 (E) and significant thinning at 9:00 to 3:00 in the left eye, except at 11:00, where the thinning was borderline (F). The average retinal NFL thickness for both eyes was reduced. The macular maps were similar for both eyes with slight superior retinal thinning (G and H). The ONH size was larger in the left eye (I), but there was more cupping in the right eye (J).

Comment

There was excellent correspondence between the VF defects and the OCT circumpapillary and macular findings. Both OCT and HRT demonstrated that the disc area was larger in the left eye with more cupping in the right eye. It was important to note that while the HRT analysis required manual tracing of the ONH margin, the OCT defined this margin automatically by detecting the termination of the RPE/choriocapillaris layer.

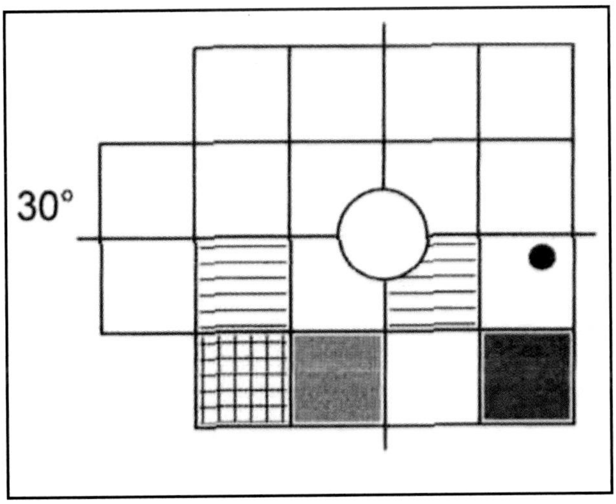

A

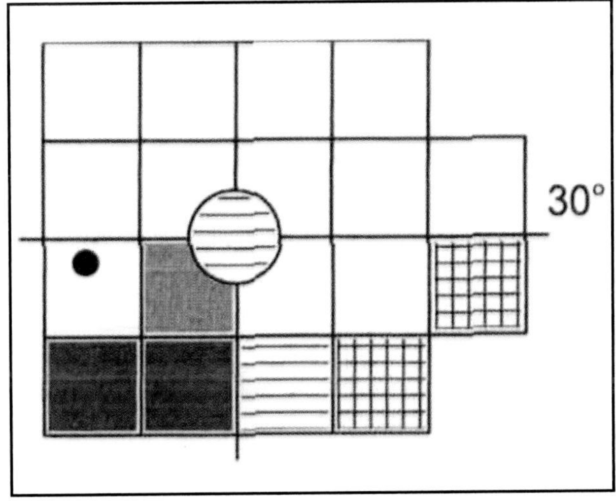

B

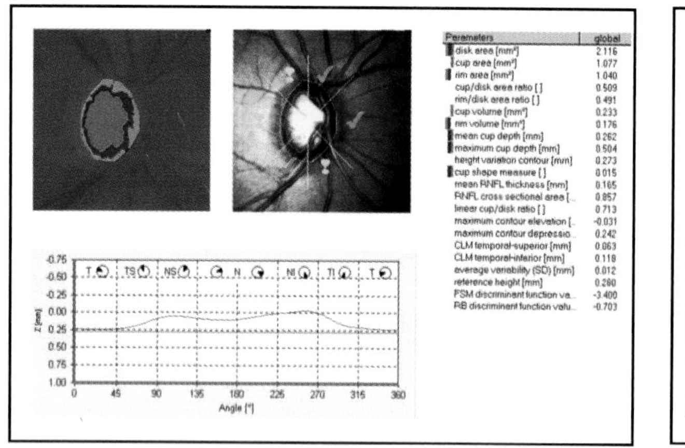
Parameters global
disk area [mm²] 2.116
cup area [mm²] 1.077
rim area [mm²] 1.040
cup/disk area ratio [] 0.509
rim/disk area ratio [] 0.491
cup volume [mm³] 0.233
rim volume [mm³] 0.176
mean cup depth [mm] 0.262
maximum cup depth [mm] 0.504
height variation contour [mm] 0.273
cup shape measure [] 0.015
mean RNFL thickness [mm] 0.165
RNFL cross sectional area [... 0.857
linear cup/disk ratio [] 0.713
maximum contour elevation [... -0.031
maximum contour depressio... 0.242
CLM temporal-superior [mm] 0.063
CLM temporal-inferior [mm] 0.118
average variability (SD) [mm] 0.012
reference height [mm] 0.280
FSM discriminant function va... -3.400
RB discriminant function valu... -0.703
T TS NS N NI TI T
Z [mm]
Angle [°]

C

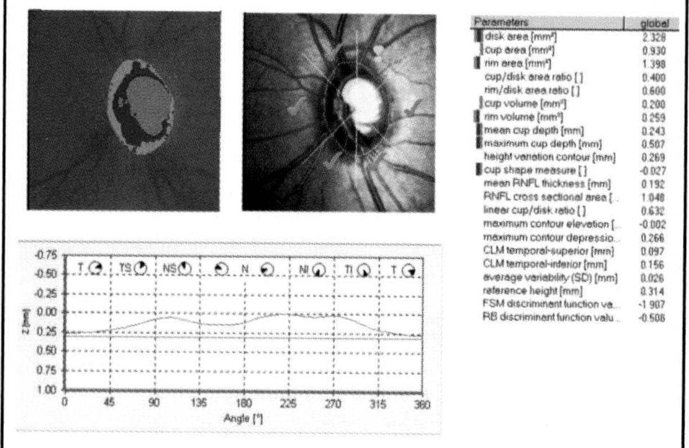
Parameters global
disk area [mm²] 2.328
cup area [mm²] 0.930
rim area [mm²] 1.398
cup/disk area ratio [] 0.400
rim/disk area ratio [] 0.600
cup volume [mm³] 0.200
rim volume [mm³] 0.259
mean cup depth [mm] 0.243
maximum cup depth [mm] 0.507
height variation contour [mm] 0.269
cup shape measure [] -0.027
mean RNFL thickness [mm] 0.192
RNFL cross sectional area [... 1.048
linear cup/disk ratio [] 0.632
maximum contour elevation [... -0.002
maximum contour depressio... 0.266
CLM temporal-superior [mm] 0.097
CLM temporal-inferior [mm] 0.156
average variability (SD) [mm] 0.026
reference height [mm] 0.314
FSM discriminant function va... -1.907
RB discriminant function valu... -0.508
T TS NS N NI TI T
Z [mm]
Angle [°]

D

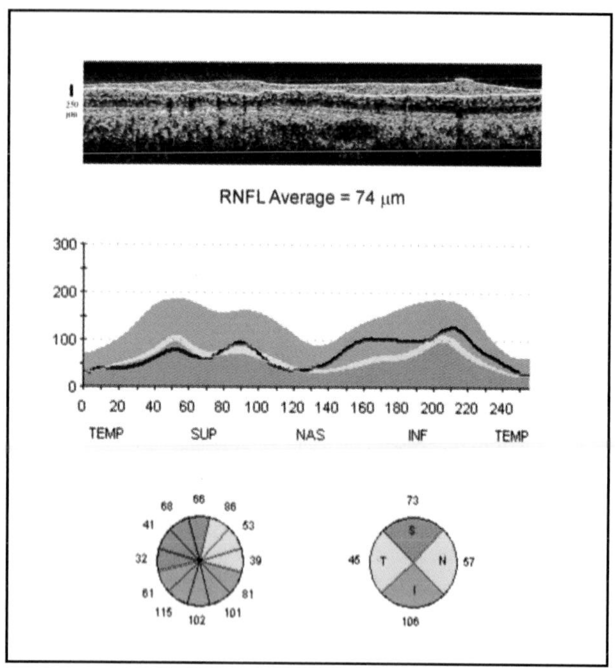
RNFL Average = 74 μm
TEMP
SUP
NAS
INF
TEMP
S
T
N
I
73
45
57
106

E

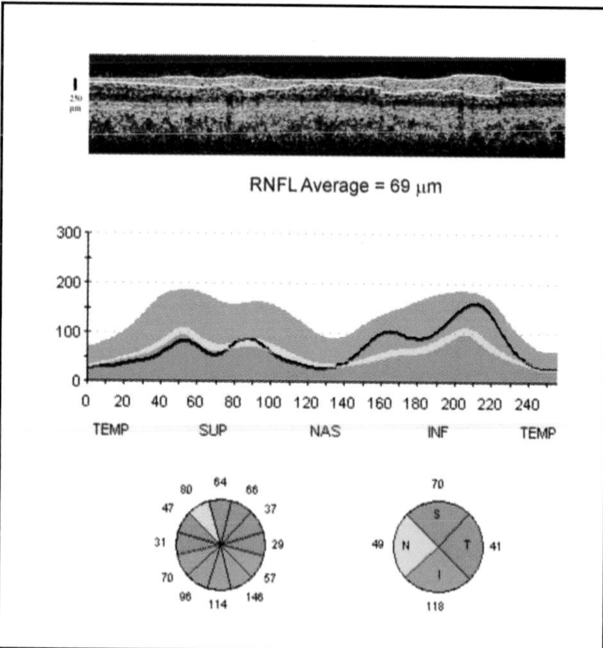
RNFL Average = 69 μm
TEMP
SUP
NAS
INF
TEMP
S
N
T
I
70
49
41
118

F

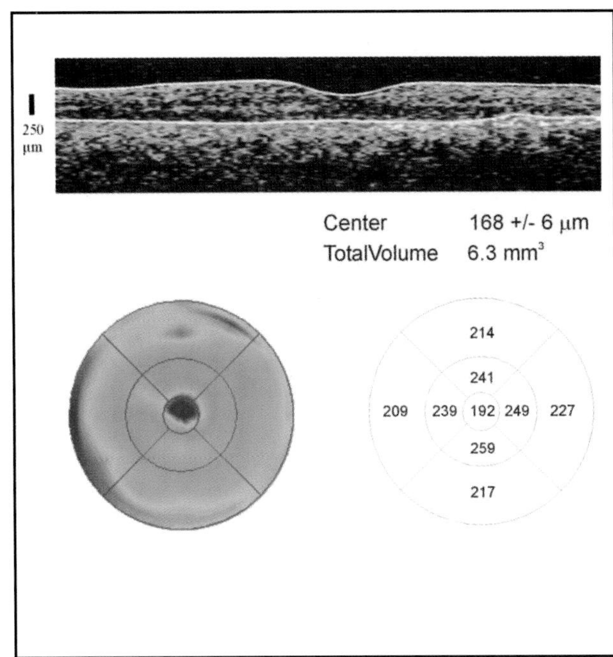
250 µm
Center 168 +/- 6 µm
TotalVolume 6.3 mm³
214
241
209 239 192 249 227
259
217

G

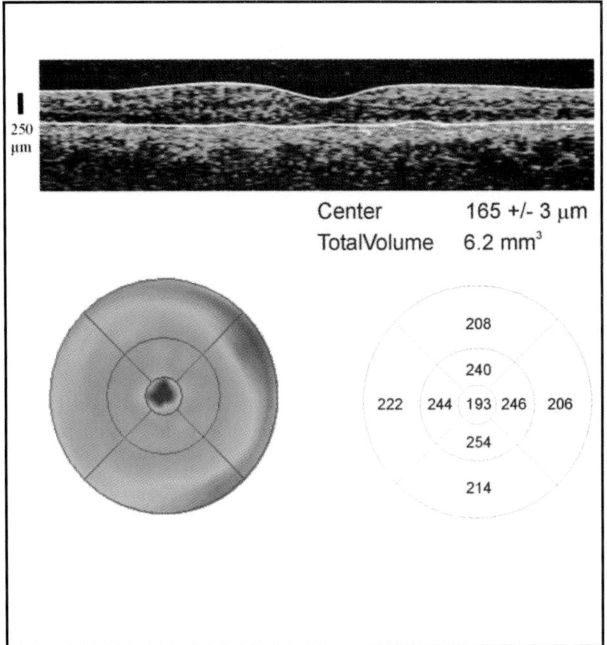
250 µm
Center 165 +/- 3 µm
TotalVolume 6.2 mm³
208
240
222 244 193 246 206
254
214

H

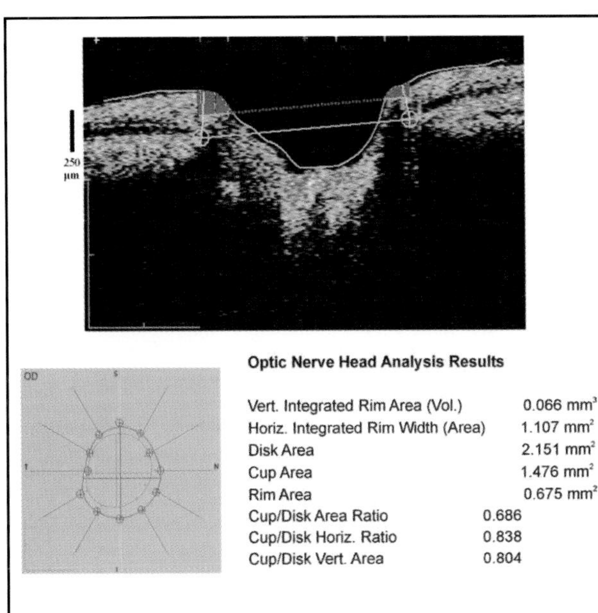
250 µm
OD
Optic Nerve Head Analysis Results
Vert. Integrated Rim Area (Vol.) 0.066 mm³
Horiz. Integrated Rim Width (Area) 1.107 mm²
Disk Area 2.151 mm²
Cup Area 1.476 mm²
Rim Area 0.675 mm²
Cup/Disk Area Ratio 0.686
Cup/Disk Horiz. Ratio 0.838
Cup/Disk Vert. Area 0.804

I

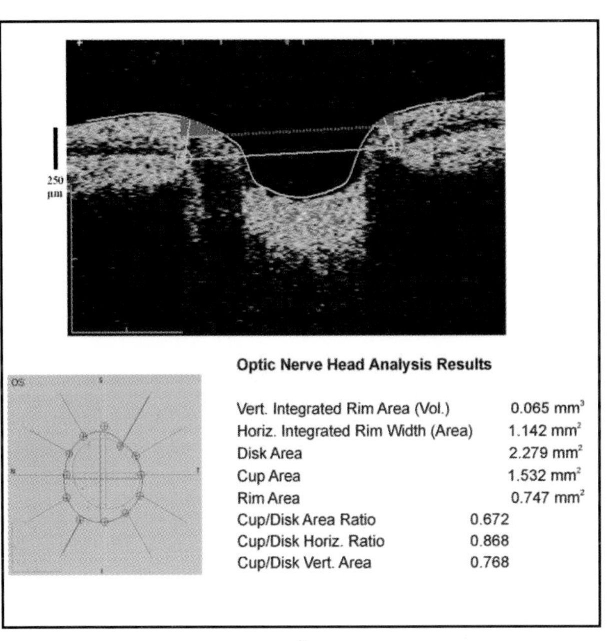
250 µm
OS
Optic Nerve Head Analysis Results
Vert. Integrated Rim Area (Vol.) 0.065 mm³
Horiz. Integrated Rim Width (Area) 1.142 mm²
Disk Area 2.279 mm²
Cup Area 1.532 mm²
Rim Area 0.747 mm²
Cup/Disk Area Ratio 0.672
Cup/Disk Horiz. Ratio 0.868
Cup/Disk Vert. Area 0.768

J

Case 12-25. Good Correspondence Among Visual Field Damage and Retinal Nerve Fiber Layer, Macular, and Optic Nerve Head Measurements

A 41-year-old Caucasian man with juvenile open-angle glaucoma underwent trabeculectomy with local application of 5-flourouracil (5-FU) in both eyes. The patient was treated with bimatoprost 0.03%, and a combination of timolol and dorzolamide. The visual acuities were 20/16 in both eyes, and the IOPs were 16 mmHg bilaterally. Slit-lamp examination revealed prominent superior blebs, quiet anterior segments, patent peripheral iridectomies, and open angles in both eyes. Dilated fundus examination disclosed advanced cupping of the optic disc bilaterally (A and B). Humphrey VFs showed superior central and nasal defects in the right eye (C) and superior and inferior nasal and paracentral defects in the left eye (D). HRT showed abnormally thin neuroretinal rim in all sectors except for nasal superior in the right eye (E) and nasal sector in the left eye (F).

Optical Coherence Tomography

The circumpapillary scan showed thinning of the retinal NFL in the right eye, mainly in the inferior and temporal quadrants, most pronounced at 7:00 to 8:00 (G). Similar average retinal NFL thickness was noted in the left eye with thinning throughout most of the clock hours (H). Macular thinning was noted in the inferior outer sector in the right eye (I). On the left, there was inferior outer macular thinning, with slightly less thinning in the temporal and superior outer regions (J). A small optic disc area was noted in the right eye with large cupping mainly in the temporal inferior sector (K). The left optic disc had a large cup and thinning of the neuroretinal rim in the temporal and the inferior-temporal sectors (L).

Comment

The NFL thickness measurements showed good correspondence with ONH appearance and VFs in each eye. Macular thickness corresponded better on the right than the left, although there was evidence of algorithm failure in the right eye macular scan, where the anterior border of the retina was misidentified on the right of the scan.

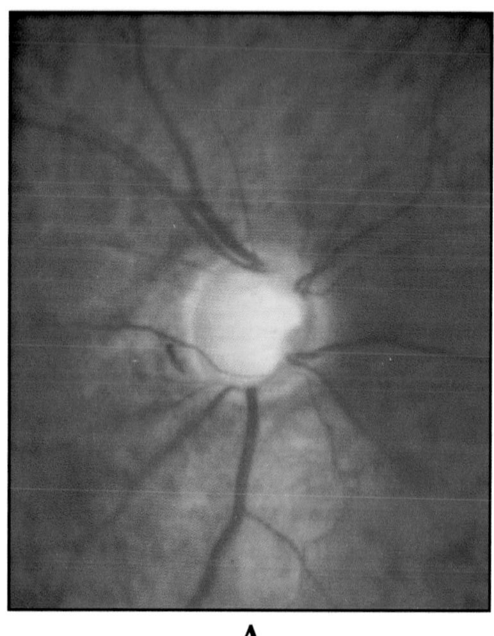

A

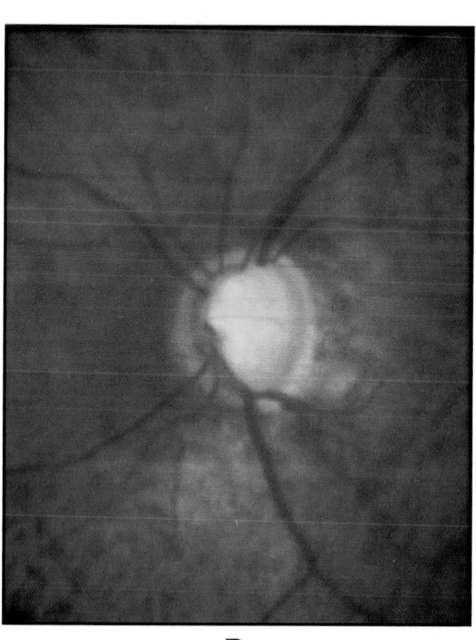

B

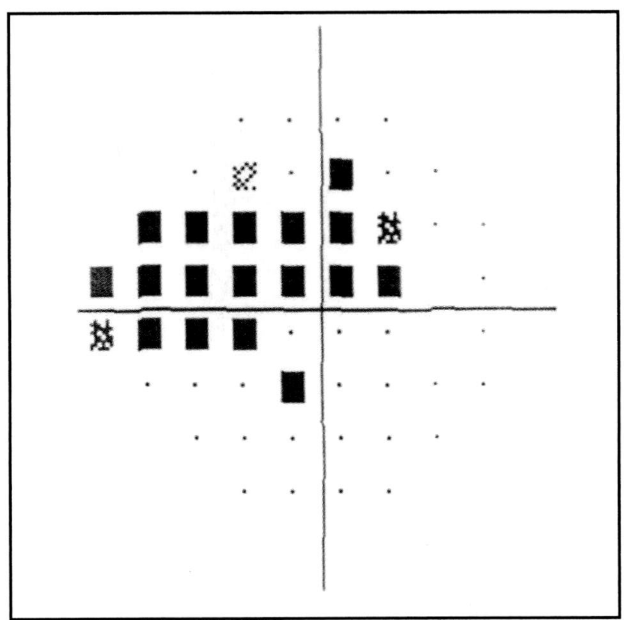

C

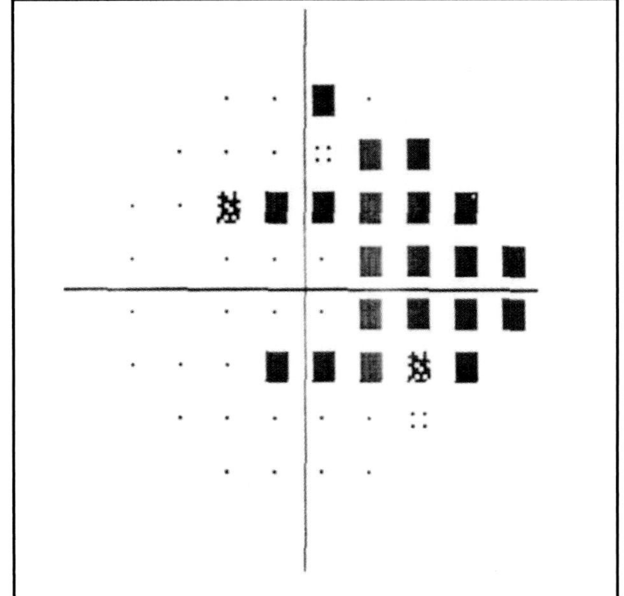

D

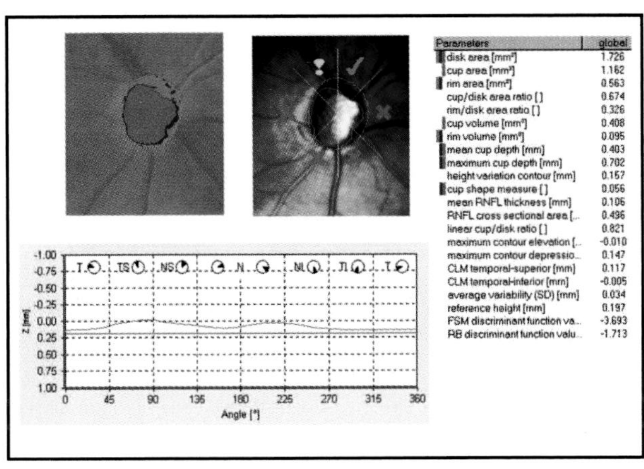

Parameters	global
disk area [mm²]	1.726
cup area [mm²]	1.162
rim area [mm²]	0.563
cup/disk area ratio [ ]	0.674
rim/disk area ratio [ ]	0.326
cup volume [mm³]	0.408
rim volume [mm³]	0.095
mean cup depth [mm]	0.403
maximum cup depth [mm]	0.702
height variation contour [mm]	0.157
cup shape measure [ ]	0.056
mean RNFL thickness [mm]	0.106
RNFL cross sectional area [...	0.496
linear cup/disk ratio [ ]	0.821
maximum contour elevation [...	-0.010
maximum contour depressio...	0.147
CLM temporal-superior [mm]	0.117
CLM temporal-inferior [mm]	-0.005
average variability (SD) [mm]	0.034
reference height [mm]	0.197
FSM discriminant function va...	-3.693
RB discriminant function valu...	-1.713

E

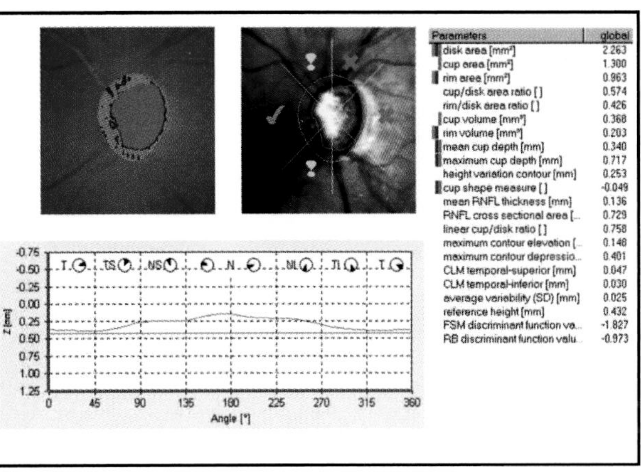

Parameters	global
disk area [mm²]	2.263
cup area [mm²]	1.300
rim area [mm²]	0.963
cup/disk area ratio [ ]	0.574
rim/disk area ratio [ ]	0.426
cup volume [mm³]	0.368
rim volume [mm³]	0.203
mean cup depth [mm]	0.340
maximum cup depth [mm]	0.717
height variation contour [mm]	0.253
cup shape measure [ ]	-0.049
mean RNFL thickness [mm]	0.136
RNFL cross sectional area [...	0.729
linear cup/disk ratio [ ]	0.758
maximum contour elevation [...	0.148
maximum contour depressio...	0.401
CLM temporal-superior [mm]	0.047
CLM temporal-inferior [mm]	0.030
average variability (SD) [mm]	0.025
reference height [mm]	0.432
FSM discriminant function va...	-1.827
RB discriminant function valu...	-0.973

F

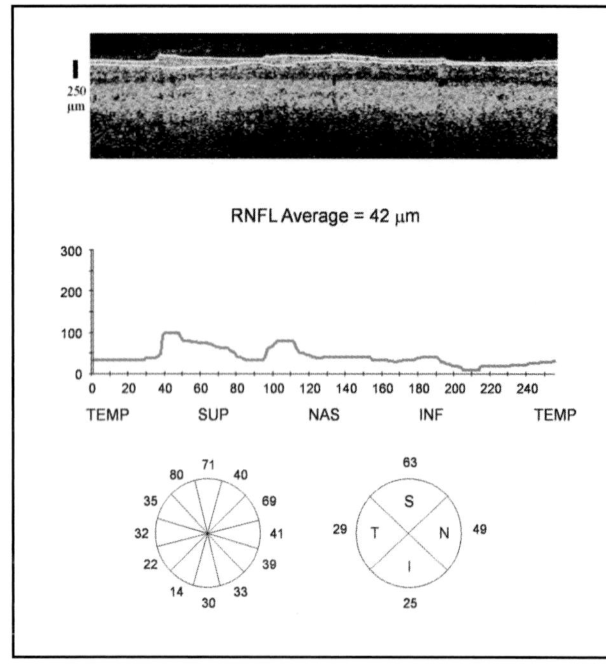
250 µm
RNFL Average = 42 µm
300
200
100
0
0 20 40 60 80 100 120 140 160 180 200 220 240
TEMP SUP NAS INF TEMP
71 40 69 41 39 33 30 14 22 32 35 80
63
S
T N
29 49
I
25

G

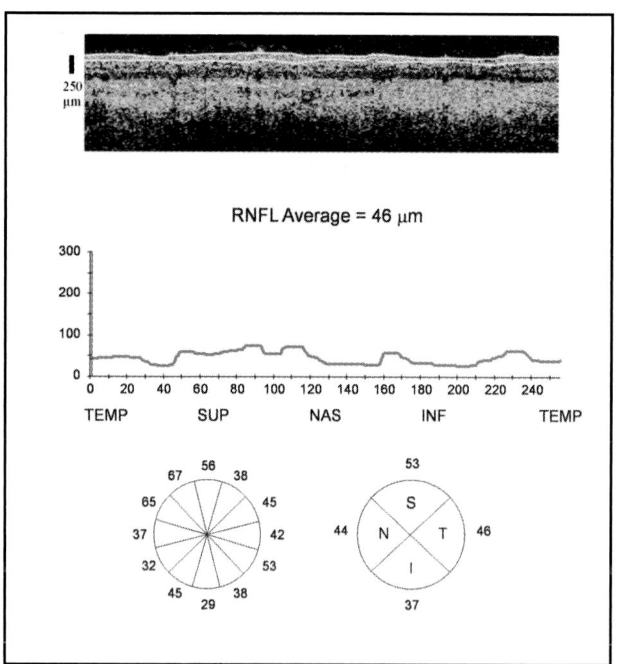
250 µm
RNFL Average = 46 µm
300
200
100
0
0 20 40 60 80 100 120 140 160 180 200 220 240
TEMP SUP NAS INF TEMP
56 38 45 42 53 38 29 45 32 37 65 67
53
S
N T
44 46
I
37

H

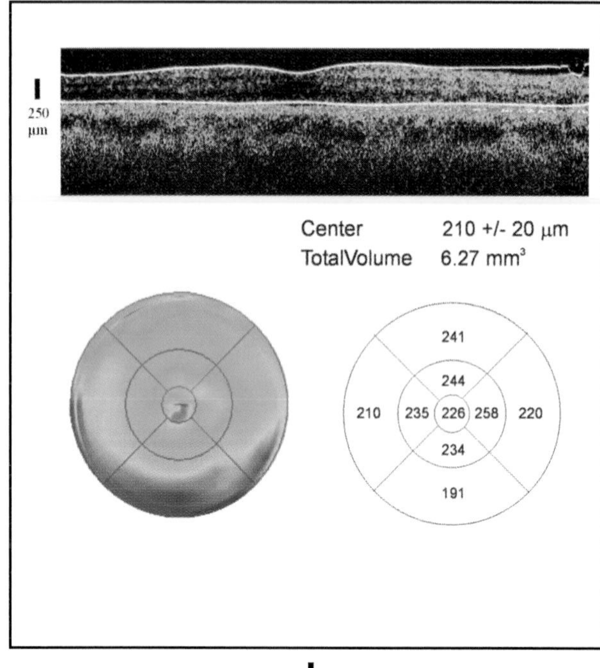
250 µm
Center 210 +/- 20 µm
TotalVolume 6.27 mm³
241
244
210 235 226 258 220
234
191

I

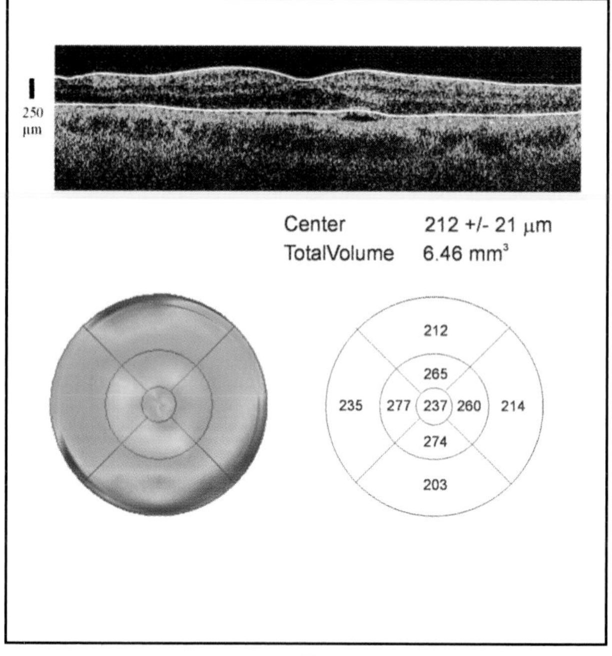
250 µm
Center 212 +/- 21 µm
TotalVolume 6.46 mm³
212
265
235 277 237 260 214
274
203

J

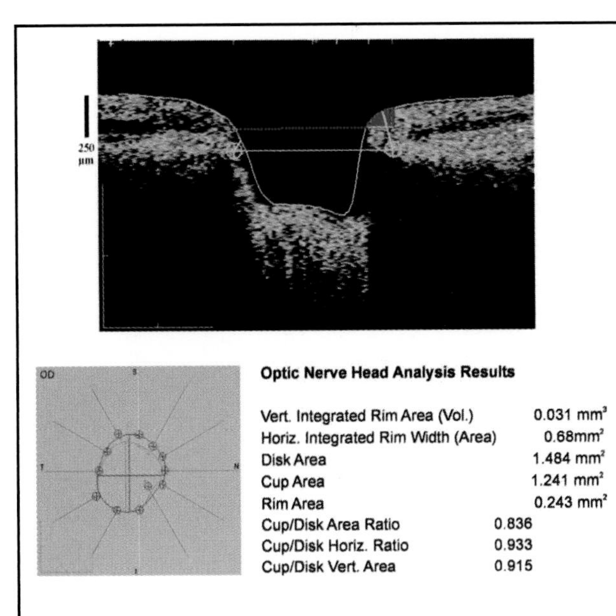
250 µm
OD
Optic Nerve Head Analysis Results
Vert. Integrated Rim Area (Vol.) 0.031 mm³
Horiz. Integrated Rim Width (Area) 0.68mm²
Disk Area 1.484 mm²
Cup Area 1.241 mm²
Rim Area 0.243 mm²
Cup/Disk Area Ratio 0.836
Cup/Disk Horiz. Ratio 0.933
Cup/Disk Vert. Area 0.915

K

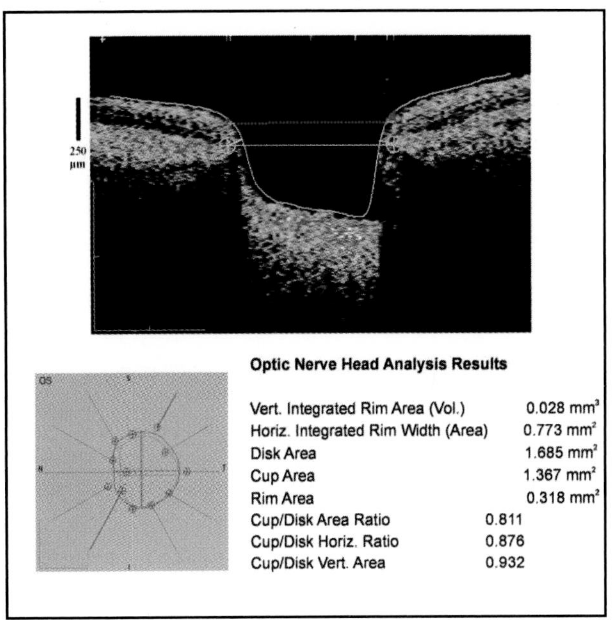
250 µm
OS
Optic Nerve Head Analysis Results
Vert. Integrated Rim Area (Vol.) 0.028 mm³
Horiz. Integrated Rim Width (Area) 0.773 mm²
Disk Area 1.685 mm²
Cup Area 1.367 mm²
Rim Area 0.318 mm²
Cup/Disk Area Ratio 0.811
Cup/Disk Horiz. Ratio 0.876
Cup/Disk Vert. Area 0.932

L

Case 12-26. Retinal Nerve Fiber Layer Assessment Corresponded to Visual Field Findings, but the Optic Nerve Head and Macular Measures Missed the Superior Temporal Loss of Tissue

A 67-year-old Caucasian woman with normal tension glaucoma in the right eye was treated with levobunolol 0.25% and bimatoprost 0.03%. On examination, the visual acuity was 20/25 and the IOP was 13 mmHg. Slit-lamp examination was unremarkable, and there was moderate to marked ONH cupping on the right (A). Superior paracentral and superior and inferior nasal defects were observed in the VF (B). An abnormally thin neuroretinal rim was noted in the inferior temporal sector with the HRT (C).

Optical Coherence Tomography

Reduced retinal NFL thickness was observed at 7:00 and 8:00 in the circumpapillary scan (D). Macular thickness was diminished in the temporal and inferior regions (E). The ONH scan showed attenuation of the neuroretinal rim in the inferior temporal area (F).

Comments

Retinal NFL thinning corresponded to VF findings. HRT detected the inferior temporal ONH abnormality, but the superior temporal defect was not detected. Similarly, superior temporal macular thinning was not seen. These findings underscored the sensitivity of retinal NFL measures compared to ONH and macular assessments.

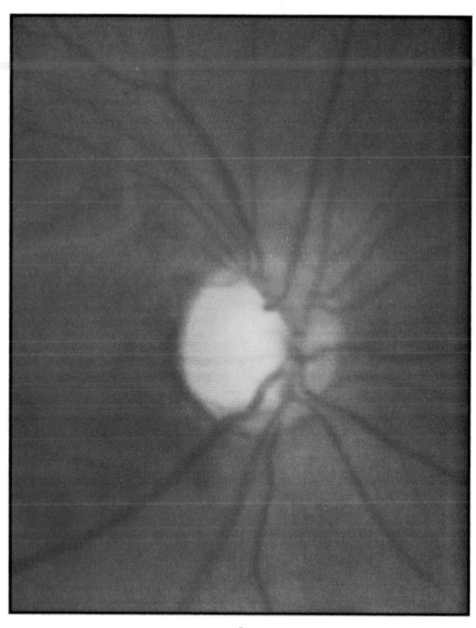

A

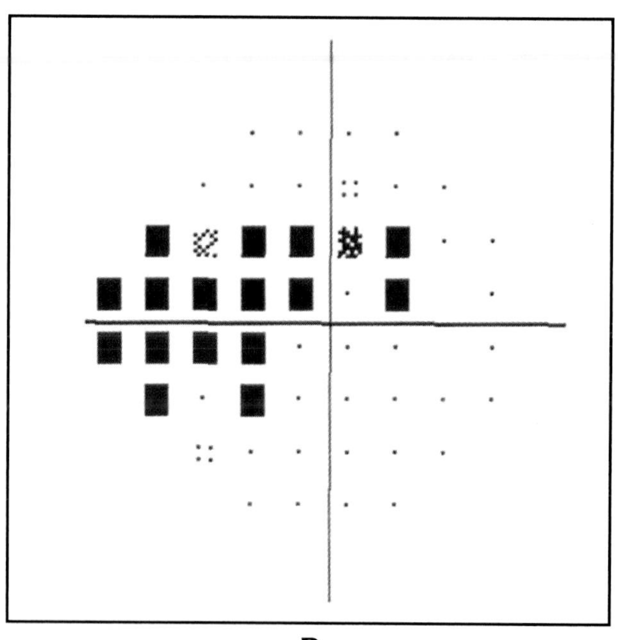

B

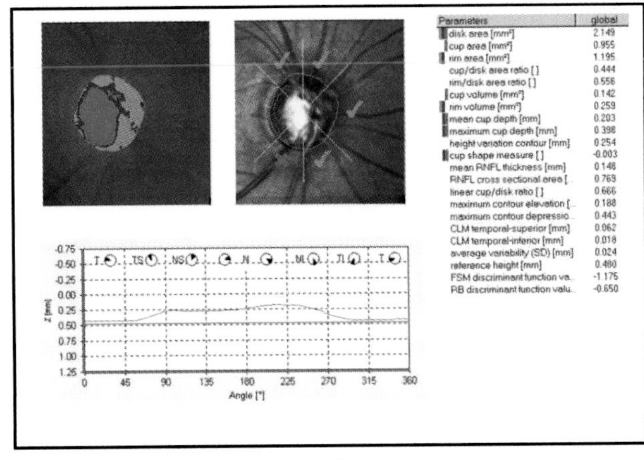
Parameters | global
disk area [mm²] 2.149
cup area [mm²] 0.955
rim area [mm²] 1.195
cup/disk area ratio [ ] 0.444
rim/disk area ratio [ ] 0.556
cup volume [mm³] 0.142
rim volume [mm³] 0.259
mean cup depth [mm] 0.203
maximum cup depth [mm] 0.398
height variation contour [mm] 0.254
cup shape measure [ ] -0.003
mean RNFL thickness [mm] 0.148
RNFL cross sectional area [... 0.763
linear cup/disk ratio [ ] 0.666
maximum contour elevation [... 0.188
maximum contour depressio... 0.443
CLM temporal-superior [mm] 0.062
CLM temporal-inferior [mm] 0.018
average variability (SD) [mm] 0.024
reference height [mm] 0.480
FSM discriminant function va... -1.175
RB discriminant function valu... -0.650
Angle [°]

C

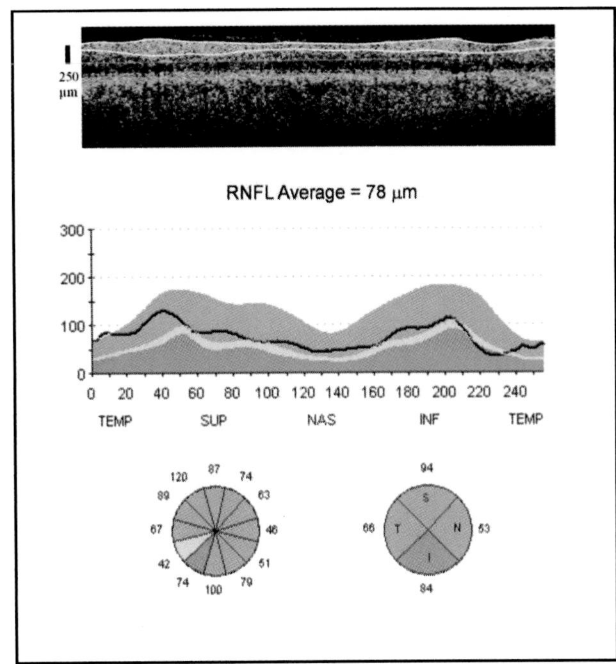
250 µm
RNFL Average = 78 µm
300
200
100
0
0 20 40 60 80 100 120 140 160 180 200 220 240
TEMP SUP NAS INF TEMP
120 87 74
89 63
67 46
42 51
74 100 79
94
S
66 T N 53
I
84

D

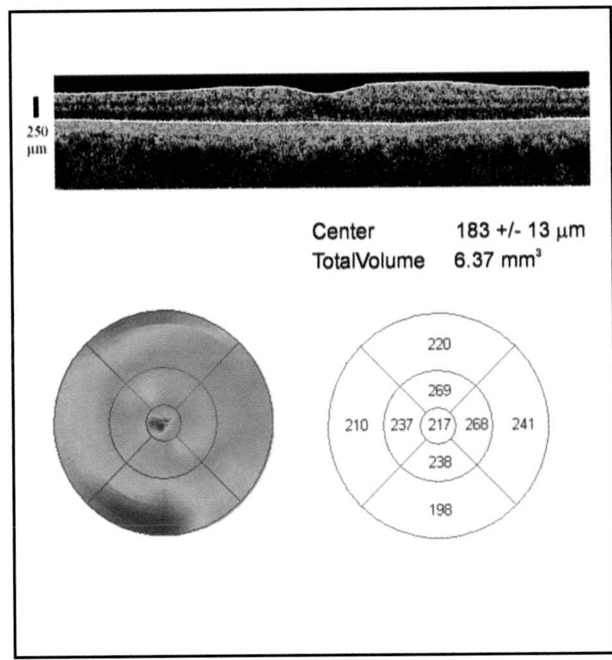
250 µm
Center 183 +/- 13 µm
TotalVolume 6.37 mm³
220
269
210 237 217 268 241
238
198

E

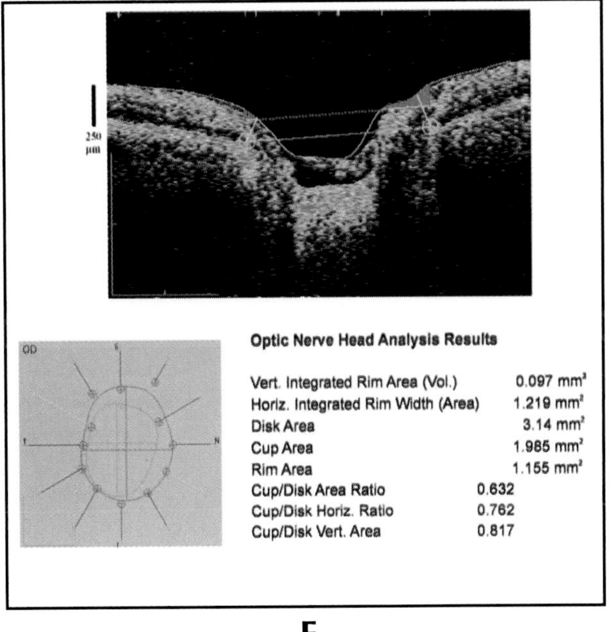
250 µm
Optic Nerve Head Analysis Results
Vert. Integrated Rim Area (Vol.) 0.097 mm³
Horiz. Integrated Rim Width (Area) 1.219 mm²
Disk Area 3.14 mm²
Cup Area 1.985 mm²
Rim Area 1.155 mm²
Cup/Disk Area Ratio 0.632
Cup/Disk Horiz. Ratio 0.762
Cup/Disk Vert. Area 0.817

F

12-27. Retinal Nerve Fiber Layer Measurements Corresponded to Functional Loss. A Small Disc on the Right Confounded Optic Nerve Head Analysis. Macular Thickness Was Reduced in Accordance With Functional Loss

A 56-year-old Caucasian woman with high myopia and primary open-angle glaucoma was referred for a second opinion. Visual acuity was 20/25 OD and 20/20 OS with a refractive error of -8.50 D OU. IOPs were 25 mmHg in the right eye and 19 mmHg on the left. Slit-lamp examination was unremarkable and dilated fundus examination showed a small optic disk size in the right eye with more cupping in the left eye and a NFL defect at 6:30 in the right eye (A and B). NFL photography disclosed a wedge-shaped defect from 6:00 to 6:30 in the right eye. Humphrey VF testing showed an early superior nasal defect in the right eye (C) and superior and inferior nasal defects in the left eye (D). Small disc with normal rim size was detected with the HRT in the right eye and thinning of the rim in the inferior, nasal, and temporal sectors in the left eye (E and F).

Optical Coherence Tomography

A slight reduction in the average retinal NFL thickness was noted in the right eye circumpapillary scan, with focally reduced thickness inferior temporally when compared with the corresponding superior clock hours (G). In the left eye, the average retinal NFL thickness was severely reduced from normal at 37 µm, with marked thinning from 8:00 to 11:00 (H). The macular volume was lower in the left than the right eye, most of which was due to thinning in the outer inferior and temporal sectors in the left eye (I and J). Both eyes had small ONH areas with a larger cup in the left eye and with inferior temporal neuroretinal rim thinning (K and L).

Comments

Retinal NFL measurements corresponded to functional loss, although retinal NFL thickness in both eyes may have been reduced out of proportion to the visual field defects because of measurement artifact due to the patient's high myopia. Eight to 10 D of myopia may reduce the OCT measured average NFL thickness by about 10 µm. This should be considered when evaluating highly myopic individuals. The ONH evaluation with both the OCT and HRT on the right showed the patient's small cup, and the HRT called the ONH normal. This is related to the small disc size, and the artifact induced by disc size with this technology. In the left eye, the HRT detected the inferior but not the superior ONH abnormality. Macular thickness reflected the loss of retinal ganglion cells, but algorithm failure was evident in the right eye, perhaps due to a borderline poor signal-to-noise ratio on these scans.

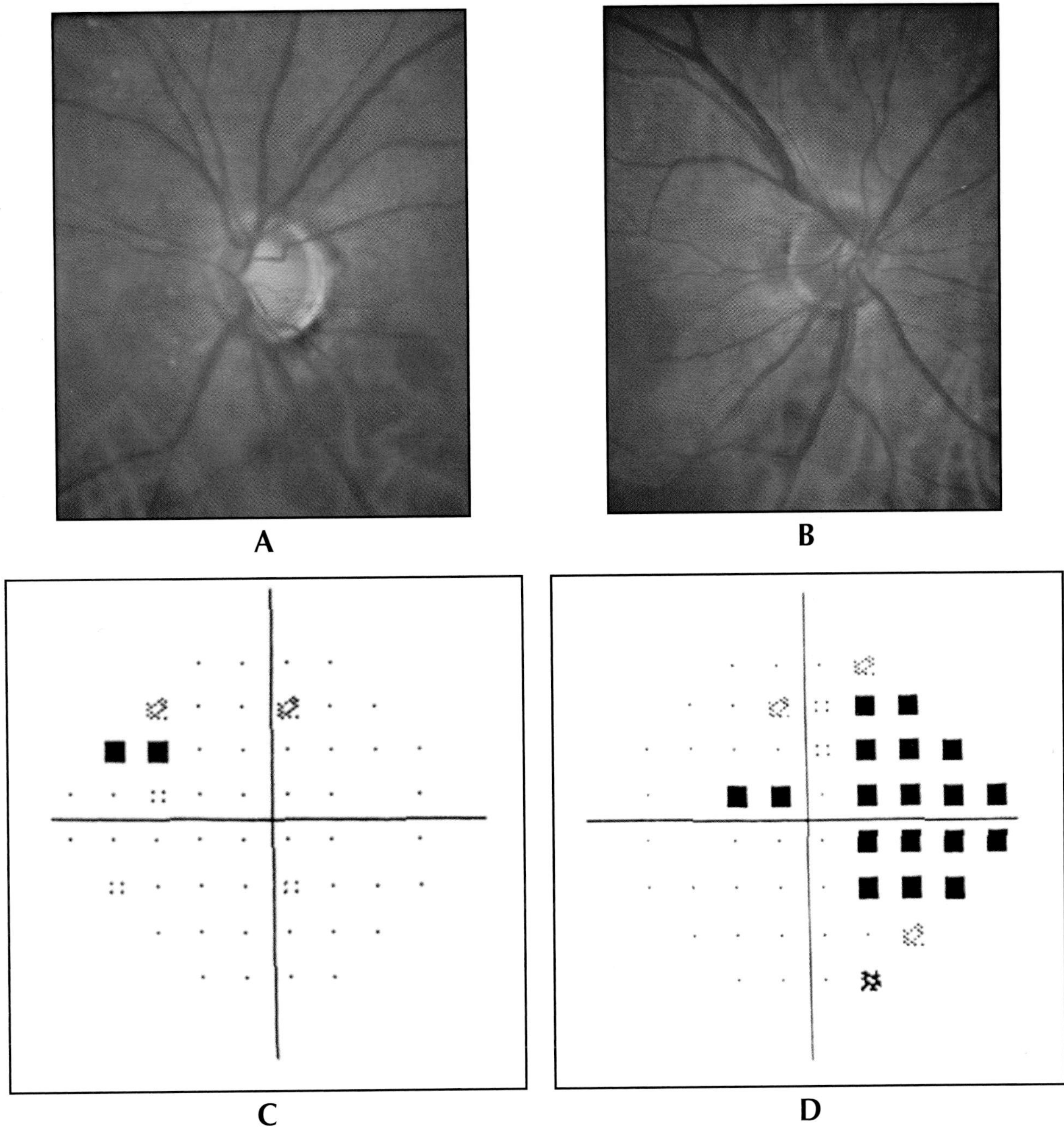
A
B
C
D

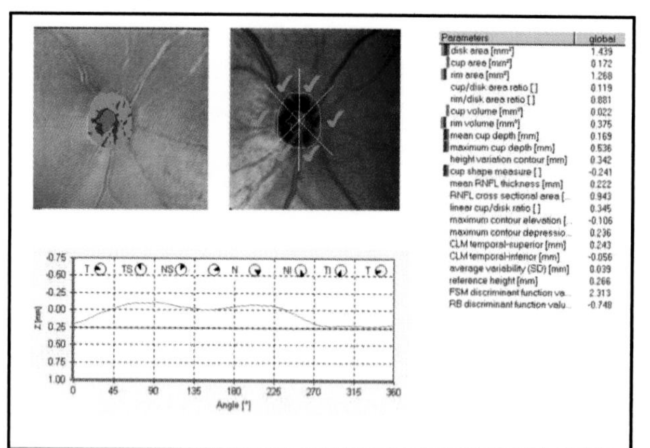
Parameters | global
disk area [mm^2] 1.439
cup area [mm^2] 0.172
rim area [mm^2] 1.268
cup/disk area ratio [] 0.119
rim/disk area ratio [] 0.881
cup volume [mm^3] 0.022
rim volume [mm^3] 0.375
mean cup depth [mm] 0.169
maximum cup depth [mm] 0.536
height variation contour [mm] 0.342
cup shape measure [] -0.241
mean RNFL thickness [mm] 0.222
RNFL cross sectional area [... 0.943
linear cup/disk ratio [] 0.345
maximum contour elevation [... -0.106
maximum contour depressio... 0.236
CLM temporal-superior [mm] 0.243
CLM temporal-inferior [mm] -0.056
average variability (SD) [mm] 0.039
reference height [mm] 0.266
FSM discriminant function va... 2.313
RB discriminant function valu... -0.748
T TS NS N NI TI T
Z [mm]
Angle [°]

E

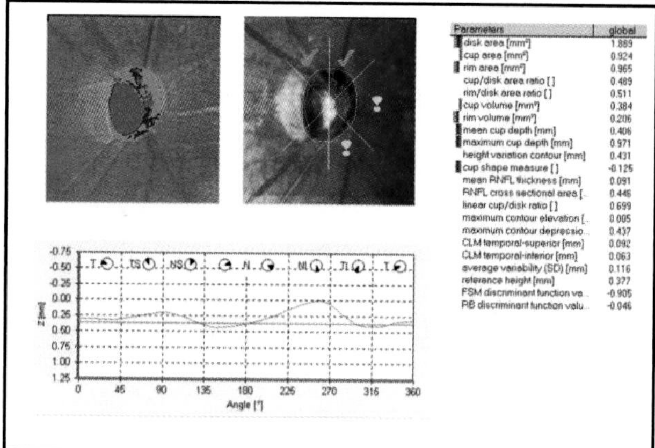
Parameters | global
disk area [mm^2] 1.889
cup area [mm^2] 0.924
rim area [mm^2] 0.965
cup/disk area ratio [] 0.489
rim/disk area ratio [] 0.511
cup volume [mm^3] 0.384
rim volume [mm^3] 0.206
mean cup depth [mm] 0.406
maximum cup depth [mm] 0.971
height variation contour [mm] 0.431
cup shape measure [] -0.125
mean RNFL thickness [mm] 0.091
RNFL cross sectional area [... 0.446
linear cup/disk ratio [] 0.699
maximum contour elevation [... 0.005
maximum contour depressio... 0.437
CLM temporal-superior [mm] 0.092
CLM temporal-inferior [mm] 0.063
average variability (SD) [mm] 0.116
reference height [mm] 0.377
FSM discriminant function va... -0.905
RB discriminant function valu... -0.046
T TS NS N NI TI T
Z [mm]
Angle [°]

F

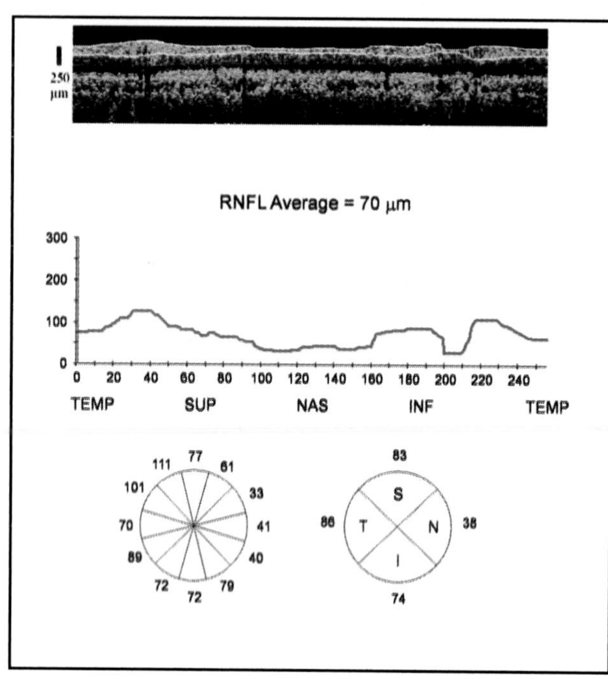
250 µm
RNFL Average = 70 µm
TEMP SUP NAS INF TEMP
111 77 61 101 33 70 41 89 40 72 72 79
83
S
T N
I
86 38
74

G

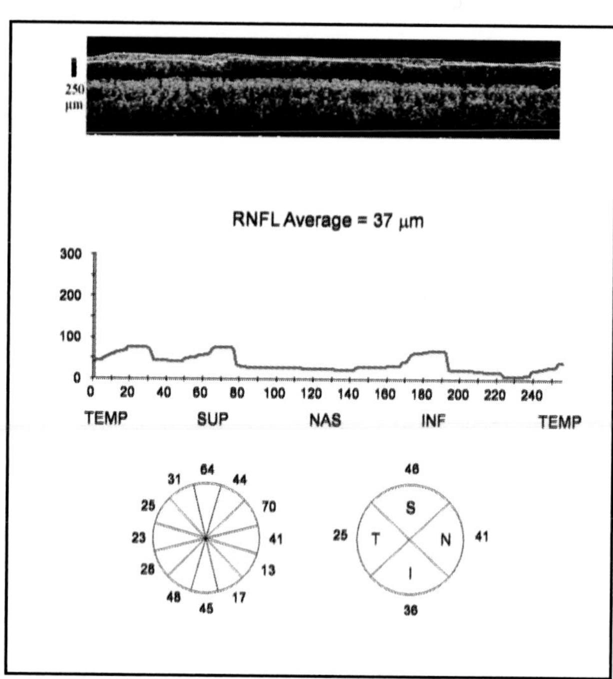
250 µm
RNFL Average = 37 µm
TEMP SUP NAS INF TEMP
31 64 44 25 70 23 41 28 13 48 45 17
46
S
T N
I
25 41
36

H

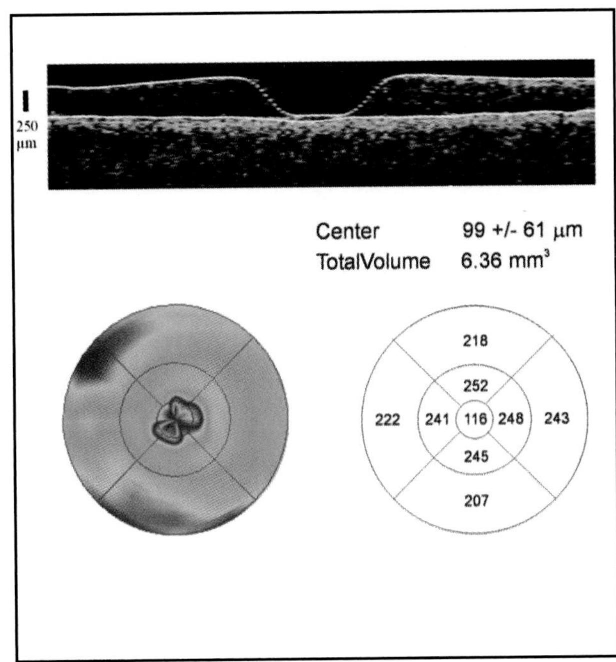

I

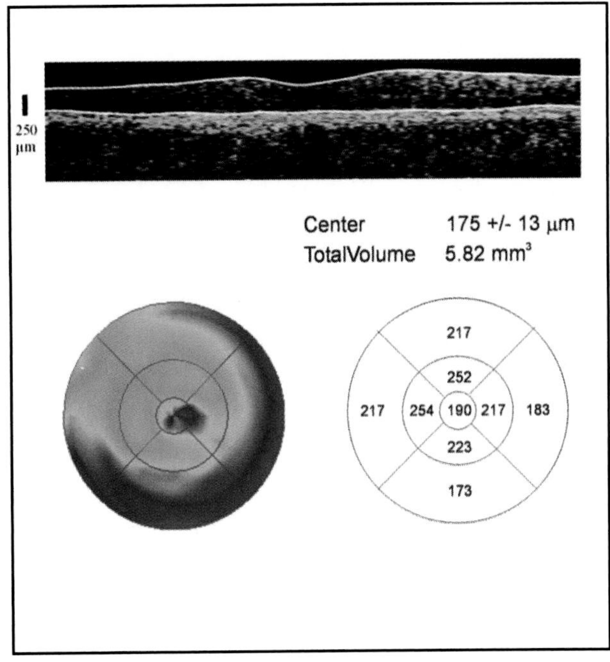

J

250 μm

OD

Optic Nerve Head Analysis Results

Vert. Integrated Rim Area (Vol.)	0.317 mm³
Horiz. Integrated Rim Width (Area)	1.452 mm²
Disk Area	1.401 mm²
Cup Area	0.258 mm²
Rim Area	1.143 mm²
Cup/Disk Area Ratio	0.184
Cup/Disk Horiz. Ratio	0.467
Cup/Disk Vert. Area	0.42

K

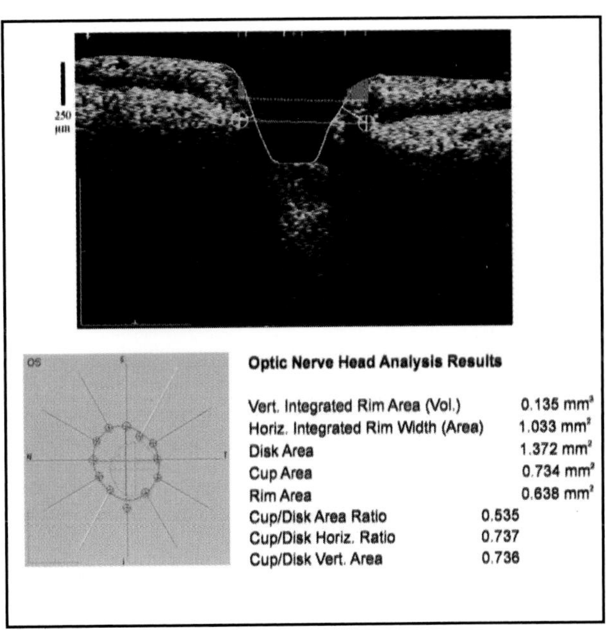

250 μm
OS
Optic Nerve Head Analysis Results
Vert. Integrated Rim Area (Vol.) 0.135 mm³
Horiz. Integrated Rim Width (Area) 1.033 mm²
Disk Area 1.372 mm²
Cup Area 0.734 mm²
Rim Area 0.638 mm²
Cup/Disk Area Ratio 0.535
Cup/Disk Horiz. Ratio 0.737
Cup/Disk Vert. Area 0.736

L

Case 12-28. A Focal Nerve Fiber Layer Defect Was Demonstrated on Optical Coherence Tomography, Nerve Fiber Layer, Macular Imaging, and Perimetry, But Not by Optic Nerve Head Analysis

A 47-year-old Caucasian woman with pseudoexfoliation glaucoma in the right eye was treated with a combination of timolol 0.5% and dorzolamide 2%. The visual acuity was 20/20 and the IOP was 13 mmHg. Slit-lamp examination disclosed pseudoexfoliation material on the iris, anterior capsule of the lens, and in the angle (A). Red-free photos of the fundus revealed a wedge-shaped NFL defect from 6:00 to 8:30 (B). Frequency-doubling technology showed superior paracentral and nasal defects in the right eye (C). HRT revealed a small optic disc with borderline thinning of the neuroretinal rim superior nasally (D).

Optical Coherence Tomography

Pronounced localized thinning of the retinal NFL was noted at 7:00 and 8:00 in the circumpapillary scan, with borderline thinning at 11:00 (E). The macular scan showed thinning of the retina inferiorly and in the outer temporal region (F). The ONH analysis was unremarkable (G).

Comments

The marked localized thinning in the retinal NFL was shown by loss of the red upper band on the right side of the circumpapillary scan.

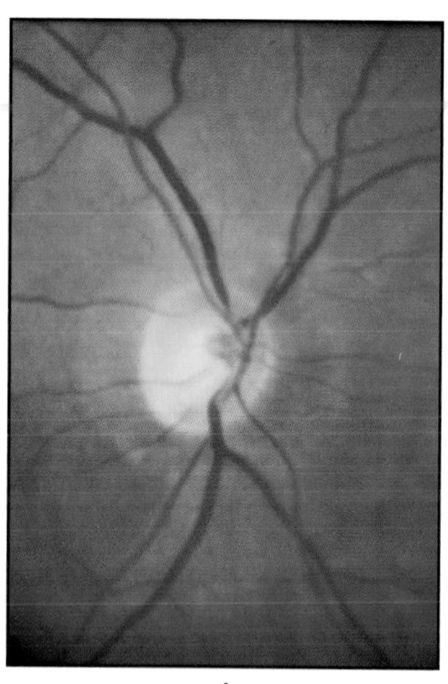

A

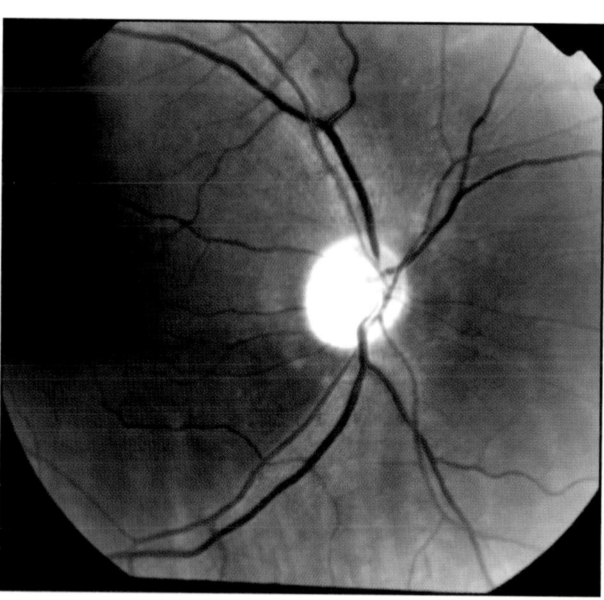

B

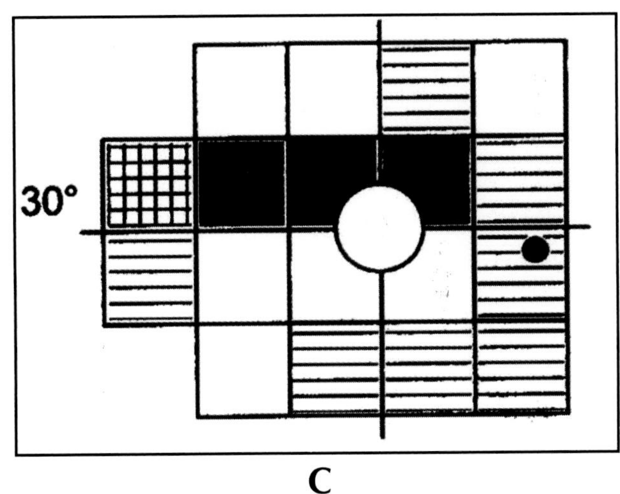
30°

C

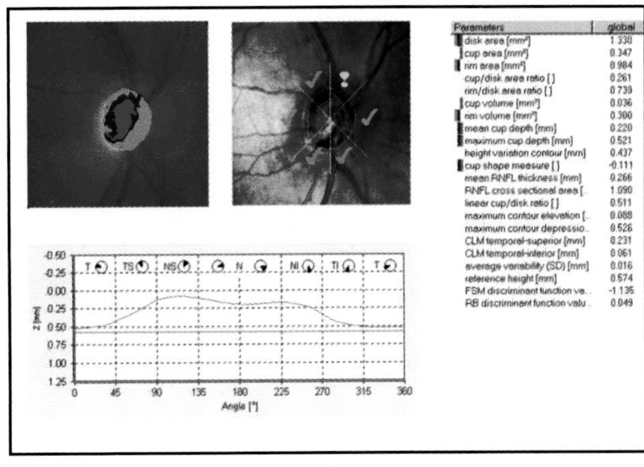
Parameters global
disk area [mm²] 1.330
cup area [mm²] 0.347
rim area [mm²] 0.984
cup/disk area ratio [] 0.261
rim/disk area ratio [] 0.739
cup volume [mm³] 0.036
rim volume [mm³] 0.390
mean cup depth [mm] 0.220
maximum cup depth [mm] 0.521
height variation contour [mm] 0.437
cup shape measure [] -0.111
mean RNFL thickness [mm] 0.266
RNFL cross sectional area [... 1.090
linear cup/disk ratio [] 0.511
maximum contour elevation [... 0.088
maximum contour depressio... 0.526
CLM temporal-superior [mm] 0.231
CLM temporal-inferior [mm] 0.061
average variability (SD) [mm] 0.016
reference height [mm] 0.574
FSM discriminant function va... -1.135
RB discriminant function valu... 0.049
T TS NS N NI TI T
Angle [°]

D

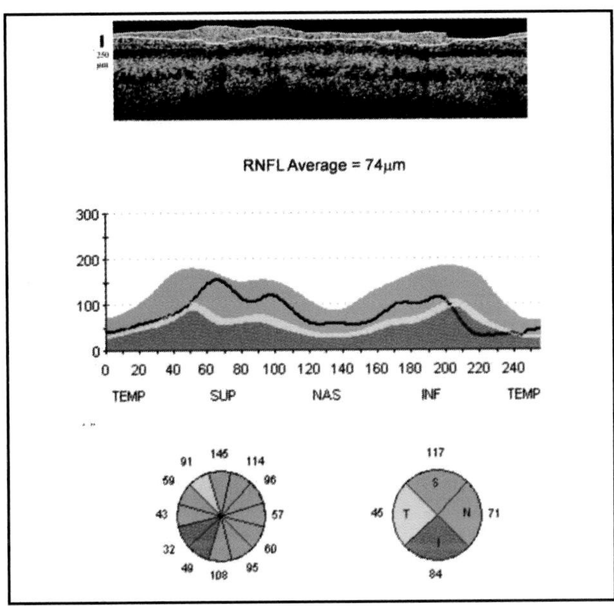
250 μm
RNFL Average = 74μm
300
200
100
0
0 20 40 60 80 100 120 140 160 180 200 220 240
TEMP SUP NAS INF TEMP
145 114 96 57 60 95 108 49 32 43 59 91
117 S N 71 84 I T 46

E

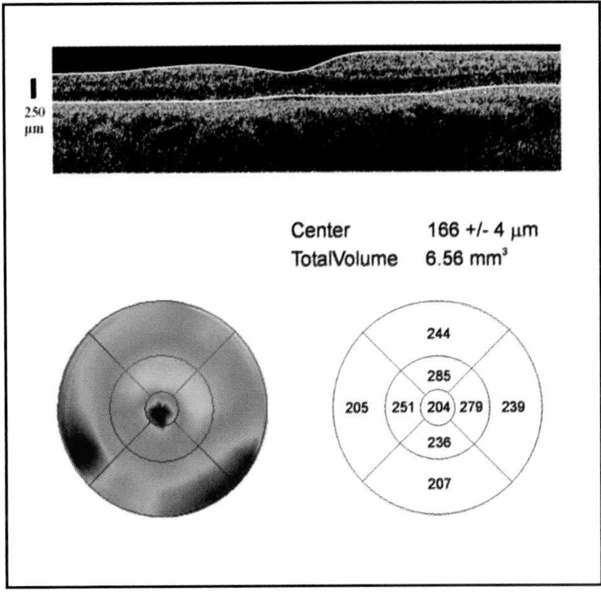
250 μm
Center 166 +/- 4 μm
TotalVolume 6.56 mm³
244
285
205 251 204 279 239
236
207

F

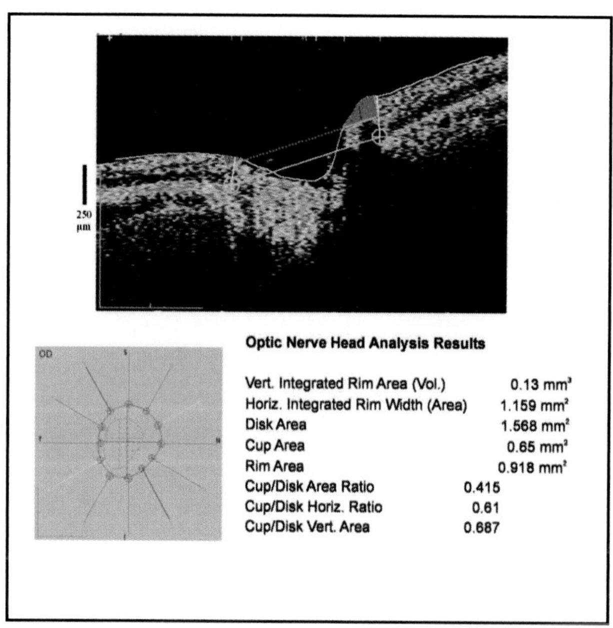
250 µm
OD
Optic Nerve Head Analysis Results
Vert. Integrated Rim Area (Vol.) 0.13 mm^3
Horiz. Integrated Rim Width (Area) 1.159 mm^2
Disk Area 1.568 mm^2
Cup Area 0.65 mm^2
Rim Area 0.918 mm^2
Cup/Disk Area Ratio 0.415
Cup/Disk Horiz. Ratio 0.61
Cup/Disk Vert. Area 0.687

G

Case 12-29. Nerve Fiber Layer and Macular Scans Showed Excellent Correspondence With Visual Fields, But Small Optic Nerves Confounded Optic Nerve Head Analysis

A 73-year-old Caucasian woman with primary open-angle glaucoma in both eyes was treated with trabeculectomy with mitomycin C. She developed chronic ocular hypotony. The visual acuity was 20/25 OD and 20/32 OS and the IOPs were 6 and 4 mmHg, respectively. A succulent bleb was noted in the right eye, and there was a diffuse bleb in the left eye with no sign of a leak. The anterior chambers were deep and quiet, and there were patent peripheral iridectomies in both eyes. The posterior segment examination showed asymmetric optic disc cupping with a larger cup in the left eye as well as peripapillary atrophy (A and B). No signs of hypotony maculopathy were present. VF testing showed a superior paracentral defect in the right eye (C) and superior paracentral and nasal defects in the left eye (D). HRT scanning disclosed a normal-sized optic disc in the right eye with borderline thinning of the rim inferior temporally (E). In the left eye, a small-sized disc was seen with a rim notch (F).

Optical Coherence Tomography

Reduced average NFL thickness was found in both eyes in the circumpapillary scan; this was more pronounced in the left eye. In the right eye, the thinning was located at 6:00 and 7:00 (G). In the left eye, the thinning spanned nearly throughout the scan (H). The macular scan showed an overall reduction in the macular volume more pronounced in the left eye (I and J). The ONH scan showed normal-sized discs with bilateral rim notches inferior temporally (K and L).

Comment

Circumpapillary NFL and macular scans correspond best with the VF abnormalities. The small ONHs confounded analysis, which underrepresented the actual damage that has occurred in the optic nerve.

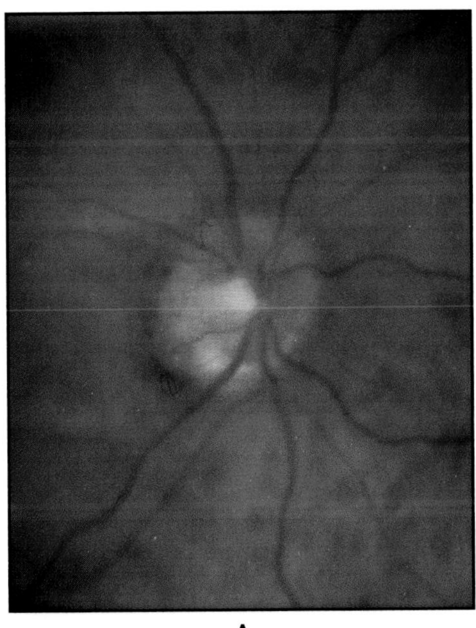

A

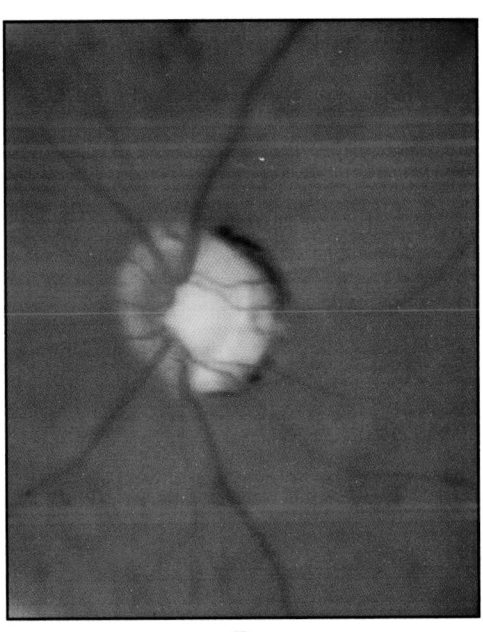

B

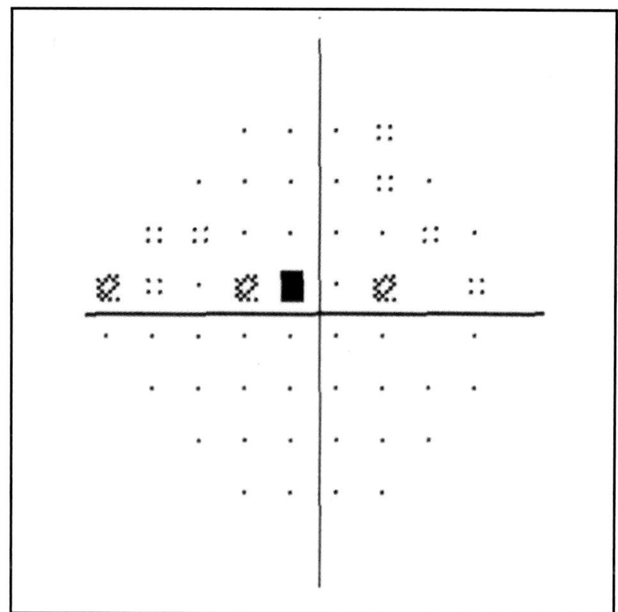

C

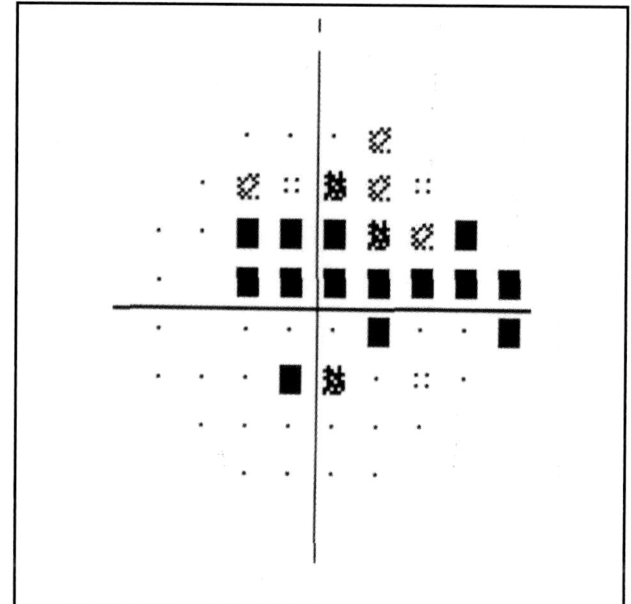

D

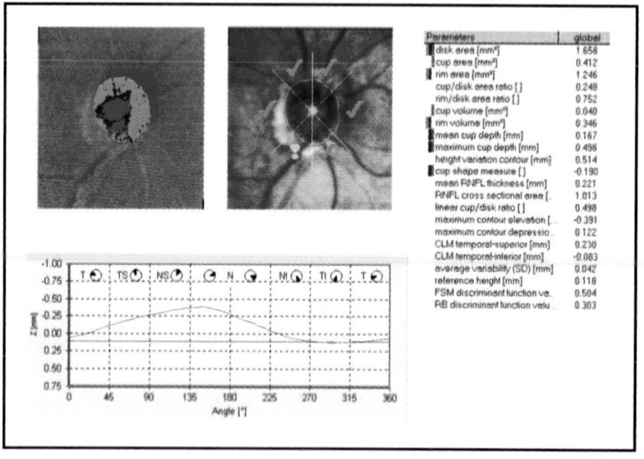
Parameters | global
disk area [mm²] 1.658
cup area [mm²] 0.412
rim area [mm²] 1.246
cup/disk area ratio [] 0.248
rim/disk area ratio [] 0.752
cup volume [mm³] 0.040
rim volume [mm³] 0.346
mean cup depth [mm] 0.167
maximum cup depth [mm] 0.498
height variation contour [mm] 0.514
cup shape measure [] -0.190
mean RNFL thickness [mm] 0.221
RNFL cross sectional area [... 1.013
linear cup/disk ratio [] 0.498
maximum contour elevation [... -0.391
maximum contour depressio... 0.122
CLM temporal-superior [mm] 0.230
CLM temporal-inferior [mm] -0.083
average variability (SD) [mm] 0.042
reference height [mm] 0.118
FSM discriminant function va... 0.504
RB discriminant function valu... 0.303
T TS NS N NI TI T
Z [mm]
Angle [°]

E

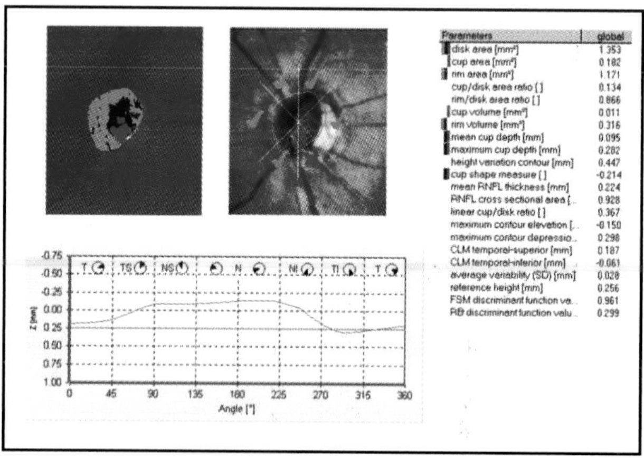
Parameters | global
disk area [mm²] 1.353
cup area [mm²] 0.182
rim area [mm²] 1.171
cup/disk area ratio [] 0.134
rim/disk area ratio [] 0.866
cup volume [mm³] 0.011
rim volume [mm³] 0.316
mean cup depth [mm] 0.095
maximum cup depth [mm] 0.282
height variation contour [mm] 0.447
cup shape measure [] -0.214
mean RNFL thickness [mm] 0.224
RNFL cross sectional area [... 0.928
linear cup/disk ratio [] 0.367
maximum contour elevation [... -0.150
maximum contour depressio... 0.298
CLM temporal-superior [mm] 0.187
CLM temporal-inferior [mm] -0.061
average variability (SD) [mm] 0.028
reference height [mm] 0.256
FSM discriminant function va... 0.961
RB discriminant function valu... 0.299
T TS NS N NI TI T
Z [mm]
Angle [°]

F

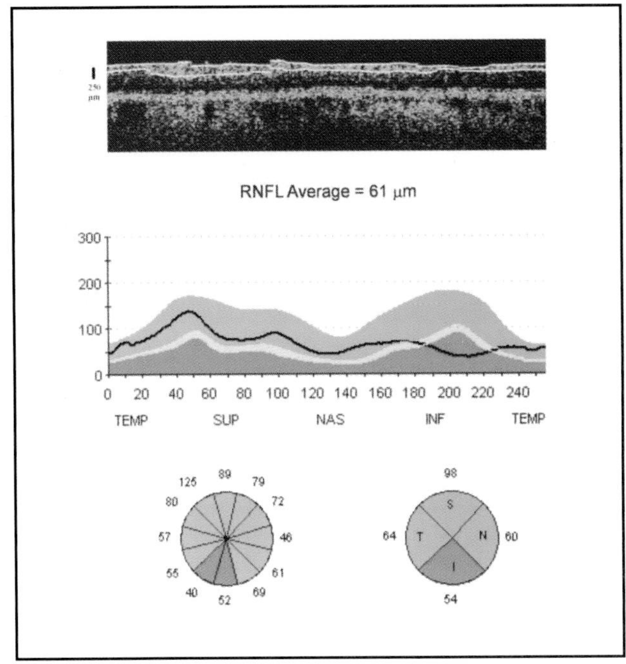
250 µm
RNFL Average = 61 µm
300
200
100
0
0 20 40 60 80 100 120 140 160 180 200 220 240
TEMP SUP NAS INF TEMP
89 79 72 46 61 69 52 40 55 57 80 125
98
S
T
N
I
64 60
54

G

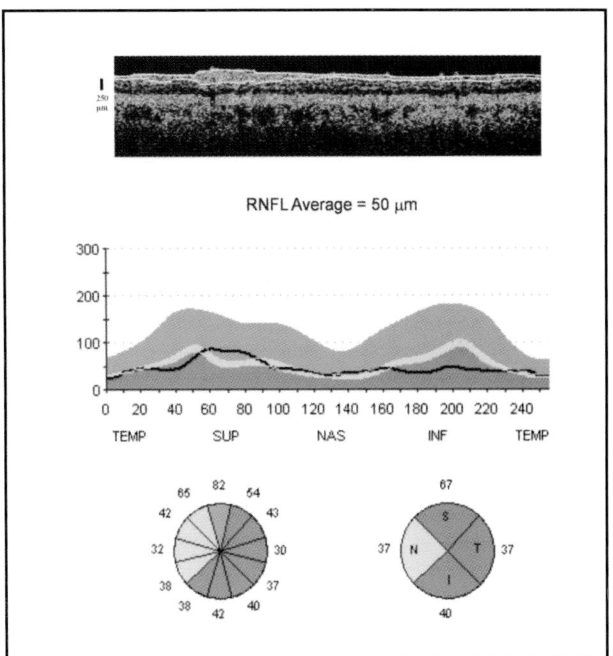
250 µm
RNFL Average = 50 µm
300
200
100
0
0 20 40 60 80 100 120 140 160 180 200 220 240
TEMP SUP NAS INF TEMP
82 54 43 30 37 40 42 38 38 32 42 65
67
S
N
T
I
37 37
40

H

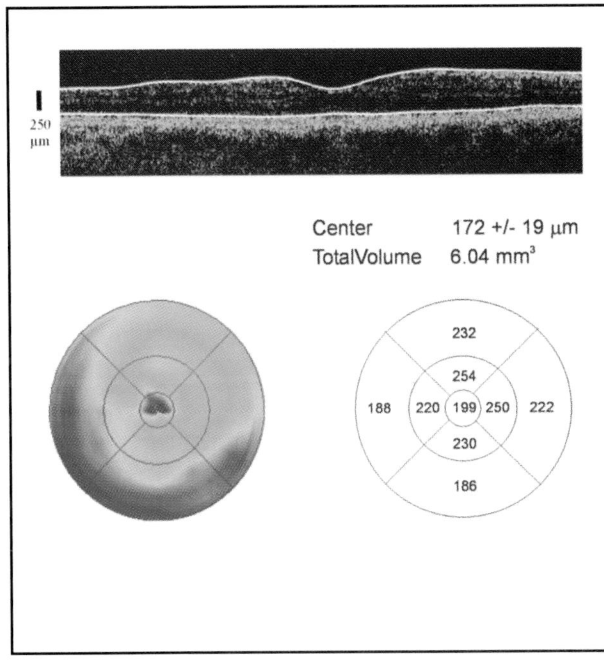
250 µm
Center 172 +/- 19 µm
TotalVolume 6.04 mm³
232
254
188 220 199 250 222
230
186

I

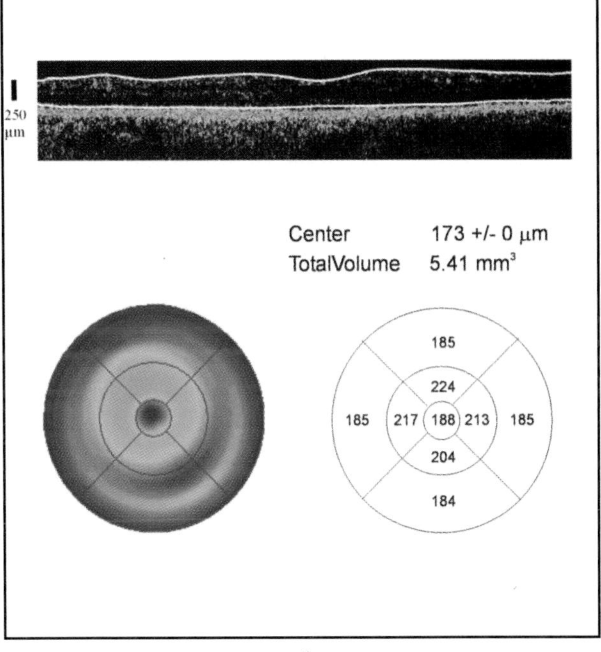
250 µm
Center 173 +/- 0 µm
TotalVolume 5.41 mm³
185
224
185 217 188 213 185
204
184

J

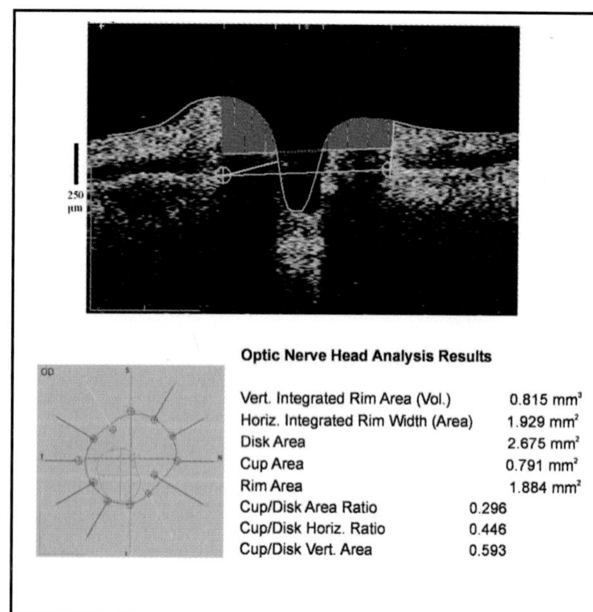
250 µm
OD
Optic Nerve Head Analysis Results
Vert. Integrated Rim Area (Vol.) 0.815 mm³
Horiz. Integrated Rim Width (Area) 1.929 mm²
Disk Area 2.675 mm²
Cup Area 0.791 mm²
Rim Area 1.884 mm²
Cup/Disk Area Ratio 0.296
Cup/Disk Horiz. Ratio 0.446
Cup/Disk Vert. Area 0.593

K

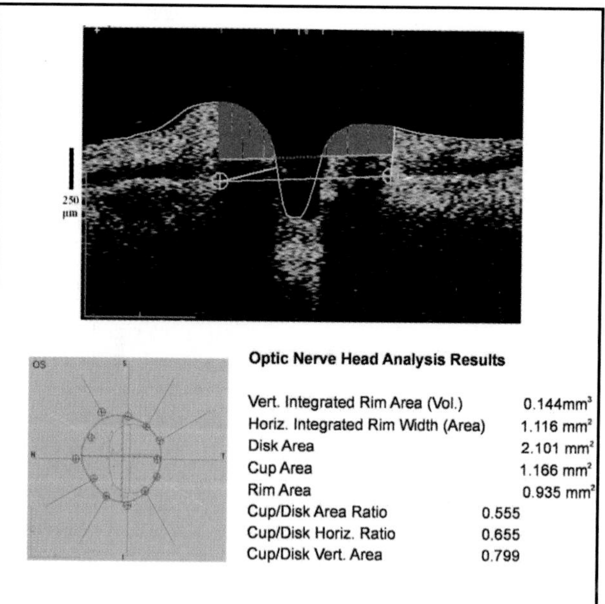
250 µm
OS
Optic Nerve Head Analysis Results
Vert. Integrated Rim Area (Vol.) 0.144mm³
Horiz. Integrated Rim Width (Area) 1.116 mm²
Disk Area 2.101 mm²
Cup Area 1.166 mm²
Rim Area 0.935 mm²
Cup/Disk Area Ratio 0.555
Cup/Disk Horiz. Ratio 0.655
Cup/Disk Vert. Area 0.799

L

Case 12-30. Nerve Fiber Layer Proved to Correspond Better to Visual Field Abnormalities Than Optic Nerve Head or Macular Imaging

A 71-year-old Caucasian man had pseudoexfoliation glaucoma in the left eye. The patient underwent trabeculectomy with application of mitomycin C and thereafter developed ocular hypotony. The visual acuity was 20/40 in the left eye with an IOP of 4 mmHg. On examination, a large avascular bleb was noted; the anterior chamber was deep with patent peripheral iridectomy and open angle. Nuclear cataract was found and marked cupping of the optic disc with neuroretinal rim thinning temporally (A and B). VF testing disclosed superior paracentral and inferior nasal defects in the left eye (C and D). HRT showed rim thinning particularly inferior temporally (E and F).

Optical Coherence Tomography

The circumpapillary scan showed a generalized thinning of the retinal NFL (G and H). The macular retinal thickness was reduced inferiorly and temporally in the left eye; macular edema was present on the right, precluding assessment for glaucoma (I and J). Diminished temporal neuroretinal rim was noted on examination of the ONH (K and L).

Comments

The left macular OCT findings closely correspond to the superior paracentral defect seen in the VF test. The macular scan on the right is confounded by macular edema. NFL findings correspond with the VFs, but ONH findings failed to detect the superior NFL loss.

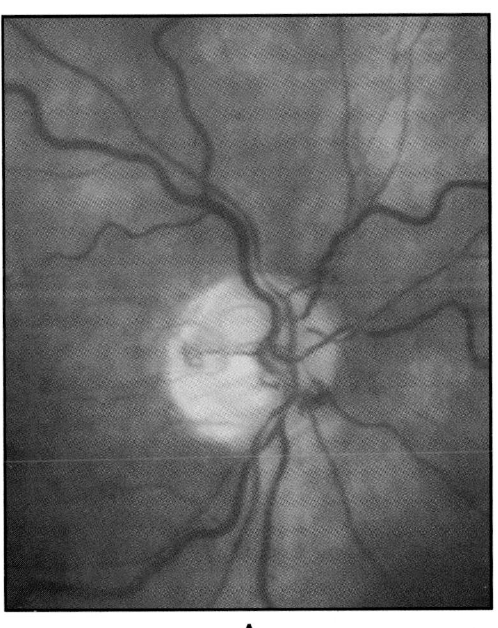

A

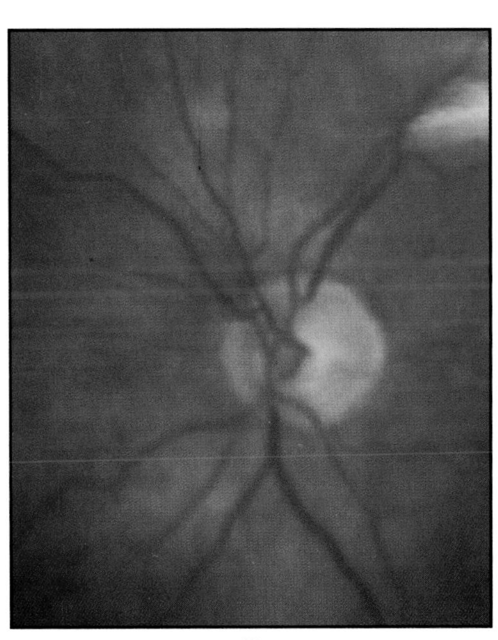

B

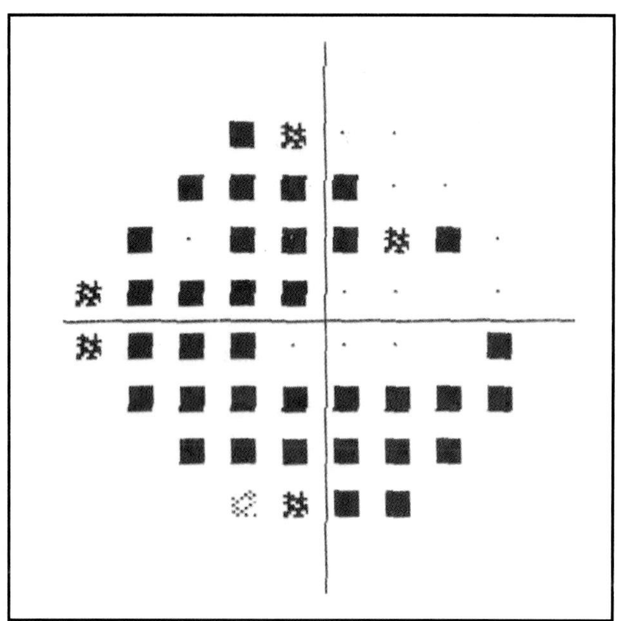

C

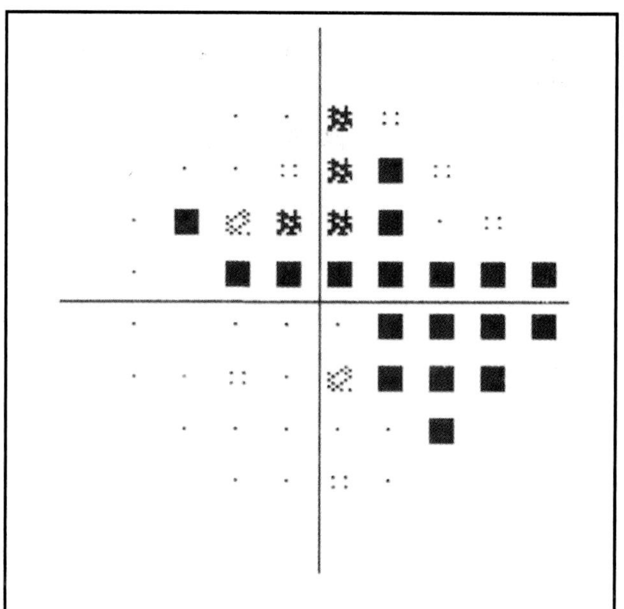

D

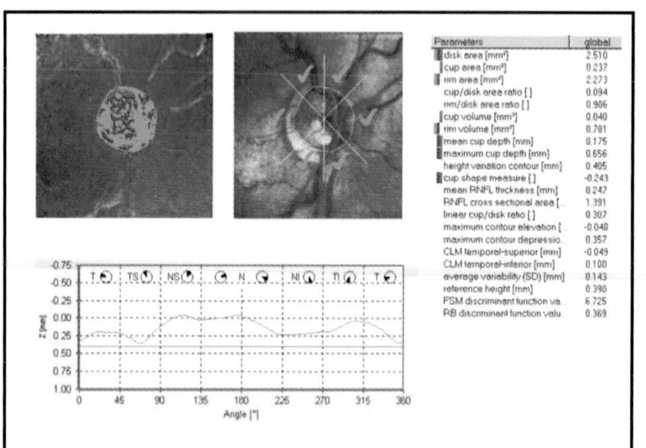
Parameters global
disk area [mm^2] 2.510
cup area [mm^2] 0.237
rim area [mm^2] 2.273
cup/disk area ratio [ ] 0.094
rim/disk area ratio [ ] 0.906
cup volume [mm^3] 0.040
rim volume [mm^3] 0.781
mean cup depth [mm] 0.175
maximum cup depth [mm] 0.656
height variation contour [mm] 0.405
cup shape measure [ ] -0.243
mean RNFL thickness [mm] 0.247
RNFL cross sectional area [... 1.391
linear cup/disk ratio [ ] 0.307
maximum contour elevation [... -0.048
maximum contour depressio... 0.357
CLM temporal-superior [mm] -0.049
CLM temporal-inferior [mm] 0.100
average variability (SD) [mm] 0.143
reference height [mm] 0.390
FSM discriminant function va... 6.725
RB discriminant function valu... 0.369
Angle [°]

E

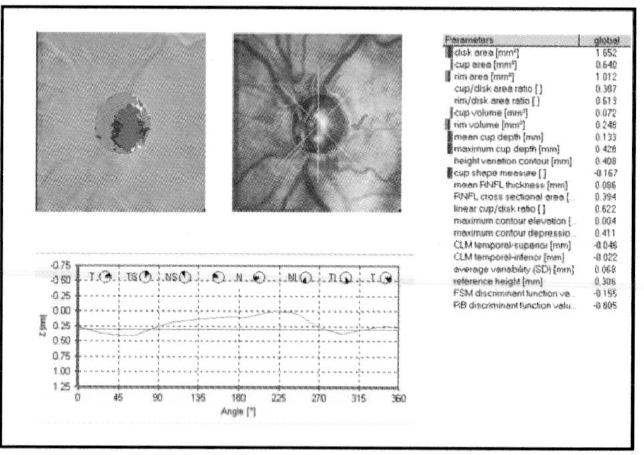
Parameters global
disk area [mm^2] 1.652
cup area [mm^2] 0.640
rim area [mm^2] 1.012
cup/disk area ratio [ ] 0.387
rim/disk area ratio [ ] 0.613
cup volume [mm^3] 0.072
rim volume [mm^3] 0.248
mean cup depth [mm] 0.133
maximum cup depth [mm] 0.428
height variation contour [mm] 0.408
cup shape measure [ ] -0.167
mean RNFL thickness [mm] 0.086
RNFL cross sectional area [... 0.394
linear cup/disk ratio [ ] 0.622
maximum contour elevation [... 0.004
maximum contour depressio... 0.411
CLM temporal-superior [mm] -0.046
CLM temporal-inferior [mm] -0.022
average variability (SD) [mm] 0.068
reference height [mm] 0.306
FSM discriminant function va... -0.155
RB discriminant function valu... -0.805
Angle [°]

F

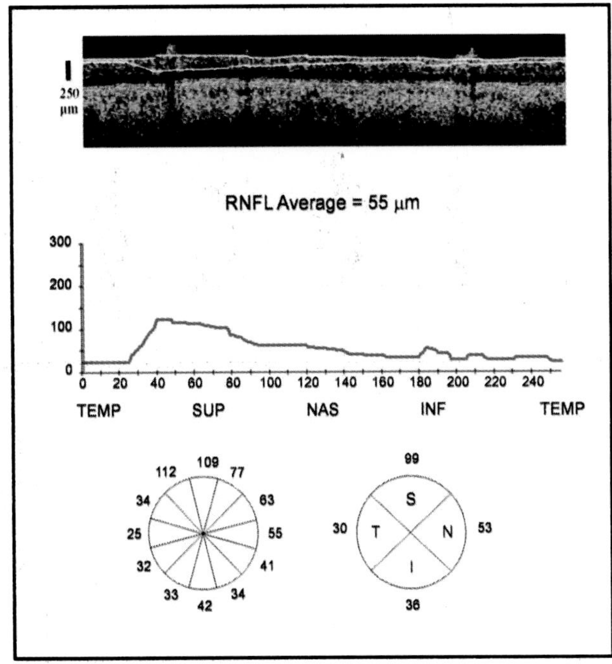
250 µm
RNFL Average = 55 µm
TEMP
SUP
NAS
INF
TEMP
99
S
T
N
I
30
53
36

G

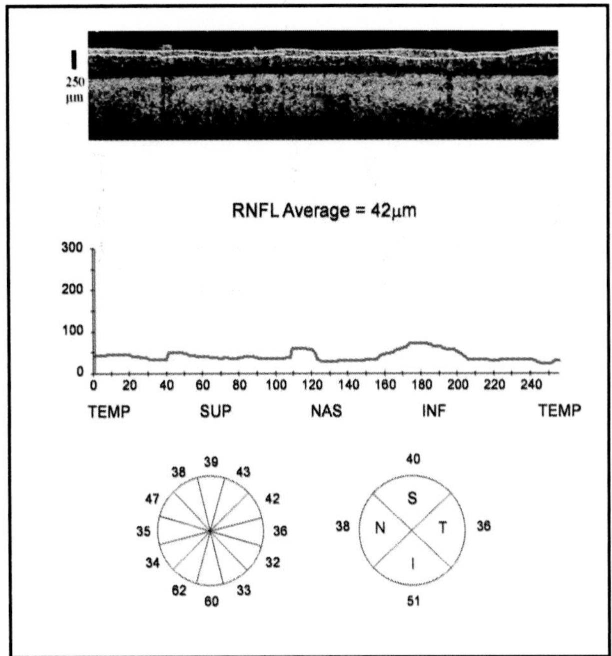
250 µm
RNFL Average = 42µm
TEMP
SUP
NAS
INF
TEMP
40
S
N
T
I
38
36
51

H

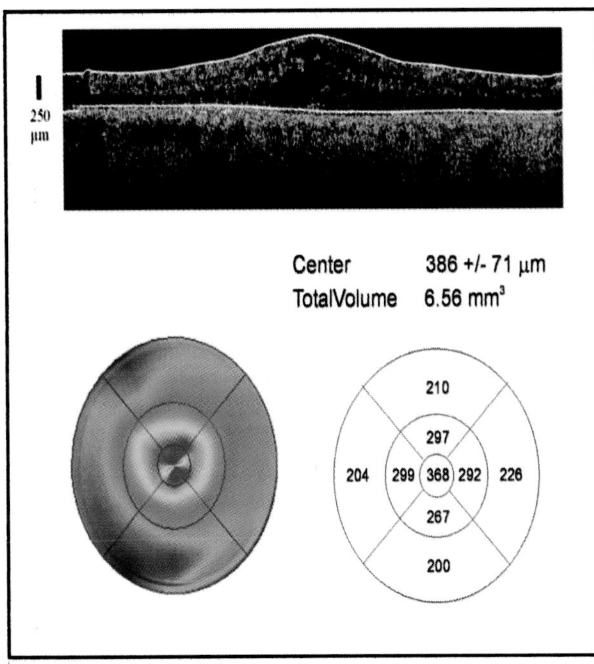
250 µm
Center 386 +/- 71 µm
TotalVolume 6.56 mm³
210
297
204
299
368
292
226
267
200

I

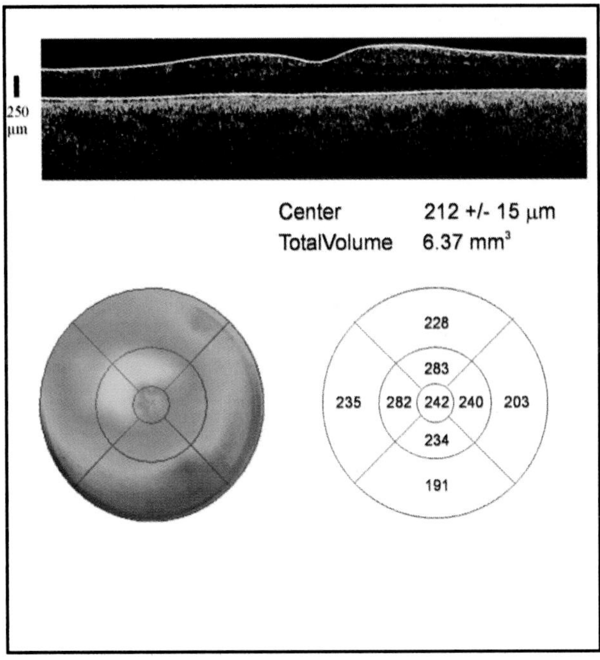
250 µm
Center 212 +/- 15 µm
TotalVolume 6.37 mm³
228
283
235
282
242
240
203
234
191

J

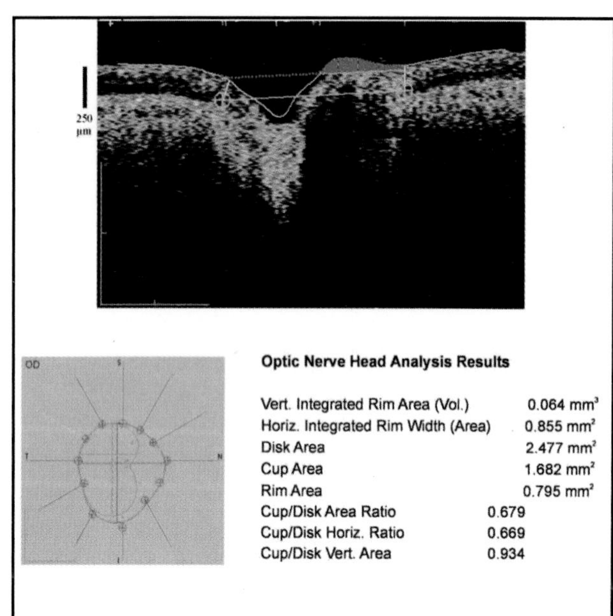
250 µm
OD
Optic Nerve Head Analysis Results
Vert. Integrated Rim Area (Vol.) 0.064 mm³
Horiz. Integrated Rim Width (Area) 0.855 mm²
Disk Area 2.477 mm²
Cup Area 1.682 mm²
Rim Area 0.795 mm²
Cup/Disk Area Ratio 0.679
Cup/Disk Horiz. Ratio 0.669
Cup/Disk Vert. Area 0.934

K

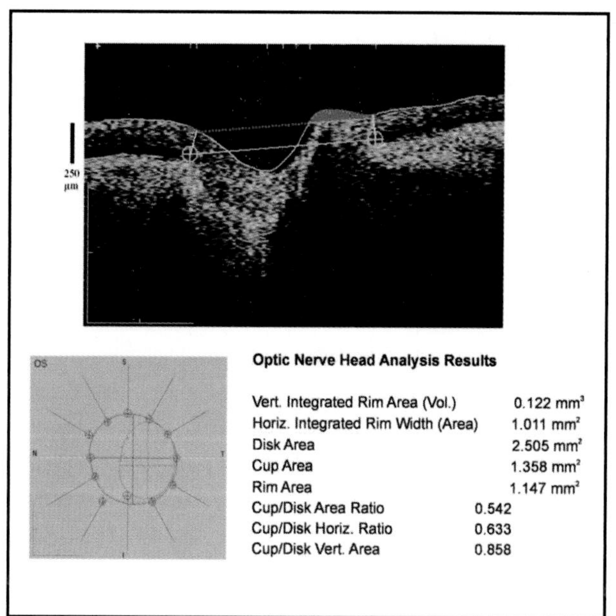
250 µm
OS
Optic Nerve Head Analysis Results
Vert. Integrated Rim Area (Vol.) 0.122 mm³
Horiz. Integrated Rim Width (Area) 1.011 mm²
Disk Area 2.505 mm²
Cup Area 1.358 mm²
Rim Area 1.147 mm²
Cup/Disk Area Ratio 0.542
Cup/Disk Horiz. Ratio 0.633
Cup/Disk Vert. Area 0.858

L

Case 12-31. Structure and Function Corresponded, With Retinal Nerve Fiber Layer Having the Closest Relationship to Visual Field Loss

A 62-year-old Caucasian female with normal tension glaucoma was treated with bimatoprost 0.03% in both eyes. On examination, the visual acuity was 20/16 in the right eye and 20/25 in the left eye and the IOP was 15 mmHg and 18 mmHg, respectively. Anterior chambers were unremarkable with open angles on gonioscopy; the posterior segment examination revealed a tilted disc with peripapillary atrophy in the right eye (A) and a normal appearing optic disc in the left eye with large cup (B). Humphrey VFs showed a superior hemifield defect with preserved central field in the right eye (C) and superior paracentral and nasal defects in the left eye (D). HRT scans revealed bilateral small disc areas with a tilted disc on the right. All segments had abnormally thin neuroretinal rim except the temporal segment in the right eye (E); the temporal segment was the only abnormal segment in the left eye (F).

Optical Coherence Tomography

The retinal NFL thickness was reduced in both eyes with thinner tissue in the left eye. The thickness measurements in the right eye in the superior half of the peripapillary region were near normal while the inferior part showed marked reduction (G). In the left eye, there was an overall reduction in thickness, most pronounced in the 5:00 to 7:00 sectors (H). The macular scans showed marked thinning of the retina in the outer temporal and inferior regions bilaterally (I and J). The disc scans revealed small discs with marked cupping in both eyes (K and L).

Comment

Retinal NFL thickness most closely corresponded with VF abnormalities, but the functional loss was reflected in the macular and ONH scanning as well.

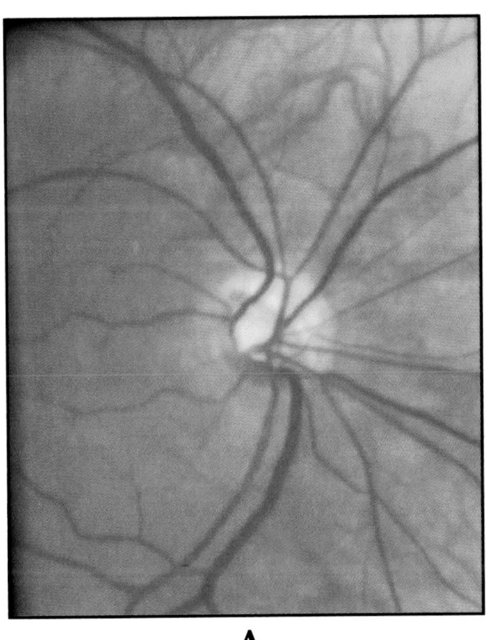

A

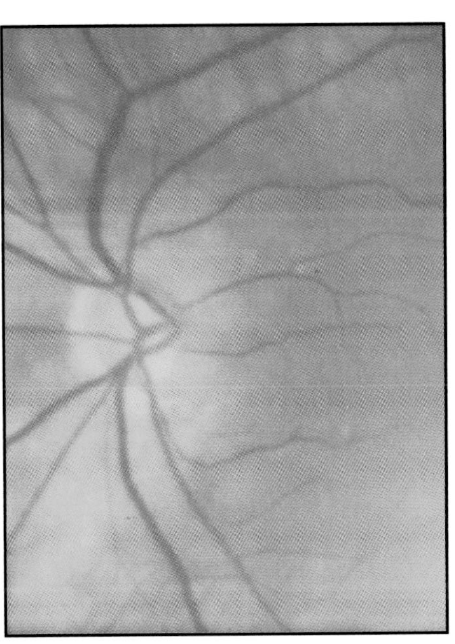

B

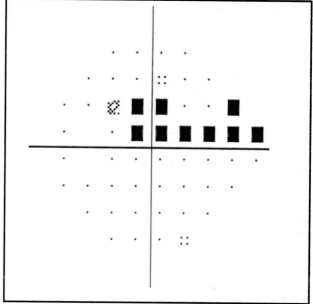

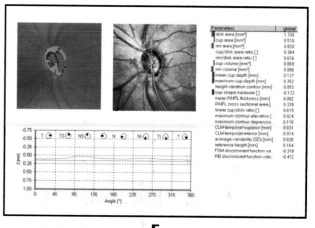

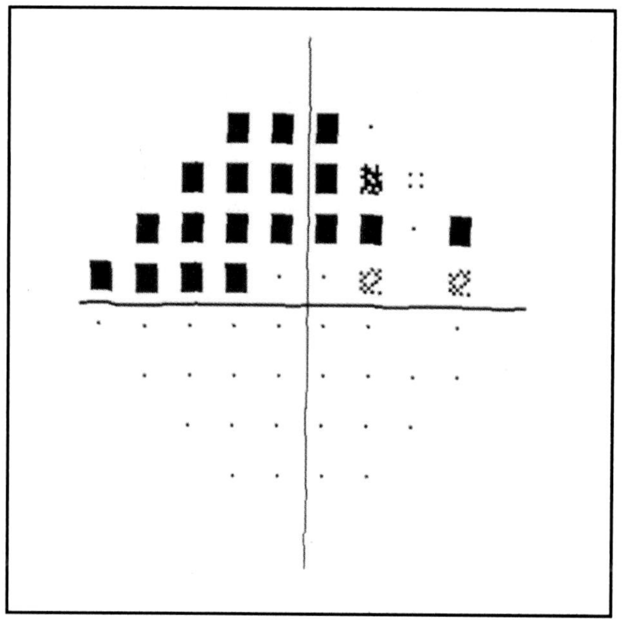

C

D

E

F

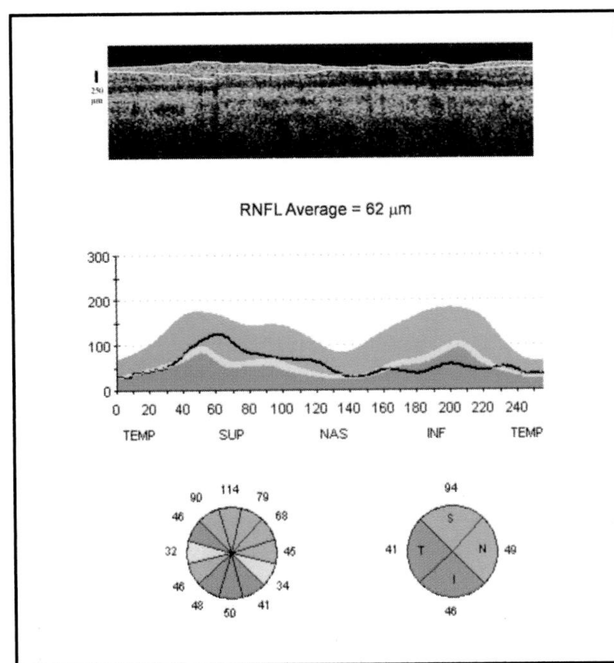

250 µm
RNFL Average = 62 µm
300
200
100
0
0 20 40 60 80 100 120 140 160 180 200 220 240
TEMP SUP NAS INF TEMP
90 114 79
46 68
32 45
46 34
48 50 41
94
S
41 T N 49
I
46

G

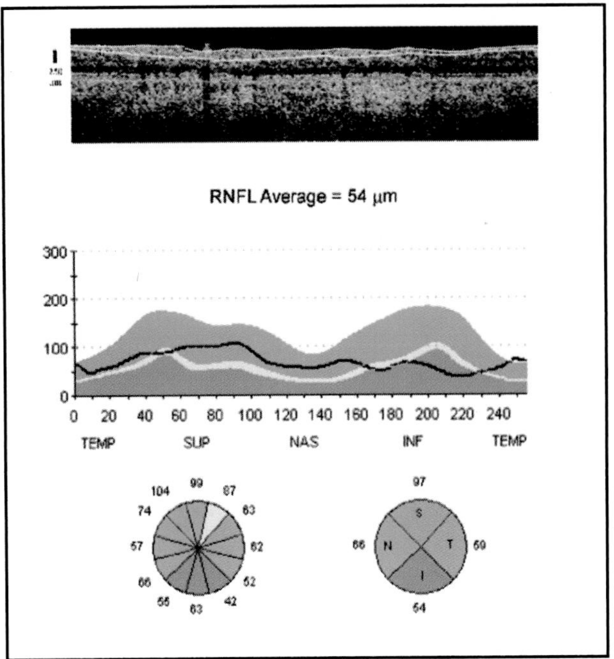

RNFL Average = 54 µm
300
200
100
0
0 20 40 60 80 100 120 140 160 180 200 220 240
TEMP SUP NAS INF TEMP
104 99 87
74 63
57 62
66 52
55 63 42
97
S
66 N T 69
I
54

H

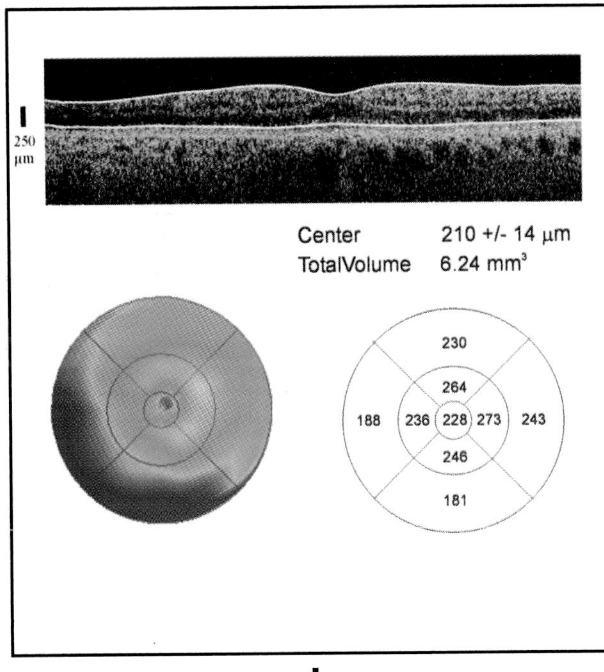

250 µm
Center 210 +/- 14 µm
TotalVolume 6.24 mm³
230
264
188 236 228 273 243
246
181

I

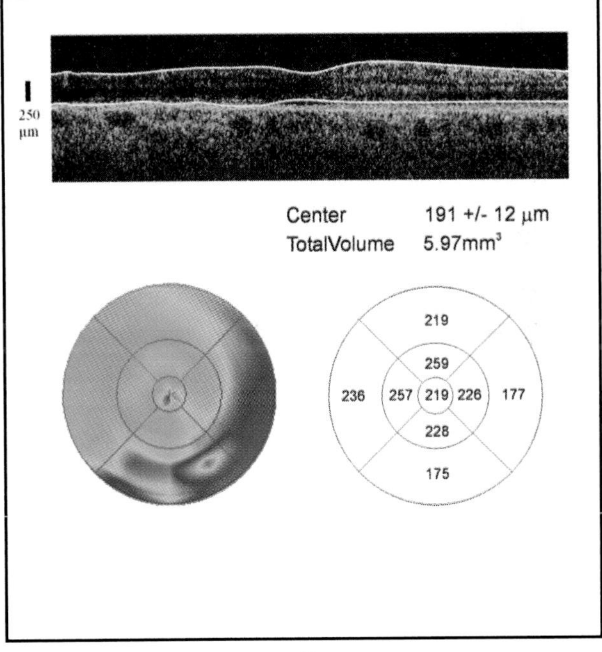

250 µm
Center 191 +/- 12 µm
TotalVolume 5.97mm³
219
259
236 257 219 226 177
228
175

J

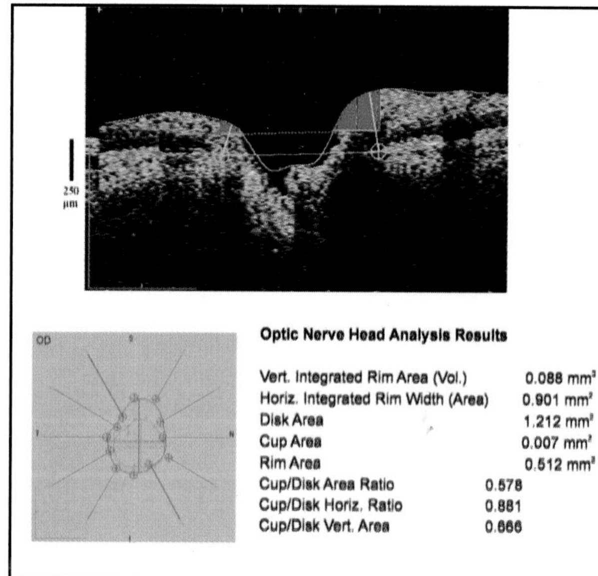
250 µm
OD
Optic Nerve Head Analysis Results
Vert. Integrated Rim Area (Vol.) 0.088 mm³
Horiz. Integrated Rim Width (Area) 0.901 mm²
Disk Area 1.212 mm²
Cup Area 0.007 mm²
Rim Area 0.512 mm²
Cup/Disk Area Ratio 0.578
Cup/Disk Horiz. Ratio 0.881
Cup/Disk Vert. Area 0.666

K

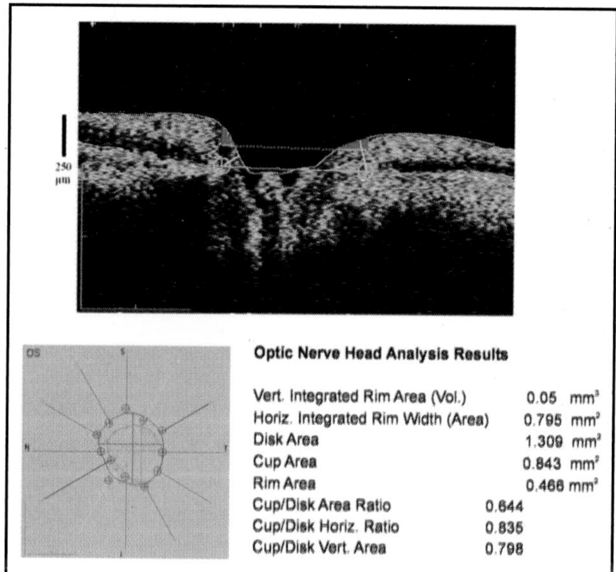
250 µm
OS
S
Optic Nerve Head Analysis Results
Vert. Integrated Rim Area (Vol.) 0.05 mm³
Horiz. Integrated Rim Width (Area) 0.795 mm²
Disk Area 1.309 mm²
Cup Area 0.843 mm²
Rim Area 0.466 mm²
Cup/Disk Area Ratio 0.644
Cup/Disk Horiz. Ratio 0.835
Cup/Disk Vert. Area 0.798

L

Case 12-32. Nerve Fiber Layer Thinning Corresponded to Severe Visual Field Loss in Advanced Glaucoma. Macular Thickness Was Normal, Which Suggested Confounding by Another Macular Disease

A 75-year-old Caucasian man underwent trabeculectomy with mitomycin C application for advanced primary open-angle glaucoma in the left eye. Ocular medication included latanoprost 0.005% once daily. Visual acuity in the left eye was 20/40 and IOP was 14 mmHg. A functioning superior bleb was noted with a deep and quiet anterior chamber. There was marked ONH cupping with thinning of the temporal neuroretinal rim and peripapillary atrophy (A). VF testing disclosed advanced generalized VF loss with preservation of a central island (B). HRT showed thinning of the neuroretinal rim in the entire temporal aspect of the ONH (C).

Optical Coherence Tomography

Remarkable retinal NFL thinning was noted in the entire circumpapillary scan with an average retinal NFL of only 16 µm (D). Surprisingly, the macular scan revealed a near normal retinal thickness (E); the ONH scan demonstrated obliteration of the rim in the entire temporal aspect of the disc (F).

Comment

Advanced damage was clearly shown by the severe NFL loss in the peripapillary region. The normal macular thickness may have been related to other retinal diseases, such as macular edema. Note the loss of the normal foveal contour, indicating macular thickening. This demonstrated one of the shortcomings of measuring macular thickness to assess glaucoma.

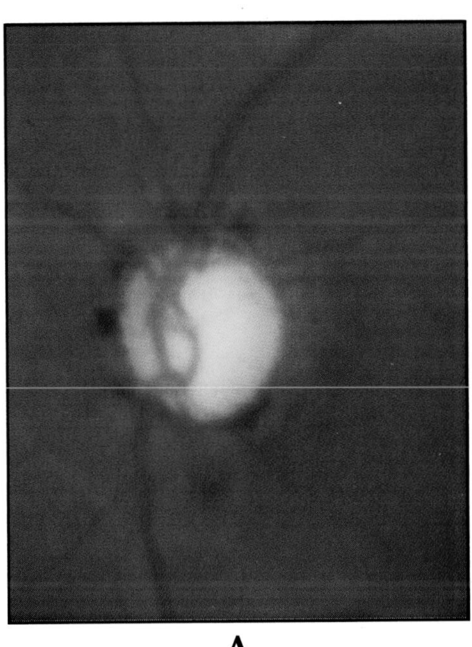

A

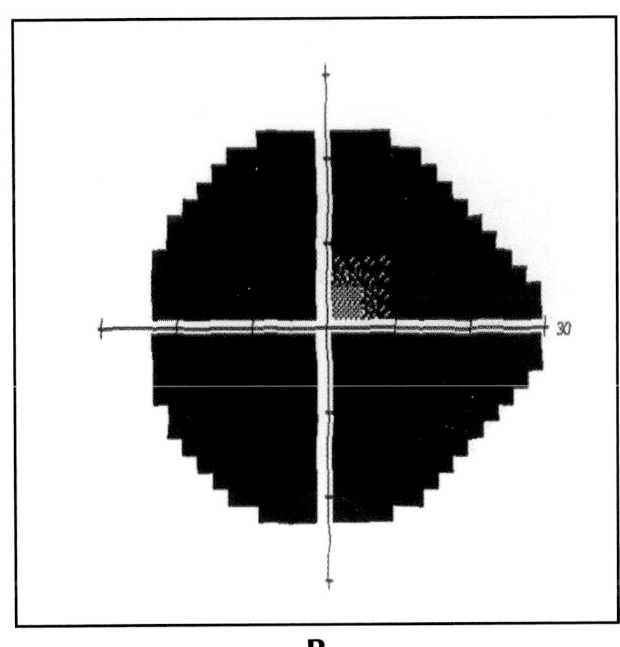

B

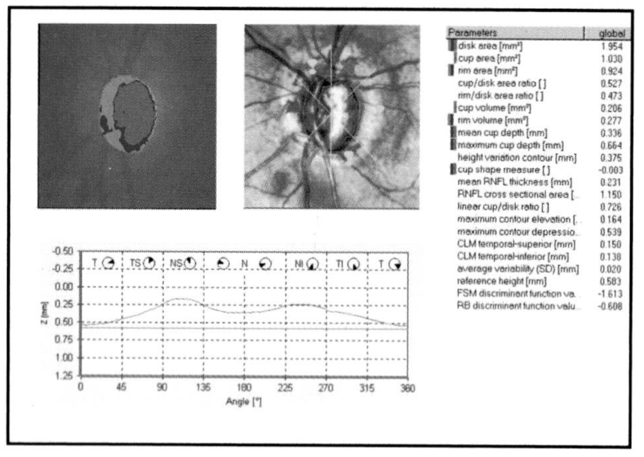

Parameters	global
disk area [mm²]	1.954
cup area [mm²]	1.030
rim area [mm²]	0.924
cup/disk area ratio [ ]	0.527
rim/disk area ratio [ ]	0.473
cup volume [mm³]	0.206
rim volume [mm³]	0.277
mean cup depth [mm]	0.336
maximum cup depth [mm]	0.664
height variation contour [mm]	0.375
cup shape measure [ ]	-0.003
mean RNFL thickness [mm]	0.231
RNFL cross sectional area [...	1.150
linear cup/disk ratio [ ]	0.726
maximum contour elevation [...	0.164
maximum contour depressio...	0.539
CLM temporal-superior [mm]	0.150
CLM temporal-inferior [mm]	0.138
average variability (SD) [mm]	0.020
reference height [mm]	0.583
FSM discriminant function va...	-1.613
RB discriminant function valu...	-0.608

C

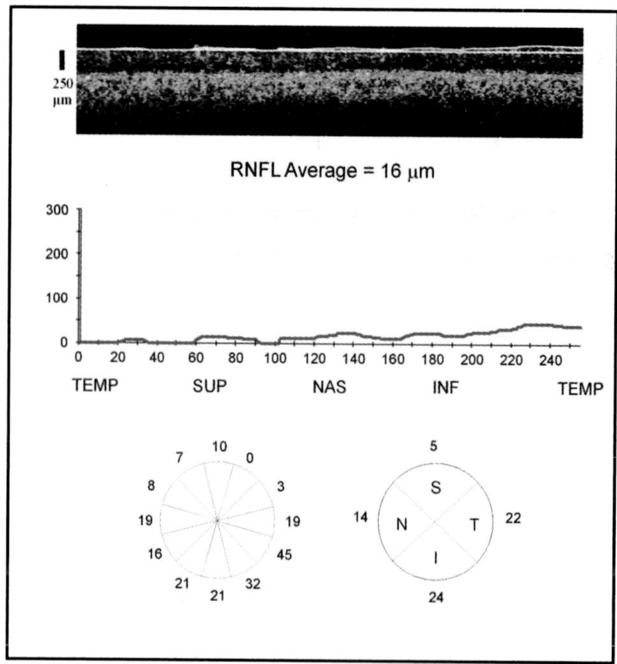

D

250 µm

Center 209 +/- 8 µm

TotalVolume 6.72 mm³

232

243

233 249 218 259 261

253

212

E

250 µm

OS

Optic Nerve Head Analysis Results

Vert. Integrated Rim Area (Vol.)	0.086 mm³
Horiz. Integrated Rim Width (Area)	0.818 mm²
Disk Area	2.71 mm²
Cup Area	1.438 mm²
Rim Area	0.633 mm²
Cup/Disk Area Ratio	0.694
Cup/Disk Horiz. Ratio	0.77
Cup/Disk Vert. Area	0.897

F

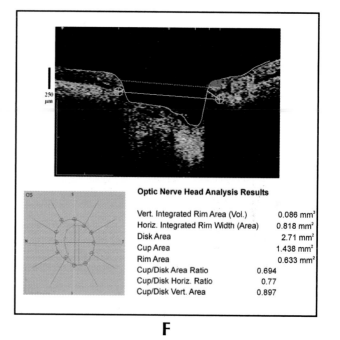

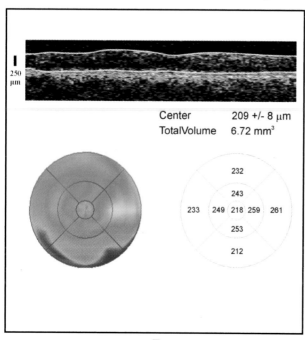

Case 12-33. Good Structure-Function Correspondence of Glaucomatous Damage on the Right With Borderline Abnormal Structure on the Left Suggested That Functional Loss May Develop on the Left

A 50-year-old African-American man with primary open-angle glaucoma in the right eye was treated with selective laser trabeculoplasty as well as bimatoprost 0.03% and brinzolamide 1%. On examination, the visual acuity was 20/25 and the IOP was 14 mmHg. The anterior segment was normal, and posterior segment examination disclosed asymmetric optic nerve cupping (A and B); the cup was larger in the right eye and there was peripapillary atrophy. Frequency doubling technology showed superior nasal and paracentral central defects (C and D). HRT showed inferior rim notching (E and F).

Optical Coherence Tomography

The right eye circumpapillary scan had an overall reduction in the retinal NFL thickness with damping of the inferior hump of the "double hump" pattern (G). Marked thinning was evident between 6:00 and 8:00 and also at 1:00. The circumpapillary scan on the left had a lower than normal average NFL thickness, although no frank VF defects were present (H). Macular thickness was reduced in the inferior and temporal outer sectors on the right (I), and there was a suggestion of macular thinning in the outer temporal and inferior regions on the left (J). ONH analysis revealed a normal sized disc with a large cup on the right (K). ONH size on the left was small with a smaller cup (L).

Comment

There was good structure-function correspondence on the right. The structural measures suggested that functional loss may develop on the left at some future time.

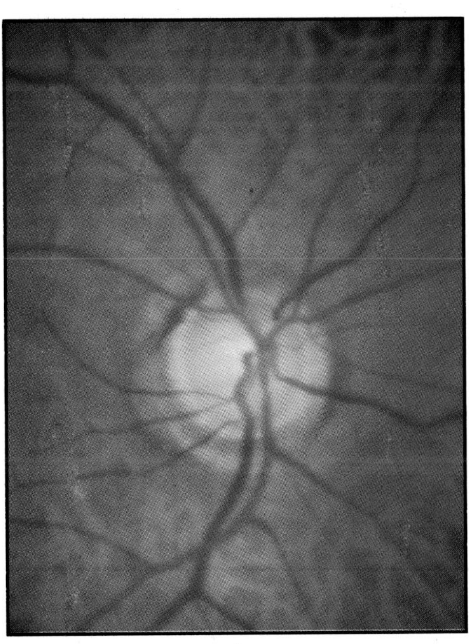

A

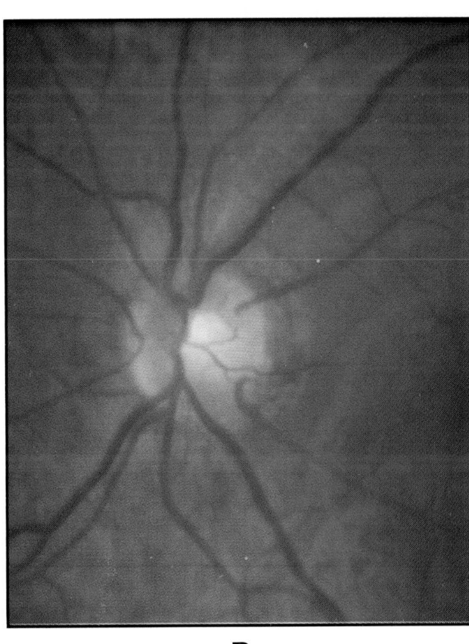

B

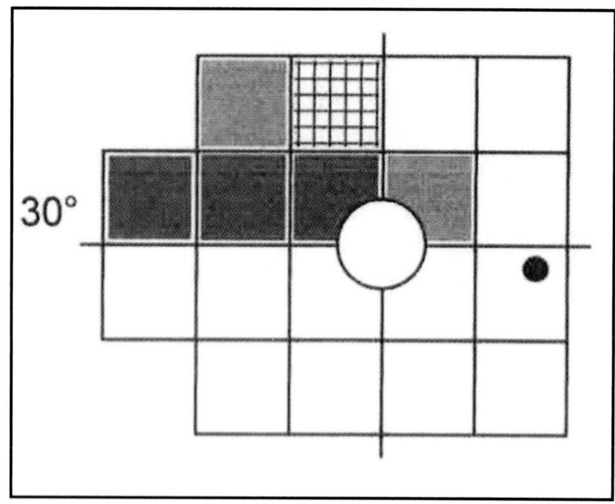

C

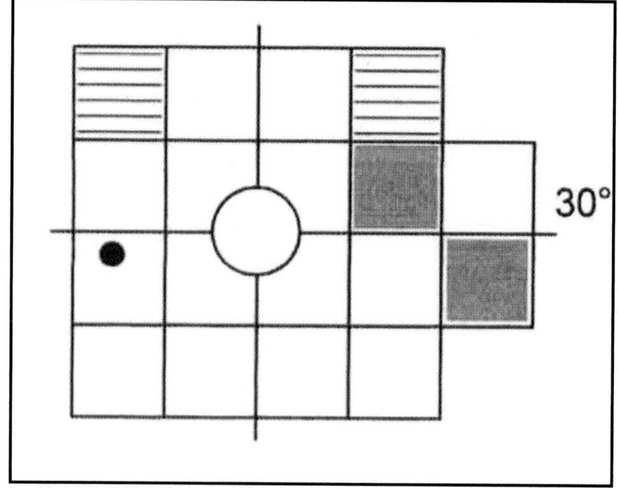

D

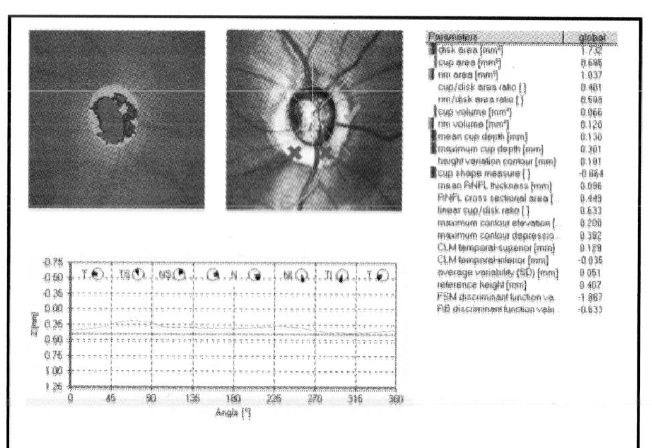

Parameters	global
disk area [mm²]	1.732
cup area [mm²]	0.695
rim area [mm²]	1.037
cup/disk area ratio [ ]	0.401
rim/disk area ratio [ ]	0.599
cup volume [mm³]	0.066
rim volume [mm³]	0.120
mean cup depth [mm]	0.130
maximum cup depth [mm]	0.301
height variation contour [mm]	0.191
cup shape measure [ ]	-0.064
mean RNFL thickness [mm]	0.096
RNFL cross sectional area [...	0.449
linear cup/disk ratio [ ]	0.633
maximum contour elevation [...	0.200
maximum contour depressio...	0.392
CLM temporal-superior [mm]	0.129
CLM temporal-inferior [mm]	-0.035
average variability (SD) [mm]	0.051
reference height [mm]	0.407
FSM discriminant function va...	-1.867
RB discriminant function valu...	-0.633

E

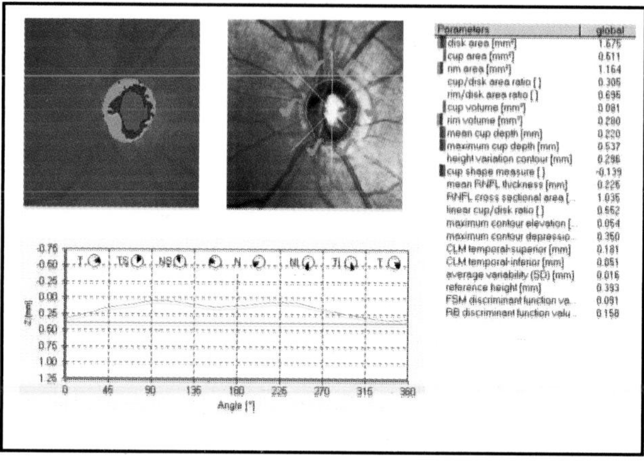

Parameters	global
disk area [mm²]	1.675
cup area [mm²]	0.511
rim area [mm²]	1.164
cup/disk area ratio [ ]	0.305
rim/disk area ratio [ ]	0.695
cup volume [mm³]	0.081
rim volume [mm³]	0.280
mean cup depth [mm]	0.220
maximum cup depth [mm]	0.537
height variation contour [mm]	0.298
cup shape measure [ ]	-0.139
mean RNFL thickness [mm]	0.226
RNFL cross sectional area [...	1.035
linear cup/disk ratio [ ]	0.552
maximum contour elevation [...	0.064
maximum contour depressio...	0.350
CLM temporal-superior [mm]	0.181
CLM temporal-inferior [mm]	0.051
average variability (SD) [mm]	0.016
reference height [mm]	0.393
FSM discriminant function va...	0.091
RB discriminant function valu...	0.158

F

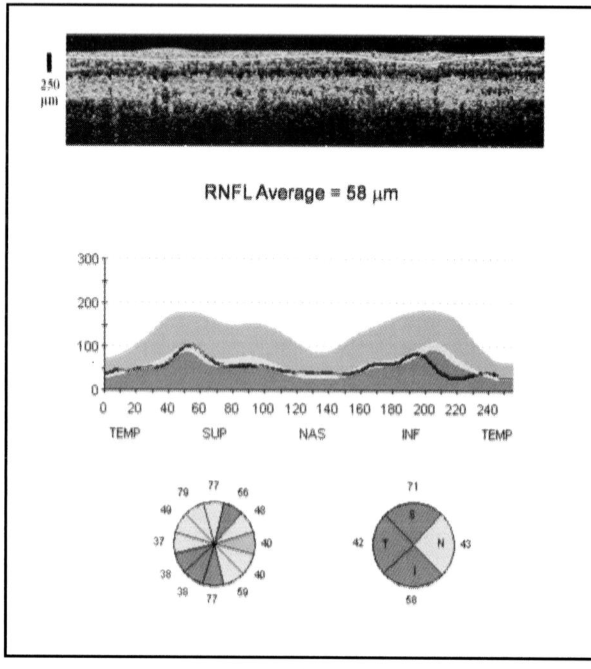

G

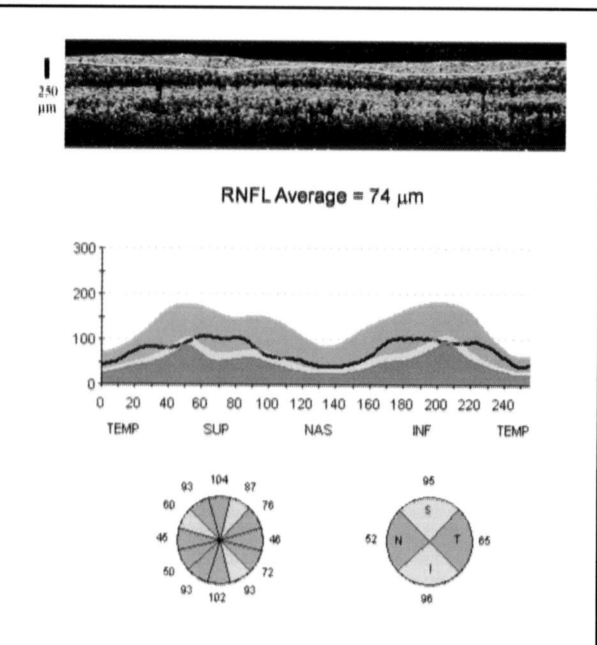

H

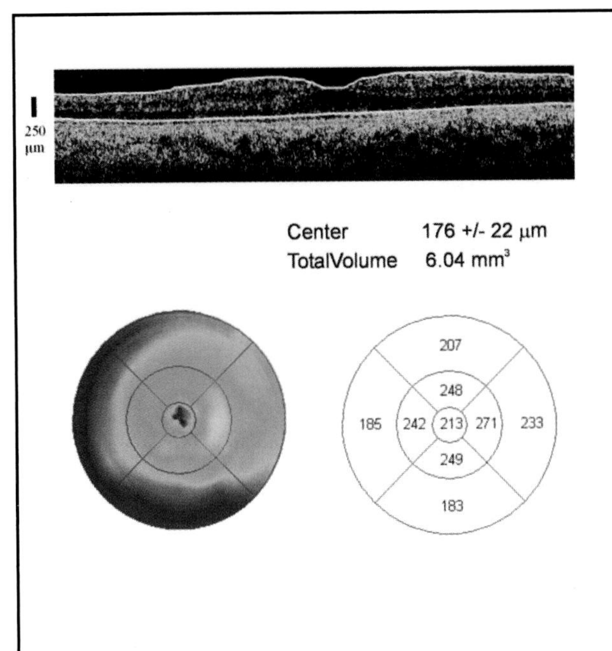

250
µm
Center 176 +/- 22 µm
TotalVolume 6.04 mm³
207
248
185
242
213
271
233
249
183

I

250
µm
Center 197 +/- 9 µm
TotalVolume 6.85 mm³
240
285
261
297
233
274
209
289
209

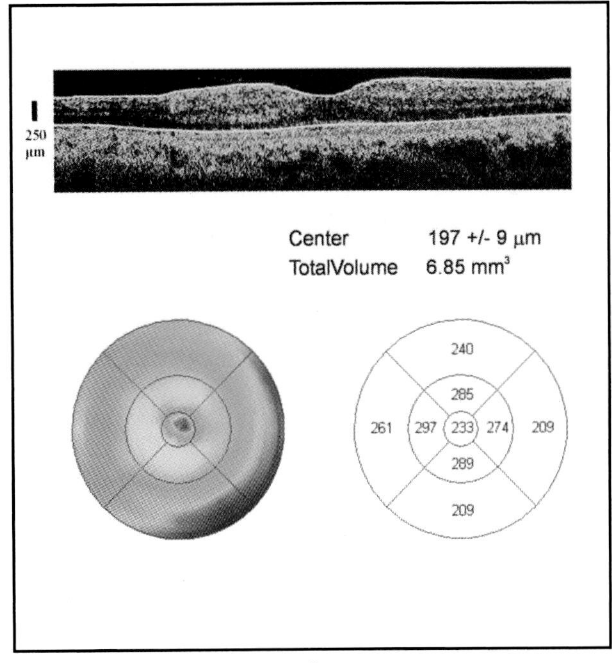

J

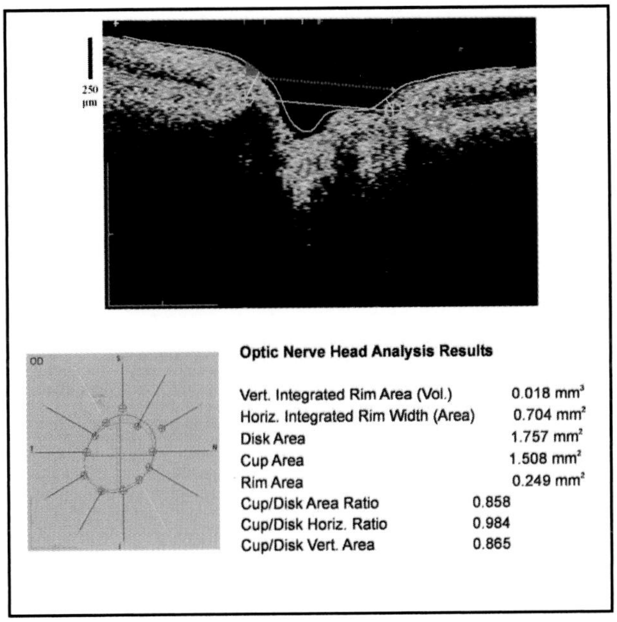

250
µm
OD
Optic Nerve Head Analysis Results
Vert. Integrated Rim Area (Vol.) 0.018 mm³
Horiz. Integrated Rim Width (Area) 0.704 mm²
Disk Area 1.757 mm²
Cup Area 1.508 mm²
Rim Area 0.249 mm²
Cup/Disk Area Ratio 0.858
Cup/Disk Horiz. Ratio 0.984
Cup/Disk Vert. Area 0.865

K

250
µm
OS
Optic Nerve Head Analysis Results
Vert. Integrated Rim Area (Vol.) 0.208 mm³
Horiz. Integrated Rim Width (Area) 1.409 mm²
Disk Area 1.984 mm²
Cup Area 0.683 mm²
Rim Area 1.301 mm²
Cup/Disk Area Ratio 0.344
Cup/Disk Horiz. Ratio 0.611
Cup/Disk Vert. Area 0.628

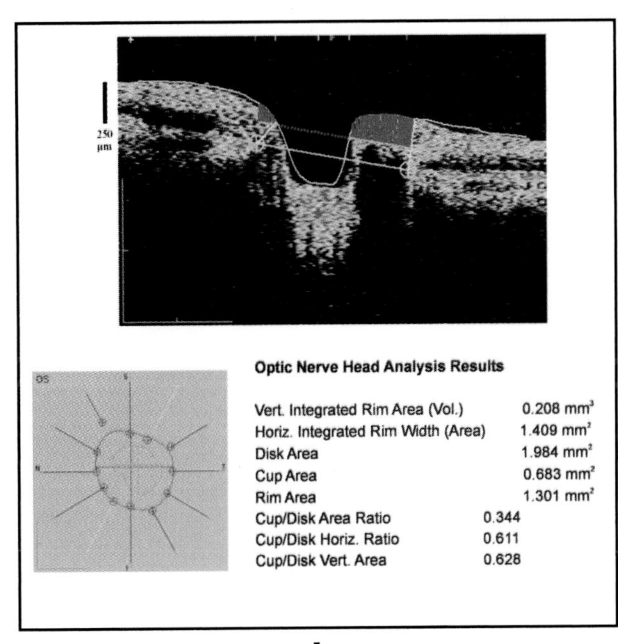

L

Case 12-34. Structural Damage on Optical Coherence Tomography May Be Harbinger of Future Further Visual Field Loss

An 85-year-old Caucasian man with ARMD and primary open-angle glaucoma in both eyes was treated with trabeculectomies. The visual acuity was 20/25 in the right eye and 20/30 on the left and the IOPs were 5 mmHg and 8 mmHg, respectively. Anterior chamber examination was normal with open angles on gonioscopy. Multiple hard drusen were noted in both maculae, and the ONHs had small central cups (A and B). Visual fields showed an early superior nasal defect in the right eye (C) and early superior arcuate and nasal defects in the left eye (D). The HRTs were of marginal quality (E and F).

Optical Coherence Tomography

Peripapillary OCT scanning showed marked thinning of the retinal NFL in the right eye between 5:00 and 8:00 (G). The left eye had thinner average retinal NFL thickness than that of the right eye with marked damage from 1:00 to 7:00 (H). In both eyes, there was total elimination of the inferior hump from the "double hump" pattern. The macular scan of the right eye showed mild reduction of the retinal thickness in the outer inferior and temporal sectors (I). Similar to the findings in the peripapillary scan, the macular scan of the left eye showed more pronounced damage than the right eye mainly in the inferior and temporal regions (J). There was no evidence of confounding of the macular scans by the patient's ARMD. A larger optic disc cup was found in the right eye compared to the left eye, and in both eyes there was thinning of the neuroretinal rim in the temporal inferior sector (K and L). OCT described larger cups than did HRT.

Comments

The VF test showed early damage that was similar in both eyes; possibly deeper on the right and broader on the left. The OCT scans showed more pronounced tissue damage in the peripapillary NFL and the macula in the left eye. This suggested that the left eye would be more likely to show further glaucomatous damage on VF testing in the future.

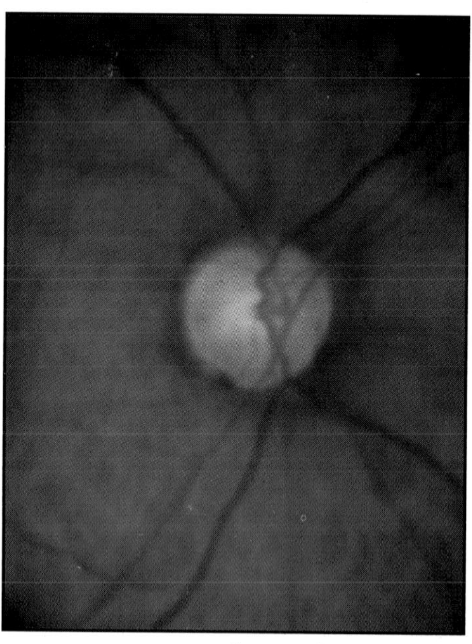

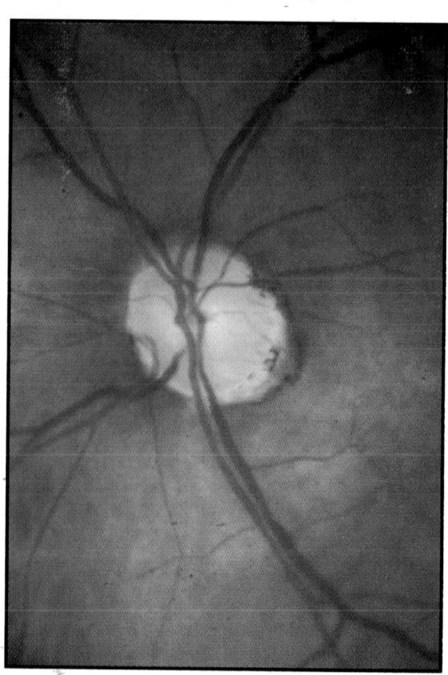

B

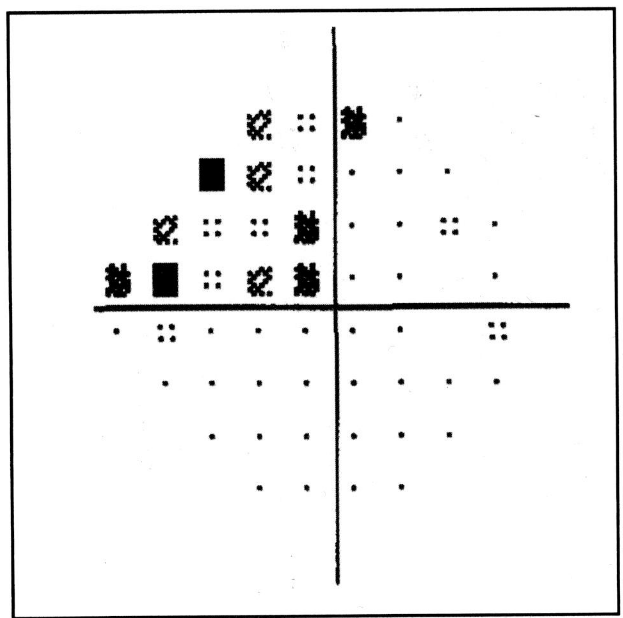

C

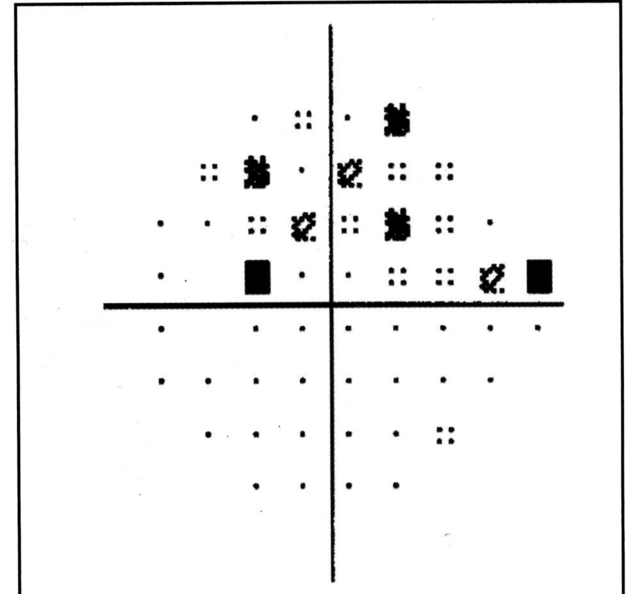

D

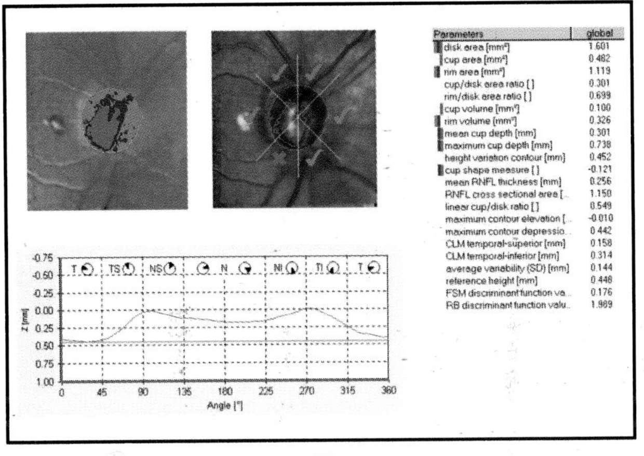

Parameters	global
disk area [mm²]	1.601
cup area [mm²]	0.482
rim area [mm²]	1.119
cup/disk area ratio [ ]	0.301
rim/disk area ratio [ ]	0.699
cup volume [mm³]	0.100
rim volume [mm³]	0.326
mean cup depth [mm]	0.301
maximum cup depth [mm]	0.738
height variation contour [mm]	0.452
cup shape measure [ ]	-0.121
mean RNFL thickness [mm]	0.256
RNFL cross sectional area [...	1.150
linear cup/disk ratio [ ]	0.549
maximum contour elevation [...	-0.010
maximum contour depressio...	0.442
CLM temporal-superior [mm]	0.158
CLM temporal-inferior [mm]	0.314
average variability (SD) [mm]	0.144
reference height [mm]	0.448
FSM discriminant function va...	0.176
RB discriminant function valu...	1.989

E

Parameters	global
disk area [mm²]	1.657
cup area [mm²]	0.189
rim area [mm²]	1.468
cup/disk area ratio [ ]	0.114
rim/disk area ratio [ ]	0.886
cup volume [mm³]	0.008
rim volume [mm³]	0.289
mean cup depth [mm]	0.085
maximum cup depth [mm]	0.262
height variation contour [mm]	0.290
cup shape measure [ ]	-0.171
mean RNFL thickness [mm]	0.174
RNFL cross sectional area [...	0.799
linear cup/disk ratio [ ]	0.338
maximum contour elevation [...	-0.115
maximum contour depressio...	0.176
CLM temporal-superior [mm]	0.165
CLM temporal-inferior [mm]	0.019
average variability (SD) [mm]	0.114
reference height [mm]	0.223
FSM discriminant function va...	1.586
RB discriminant function valu...	0.495

F

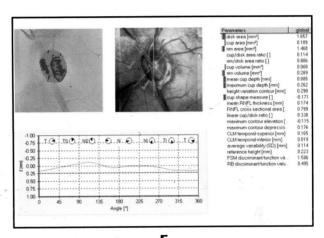

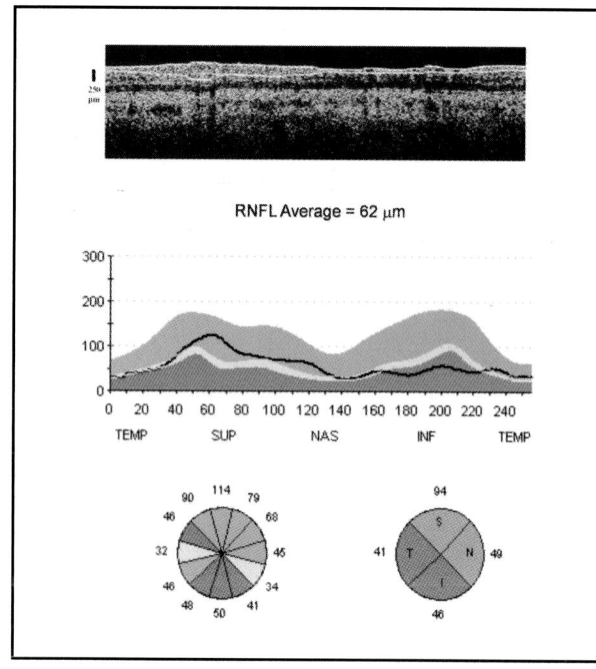

RNFL Average = 62 µm
300
200
100
0
0 20 40 60 80 100 120 140 160 180 200 220 240
TEMP SUP NAS INF TEMP
114 79 68 45 34 41 50 48 46 32 46 90
94 49 46 41
S N I T

G

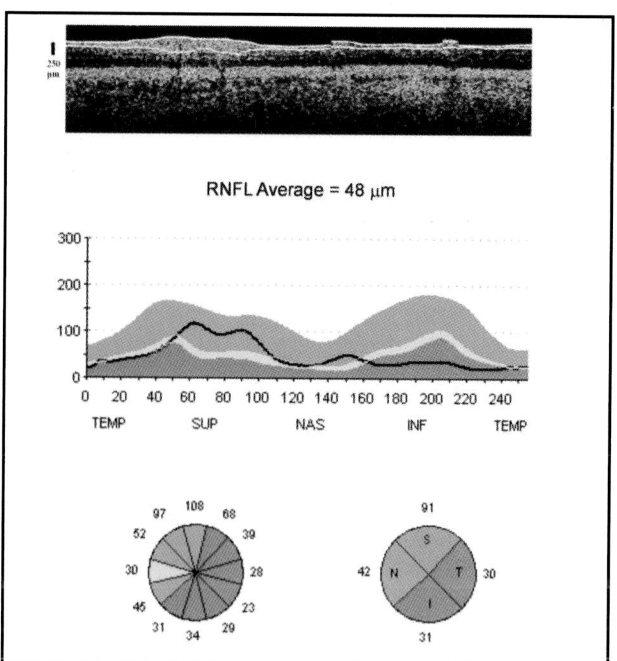

RNFL Average = 48 µm
300
200
100
0
0 20 40 60 80 100 120 140 160 180 200 220 240
TEMP SUP NAS INF TEMP
108 68 39 28 23 29 34 31 45 30 52 97
91 30 31 42
S T I N

H

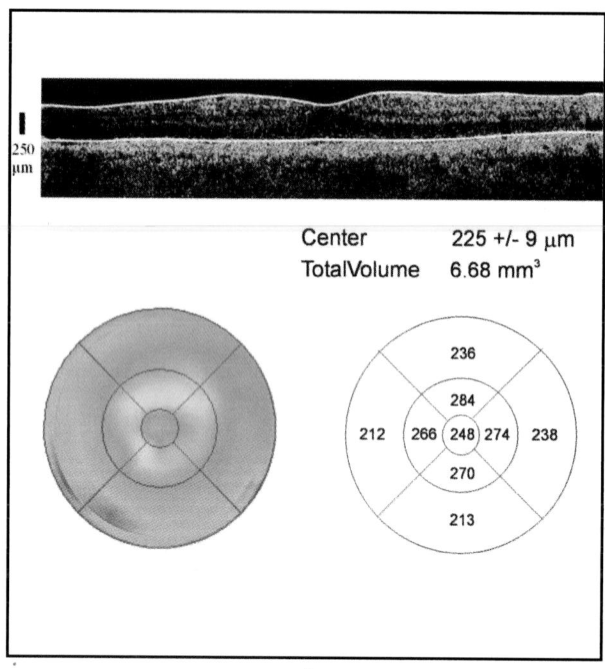

250 µm
Center 225 +/- 9 µm
TotalVolume 6.68 mm³
236
284
212 266 248 274 238
270
213

I

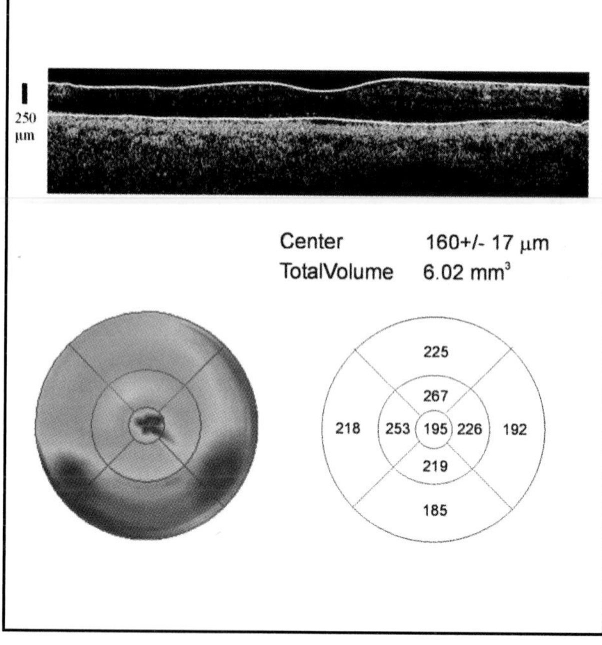

250 µm
Center 160+/- 17 µm
TotalVolume 6.02 mm³
225
267
218 253 195 226 192
219
185

J

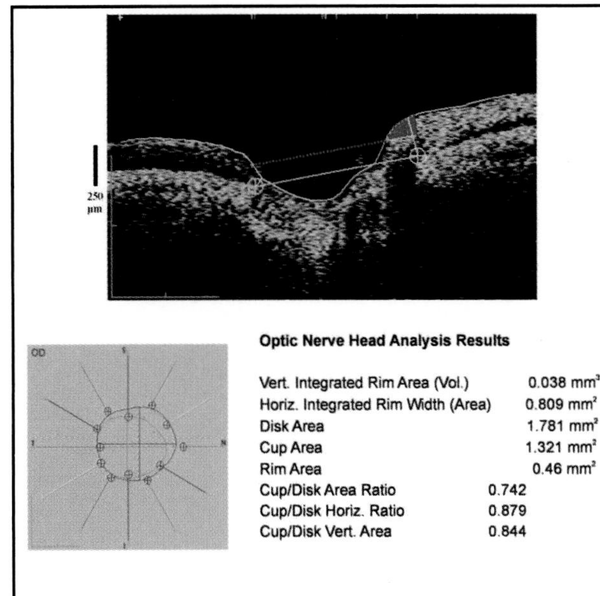
250 µm
OD
Optic Nerve Head Analysis Results
Vert. Integrated Rim Area (Vol.) 0.038 mm³
Horiz. Integrated Rim Width (Area) 0.809 mm²
Disk Area 1.781 mm²
Cup Area 1.321 mm²
Rim Area 0.46 mm²
Cup/Disk Area Ratio 0.742
Cup/Disk Horiz. Ratio 0.879
Cup/Disk Vert. Area 0.844

K

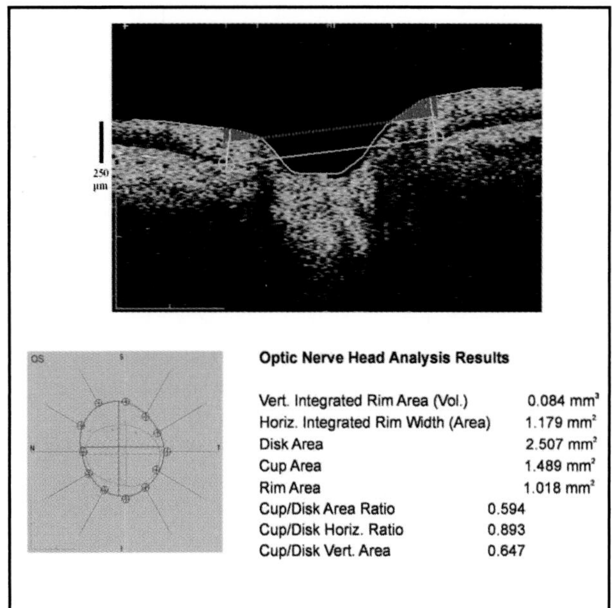
250 µm
OS
Optic Nerve Head Analysis Results
Vert. Integrated Rim Area (Vol.) 0.084 mm³
Horiz. Integrated Rim Width (Area) 1.179 mm²
Disk Area 2.507 mm²
Cup Area 1.489 mm²
Rim Area 1.018 mm²
Cup/Disk Area Ratio 0.594
Cup/Disk Horiz. Ratio 0.893
Cup/Disk Vert. Area 0.647

L

Case 12-35. Nerve Fiber Layer, Optic Nerve Head, and Macula Corresponded With Visual Field; Superior Structural Abnormalities May Presage Inferior Visual Field Loss

A 28-year-old Caucasian man with juvenile open-angle glaucoma underwent trabeculectomy with local application of 5-FU to the right eye. The patient resumed treatment with timolol 0.5% due to postoperative high IOP. On examination, the visual acuity was 20/30 and the IOP was 14 mmHg. A functional bleb was noted. The anterior chamber was deep and quiet and there was a patent peripheral iridectomy. An epiretinal membrane was noted in the right macula, and there was marked optic disc cupping with peripapillary atrophy (A and B). Humphrey VFs disclosed superior nasal and central defects in the right eye (C).

Optical Coherence Tomography

Retinal NFL thickness was reduced on the circumpapillary scan from 6:00 to 8:00 and 10:00 (D). Thinning of the macular retina was noted in the outer inferior region (E). Optic disc analysis showed thinned neuroretinal rim inferior temporally (F).

Comments

The thinnest retinal NFL was noted inferior temporally corresponding to the superior VF defect and the ONH and macula. Note that borderline thinning was also noted in the outer temporal superior macula, which is not yet evident in the inferior part of the VF.

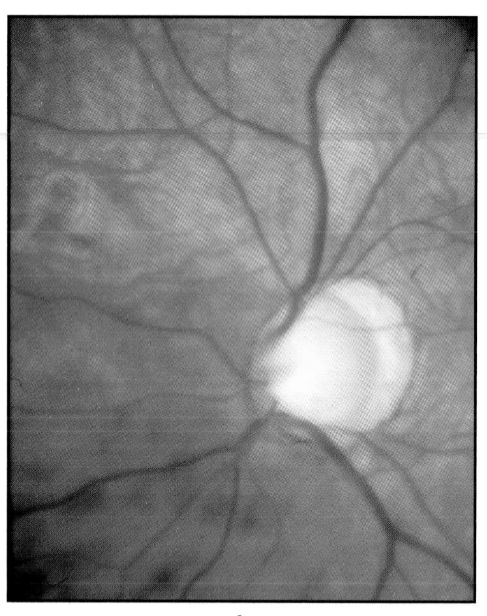

A

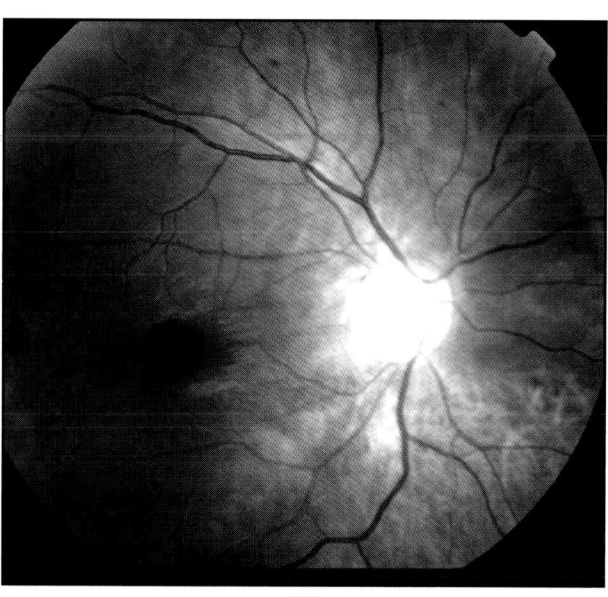

B

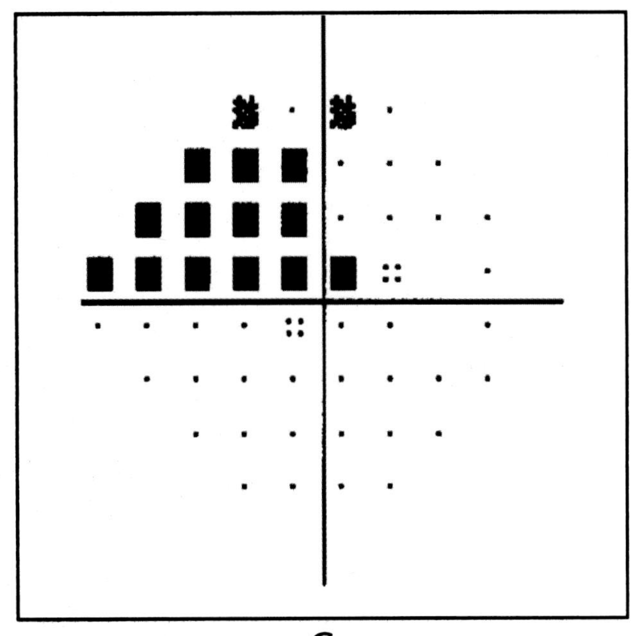

C

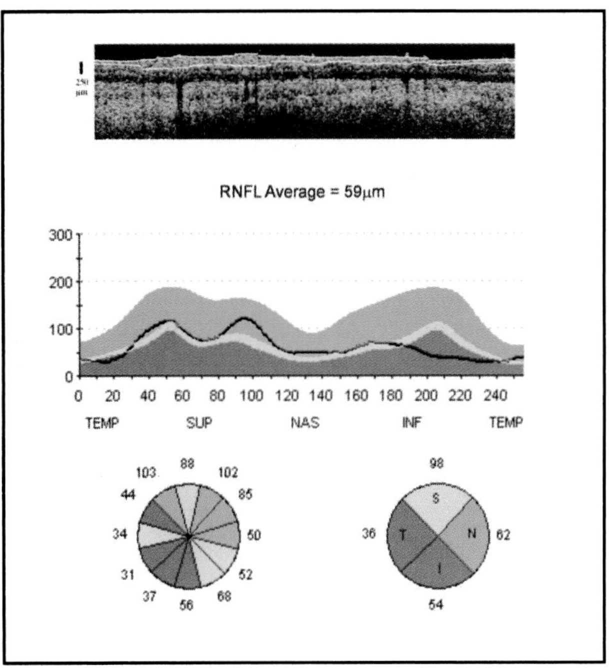
250 µm
RNFL Average = 59µm
300
200
100
0
0 20 40 60 80 100 120 140 160 180 200 220 240
TEMP SUP NAS INF TEMP
103 88 102
44 85
34 50
31 52
37 56 68
98
S
36 T N 62
I
54

D

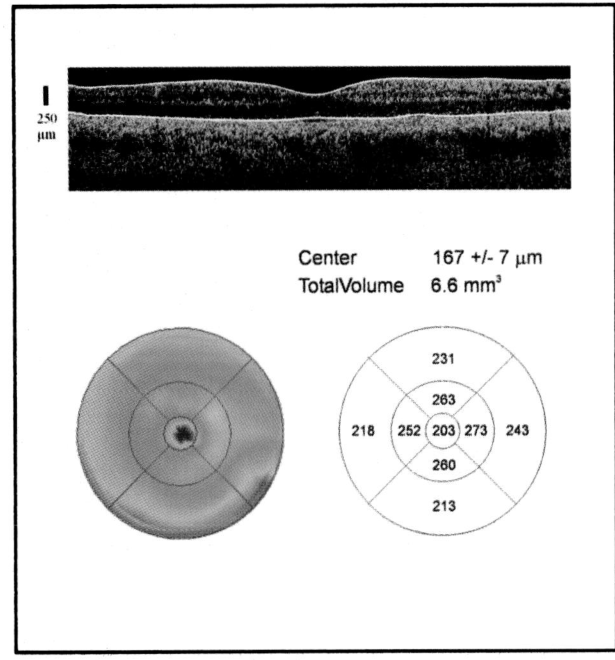
250 µm
Center 167 +/- 7 µm
TotalVolume 6.6 mm³
231
263
218 252 203 273 243
260
213

E

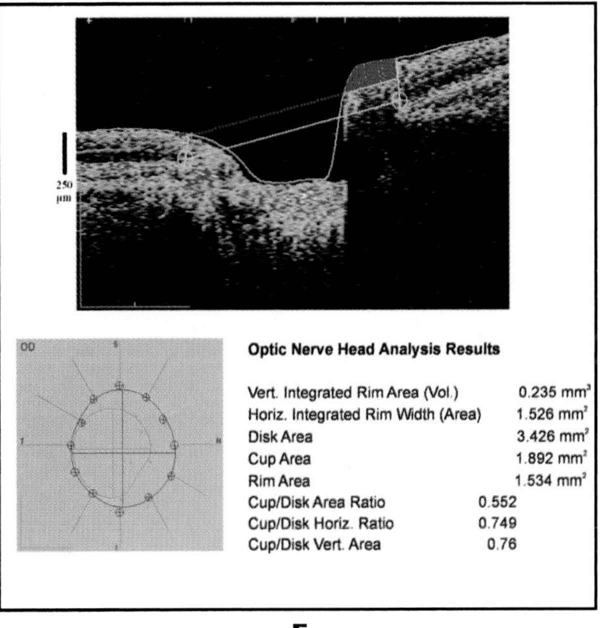
250 µm
OD
Optic Nerve Head Analysis Results
Vert. Integrated Rim Area (Vol.) 0.235 mm³
Horiz. Integrated Rim Width (Area) 1.526 mm²
Disk Area 3.426 mm²
Cup Area 1.892 mm²
Rim Area 1.534 mm²
Cup/Disk Area Ratio 0.552
Cup/Disk Horiz. Ratio 0.749
Cup/Disk Vert. Area 0.76

F

Case 12-36. A Patient With Narrow Angles But No Glaucoma Was Stable by Nerve Fiber Layer and Visual Field Throughout Follow-Up

A 64-year-old Asian woman had narrow, occludable angles treated with laser peripheral iridectomies bilaterally. The visual acuity of the right eye was 20/70 and the IOP was 22 mmHg. Upon examination, the anterior chamber depth was intermediate with a patent peripheral iridectomy. Gonioscopy revealed an open angle. The posterior segment examination was normal. There was no evidence of glaucomatous damage in the right eye.

VF were full (A and B), although there was a possible inferior temporal wedge defect on the final field (C).

Optical Coherence Tomography

Circumpapillary scans demonstrated stable peripapillary retinal NFL thickness throughout the follow-up period (D, E, and F). Note that the final scan included an area of software failure in the detection of the NFL in the nasal sector (center of the scan). Due to this failure, the average and the nasal thicknesses were reduced compared to subsequent visits.

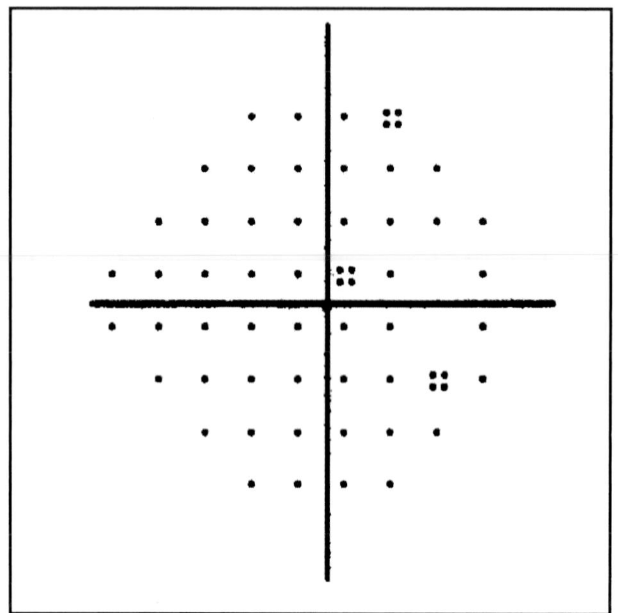

A—June 1996

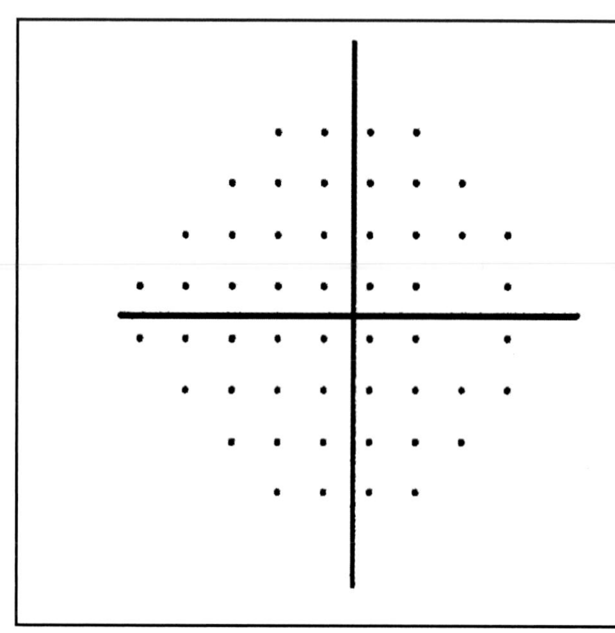

B—June 1997

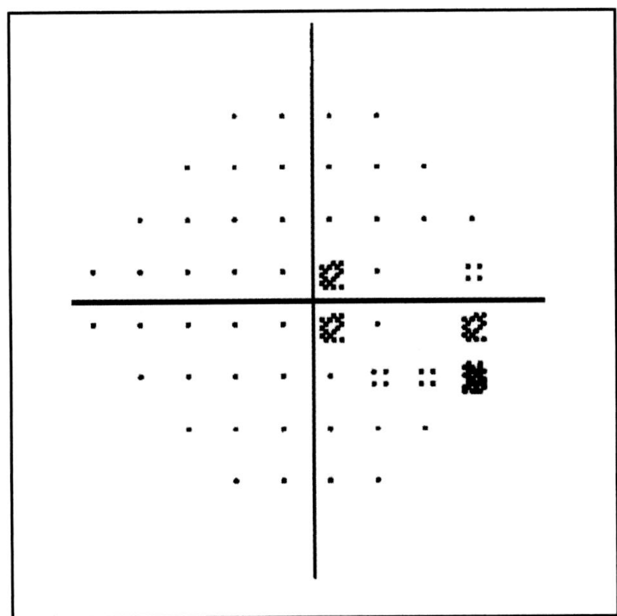

C—November 1998

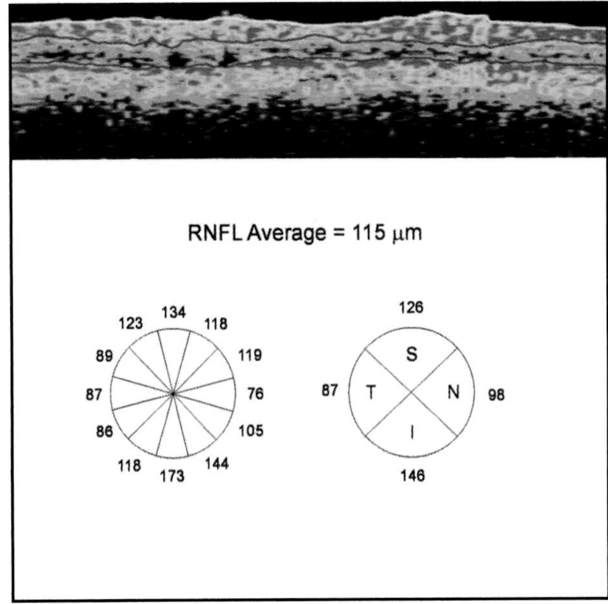

D—June 1996

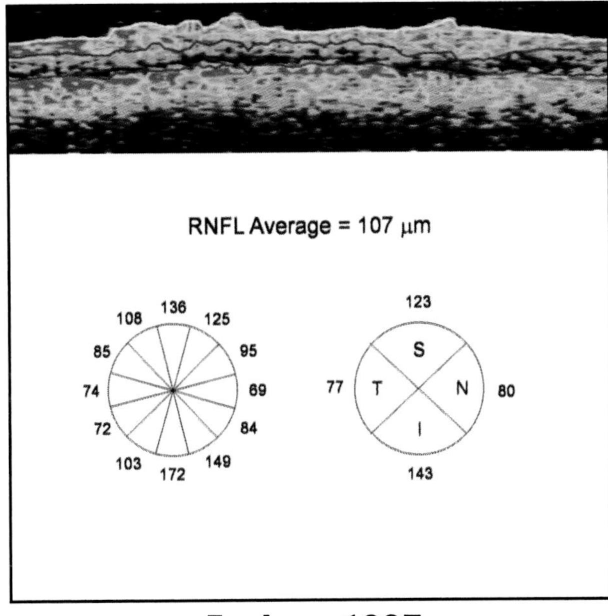

E—June 1997

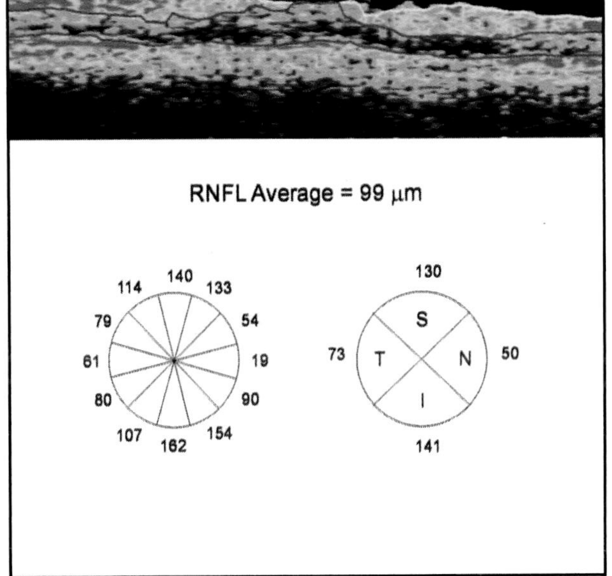

F—November 1998

Case 12-37. A Normal and Stable Circumpapillary Nerve Fiber Layer Suggested the Absence of Glaucoma in the Presence of Pseudoexfoliation and Fluctuating Visual Field Defects

A 72-year old Caucasian woman with pseudoexfoliation had suspected open-angle glaucoma in the left eye. The visual acuity was 20/20 and the IOP was 12 mmHg. The anterior segment examination revealed an open angle with pseudoexfoliation material on the anterior surface of the lens. The posterior segment was normal.

VFs showed fluctuating nonspecific abnormalities, primarily in the superior hemifield (A, B, and C).

Optical Coherence Tomography

The average retinal NFL thickness remained stable throughout follow-up, although some fluctuation was evident (D, E, and F).

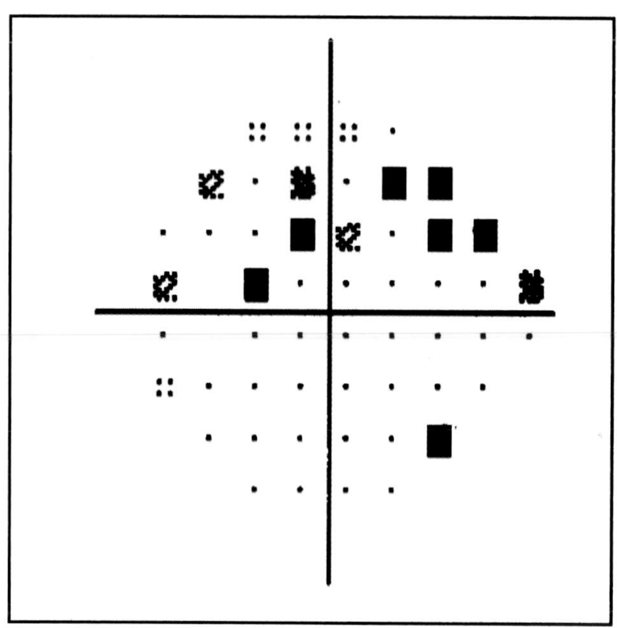

A—March 1996

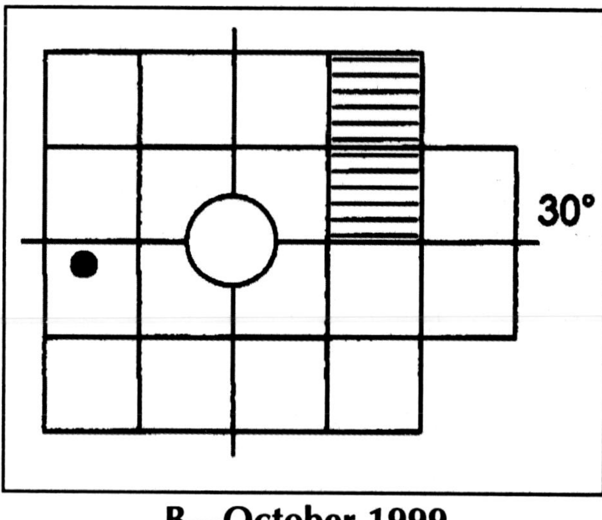

B—October 1999

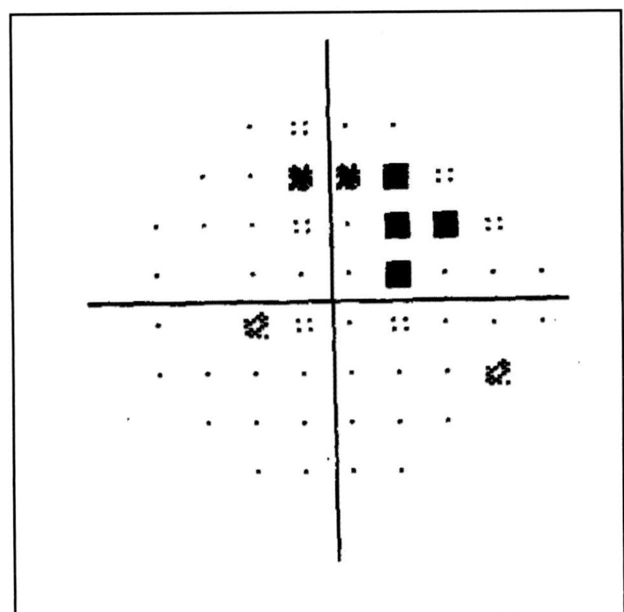

C—October 2000

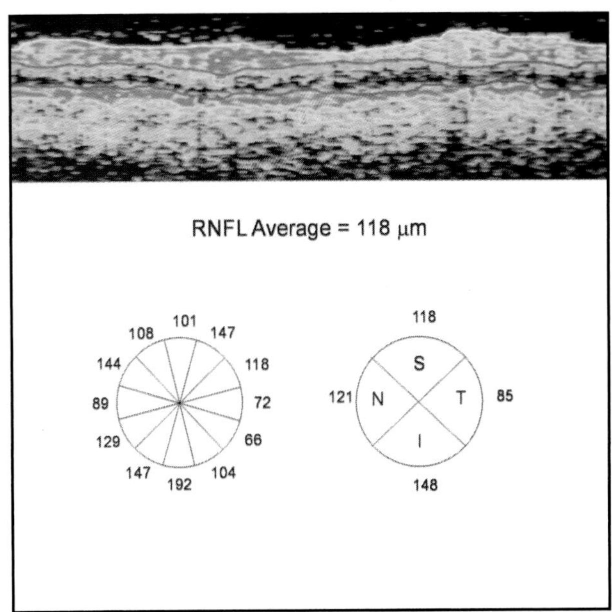

D—March 1996

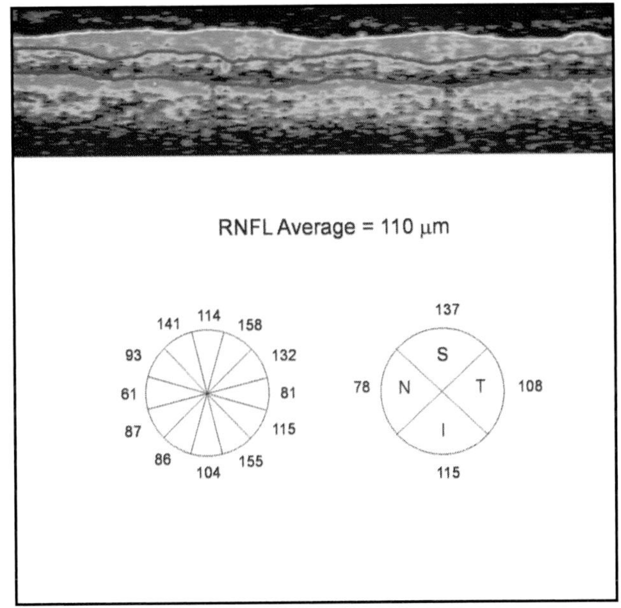

E—October 1999

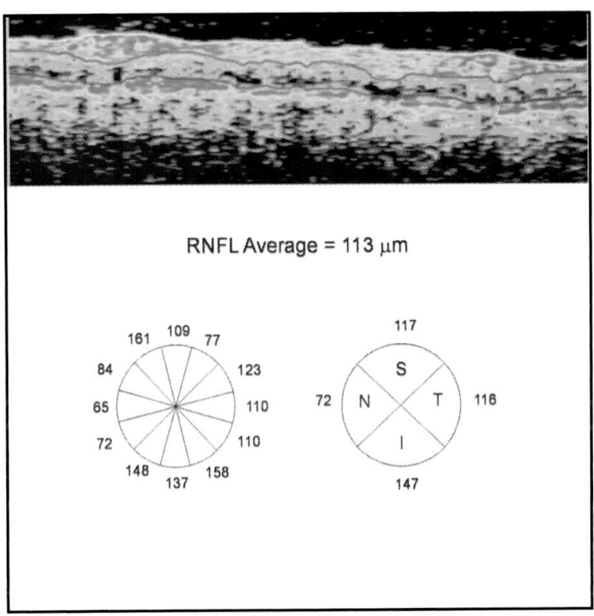

F—October 2000

Case 12-38. Longitudinal Evaluation of Optical Coherence Tomography and Visual Fields Demonstrated Loss of Nerve Fiber Layer Prior to Development of Visual Field Defect

An 86-year-old Caucasian man had primary open-angle glaucoma treated surgically with combined cataract extraction and trabeculectomy in the left eye. The visual acuity was 20/30 and the IOP was 8 mmHg. A high and functioning superior bleb was noted and the anterior chamber was deep and quiet with a patent peripheral iridectomy. A posterior chamber intraocular lens was well positioned and a marked cupping of the ONH was noted, with loss of the inferior temporal neuroretinal rim.

VFs showed initial fluctuation in the superior hemifield (A and B), which gradually consolidated as an early superior hemifield defect (C and D).

Scanning of the peripapillary retina with OCT version 1 demonstrated gradual and constant thinning of the retinal NFL mainly in the inferior quadrant (E, F, G, and H).

Note that the OCT demonstrated tissue loss prior to the appearance of the VF defect.

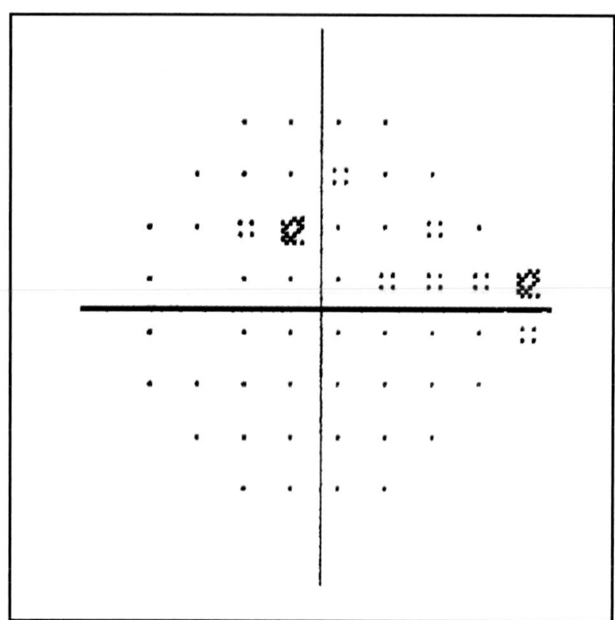

A—July 1996

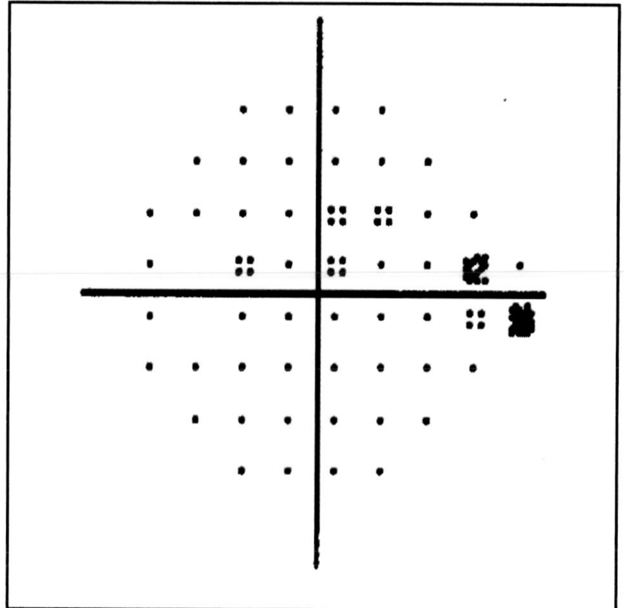

B—January 1997

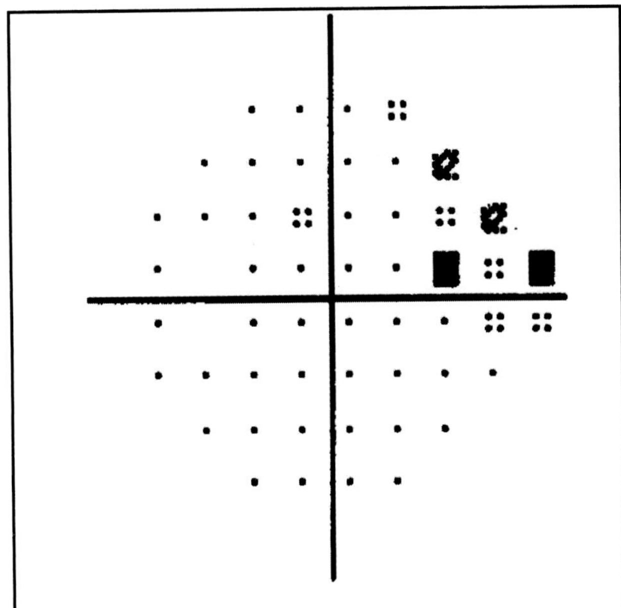

C—June 1997

D—March 1999

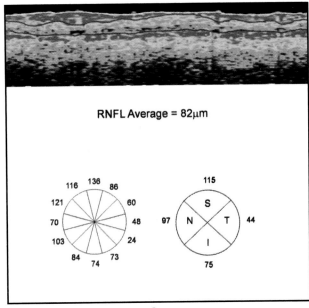

RNFL Average = 82µm

116 136 86 60 48 24 73 74 84 103 70 121

115 S 97 N T 44 I 75

E—July 1996

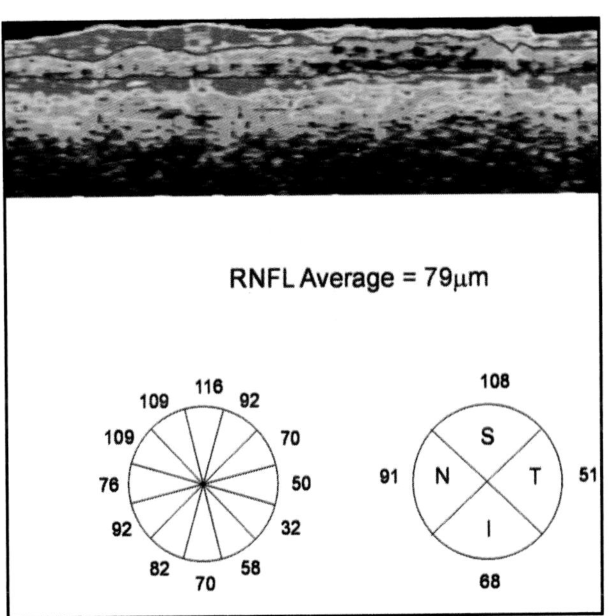

F—January 1997

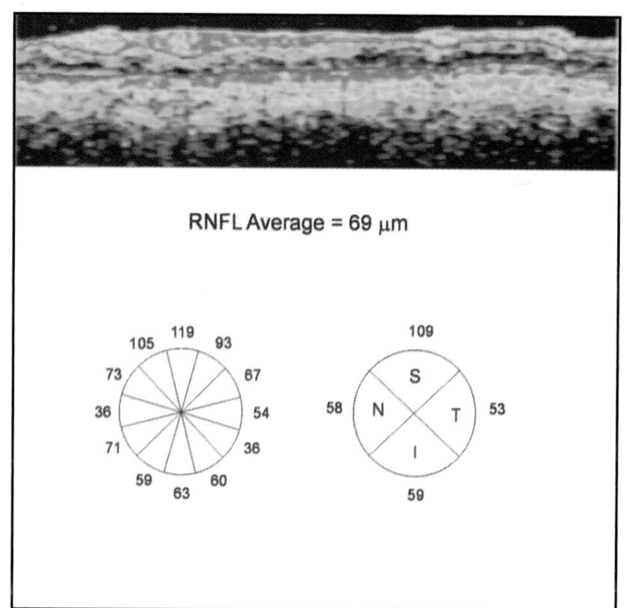

G—June 1997

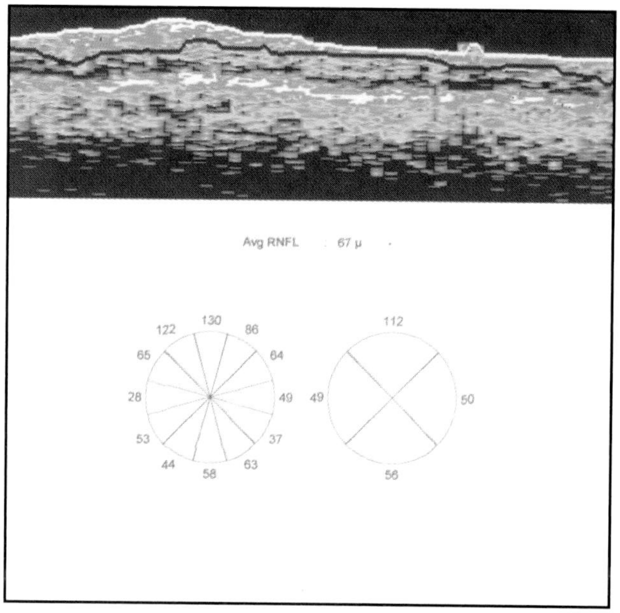

Avg RNFL 67 µ

122
130
86
65
64
28
49
49
50
53
37
44
58
63
112
56

H—March 1999

Case 12-39. Progressive Nerve Fiber Layer and Visual Field Loss Went Hand-in-Hand

An 80-year-old Caucasian woman had primary open-angle glaucoma treated with trabeculectomy in the right eye. Visual acuity was 20/25 and the IOP was 7 mmHg. A functioning bleb was noted with a deep and quiet anterior chamber and a patent peripheral iridectomy. There was a vertically elongated ONH cup with pronounced peripapillary atrophy.

VFs initially showed an inferior nasal defect (A). This gradually deteriorated to inferior and superior nasal, paracentral, and inferior arcuate defects (B, C, and D).

Optical Coherence Tomography

The OCT scans showed a constant deterioration of the retinal NFL thickness. The progressive thinning was noted in all quadrants except the superior (E, F, G, and H).

Comment

Note the relative initial thinness of the superior quadrant corresponding to the inferior VF on the initial scan. The progressive retinal NFL deterioration in all segments other than the superior corresponded with the visual field changes. The lack of progressive loss in the superior quadrant may have indicated that the VF loss lagged behind the structural damage that had already occurred in the superior quadrant or may have shown a relative insensitivity of OCT in this patient.

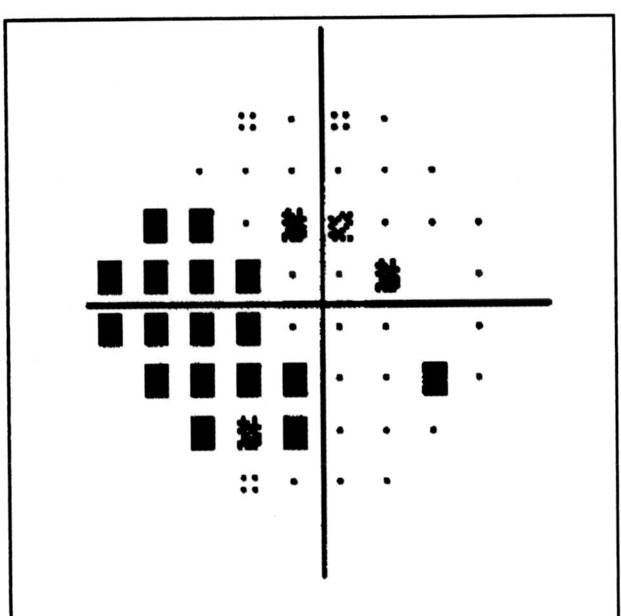

A—October 1996

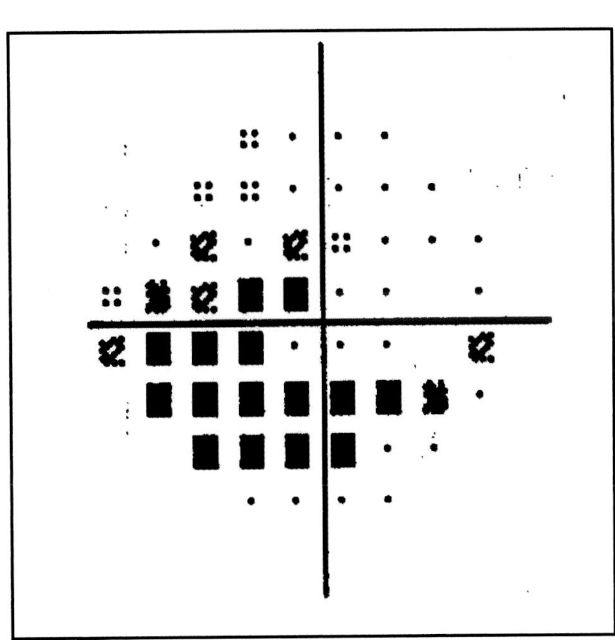

B—February 1997

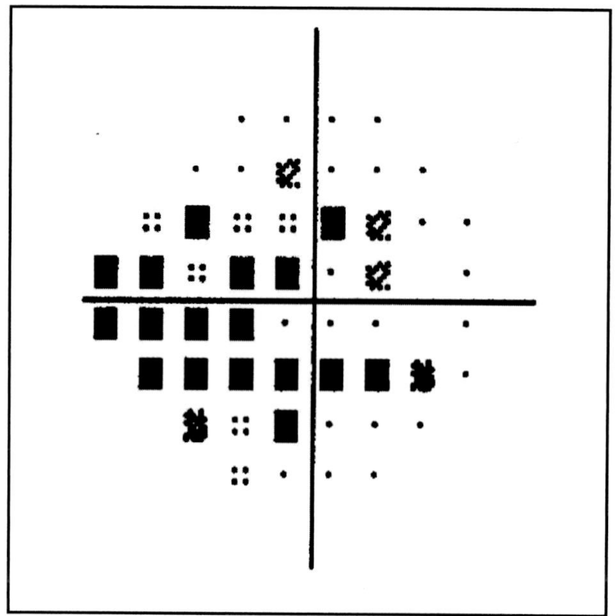

C—November 1998

D—October 1999

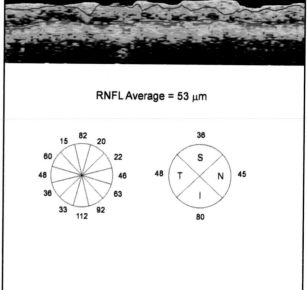

RNFL Average = 73 μm

43 35 56
89 89
47 44
73 72
61 128 130

41
70 T S N I 72
108

E—October 1996

RNFL Average = 53 μm

15 82 20
60 22
48 46
36 63
33 112 92

36
48 T S N I 45
80

F—February 1997

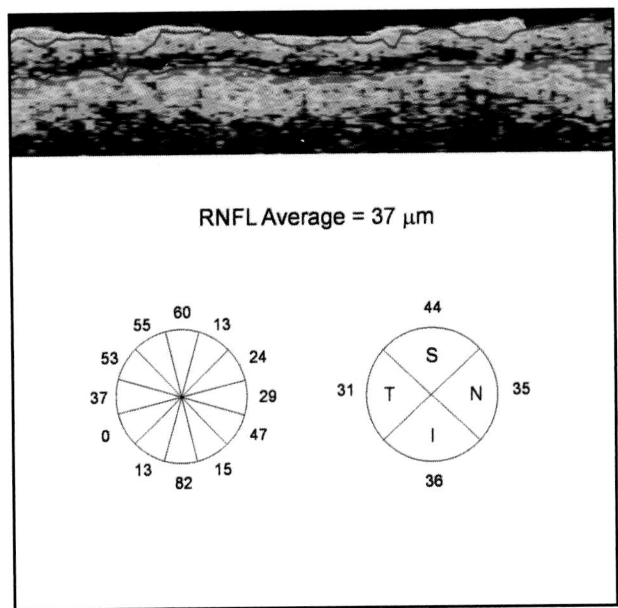

G—November 1998

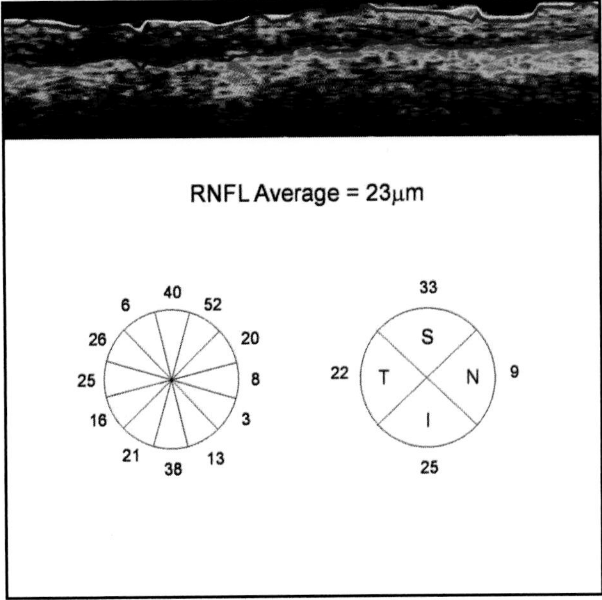

H—October 1999

Case 12-40. Loss of Nerve Fiber Layer Paralleled Visual Field Loss

A 77-year-old Caucasian woman with diabetes mellitus, ARMD, and primary open-angle glaucoma was treated with combined cataract extraction and trabeculectomy with mitomycin C in the right eye. On the final examination, the visual acuity was 20/30 and the IOP was 12 mmHg. A functioning bleb was noted with a deep and quiet anterior chamber and a patent peripheral iridectomy. A posterior chamber IOL, macular drusen, and marked ONH cupping were noted.

VFs showed reproducible superior and inferior nasal, arcuate, and paracentral defects with gradual deterioration (A, B, and C).

Optical Coherence Tomography

The deterioration of the peripapillary NFL appeared to parallel the VF loss (D, E, and F).

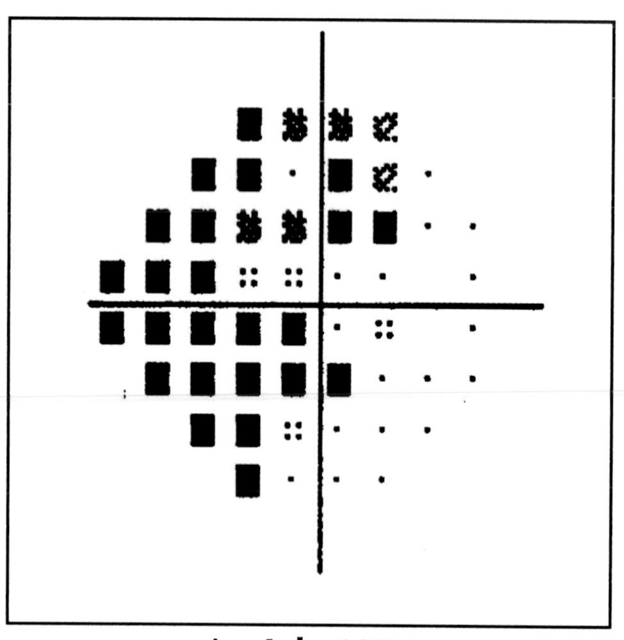

A—July 1997

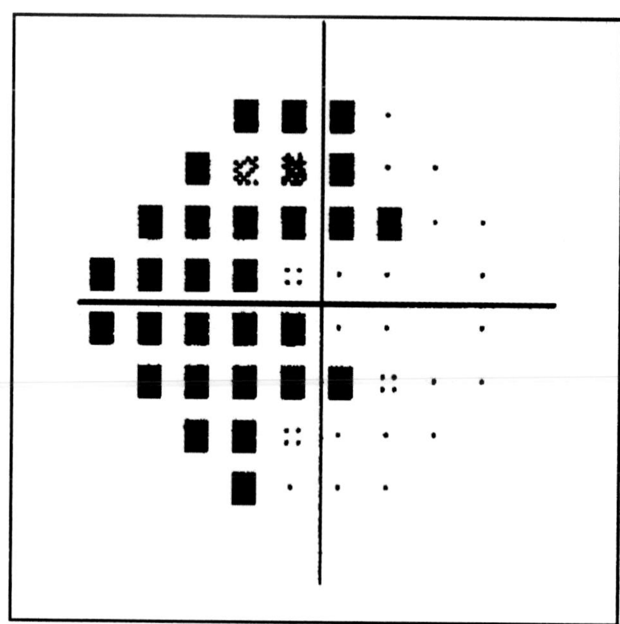

B—May 1998

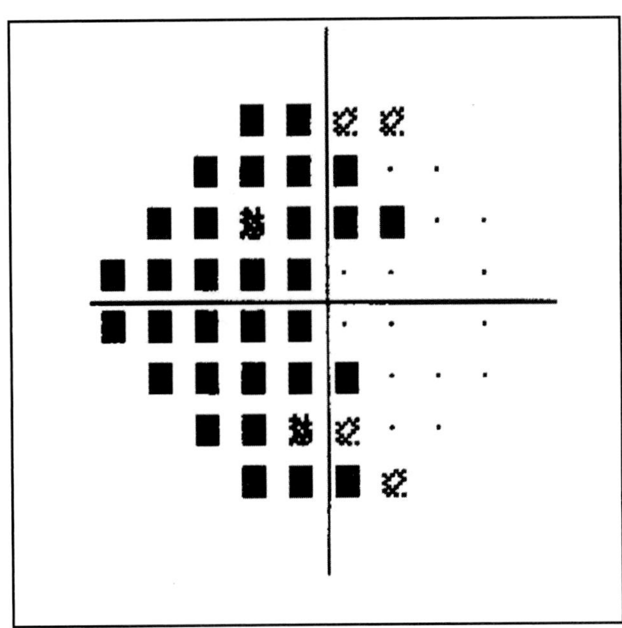

C—July 2000

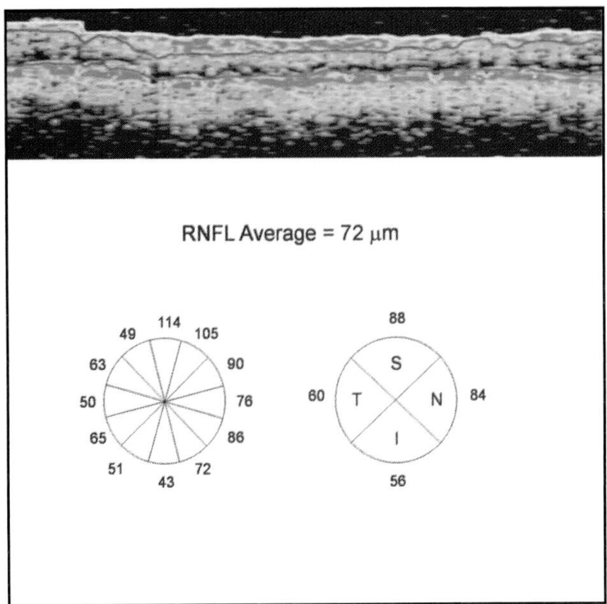

D—July 1997

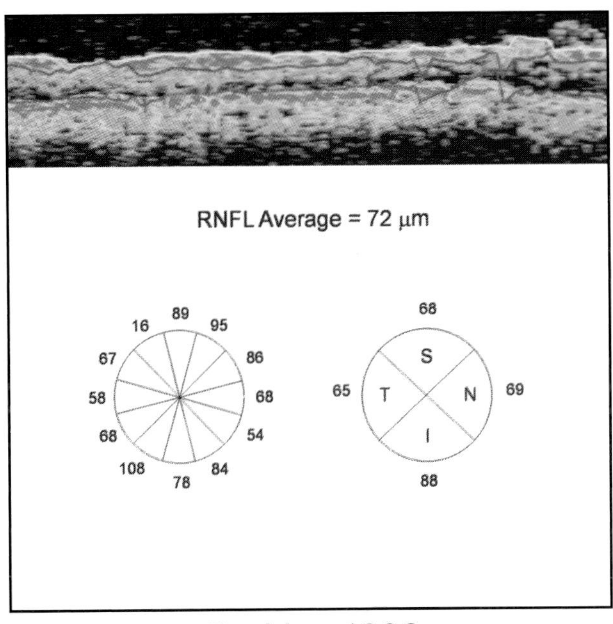

E—May 1998

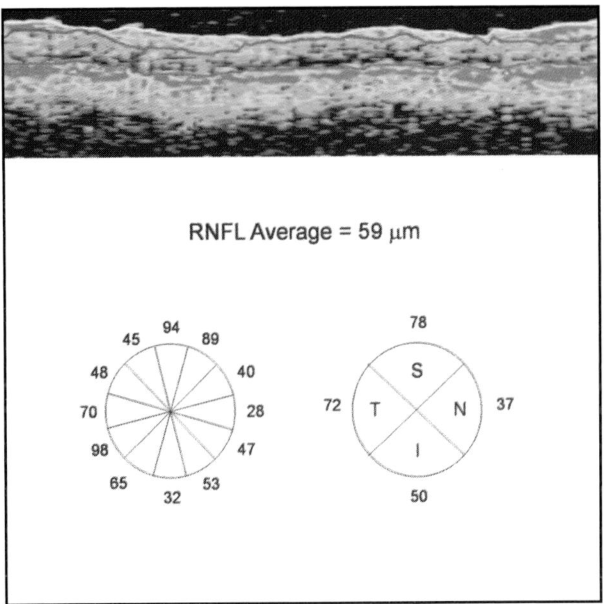

F—July 2000

Chapter 13

Optical Coherence Tomography in Neuro-Ophthalmology

Thomas R. Hedges III, MD

In neuro-ophthalmology, optical coherence tomography (OCT) can be useful for cross-section profiling of the optic nerve head, but more importantly it is useful in quantifying the status of the retinal nerve fiber layer (NFL). This is done with circular scans around the optic nerve head. Relative areas of retinal NFL drop-out and areas of NFL thickening can be assessed and correlated with a patient's visual status. Also, the relationship between the optic nerve head and the macula can be determined using cross-sectional imaging from disc to macula. One of the best uses of OCT for neuro-ophthalmologists is in dealing with those patients who are thought to have optic nerve disease but actually turn out to have retinal disease. OCT can show subtle areas of subretinal fluid that may be missed on ophthalmoscopy and may be considered insignificant on fundus fluorescein angiography (FA). Secondary effects on the macula from optic nerve head disease can also be detected. For example, we have identified subretinal fluid accumulations not seen on FA that appear to extend from the optic disc margin to the macula in patients with decreased visual acuity from papilledema (see Case 13-8).

OCT can identify permanent retinal NFL damage in cases of compressive optic neuropathy. This can be useful in following such individuals and may be helpful with regard to prognosis (see Case 13-1). In patients with nutritional, toxic, or hereditary optic neuropathy, characteristic maculopapillary NFL dropout can be identified with OCT. This can be confirmatory in individuals who have subtle, bilateral decreases in visual acuity and mild central visual field (VF) loss (see Cases 13-3 and 13-4).

OCT can help distinguish NFL swelling in patients with papilledema from congenital crowing of the optic nerve head. This still does depend on serial observations because we have found that patients who have congenitally crowded optic nerve heads have slightly thickened NFL when compared to normal control subjects. Therefore, on initial evaluation, the NFL thickness measurements from patients with congenitally crowded optic nerves may be difficult to distinguish from NFL thickening from very mild papilledema. However, the objective quantification that is provided by OCT allows for observation of changes in the NFL that occur over time from pathologic optic disc swelling as opposed to the relatively static nature of the NFL in patients who have congenitally anamolous optic nerve heads. In patients with nerves that are crowded enough to lead to optic disc drusen, the NFL will be thinner, and OCT allows for follow-up of patients who may develop slowly progressive NFL dropout from optic disc drusen (see Cases 13-19 and 13-20). OCT can be used to follow the course of papilledema. OCT may not distinguish between the resolution of NFL swelling and attrition of nerve fibers from chronic papilledema. However, when OCT is correlated with other clinical findings, such as VFs, it can be quite useful in measuring changes during follow-up of patients with papilledema, especially those with idiopathic increased intracranial pressure.

We have been able to identify retinal NFL thickening in patients with incipient anterior ischemic optic neuropathy before symptoms occur (see Case 13-11). Once optic nerve infarction has occurred, OCT shows NFL thickening that accompanies the acute phase of the disease. OCT correlates with VF loss in terms of retinal NFL loss as optic atrophy develops (see Case 13-12).

The phenomenon of apparent optic disc swelling caused by vitreous traction on the optic disc can be demonstrated by OCT (see Case 13-16). Various anomalies can be demonstrated by OCT with findings that one would expect based on clinical examination. In some cases, OCT can help follow the occasional complications that may accompany anomalies, especially subretinal fluid from optic disc pits.

The new generation of the commercial OCT system allows imaging with high resolution, which is on the order of 8 to 10 microns (μm) in the longitudinal direction, with a maximum of 512 A-scans per image acquired in 1.25 seconds. This technology generates 10 to 15 times finer images than ultrasound. The ability of OCT to perform high resolution imaging as well as quantitative morphometry is advantageous for measurement of the retinal layers, including the NFL, as well as for optic nerve head analysis. Normative data, not available for previous generations of OCT technology, have been generated for a middle-aged population for the third generation of OCT technology. The clinical relevance of the NFL measurements are displayed in comparison with this normative data, which give more information about the normal and abnormal regions. More detailed information regarding this approach is presented in Chapter 2.

References

1. Hoye VJ, Berrocal AN, Hedges TR, Amaro-Quireza ML. Optical coherence tomography demonstrates subretinal macular edema from papilledema. *Arch Ophthalmol.* 2001;119:1287-1290.
2. Roh S, Noecker RJ, Schuman JS, Hedges TR, Weiter JJ, Mattox C. Effect of optic nerve head drusen on nerve fiber layer thickness. *Ophthalmology.* 1998;105:878-885.
3. Theodossiadis GP, Theodossiadis P. Optical coherence tomography in optic disc pit maculopathy treated by macular buckling procedure. *Am J Ophthalmol.* 2001;132:184-190.
4. Medeiros FA, Moura FC, Vessani RM, Susanna R. Axonal loss after traumatic optic neuropathy documented by optical coherence tomography. *Am J Ophthalmol.* 2001;135:406-408.
5. Lincoff H, Kreissig I. Optical coherence tomography of pneumatic displacement of optic disc maculopathy. *Am J Ophthalmol.* 1998;82:367-372.
6. Unoki K, Ohba N, Hoyt WF. Optical coherence tomography of superior segmental optic hypoplasia. *Br J Ophthalmol.* 2002;86:910-914.

Index to Cases

Optic Atrophy

Case 13-1 Compressive Optic Neuropathy . . 613
Case 13-2 Optic Neuritis 615
Case 13-3 Nutritional/Toxic/Hereditary Optic Neuropathy 617
Case 13-4 Nutritional/Toxic/Hereditary Optic Neuropathy 619

Optic Disc Swelling

Case 13-5 Mild Papilledema 621
Case 13-6 Moderate Papilledema 625
Case 13-7 Severe Papilledema 627
Case 13-8 Papilledema With Subretinal Fluid 629
Case 13-9 Hypotony With Papilledema 631
Case 13-10 Optic Nerve Compression With Optic Disc Swelling 633
Case 13-11 Anterior Ischemic Optic Neuropathy (Presymptomatic/Progressive) . . . 635
Case 13-12 Acute and Remote Anterior Ischemic Optic Neuropathy: Pseudo-Foster-Kennedy Syndrome 638
Case 13-13 Juvenile Diabetic Papillopathy . . . 640
Case 13-14 Papillitis 642
Case 13-15 Neuroretinitis 643
Case 13-16 Vitreopapillary Traction 644
Case 13-17 Papillophlebitis 645

Anomalies

Case 13-18 Congenitally Crowded Optic Nerves 646
Case 13-19 Mild Optic Disc Drusen 648
Case 13-20 Severe Optic Disc Drusen 650
Case 13-21 Morning Glory Anomaly 652
Case 13-22 Myelinated Nerve Fibers 653
Case 13-23 Tilted Optic Discs 654
Case 13-24 Optic Nerve Hypoplasia 656
Case 13-25 Optic Disc Pit 658
Case 13-26 Bergmeister's Papilla Anomaly . . . 660

Case 13-1. Compressive Optic Neuropathy

A 56-year-old man underwent resection of a pituitary adenoma after he was found to have bitemporal hemianopia 3 years previously. Two years later, he had a second resection and required radiation for a residual tumor. On examination at that time, visual acuities were 20/25 OD and 20/40 OS. The optic nerve heads appeared mildly pale, more so on the right (A) than on the left (D).

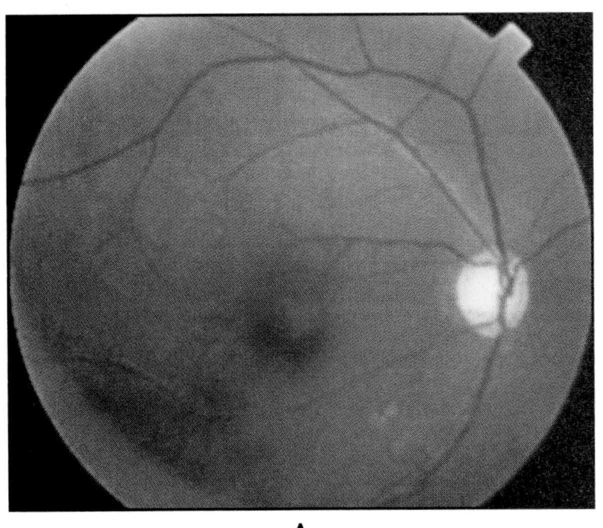

A

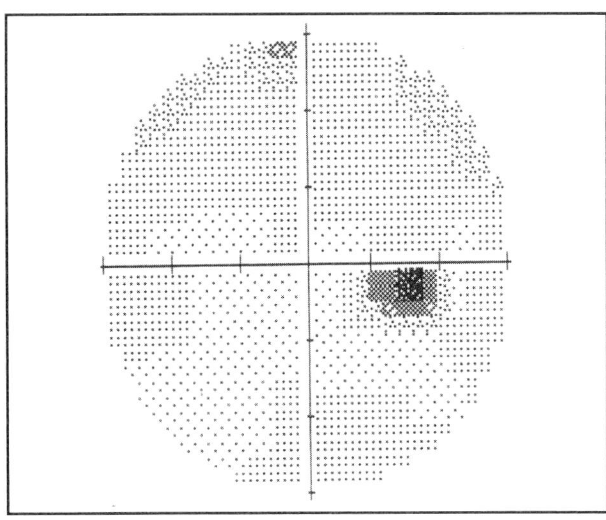

B

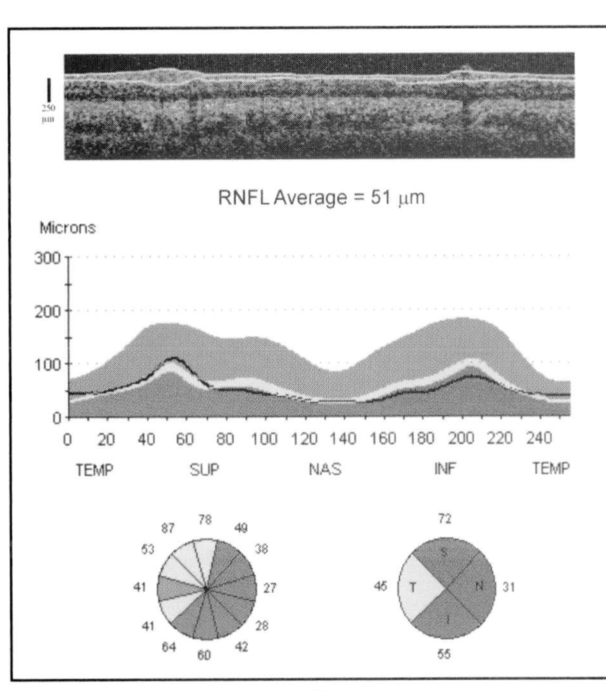

C

There was mild superotemporal depression in the right VF (B) and patchy temporal loss in the left VF (E) (Humphrey 24-2). OCT showed generalized thinning of the NFLs with greatest attenuation nasally on both sides (C and F). The VF defects remained stable over the ensuing months.

Comment

OCT reflects permanent nerve fiber damage from compressive optic neuropathy.

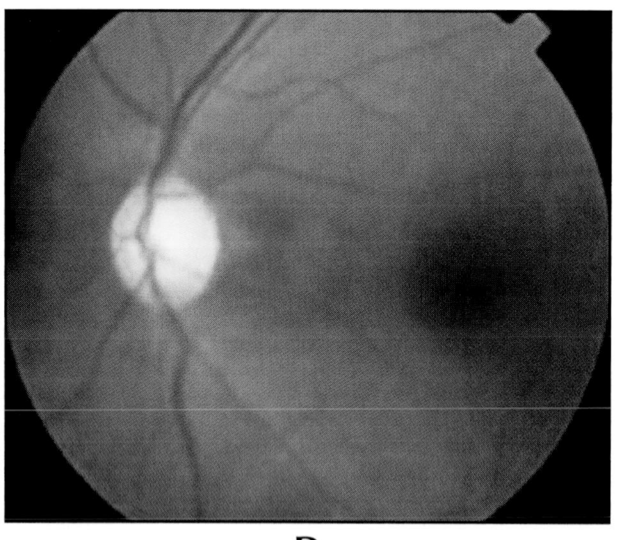

D

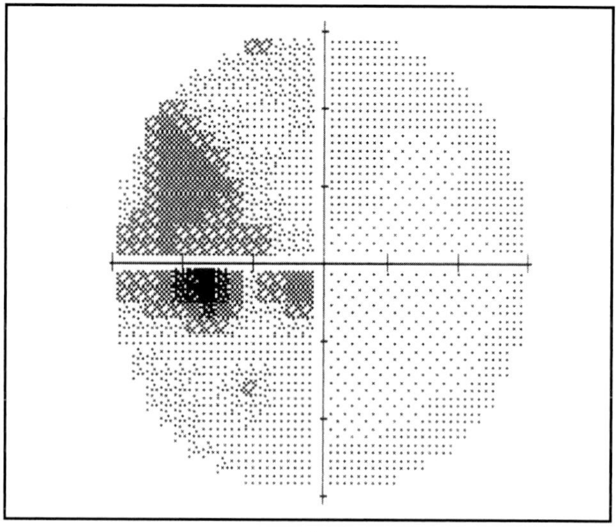

E

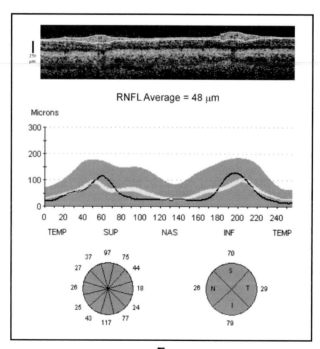

RNFL Average = 48 μm

F

Case 13-2. Optic Neuritis

A 28-year-old woman lost vision in her right eye 2 weeks before she was referred for further evaluation. She had pain with eye movement. Magnetic resonance imaging (MRI) showed typical demyelinating plaques extending into the white matter above the corpus callosum. Visual acuities were 1/200 OD and 20/20 OS. Color vision was reduced, and there was a relative afferent pupillary defect OD. The right VF (Humphrey 24-2) showed severe central loss (B). The optic disc was relatively normal (A).

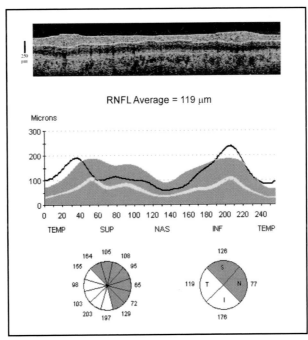

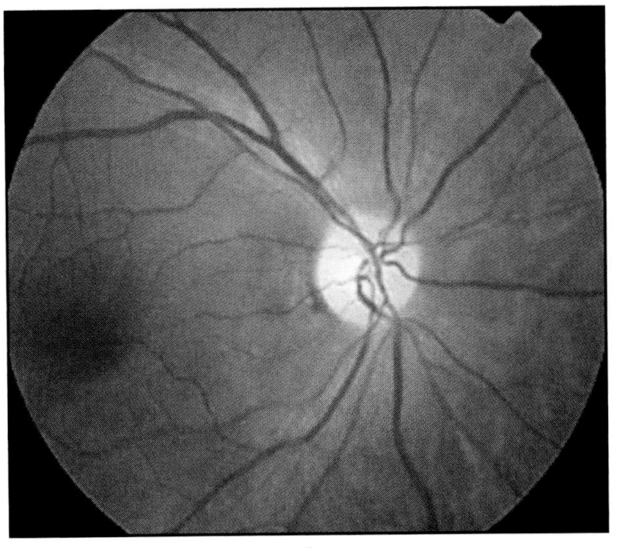

A

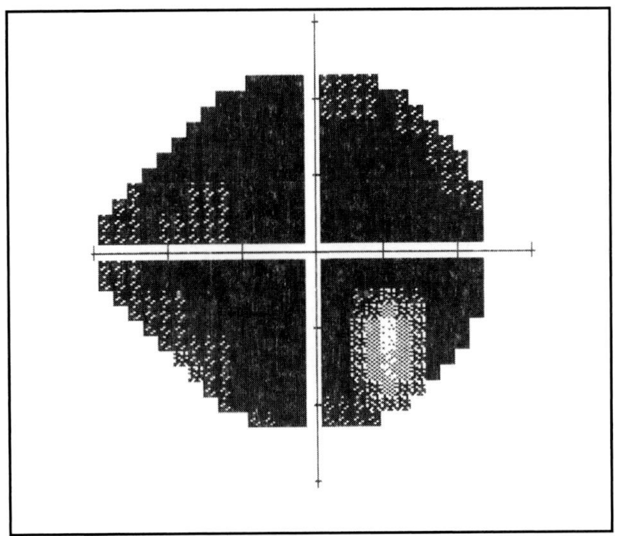

B

C

Optic Neuritis—1-Month Follow-Up

OCT showed slightly thickened retinal NFL OD initially (C). One month later, as her vision returned, OCT showed less NFL thickening (D).

Comment

In retrobulbar, demyelinating optic neuritis, OCT shows normal or slightly thickened retinal NFL initially that can remain normal, return to normal, or become thinner, depending on the extent of optic nerve damage.

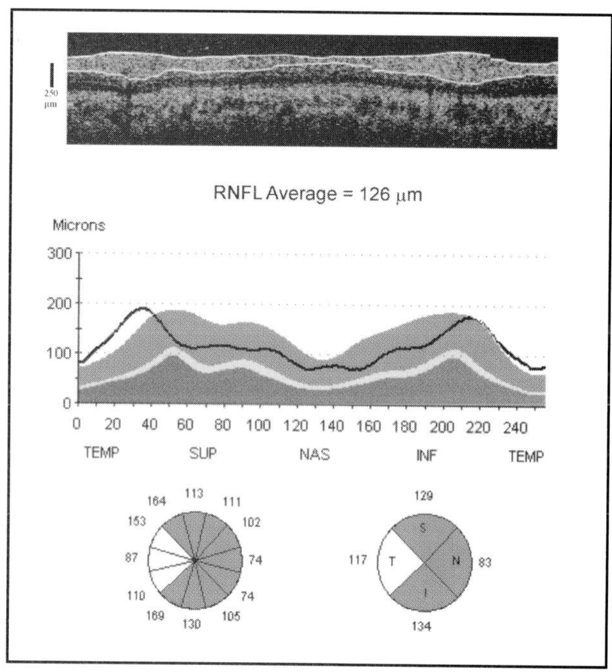

D

Case 13-3. Nutritional/Toxic/Hereditary Optic Neuropathy

A 59-year-old woman (and mother of the patient in Case 13-4) was seen because of poor central vision of many years duration. She used tobacco heavily (up to three packs/day). She became aware of poor vision in both eyes at age 16 when she could not pass a driver's test. Over the past 5 years, she noted a steady decline in central vision. Mitochondrial DNA testing for Leber's hereditary optic neuropathy was normal.

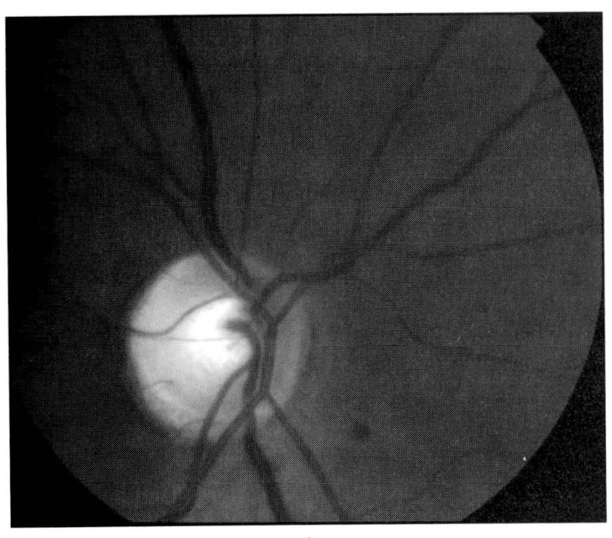

A

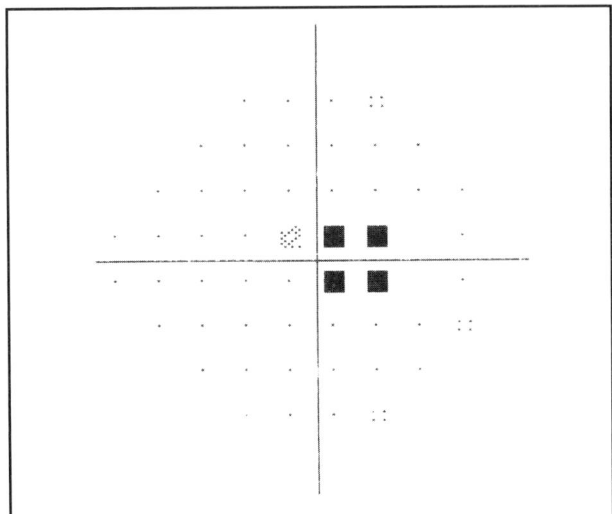

B

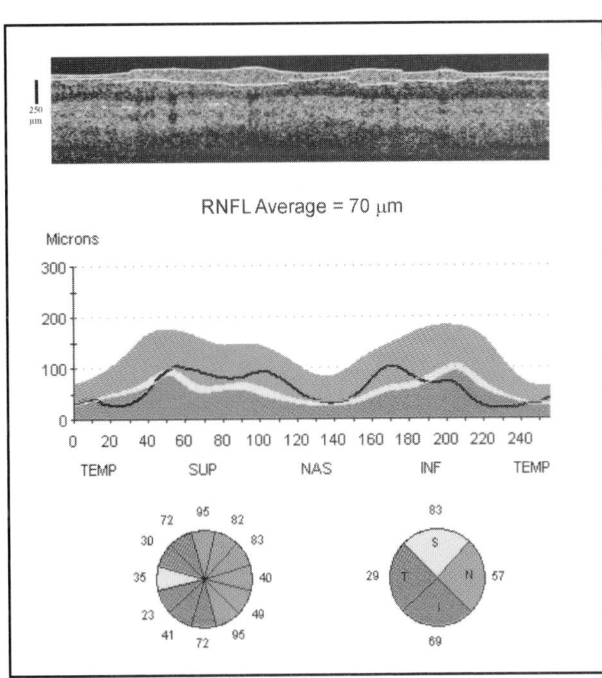

C

Visual acuities were 20/200 OD and 20/200 OS. There were central scotomas (Humphrey 24-2) (B and E) and temporal pallor of both optic discs (A and D). OCT showed temporal thinning of the retinal NFLs OU (C and F).

Comment

OCT shows primary involvement of the maculopapillary bundle of nerve fibers in nutrition/toxic/hereditary optic neuropathy.

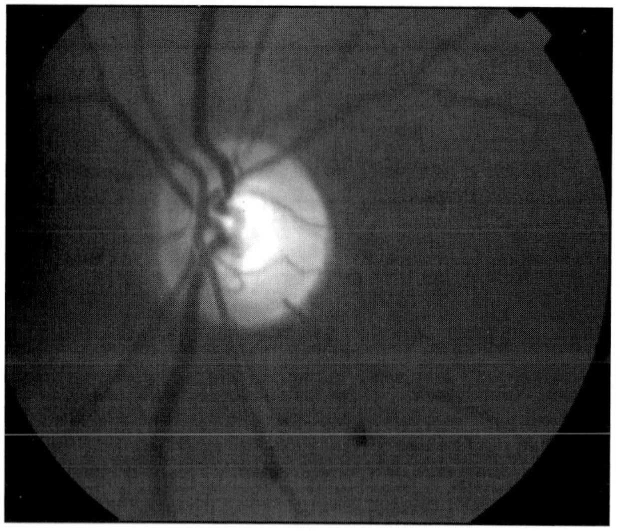

D

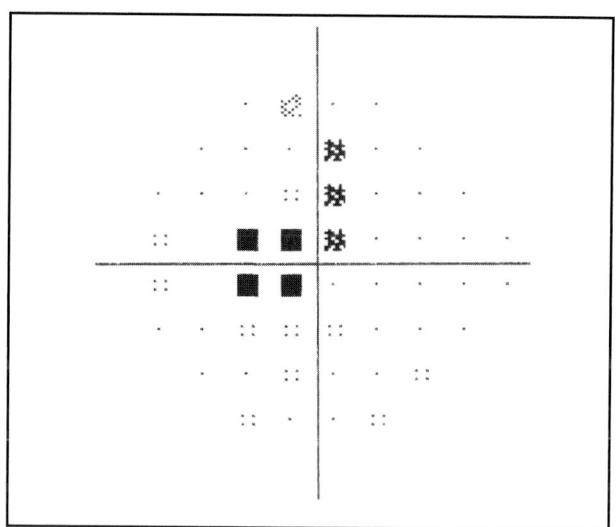

E

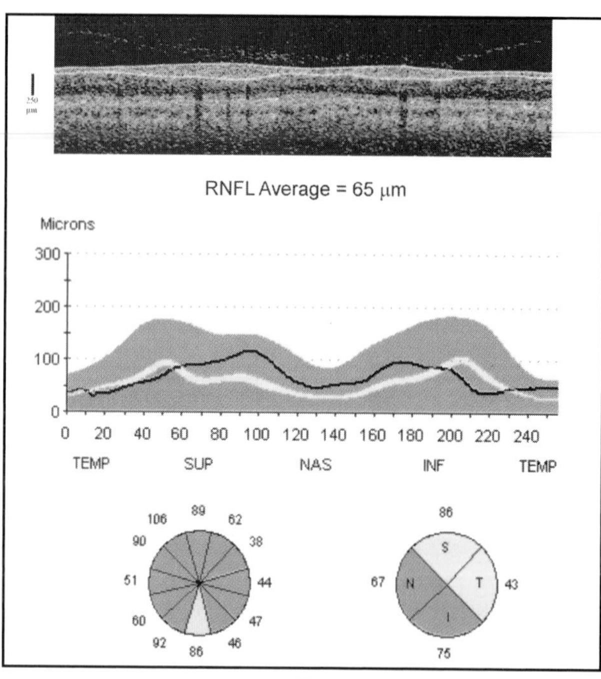

F

Case 13-4.
Nutritional/Toxic/Hereditary Optic Neuropathy

A 28-year-old woman developed blurred vision in both eyes over a period of weeks. She had used alcohol and tobacco in excess and had not been eating a balanced diet for years. Her mother was diagnosed with tobacco/alcohol amblyopia (see Case 13-3). Mitochondrial DNA testing did not show Leber's mutations. Visual acuities were 20/50 OD and 20/70 OS. VFs showed central loss on the right (B) and on the left (E) (Humphrey 24-2 pattern deviation). Both optic nerves showed temporal pallor and mild NFL thinning (A and D).

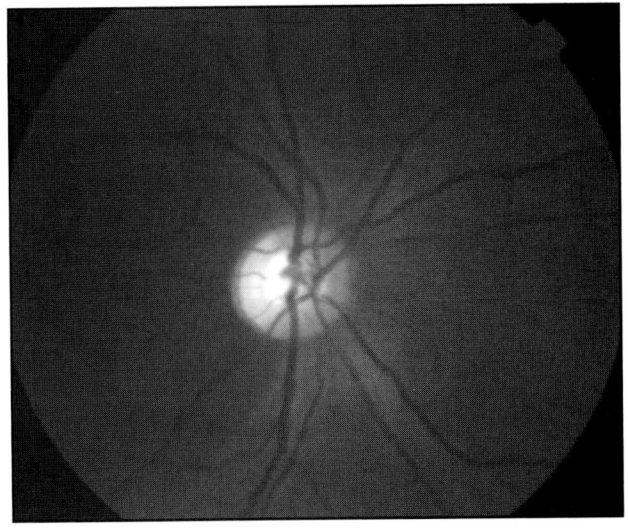

A

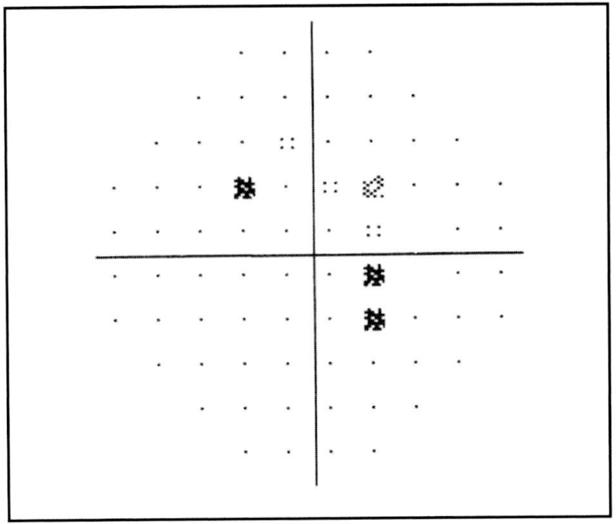

B

C

OCT showed thinning of the NFL temporally (C and F). Visual acuities improved slightly after discontinuing alcohol, reducing cigarette comsumption, and resuming a more balanced diet with vitamin supplements.

Comment

OCT can show retinal NFL thinning in nutritional/tobacco/alcohol amblyopia with loss of visual acuity when there are few changes in the fundi or in the VFs.

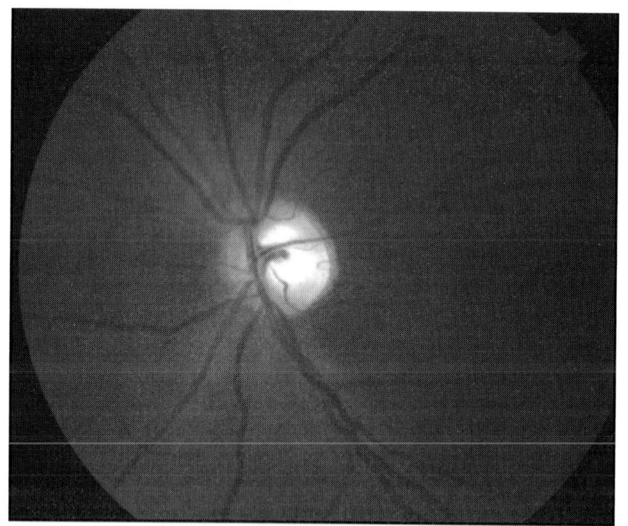

D

E

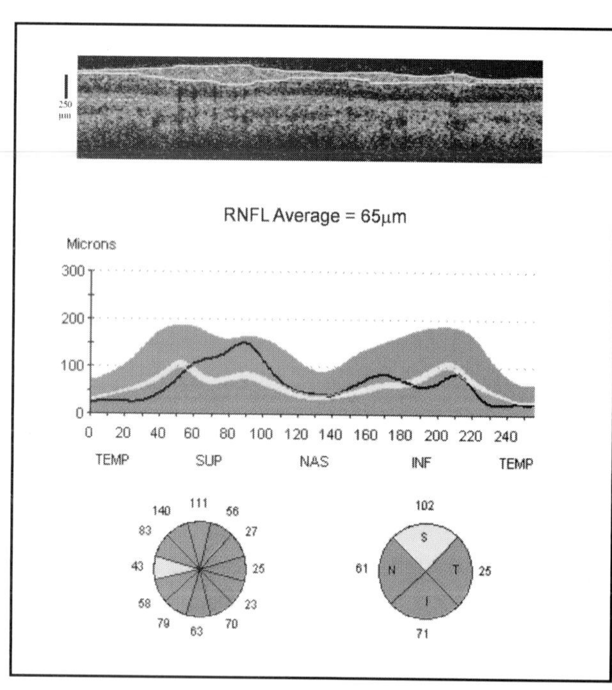

F

Case 13-5. Mild Papilledema

An 18-year-old woman underwent ventriculostomy for obstructive hydrocephalus from a third ventricular cyst. When she was evaluated, the papilledema was resolving. Visual acuities were 20/20 OD and 20/20 OS. Her VFs were normal. Optic disc photos showed swelling (A and D). OCT showed mild swelling of the optic discs (B and E) and thickening of the NFLs (C and F).

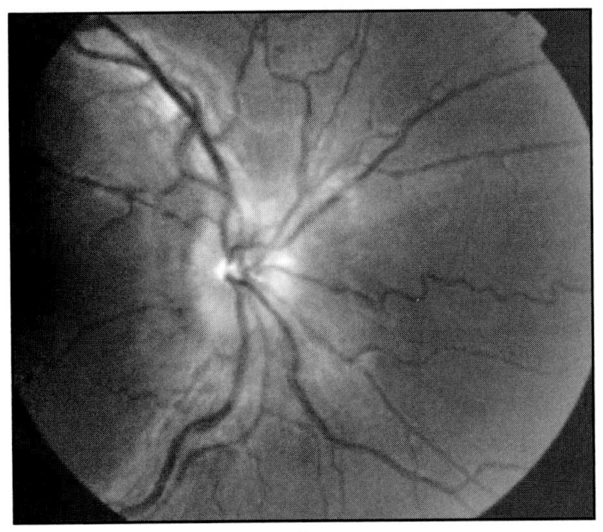

A

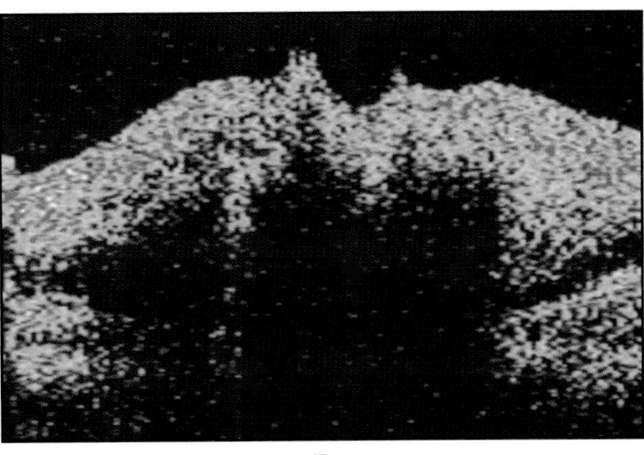

B

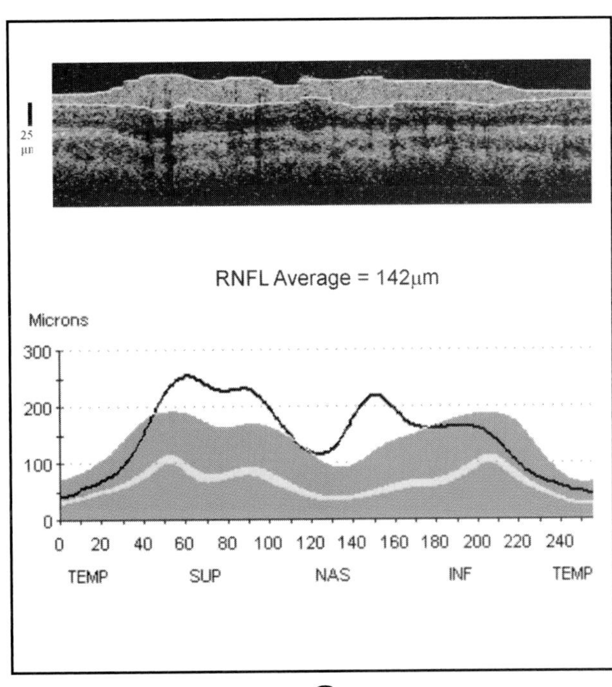

C

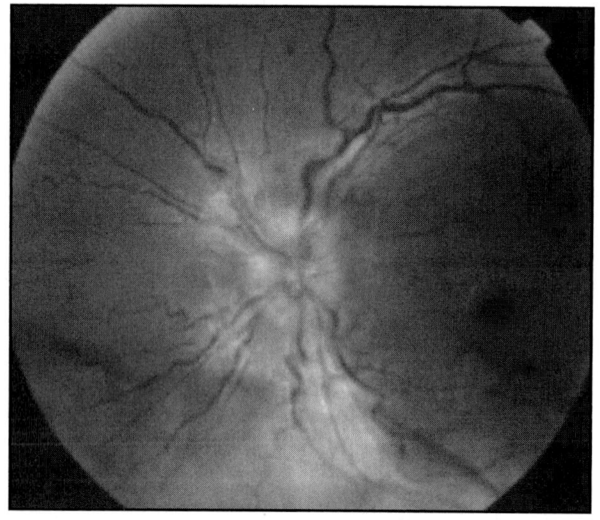

D

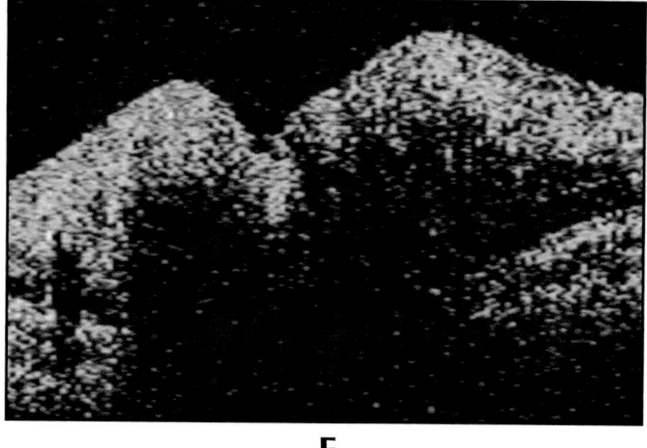

E

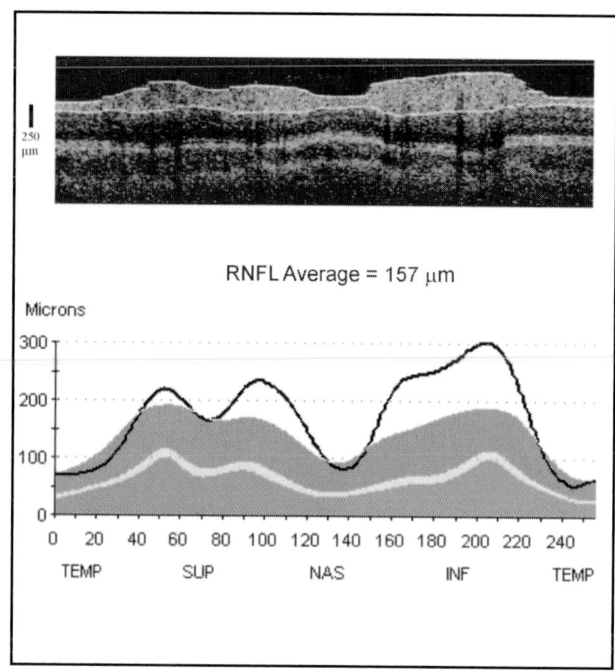
250 µm
RNFL Average = 157 µm
Microns
300
200
100
0
0 20 40 60 80 100 120 140 160 180 200 220 240
TEMP SUP NAS INF TEMP

F

Papilledema—2-Month Follow-Up

As the optic nerve heads returned to normal (G and J), the retinal NFLs also became normal on OCT. Two months later, the optic nerves appeared less elevated (H and K) and OCT showed normal average NFL thicknesses bilaterally (I and L).

Comment

OCT can be used to identify pathologic optic disc swelling and monitor changes in NFL thickness over time.

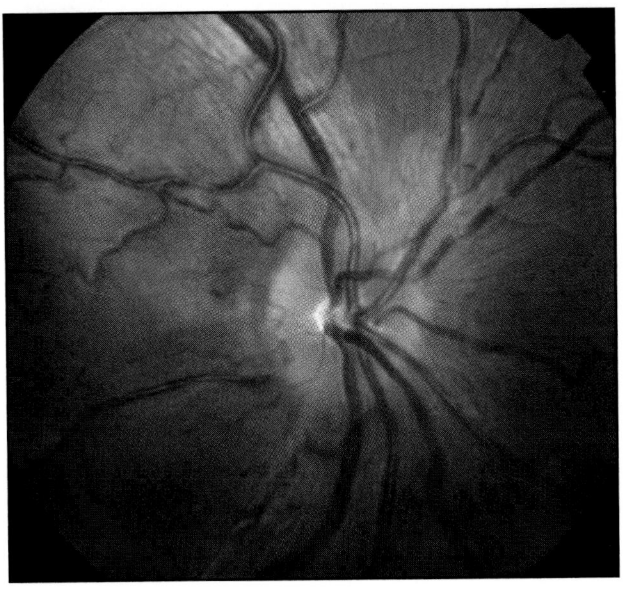

G

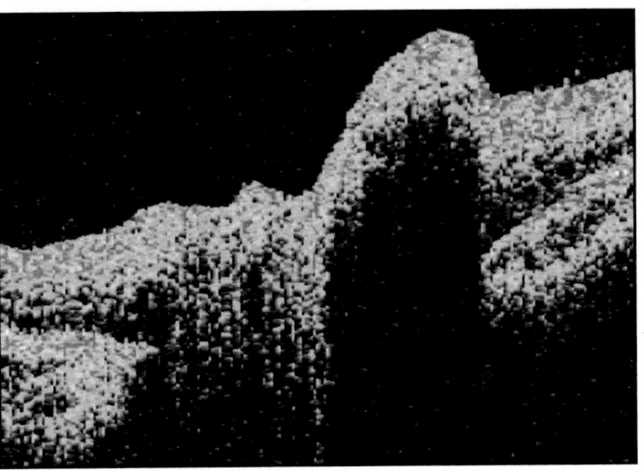

H

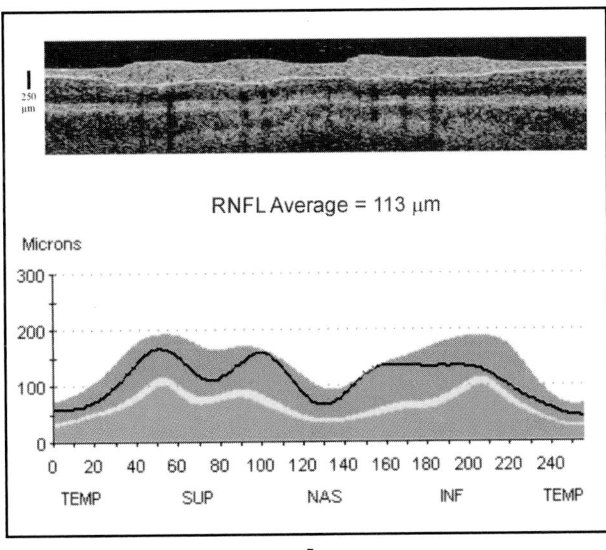

I

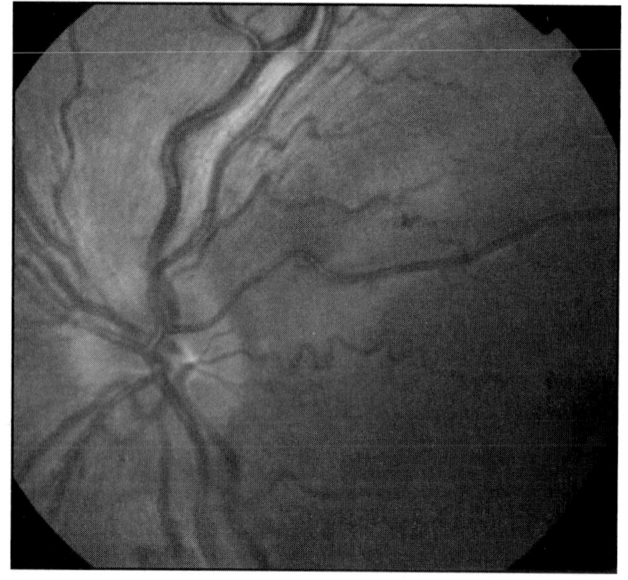

J

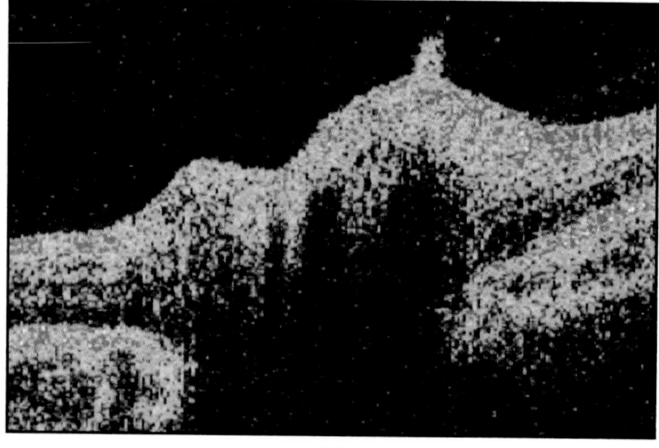

K

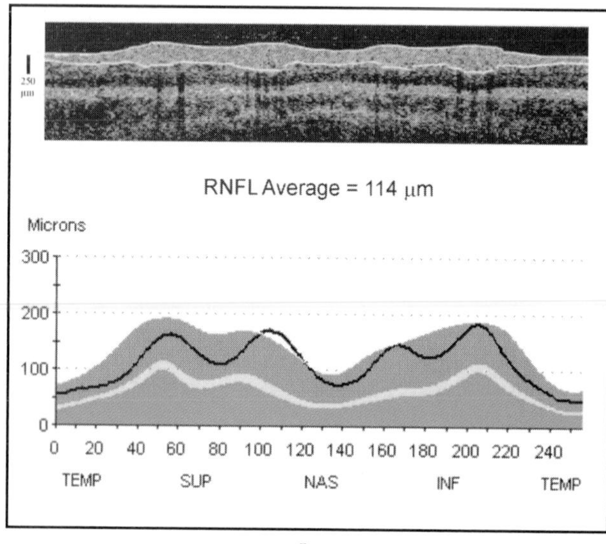
250 µm
RNFL Average = 114 µm
Microns
300
200
100
0
0 20 40 60 80 100 120 140 160 180 200 220 240
TEMP
SUP
NAS
INF
TEMP

L

Case 13-6. Moderate Papilledema

A 63-year-old woman was found to have papilledema associated with a meningioma of the tentorium apparently blocking the straight sinus and causing increased intracranial pressure to 380 mm H_2O. She was also obese.

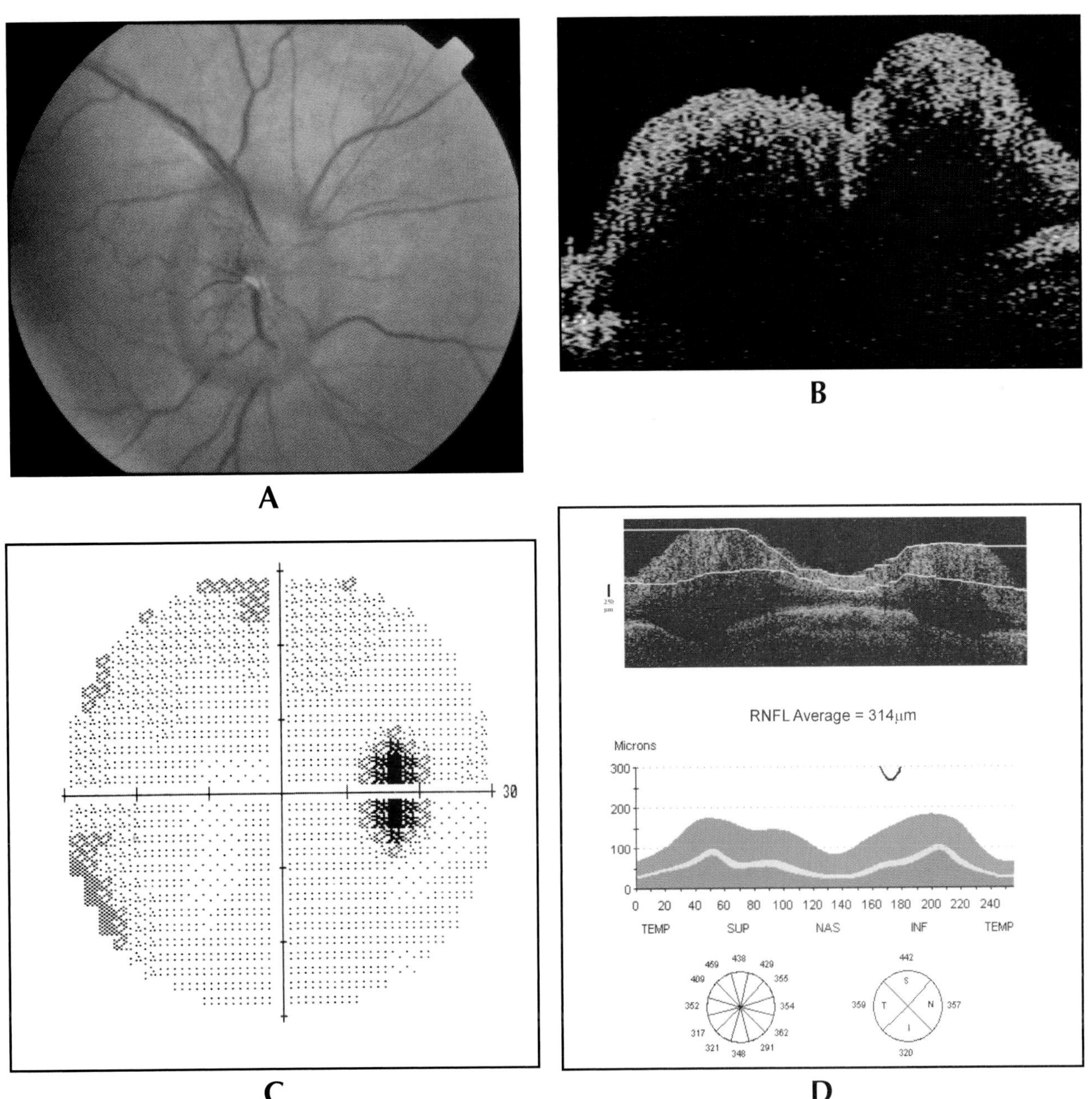

Visual acuities were 20/25 OD and 20/25 OS. VFs showed enlargement of the blind spots (C and G). The optic discs showed well-established, moderate papilledema (A and E). OCT showed optic disc swelling (B and F) and thickening of the NFLs on both sides (D and H). NFL thickening of this degree might cause artifact with the circular measurements at 3.5 mm in diameter (D).

Comment

OCT can quantitate the degree of papilledema.

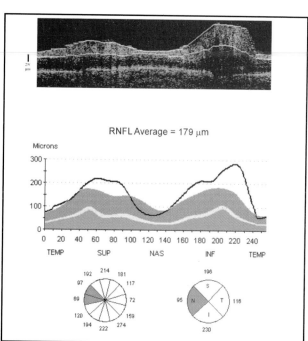

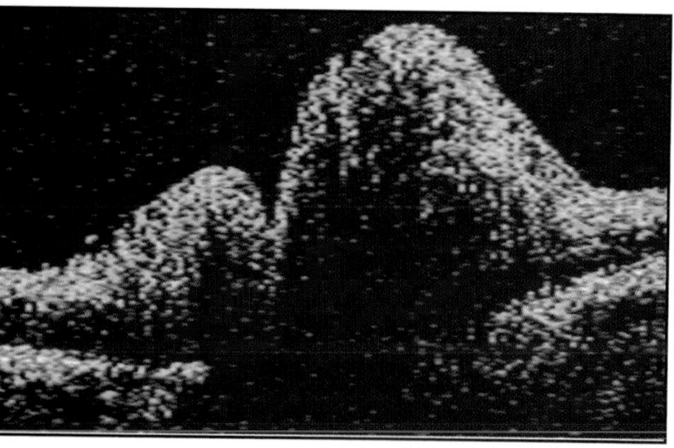

F

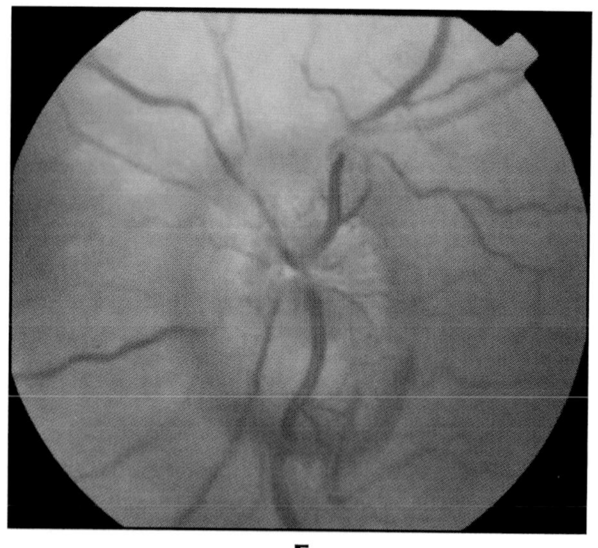

E

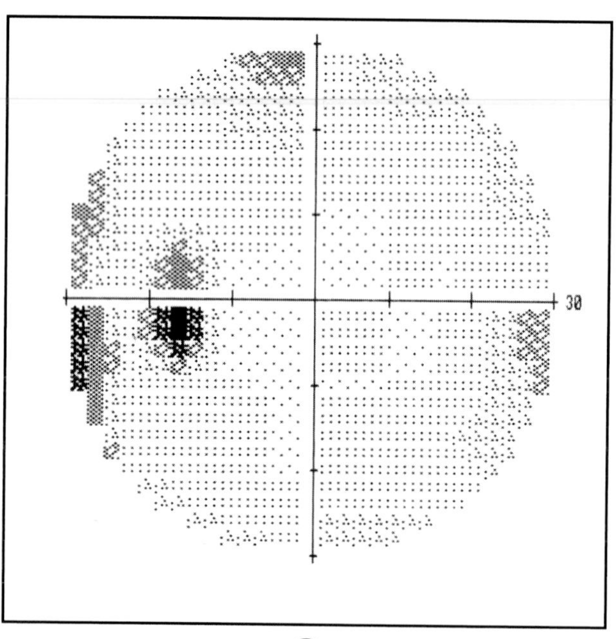

G

H

Case 13-7. Severe Papilledema

A 22-year-old, obese woman developed rapid onset of headaches and blurred vision. She was found to have cerebral venous sinus thrombosis. Intracranial pressure was measured from a lumbar puncture as greater than 500 mm H_2O. She was very uncooperative, and visual acuities could only be estimated as 20/200 in both eyes. VFs were grossly full but automated perimetry showed severe loss (C and G). She underwent lysis of the clot in the straight and sigmoid venous sinuses and placement of a ventriculoperitoneal shunt.

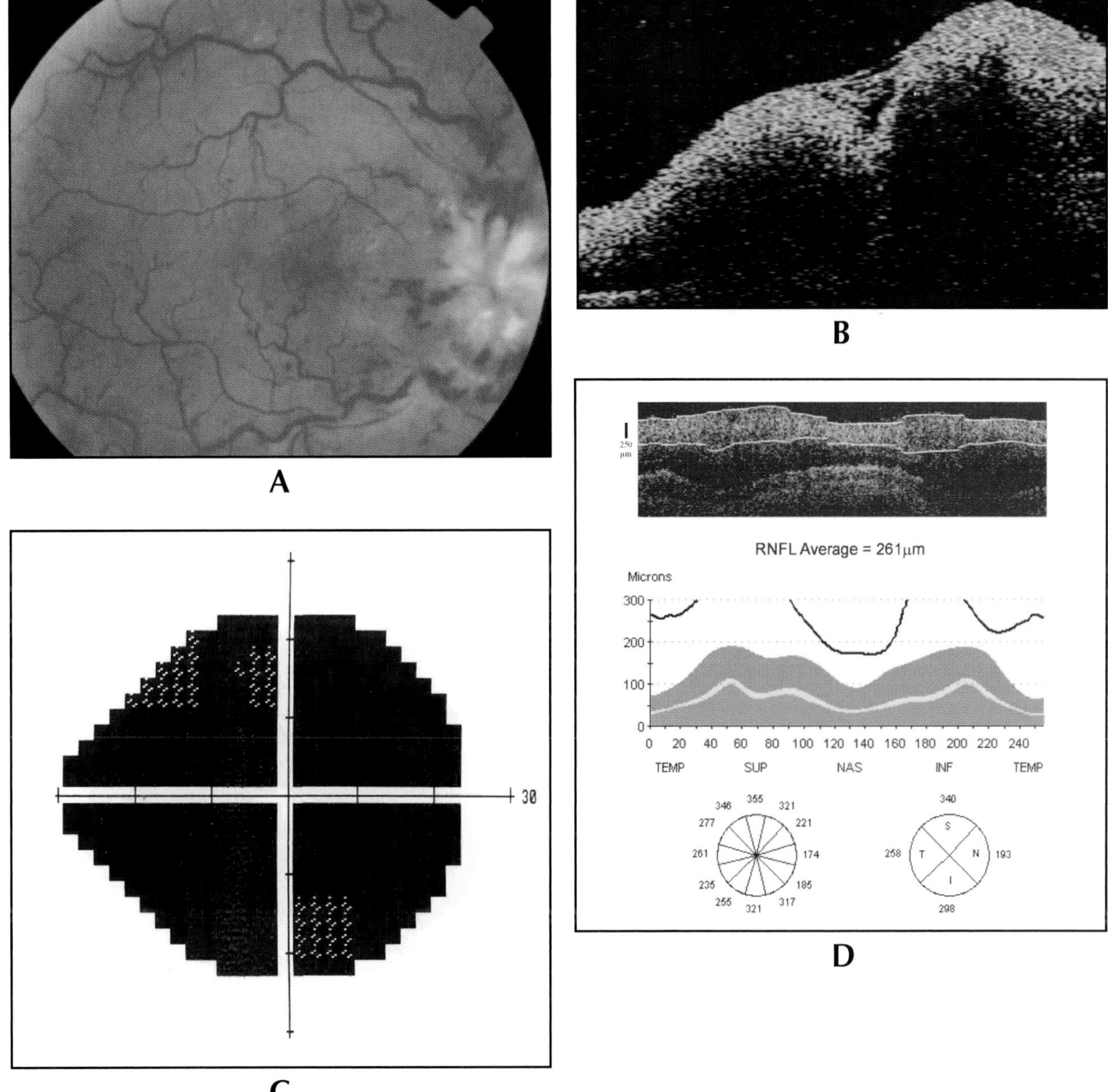

The optic nerves appeared swollen and pale with surrounding hemorrhages (A and E). There were residual intraretinal accumulations of exudate nasal to the maculas. OCT showed swollen optic nerve heads (B and F) and retinal NFL thickening (D and H). Ultimately, optic atrophy became more profound. However, visual acuities slowly recovered to 20/200 OD and 20/40 OS. VFs were constricted.

Comment

OCT cannot differentiate between residual optic nerve swelling that may be resolving and swelling with the development of optic atrophy in severe papilledema.

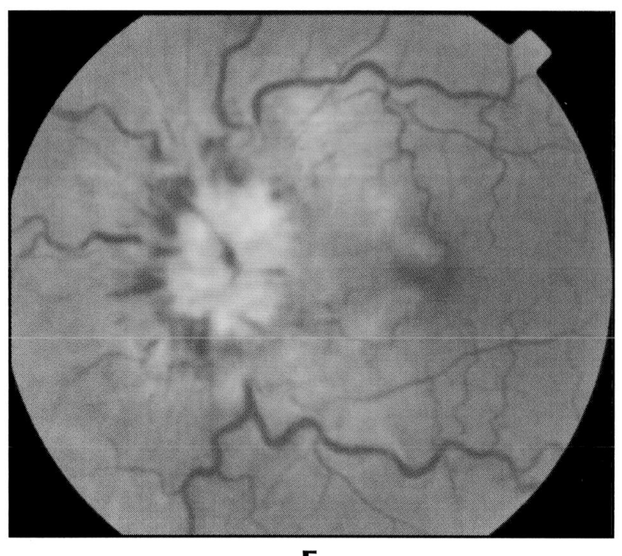

E

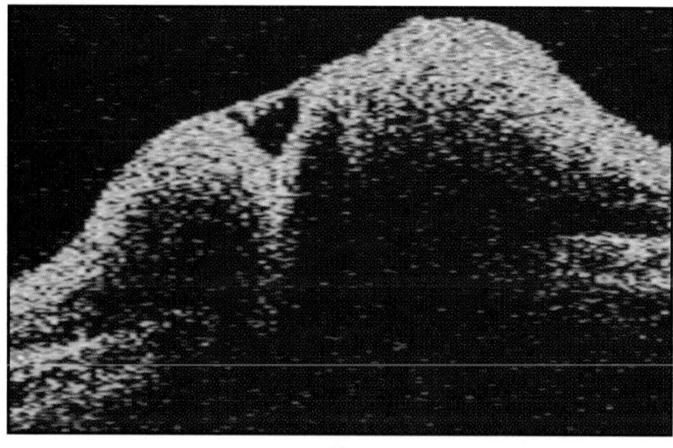

F

30

G

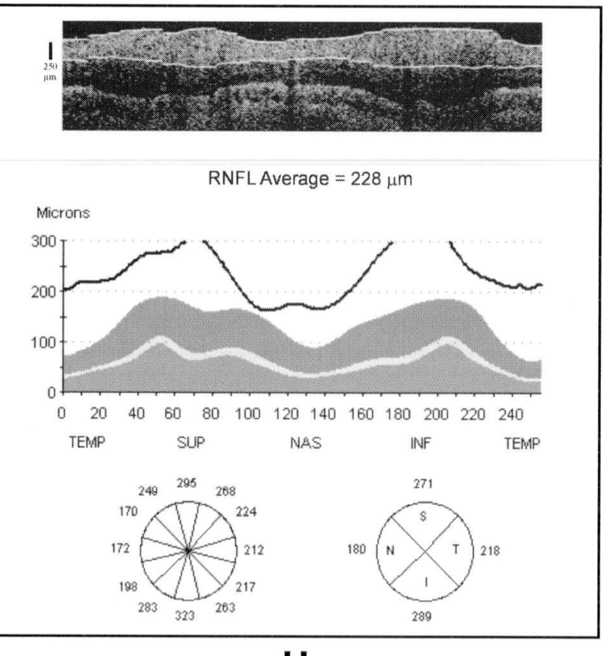

H

Case 13-8. Papilledema With Subretinal Fluid

A 22-year-old woman developed severe headaches, double vision, and intermittent blurred vision. Intracranial pressure was 450 mm H_2O by lumbar puncture. Visual acuities were 20/30 OD and 20/200 OS. VF testing showed central as well as peripheral loss in both eyes, left greater than right (D and H). There was marked optic disc swelling with hemorrhages and exudates (A and E).

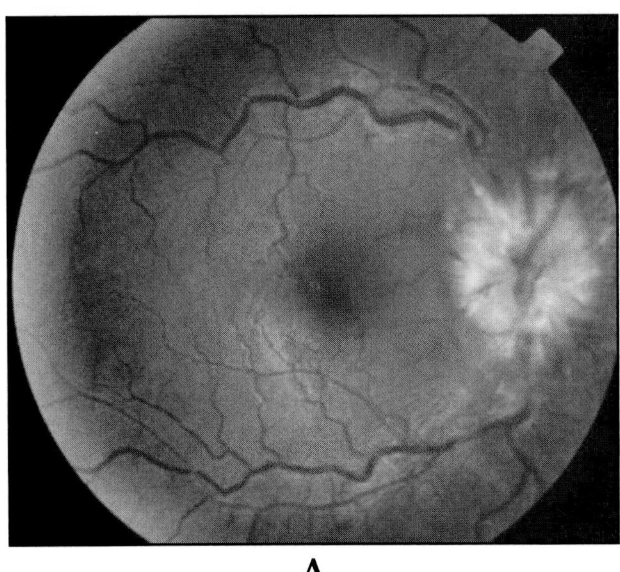

A

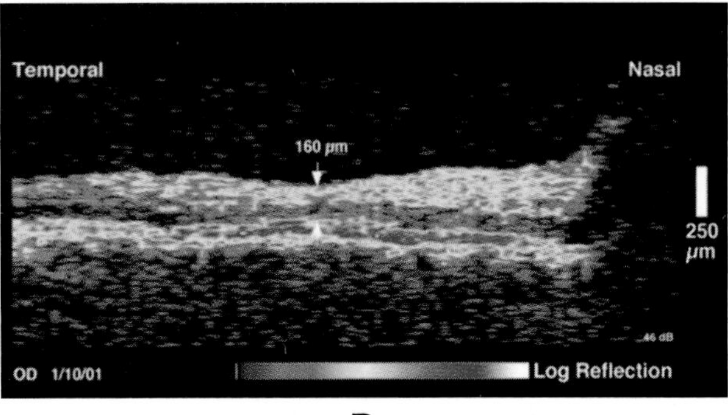

B

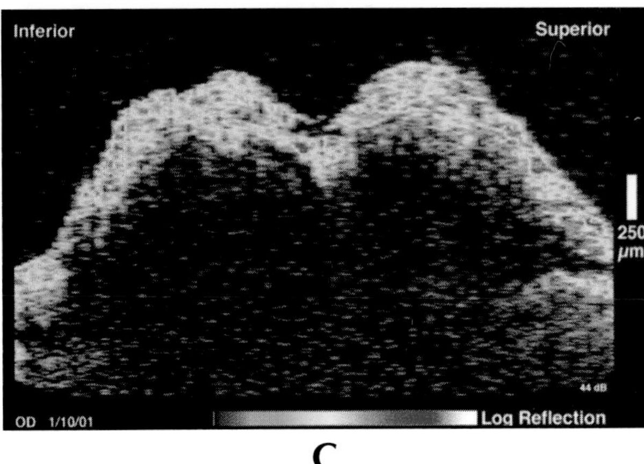

C

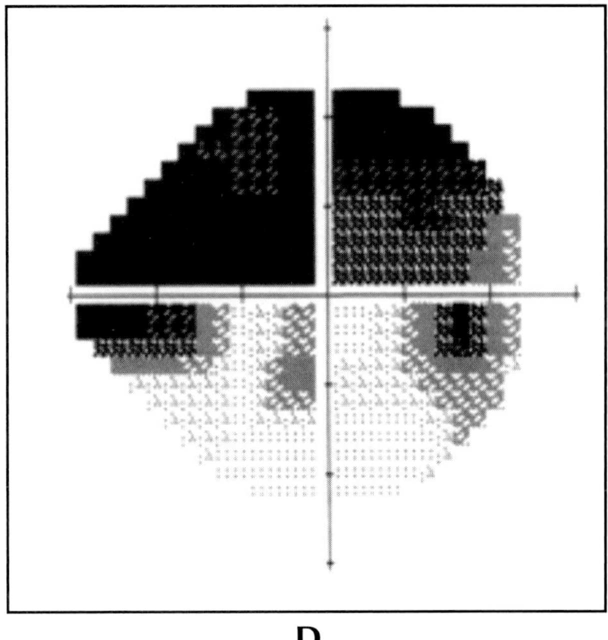

D

OCT showed elevation of both optic discs (C and F), and macular scans (B and G) showed elevation of the left macular region from apparent subretinal fluid. This resolved and vision improved after administration of acetazolamide, optic nerve sheath fenestration OS, and weight loss.

Comment

OCT shows subretinal fluid as a cause of decreased central vision in some patients with papilledema.

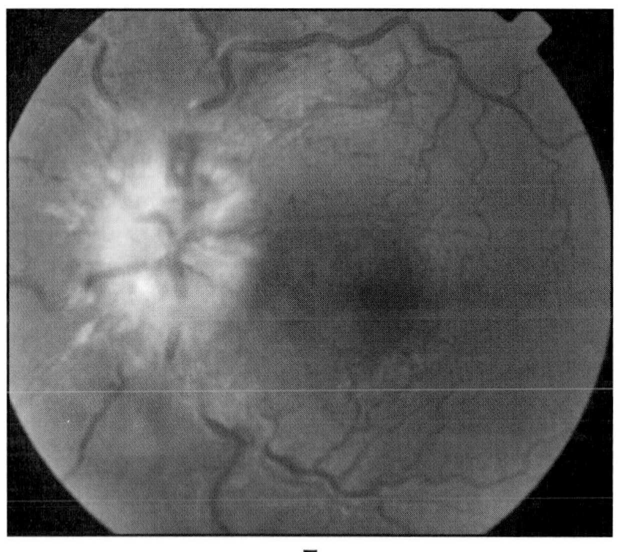

E

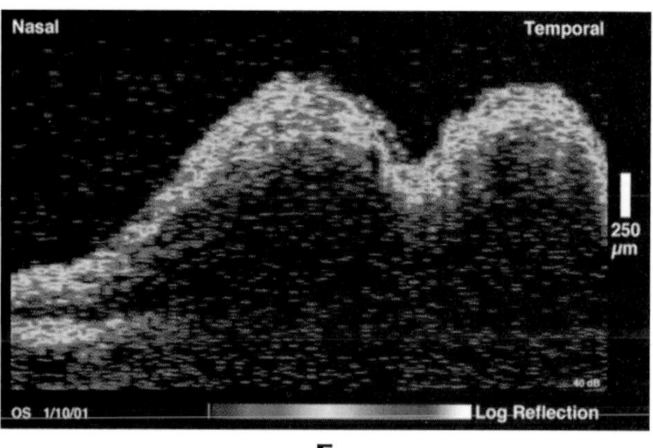

F

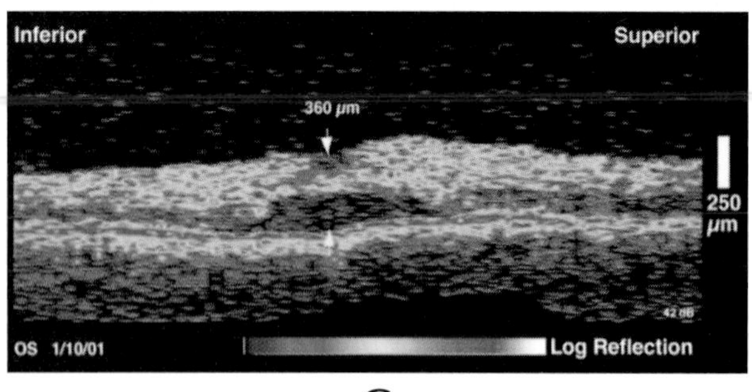

G

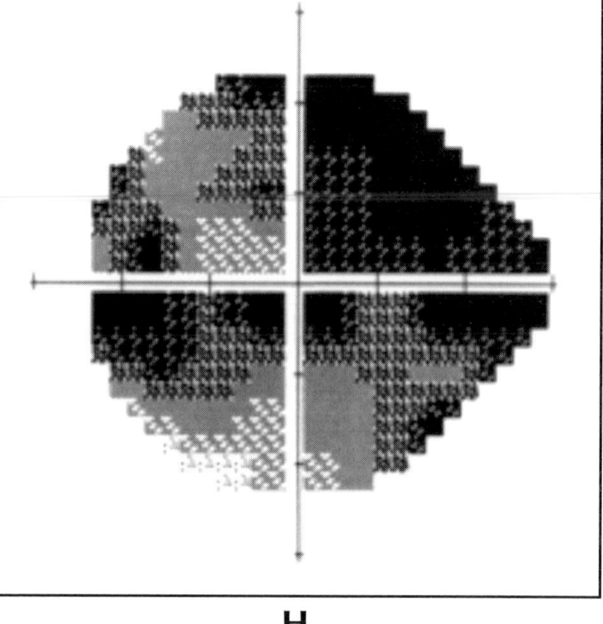

H

Case 13-9. Hypotony With Papilledema

A 38-year-old man had right eye hypotony due to car airbag trauma 2 years earlier. The visual acuity was 20/70 and the IOP was 6 mmHg. A cyclodialysis cleft of two clock hours was found by gonioscopy. Indirect funduscopy revealed an elevated disc with engorgement and tortuosity of the veins, a macular star, and choroidal folds (A). OCT showed thickening of the macula (C). The optic nerve head OCT image showed elevation of the disc (B).

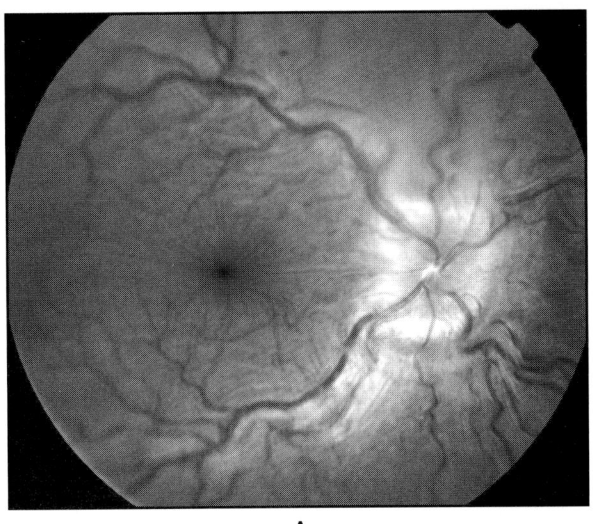

A

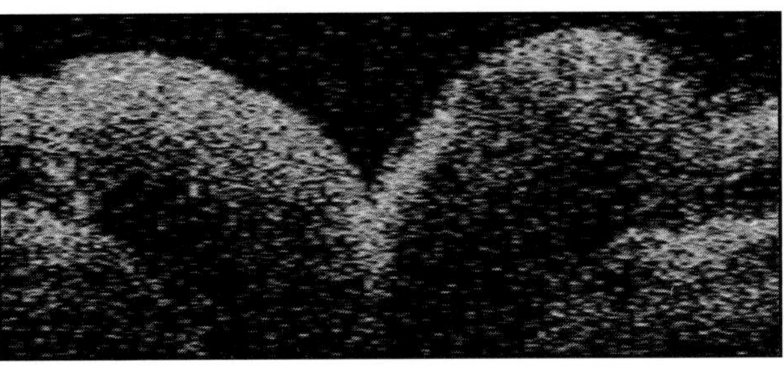

B

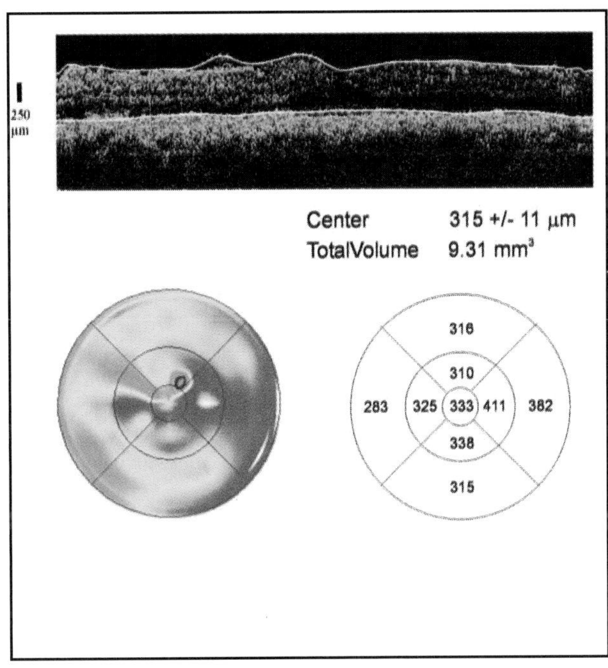

C

OCT showed thickening of the retinal NFL (D). The retinal pigment epithelium (RPE) appeared discontinuous in the OCT image because of the weak OCT signal due to elevation of the disc.

Comments

The OCT is customized to align the RPE. Retinal folds, which are apparent on clinical examination, appear to be flattened on the OCT.

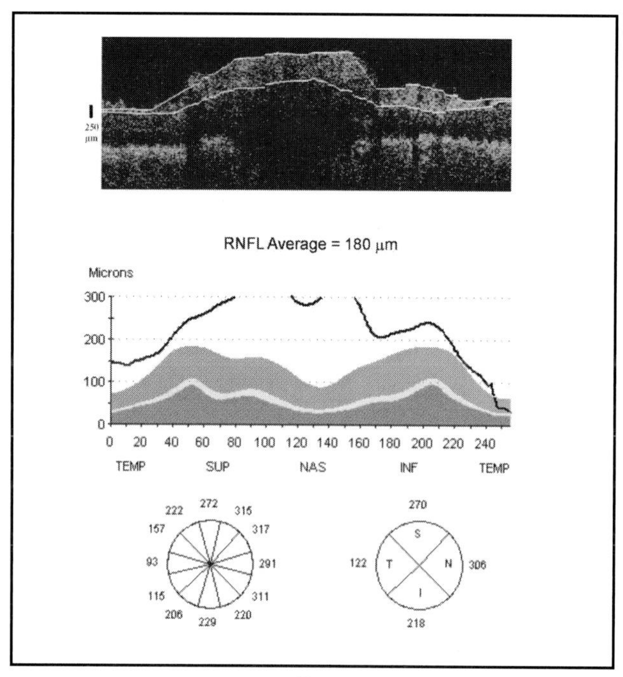

D

Case 13-10. Optic Nerve Compression With Optic Disc Swelling

A 34-year-old woman noted brief spells of visual dimming in her left eye over 1 year. Her visual acuities were 20/15 OD and 20/20 OS. The right VF was normal (C). The left VF showed blind spot enlargement and generalized constriction. There was a relative afferent pupillary defect OS. The right optic disc was normal (A), but the left one was swollen (E), appearing very much like papilledema.

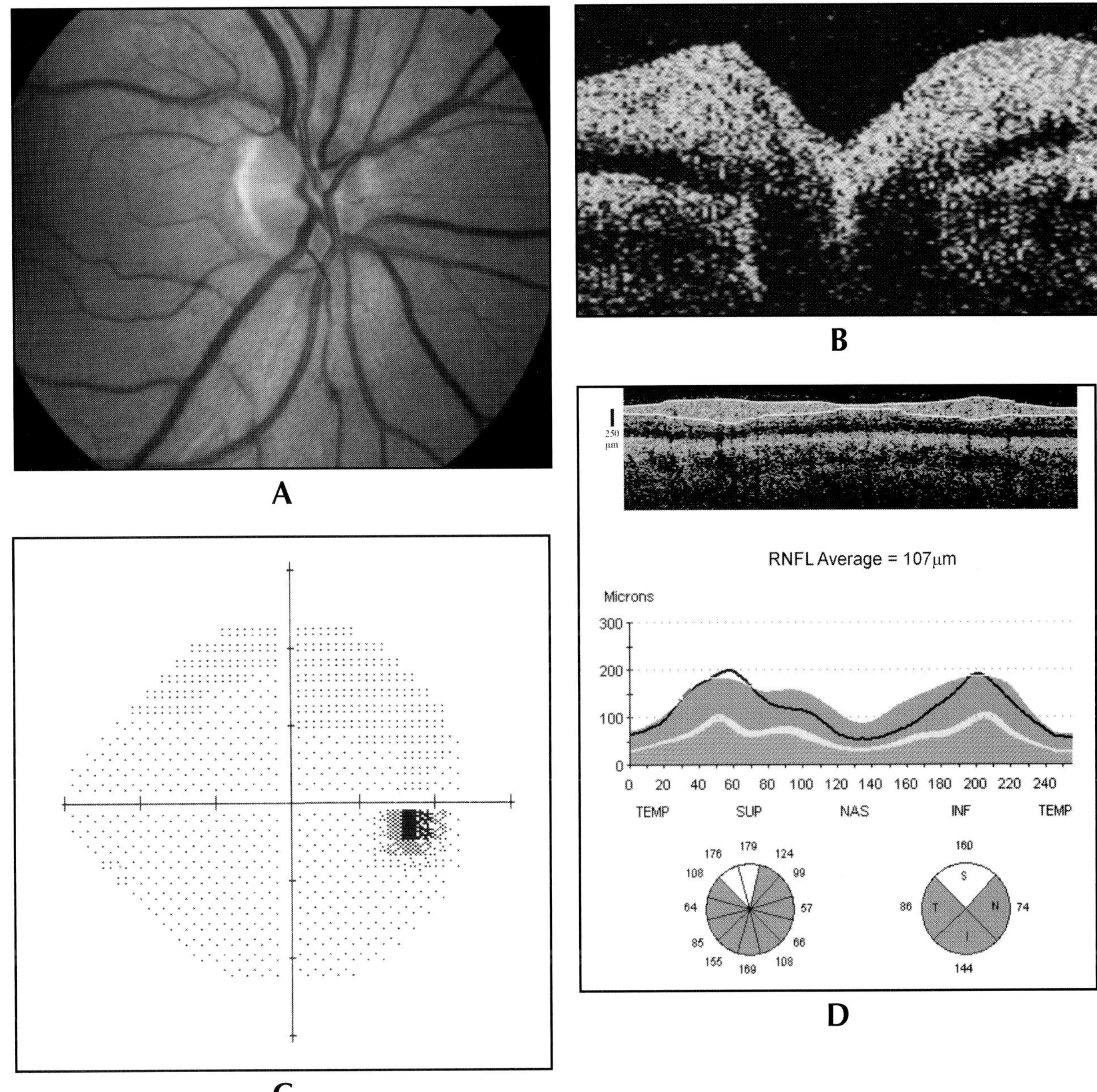

OCT showed optic disc swelling (F) and generalized thickening of the NFL OS (H). The right eye showed normal OCT of the optic disc (B) and NFL (D). MRI showed a small meningioma in the orbital apex extending intracranially. The tumor was surgically excised. Vision remained stable, and the optic disc swelling slowly resolved.

Comment

OCT shows optic disc swelling, which resembles papilledema, in patients with circumferential compression of the optic nerve from meningioma.

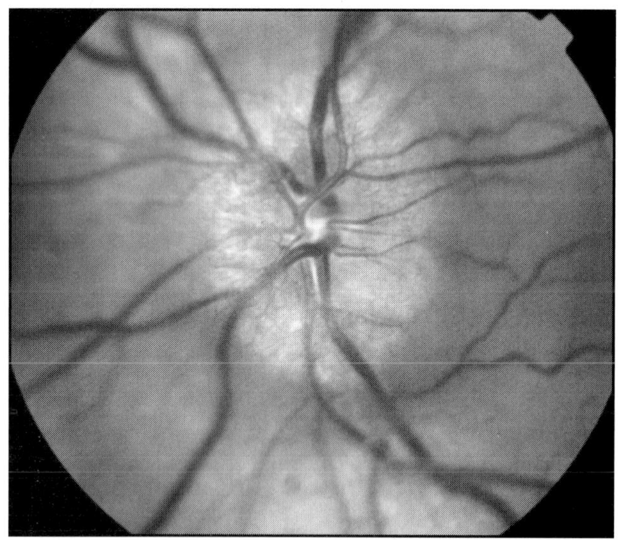

E

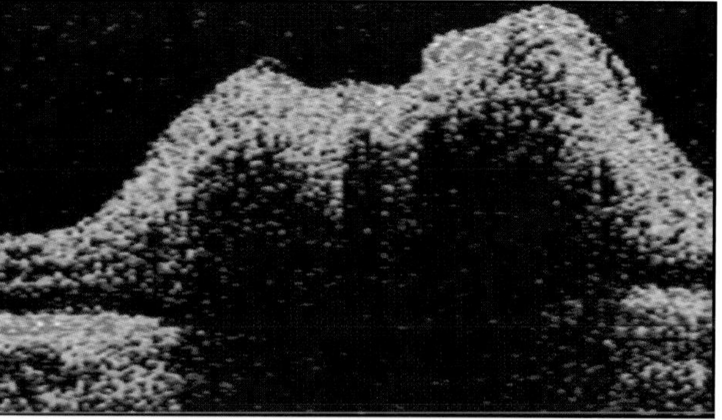

F

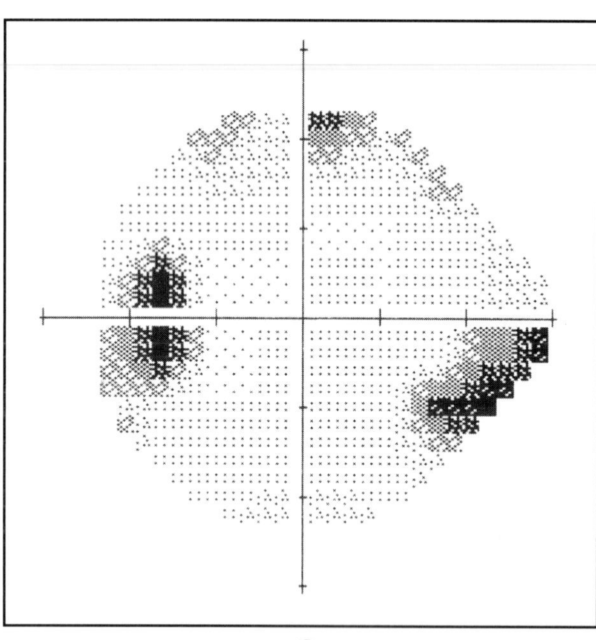

G

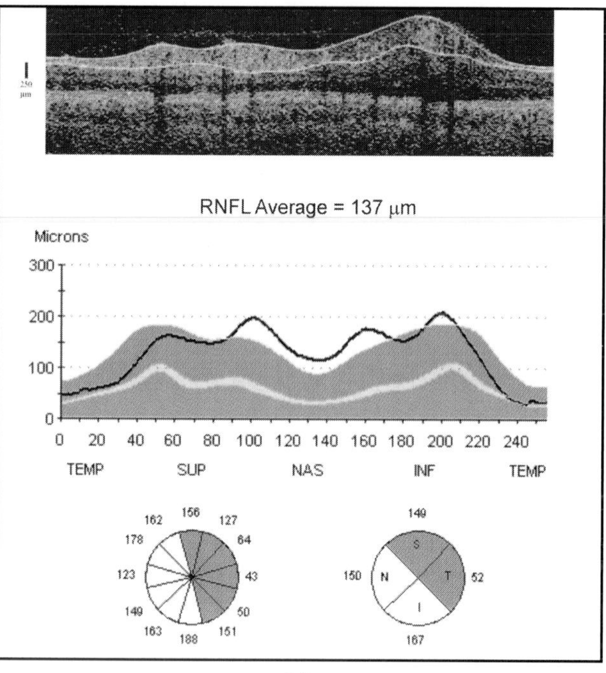

H

Case 13-11. Anterior Ischemic Optic Neuropathy (Presymptomatic/Progressive)

A 51-year-old woman with diabetes and hypertension developed typical anterior ischemic optic neuropathy (AION) in her right eye. When she was initially evaluated, she had no symptoms in her left eye. Visual acuity in the left eye was 20/25 and there was minimal VF change (B). The left optic nerve head showed crowding; minimal swelling; and a small, peripapillary, flame-shaped hemorrhage (A). Three weeks later, she lost vision in this previously asymptomatic left eye to 20/40 and there was inferior and paracentral VF loss (E). The optic disc was now quite swollen (D). About 9 weeks later, visual acuity and the VF were about the same (H). However, the optic disc was becoming atrophic superiorly (G). Sequential OCTs showed retinal NFL swelling at the first evaluation when the patient was asymptomatic (C) and had relatively normal visual acuity and VF. There was marked RNFL thickening (F) when the vision was lost, and thinning of the retinal NFL superiorly after several weeks (I) when there was persistent inferior VF loss. No normative data were available for this case imaged with the first generation of commercial OCT.

Comment

OCT can show retinal NFL thickening in the presymptomatic phase of AION.

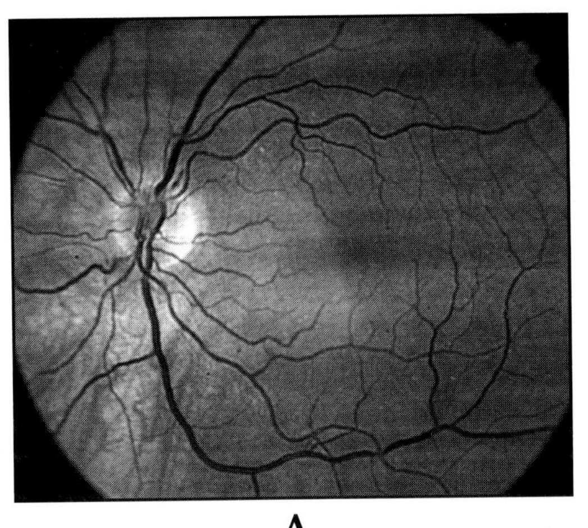

A

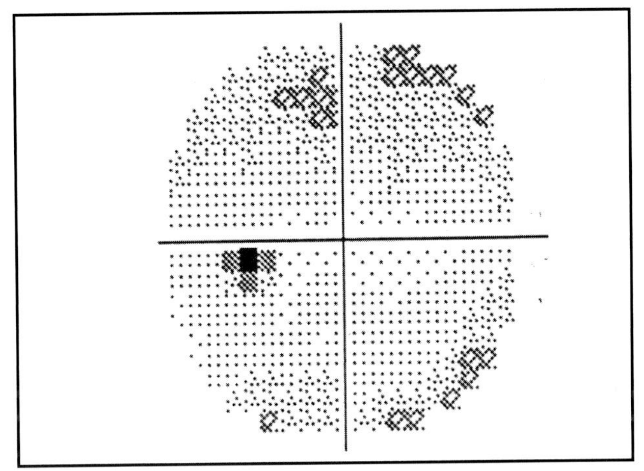

B

C

3-Week Follow Up

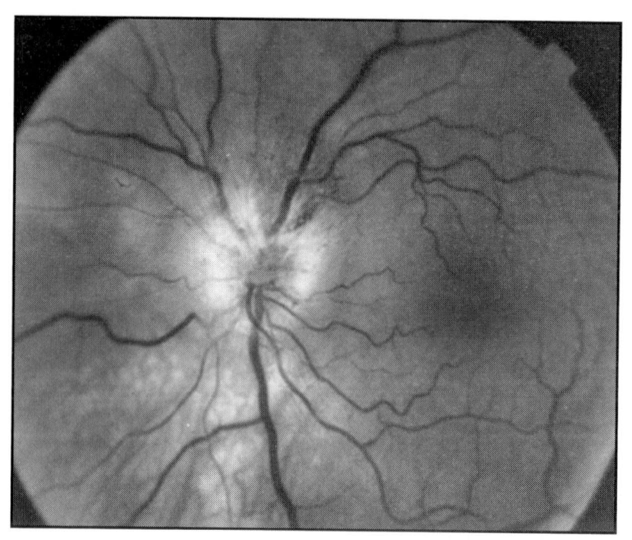

D

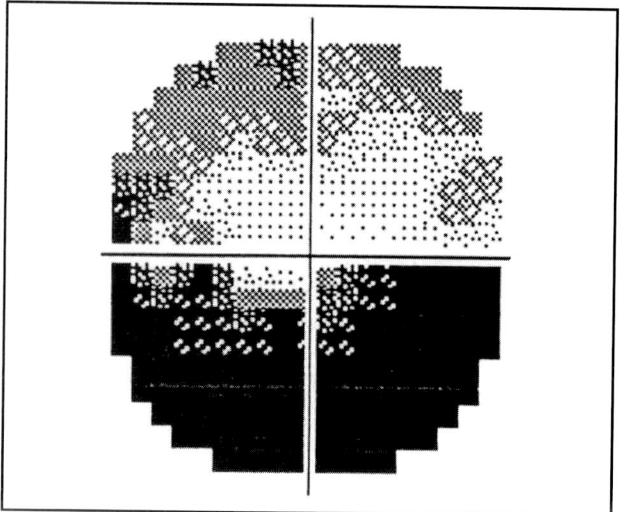

E

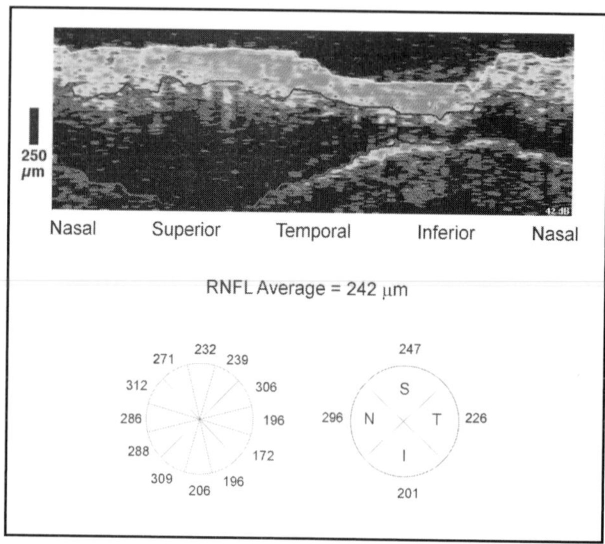

F

9-Week Follow-Up

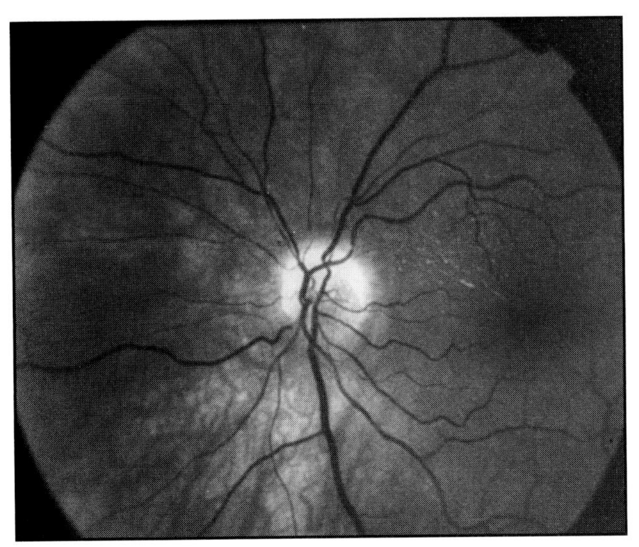

G

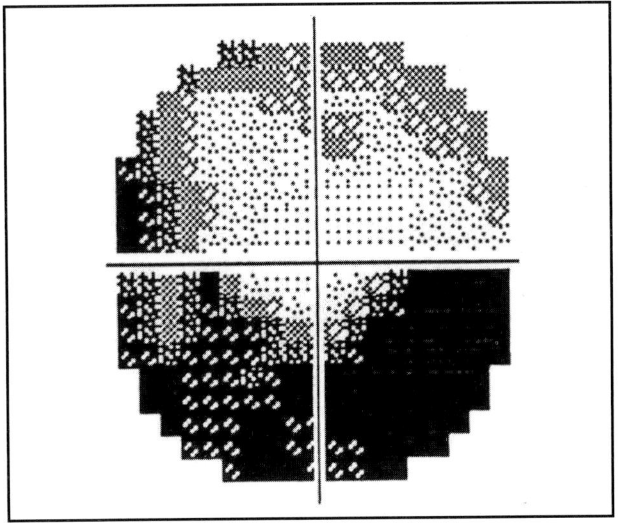

H

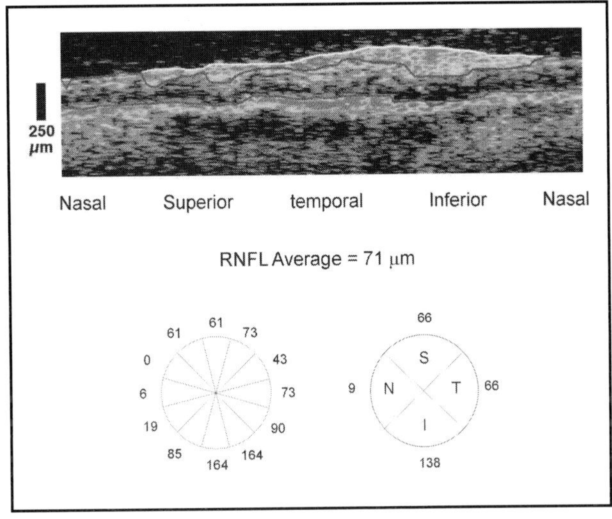

I

Case 13-12. Acute and Remote Anterior Ischemic Optic Neuropathy: Pseudo-Foster-Kennedy Syndrome

A 61-year-old man suddenly lost vision in his left eye 9 years previously without any significant recovery. He was referred for further evaluation when he awoke with loss of vision in his right eye. He was hypertensive. Visual acuities were 20/40 OD and 20/400 OS.

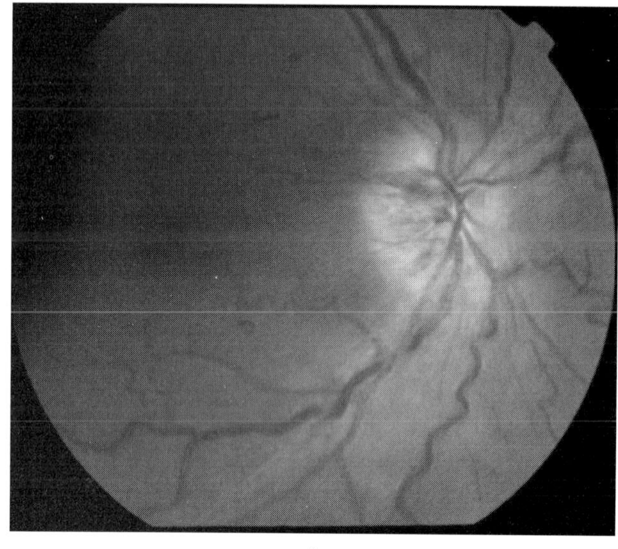

A

B

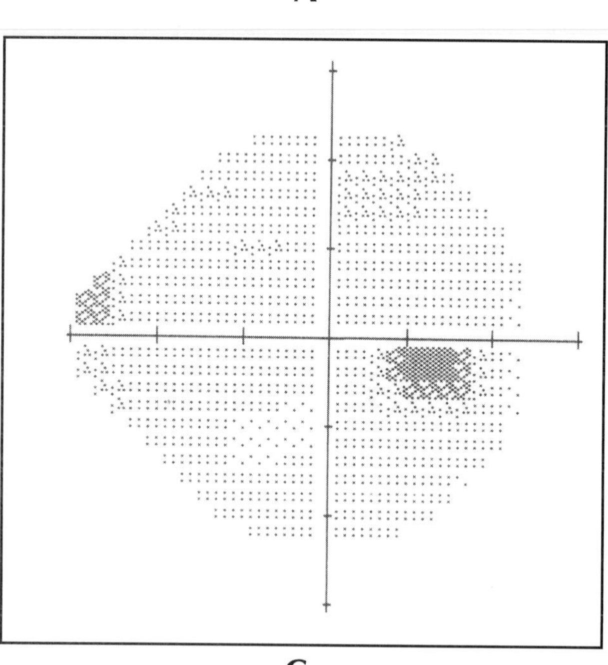

C

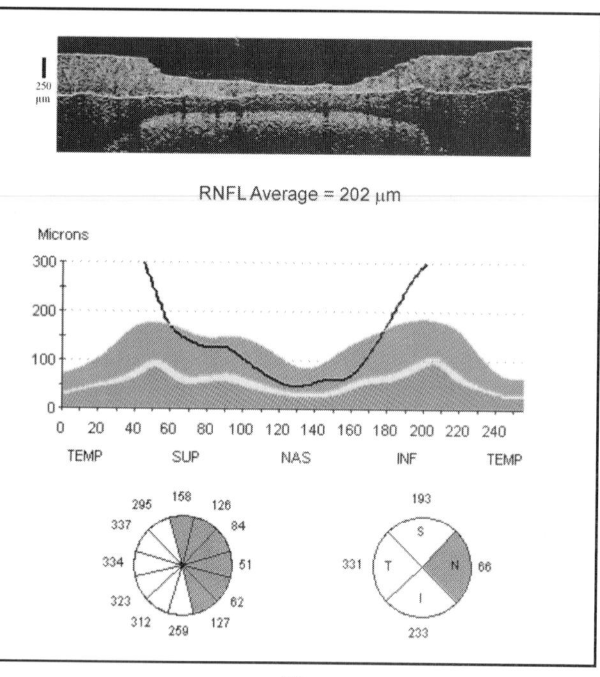

D

VF testing showed a small superior arcuate defect on the right (C) and dense, inferior, acuate loss with inferior and superior nasal steps on the left (G). The right optic disc was swollen with flame hemorrhages and evidence of congenital crowding (A). The left optic nerve head was atrophic (E). OCT showed elevation of the optic nerve head (B) with diffuse swelling of the NFL (D). OCT of the left eye showed crowding of the optic nerve head (F) and diffuse thinning of the retinal NFL (H).

F

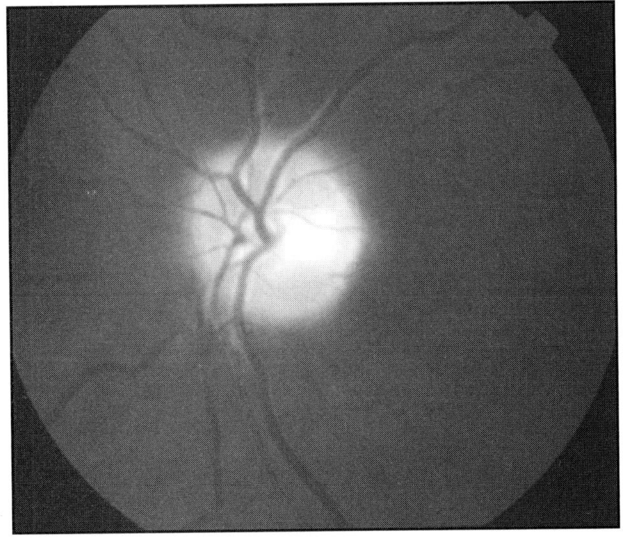

E

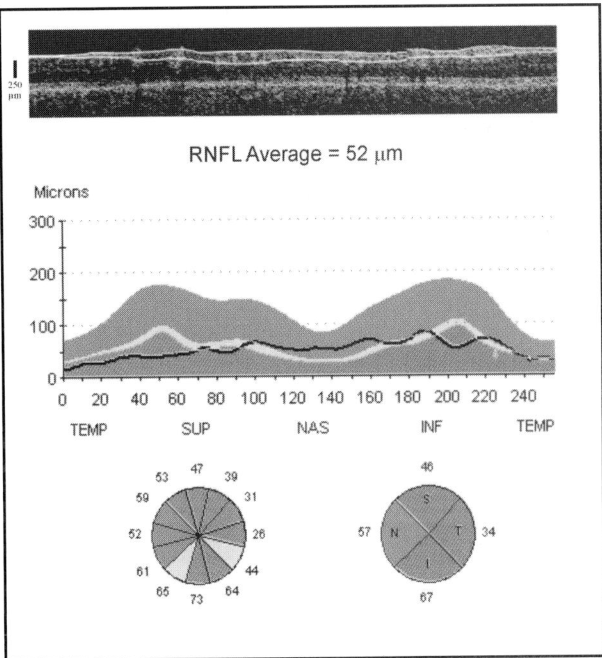

H

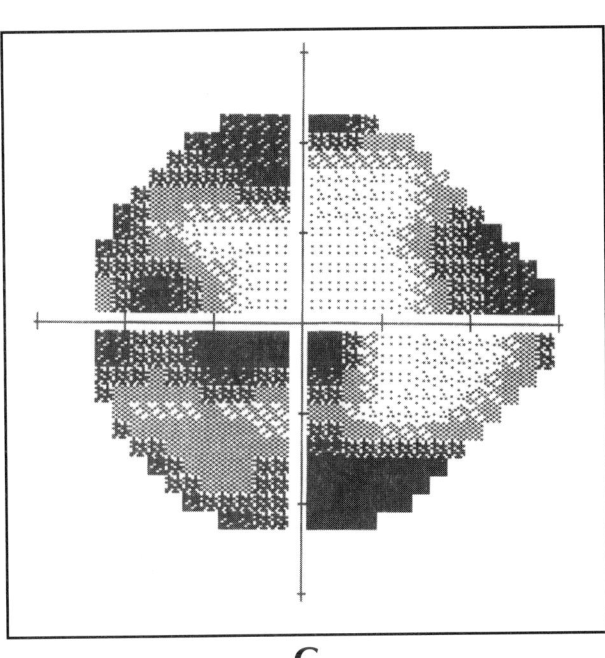

G

Case 13-13. Juvenile Diabetic Papillopathy

A 24-year-old woman who had been insulin dependent for 15 years developed blurred vision in her left eye. This had been present for 3 months when she was evaluated. Visual acuities were 20/20 OD and 20/30 OS. VF testing showed enlargement of the blind spot OS (D). The right fundus showed minimal background diabetic microvascular changes. The left optic disc was swollen (A). OCT showed elevation of the optic nerve head (B), NFL thickening (C), and macular thickening with apparent intra- and subretinal fluid (E).

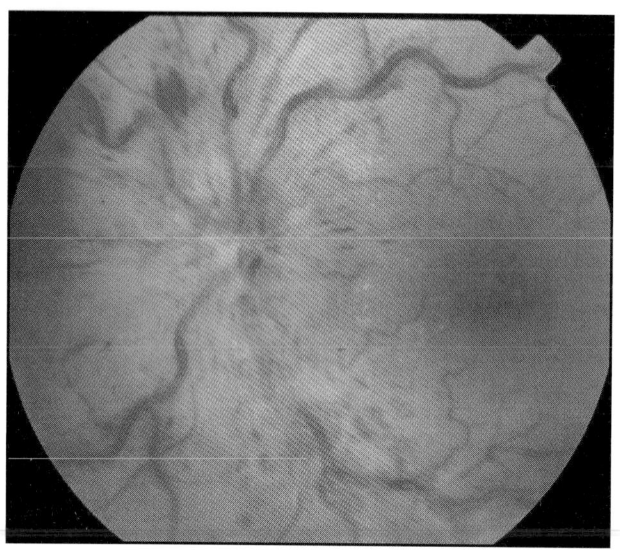

A

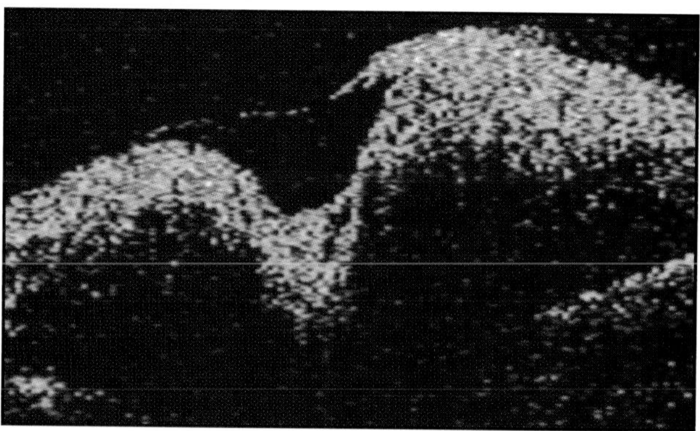

B

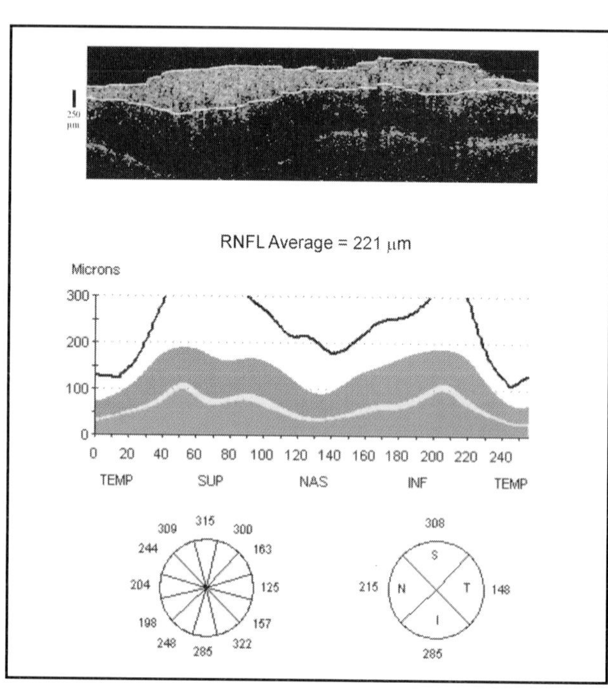

C

Comment

OCT shows the swelling of the optic disc and retina in juvenile diabetics who develop visual loss with optic disc swelling and can be used to monitor affected patients. OCT shows macular involvement.

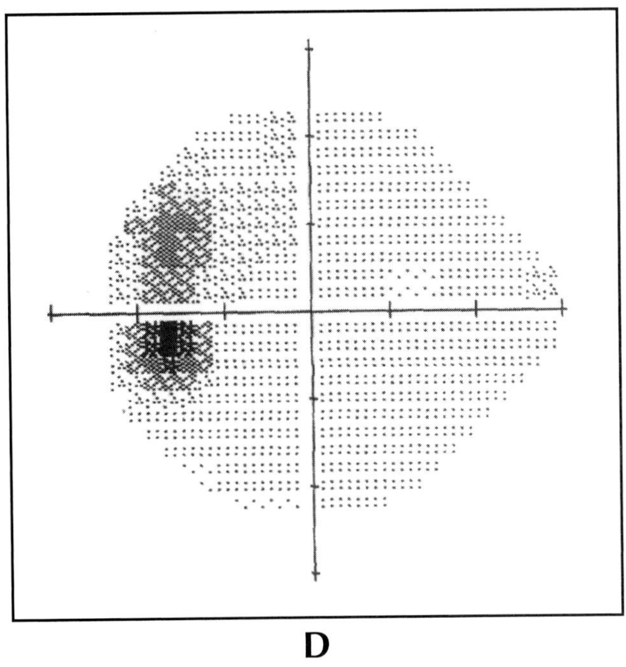

D

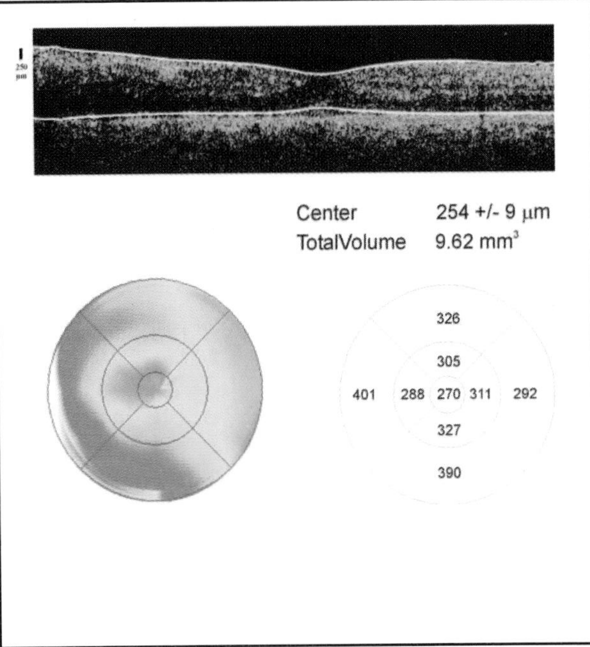

E

Case 13-14. Papillitis

A 30-year-old woman developed painful loss of vision in her right eye. She had aches and pains in several joints over the previous years, and a rheumatological evaluation had shown an increased rheumatoid factor. MRI showed no abnormalities in the orbits or brain. Visual acuity was reduced to 20/40, and there was an inferior VF defect (C). The right optic disc was swollen (A). OCT showed optic nerve head swelling (B), retinal NFL thickening (D), and macular thickening OD.

Comment

OCT can show retinal thickening (edema) associated with papillitis.

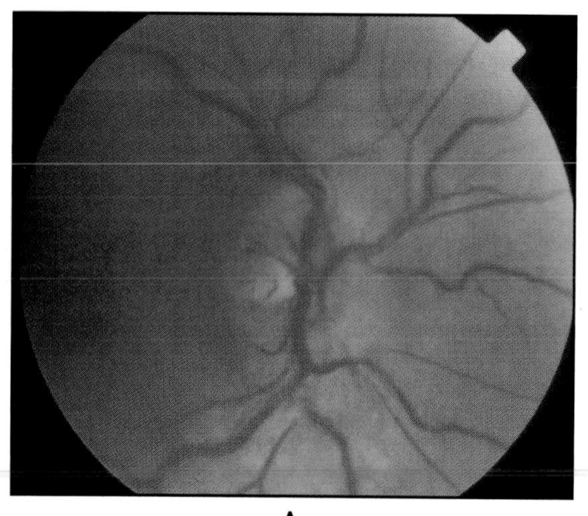

A

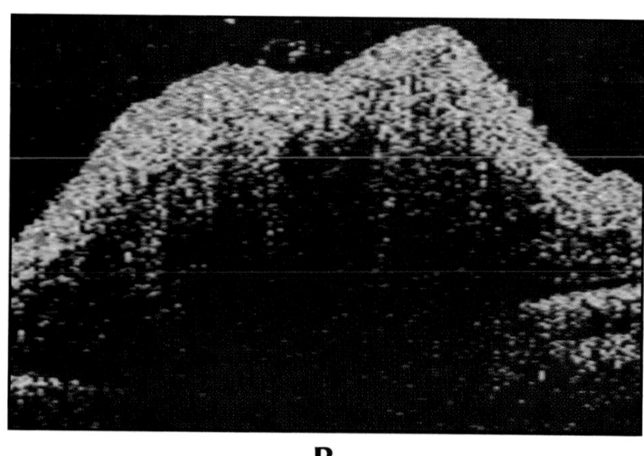

B

C

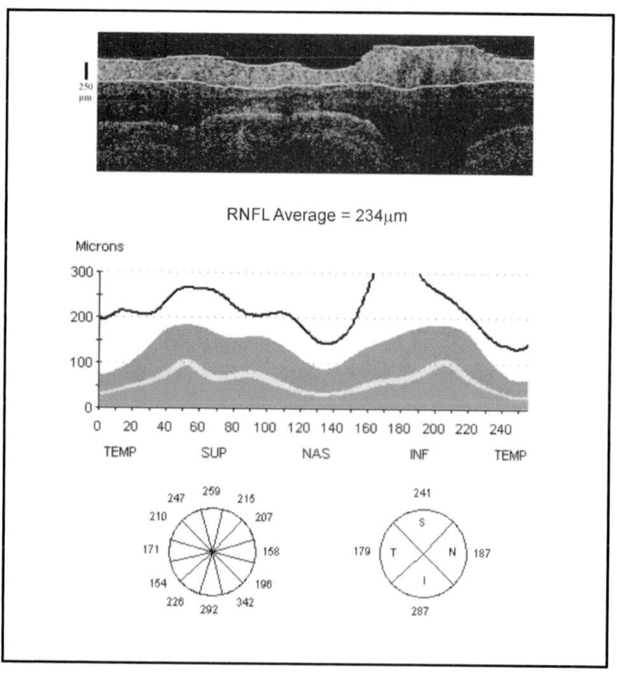

D

Case 13-15. Neuroretinitis

A 12-year-old girl noted blurred vision in her right eye. Bartonella hesilae IgG titer was >1024 and IgM titer was 64. Visual acuities were 20/40 OD and 20/20 OS. The right VF showed enlargement of the blind spot (C). The right optic disc was slightly swollen, and there were exudates inferior to the optic disc and in the macular region in a star pattern (A). OCT showed elevation of the optic nerve head and areas of increased reflectance near the fovea (B). Thickening of NFL and presence of the high-reflectant posterior hyaloid membrane caused artifact of the OCT NFL detection (D). The normative data were not available for patients below 18 years of age.

Comment

OCT can show the swelling of the optic disc, which accompanies neuroretinitis and perifoveal thickening of the retina.

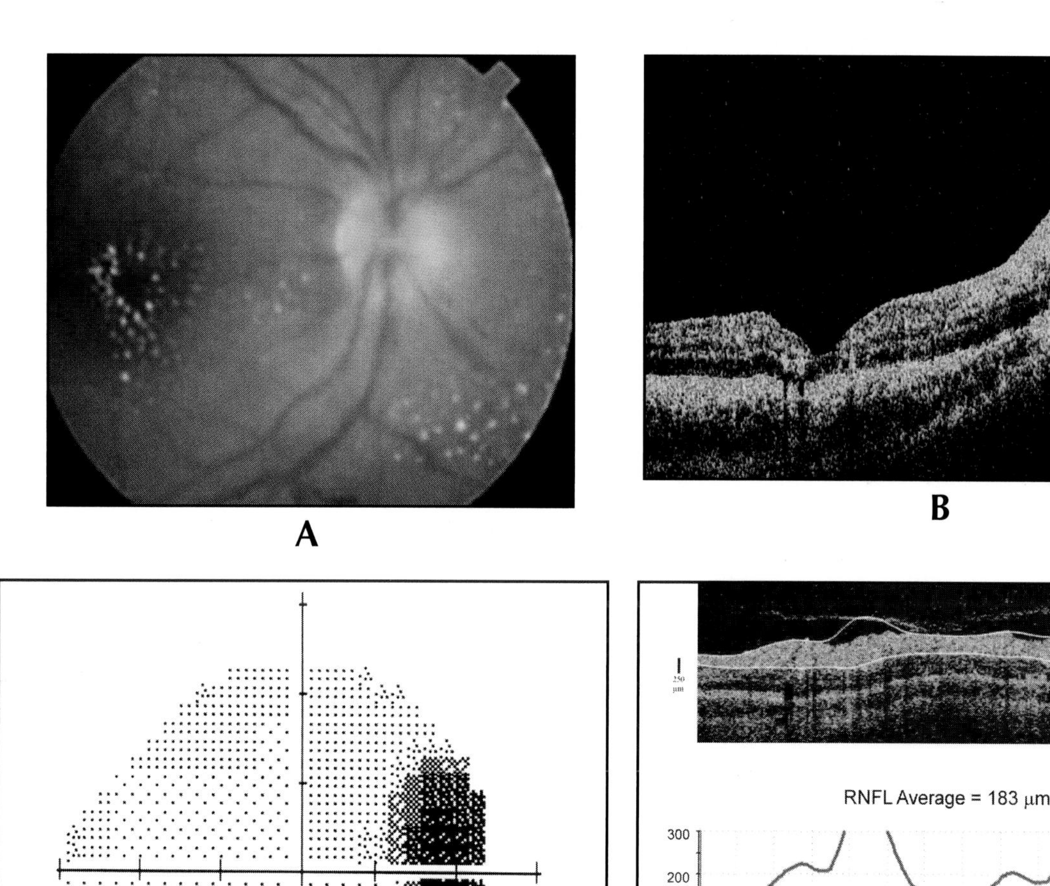

B

A

C

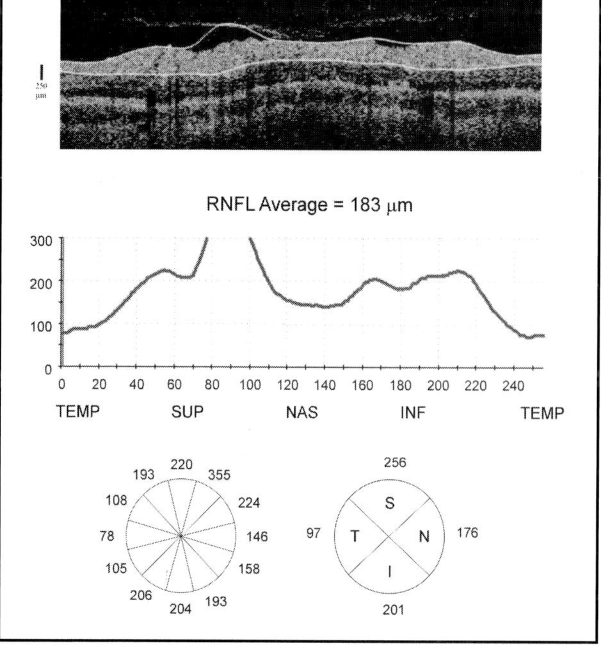

D

Case 13-16. Vitreopapillary Traction

An 87-year-old woman was found to have optic disc swelling in her right eye during a routine preoperative visit before cataract surgery. Visual acuities were 20/40 OD and 20/40 OS. VF testing showed mild, nonspecific depression in both eyes (B). The right optic nerve head was slightly elevated without definite edema or hemorrhage (A). The left optic disc appeared unremarkable. OCT showed elevation of the optic nerve head with apparent vitreous attachments causing the optic disc margins to appear "tented," forming the appearance of a suspension bridge (C). She underwent uneventful cataract surgery. The vitreous-optic traction did not change after cataract surgery.

Comment

OCT can demonstrate traction on the optic disc from adherent vitreous and helps rule out pathological swelling of the optic nerve.

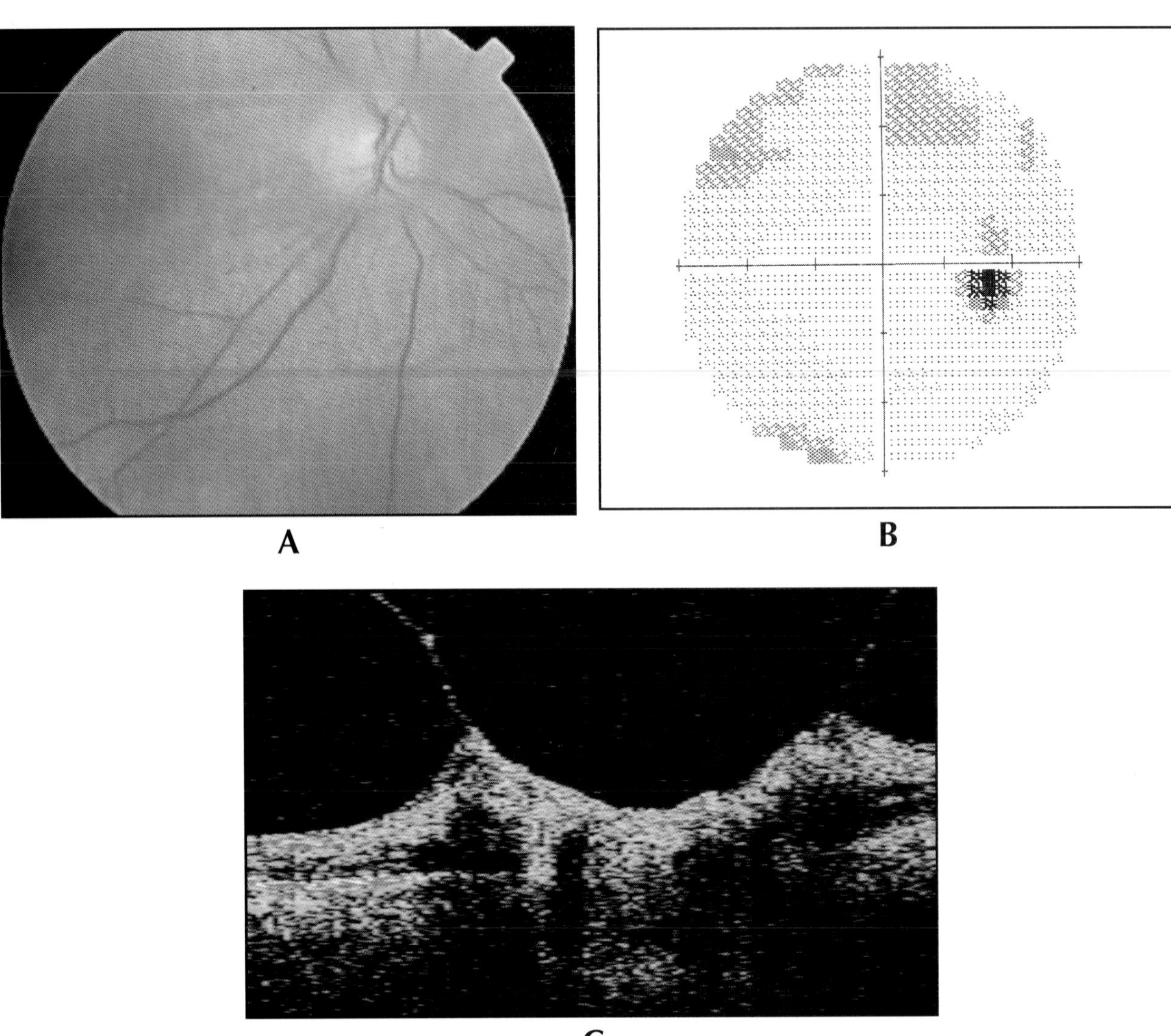

Case 13-17. *Papillophlebitis*

A 27-year-old woman saw her optometrist because she thought that she needed a new prescription. Optic disc swelling was noted. She was otherwise healthy. Visual acuities were 20/20 OD and 20/20 OS. The right blind spot was enlarged (A). The right optic disc was swollen and there were multiple hemorrhages and some cotton wool spots in the posterior pole (B). OCT showed elevation of the optic nerve head and thickening of the retinal NFL (C).

Comment

OCT shows retinal NFL thickening in papillophlebitis and can be used for follow-up in affected patients.

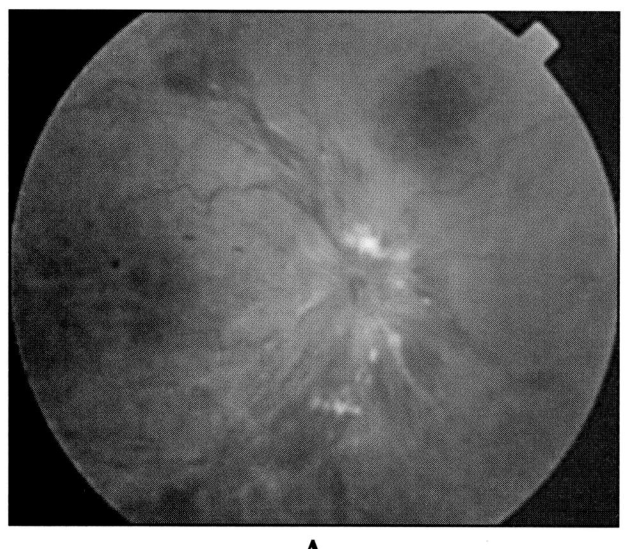

A

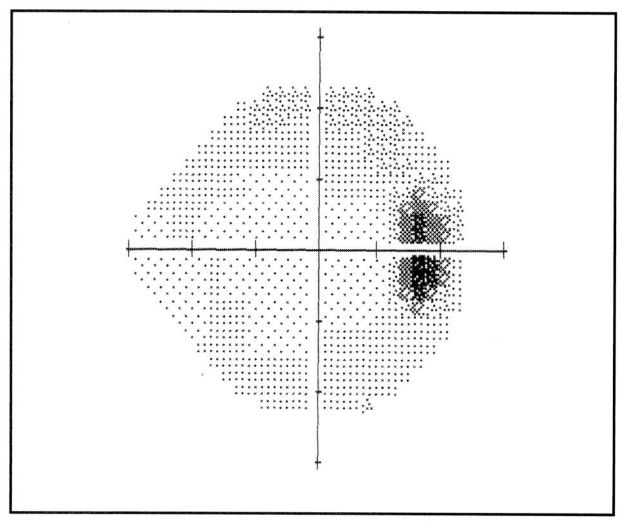

B

250 µm

RNFL Average = 226 µm

Microns

300

200

100

0

0 20 40 60 80 100 120 140 160 180 200 220 240

TEMP SUP NAS INF TEMP

372 351 243 208 242 291 281 273 237 186 217 303

342 231 282 214

S N I T

C

Case 13-18. Congenitally Crowded Optic Nerves

A 21-year-old woman was referred to rule out papilledema. Visual acuities were 20/20 OD and 20/20 OS. VFs were normal. The optic discs appeared crowded without evidence of pathological swelling (A and D).

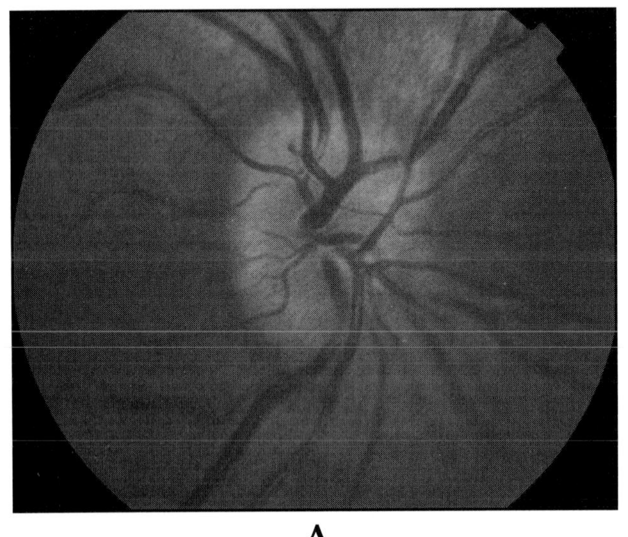

A

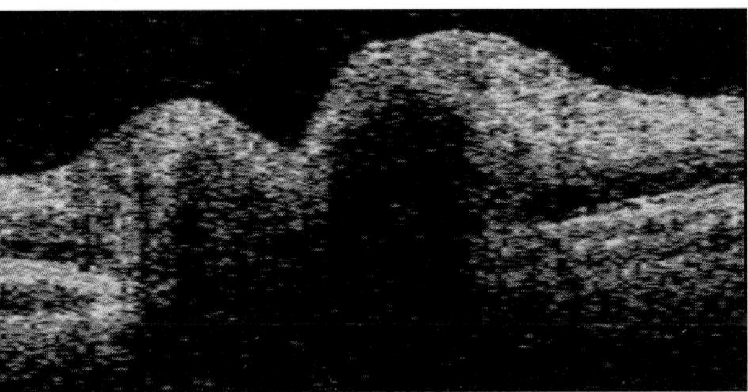

B

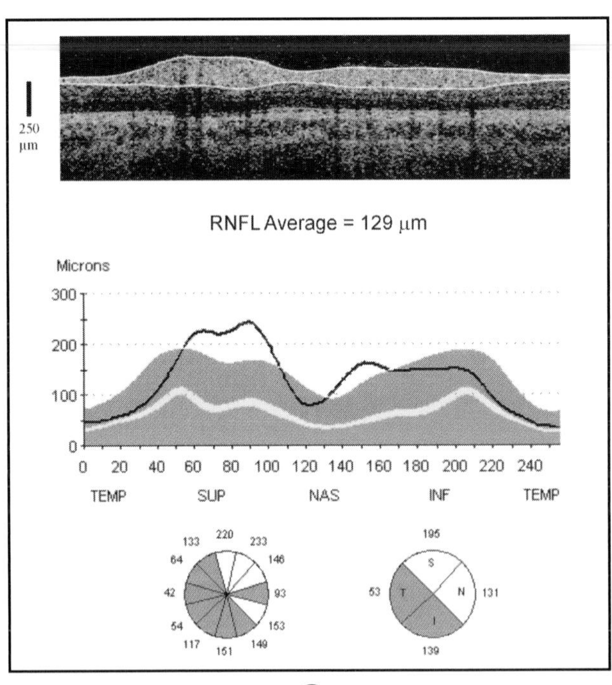

C

OCT showed elevated optic nerve heads (B and E), and NFLs were slightly thicker than normal (C and F). Follow-up 4 months later showed no change in the appearance of the nerves or in the OCT measurements of the NFL in both eyes.

Comment

OCT shows that the retinal NFL may be slightly thicker than normal in patients with congenital crowding of the optic nerves. Follow-up of OCTs can compliment serial observation to ensure that there is no change over time and can help confirm that nerves suspected of being swollen are actually congenitally anomalous.

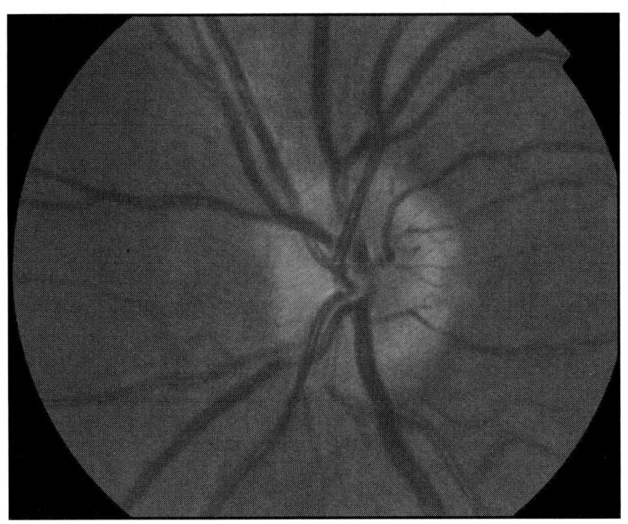

D

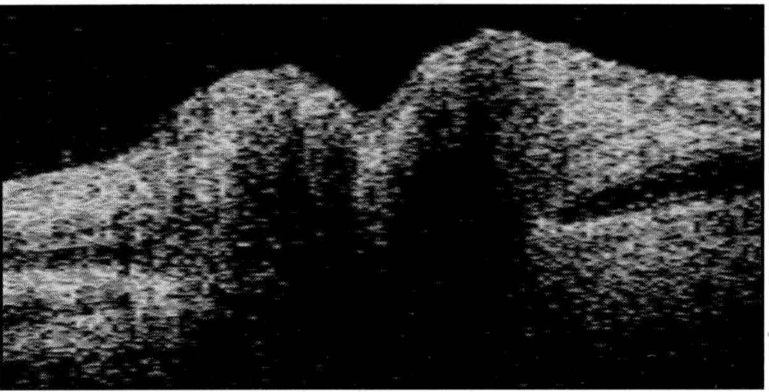

E

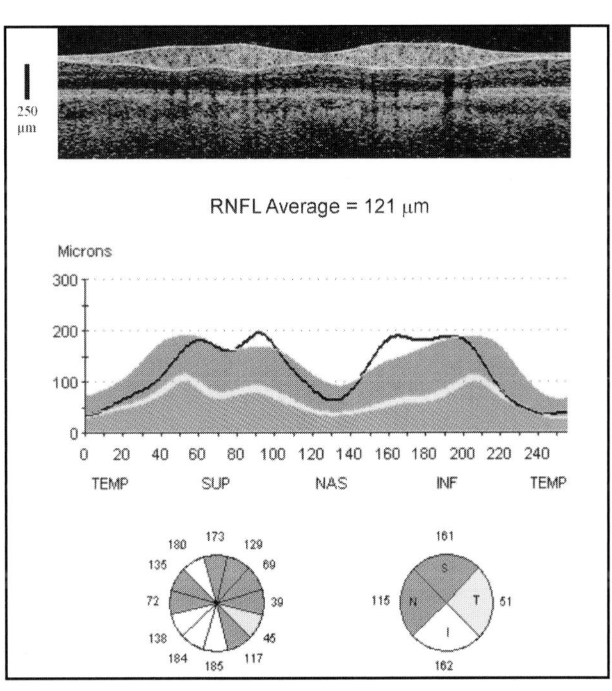

F

Case 13-19. Mild Optic Disc Drusen

A 40-year-old man had been followed because of optic disc drusen for 14 years. He was aware of a small VF defect in his right lower VF, but it had not changed. Visual acuities were 20/20 OD and 20/20 OS.

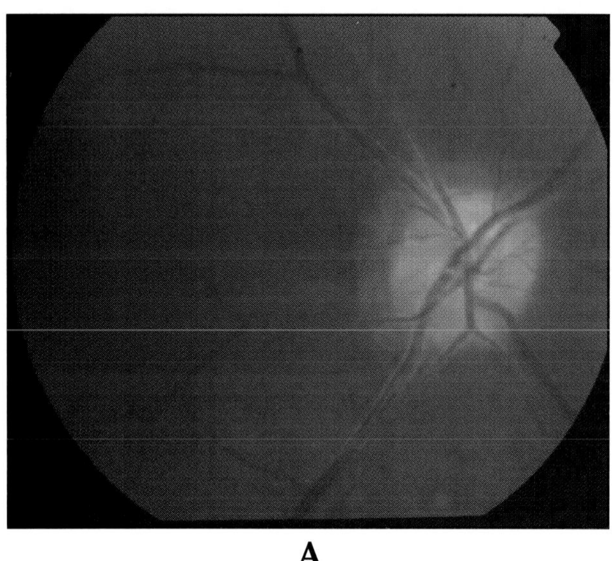

A

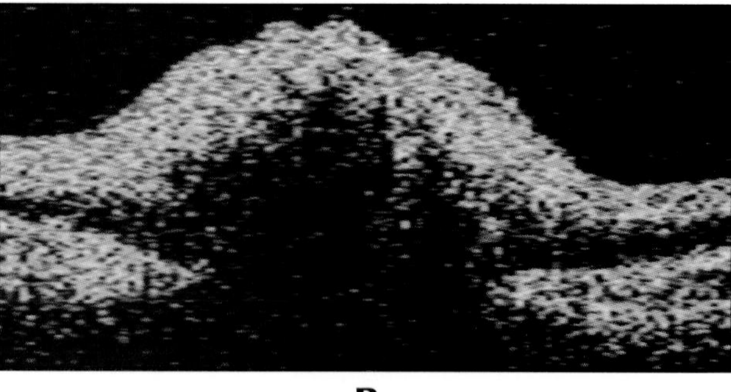

B

C

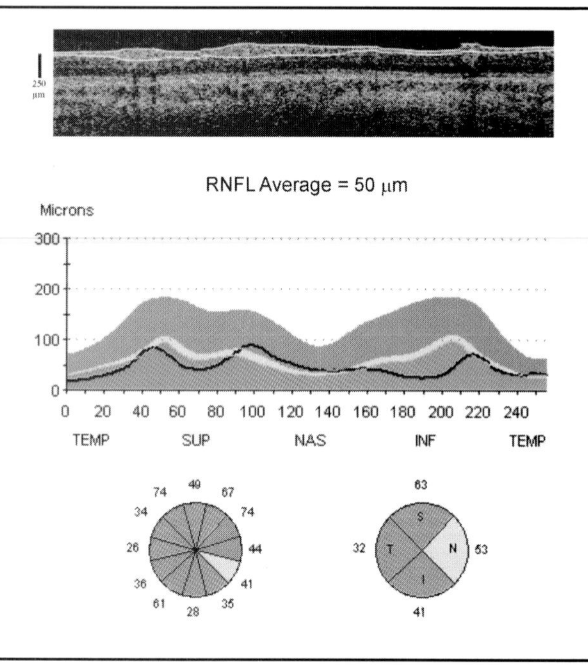

D

There was inferior VF loss OD (C) and patchy loss OS (G). Optic disc drusen were barely visible bilaterally (A and E). OCT showed full optic nerve heads with shadows caused by drusen (B and F) and thinning of the NFL (D and H).

Comment

OCT of the optic disc may demonstrate shadows, indicating buried drusen.

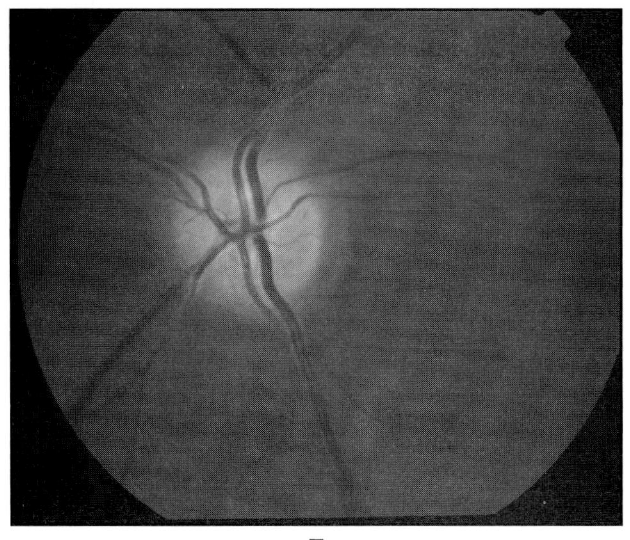

E

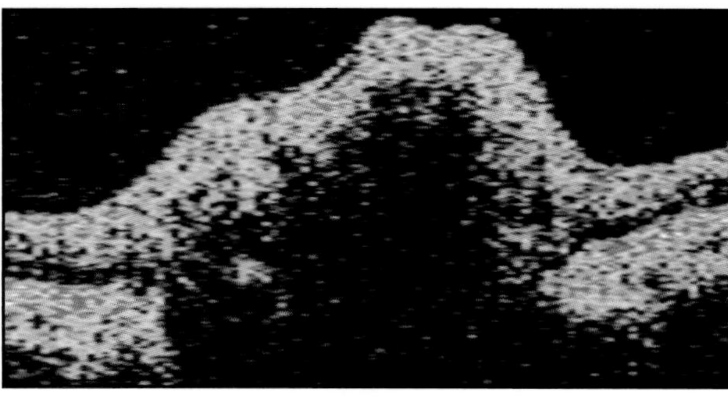

F

G

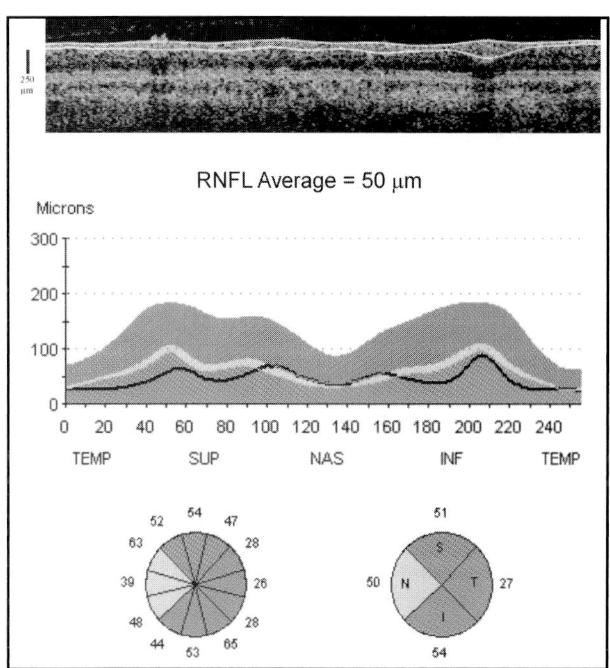

H

Case 13-20. Severe Optic Disc Drusen

A 44-year-old woman was told that she had optic disc drusen when she was 17 years of age. Her VF defects had progressed somewhat since, but she remained without visual disability. Visual acuities at the time of evaluation were 20/20 OD and 20/30 OS.

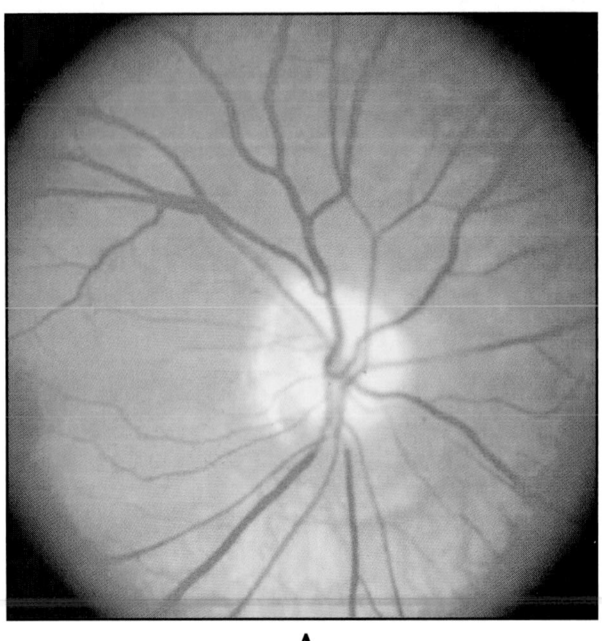

A

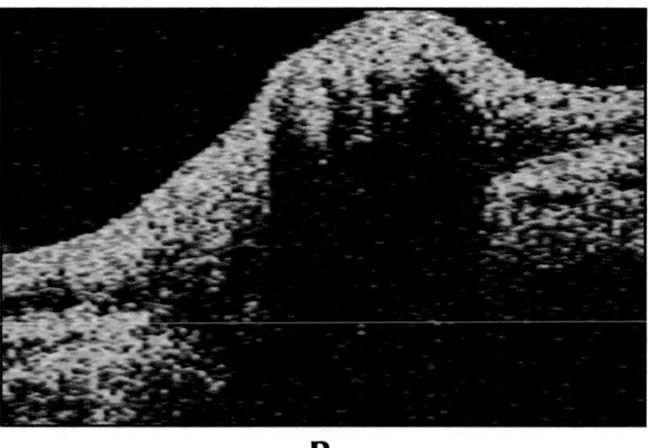

B

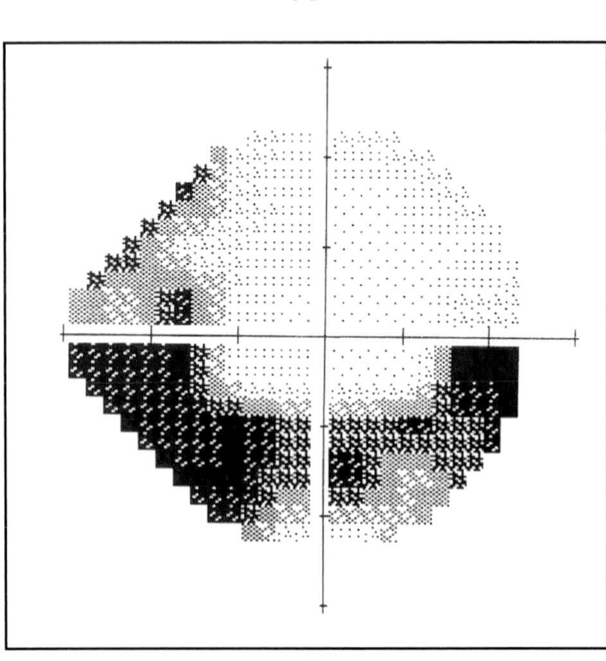

C

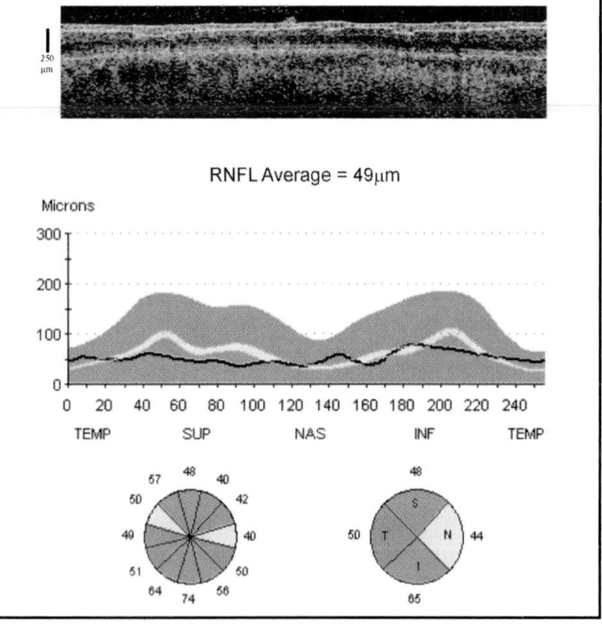

D

VFs showed inferior arcuate loss OD (C) and inferior with paracentral loss OS (G). The optic discs contained multiple drusen (A and E). OCT showed elevation of the optic discs, dense shadowing (B and F), and thinning of the NFLs (D and H).

Comment

OCT can be used to objectively follow NFL changes in patients with optic disc drusen.

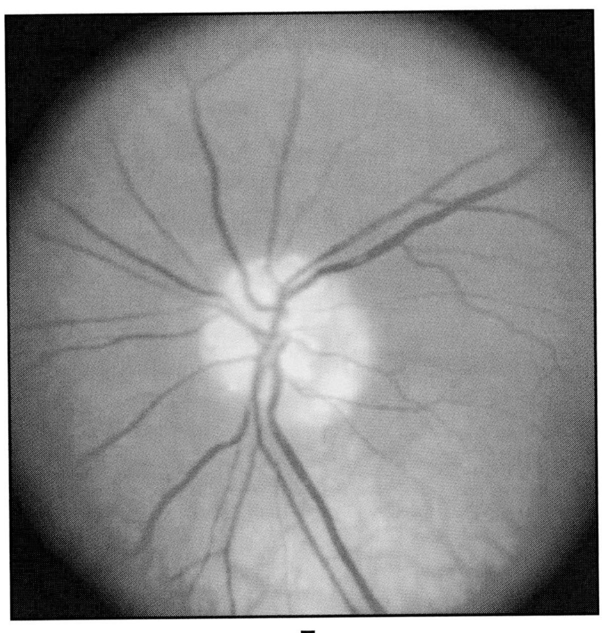

E

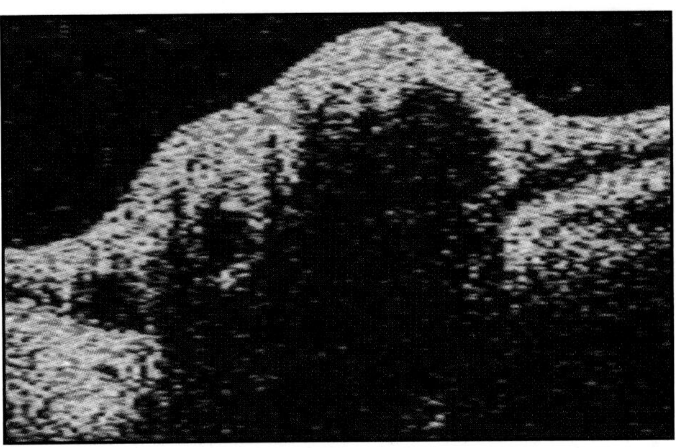

F

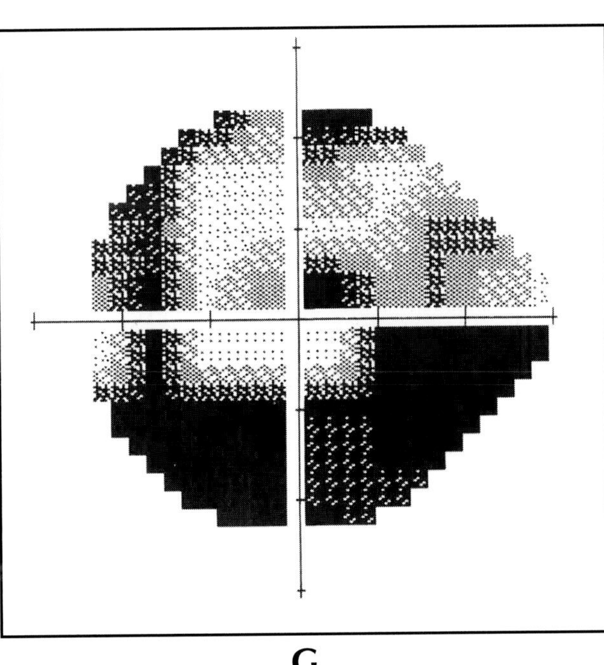

G

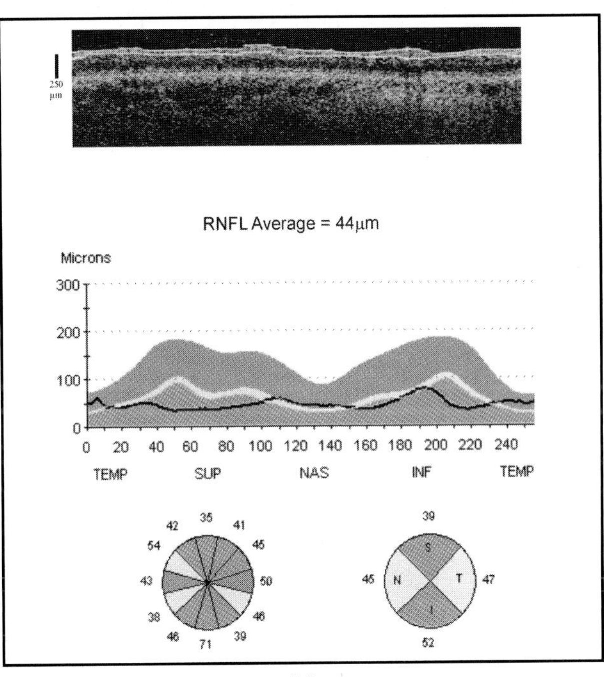

H

Case 13-21. Morning Glory Anomaly

A 61-year-old man was found to have an anomalous optic disc in the left eye as an infant when he was evaluated for amblyopia in the opposite right eye. He had hyperopic astigmatism in both eyes. Visual acuities were 20/200 OD and 20/30 OS when he was evaluated. VFs showed enlargement of the blind spot OS. The right optic disc appeared relatively normal, but the left one showed typical morning glory appearance (A). OCT showed a normal optic nerve configuration OD and generalized depression of an enlarged nerve with lacey defects within the anterior portion OS (B).

Comment

OCT provides images of this anomaly similar to what has been reported histopathologically. It is surprising that it was present in the patient's nonamblyopic eye.

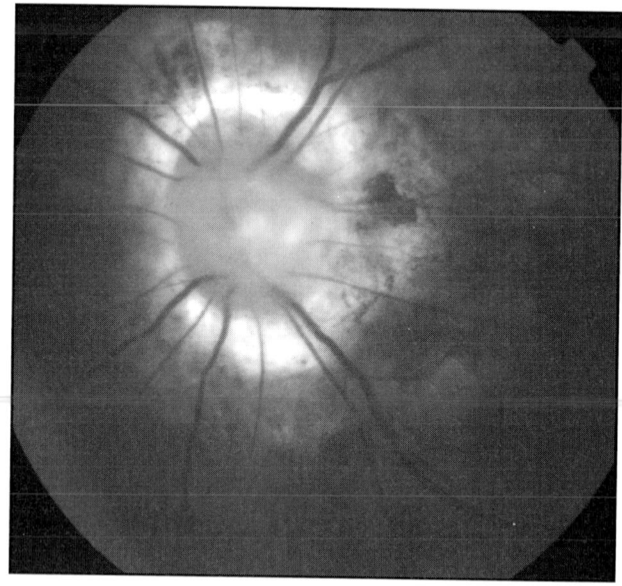

A

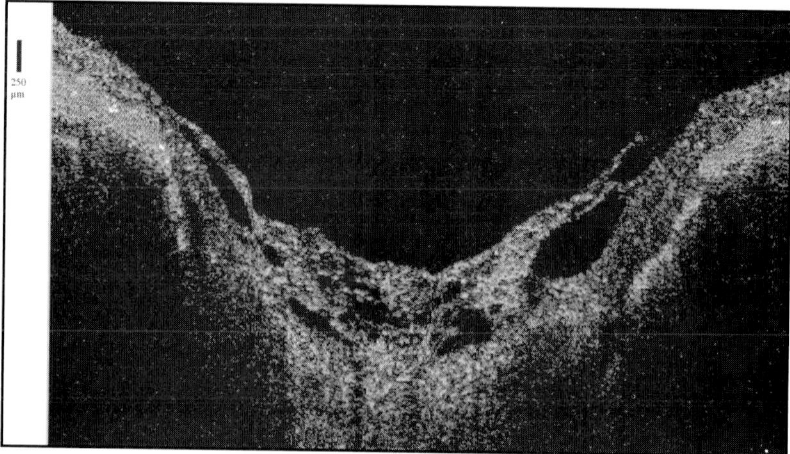

B

Case 13-22. Myelinated Nerve Fibers

A 27-year-old woman was evaluated because of a possible optic nerve head tumor noted by an optometrist 2 years previously. She was asymptomatic. Visual acuities were 20/20 OD and 20/15 OS. VFs showed enlargement of the blind spot in the left eye only (C). The right fundus showed a small cup and some blurring of the margins. The left disc showed exuberant myelin and possibly additional glial proliferation extending superiorly and inferiorly (A). OCT showed thickening of the nerve fibers in the region of the apparent myelinated regions without evidence of more solid areas, which might represent tumor (B and D).

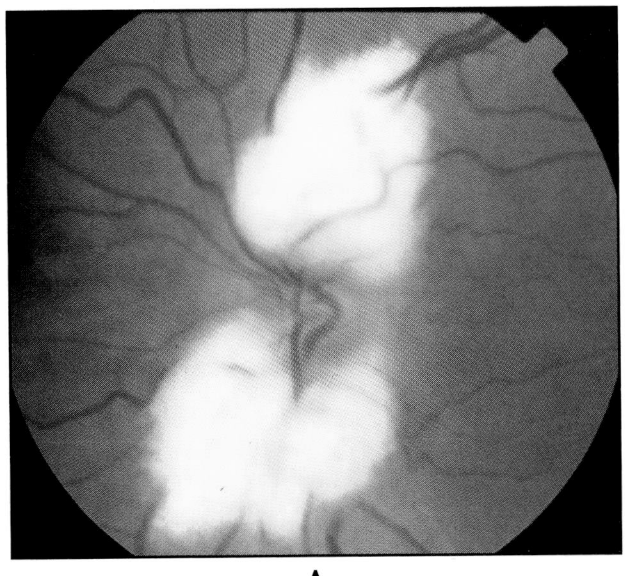

A

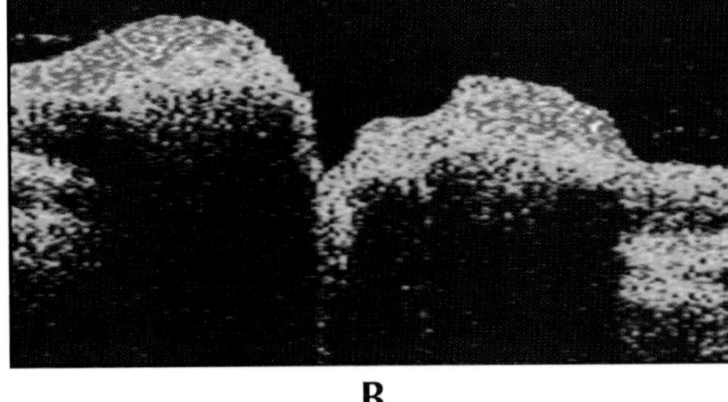

B

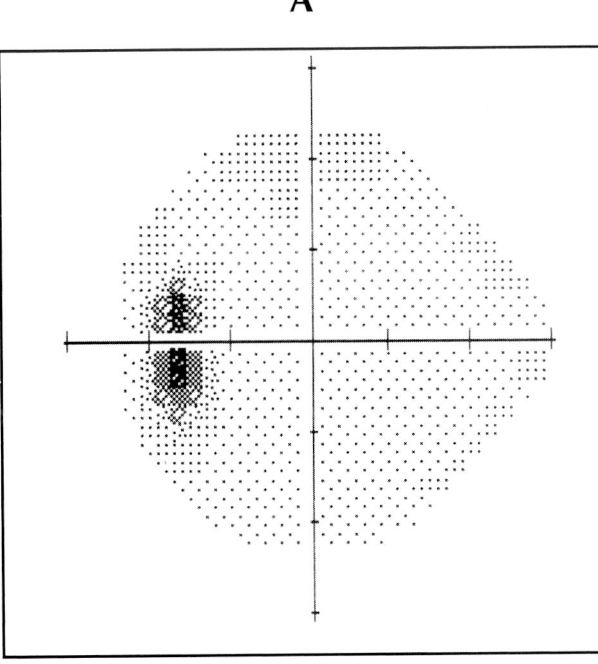

C

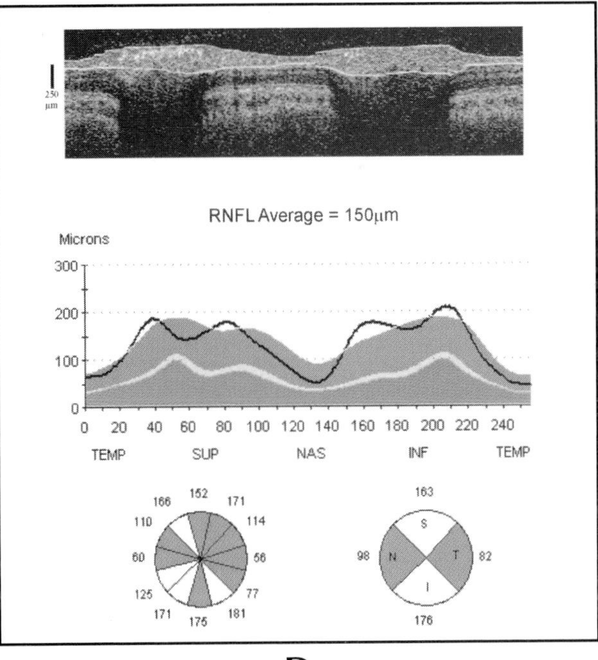

D

Case 13-23. Tilted Optic Discs

A 27-year-old woman was noted to have abnormal optic nerves 7 years before she was referred because of awareness of a shadow obscuring vision in the left eye. A peripapillary hemorrhage was observed (A). The blood cleared after several months. Visual acuities remained 20/20 OD and 20/20 OS. VFs initially showed an enlarged blind spot OS (C), which reverted to normal after the peripapillary hemorrhage cleared (G). The optic nerve head was tilted along an oblique axis (A and E).

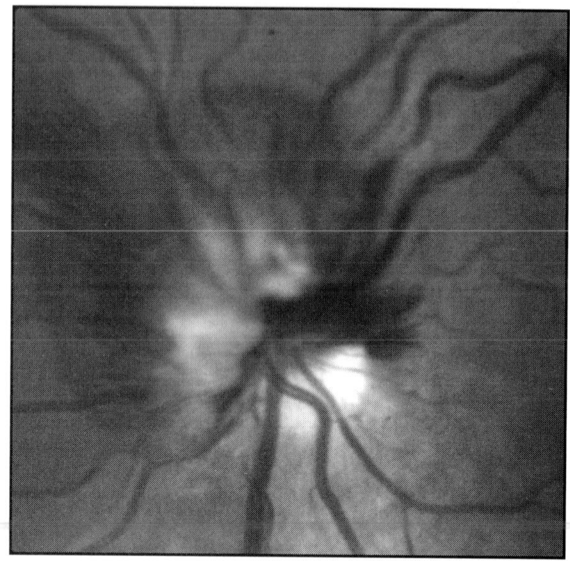

A

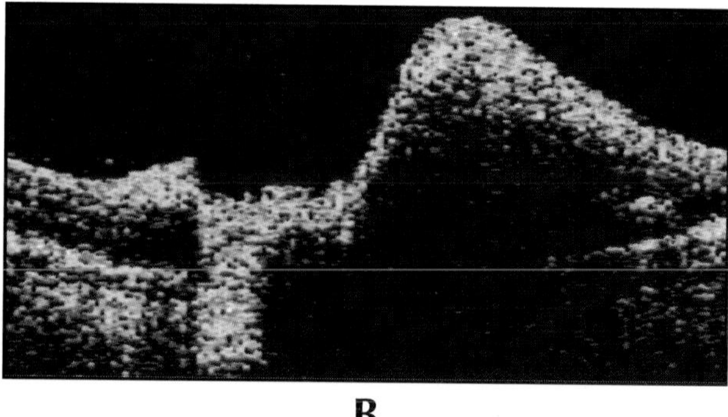

B

C

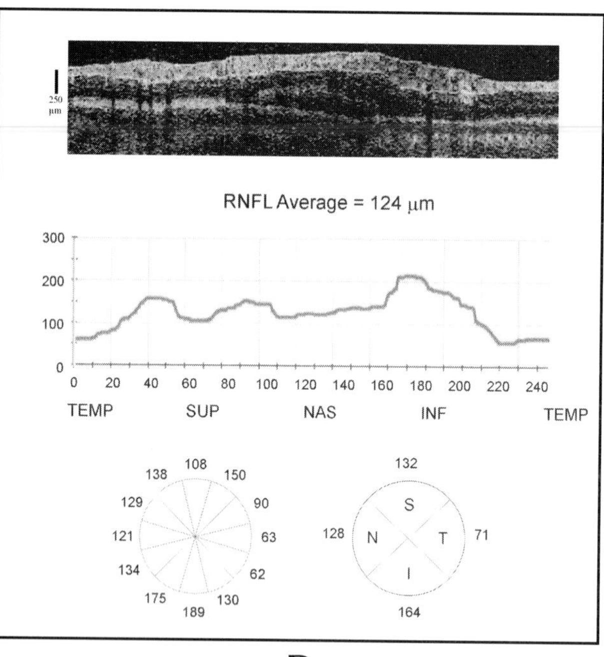

D

Tilted Optic Disc—1-Month Follow-Up

OCT showed the tilting of the optic disc OS (B and F). OCT showed apparent thickening and elevation of the NFL (D), which reverted toward normal (H) as the peripapillary hemorrhage resolved (E).

Comment

Tilted optic nerves may give the appearance of optic disc swelling, but OCT demonstrates that the NFL is normal or thinner in areas of dysplasia. However, these findings may be altered when there is associated peripapillary hemorrhage, which may occur spontaneously in some patients with tilted discs.

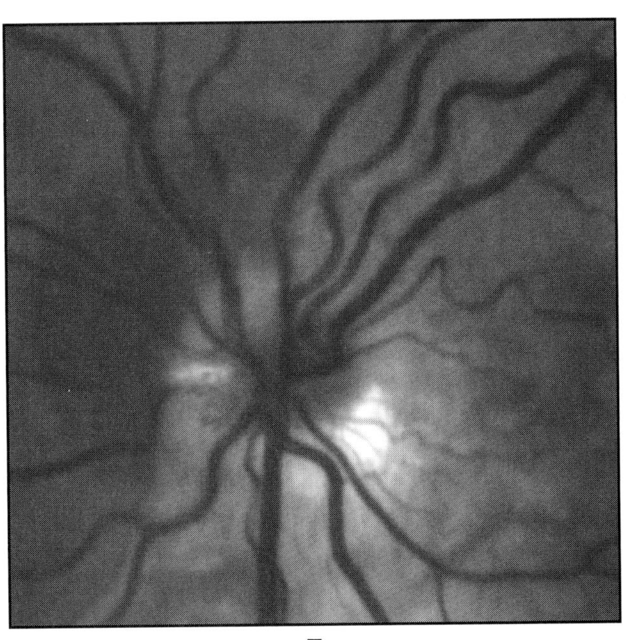

E

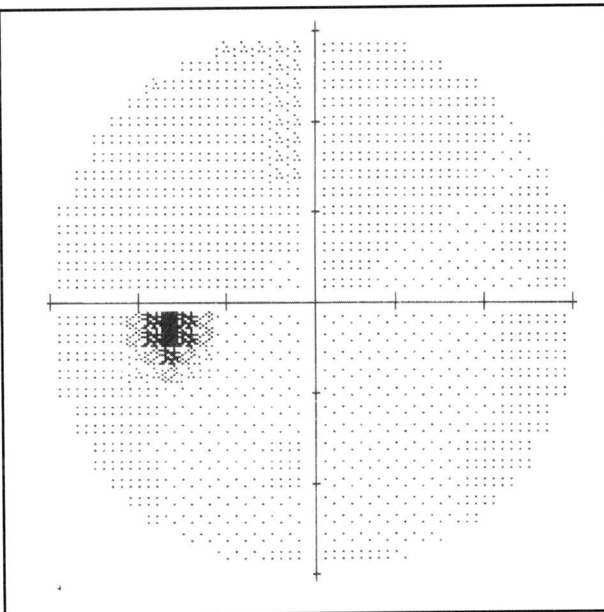

G

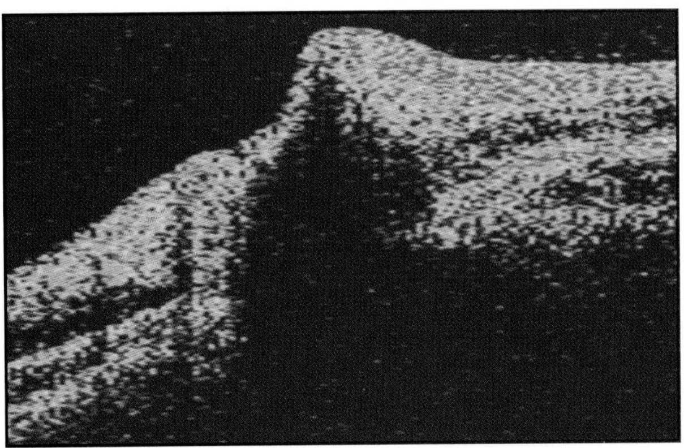

F

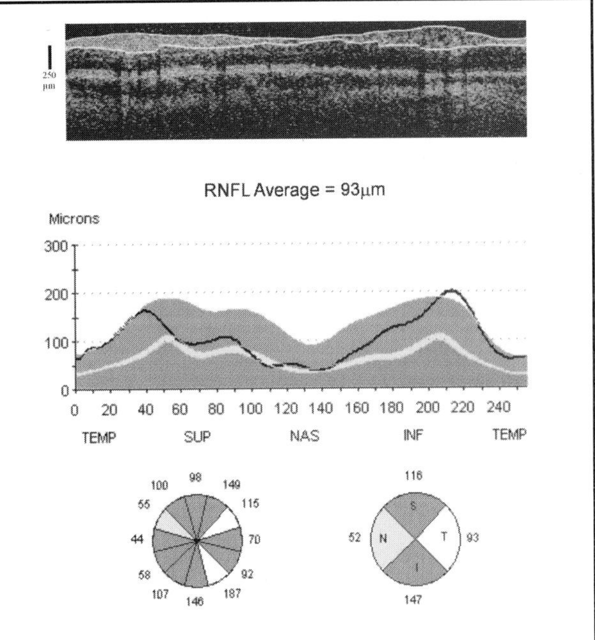

H

Case 13-24. Optic Nerve Hypoplasia

A 34-year-old man was found to have inferior VF defects by his optometrist. He was unaware of any visual problems. His mother was diabetic and had been insulin dependent when pregnant with the patient. Visual acuities were 20/25 OD and 20/20 OS. VF testing showed inferior depression, more on the right (C) than the left (G).

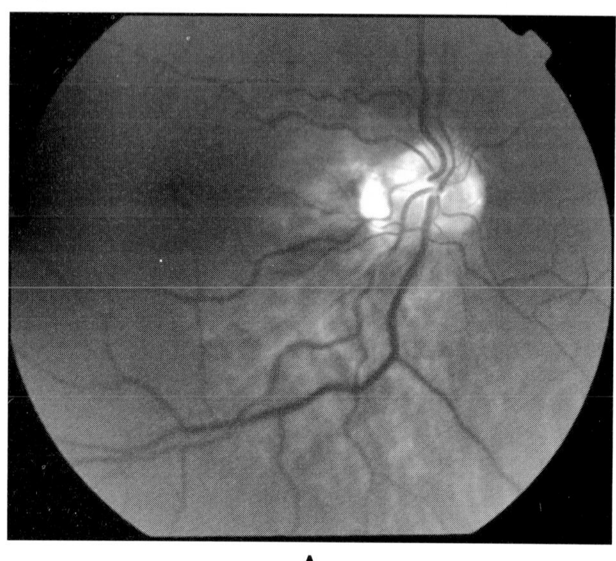

A

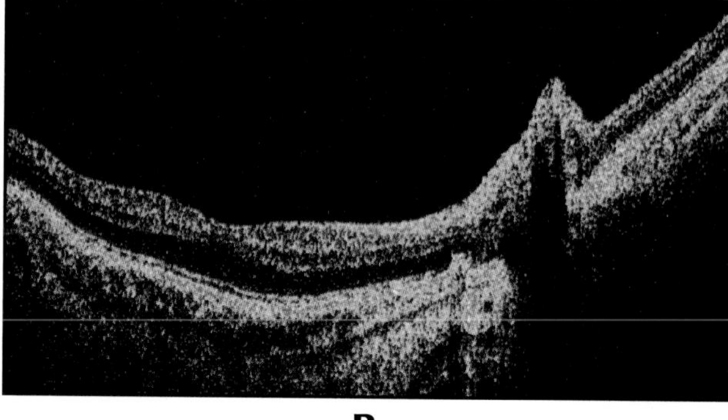

B

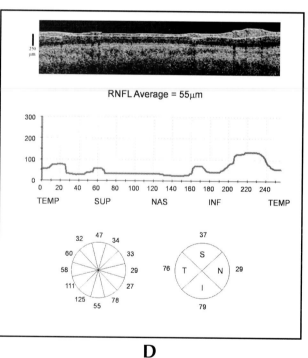

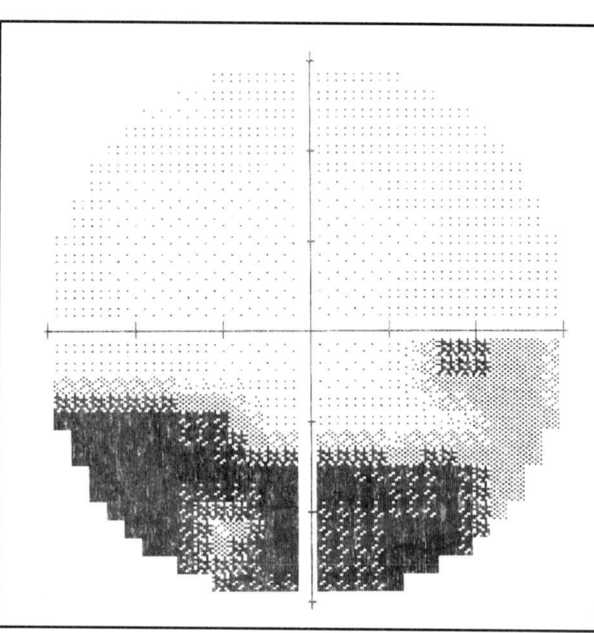

C

250 μm

RNFL Average = 55μm

300
200
100
0
0 20 40 60 80 100 120 140 160 180 200 220 240
TEMP SUP NAS INF TEMP

47 32 34 60 33 58 29 111 27 125 78 55

37 S 76 T N 29 I 79

D

Both optic nerve heads were small with areas of incomplete pigmentation surrounding them (A and E). Circumferential OCT showed thinning of the retinal NFLs, especially superiorly, on both sides (D and H). Cross-sectional OCT also showed small optic nerves (B and F). No normative data were available for this patient.

Comment

OCT shows NFL thinning, especially inferiorly in optic nerve hypoplasia.

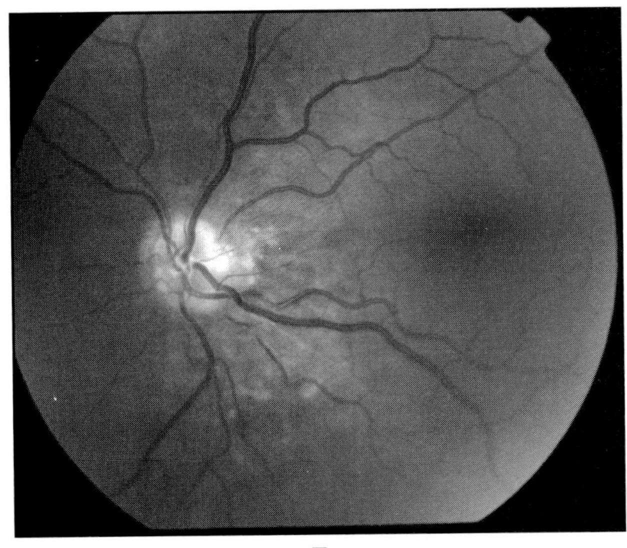

E

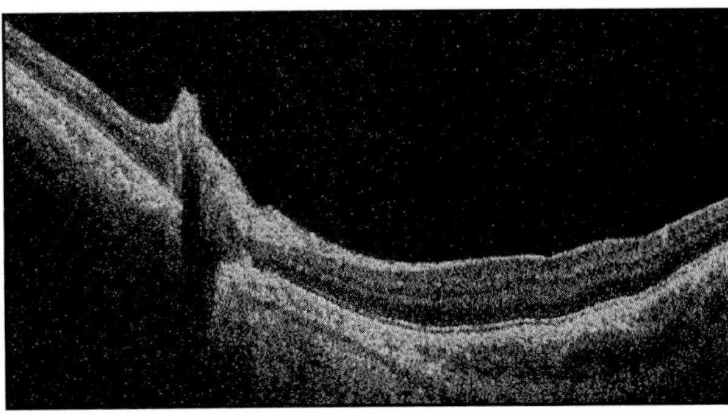

F

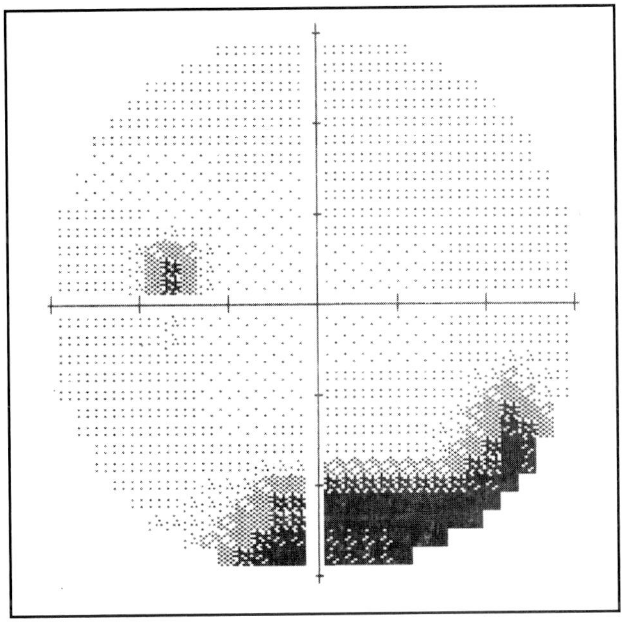

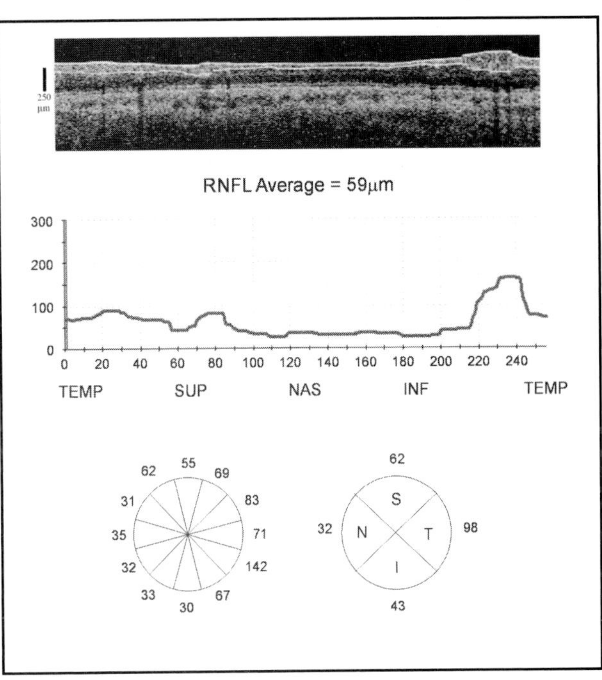

H

G

Case 13-25. Optic Disc Pit

A 13-year-old girl was found to have a right optic nerve pit and serous retinal detachment. Prior surgical attempts (vitrectomy with gas injection and two laser treatments) to eliminate the serous detachment were unsuccessful. On examination, visual acuity was 20/20 and IOP was 16 mmHg. The anterior segment was normal, and fundus examination showed a temporal inferior optic nerve pit with retinal serous detachment extending from the optic disc temporal to the macula. Hyperpigmented regions were noted temporal to the disc margin (A and D).

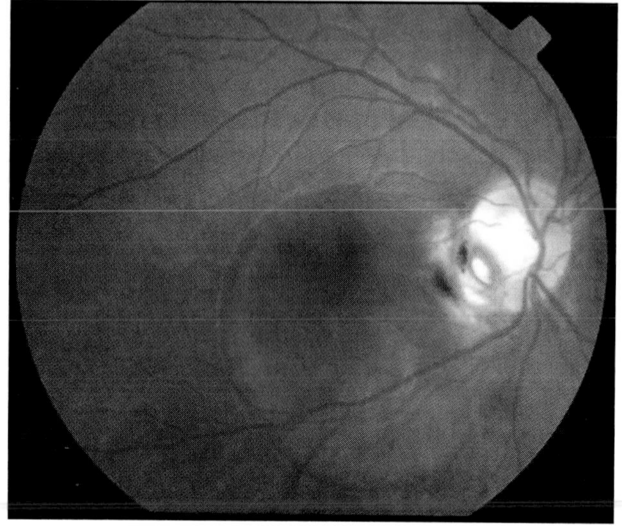

A

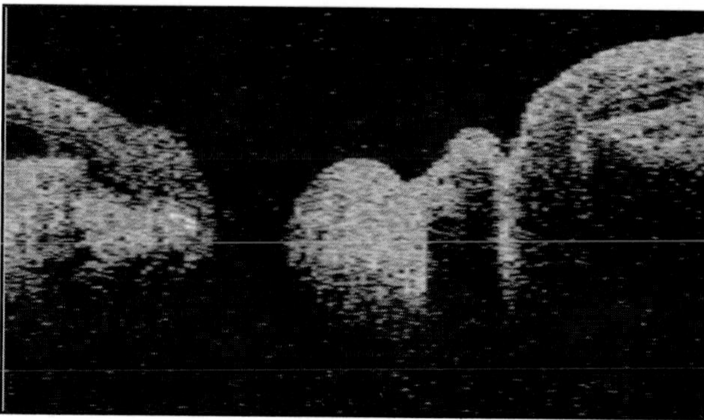

B

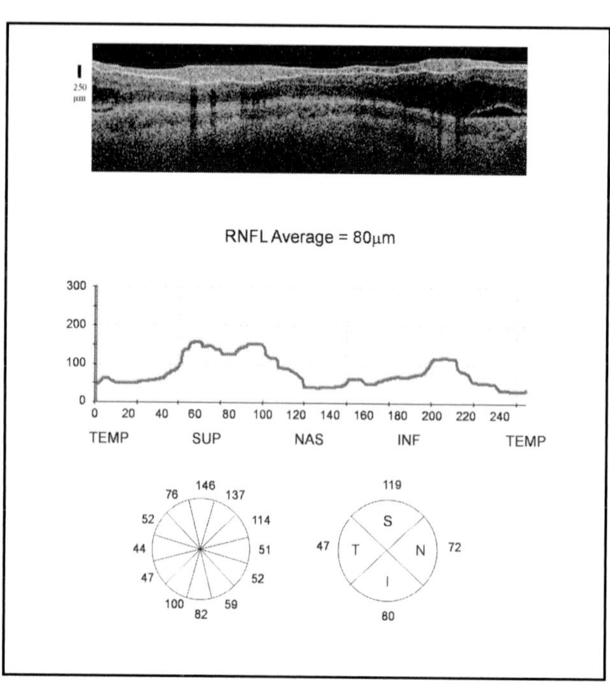

C

In the OCT images, fluid was noted within and underneath the temporal inferior retina in the peripapillary scan (C). The fluid was detected also in the retina and underneath the RPE extending throughout the nasal part of the macula and toward the temporal side of the fovea (E). Optic nerve head scan showed the pit and fluid in the retina (B). An extended linear OCT image from the macula through the optic disc showed the fluid extending underneath the retina through the optic disc and the full pit (F). No normative data were available for patients below 18 years of age.

Comment

OCT can confirm the presence of an optic disc pit and can demonstrate subretinal fluid as the cause of visual loss in affected patients.

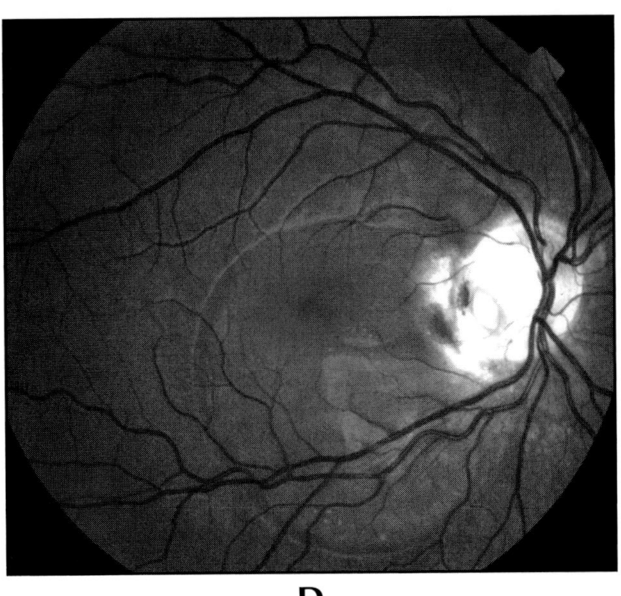

D

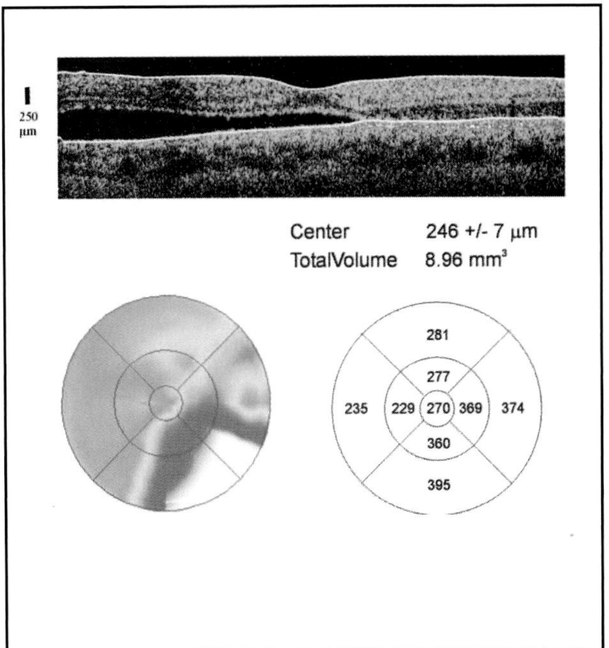

E

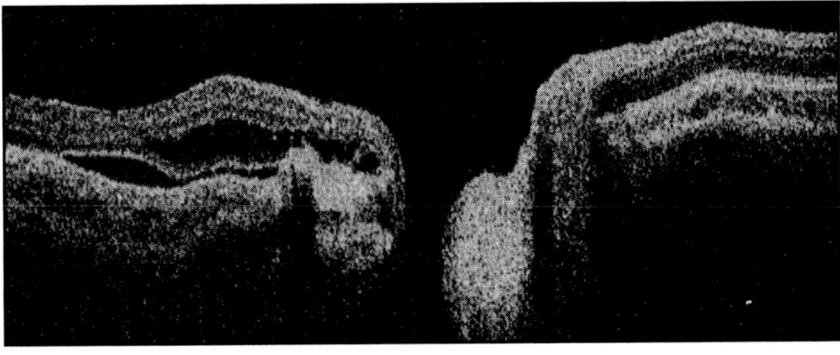

F

Case 13-26. Bergmeister's Papilla Anomaly

A 25-year-old woman was found to have tissue protruding from the optic disc in the right eye representing Bergmeister's papilla anomaly. She had myopia with visual acuities of 20/25 and normal VFs in both eyes. The optic discs appeared normal but tilted and the right one showed typical Bergmeister's papilla appearance (A). OCT showed a normal optic nerve configuration with a highly reflective area representing glial remnants of the posterior primary vitreous (B).

Comment

OCT provides images of this anomaly similar to what has been reported histopathologically.

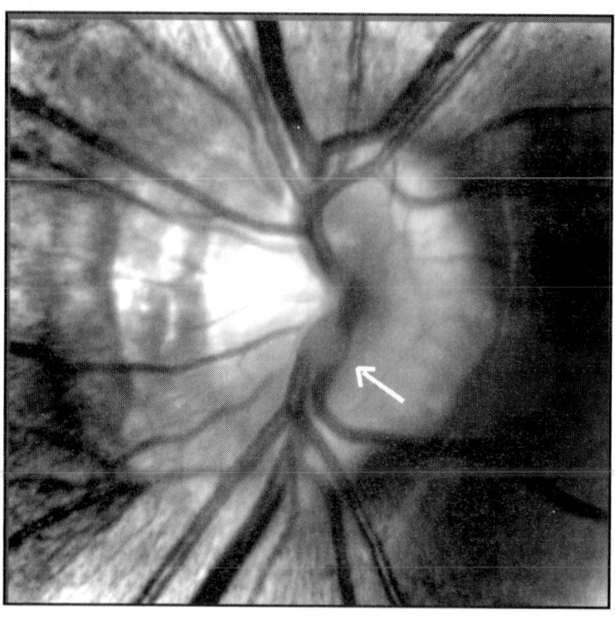

A

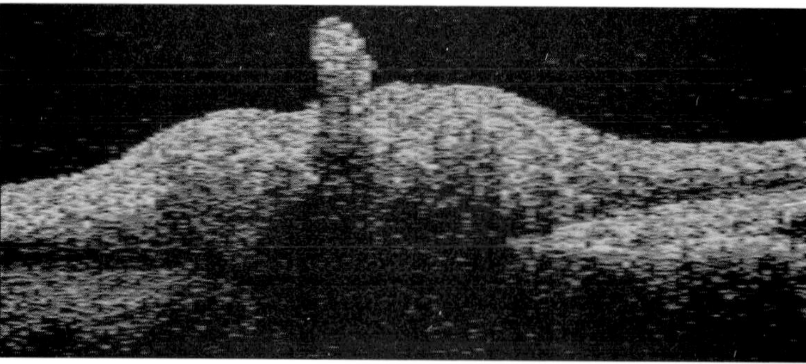

B

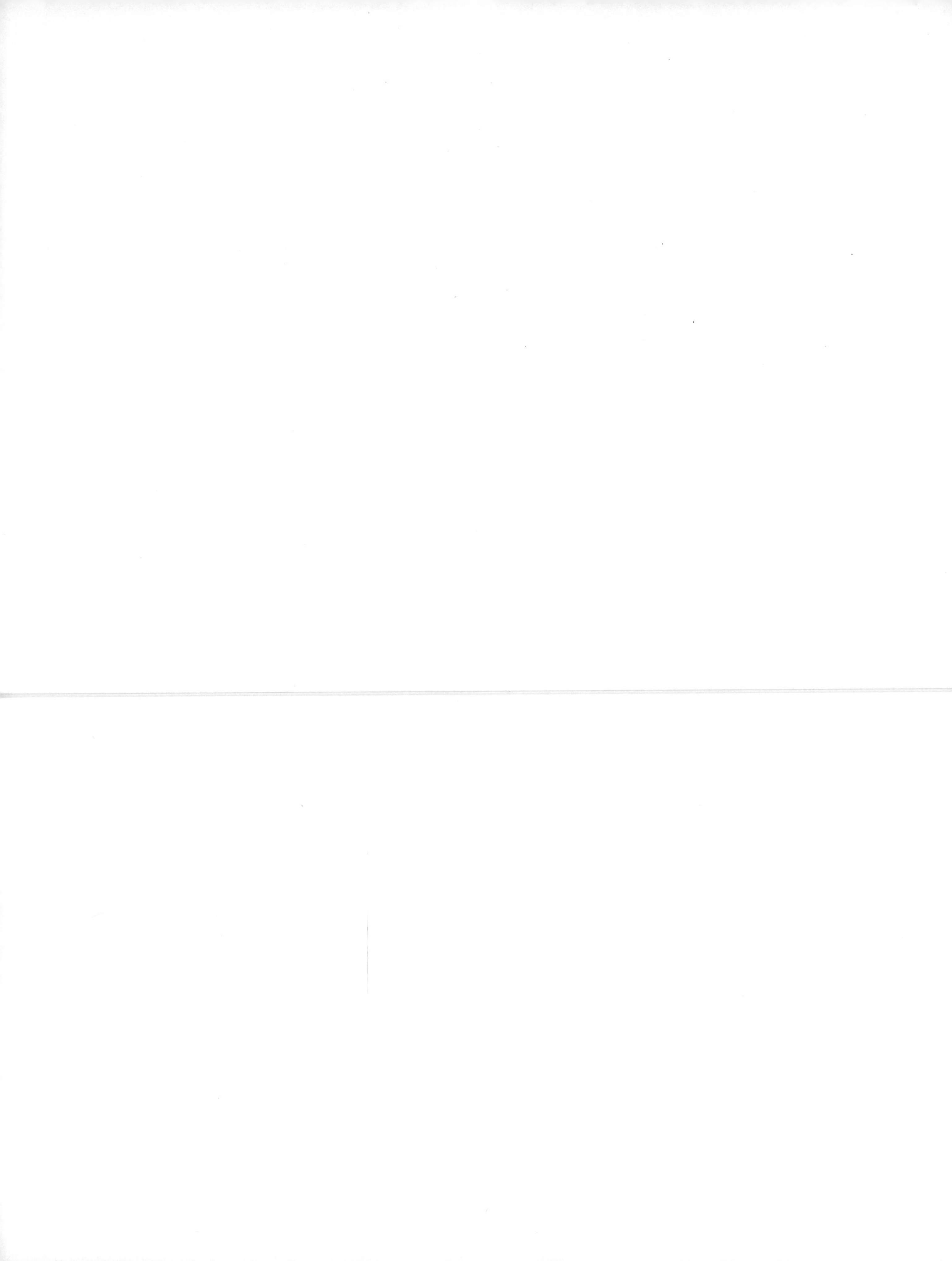

Chapter 14

Corneal and Anterior Segment Optical Coherence Tomography

David Huang, MD, PhD; Yan Li, MS;
Sunita Radhakrishnan, MD; and Maria Regina Chalita, MD, PhD

Background

The precursor technology of optical coherence tomography (OCT)[1], optical coherence domain reflectometry (OCDR), was first applied to the measurement of corneal thickness[2] before any other biomedical application. The first report of OCT for corneal and anterior segment imaging was published by Izatt et al in 1994.[3] After that, there was an interlude in which attention in the OCT field was concentrated on retinal applications. Little attention was paid to anterior segment applications until the Lubeck group described OCT imaging of laser thermokeratoplasty (LTK) lesions in 1997[4,5] and Maldonado et al reported imaging of the LASIK flap in 1998.[6-8] Since then, the rapid popularization of corneal refractive surgery has spurred more investigators to apply OCT to corneal imaging and refine the instrumentation for anterior segment OCT.

The commercial retinal OCT scanners (Carl Zeiss Meditec, Inc, Dublin, Calif) have been used by several investigators for corneal and anterior segment imaging.[6-23] These scanners are intended for retinal imaging and are not optimized for anterior segment scanning. To focus these retinal scanners on the anterior segment, the objective lens is moved forward. This results in the OCT beam being scanned in the fashion of a diverging fan. For corneal imaging, the diverging beam path can only capture strong signal within approximately 1 mm from the apex. Beyond that, reflections from the corneal surfaces and lamellae become very weak due to off-normal incidence angles. The peripheral signal fade becomes evident when one attempts a scan only as wide as 4 mm (Figure 14-1). The image acquisition rate (1 second) is too slow to allow accurate surface contour or width measurements in the presence of biological motion. The relatively short wavelength (0.8 micron [μm]) used in retinal OCT does not allow penetration through the limbus, sclera, and iris. These limitations have been overcome by more recent developments.

The research group in Lubeck developed a slit-lamp-adapted OCT system[24] that enabled wider scan width and was tested in several applications.[25-29] They also demonstrated transscleral imaging with a 1.3-μm wavelength system.[30,31] Ocular imaging with the 1.3-μm wavelength was first reported by Radhakrishnan et al using a system developed at the Case Western Reserve University by Professor Joseph Izatt's group.[32] The Izatt system took full advantage of the higher power that can be safely used at the longer wavelength to achieve a very high acquisition rate of 4000 axial scans per second. The high-speed implementation is essential for accurate biometry and three-dimensional (3-D) imaging.

In this chapter, we present the results of corneal and anterior segment OCT development at the Cleveland Clinic. We began with an arc-scanning OCT system at 0.8 μm wavelength. The system scanned in an arc concentric to the cornea, and we gained valuable experience with laser in-situ keratomileusis (LASIK) anatomy with it. Subsequently, we developed and tested a telecentric (rectangular scan geometry) system based on the high-speed OCT engine designed at Professor Joseph Izatt and Andrew Rollins' laboratory at the Case Western Reserve University. The system was applied to LASIK anatomy, anterior chamber biometry, angle assessment, and imaging of anterior segment pathologies and surgical anatomy in general. We believe that high-speed imaging at 1.3 μm wavelength with the telecentric scan geometry has great versatility and will become the preferred instrument for corneal and anterior segment OCT (CAS OCT).

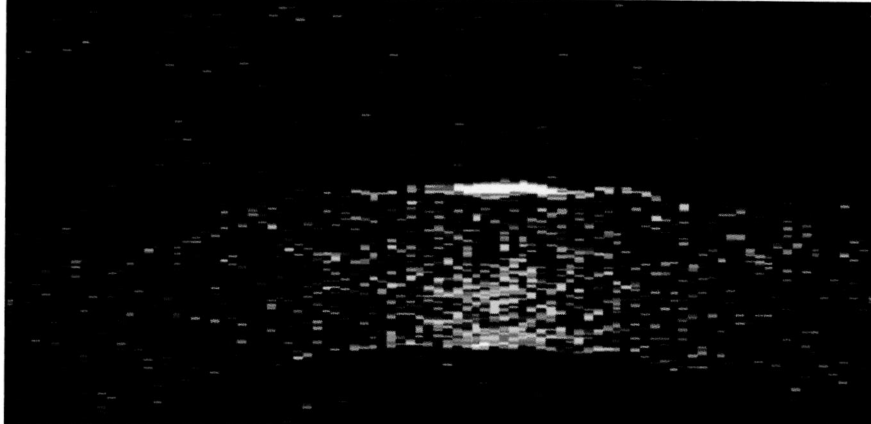

Figure 14-1. OCT of the cornea with 4-mm scan width performed with the Zeiss OCT system. The image has not been corrected for the divergent fan shape of the beam scan path; therefore, the corneal curvature is exaggerated.

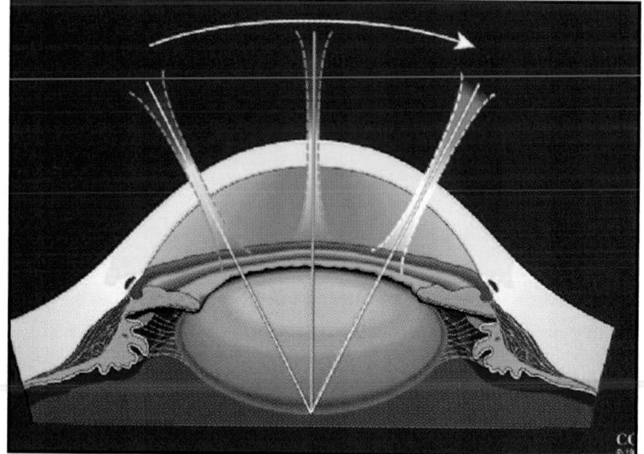

Figure 14-2. Illustration of arc-scanning on cornea.

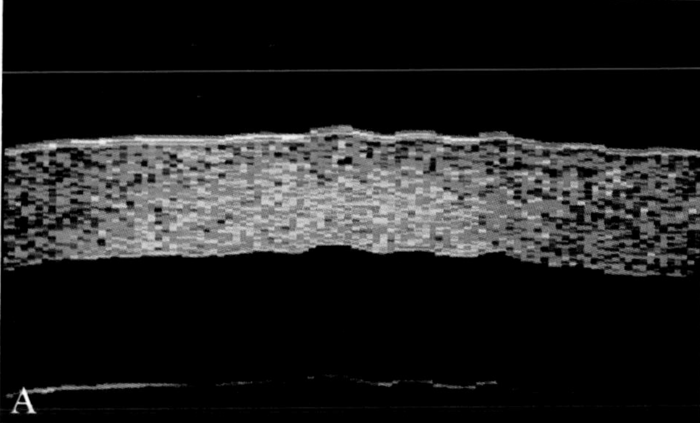

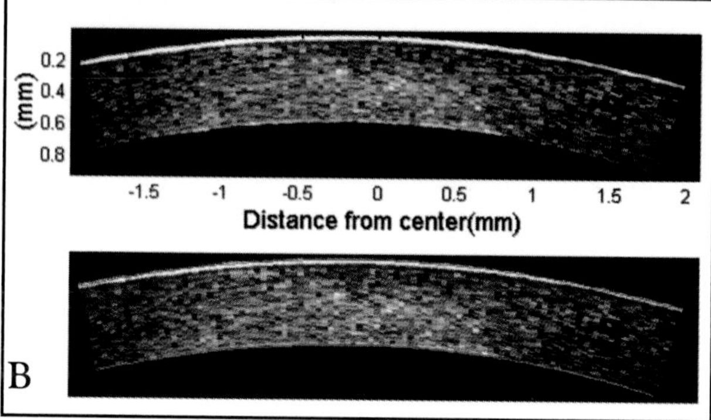

Figure 14-3. Arc-scanning OCT of cornea. (A) Unprocessed image in color scale. (B) The gray-scale image is aligned at the anterior surface with correct curvature (top) and the surface boundaries are overlaid in red (bottom).

Arc-Scanning Optical Coherence Tomography

The reflected signal from the corneal surfaces and lamellae are stronger when the OCT beam's incidence angle is near perpendicular. We have tested an OCT prototype that scans an arc concentric with the cornea and thereby maintains perpendicular incidence (Figure 14-2). The system obtains relatively uniform corneal signal over a 4-mm scan width (Figure 14-3). The prototype was provided by the Humphrey Division of Carl Zeiss Meditec Inc. This system used the interferometer and control unit of a commercial OCT unit and therefore had the same basic performance. It used 830-nm wavelength light and provided one image frame per second with 100 axial scans in each image. The axial resolution is approximately 12 μm (corneal index of 1.38 is assumed). The raw image (see Figure 14-3A) shows undulation of the corneal contour due to motion. We developed image-processing software to automatically identify the anterior and posterior corneal boundaries and align the corneal image at the anterior boundary (see Figure 14-3B).

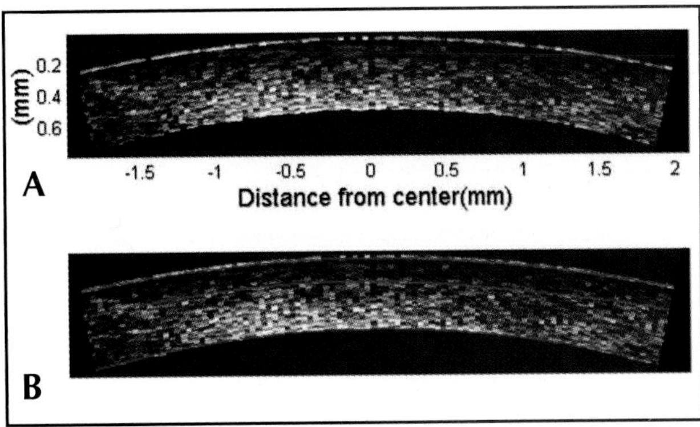

Figure 14-4. Arc-scanning OCT of cornea 1 day after LASIK (A) with overlay of corneal and flap boundary overlaid in red (B). Central flap thickness was 153 μm and posterior stromal thickness was 307 μm.

Longitudinal Laser In-Situ Keratomileusis Study

We performed a longitudinal LASIK study[33] to compare arc-scanning OCT with ultrasonic pachymetry, the current clinical standard for corneal thickness measurement. Thirty eyes from 17 patients who had LASIK for myopia had corneal measurements on preoperative and postoperative visits. High-frequency (50 MHz) ultrasound pachymetry (CorneoGage 2, Sonogage, Cleveland, Ohio) was also used for subtractive flap thickness and ablation depth measurements during the LASIK procedure. OCT images were obtained by scanning 4 mm along the horizontal meridian on central cornea. On post-LASIK OCT, the flap has relatively low internal reflectivity compared to the posterior stroma (Figure 14-4). There are small reflectivity peaks at the flap lamellar interface that also aid in the delineation of the boundary.

We developed automated image-processing to locate both corneal surfaces and the flap interface from OCT images (Figure 14-4B). The thickness profiles for the cornea, flap, and posterior stroma are then computed.[34] The central thickness measurements were compared with ultrasonic pachymetry. Corneal and flap thickness measurement by OCT agreed well with ultrasound. OCT and ultrasound had similar repeatability (pooled standard deviation [SD] = 4 μm), but OCT may be more accurate. Although we had no gold standard reference for absolute corneal thickness, the programmed laser ablation depth served as a relative standard for comparison with subtractive ablation depth measurement on both OCT and ultrasound. OCT measurements agreed well, while ultrasound measurements had poor agreement and correlation with the programmed depths.

Differential Diagnosis of Keratoconus and Post-Laser In-Situ Keratomileusis Keratectasia

The ability to profile or map corneal thickness is useful in the prevention and diagnosis of post-LASIK keratectasia.[35] Both keratoconus and post-LASIK keratectasia are characterized by progressive focal bulging and thinning of the cornea. While keratoconus is naturally occurring, keratectasia is associated with weakening of the corneal structure due to LASIK. The known causes of keratectasia include pre-existing keratoconus and excessive laser ablation. Both keratoconus and keratectasia appear on corneal topography focal steepening, usually in an inferior location (Figure 14-5A). However, inferior or focal steepening after LASIK can also be caused by irregular ablation (steep central island), decentered ablation, asymmetric healing, or tear film instability.

OCT corneal thickness profiling or mapping would show focal thinning in the area of steepening in a keratectasia case (Figures 14-5B and 14-5C). In the other conditions, OCT should show relatively thicker cornea in the area of steepening. In pre-LASIK examinations, OCT may be helpful in preventing keratectasia by providing more accurate diagnosis of keratoconus and more accurate measurements of corneal thickness.

OCT is able to detect the lamellar interface and directly measure the thickness of the flap and posterior stroma. This is not possible with conventional Placido-ring corneal topography or slit-scanning topography (Orbscan, Bausch & Lomb, Rochester, NY). Although flap imaging is possible with very high-frequency ultrasound biomicroscopy (UBM),[36] the immersion requirement makes UBM relatively impractical for routine LASIK practice. The ability to routinely measure flap and posterior stromal thicknesses is useful for the calculation of available potential ablation depth, particularly for LASIK enhancements. It is also useful in determining the cause of keratectasia. Figure 14-6 shows a case of suspected keratectasia associated with unexpectedly thick flap. The patient was a young adult male who had normal topography and central corneal thickness preoperatively. He underwent bilateral LASIK for moderate myopia using the LADARVision system (Alcon Laboratories, Inc, Orlando, Fla) and a manually operated Moria CB microkeratome (Moria Instruments, Antony, France) with 160-μm plate setting. The patient complained of deterioration in vision in both eyes 2 weeks later. Topography showed inferior steepening, which changed over time. Arc-scanning OCT was performed in both eyes 40 days after LASIK (see Figure 14-6). In both eyes, the flap thicknesses were found to be abnormally thick (295 to 310 μm) compared with the expected value of 160 μm. The residual posterior stromal thickness was slightly less

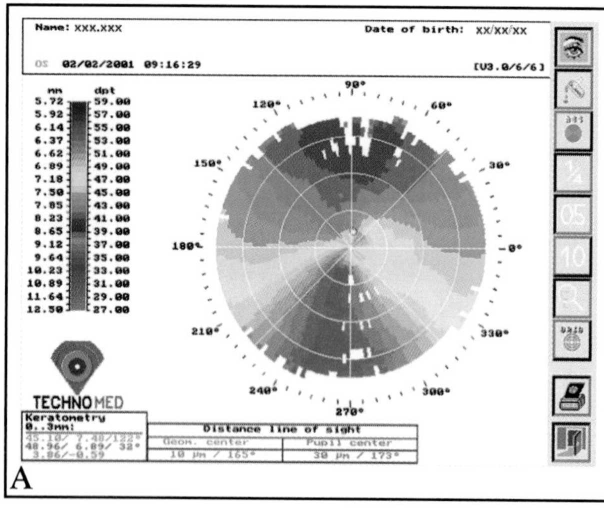

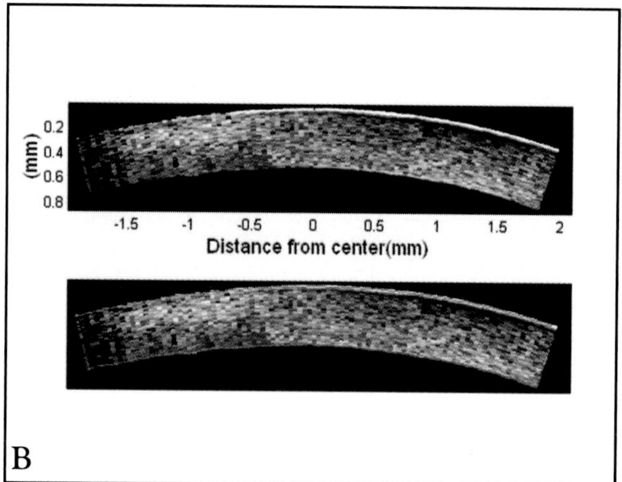

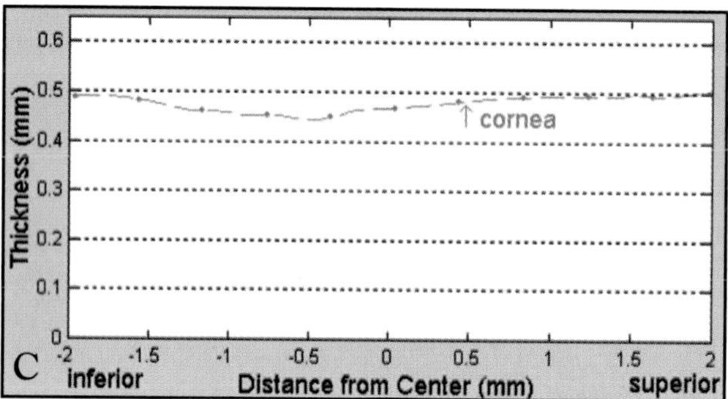

Figure 14-5. A case of keratectasia after LASIK. (A) Topography showing inferior steepening. (B) OCT with (bottom) and without (top) overlay of corneal surfaces. (C) Vertical thickness profile derived from OCT showing inferior thinning.

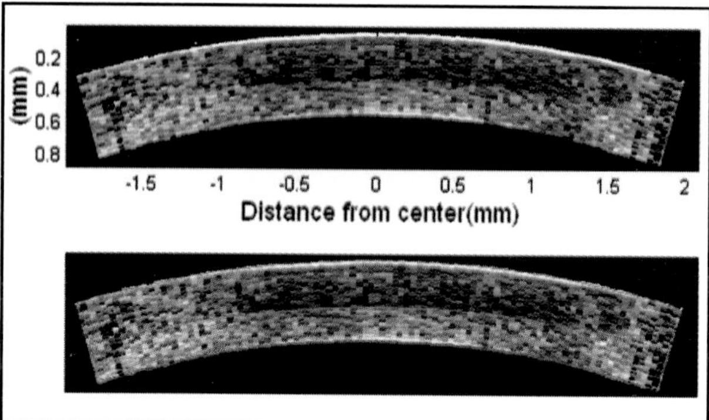

Figure 14-6. Arc-scanning OCT of cornea 40 days after LASIK for the evaluation of possible keratectasia. Central flap thickness was 305 µm and residual posterior stromal thickness was 198 µm.

than 200 µm at the thinnest points. Residual posterior stromal thickness of less than 250 µm is considered a risk factor for keratectasia.[35] The OCT images were helpful in establishing the unusual cause of the problem as excessively thick flap cut.

Disadvantages of Arc-Scanning

We eventually decided to develop rectangular scanning geometry instead of the arc-scanning geometry for several reasons. It is more difficult to detect the signal peak at the lamellar flap interface with arc-scanning because normal corneal lamellar reflections are nearly as strong near normal incidence. The anterior air-tear interface reflection is very strong compared to internal reflections, and this necessitated an adjustment to the system to obtain a slight off-normal incidence angle. The converging beam path means that the scan width at the cornea is much smaller than the width of the objective lens. Thus, it is difficult to scan across the entire cornea without a very large lens or very small working distance. Accurate calibration of the scan width is also more difficult because it varied with working distance. Due to all these concerns, we decided to implement a rectangular (also called *telecentric*) scan geometry in which the scanned beam paths are parallel. Those results are shown in the following sections.

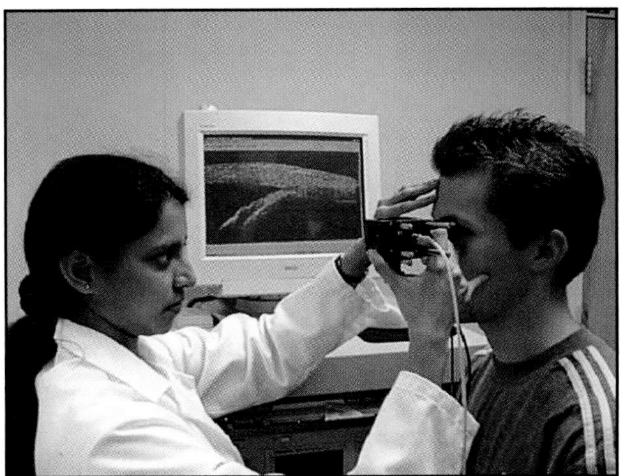

Figure 14-7. The handheld high-speed 1.3 μm wavelength CAS OCT system in action. Note real-time display of color OCT image in background. (Courtesy of Radhakrishnan S, Rollins AM, Roth JE, et al. Real-time optical coherence tomography of the anterior segment at 1310 nm. *Arch Ophthalmol.* 2001;119: 1181. © 2001 American Medical Association.

High-Speed Corneal and Anterior Segment Optical Coherence Tomograph at 1.3-μm Wavelength

There are important advantages of using a longer wavelength of 1.3 μm for CAS OCT compared to the 0.8-μm wavelength that is commonly used for retinal imaging. Because scattering loss is much lower at the longer wavelength, 1.3-μm OCT is able to penetrate the limbus and sclera to provide a view of the angle. Absorption by water is also much stronger at 1.3 μm (9.3 mm absorption length).[37] For an eye of average length, 91% of 1.3-μm light that falls on the cornea would be absorbed by the ocular media, leaving only 9% to reach the retina. This allows much higher optical power to be used without damaging the retina. The permissible exposure level at 1.3-μm wavelength is 15 milliwatts (mW) according to the current standard set by the American Laser Institute and the American National Standards Institute (ANSI).[38] This is 20 times higher than the 0.7 mW limit at 0.8-μm wavelength.[38] This means that anterior segment OCT can use much higher power and achieve much higher scan rates. This potential was demonstrated in a high-speed prototype[32] that is capable of 4000 axial scans per second (40 times the speed of Zeiss OCT1). We describe below the clinical results obtained with two generations of the high-speed OCT system.

Handheld Scanner

The initial high-speed CAS OCT system utilized a hand-held probe to scan subjects. This unit was used in the initial studies that demonstrated the high speed and superior penetration of CAS OCT at 1.3-μm wavelength.[32] The scan depths were 3.25 or 6 mm and the width was up to 5 mm. The scanned beam paths were slightly divergent. The imaging rate was adjustable between 4 to 16 frames per second to provide 1000 to 250 axial scans per image. The OCT probe is held in both hands with the examiner's fingers resting on the subject's face for support (Figure 14-7). Different structures in the anterior segment can be imaged by either moving the probe itself or by asking the subject to move the eyes. Positioning of the probe is adjusted as the operator looks at the real-time display of OCT images. The operator can freeze and save selected image frames during scanning by using foot pedals.

The hand-held probe enables great flexibility in anterior segment examination. Scanning in any meridian is easily performed. Also, subject positioning is not critical and examinations can be performed in a standing, sitting, or supine position. This may prove useful in the elderly population, children, and others with difficulties in holding particular positions. In such a setting, the handheld OCT would be an excellent "quick-look" modality for assessment of the anterior chamber (AC) angle.

The main limitations of the handheld OCT system are that fine adjustment and stabilization of the scan position are difficult. Also, the width of scan was not sufficient to accommodate the entire AC in one frame in this particular prototype. This prompted the development of a second prototype that is slit-lamp mounted.

Slit-Lamp-Mounted Scanner

We developed a slit-lamp-mounted CAS OCT system to replace the handheld scanner for most clinical studies. The new system has several improved features. The system is mounted on the sliding slit-lamp platform and the patient's head is stabilized on the usual chin and forehead rest. The scan area is visualized in real-time using a charged-coupled device (CCD) camera (Figure 14-8). The scan geometry is telecentric (ie, rectangular) with adjustable scan widths of 4 to 15 mm and scan depths of 3.25 or 6 mm. The interferometer engine is similar to that of the handheld system except that a lower power of 2.5 mW is used. The wavelength remains at 1.31 μm and the axial scan rate was 4000/s. Eight frame images are acquired and displayed per second in real time, each with 500 axial scans. The axial resolution was 14 μm full-width-half-maximum in cornea. The system was utilized to conduct most of the following studies.

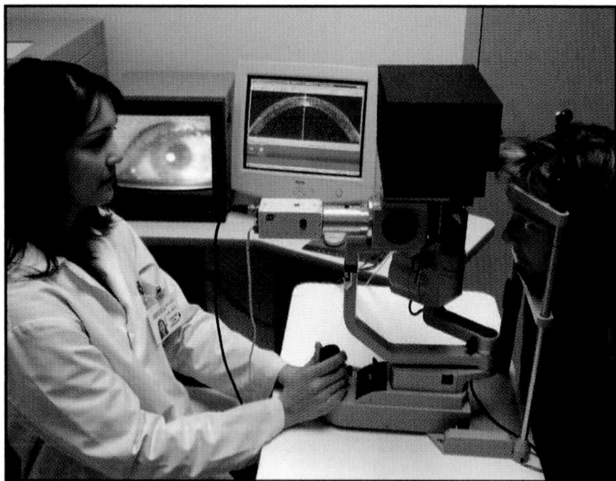

Figure 14-8. The slit-lamp-mounted high-speed 1.3-μm wavelength CAS OCT system in action. Note simultaneous real-time display of OCT and CCD camera images.

Laser In-Situ Keratomileusis Anatomy

We used the 1310 nm slit-lamp-mounted CAS OCT system to examine post-LASIK eyes. The scan dimensions are 12 mm wide and 3.25 mm deep (in air). There is no apparent motion artifact at the higher image acquisition rate of 8 frames/s (Figure 14-9) compared to the image from the 0.8-μm prototype (see Figure 14-3). The image detail is also much finer with 500 axial scans per frame (see Figure 14-9) compared to 100 axial scans per frame (see Figure 14-3). The anterior surface reflection is so strong at perpendicular incidence that it produces a vertical flare that helps localize the apex (see Figure 14-9). Finer features such as the epithelial-Bowman and the flap lamellar boundaries are best visualized with a slight off-normal beam incidence angle in the midperiphery. The flap internal reflectivity is stronger than that of the posterior stroma (see Figure 14-9), which reverses the contrast seen at 0.8-μm wavelength (see Figure 14-4). The flap interface also has stronger reflectivity at 1.3-μm wavelength and can often be visualized from edge to edge. At 1 week after LASIK, we find that the flap interface could be visualized in 91% of 1.3-μm OCT compared to 21% of 0.8-μm OCT. The improved flap interface detection is due to both the 1.3-μm wavelength and the telecentric scanning geometry.

Angle Assessment

Gonioscopy is the gold standard for evaluation of the AC angle. It is, however, highly subjective and requires specialized training. Cross-sectional imaging of the AC angle with either UBM or OCT is easier to interpret.

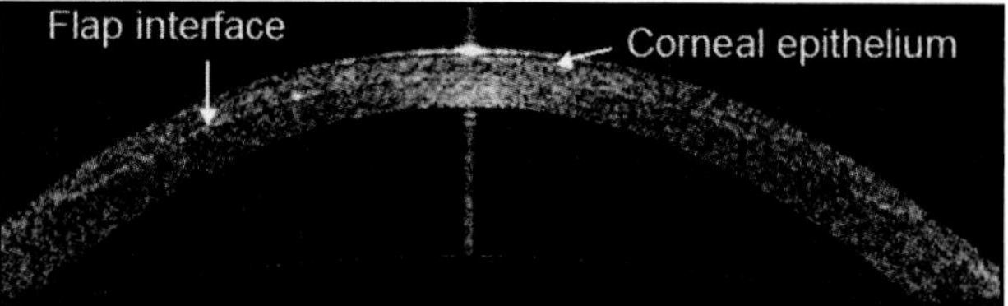

Figure 14.9. OCT of an eye 1 day after LASIK with the 1.3-μm wavelength slit-lamp-mounted system. Central corneal thickness was 529 μm and the flap thickness was 195 μm.

Furthermore, objective quantification of the angle can be obtained from a cross section. UBM[39] and Scheimpflug photography[40] have been used for quantitative angle evaluation. OCT can provide the same detailed angle anatomy with the further advantage of being noncontact and easy to perform.

We developed a system to assess the angle with the 1.3-μm wavelength high-speed CAS OCT. Either the handheld or the slit-lamp-mounted scanner was used. Computer image processing was used to obtain correct dimension images with adjustments for the scan geometry and refraction of OCT beam at the anterior eye surface. Images of an open angle and an occludable angle are shown in Figures 14-10 and 14-11, respectively. Corneal, scleral, and iris anatomy are visualized in detail. Features in the limbus and angle are clearly shown, including the scleral spur, ciliary body band, angle recess, and iris root. For angle measurements, it is particularly useful that the scleral spur is highly reflective and easily identified on OCT. In some images, Schlemm's canal can be identified as well (Figure 14-12). To take advantage of the highly contrasted scleral spur, we devised a diagnostic parameter called the trabeculo-iris space area (TISA) to quantify the angle opening. TISA-X is defined as the aqueous space bounded by a roughly trapezoidal shape between the scleral spur, a point on the corneal endothelium X μm anteromedial from the scleral spur, and the intersections of the anterior iris surface with perpendicular lines drawn from the first two landmarks (see Figure 14-10B). We tested both TISA-500 and TISA-750. The 500-μm figure is anatomically meaningful because the average trabecular meshwork extends approximately 500 μm anteromedially from the scleral spur. The 750-μm figure utilized a greater portion of the images.

We performed a clinical study to compare OCT and UBM parameters against gonioscopic grading by glaucoma specialists. Thirty-one eyes of 28 subjects were examined. Eight eyes were judged to be occludable by gonioscopy. Subjects underwent OCT and UBM imaging of the nasal and temporal AC angles. Both OCT and UBM had excellent correlation with gonioscopy in terms

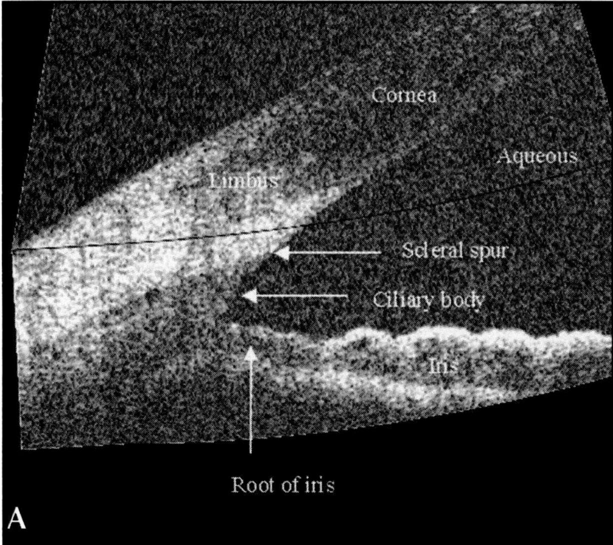

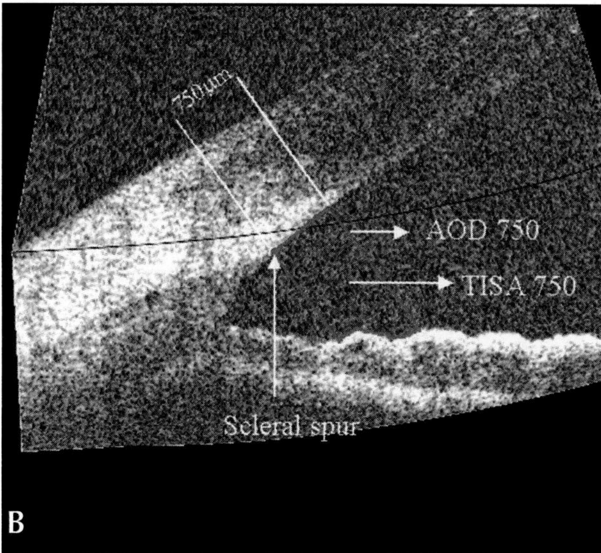

Figure 14-10. High-speed 1.3-μm wavelength OCT of an open angle, with (A) annotated landmarks and (B) overlay of the boundaries for measuring the TISA-750.

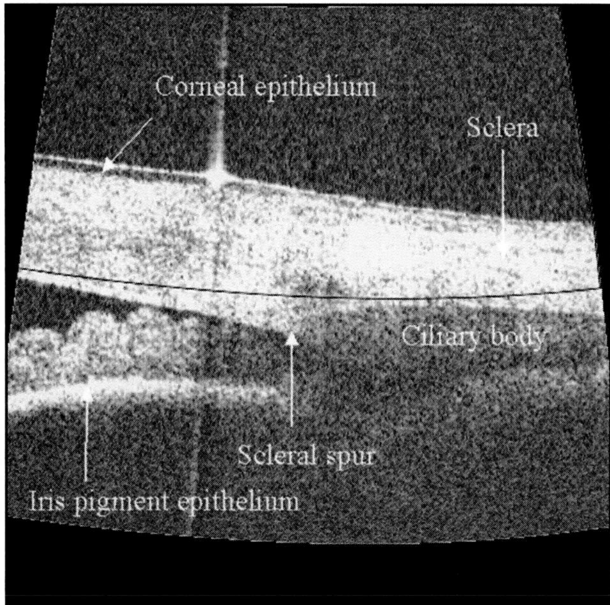

Figure 14-11. High-speed 1.3-μm wavelength OCT of an occludable angle.

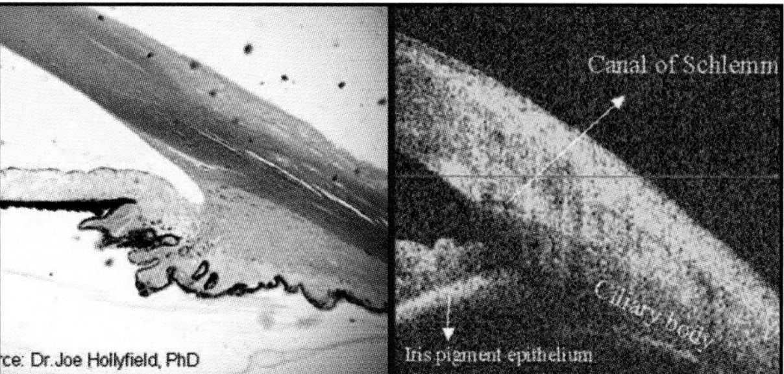

Figure 14-12. Correlation between histology (left) and high-speed 1.3-μm wavelength in vivo OCT (right) of the angle showing Schlemm's canal. The images were from different eyes. (Courtesy of Joe G. Hollyfield, PhD).

of the identification of occludable angles. TISA-750 was the best OCT parameter for identifying gonioscopically occludable angles with a cut-off value of 0.12 mm². TISA-750 had 100% sensitivity and 95.7% specificity.

In a separate CAS OCT study to measure AC width, we incidentally detected occludable angles in one subject. The image was obtained with a 15-mm linear scanning laser beam oriented horizontally across the center of the pupil (Figure 14-13A). TISA-750 values were 0.054 mm² nasally and 0.099 mm² temporal in the right eye, and 0.064 mm² nasally and 0.089 mm² temporally in the left eye. These TISA-750 values showed occludable angle according to our cutoff value of 0.12 mm². Five days later, the patient underwent successful neodymium:yttrium-aluminum-garnet (Nd:YAG) iridotomy in both eyes. One week after laser iridotomy, CAS OCT of the angles was performed. One OCT image showed the patent iridotomy (Figure 14-13B), as well as the widened angle. TISA-750 increased to 0.268 mm² nasally and 0.291 mm² temporally in the right eye, and 0.342 mm² nasally and 0.354 mm² temporally in the left eye. These TISA-750 values fell comfortably in the nonoccludable range. This case demonstrates the utility of OCT in detecting occludable angles and monitoring the results of treatment.

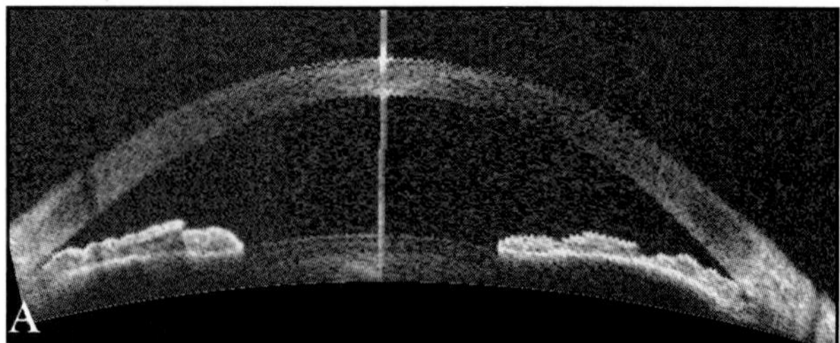

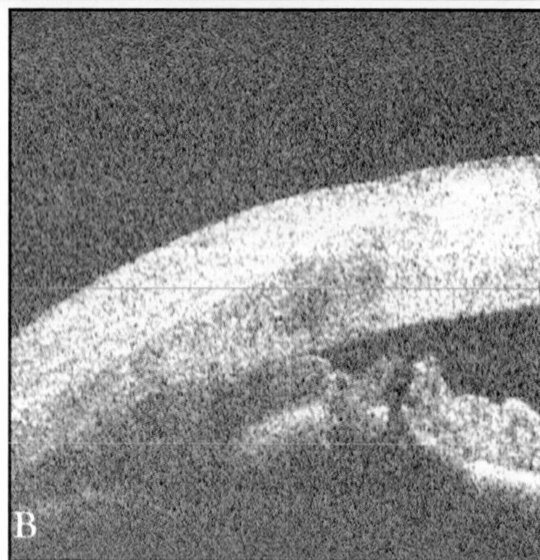

Figure 14-13. CAS OCT of an eye with occludable angle necessitating laser peripheral iridotomy. (A) Horizontal scan of anterior segment (15 mm wide) before laser iridotomy. (B) OCT (4 mm wide) showing widened angle and patent iridotomy after laser iridotomy.

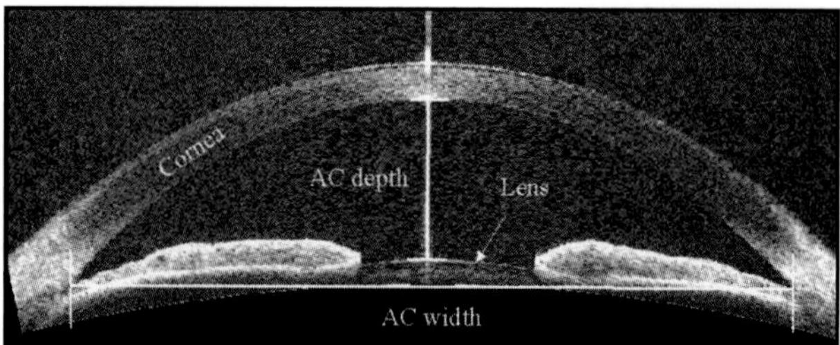

Fig. 14-14. AC imaged with the wide-field (15 mm) setting on the slit-lamp–mounted high-speed CAS OCT system. The AC width is measured between angle recesses and its depth is measured from corneal apex to lens apex.

Anterior Chamber Width and Other Biometric Parameters

OCT is well suited for ocular biometry due to its high image resolution. Compared to ultrasound, OCT's noncontact nature eliminates discomfort and distortion from probe contact or immersion. Our slit-lamp-mounted OCT prototype had sufficient speed and field width to produce detailed images of the entire AC without any visible motion artifact (Figure 14-14). This makes the accurate measurement of AC width and other biometric parameters possible. AC width (ACW) measurement is clinically important for sizing angle-supported anterior chamber intraocular lenses (IOLs). With the increasing use of refractive phakic IOLs, accurate sizing becomes an important issue. An IOL that is too large can press on the iris root and produce pupil ovalization, while an IOL that is too small can lead to IOL movement, decentration, corneal endothelial damage, and iritis.[41] The traditional method for IOL sizing utilizes the external corneal diameter, which was assumed to correspond to the internal ACW. Typically, the IOL length is chosen to be the corneal diameter (CD) plus a constant such as 1 mm.

With the slit-lamp–mounted, high-speed CAS OCT system, it is possible to directly measure the internal width of the AC (see Figure 14-14). We compared ACW measurement by OCT with CD measured by a Holladay cornea gauge in 20 normal subjects. The ACW was 12.53 ± 0.47 mm (mean ± SD). The difference ACW-CD was 0.75 ± 0.44 mm with a range of 1.84 mm. The improvement of SD from 0.47 mm to 0.44 mm was minimal and showed that IOL sizing with CD would be only marginally better than using the same size for all eyes. OCT can potentially increase the accuracy of IOL sizing several folds. The reproducibility of ACW measurements from OCT images was assessed by analysis of variance. The variation of ACW between images was small (SD = 0.10 mm), but disagreement between the three human graders was larger (SD = 0.29 mm). We are developing an automated ACW measurement software that would remove the need for a human grader to place cursors at the angle recesses. AC depth and the crystalline lens vault were also measured from the OCT images with very high reproducibility.

OCT appears to be a reproducible, convenient, and noncontact technique to perform biometry of AC dimensions. Further studies are needed to see if it can contribute to reduction of complications through better fitting of AC IOLs.

Surgical Anatomy

The slit-lamp-mounted, high-speed CAS OCT system was used to survey a number of corneal and anterior segment surgical results. In OCT of a corneal transplant (Figure 14-15), the junction of the thinner graft and thicker host bed can be visualized. Scarring on the anterior and posterior aspects of the host corneal rim can be appreciated. The outline of an AC IOL is faintly seen. Reflected signal strength from the IOL surfaces is highly dependent on the incidence angle of the OCT beam.

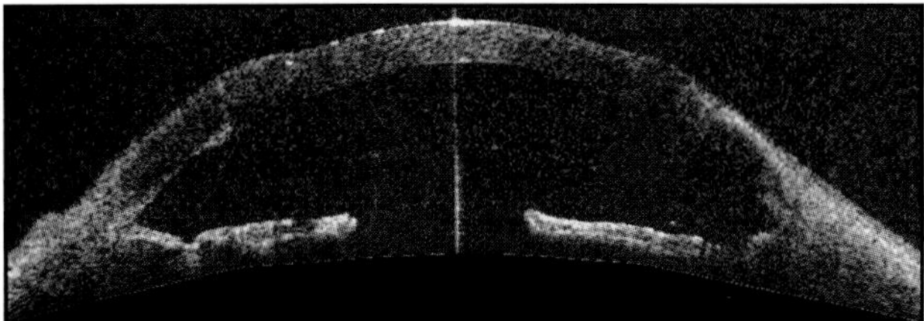

Figure 14-15. Corneal graft 2 years after transplantation. The OCT scan width was 15 mm.

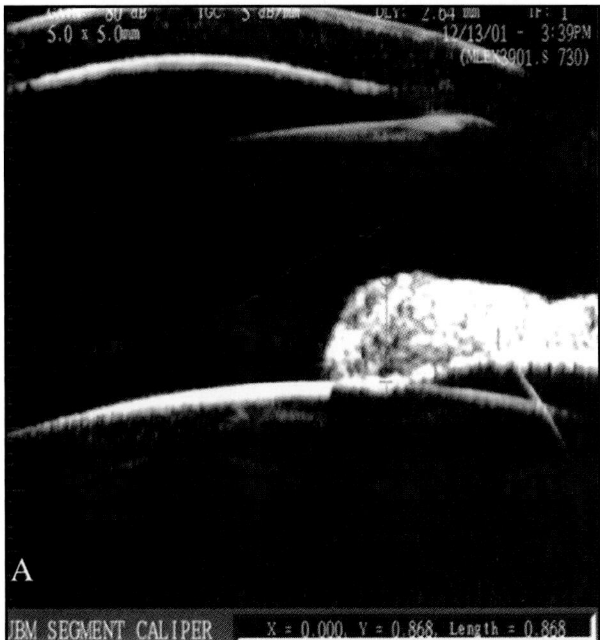

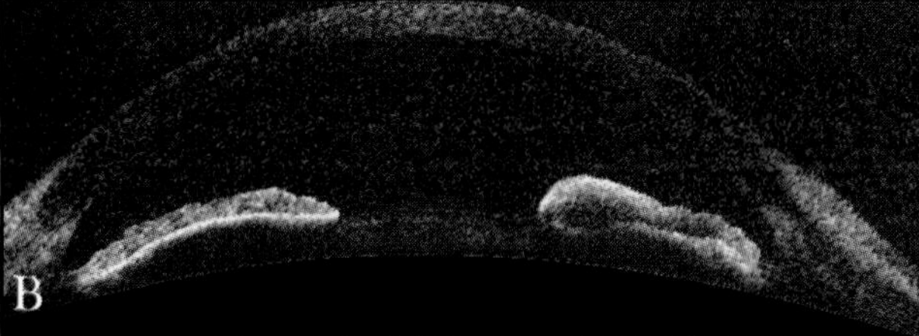

Figure 14.17 An iris nevus. (A) UBM and (B) OCT (nevus on right).

Trabeculectomy site can be visualized with OCT (Figure 14-16). The thickness of the bleb wall and the height of the fluid space can be evaluated (see Figure 14-16A). The sclerotomy channel can be visualized (see Figure 14-16B). We do not yet have experience in correlating the function and OCT anatomy of trabeculectomy. But a potential application for OCT is assessing the cause of a filtration failure to guide the planning of surgical revision.

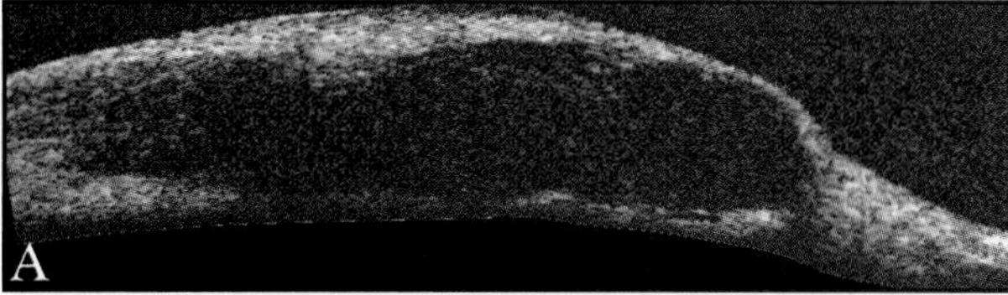

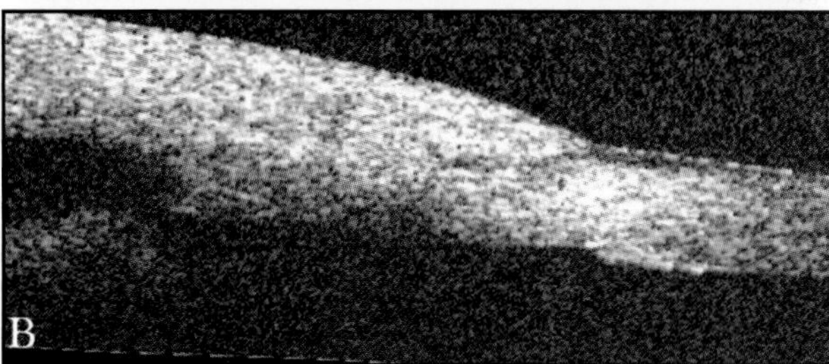

Figure 14-16 A functioning trabeculectomy site 7 months after surgery. (A) Transverse (horizontal) OCT section of bleb. (B) Sagittal (vertical) OCT section showing cornea and iris on left and sclera on right with sclerotomy near the junction.

Pathologies

We also used the slit-lamp-mounted, high-speed CAS OCT system to survey several types of ocular pathologies. Iris nevus and masses are often followed for growth over the long term to assess their malignant potential. OCT is an alternative to UBM for measuring the thickness of iris masses. The UBM and OCT of an iris mass are shown in Figure 14-17. OCT provides a detailed cross-sectional view of iris anatomy and the angle. The iris pigment epithelium appears as a bright band on the posterior surface of the iris. The nevus also appears bright on the anterior surface of the iris, presumably due to reflections from the melanin granules.

Compared to UBM, the OCT image has both higher resolution and wider field. OCT is also much more comfortable due to its noncontact nature. However, OCT is not able to penetrate and visualize structures behind the iris as well as UBM.

Cataracts can also be evaluated with OCT. The dimensions, density, and capsular proximity of a polar cataract can be closely examined in Figure 14-18. Because OCT penetrates poorly behind the iris, pharmacologic pupillary dilation is required to visualize the crystalline lens over a wide area.

Future Developments

CAS OCT is a versatile tool for visualization and measurement of CAS anatomy. It has the potential for improving upon the functions currently served by Placido-ring corneal topography, slit-scanning corneal topography, ultrasound imaging, and ultrasound pachymetry. Compared with current optical topography methods, OCT is unique in the ability to delineate the LASIK flap interface, in addition to the anterior and posterior interfaces and the epithelium-Bowman's interface. Compared to ultrasound techniques, OCT has the advantages of higher resolution and noncontact measurement

We are working to develop and demonstrate 3-D scanning capabilities for CAS OCT. The high speed that has been demonstrated is already sufficient for 3-D imaging. But software tools for scanning, displaying, measuring, and mapping from 3-D OCT need to be developed. For the cornea, the most useful application may be the mapping of multiple surfaces and thicknesses, including the LASIK flap. Imaging of surgical anatomy and pathologies will benefit from multi-cross-sectional imaging and display.

Refractive surgery, AC biometry, angle assessment, trabeculectomy, and tumors are some of the applications that we believe will benefit from CAS OCT. The commercialization and general availability of this technology will bring forth more applications through the ingenuity of many practitioners, and we are working to help bring this to fruition soon.

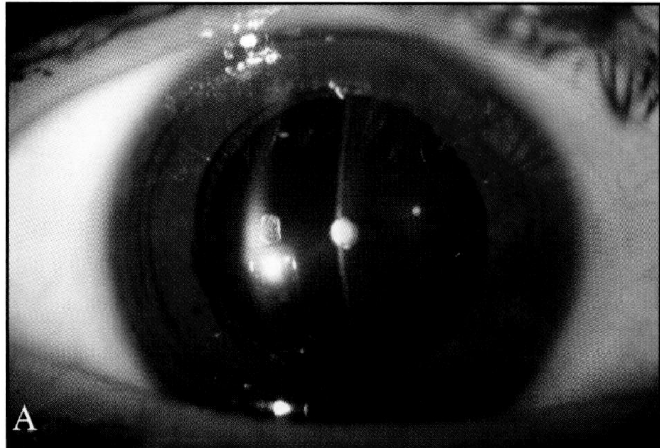

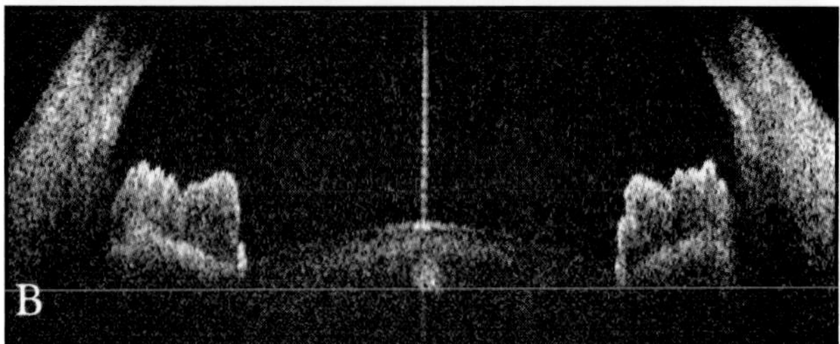

Figure 14.18 An anterior polar cataract viewed with (A) slit-lamp and (B) OCT.

References

1. Huang D, Swanson EA, Lin CP, et al. Optical coherence tomography. *Science*. 1991;254(5035):1178-1181.
2. Huang D, Wang J, Lin CP, Puliafito CA, Fujimoto JG. Micron-resolution ranging of cornea anterior chamber by optical reflectometry. *Lasers Surg Med.* 1991;11(5):419-425.
3. Izatt JA, Hee MR, Swanson EA, et al. Micrometer-scale resolution imaging of the anterior eye in vivo with optical coherence tomography. *Arch Ophthalmol.* 1994;112(12):1584-1589.
4. Koop N, Brinkmann R, Lankenau E, Flache S, Engelhardt R, Birngruber R. Optical coherence tomography of the cornea and the anterior eye segment. *Ophthalmologe*. 1997;94(7):481-486.
5. Asiyo-Vogel MN, Koop N, Brinkmann R, et al. Imaging of laser thermokeratoplasty lesions by optical low coherence tomography and polarization microscopy after Sirius Red staining. *Ophthalmologe*. 1997;94(7):487-491.
6. Maldonado MJ. Undersurface ablation of the flap for laser in situ keratomileusis retreatment. *Ophthalmology*. 2002;109(8):1453-1464.
7. Maldonado MJ, Munuera JM, Garcia-Layana A, Moreno J, Aliseda D. Optical coherence tomography (OCT) evaluation of the corneal cap and stromal bed features after LASIK for high myopia. Paper presented at: American Academy of Ophthalmology Annual Meeting; November 8-11, 1998; New Orleans, La.
8. Maldonado MJ, Ruiz-Oblitas L, Munuera JM, Aliseda D, Garcia-Layana A, Moreno-Montanes J. Optical coherence tomography evaluation of the corneal cap and stromal bed features after laser in situ keratomileusis for high myopia and astigmatism. *Ophthalmology*. 2000;107(1):81-87; discussion 88.
9. Muscat S, McKay N, Parks S, Kemp E, Keating D. Repeatability and reproducibility of corneal thickness measurements by optical coherence tomography. *Invest Ophthalmol Vis Sci*. 2002;43(6):1791-1795.
10. Neubauer AS, Priglinger SG, Thiel MJ, May CA, Welge-Lussen UC. Sterile structural imaging of donor cornea by optical coherence tomography. *Cornea*. 2002;21(5):490-494.
11. Nozaki M, Kimura H, Kojima M, Ogura Y. Optical coherence tomographic findings of the anterior segment after nonpenetrating deep sclerectomy. *Am J Ophthalmol*. 2002;133(6):837-839.
12. Priglinger SG, Neubauer AS, May CA, et al. Optical coherence tomography for the detection of laser in situ keratomileusis in donor corneas. *Cornea*. 2003;22(1):46-50.
13. Toth CA, Chiu EK, Winter KP, et al. In-vivo response to free electron laser incision of the rabbit cornea. *Lasers Surg Med*. 2001;29(1):44-52.

14. Ucakhan OO, Tello C, Liebmann JM, Ritch R, Asbell PA. Optical coherence tomography of Intacs. *J Cataract Refract Surg.* 2001;27(10):1535.
15. Ustundag C, Bahcecioglu H, Ozdamar A, Aras C, Yildirim R, Ozkan S. Optical coherence tomography for evaluation of anatomical changes in the cornea after laser in situ keratomileusis. *J Cataract Refract Surg.* 2000;26(10):1458-1462.
16. Wang J, Fonn D, Simpson TL, Jones L. Relation between optical coherence tomography and optical pachymetry measurements of corneal swelling induced by hypoxia. *Am J Ophthalmol.* 2002;134(1):93-98.
17. Wang J, Fonn D, Simpson TL, Jones L. The measurement of corneal epithelial thickness in response to hypoxia using optical coherence tomography. *Am J Ophthalmol.* 2002;133(3):315-319.
18. Wong AC, Wong CC, Yuen NS, Hui SP. Correlational study of central corneal thickness measurements on Hong Kong Chinese using optical coherence tomography, Orbscan and ultrasound pachymetry. *Eye.* 2002;16(6):715-721.
19. Bagayev SN, Gelikonov VM, Gelikonov GV, et al. Optical coherence tomography for in situ monitoring of laser corneal ablation. *J Biomed Opt.* 2002;7(4):633-642.
20. Bechmann M, Thiel MJ, Neubauer AS, et al. Central corneal thickness measurement with a retinal optical coherence tomography device versus standard ultrasonic pachymetry. *Cornea.* 2001;20(1):50-54.
21. Feng Y, Varikooty J, Simpson TL. Diurnal variation of corneal and corneal epithelial thickness measured using optical coherence tomography. *Cornea.* 2001;20(5):480-483.
22. Hirano K, Ito Y, Suzuki T, Kojima T, Kachi S, Miyake Y. Optical coherence tomography for the noninvasive evaluation of the cornea. *Cornea.* 2001;20(3):281-289.
23. Hirano K, Kojima T, Nakamura M, Hotta Y. Triple anterior chamber after full-thickness lamellar keratoplasty for lattice corneal dystrophy. *Cornea.* 2001;20(5):530-533.
24. Hoerauf H, Wirbelauer C, Scholz C, et al. Slit-lamp-adapted optical coherence tomography of the anterior segment. *Graefes Arch Clin Exp Ophthalmol.* 2000;238(1):8-18.
25. Wirbelauer C, Scholz C, Engelhardt R, Laqua H, Pham DT. Biomorphometry of corneal epithelium with slit-lamp-adapted optical coherence tomography. *Ophthalmologe.* 2001;98(9):848-852.
26. Wirbelauer C, Scholz C, Haberle H, Laqua H, Pham DT. Corneal optical coherence tomography before and after phototherapeutic keratectomy for recurrent epithelial erosions(2). *J Cataract Refract Surg.* 2002;28(9):1629-1635.
27. Wirbelauer C, Scholz C, Hoerauf H, Engelhardt R, Birngruber R, Laqua H. Corneal optical coherence tomography before and immediately after excimer laser photorefractive keratectomy. *Am J Ophthalmol.* 2000;130(6):693-699.
28. Wirbelauer C, Scholz C, Hoerauf H, Pham DT, Laqua H, Birngruber R. Noncontact corneal pachymetry with slit-lamp-adapted optical coherence tomography. *Am J Ophthalmol.* 2002;133(4):444-450.
29. Wirbelauer C, Winkler J, Bastian GO, Haberle H, Pham DT. Histopathological correlation of corneal diseases with optical coherence tomography. *Graefes Arch Clin Exp Ophthalmol.* 2002;240(9):727-734.
30. Hoerauf H, Scholz C, Koch P, Engelhardt R, Laqua H, Birngruber R. Transscleral optical coherence tomography: a new imaging method for the anterior segment of the eye. *Arch Ophthalmol.* 2002;120(6):816-819.
31. Hoerauf H, Winkler J, Scholz C, et al. Transscleral optical coherence tomography—an experimental study in ex-vivo human eyes. *Lasers Surg Med.* 2002;30(3):209-215.
32. Radhakrishnan S, Rollins AM, Roth JE, et al. Real-time optical coherence tomography of the anterior segment at 1310 nm. *Arch Ophthalmol.* 2001;119(8):1179-1185.
33. Li Y, Shekhar R, Huang D. Corneal anatomic changes after LASIK measured by arc-scanning optical coherence tomography and ultrasonic pachymetry. *ARVO Meeting Abstracts.* 2002;43(12):153.
34. Li Y, Shekhar R, Huang D. Segmentation of 830- and 1310-nm LASIK corneal optical coherence tomography images. Paper presented at: SPIE Medical Imaging 2002: Image Processing; May 2002; San Diego, Calif.
35. Seiler T, Quurke AW. Iatrogenic keratectasia after LASIK in a case of forme fruste keratoconus. *J Cataract Refract Surg.* 1998;24(7):1007-1009.
36. Reinstein DZ, Silverman RH, Sutton HF, Coleman DJ. Very high-frequency ultrasound corneal analysis identifies anatomic correlates of optical complications of lamellar refractive surgery: anatomic diagnosis in lamellar surgery. *Ophthalmology.* 1999;106(3):474-482.
37. van den Berg TJ, Spekreijse H. Near infrared light absorption in the human eye media. *Vision Res.* 1997;37(2):249-253.
38. American National Standard for Safe Use of Lasers. Orlando: Laser Institute of America, American National Standards Institute, Inc.; June 28, 2000. ANSI Z136.1-2000.
39. Pavlin CJ, Harasiewicz K, Sherar MD, Foster FS. Clinical use of ultrasound biomicroscopy. *Ophthalmology.* 1991; 98(3):287-295.
40. Chen HB, Kashiwagi K, Yamabayashi S, Kinoshita T, Ou B, Tsukahara S. Anterior chamber angle biometry: quadrant variation, age change and sex difference. *Curr Eye Res.* 1998;17(2):120-124.
41. Saragoussi JJ, Othenin-Girard P, Pouliquen YJ. Ocular damage after implantation of oversized minus power anterior chamber intraocular lenses in myopic phakic eyes: case reports. *Refract Corneal Surg.* 1993;9(2):105-109.

SECTION IV

APPENDICES

Appendix A

Physical Principles of Optical Coherence Tomography

James G. Fujimoto, PhD; David Huang, MD, PhD; Michael R. Hee, MD, PhD; Tony Ko, MS; Eric Swanson, MS; Carmen A. Puliafito, MD; and Joel S. Schuman, MD

- Introduction
- Optical Interferometry
- Low-Coherence Interferometry Measurement of Light Echoes
- Sensitivity
- Spatial Resolution
- Pixel Density and Image Acquisition Time
- Advances in Optical Coherence Tomography Technology
- Summary

Introduction

Optical coherence tomography (OCT) is analogous to ultrasound imaging, except that it measures the echo time delay and magnitude of light rather than sound.[1-3] OCT can achieve axial image resolutions of 1 to 15 microns (μm), which is one to two orders of magnitude finer than standard clinical ultrasound. In tissues other than the eye, the maximum imaging depth is limited to approximately 2 to 3 mm by attenuation from light scattering. Although this depth is shallow when compared to other clinical imaging techniques, OCT can achieve resolutions 10x to 100x finer than conventional ultrasound, magnetic resonance imaging (MRI), or computer tomography (CT). OCT imaging has been termed *optical biopsy* because it provides images of tissue pathology in situ and in real time, without the need to remove and process specimens, which is required in excisional biopsy and histopathology.[4,5]

OCT imaging has several features that are attractive for medical imaging:

1. OCT can perform imaging with resolutions approaching conventional histopathology
2. Imaging can be performed in situ and in real time
3. Imaging may be performed using a wide range of instruments, such as ophthalmoscopes, microscopes, handheld probes, endoscopes, catheters, laparoscopes, and needles
4. OCT can perform functional imaging such as spectroscopic imaging, Doppler blood flow imaging, and the measurement of blood oxygenation or tissue birefringence
5. Computer image-processing algorithms can be used to quantitatively assess OCT images and to generate objective diagnostic information

Figure A-1 shows a collage of OCT images illustrating different applications.[6-9] OCT promises to have clinical applications in three general scenarios:

1. To image tissue pathology when excisional biopsy is hazardous or impossible, such as in the eye
2. To guide surgical procedures
3. To reduce sampling errors and associated false negatives that can occur with excisional biopsy

Figure A-2 shows a schematic of the principles of OCT imaging. A beam of light is directed onto the tissue or specimen to be imaged. The internal structure is measured noninvasively by measuring the echo delay time and magnitude of light, which is backreflected or backscattered from microstructural features at different depths. Two-dimensional imaging is accomplished by performing successive axial (longitudinal) measurements at different transverse positions and by displaying the results as a two-dimensional cross-sectional image.[1,10-12] This appendix provides detailed information on the physical principles of OCT, including how low-coherence interferometry works, as well as what determines the resolution, sensitivity, and speed of OCT imaging systems.

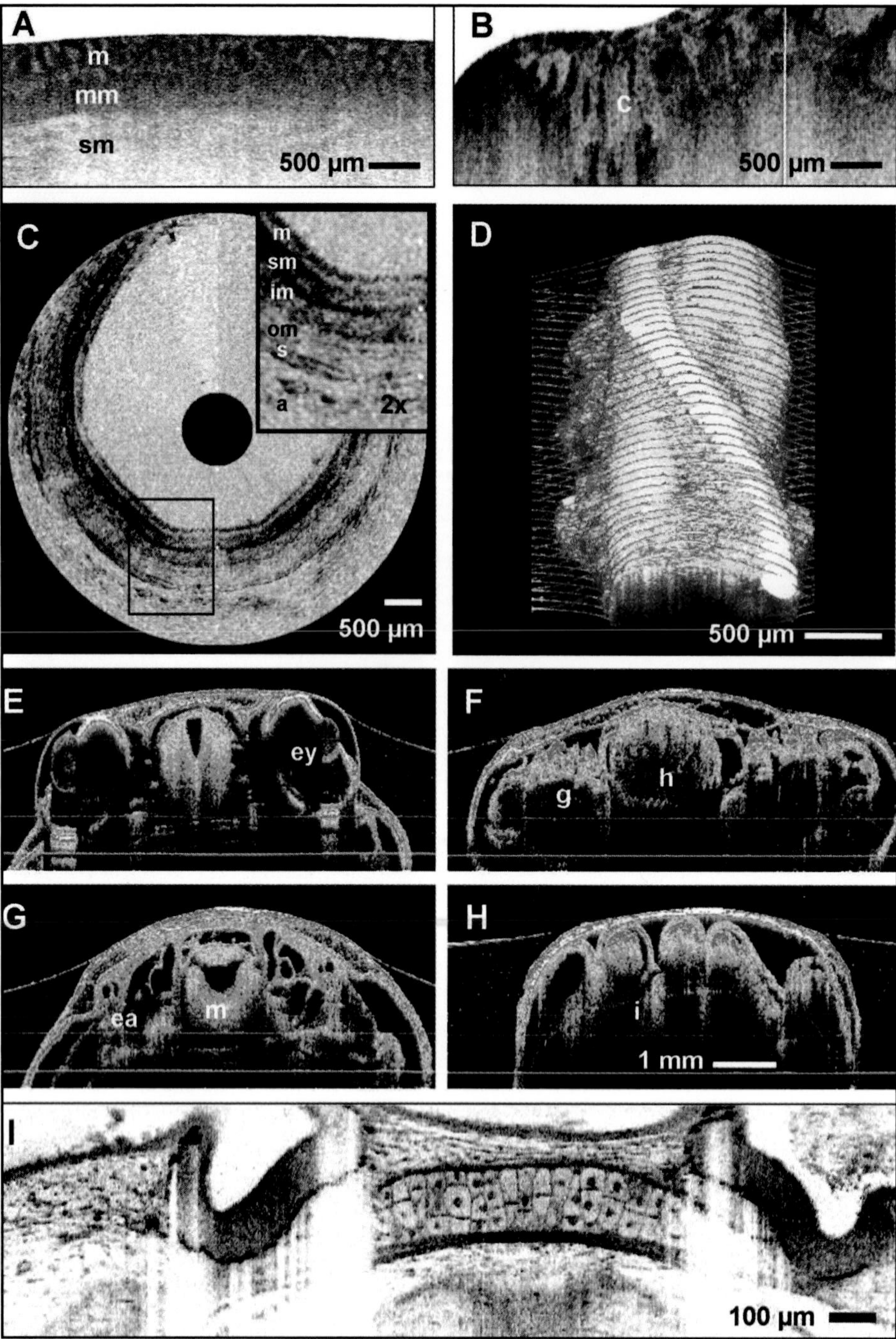

Figure A-1. Examples of OCT images illustrating the broad range of OCT applications. (A and B) Normal colonic mucosa versus adenocarcinoma ex vivo. (Reproduced from Pitris C, Jesser C, Boppart SA, Stamper D, Brezinski ME, Fujimoto JG. Feasibility of optical coherence tomography for high-resolution imaging of human gastrointestinal tract malignancies. *J Gastroenterol.* 2000;35(2):87-92.) (C) Endoscopic OCT of the esophagus in vivo in the rabbit. (Reproduced from Tearney GJ, Brezinski ME, Bouma BE, et al. In vivo endoscopic optical biopsy with optical coherence tomography. *Science.* 1997;276(5321):2037-2039.) (D) Three-dimensional display of a peripheral nerve ex vivo. (Reproduced from Boppart SA, Bouma BE, Pitris C, et al. Intraoperative assessment of microsurgery with three-dimensional optical coherence tomography. *Radiology.* 1998;208(1):81-86.) (E to H) Developmental biology image of the Rana pipiens tadpole in vivo. (Reproduced from Boppart SA, Brezinski ME, Bouma BE, Tearney GJ, Fujimoto JG. Investigation of developing embryonic morphology using optical coherence tomography. *Dev Biol.* 1996;177(1):54-63, with permission from Elsevier.) (I) Ultrahigh-resolution cellular imaging of the Xenopus laevis tadpole in vivo.

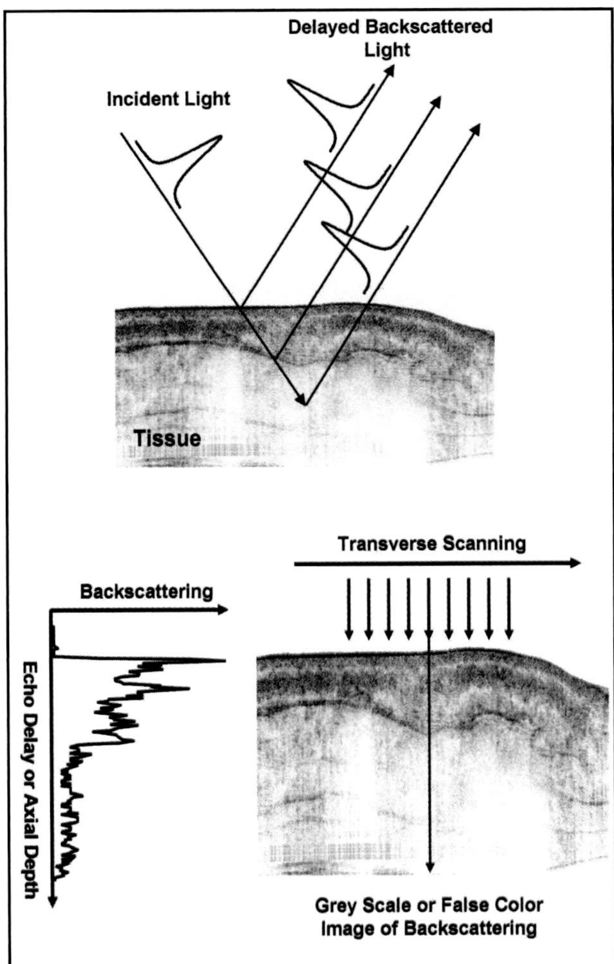

Figure A-2. OCT performs high-resolution cross-sectional imaging of the internal structure in tissue by measuring the echo time delay and intensity of backscattered or backreflected light. High image resolution is achieved and it is possible to perform imaging in situ and in real time without the need to remove and process specimens, as in conventional biopsy. For this reason, OCT imaging has been termed *optical biopsy*.

Optical Interferometry

In order to perform OCT imaging, it is first necessary to perform high-resolution measurements of the echo delay time of backreflected or backscattered light from inside tissue. Because light travels much faster than sound, a direct measurement of optical echoes is not possible. In OCT, measurements of optical echoes are performed using a correlation technique known as *low-coherence interferometry*. Low-coherence interferometry is a simple method that can measure distances to objects with high precision by measuring light reflected from them and correlating it with light that travels a known reference path delay.[13-15]

Light is a wave. A beam of light is composed of electric and magnetic fields that oscillate or periodically vary in time and in space.[13] Light can be characterized by its frequency, υ, or its wavelength, λ. Light propagates with a characteristic velocity that varies according to the medium in which it is propagating. In a vacuum, the velocity of light is $c = 3 \times 10^8$ m/s. In different media, such as water, vitreous, or glass, the velocity of propagation of light is reduced from its speed in vacuum. The velocity of light in a medium is c/n, where n is the index of refraction of the medium. Because OCT measures echo time delays, the axial delay in an OCT image is adjusted by 1/n in order to obtain the physical dimension. This is analogous to ultrasound in which measurements of dimensions require a knowledge of the sound-wave velocity.

Equation A-1 describes the functional form of the oscillating electric field in a light wave as:

$$E(t) = E \cos[(2\pi\upsilon)t - (2\pi/\lambda)z] \qquad \text{(A-1)}$$

Because light is a wave composed of oscillating electrical and magnetic fields, a phenomena known as *interference* can occur when two beams of light are combined. The electric and magnetic fields that compose the two beams can add either constructively or destructively according to the relative phase of their oscillations. When two beams of light are added so that their fields are in phase, constructive interference occurs and the resulting light is more intense. Conversely, when beams of light are added, so that their fields are out of phase, destructive interference occurs where the fields tend to cancel and the resulting light is less intense.

An optical interferometer functions by adding or by interfering the light waves in two light beams.[13] Figure A-3 shows a schematic diagram of a simple Michelson-type interferometer. A light wave is incident onto a partially reflecting mirror or beamsplitter that splits the light into two beams: one functioning as a reference beam and the other as a measurement or signal beam. The beams travel given distances in the two paths or arms of the interferometer. The measurement beam is backreflected or backscattered from the tissue being imaged to the signal beam $E_{Sig}(t)$, while the reference beam $E_{Ref}(t)$ is reflected from a reference mirror.

The signal and reference beams are then interfered or added at the partially reflecting mirror (beamsplitter), and the intensity of the resulting interferometer output beam is measured by a photodetector. The output of the interferometer is an optical beam with an electric field $E_{Out}(t)$ that is the sum of the fields from the signal and reference optical beams. Equation A-2 gives the mathematical form of the electric field output of the interferometer $E_{Out}(t)$:

$$E_{Out}(t) \sim E_{Ref}(t) + E_{Sig}(t) \qquad \text{(A-2)}$$

The detector measures the intensity of the output light from the interferometer. The intensity is proportional to the square of the electric field. For the purposes of this analysis, let us assume that the reflected signal beam consists of a single reflection at a given distance rather than multiple echoes, as would be the case in an actual imaging measurement. If the length of the signal path is L_{Sig} and the length of the reference path is L_{Ref}, then the path difference is $\Delta L = L_{Sig} - L_{Ref}$. The output intensity from the interferometer will oscillate as a function of the path difference ΔL because of interference effects. Equation A-3 gives the output intensity of the interferometer as a function of E_{Sig}, E_{Ref}, and ΔL as:

$$I_{Out}(t) \sim (1/4)\,|E_{Ref}|^2 + (1/4)\,|E_{Sig}|^2 + (1/2)\,E_{Ref}E_{Sig}\cos[2\,(2\pi/\lambda)\,\Delta L] \qquad \text{(A-3)}$$

If the position of the reference mirror is varied or scanned, the path length that the light travels in the reference arm will change and the reference light will have a variable time delay. The reference beam can add either destructively or constructively to the measurement beam from the specimen. Interference effects will be observed in the output intensity as the length of the reference path is changed by translating the reference mirror. This is shown schematically in Figure A-3. The output signal oscillates between maximum and minimum each time the total path difference travelled changes by one optical wavelength or the position of the reference mirror changes by one-half an optical wavelength.

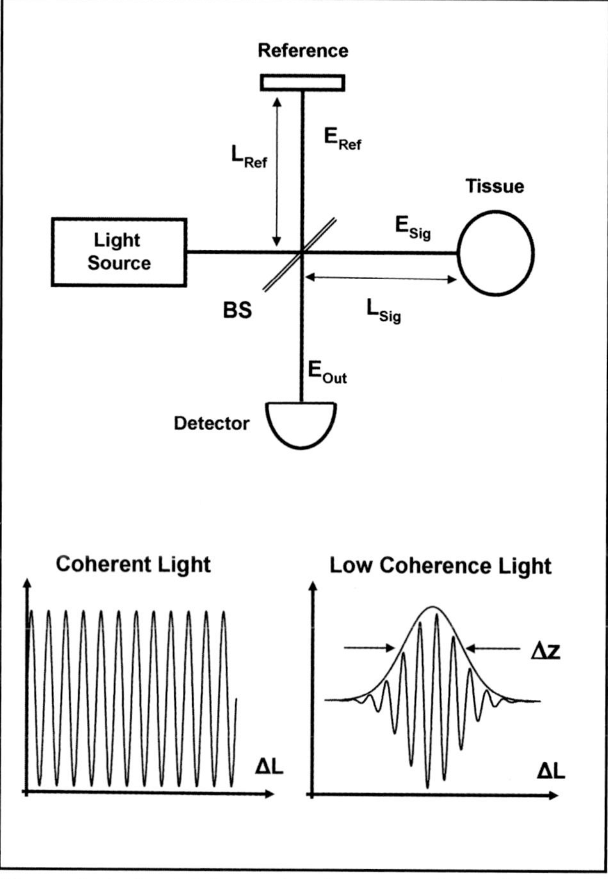

Figure A-3. (Top) Schematic of an optical interferometer for low-coherence interferometry measurement of echo delay. A beam from a light source is split into a reference beam and a measurement beam by a partially reflecting mirror (beamsplitter). The measurement beam is backscattered or backreflected from tissue at a distance L_{Sig} to produce an optical echo signal, while the reference beam is reflected from a mirror at a variable distance L_{Ref}. The reference and signal light waves are combined and interfere. The interferometer output intensity is measured by a photodetector. (Bottom) If coherent light is used, then interference occurs between the reference and the signal light beams. The output intensity oscillates as the length difference $\Delta L = L_{Sig} - L_{Ref}$ between the reference and signal paths is varied by multiples of one-half the wavelength of light. These interference effects are observed for all relative delays between the reference and measurement beam. In contrast, if low-coherence light is used, interference effects are only observed when the path length difference is less than the coherence length of the light. The coherence length is a statistical property of the light and is related to statistical phase changes in the light waves. Because interference is only observed when the reference delay matches the echo delay in the signal light, low-coherence interferometry enables precise measurement of the echo time delay of backscattered or backreflected light.

Low-Coherence Interferometry Measurement of Light Echoes

If the light beam is coherent and has a long coherence length, then interference oscillations will be observed for a wide range of relative path length differences, ΔL, of the reference and signal paths. For applications in optical ranging or OCT, it is necessary to precisely measure absolute position of a structure within the tissue. In this case, light with a short coherence length, or low-coherence light, is used. The property of coherence is a statistical property of light. Low-coherence light is composed of an oscillating electric field that has statistical changes in phase as a function of time and space. Low-coherence

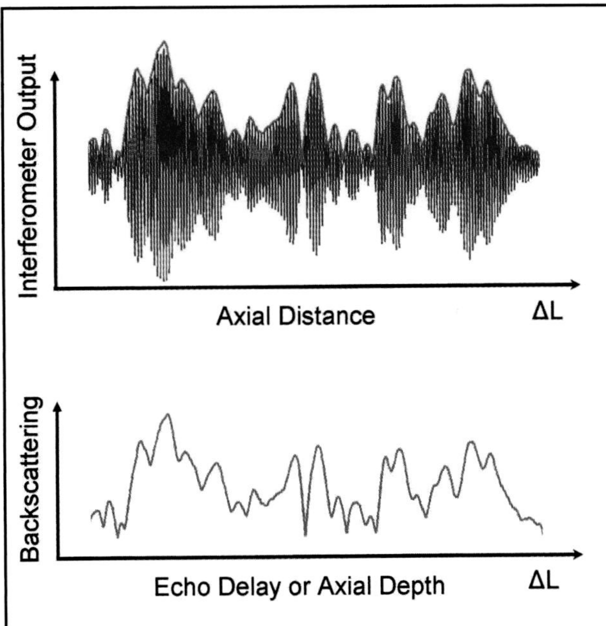

Figure A-4. Measurement of backscattering echoes from the interferometer output signal. The echo signal can be measured by demodulating or extracting the envelope of the interference signal. The interferometer output is proportional to the product of the signal and reference fields, so the interferometer measures the field of the echo light wave. The measurement is closely related to a technique known as *optical heterodyne detection,* which is used in optical communications.

light is not a single frequency or wavelength, but is composed of a spread or bandwidth of several different frequencies and wavelengths. The coherence of light can be characterized by a distance, the coherence length, over which the light is coherent and does not have statistical phase discontinuities. The coherence length is inversely proportional to its frequency content or bandwidth. Conceptually, it is also possible to think of low-coherence light as being composed of a continuous series of short optical pulses or fluctuations that have a duration equal to the coherence length. This coherence length determines the axial resolution of OCT imaging.

When low-coherence light is used in the interferometer, interference is only observed when the path lengths of the reference and signal paths are closely matched to within the coherence length of the light (ΔL less than the coherence length). If the path lengths differ by a larger amount, then the fields from the two beams are not coherent or correlated, and there is no interference. This is shown schematically in Figure A-3 (Bottom). When the interferometer paths are nearly matched in length, ΔL small, complete destructive or constructive interference between the reference and signal beams is observed when the reference mirror position is scanned. However, when the path length difference, and hence the time delay difference, between the reference beam and the measurement beam is large, no interference occurs. The length Δz over which interference occurs is determined by the coherence length of the light.

Thus, the echo time delay of light can be determined by measuring the interference at the output of the interferometer as the reference arm path length is scanned. The interferometer effectively measures the echo delay and magnitude of light by correlating the backreflected or backscattered light with reference light that has a known delay.

Sensitivity

In order to obtain high-quality OCT images, it is necessary to achieve extremely high detection sensitivities. For ophthalmic imaging, high sensitivity is required because the retina is nominally transparent and the intensity of weak backreflections and backscattering is extremely weak. For imaging other tissues that are optically scattering, the sensitivity determines the imaging depth because the incident light is attenuated by absorption and scattering in tissue. OCT uses a technique known as *optical heterodyne detection*, the same detection technique developed for optical communications systems. OCT can achieve high detection sensitivity to weak backreflected or backscattered light approaching the quantum mechanical detection limit. The process of performing interferometry provides an amplification of weak optical signals. This can be seen by examining the expression (see Equation A-3) for the interferometer output intensity. The interference term of the output signal is proportional to $E_{Ref}E_{Sig}$. The is the result of interference of the electric field E_{Sig} from the backreflected or backscattered beam from the tissue, multiplied by the electric field E_{Ref} of the reference beam. The signal from the tissue E_{Sig} can be weak, but it is multiplied by the strong electric field E_{Ref} from the reference beam, thereby increasing the magnitude of the oscillating interference term measured by the photodetector. In addition, since the interferometer measures the field of the backscattered or backreflected light rather than the intensity, which is the square of the field, a high dynamic range can be achieved.

Figure A-4 shows a schematic of how the echo time delay and magnitude are extracted from the interferometer output signal as the path length difference is scanned.[16] The reference mirror is usually scanned at a constant velocity v, which causes interference to be generated at a frequency $2v/\lambda$. The scanning reference mirror can also be thought of as Doppler shifting the reflected reference beam light. When this reference light interferes with the signal light, interference at the Doppler frequency $2v/\lambda$ is produced. The profile of the echo time delay can be measured by electronically filtering and demodulating the photodetector signal. The process of demodulation corresponds to taking the envelope of the interference signal. Finally, the interferometer measures the field of the backscattered or backreflected signal versus delay or depth so that the intensity is the square of the envelope.

Since the principles of operation of OCT are similar to optical communications systems, the performance of OCT systems can be calculated using well established methods in optical communications theory.[16] The signal-to-noise ratio (SNR) in the detected signal is given by:

$$SNR = 10\,\mathrm{Log}(\eta P/2h\upsilon\,NEB) \qquad \text{(A-4)}$$

In this equation, η is the photodetector quantum efficiency, $2h\upsilon$ is the photon energy, P is the power in the detected signal, and *NEB* is the noise equivalent bandwidth of detection system. The sensitivity of the OCT imaging is proportional to the amount of available power in the signal and is inversely proportional to the bandwidth of the detection. Faster image acquisition or higher resolution imaging requires a broader detection bandwidth since there is more data. Therefore, there is a tradeoff in signal-to-noise performance or sensitivity. For typical measurement parameters, OCT systems have a signal-to-noise performance of ~95 dB, which means that backscattered or backreflected intensities as small as -95 dB of the incident intensity can be detected. In ophthalmic imaging, high sensitivity is required in order to visualize weak backscattering or backreflecting structures in the retina and vitreous. A decrease in signal-to-noise performance means that structures such as the nuclear layer or reflections from subtle vitreal anomalies appear dark and are difficult to visualize.

Spatial Resolution

Image resolution is also an important parameter that governs OCT system performance. In OCT, the axial (longitudinal) and transverse resolutions are determined by completely different physical mechanisms. The axial image resolution depends upon the coherence length of the light source, which determines the resolution or accuracy Δz with which distance can be measured. Because low-coherence length light contains a spread of frequencies or wavelengths, it can also be characterized by its frequency or wavelength bandwidth. Theoretical calculations show that the axial resolution Δz is related to the wavelength bandwidth Δl by the formula:

$$\Delta z = (2\ln 2/\pi)(\lambda^2/\Delta\lambda) \qquad \text{(A-5)}$$

Equation A-5 shows that the axial resolution Δz is inversely proportional to the full-width at half-maximum of the wavelength bandwidth $\Delta\lambda$ of the light source. A typical superluminescent diode light source for OCT operates in near-infrared wavelengths at ~800 nm and has a wavelength bandwidth of 20 nm. This yields an axial resolution of ~15 µm in air. Because the speed of light is slower in tissue, the axial dimension is divided by the index of refraction of the tissue to give an axial resolution of ~10 µm.

The transverse resolution in OCT imaging is determined by the same principles as the transverse resolution in conventional optical microscopy. The transverse resolution is determined by the spot size of the focused OCT imaging beam. The minimum focal spot size Δx of an optical beam is determined by the diffraction properties of light and the focusing parameters being used. Equation A-6 gives an expression for the focused spot size Δx in terms of the diameter d of an optical beam incident upon a lens of focal length f:

$$\Delta x = (4\lambda/\pi)(f/d) \qquad \text{(A-6)}$$

This result follows from optical diffraction theory and is well known in microscopy. The focused spot size is proportional to the focal length of the focusing lens and inversely proportional to the diameter of the incident beam. Stated another way, the focused spot size is inversely proportional to the numerical aperture of the beam. This means, in order to achieve an extremely small spot size, it is necessary to have a large beam diameter and a short focal length lens or a high numerical aperture. Figure A-5 shows two different focusing conditions with large and small transverse spot sizes, which correspond to low and high numerical aperture focusing conditions, respectively.

There is a tradeoff between the transverse resolution and the depth of field in OCT imaging. This is similar to microscopy in which higher magnifications have very short depths of field. The depth of field is characterized by a parameter known as the confocal parameter b:

$$b = \pi(\Delta x)^2/2\lambda \qquad \text{(A-7)}$$

Smaller spot sizes, which improve the transverse resolution, are shallower in depth of focus. The depth of field decreases with the square of the focused spot size.

Figure A-5 shows schematically the relationship between focused spot size and depth of field for low and high numerical aperture focusing. The focusing conditions define two limiting cases for OCT imaging. Typically, OCT is performed with low numerical aperture focusing because it is desirable to have a large depth of

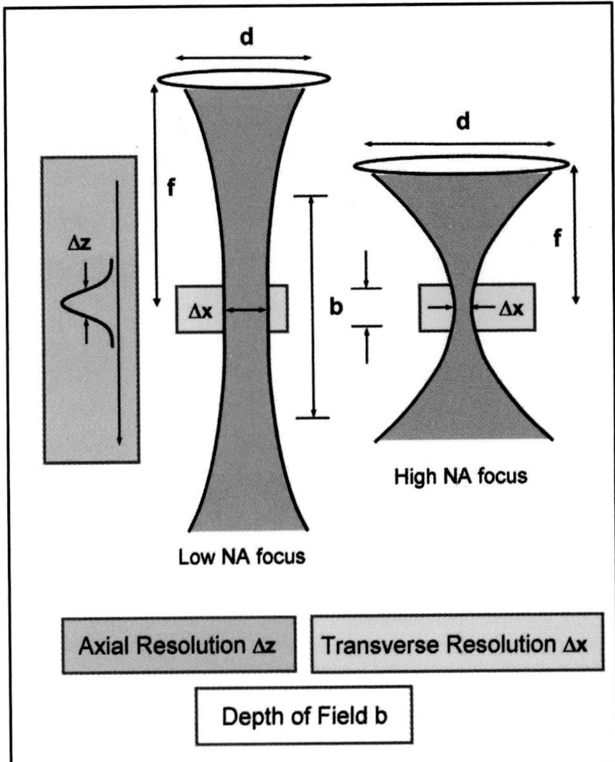

Figure A-5. Image resolution in OCT. The transverse resolution in OCT imaging is determined by the transverse spot size of the optical beam. This spot size is determined by the focusing optics, the diameter d of the incident beam, and the focal length f of the focusing lens. A small focusing angle or small numerical aperture NA gives a large transverse spot size Δx and a long depth of focus b. A large focusing angle or large numerical aperture NA gives a small transverse spot size Δx, but a short depth of focus b. The axial or longitudinal resolution is given by the coherence length of the light source and is independent of the focusing. In ophthalmology, this enables OCT imaging to achieve extremely high axial resolutions despite the limited pupil size of the eye.

field and to use low-coherence interferometry to achieve axial (longitudinal) resolution. Within this limit, the depth of field is longer than the coherence length. In contrast to conventional microscopy, OCT can achieve high axial resolution independently of the focusing conditions and depth of field. This feature is particularly powerful in ophthalmic applications where the available numerical aperture is limited by the pupil of the eye. The smallest spot size that can be achieved on the retina is also limited by optical aberrations in the eye. Typical ophthalmic OCT systems have a ~20 μm spot size on the retina. In other applications, it is also possible to focus with high numerical aperture and to achieve high-transverse resolutions at the expense of a reduced depth of focus. This operating regime is typical for conventional microscopy or confocal microscopy. Depending upon the coherence length of the light, the depth of field can be shorter than the coherence length. In this case, the depth of field can be used to differentiate backscattered or backreflected signals from different depths. This regime of operation is called *optical coherence microscopy* (OCM).[17]

As noted previously, standard OCT imaging systems use superluminescent diode light sources that have an axial resolution of 15 μm in air, which corresponds to 10 μm in tissue. However, it is possible to significantly improve the axial resolution of OCT by using new light sources that have broader bandwidths and shorter coherence lengths. Axial image resolutions as fine as 1 to 3 μm have been achieved in research OCT systems using short-pulse laser light sources with bandwidths of 100 to 200 nm.[18,19]

Pixel Density and Image Acquisition Time

It is important to note that the fundamental resolution of an OCT instrument is different from the pixel size or density in an OCT image. The pixel density in an OCT image is analogous to pixel density in digital photography. The image must have sufficient pixel density in order to be able to visualize small features with a given resolution. Figure A-6 shows a schematic describing pixel density and size in the axial and transverse directions.

OCT images are generated by acquiring successive axial measurements (axial scans) of backreflection or backscattering versus depth at different transverse positions. Therefore, the number of pixels in the transverse direction is equal to the number of axial scans. If the OCT image has N_x transverse pixels (axial scans) and is L_x wide in the transverse direction, then the pixel size in the transverse direction is L_x/N_x. For example, a typical OCT retinal image is 6 mm wide in the transverse direction and has 512 transverse pixels (axial scans), so the pixels are 6 mm/512 = 11.7 μm wide. In contrast, the transverse resolution for a typical retinal image is determined by the focused spot size and is typically ~20 μm. In order to utilize the full instrumental resolution, the size of the pixels must be smaller than the instrument resolution.

The pixel density in the axial (longitudinal) direction is governed by a different mechanism than in the transverse direction. In this case, the number of pixels N_z is determined by the speed at which the computer can record the electronic signal from the axial scan of backscattering, or backreflection, versus depth. This speed is governed by the analog-to-digital conversion rate

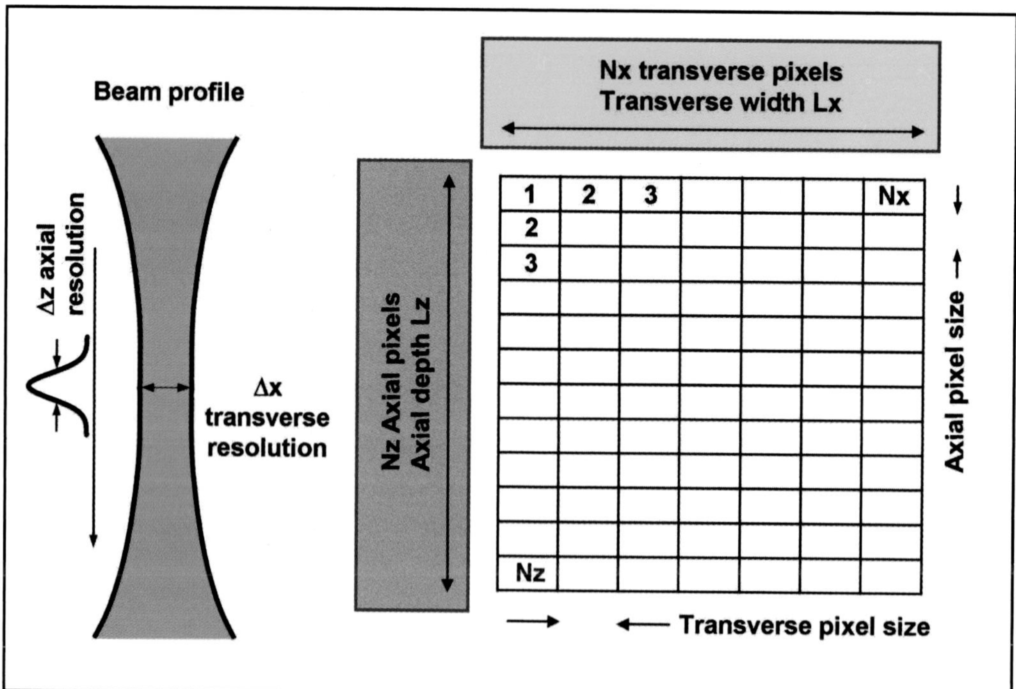

Figure A-6. OCT image resolution and pixel density. The fundamental resolution of the OCT instrument can be different from the pixel density in an image. The number and size of the pixels in the transverse direction is determined by the number of axial scans in the OCT image. Since the axial scan rate in an OCT instrument is limited, there is a tradeoff between the axial pixel density and image acquisition time. The number of pixels in the axial direction is determined by other factors, such as computer data acquisition speed, which can be very high. In order to resolve a small feature in an image, the pixel size must be sufficiently small or there must be a large enough number of pixels in the image.

and can be very rapid. If the OCT image has N_z axial pixels and is L_z deep in the axial direction, then the pixel size is L_z/N_z in the axial direction. For example, a typical OCT retinal image is 2 mm deep in the axial direction, and the instrument acquires 1024 pixels in the axial direction. Therefore, the pixel size is 2 mm/1024 = 1.9 µm in axial depth. In contrast, the axial (longitudinal) resolution of the typical retinal image is ~10 µm.

Achieving rapid image acquisition time is important for clinical imaging applications. Rapid image acquisition in ophthalmic imaging is important in order to minimize image distortion artifacts from residual eye motion, as well as to improve patient comfort during the examination. The image acquisition time is directly related to the sensitivity of the measurement, since imaging more rapidly (ie, increasing the noise equivalent detection bandwidth NEB) reduces signal-to-noise performance. The signal-to-noise performance could, in principle, be improved by using higher incident optical power, as shown in Equation A-4. However, the maximum permissible light exposure is determined by safety standards, such as the American National Standards Institute (ANSI) standards, for laser exposure. Thus, the image acquisition time is determined by a combination of the safe incident power and the signal-to-noise requirements that are necessary to achieve sufficient quality images for clinical applications.

Image acquisition time also increases in proportion to the number of transverse pixels in an image. If the instrument can generate axial measurements at a scan repetition rate of R, then the image acquisition time T is given by $T = N_x / R$. The acquisition time is the number of axial scans or transverse pixels N_x in the image divided by the axial scan repetition rate R of the instrument. If higher transverse pixel resolution is desired, more axial scans are necessary and the image acquisition time increases proportionally. Conversely, if only low-transverse resolution imaging is necessary (eg, if only topographic information is required), then the number of transverse pixels may be reduced and the image acquisition time will be proportionally faster.

OCT instruments have a maximum rate of axial scans per second, so that the tradeoff between the pixel density and acquisition speed is an important factor in determining the imaging protocols. Figure A-7 shows OCT high-

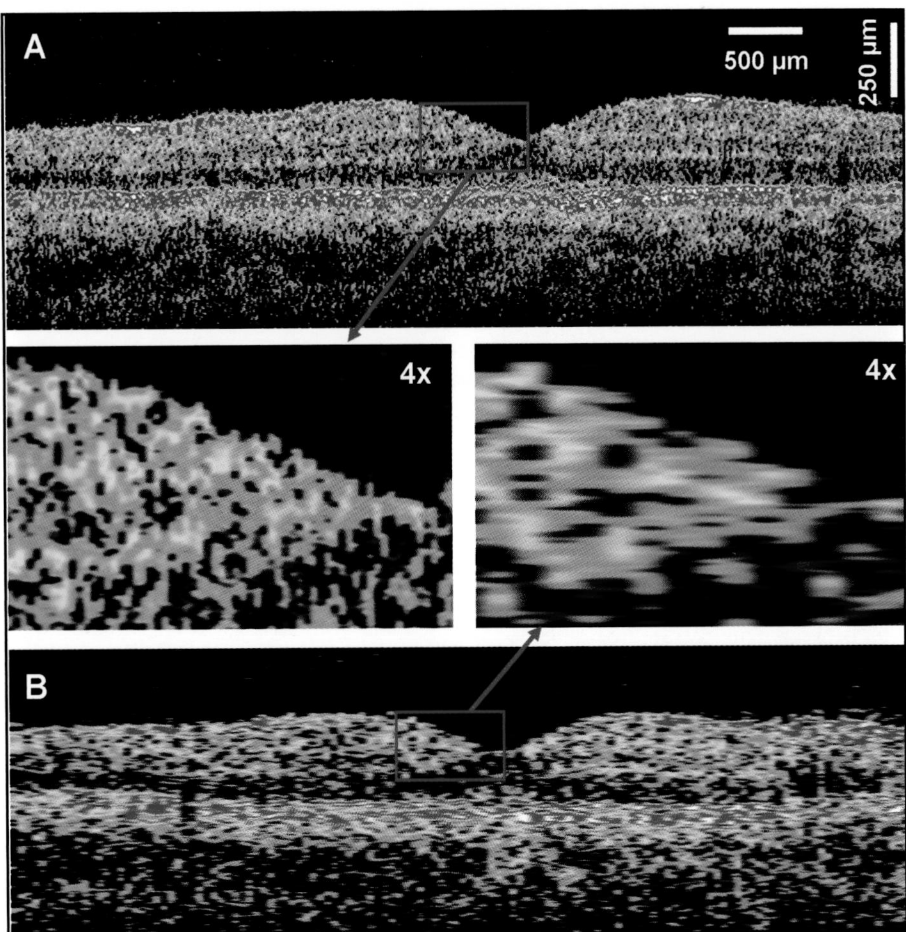

Figure A-7. Tradeoff between transverse pixel density and image acquisition speed. (Top) High-transverse pixel density image of the macula with 512 transverse pixels requires slower image acquisition speed. (Bottom) Low-transverse pixel density image with 128 transverse pixels. This image can be acquired four times faster than the high-pixel density image. Enlargements of foveal area show that the pixels are wider in the low-transverse pixel density rapid-acquisition image when compared to the high-pixel density slow-acquisition image.

transverse pixel density versus low-transverse pixel density images with 512 versus 128 transverse pixels, respectively. Current ophthalmic OCT instruments have an axial scan repetition rate R of approximately 400 axial scans per second. The high-transverse pixel density slow-acquisition image (A) of Figure A-7 is 6 mm wide and has 512 transverse pixels, thus the transverse pixel spacing is 6 mm/512 = 11.7 μm and the image is acquired in T = 512/400 = 1.28 seconds. The low-transverse pixel density, fast acquisition, image (B) of Figure A-7 is 6 mm wide and has 128 transverse pixels, so the transverse pixel spacing is 6 mm/128 = 48 μm and the image is acquired in T = 128/400 = 0.32 seconds. Note the grainier appearance of the low-transverse pixel density image. Images with higher or lower numbers of transverse pixels can also be acquired, and acquisition times will vary accordingly. In nonophthalmic imaging applications, higher incident optical powers can be used so that image acquisition speeds can be dramatically increased.

These examples illustrate an important fundamental tradeoff between the transverse pixel density of the image and the acquisition speed. In ophthalmic imaging, a larger number of transverse pixels is desirable in order to improve the visualization of retinal features; however, this high-density image requires a longer time, thus artifacts from eye motion can increase. A more precise registration of an OCT image to the fundus position is possible by acquiring images rapidly, and eye motion artifacts are reduced. However, because of a corresponding reduction in the transverse pixel density, the image appears grainier.

Advances in Optical Coherence Tomography Technology

OCT technology is closely related to photonics and fiberoptics, and it can utilize many of the recent technological advances in these areas. Research on OCT technology has developed into an active area of biomedical optics.[3] The development of technology for high-speed, real-time imaging, which reduces motion artifacts, has enabled many clinical applications.[7,20,21] OCT has been integrated with a wide range of imaging devices, including slit-lamp biomicroscopes and microscopes; handheld imaging probes, catheters, and endoscopes that enable intraluminal imaging; and needles that can image inside solid organs.[7,10,12,22-24] Short-pulse laser light sources have dramatically improved axial image resolution from 10 to 15 μm to 1 to 5 μm.[18,25,26] Cellular-level image resolutions as fine as 1 μm were demonstrated in developmental biology specimens, thus allowing the visualization of the miotic cycle and tracking cell migration.[18,27] OCT has been combined with confocal microscopy to achieve cellular-level imaging in human tissues.

In ophthalmic imaging, axial resolutions of 3 μm have been achieved.[19] Figure A-8 shows an example of a standard OCT image with 10 μm axial resolution and an ultrahigh-resolution image with 3 μm axial resolution. Enlargements of the ultrahigh-resolution image in the foveola and parafoveal regions are also shown. Ultrahigh-resolution improves the visualization of internal retinal architectural morphology and provides additional confirmation to interpret standard-resolution OCT images.

Other areas of OCT research involve functional imaging. Spectroscopically resolved OCT enables the measurement of the spectrum of backscattered or backreflected light from each pixel.[28] Spectroscopic OCT allows tissue contrast to be enhanced based upon their different optical properties. The spectroscopic indicators of tissue hydration or hemoglobin oxygenation can be measured and imaged.[29,30] Functional imaging of brain activity has been demonstrated in animal models.[31] Properties such as tissue birefringence can be imaged and assessed.[32,33] Tissue birefringence can be used to assess the retinal NFL and degenerative effects in osteoarthritic cartilage and to determine burn depth.[34-36] Doppler flow imaging and measurement using OCT is also an active research area.[37-45] Doppler OCT enables quantitative measurement of blood flow with high flow sensitivities, as well as the measurement of capillary density, which may be important in assessing angiogenesis and neovascularization.

Summary

OCT is a powerful imaging modality that can have applications in a wide range of areas in addition to ophthalmology. The ability to perform "optical biopsy" (ie, visualizing tissue morphology in situ and in real time) promises to improve not only the understanding of disease pathogenesis, but also the sensitivity and specificity of diagnosis and interventional procedures. The realization of the full clinical potential of this exciting technology relies on the structured and systemic clinical studies that will determine its applications and efficacy.

References

1. Huang D, Swanson EA, Lin CP, et al. Optical coherence tomography. *Science*. 1991;254(5035):1178-1181.
2. Fujimoto JG, Pitris C, Boppart SA, Brezinski ME. Optical coherence tomography: an emerging technology for biomedical imaging and optical biopsy. *Neoplasia*. 2000;2(1-2):9-25.
3. Fujimoto JG. Optical coherence tomography for ultrahigh resolution in vivo imaging. *Nat Biotechnol*. 2003;21(11):1361-1367.
4. Fujimoto JG, Brezinski ME, Tearney GJ, et al. Optical biopsy and imaging using optical coherence tomography. *Nat Med*. 1995;1(9):970-972.
5. Brezinski ME, Tearney GJ, Bouma BE, et al. Optical coherence tomography for optical biopsy. Properties and demonstration of vascular pathology. *Circulation*. 1996;93(6):1206-1213.
6. Boppart SA, Brezinski ME, Bouma BE, Tearney GJ, Fujimoto JG. Investigation of developing embryonic morphology using optical coherence tomography. *Dev Biol*. 1996;177(1):54-63.
7. Tearney GJ, Brezinski ME, Bouma BE, et al. In vivo endoscopic optical biopsy with optical coherence tomography. *Science*. 1997;276(5321):2037-2039.
8. Boppart SA, Bouma BE, Pitris C, et al Intraoperative assessment of microsurgery with three-dimensional optical coherence tomography. *Radiology*. 1998;208(1):81-86.
9. Pitris C, Jesser C, Boppart SA, Stamper D, Brezinski ME, Fujimoto JG. Feasibility of optical coherence tomography for high-resolution imaging of human gastrointestinal tract malignancies. *J Gastroenterol*. 2000;35(2):87-92.
10. Swanson EA, Izatt JA, Hee MR, et al. In vivo retinal imaging by optical coherence tomography. *Optics Letters*. 1993;18(21):1864-1866.
11. Izatt JA, Hee MR, Swanson EA, et al. Micrometer-scale resolution imaging of the anterior eye in vivo with optical coherence tomography. *Arch Ophthalmol*. 1994;112(12):1584-1589.

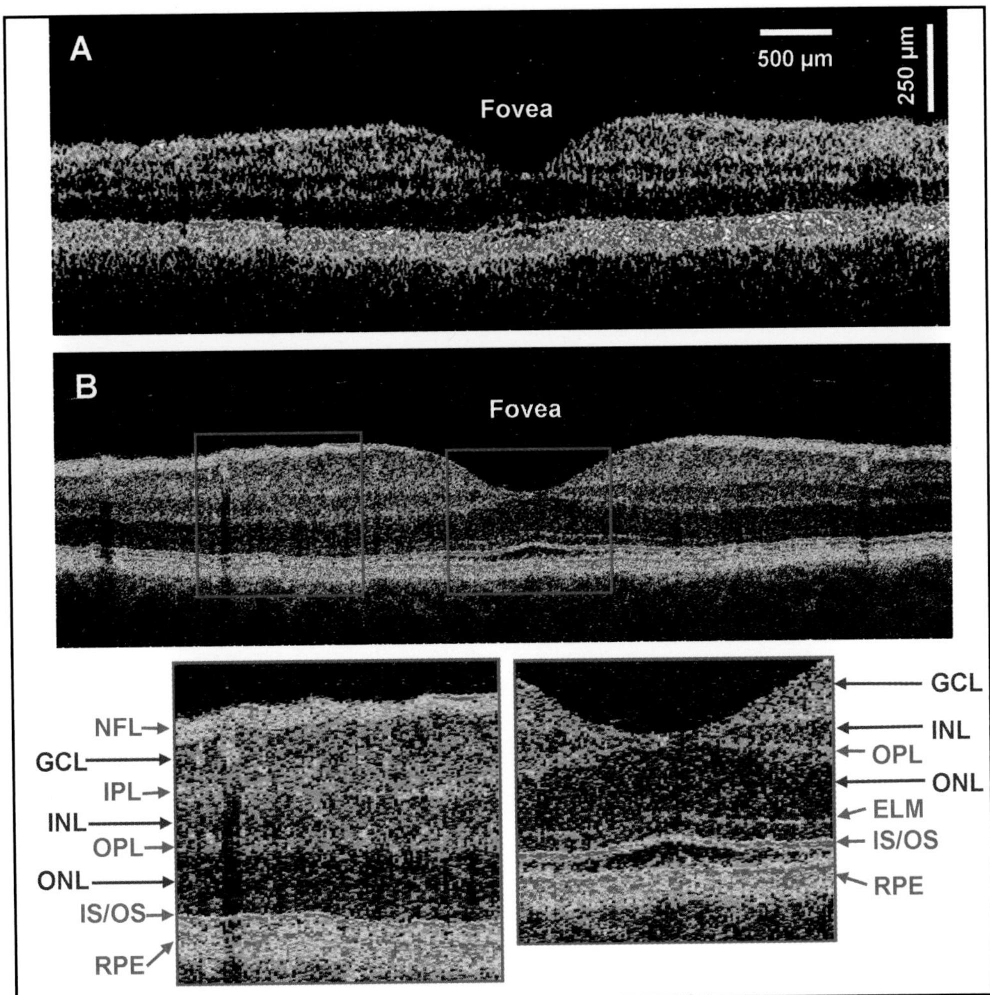

Figure A-8. Ultrahigh-resolution OCT imaging. Standard-resolution image of the macula (A) with 10 μm axial resolution versus ultrahigh-resolution image (B) with 3 μm axial resolution. Enlargements of foveola and parafoveal regions are also shown. (Bottom). Nuclear layers have lower backscattering, while the nerve fiber layer (NFL) and plexiform layers have higher backscattering. Visible features include the NFL, ganglion cell layer (GCL), inner plexiform layer (IPL), inner nuclear layer (INL), outer plexiform layer (OPL), outer nuclear layer (ONL), external limiting membrane (ELM), boundary between the inner (IS) and outer segments (OS) of the photoreceptors, and retinal pigment epithelium (RPE). Ultrahigh-resolution imaging enables excellent visualization of retinal microstructure and provides additional confirmation for the interpretation of standard-resolution images.[19]

12. Hee MR, Izatt JA, Swanson EA, et al. Optical coherence tomography of the human retina. *Arch Ophthalmol.* 1995;113(3):325-332.
13. Born M, Wolf E, Bhatia AB. *Principles of Optics: Electromagnetic Theory of Propagation, Interference and Diffraction of Light.* 7th (expanded) ed. Cambridge, England: Cambridge University Press; 1999.
14. Youngquist R, Carr S, Davies D. Optical coherence-domain reflectometry: a new optical evaluation technique. *Optics Letters.* 1987;12(3):158.
15. Gilgen HH, Novak RP, Salathe RP, Hodel W, Beaud P. Submillimeter optical reflectometry. *IEEE Journal of Lightwave Technology.* 1989;7:1225-1233.
16. Swanson EA, Huang D, Hee MR, Fujimoto JG, Lin CP, Puliafito CA. High-speed optical coherence domain reflectometry. *Optics Letters.* 1992;17:151-153.
17. Izatt JA, Hee MR, Owen GM, Swanson EA, Fujimoto JG. Optical coherence microscopy in scattering media. *Optics Letters.* 1994;19(8):590-592.

18. Drexler W, Morgner U, Kartner FX, et al. In vivo ultrahigh-resolution optical coherence tomography. *Optics Letters*. 1999;24(17):1221-1223.

19. Drexler W, Morgner U, Ghanta RK, Kärtner FX, Schuman JS, Fujimoto JG. Ultrahigh-resolution ophthalmic optical coherence tomography. *Nat Med*. 2001;7(4):502-507.

20. Tearney GJ, Bouma BE, Fujimoto JG. High-speed phase- and group-delay scanning with a grating-based phase control delay line. *Optics Letters*. 1997;22(23):1811-1813.

21. Rollins AM, Kulkarni MD, Yazdanfar S, Ung-arunyawee R, Izatt JA. In vivo video rate optical coherence tomography. *Optics Express*. 1998;3(6).

22. Boppart SA, Bouma BE, Pitris C, Tearney GJ, Fujimoto JG, Brezinski ME. Forward-imaging instruments for optical coherence tomography. *Optics Letters*. 1997;22(21):1618-1620.

23. Tearney GJ, Bouma BE, Boppart SA, Golubovic B, Swanson EA, Fujimoto JG. Rapid acquisition of in vivo biological images by use of optical coherence tomography. *Optics Letters*. 1996;21(17):1408-1410.

24. Li X, Chudoba C, Ko T, Pitris C, Fujimoto JG. Imaging needle for optical coherence tomography. *Optics Letters*. 2000;25(20):1520-1522.

25. Bouma B, Tearney GJ, Boppart SA, Hee MR, Brezinski ME, Fujimoto JG. High-resolution optical coherence tomographic imaging using a mode-locked Ti:Al/sub 2/O/sub 3/ laser source. *Optics Letters*. 1995;20(13):1486-1488.

26. Bouma BE, Tearney GJ, Bilinsky IP, Golubovic B, Fujimoto JG. Self-phase-modulated Kerr-lens mode-locked Cr:forsterite laser source for optical coherence tomography. *Optics Letters*. 1996;21(22):1839-1841.

27. Boppart SA, Bouma BE, Pitris C, Southern JF, Brezinski ME, Fujimoto JG. In vivo cellular optical coherence tomography imaging. *Nat Med*. 1998;4(7):861-865.

28. Morgner U, Drexler W, Kartner FX, et al. Spectroscopic optical coherence tomography. *Optics Letters*. 2000;25(2):111-113.

29. Schmitt JM, Xiang SH, Yung KM. Differential absorption imaging with optical coherence tomography. *J Opt Soc Am A Opt Image Sci Vis*. 1998;15(9):2288-2296.

30. Faber DL, Mik EG, Aalders MCG, van Leeuwen TG. Light absorption of (oxy-)hemoglobin assessed by spectroscopic optical coherence tomography. *Optics Letters*. 2003;28(16):1436-1438.

31. Maheswari RU, Takaoka H, Kadono H, Homma R, Tanifuji M. Novel functional imaging technique from brain surface with optical coherence tomography enabling visualization of depth resolved functional structure in vivo. *J Neurosci Methods*. 2003;124(1):83-92.

32. De Boer JF, Milner TE, van Gemert MJC, Nelson JS. Two-dimensional birefringence imaging in biological tissue by polarization-sensitive optical coherence tomography. *Optics Letters*. 1997;22(12):934-936.

33. de Boer JF, Milner TE. Review of polarization sensitive optical coherence tomography and Stokes vector determination. *J Biomed Opt*. 2002;7(3):359-371.

34. Cense B, Chen TC, Hyle Park B, Pierce MC, de Boer JF. In vivo depth-resolved birefringence measurements of the human retinal nerve fiber layer by polarization-sensitive optical coherence tomography. *Optics Letters*. 2002;27(18):1610-1612.

35. Herrmann JM, Pitris C, Bouma BE, et al. High resolution imaging of normal and osteoarthritic cartilage with optical coherence tomography. *J Rheumatol*. 1999;26(3):627-635.

36. de Boer JF, Srinivas SM, Malekafzali A, Chen Z, Nelson JS. Imaging thermally damaged tissue by polarization sensitive optical coherence tomography. *Optics Express*. 1998;3(6).

37. Izatt JA, Kulkami MD, Yazdanfar S, Barton JK, Welch AJ. In vivo bidirectional color Doppler flow imaging of picoliter blood volumes using optical coherence tomography. *Optics Letters*. 1997;22(18):1439-1441.

38. Westphal V, Yazdanfar S, Rollins AM, Izatt JA. Real-time, high velocity-resolution color Doppler optical coherence tomography. *Optics Letters*. 2002;27(1):34-36.

39. Wong RC, Yazdanfar S, Izatt JA, et al. Visualization of subsurface blood vessels by color Doppler optical coherence tomography in rats: before and after hemostatic therapy. *Gastrointest Endosc*. 2002;55(1):88-95.

40. Yazdanfar S, Rollins AM, Izatt JA. In vivo imaging of human retinal flow dynamics by color Doppler optical coherence tomography. *Arch Ophthalmol*. 2003;121(2):235-239.

41. Chen Z, Milner TE, Dave D, Nelson JS. Optical Doppler tomographic imaging of fluid flow velocity in highly scattering media. *Optics Letters*. 1997;22(1):64-66.

42. Zhao Y, Chen Z, Saxer C, Xiang S, de Boer JF, Nelson JS. Phase-resolved optical coherence tomography and optical Doppler tomography for imaging blood flow in human skin with fast scanning speed and high velocity sensitivity. *Optics Letters*. 2000;25(2):114-116.

43. Ding Z, Zhao Y, Ren H, Nelson JS, Chen Z. Real-time phase-resolved optical coherence tomography and optical Doppler tomography. *Optics Express*. 2002;10(5).

44. Ren H, Ding Z, Zhao Y, Miao J, Nelson JS, Chen Z. Phase-resolved functional optical coherence tomography: simultaneous imaging of in situ tissue structure, blood flow velocity, standard deviation, birefringence, and Stokes vectors in human skin. *Optics Letters*. 2002;27(19):1702-1704.

45. Li X, Ko TH, Fujimoto JG. Intraluminal fiber-optic Doppler imaging catheter for structural and functional optical coherence tomography. *Optics Letters*. 2001;26(23):1906-1908.

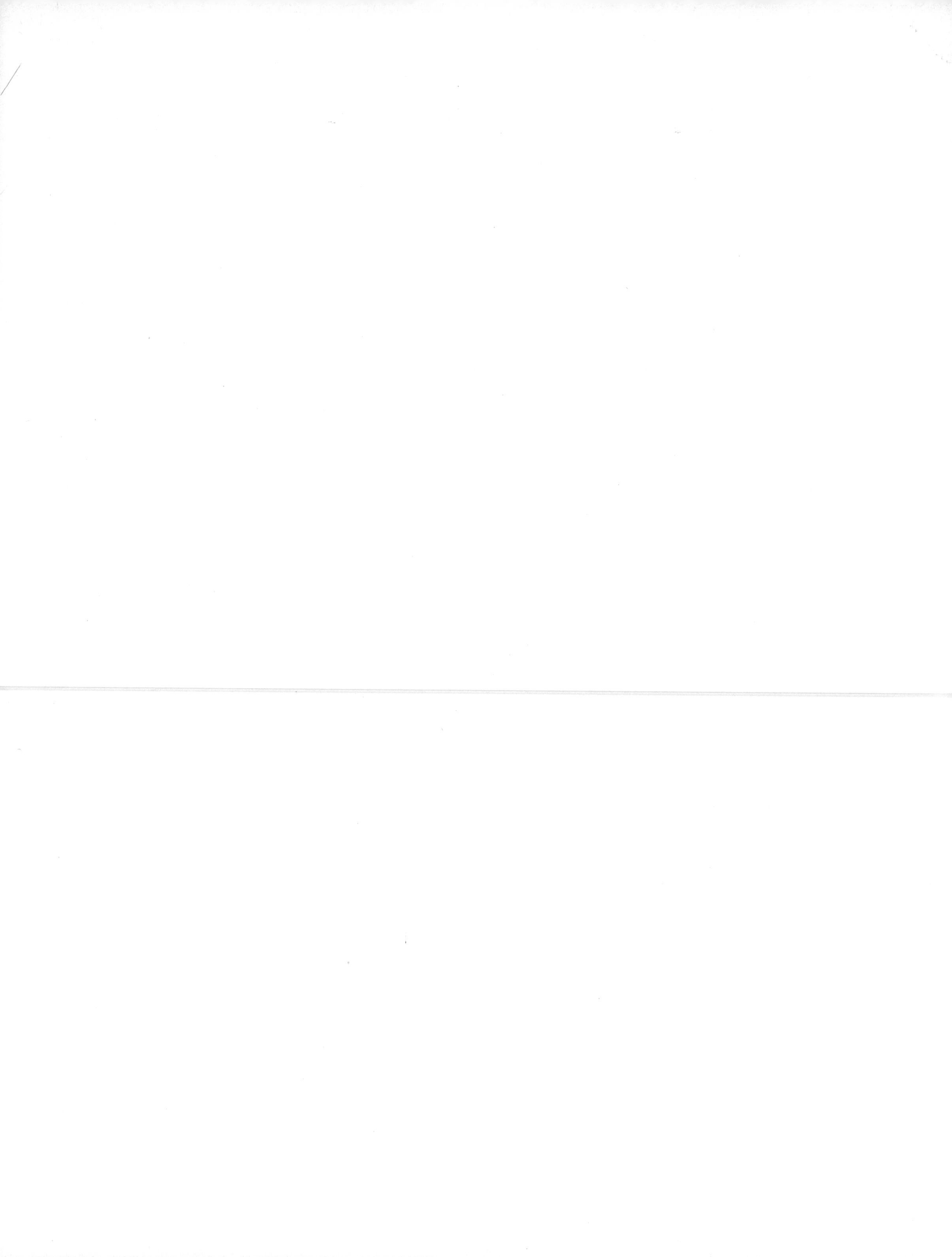

Appendix B

Optical Coherence Tomography Scanning and Image-Processing Protocols

Ji Eun Lee, MD; Joel S. Schuman, MD; James G. Fujimoto, PhD; and Carmen A. Puliafito, MD

- Line Scan Protocols
- Circle Scan Protocols
- Time-Efficient or Fast Scans
- Image-Processing Protocols
- Retinal Thickness and Retinal Thickness Map
- Nerve Fiber Layer
- Optic Disc

Commercially available optical coherence tomography (OCT) machines have various scan protocols. They are composed of two basic types of scans: line and circle. Each protocol is composed of line or circle scans with different parameters (ie, number, angle, length, and diameter). Some protocols have characteristic directions, so attention should be paid to the parameters when interpreting a scanned image. Furthermore, there are some changes in scan directions between the older model OCT machines (OCT 1 and OCT 2) and the newer model machine (OCT 3) (Carl Zeiss Meditec, StratusOCT, Model 3000 or later). The following protocols refer mainly to the OCT 3 unless otherwise specified.

Line Scan Protocols

The *line* is a basic scan protocol of OCT to get a linear scan. The length and angle can be adjusted. To interpret a scanned image, it is important to orient the direction that the scan preceded. A scan direction legend is provided for a linear scan, including scans of the following protocols with new software (version 2.0 or later). The legend enables you to orient the scan image with respect to the scan path. The default pattern is a horizontal line (0) 5 mm in length. It is possible to get multiple line scans without returning to the main window. The *line group* protocol of OCT 2 is an analogue of the line protocol.

The *raster lines* protocol consists of a series of six to 24 equally spaced parallel line scans over a rectangular region.[1] The default pattern has six lines over a 3-mm square and the scan series proceeds from superior to inferior, each scan proceeds from nasal to temporal. The height and width of the aiming box can be adjusted. The height of the aiming box affects the spacing between the lines, and the width of the aiming box determines the line scan length. The *raster six lines* protocol is OCT 2's version and the number of lines is fixed at six. The default scan region is 4.52 mm long and is approximately square.

The *cross hair* protocol consists of two perpendicular line scans that intersect at their centers to form a cross. The default line scan is 3 mm long and the height (ie, the length of the vertical line) and width (ie, the length of the horizontal line) can be adjusted.

The *radial lines* protocol consists of a series of six to 24 equally spaced line scans through a common center. The default pattern has six lines 6 mm in length. The length of the scan line can be adjusted by adjusting the aiming circle size. In OCT 2, the number of lines is fixed at six and the default radius (equal to one-half the line scan length) is 3 mm. The scan process directions are different between the OCT 2 and the OCT 3. In the OCT 2, the six line scans proceed clockwise in order from 6:00 to 12:00, 7:00 to 1:00, 8:00 to 2:00, 9:00 to 3:00, 10:00 to 4:00, and 11:00 to 5:00, regardless of which side of the eye is being scanned. In the OCT 3, the scans proceed from temporal to nasal basis. In other words, the directions of the scans are the same as the OCT 2 in the right eye, but they proceed counterclockwise in the left eye (ie, 6:00 to 12:00, 5:00 to 11:00, 4:00 to 10:00, 3:00 to 9:00, 2:00 to 8:00, and 1:00 to 7:00).

The *macular thickness map* protocol is a version of the radial lines protocol and is available only with the OCT 3. It consists of a series of six to 24 equally spaced line scans through a common center. The diameter of the aiming circle is fixed at 6 mm.[2]

The *optical disc (disc topography* of the OCT 2) protocol is a 4-mm version of the radial lines pattern. The scans created with this protocol are used with the optic nerve head analysis protocol.

The *x-line* protocol consists of two line scans that intersect at their center to form an X. The default X pattern consists of two perpendicular lines 3 mm in length. The height and width of the imaginary box surrounding the X can be adjusted.

Circle Scan Protocols

The *circle* protocol is a basic scan form used to acquire multiple circle scans.[3,4] This is an analogue of the *circle group* protocols of the OCT 2. The OCT 3 does not have the *single circle* protocol. The default pattern is a circle with a diameter of 3.46 mm and a radius of 1.73 mm. The radius of each scan can be adjusted. The scan proceeds from 9:00 clockwise in the right eye and from 3:00 counterclockwise in the left eye. A scan direction legend including a TSNI label is provided for a circle scan as well as scans of the following protocols with new version 2.0 software.

The *proportional circle* protocol enables the operator to tailor a circle scan to account for the variability in size of the optic disk. The default pattern provides an aiming circle of 1.5 mm radius and a multiplication factor of 1. The aiming circle is supposed to be matched with the optic disk size. This protocol is available only with the OCT 3.

The *concentric 3 rings* protocol consists of three equally spaced concentric circle scans with radii in the ratio of 1:2:3. The default radii of the three circles are 0.9 mm, 1.81 mm, and 2.71 mm. The scans proceed from smallest to largest. The ratio is not fixed. It is also possible to render the circles nonconcentric by adjusting the placement of the second and third scans.

The *retinal nerve fiber layer (RNFL) thickness* (3.4) protocol is designed to acquire three circle scans of diameter of 3.4 mm around the optic disk. No parameters are alterable.

The *nerve head circle* protocol is used to acquire a single circle scan around the optic disk. The default pattern has an aiming circle diameter of 1.5 mm (radius 1) and a scanning circle diameter of 3.46 mm (radius 2). Both radii can be adjusted.

The *RNFL thickness* (2.27 x disc) is used to acquire a single circle scan that is 2.27 times the radius of the aiming circle. The default pattern has an aiming circle of 1.5 mm radius. The multiplication factor is fixed at 2.27, and the aiming circle size can be adjusted. The last three protocols are used to measure RNFL thickness. In order to perform scans with the above three protocols without changing the default settings, the same results would be acquired (1.5 x 2.27 = 3.4).

The *nerve head 1.5R* and *nerve head 2.0R* protocols are the OCT 2's version of the above protocols. The default diameter of the nerve head is set as 1.73 mm and the scanner traces a circle scan with radius multiplied by 1.5 and 2.0 times, respectively.

The *RNFL map (NFL map circles of the OCT 2)* protocol consists of a set of six concentric circle scans of predetermined radius. The scans proceed in order of increasing radius as follows, in mm, from 1.44 to 1.69 to 1.90 to 2.25 to 2.73 to 3.40. The predetermined scan sizes provide optimum results for the RNFL thickness map analysis protocol.

Time-Efficient or Fast Scans

The three time-efficient or fast scan protocols are designed to simplify the process and shorten the time to acquire the scan series used most frequently to detect glaucoma or other retinal pathologies. They are available only with the OCT 3. All three protocols share the following characteristics and advantages:

- They compress a scan series into one scan acquired in 1.92 seconds
- All parameter areas are fixed
- The scan alignment and placement area is required only once
- They tend to improve accuracy of relative scan placement among the lines or circles compared to their one-by-one siblings
- They each acquire 768 A-scans—6 x 128 A-scans per radial line or 3 x 256 A-scans per circle compared to the scans one by one at 512 A-scans per line or circle. The resolution is lower but the chance of error from patient movement is less

The *fast macular thickness map* protocol consists of six 6-mm radial line scans that compress the six macular thickness map scans into one scan.

The *fast optical disc protocol* compresses the six optical disc scans into one scan. This protocol consists of six 4-mm radial line scans.

The *fast RNFL thickness* (3.4) protocol compresses the three RNFL thickness (3.4) circle scans into one scan.

Image-Processing Protocols

Commercially available OCT software offers seven image-processing protocols to enhance the scan image. These protocols apply mathematical algorithms to change the appearance of the scan image and do not change the raw scan data.

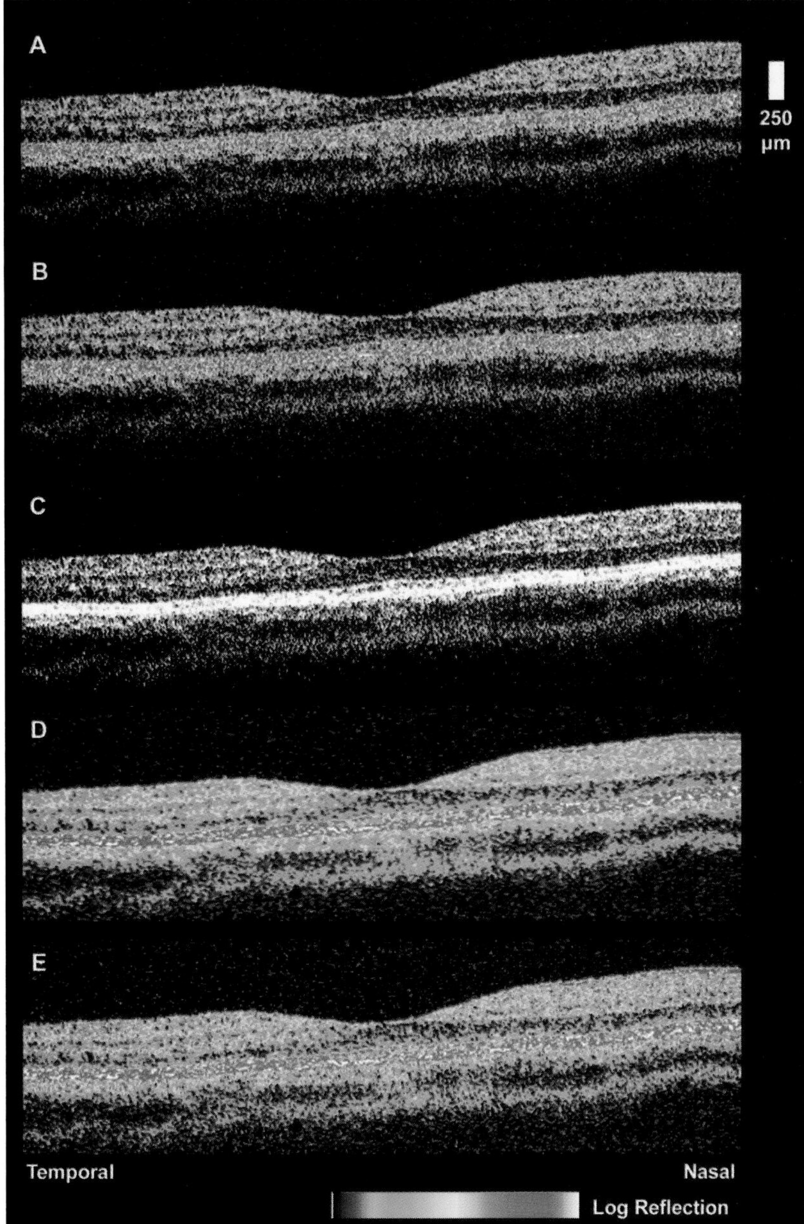

Figure B-1. Original scanned image (A) and processed image by mathematical algorithms (B to E). Align is used to remove artifacts from patient eye motion (B). Normalized image shows the whole color range of log reflection (C). Median smoothing (E) removes noise while preserving small details compared to Gaussian smoothing (D).

As mentioned in the previous chapter, *align* (Figure B-1B) uses image processing to correct the effects due to patient motion in the axial direction.[5] Although the align function is a powerful tool to remove "wiggles" from patient eye motion, it may introduce artifacts in the scan image since it cannot distinguish true retinal height changes from apparent changes due to patient motion.

Normalize (Figure B-1C) is used to eliminate background noise and to utilize the whole color scale in the processed scan image. The scan image false-color scale operates in a signal value range of 0 to 255. Normalize displays data points with values less than or equal to the average noise level as zero (black) and data points with values greater than or equal to the maximum signal value minus a fixed constant as 255 (white). It adjusts intervening signal values to maintain their relative position in the new range. The resulting images use the entire color scale between the noise and saturation signal levels and appear equally bright and normalized in regard to noise and signal strength. Normalize and align can be applied at the same time on an image.

Gaussian smoothing (Figure B-1D) averages out noise and blends the colors of the scan image by calculating a moving average of signal values of a 3 x 3 region according to a Gaussian function. The outer points in the region are weighted less than the center point, and some small details may be lost.

Median smoothing (Figure B-1E) is similar to Gaussian smoothing except that it uses the median value of the 3 x 3 region. It removes noise while preserving small details in the data.

Proportional is used to obtain a scan image that is true in its horizontal and vertical proportions. The usual presented images are elongated vertically to allow the viewer more detail throughout the plane. As a result, the proportional scan image appears compressed vertically compared to the usual image and may appear either horizontally elongated or compressed depending on the actual scan length.

Scan profile is used to display an interactive profile of all signal values for any single scan group. You can calculate the distance and difference between two points on single A-scan.

with retinopathy tend to exhibit larger standard deviations, which suggests low consistency of fixation.[2]

Retinal thickness/volume tabular (Figure B-2) provides all the output of the retinal thickness/volume analysis and a data table that includes thickness and volume quadrant averages, ratios, and differences among the quadrants and between the eyes.

Retinal thickness/volume change calculates changes in retinal thickness or volume between examinations. This analysis protocol operates on one radial line or (fast) macular thickness map protocol.

Retinal thickness (Figure B-3) analyzes one scan image at a time. Graphs of retinal thickness for any scan can be obtained with this analysis protocol. The retinal thickness at any one of the A-scan locations can be calculated, and distances on image can be measured with the caliper function.

Retinal map (Figure B-4) displays two circular maps of retinal thickness of an eye and a scanned image. The maps are actually that of retinal thickness/volume except that they are of just one eye. This analysis protocol operates on one radial lines or (fast) macular thickness map scan group at a time. The diameters of the circles can be changed.

Retinal probability map can be used to obtain the maps that indicate the probability that areas of the retina are of a thickness that is outside the normal range.

Retinal thickness measurements may be increased with edema, retinal traction, retinoschisis, or neurosensory retinal detachment.[6,7]

Retinal Thickness and Retinal Thickness Map

Retinal thickness can be analyzed with various analysis protocols.[2]

Retinal thickness/volume analysis can be made with the radial lines or (fast) macular thickness map protocols. It consists of two circular maps divided into nine areas centered on the macula for each eye. The upper map always presents retinal thickness using a color code and the lower map shows either average retinal thickness or volume in each area. The default diameters of the map circles are 1, 3, and 6 mm. They can be changed to circle diameters of 1, 2.22, and 3.45 mm.

If patients could not maintain their fixation consistently for each radial scan, the accuracy and the reproducibility would be low. The consistency of the fixation can be checked with numeric information on the lower right corner of retinal thickness/volume analysis. Foveal thickness represents the calculation of average thickness in microns ± the standard deviation for the center point, where all the scans intersect. This figure typically varies between 5 and 20 microns (μm) for normal subjects. Eyes

Nerve Fiber Layer

The nerve fiber layer (NFL) appears in the OCT images as a highly backscattering layer in the superficial retina, exhibits increased layer in the superficial retina, and exhibits increased reflectivity compared to the deeper retinal layers. NFL thickness may be assessed at individual points on a cylindrical or linear tomogram in the peripapillary region. Alternatively, a computer algorithm can be used to evaluate both retinal and NFL thickness.[3,4,8] Computer generated profiles of the NFL and retinal boundaries are displayed by selecting the *RNFL thickness* or *RNFL thickness average* analysis protocol. The NFL thicknesses are reported as averages over either each quadrant or clock hour and as graphs of NFL thickness along the scan line (Figure B-5).[3,4] These protocols will be performed with circle or (fast) RFNL thickness scan protocols.

RNFL thickness average protocol (Figure B-6) is extremely useful in comparing the measurements of NFL between the eyes. S_{max} and I_{max} represent the maximum thickness of NFL in superior and inferior quadrant respectively. Similarly, T_{avg}, N_{avg}, S_{avg}, and I_{avg} represent the average thickness of NFL in each quadrant.

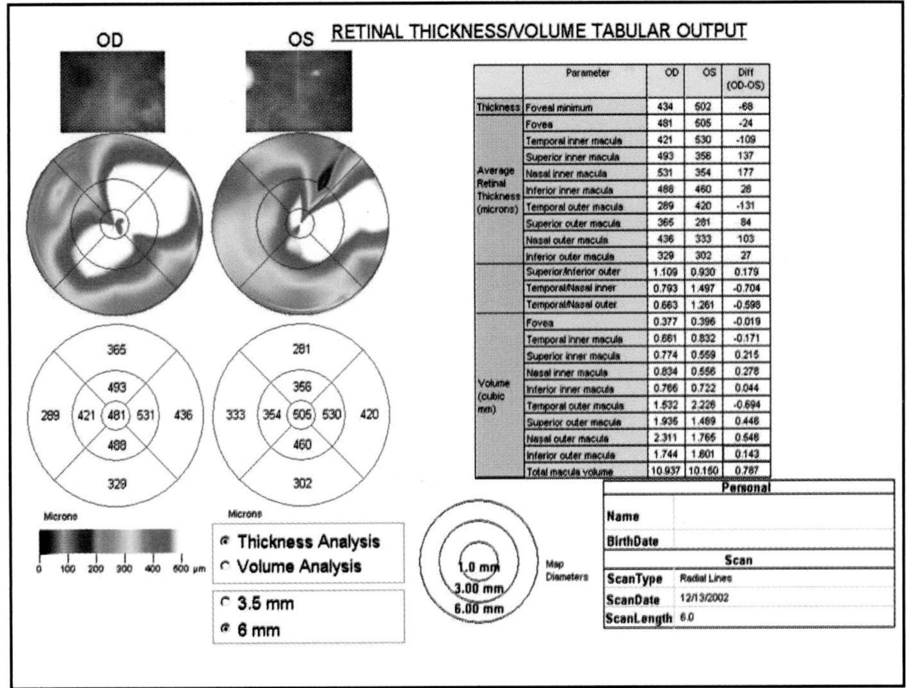

	Parameter	OD	OS	Diff (OD-OS)
Thickness	Foveal minimum	434	502	-68
Average Retinal Thickness (microns)	Fovea	481	505	-24
	Temporal inner macula	421	530	-109
	Superior inner macula	493	356	137
	Nasal inner macula	531	354	177
	Inferior inner macula	488	460	28
	Temporal outer macula	289	420	-131
	Superior outer macula	365	281	84
	Nasal outer macula	436	333	103
	Inferior outer macula	329	302	27
	Superior/Inferior outer	1.109	0.930	0.179
	Temporal/Nasal inner	0.793	1.497	-0.704
	Temporal/Nasal outer	0.663	1.261	-0.598
Volume (cubic mm)	Fovea	0.377	0.396	-0.019
	Temporal inner macula	0.661	0.832	-0.171
	Superior inner macula	0.774	0.559	0.215
	Nasal inner macula	0.834	0.556	0.278
	Inferior inner macula	0.766	0.722	0.044
	Temporal outer macula	1.532	2.226	-0.694
	Superior outer macula	1.936	1.489	0.448
	Nasal outer macula	2.311	1.765	0.546
	Inferior outer macula	1.744	1.601	0.143
	Total macula volume	10.937	10.150	0.787

Figure B-2. Retinal thickness/volume tabular output shows retinal thickness/volume maps and a data table of average thickness and volume of both eyes. Upper maps always present retinal thickness and lower maps present either average retinal thickness or volume in each area.

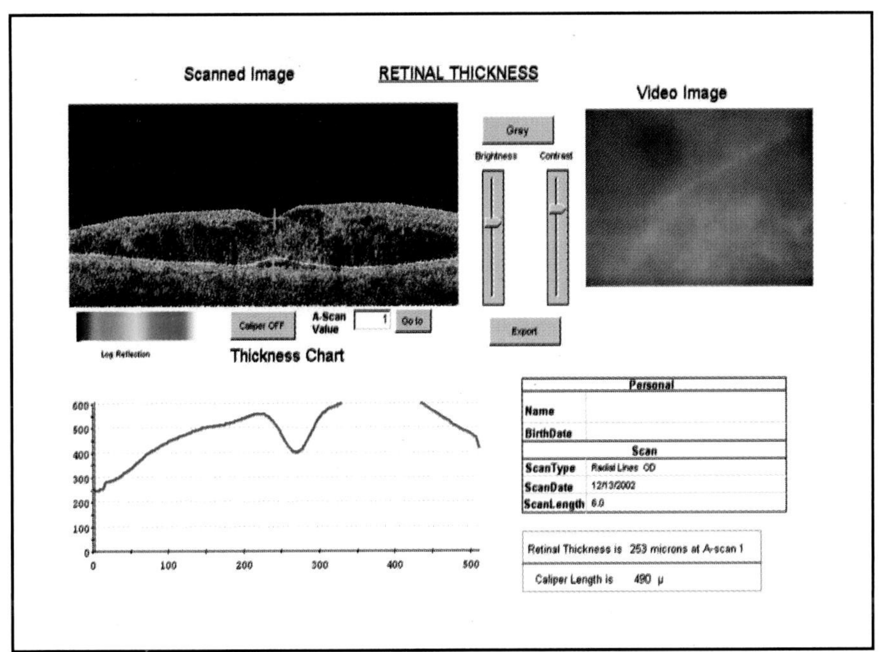

Figure B-3. Retinal thickness analysis shows a retinal thickness graph of all A-scans. The retinal thickness of each A-scan can be obtained by changing the A-scan value. A distance image is calculated with the caliper function.

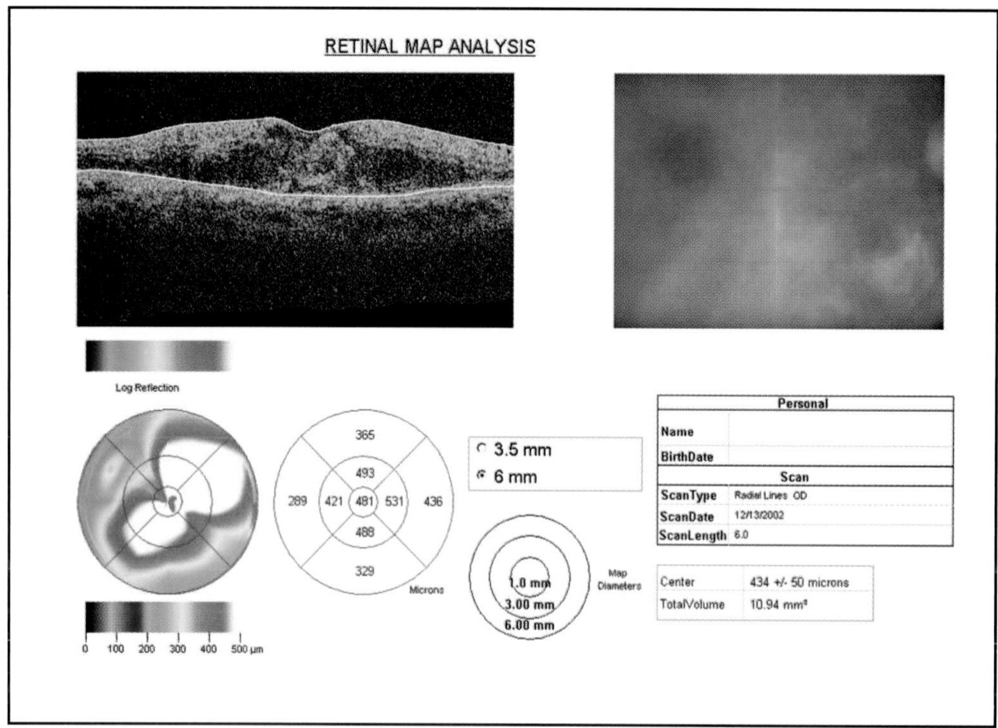

Figure B-4. Retinal map analysis displays two circular maps of retinal thickness. Each map is divided into nine areas, and the average thickness of each area is displayed on the right circular map. The foveal thickness is displayed on the right lower corner with the standard deviation. The high standard deviation value means poor fixation due to poor vision.

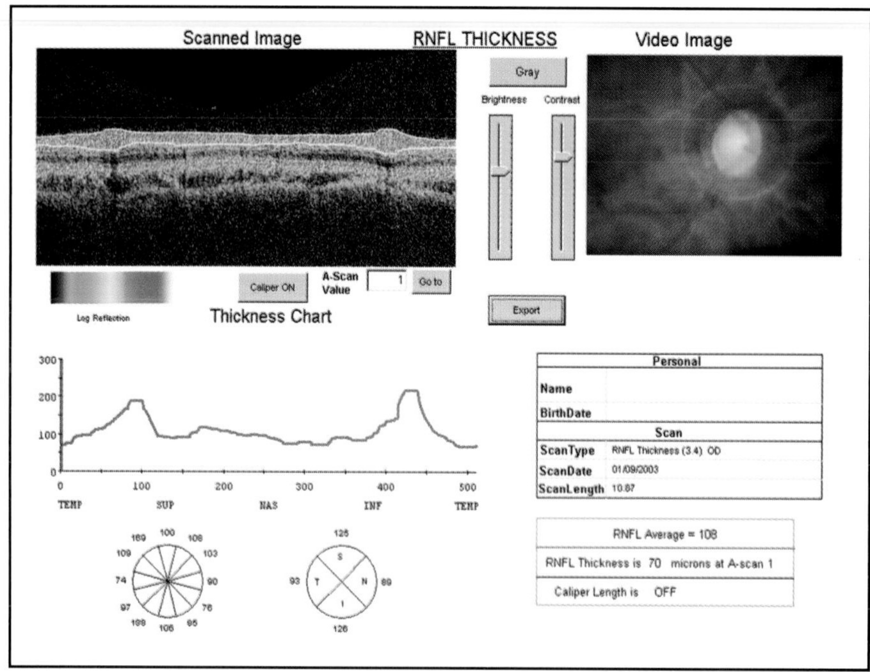

Figure B-5. RNFL thickness analysis shows a circular tomogram representing a cylindrical section around the optic disc at a diameter of 3.4 mm and thicknesses of RNFL over quadrant and clock hour. White lines on the tomogram indicate the computer generated profiles of the anterior and posterior RNFL boundaries.

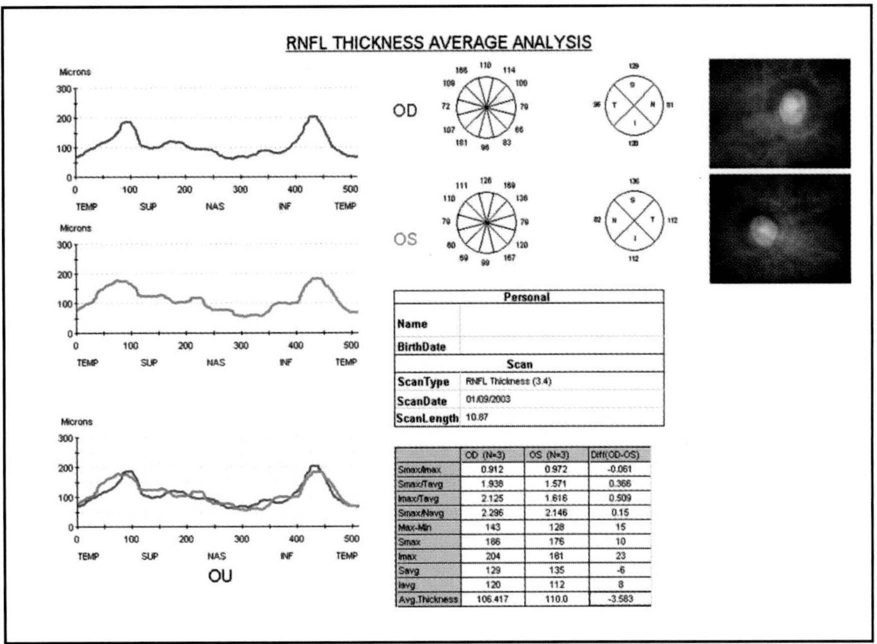

Figure B-6. RNFL thickness average analysis protocol provides graphs of NFL thickness along the scan line, various measurements, and calculated values of both eyes.

Careful inspection of the circular tomograms is required to identify focal NFL defects, which must be distinguished from normal variations in reflectivity and NFL thickness. The observation of depressions from both the anterior and posterior margins of the NFL is a helpful indicator of actual thinning. It is helpful to inspect the NFL thickness graphs. The graphs of a person with normal eyes show the typical double-hump pattern of normal NFL thickness that is thicker superiorly and inferiorly. Several spikes may be seen, and they are typically blood vessels and could be NFL defects. The best evaluation can be made by comparing the graphs with the fellow eye and clinical correlation is essential when making the correct diagnosis.

The *RNFL thickness map* analysis protocol is used to obtain a map of NFL thickness of peripapillary area. This analysis protocol is available with RNFL map or concentric 3 rings scan protocols.

To assess changes in NFL thickness between examinations, *RNFL thickness change* or *RNFL thickness serial* analysis protocol would be useful.

Optic Disc

Linear tomograms through the optic disc are useful for assessing disc and cup parameters (Figure B-7). Optic disc topography acquired by OCT shows comparative results with other optic disc analyzing instruments.[9]

By selecting (fast) optical disc scan protocol, the operator can get the cross-sectional image of optic disc along every clock hour angle. The optic nerve dead analysis protocol can be applied to one (fast) optical disc scan group. This analysis protocol provides various parameters of optic nerve configuration. The points at which the retinal pigment epithelium (RPE)/choriocapillaris terminates at the lamina cribrosa are used to determine the boundaries of the disc. In the output display, the disk reference points can be adjusted. The nerve bundle widths at the disk will be measured from each disk reference point to the nearest point on the anterior surface, and the average of the widths will be calculated. The disc diameter is determined by tracing a straight line between the two disk reference points. The cup diameter is estimated by measuring the length of a line segment parallel to the disc line and offset at a depth of 150 μm. This parameter-cup offset is adjustable. Throughout this text, we have used a depth of 140 μm to define the cup diameter.

The disc and cup diameters can provide an estimate of disc, cup, and neuroretinal rim areas. From the image measurements, composite measurements will be calculated and provided on the right lower corner—vertical integrated rim area (volume), horizontal integrated rim width (area), disk area, cup area, rim area, cup/disk area ratio, cup/disk horizontal ratio, and cup/disk vertical ratio.

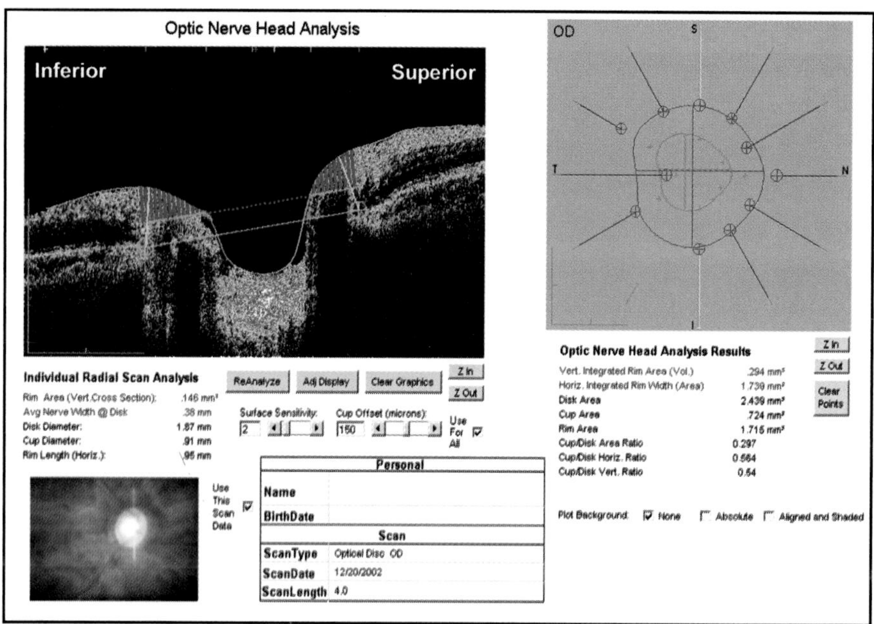

Figure B-7. Optic nerve head analysis protocol showing the cross section of the optic nerve head and the disc reference points. The reference points can be adjusted. The measurements are displayed on the left side and the composite measurements are on the right side.

References

1. Hee MR, Izatt JA, Swanson EA, et al. Optical coherence tomography of the human retina. *Arch Ophthalmol.* 1995;113:325-332.
2. Hee MR, Puliafito CA, Duker JS, et al. Topography of diabetic macular edema with optical coherence tomography. *Ophthalmology.* 1998;105:360-370.
3. Schuman S, Hee MR, Puliafito CA, et al. Quantification of nerve fiber layer thickness in normal and glaucomatous eyes using optical coherence tomography. *Arch Ophthalmol.* 1995;113:586-596.
4. Schuman S, Pedut-Kloizman T, Hertzmark E, et al. Reproducibility of nerve fiber layer thickness measurements using optical coherence tomography. *Ophthalmology.* 1996;103:1889-1898.
5. Swanson A, Izatt JA, Hee, MR, et al. In vivo retinal imaging by optical coherence tomography. *Optics Letters.* 1993; 18:1864-1866.
6. Iida T, Hagimura N, Sato T, Kishi S. Evaluation of central serous chorioretinopathy with optical coherence tomography. *Am J Ophthalmol.* 2000;129:16-20.
7. Ip M, Garza-Karren C, Duker JS, et al. Differentiation of degenerative retinoschisis from retinal detachment using optical coherence tomography. *Ophthalmology.* 1999;106: 600-605.
8. Pieroth L, Schuman JS, Hertzmark E, et al. Evaluation of focal defects of the nerve fiber layer using optical coherence tomography. *Ophthalmology.* 1999;106:570-579.
9. Zangwill LM, Bowd C, Berry CC, et al. Discriminating between normal and glaucomatous eyes using the Heidelberg Retina Tomograph, GDx Nerve Fiber Analyzer, and Optical Coherence Tomograph. *Arch Ophthalmol.* 2001;119:985-993.

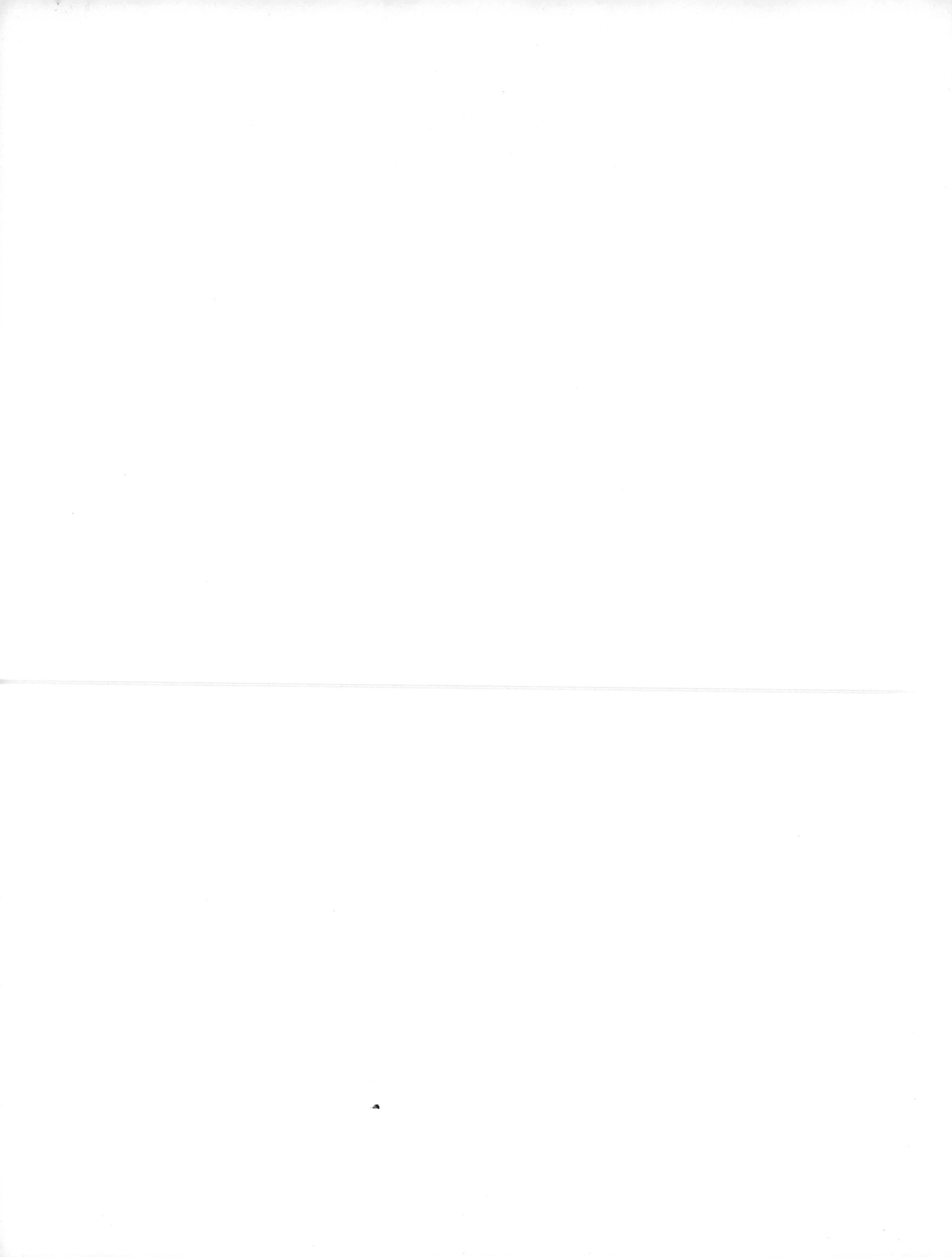

Index

A-mode scan, 11
acetazolamide
  in papilledema, 630
  for retinitis pigmentosa, 413
adventitial sheathotomy, 104
amblyopia, nutritional/toxic, 620
American Laser Institute standards, 667
American National Standards Institute standards, 667, 684
analog-to-digital conversion rate, 683-684
angioid streaks
  in choroidal neovascularization, 345
  with choroidal neovascularization, 357-359
  photodynamic therapy for, 359
angle assessment, 663, 668-669
anterior chamber
  angle assessment of, 668-669
  biometry of, 663
  cellular reaction of, 379
  depth of, 11
  interpreting OCT images of, 28
  OCT image of in vivo, 5
  width of, 670
anterior eye
  interpreting normal OCT images of, 28
  OCT imaging of, 29
anterior segment
  high-speed optical coherence tomograph of, 667-671
  instrumentation for imaging of, 17-18
  optical coherence tomographic scanning of, 663-672
arc-scanning optical coherence tomography, 664
  in differential diagnosis of keratoconus and post-LASIK keratectasia, 665-666
  disadvantages of, 666
  in longitudinal LASIK study, 665
arcuate scotoma, superior, 535-538
arterial plaque, 6
artifact
  inferior visual field loss as in glaucoma, 539-540
  in optical coherence tomography images, 46-49
  visual field defect as in glaucoma findings, 535-538
axial image resolution, 13-14, 682, 683, 686
axial scan, 10-11

backreflection, 7-8, 679, 683
  intensity of, 10, 22
backscattering, 7-8, 13, 679
  differential in, 10
  intensity of, 22
backscattering echoes, 680-681
Bartonella hesilae IgG titer, 643
beamsplitter, 15-16, 17, 679-680
Bergmeister's papilla anomaly, 660
Best's disease, 414
  clinical studies of, 446-451
bimatoprost
  for advanced glaucoma, 510
  for advanced pseudoexfoliation glaucoma, 551
  for glaucoma, 562
  for normal tension glaucoma, 566, 583
  for open-angle glaucoma, 527, 589
biometric parameters, 670
birdshot chorioretinopathy, 394-396
blind spot, enlarged, 653
blindness, in diabetic retinopathy, 157
bone-spicule formation
  in cone-rod dystrophy, 413
  in retinitis pigmentosa, 420
brimonidine, 521, 553
brinzolamide, 514, 527, 589
Bruch's membrane, 243
  choroidal neovascularization in, 265
  disruption of, 247

cancer-associated retinopathy, 478-479
Carl Zeiss Meditec, Humphrey Division of, 664
Case Western Reserve University laboratory, 663
cataract
  anterior polar, 672
  extraction of with glaucoma treatment, 602-604
  optical coherence tomography for, 671
cellular-level image resolutions, 686
central serous chorioretinopathy
  bullous, 224-227
  with choroidal neovascularization, 364
  chronic, 222-223
  clinical features of, 217-240
  fluctuating subretinal fluid in, 232-234
  focal laser treatment of, 235-236
  photodynamic therapy for, 237-240
  spontaneous resolution of, 228-229, 231
  spontaneously improved, 230
charged-coupled device (CCD) camera, 667
choriocapillaris, 25, 27
  identifying, 23
  imaging of, 24
  optical coherence tomography of, 44-46
chorioretinal colobomatous defect, 475-476
chorioretinal inflammatory disease
  inflammatory lesions of, 371-372
  multiple lesions of, 380
  optical cohesion tomography for, 373-410
  uveitis in, 371
chorioretinal scars
  multifocal, 381
  with uveitis, 371
chorioretinitis
  bilateral syphilitic, 405-408
  sclopetaria, 471-472
chorioretinopathy
  birdshot, 394-396
  central serous, 42, 215-216
choroid, 25
  imaging of, 24
  inferotemporal nevus of, 432
  post-traumatic rupture of, 469
choroidal granuloma, sarcoidosis with, 383-385
choroidal neovascularization (CNV), 45-46, 244
  in age-related macular degeneration
    classic, 279-280, 289-290, 295-296
    minimally classic, 265-272
    predominantly classic, 273-274
  angioid streaks with, 357-359
  conditions associated with, 345, 347-369
  diagnosis of, 221
  enlargement of lesion in, 349
  idiopathic, 360-362
    central serous chorioretinopathy with, 364
    photodynamic therapy for, 363
  juxtafoveal retinal telangiectasis with, 365-367
  monitoring and detection of, 5
  myopic degeneration with, 350
  occult
    in age-related macular degeneration, 260-264
    with retinal pigment epithelium tear progression, 332-333
  pathologic myopia with, 345, 347-348, 354-356
  photodynamic therapy for, 351
  with subretinal hemorrhage, 360-362
  with uveitis, 371
choroiditis, multifocal, 371
  with panuveitis, 379
    treatment of, 380
  with subretinal fibrosis, 381-382
circle group protocols, 692
circle scan protocols, 692
circular tomogram, peripapillary, 26-27
circumpapillary optic coherence tomogram, 27
  in glaucoma, 47
coagulative necrosis, 103
coherence length, 681, 683
colobomatous defect, 475-476
color vision, 413
computer image-processing, 14, 15, 36
computer tomography (CT), 3, 677
  of retinal macula, 30
cone-rod dystrophy, 413
confocal scanning laser ophthalmoscopy (CSLO), 483
cornea
  arc-scanning OCT of, 664, 665, 666
  high-speed optical coherence tomograph of, 667-671
  imaging thickness of, 3
  interpreting OCT images of, 28
  optical coherence tomogram of, 663-672, 664
corneoscleral limbus, 28
corticosteroids
  for acute sympathetic ophthalmia, 391
  for chronic sympathetic ophthalmia, 393
  for multifocal choroiditis with subretinal fibrosis, 382
  for sarcoidosis with choroidal granulomas, 385
  for Vogt-Koyanagi-Harada disease, 389-390
cotton wool spots, 119
  in central retinal vein occlusion, 136
cross-sectional imaging, 5
cupping, asymmetric, 500
  in open-angle glaucoma, 492
cyclodialysis cleft, 631
cyst. *See also* fluid accumulation, cystic
  foveal, 84-85
  intraretinal, 265, 364
  macular, 58, 211
    nonfilling, 373

cytomegalovirus retinitis, 409-410

daraprim, 397-399
demyelinating optic neuritis, 616
demyelinating plaques, 615
depth of field, 682-683
diabetic papillopathy, juvenile, 640-641
diabetic retinopathy
  blindness with, 157
  causes of, 157
  macular edema in, 43-44
  nonproliferative, 157
    diabetic macular edema and, 159-180
    with epiretinal membrane formation and macular edema, 181-182
    with macular edema and lamellar hole, 183-185
  OCT studies in, 157-213
  proliferative, 157-158
  retinal morphology in, 35
disciform scar, 340-341
  in age-related macular degeneration, 244
  fibrotic, with central atrophy, 342-343
Doppler flow imaging, 686
Doppler frequency, 681-682
Doppler shifting, 681-682
dorzolamide
  for advanced glaucoma, 510, 551
  for glaucoma, 562
  for open-angle glaucoma, 553
  for pseudoexfoliation glaucoma, 551, 572
  for rhegmatogenous retinal detachment, 465
double hump pattern, 488, 553, 557-558, 589, 592
drainage retinotomy, 467
drusen
  in age-related macular degeneration, 243, 247-255
  basal laminar, 251-255
  in foveal vitelliform lesion, 256
  macular, in open-angle glaucoma, 608
  mild optic disc, 648-649
  multiple hard, 592
  severe optic disc, 650-651
  soft, 45, 247-248
drusen-like deposits, 446, 447

echo delay, 680
echo time delay, 22, 681-682
electric field, 679
electroretinogram, rod-code dysfunction in, 432
endoscope, 686
epiretinal membrane, 5-6, 41
  contraction of, 57
  dense, with extensive macular edema, 73
  idiopathic, 57-58
  with macular edema, 68, 69
    in both eyes, 64-65, 66-67
    extensive, 70, 73
    improved after vitrectomy surgery, 71-72
    vitreomacular traction and, 74
  mild, 61
  in nonproliferative diabetic retinopathy, 181-182
  in proliferative diabetic retinopathy, 194-198
  with pseudohole, 62, 63
  retinal dystrophies and, 413
  with tractional retinal detachment, 211
  vitrectomy surgery for, 75-77
expert algorithms, 37
exudative maculopathy, 376-378
eye, light and sound reflection from, 7
eye motion, correction for, 14-15

false color map, 3
false-color optical coherence tomography, 11-13
fast optical disc protocol, 692
fast RNFL thickness protocol, 692
fast scan, 692
fiberoptic interferometer, 10
fiberoptic technology, 9-10
fibrinoplatelet embolus, 106
fibroglial tissue, preretinal, 206
fibrovascular proliferation, 40-43
fixation error, 49
flap imaging, 665-666
flap lamellar interface, 665
fluid accumulation
  cystic
    in central retinal vein occlusion, 125, 129
    in nonproliferative diabetic retinopathy, 171
  subretinal, 42
    in age-related macular degeneration, 244
    with angioid streaks, 359
    around choroidal neovascularization, 345
    in Best's disease, 446
    in central serous chorioretinopathy, 218, 220, 221, 230, 233
  diabetic, 157
  fluctuating levels of in central serous chorioretinopathy, 232-234
  in macula, 223
  in nonproliferative diabetic retinopathy, 168, 178
  with optic nerve head pits, 458
  optical coherence tomography of, 40-43
  with papilledema, 629-630
  in proliferative diabetic retinopathy, 197, 209
  quantitative measurements of, 216
  recurrent, 240
  serous, 217
  shallow, in retinal detachment, 457

fluorescein angiography, 5
for age-related macular degeneration, 243
for bilateral idiopathic juxtafoveal retinal telangiectasis, 140, 142, 144, 146
for branch retinal artery occlusion, 106, 108
for branch retinal vein occlusion, 111, 113, 123
for central retinal vein occlusion, 125, 127, 133
for central serous chorioretinopathy, 220
in central serous chorioretinopathy, 215
for chorioretinal inflammatory disease, 371
for choroidal neovascularization, 345
for cystoid macular edema, 457
for epiretinal membrane with macular edema, 66, 68
for idiopathic epiretinal membrane, 57
for impending macular hole, 79
intravenous, for retinal vein occlusion, 104
of lamellar hole, 100
for nonproliferative diabetic retinopathy, 162, 164, 166, 168, 171, 173
for retinal arterial macroaneurysm, 148-149, 151, 153
5-fluorouracil, 562, 596
fovea
cysts of, 84
resolution of, 85
detached, 222
in idiopathic macular hole, 59
normal OCT tomogram of, 23
vitelliform lesion of, 256
frequency doubling technology, 500, 514, 559, 589
Fuch's spot, 348
full visual field
in healthy eye, 488-489
fundus camera, 15
fundus examination, dilated
for branch retinal artery occlusion, 108
for branch retinal vein occlusion, 113, 123
for central retinal vein occlusion, 133
for epiretinal membrane with macular edema, 64, 66, 68, 69
for epiretinal membrane with pseudohole, 62, 63
of impending macular hole, 79
of lamellar hole, 100, 101
for mild epiretinal membrane, 61
for nonproliferative diabetic retinopathy, 162, 171
for retinal arterial macroaneurysm, 151
fundus photography, 5

geographic atrophy, 257-259

glaucoma
abnormalities in, 483-484
advanced
nerve fiber layer and macular analysis corresponding to visual field abnormality in, 508-509
nerve fiber loss, macular thinning, and central island visual field in, 510-513
clinical studies of, 488-609
early superior visual field defect in, 523-526
focal nerve fiber layer defect demonstrated in, 572-574
future functional loss in, 547-550
global damage in, 521-522
inferior visual field defects in, 545-546
interpreting OCT images in, 483-484
nerve fiber layer, macular, and optic nerve head scanning corresponding with visual field loss in, 531-534
nerve fiber layer, optic nerve head, and macula corresponding with visual fields in, 504-507
nerve fiber layer and macular findings in, 557-558, 575-578
nerve fiber layer and neuroretinal rim loss corresponding with early visual field defect in, 529-530
nerve fiber layer and visual field abnormalities in, 579-582
nerve fiber layer measurements corresponding to functional loss in, 568-570
normal tension
functional findings in, 496-499
nerve fiber layer assessment in, 566-567
structural and functional analysis in, 547-550, 583-586
OCT, Heidelberg retina tomography, and visual field findings in, 535-538
OCT and Heidelberg retina tomography in, 559-561
OCT assessment of, 24-26, 47, 483-609
open-angle
nerve fiber layer loss paralleling visual field loss in, 608-609
nerve fiber layer thinning in, 587-588
with progressive nerve fiber layer and visual field loss, 605-607
structural and functional analyses in, 492-495, 553-556
structural-functional correspondence of glaucomatous damage in, 589-591
superior structural abnormalities presaging inferior visual field loss in, 596-597

treatment of, 575
visual field testing for, 602-604
pseudoexfoliation
structural and functional analysis of, 551-552
structural and functional evaluation of, 514-516
structural damage indicating future visual field loss in, 592-595
structural imaging corresponding with visual field in early superior visual field defect findings, 527-528
structural imaging suggesting visual field abnormalities in, 541-544
structure-function correlation in diagnosis and treatment of, 500-503
superior functional loss and inferior visual field loss in, 539-540
visual field damage in, 562-565
glaucoma drops, 463-464
gonioscopy, 668-669
gray-scale imaging, 11-13

handheld imaging probes, 686
handheld scanners, 667
Heidelberg retina tomography, 488
corresponding with optical coherence tomography, 559-561
corresponding with visual field defects in glaucoma, 535-538
in glaucoma, 517-520
hemorrhage, 244
in central retinal vein occlusion, 136
dense vitreous, 138
dot and blot, 166, 206
flame-shaped, 115
in anterior ischemic optic neuropathy, 639
intraretinal, 119
peripapillary, 129, 133
in papilledema, 629
in papillophlebitis, 645
peripapillary, 654, 655
subretinal, 105
after photodynamic therapy for age-related macular degeneration, 291-292
in age-related macular degeneration, 244
with age-related macular degeneration, 336-339
with choroidal neovascularization, 345-346, 360-362
in retinal arterial macroaneurysm, 148, 151
spontaneous resolution of, 361
Henle's fiber layer, 24
high-speed optical coherence tomography, 667-671
histopathology, 677
histoplasmosis, 345
Humphrey visual field testing, 529, 531-534, 535-538, 545, 553, 568, 583

hyaloid
taut posterior, 203-205
taut premacular posterior, 204-205
hyperpigmentation, 44-45
hypopigmented scar, 368
hypotony, with papilledema, 631-632

IgG toxoplasmosis titers, 397
image acquisition
rate of, 663
speed of
versus pixel density, 30
pixel density and, 28-29
transverse pixel density and, 685
time, 683-685
image analysis errors, 50
image pixel density, 28-29
image-processing protocols, 691-698
image resolution, 682-683
of OCT images, 13-14
immune recovery vitreitis, 409-410
indocyanine green (ICG) angiography
for age-related macular degeneration, 243
for birdshot chorioretinopathy, 394, 395
for bullous central serous chorioretinopathy, 224, 226
for central serous chorioretinopathy, 215, 237, 238, 239
for choroidal neovascularization with subretinal hemorrhage, 360
inflammatory chorioretinopathy, 345
inflammatory lesions, chorioretinal, 371-372
clinical features of, 373-410
instrumentation, optical coherence tomography, 14-18
interference, 679-680
interferometer, 8-9
fiberoptic, 10
output intensity of, 681
intracranial pressure
increased, with papilledema, 625-626
in severe papilledema, 627
intraluminal imaging, 686
intraocular lens implant
fitting of, 670-671
in pseudophakic cystoid macular edema, 459
intraocular pressure
in advanced glaucoma, 508, 510
in healthy eye, 488
in papilledema, 631
intraretinal cystic edema, 265
intraretinal neovascularization stage I, 245
iris
interpreting OCT images of, 28
nevus in, 671
Izatt system, 663

juvenile diabetic papillopathy, 640-641
juxtafoveal retinal telangiectasis
  bilateral idiopathic, 104, 140-147
  with choroidal neovascularization, 365-367

keratectasia, post-LASIK, 665-666
keratoconus, 665-666

LADARVision system, 665
lamellar hole, 99-101
  in central retinal vein occlusion, 138-139
  in nonproliferative diabetic retinopathy with macular edema, 183-185
laser biomicroscopy, 483-484
laser in-situ keratomileusis (LASIK)
  anatomy of, 668
  longitudinal, 665
laser iridotomy, 669
laser peripheral iridectomy, 598
laser peripheral iridotomy, 670
laser photocoagulation
  for age-related macular degeneration, 243, 245
  for branch retinal vein occlusion, 113
  focal
    for central serous chorioretinopathy, 216, 235-236
    for nonproliferative diabetic retinopathy, 162-163
    for retinal vein occlusion, 104
  focal/grid, 194, 197-198, 199
  for nonproliferative diabetic retinopathy, 168, 175
  for proliferative diabetic retinopathy, 203, 209
  scarring from, 171, 173, 186, 201, 204, 206
  thermal, 243
laser therapy, 382
laser thermokeratoplasty (LTK), 663
laser trabeculoplasty, 541, 589
LASIK flap, imaging of, 663
latanoprost, 504, 521, 547, 553
Leber's hereditary optic neuropathy, 617-619
Leber's mutations, 619
levobunolol, 566
light
  distance and time scales for, 8
  incident onto tissue, 22
  intensity of, 680
  low-coherence, 680-681
  scattering of, 677
light echoes, 8-10, 680-681
light waves, 679
line scan protocols, 691-692
lipid exudates
  hard, 159, 178, 181, 201
    intraretinal, 157
  in retinal vasculitis and neuroretinitis, 376
lipid nodules, 378
low-coherence interferometry, 7, 680-681, 682-683
  measuring depth of anterior chamber, 11
  in measuring light echoes, 8-10
Lubeck group, 663

macroaneurysm
  near optic nerve, 378
  retinal arterial, 148-154
macula
  in advanced glaucoma, 504-507, 508-509
  age-related degeneration of, 45, 216, 592
    choroidal neovascularization in, 260-274
    classic choroidal neovascularization with, 279-280, 289-290, 295-296
    conditions associated with, 347-369
    disciform scar with, 340-341
    drusen in, 247-255
    fibrotic disciform scar and central atrophy in, 342-343
    foveal vitelliform lesion in, 256
    geographic atrophy in, 257-259
    idiopathic, 345
    intravitreal triamcinolone injection for, 322-329
    with large subretinal hemorrhages, 345-346
    nonexudative age-related, 44-45
    with normal tension glaucoma, 547
    optical coherence tomography for, 243-245, 247-343, 346
    pathologic myopia in, 345
    photodynamic therapy for, 275-278, 281-288, 291-292, 293-294, 297-309
    retinal angiomatous proliferation in, 320-329
    with retinal pigment epithelium tear progression, 330-335
    RPE abnormalities in, 345
    with subretinal hemorrhage, 336-339
    treatment of, 346
    vascularized pigment epithelial detachment in, 310-311
    in vision loss, 243
  atrophy of
    central, fibrotic disciform scar with, 342-343
    in Stargardt's disease, 437
  central
    remodeling of, 245
    thinning of, 452
  cysts of, 58, 428
    in proliferative diabetic retinopathy, 211
  discoloration and mottling of, 393
  hyperfluorescent lesions of in Vogt-Koyanagi-Harada disease, 388
  imaging of
    in advanced pseudoexfoliation glaucoma, 551-552
    corresponding with visual field loss in glaucoma, 531-534

of focal nerve fiber layer defect, 572-574
in glaucoma, 500, 502, 517
in glaucoma diagnosis, 529-530
in normal tension glaucoma, 583
in open-angle glaucoma, 575-578
visual field abnormalities and, 579
measuring thickness of, 157
monitoring and detection of disease in, 5
normal, 488-489
OCT images of, 15, 25
pigmentary atrophy of with pathologic myopia, 354
schisis formation in, 207-208
serial horizontal tomogram of, 31
serial raster scans through, 30
thickness map protocol for, 691-692
fast, 692
thinning of
in advanced glaucoma, 510-513
corresponding with visual field loss, 596
with disc hemorrhage and visual field loss in glaucoma, 557-558
functional evaluation of in glaucoma, 547-550
in glaucoma, 559-561, 568-570
in open-angle glaucoma, 589
visual field loss corresponding with, 562-565, 568-570
vitelliform lesion of, 252-255
macular edema
in age-related macular degeneration, 244
in branch retinal vein occlusion, 115
in central retinal vein occlusion, 136
cystoid (CME), 44, 58, 111, 157, 371, 457
in age-related macular degeneration, 244
cytomegalovirus retinitis with, 409-410
with glaucoma drops, 463-464
intermediate uveitis with, 373-375
postoperative, intravitreal triamcinolone for, 461-462
pseudophakic, 459-460
retinal dystrophies in, 413
topical medication for, 464
with dense epiretinal membrane, 73
diabetic, 157
retinal dystrophies in, 413
disciform scar with, 340-341
epiretinal membrane with, 64-65, 66-67, 68, 69, 70
improved after vitrectomy surgery, 71
in nonproliferative diabetic retinopathy, 159-185, 173
with nonproliferative diabetic retinopathy, 162-185
and epiretinal membrane formation, 181-182
and lamellar hole, 183-185
optical coherence tomography of, 43-44
proliferative diabetic retinopathy and, 188-193, 199-202
with epiretinal membrane formation, 194-198
retinal dystrophies and, 413
in retinitis pigmentosa, 418
macular hole, 37
bilateral full-thickness, 91-92
disrupting normal retinal structure, 39
formation and surgical management of, 82-83
full-thickness
closed with vitrectomy surgery, 94-95
with lamellar macular hole in fellow eye, 96-98
myopic degeneration with, 93
idiopathic, 58-59
impending
with spontaneous resolution, 79-81
with stage 2 hole in fellow eye, 86-87
lamellar, 99-101
in central retinal vein occlusion, 138-139
with full-thickness macular hole in fellow eye, 96-98
in nonproliferative diabetic retinopathy with macular edema, 183-185
optical coherence tomography of, 38-40
quantitative information about, 59
retinal dystrophies and, 413
spontaneous resolution of, 81
stage 1A, 78
stage 1B, vitrectomy surgery for, 84-85
stage 2 full-thickness, 86-87, 88
stage 3 full-thickness, 89-90
macular pseudohole, 39
versus macular hole, 101
macular retinoschisis, diabetic, 157
maculopathy
end-stage, 440
hereditary, 345
magnetic field, 679
magnetic resonance imaging (MRI), 3, 677
for optic neuritis, 615
of retinal macula, 30
meningioma, of tentorium, 625-626
methotrexate, 382
Michelson-type interferometer, 679
microaneurysms
in nonproliferative diabetic retinopathy, 166, 168, 171
in proliferative diabetic retinopathy, 188
micropsia, 215
mitochondrial DNA testing, 617, 619
mitomycin C, 541, 575, 579, 587
morning glory anomaly, 652
morphometry, 37-38
myelinated nerve fibers, 477, 653
myopia
in open-angle glaucoma, 568
pathologic, with choroidal neovascularization, 345, 347-348, 352-353, 354-356
myopic degeneration
with choroidal neovascularization, 350
with full-thickness macular hole, 93

myopic pigmentary atrophy, 347, 348

Nd:YAG iridotomy, 669
Nd:YAG laser posterior capsulotomy, 74
nerve fiber layer
  in advanced glaucoma, 504-507, 508-509
  analysis of in glaucoma, 517, 575-578, 598-599
  appearing thin with improper alignment, 490-491
  assessment of corresponding to visual field findings, 566-567
  atrophy of, 46
  circumpapillary thickness of, 35-37
  corresponding with visual field loss in glaucoma, 531-534
  damage to, 611
  focal defect of, 572-574
  functional evaluation of in glaucoma, 547-550
  histological evaluation of, 483
  identifying, 23-24
  imaging of, 26-27
  loss of
    with early visual field defect, 529-530
    in glaucoma, 483, 510-513, 559-561
    paralleling visual field loss, 608-609
    progressive, with visual field loss, 605-607
    visual field tests demonstrating, 602-604
  normal, 488-489
  OCT in quantifying, 611
  posterior boundary of, 35
  retinal, thickness of, 35-37
  stable circumpapillary, 600-601
  swelling of, 611
  thickening of, 611
    in anterior ischemic optic neuropathy, 635
    in neuroretinitis, 643
    in optic neuritis, 616
  thinning of
    in anterior ischemic optic neuropathy, 639
    in compressive optic neuropathy, 614
    corresponding with visual field loss, 562-565, 583-586, 596
    in glaucoma, 539, 545-546, 553, 557-558, 568-570, 587-588, 589
    in hereditary optic neuropathy, 618
    in nutritional/toxic amblyopia, 620
    with optic nerve hypoplasia, 657
    peripapillary, 514
    with severe optic disc drusen, 651
    with visual field abnormalities, 579
nerve fiber layer protocols, 694-697
nerve fiber layer thickness algorithm, 51
nerve head circle protocol, 692
neuro-ophthalmic disease, 24-26
neuro-ophthalmology
  clinical studies of, 613-660
  optical coherence tomography in, 611-660
neuroretinal rim
  atrophy of, 587
  loss of, 529-530, 539
  thinning of, 521, 547, 553, 557-558, 559
neuroretinitis, 643
  with exudative maculopathy, 376-378
neurosensory retina
  in age-related macular degeneration, 245
  detachment of, 160, 168, 209-213, 215, 237
    in central serous chorioretinopathy, 233, 239
    in cystoid macular edema, 373-374
    shallow, 236
  serous detachment of, 215
  thinning of, 453, 478-479
  thinning of in Best's disease, 450
neurosensory retina/RPE/choroid fibrosis fusing, 471
nonfilling cyst, macular, 373
nonsteroidal anti-inflammatory drugs, 464
nutritional optic neuropathy, 611, 617-620
nyctalopia, 413

OCT scanners, commercial, 663
ocular histoplasmosis, 368
  in choroidal neovascularization, 345
  photodynamic therapy for, 369
open angle without glaucoma, 598-599
operculum, 82, 87, 91
  small reflective, 98
ophthalmia
  acute sympathetic, 391-392
  chronic sympathetic, 393
optic atrophy, 613-620
optic disc
  congenital pit of, 473-476
  cupping of, 596
  diameters of, 697
  drusen of
    mild, 648-649
    severe, 650-651
  edema of in central retinal vein occlusion, 131
  in glaucoma, 500, 503, 517
  hemorrhage of with nerve fiber layer and macular thinning, 557-558
  myelinated fibers of, 477
  pitting of, 658-659
    subretinal fluid from, 611
  radial optical cohesion tomographic section through, 32
  serial radial tomograms through, 30-32
  swelling of, 621-622, 626
    in anterior ischemic optic neuropathy, 635
    in congenitally crowded optic nerve, 646
    in juvenile diabetic papillopathy, 640-641
    in neuroretinitis, 643

optic nerve compression with, 633-634
in optic neuropathy, 621-645
in papilledema, 629
tilted, 654-655
optic disc protocols, 697-698
optic nerve
anomalies of, 646-660
compression of with optic disc swelling, 633-634
congenitally crowded, 646-647
cupping of in glaucoma, 523
in glaucoma, 545
hypoplasia of, 656-657
swelling of, 407-408
in severe papilledema, 628
optic nerve head
abnormalities of
functional evaluation of in glaucoma, 547-550
with visual field loss, 562-565
in advanced glaucoma, 504-507
analysis of, 572
abnormalities in, 568-570
asymmetric cupping in, 575
corresponding with visual field loss, 596
visual field abnormalities and, 579
analysis protocol for, 698
cross-section of, 26
cupped, 523
asymmetric, 553, 559
in glaucoma, 541
edema of in central retinal vein occlusion, 133
expert algorithms in analysis of, 37
imaging of, 24-26, 539
corresponding with visual field loss in glaucoma, 531-534
in glaucoma, 559-561
in healthy eye, 488-489
pitting of, 458
tilted, 654
optic nerve sheath fenestration, 630
optic neuritis, 615
follow-up in, 616
optic neuropathy
anterior ischemic, 635-637
acute and remote, 638-639
compressive, 611, 613-614
hereditary, 611
nutritional/toxic/hereditary, 617-620
optical beam, 14
optical biopsy, 677
optical coherence, 215
optical coherence domain reflectometry (OCDR), 663
optical coherence microscopy (OCM), 683
optical coherence tomography (OCT). *See also* tomogram
advances in, 686
for age-related macular degeneration, 243-245, 247-343, 275-278, 281-288
applications of, 5-6, 677-678
arc-scanning, 664-666
axial scans and, 10-11
for bilateral idiopathic juxtafoveal retinal telangiectasis, 140-147
of branch retinal artery occlusion, 106-109
of branch retinal vein occlusion, 111-124
for central retinal vein occlusion, 125-139
for central serous chorioretinopathy, 217-240
for choroidal neovascularization in age-related macular degeneration, 260-274
computer image processing in, 14
corneal and anterior segment, 663-672
cross-sectional images of, 21
in diabetic retinopathy, 157, 159-213
for epiretinal membrane with macular edema, 64, 66, 69
in evaluating retinal diseases, 457-479
first demonstration of, 3, 4
follow-up after photodynamic therapy, 291-294, 297-309
future developments in, 672
in glaucoma, 483-609
gray-scale versus false-color images of, 11-13
Heidelberg retina tomography and, 559-561
image generation using, 12, 21-22
image resolution in, 13-14
instrumentation in, 14-18
interpretation of image in, 21-50
interpreting retinal pathologies in, 37-46
longitudinal evaluation of, 602-604
with low signal to noise, 50
for macular degenerations with choroidal neovascularization, 345-369
of macular holes, 79-81, 86-87, 91-92, 93, 94-95, 96-98, 99-101
in neuro-ophthalmology, 611-660
for nonproliferative diabetic retinopathy and macular edema, 159-185
optical properties of tissues in, 21-22
physical principles of, 677-687
precursor technology of, 663
principles and clinical impact of, 3-5
for proliferative diabetic retinopathy, 186-213, 203-208, 209-213
protocols for, 691-698
quality, artifacts, and errors in images of, 46-50
for retinal angiomatous proliferation, 312-329
for retinal arterial macroaneurysm, 148-154
for retinal dystrophies, 416-454
scanning and imaging protocols of, 28-31
supporting early visual field abnormalities, 517-520
versus ultrasound imaging, 6-8
visual field defects and, 535-538

for vitreomacular traction and epiretinal membrane, 75-77
optical disc protocol, 692
optical interferometry, 679-680
output intensity, 680

pachymetry, 514
high-frequency ultrasound, 665
panuveitis, multifocal choroiditis with, 379-380
papilledema, 611
follow-up for, 623-624
hypotony with, 631-632
mild, 621-624
moderate, 625-626
severe, 627-628
with subretinal fluid, 629-630
papillitis, 642
papillomacular axis, 22-24
papillophlebitis, 645
parallel raster scans, 245
pars plana vitrectomy
closing full-thickness macular hole, 94
persistent subfoveal fluid after, 467-468
for retinal vein occlusion, 104
pattern dystrophy, 414, 452-453
penicillin, 405, 407-408
perifoveal leakage, 104
perifoveal vitreous detachment, 86
perimetry, 572-574
peripapillary region
circular tomogram in, 26-27
radial optical cohesion tomographic section through, 32
peripheral visual loss, 413
photodetector, 679-680
photodynamic therapy
acute vision loss after, 307-309
for age-related macular degeneration
follow-up after, 293-294, 297-309
follow-up optical coherence tomography after, 275-278, 281-288
for angioid streaks with choroidal neovascularization, 359
for central serous chorioretinopathy, 216, 237-240
for choroidal neovascularization, 346, 351
for idiopathic choroidal neovascularization, 363
with intravitreal triamcinolone injection, 326-329
monitoring after, 277-278
for pathologic myopia with choroidal neovascularization, 353
for presumed ocular histoplasmosis, 369
subretinal hemorrhage after, 291-292
for toxoplasmosis with subretinal neovascularization, 403-404
verteporfin, 243
photonics communications technology, 9-10
photoreceptor cell loss, 413
photoreceptor layer, 25
in age-related macular degeneration, 250
bilateral degeneration of, 478
degeneration of, 48
discontinuity of in Best's disease, 450, 451
imaging of, 24
increased reflectivity from, 42
loss of, 257
partial, 432-433
in pattern dystrophy, 453
in Stargardt's disease, 440
partial disorganization of, 437
thinning of, 46
physical principles, 677-687
pigment epithelial defect, 224-225
in central serous chorioretinopathy, 226-228
pigment epithelial detachment (PED), 40-43
in central serous chorioretinopathy, 235
fibrovascular, 43, 260
occult choroidal neovascularization with, 260-261
ocular choroidal neovascularization with, 269-270
hyperfluorescent, 226-227
with minimally classic choroidal neovascularization, 271-272
serous, 220, 244
vascularized, 310-311
pigment metaplasia stellate pigment plaques, 140-142
pigment migration, intraretinal, 146
pigmentary mottling
with angioid streaks, 357, 358
in central serous chorioretinopathy with choroidal neovascularization, 364
with presumed ocular histoplasmosis, 369
in subretinal hemorrhage with choroidal neovascularization, 361
in Vogt-Koyanagi-Harada disease, 389
pixels, 14
density of, 28-29, 683-685
versus image acquisition speed, 30
placido-ring corneal topography, 665
point spread function, 13
posterior segment
ocular structures of, 483-484
trauma to, 458
prednisone, 397-399
preretinal fibrosis, 471
proportional circle protocol, 692
prostaglandin analog, 463-464
pseudo-Foster-Kennedy syndrome, 638-639
pseudoexfoliation
in absence of glaucoma, 600-601
in glaucoma, 572, 579-582

pseudohole, 62, 63
pseudohypopyon lesion, 451

quantitative measurement
  for idiopathic epiretinal membrane, 58
  of retinal morphology, 32-37
quantitative morphometry, 24-26

radial lines protocol, 691
raster lines protocol, 691
reference beam, 679-680, 681
refraction, index of, 10
resolution imaging, low-transverse, 684
retina
  abnormalities of, 38
  atrophy of, 37, 46
    degenerative diseases producing, 48
  boundaries of, 33
  central thickness of, 65
  characteristic features of, 30
  computer image-processing of, 36
  cross-sectional imaging o f, 5
  cystic changes of in papillomacular bundle area, 473
  dehiscence of inner layers of, 87
  diseases of, 457-479
  early OCT image of, 4
  glaucomatous damage to, 510
  gray-scale and false-color displays of, 12
  hemorrhage of, 40-43
  image resolution for, 13-14
  increased reflectivity of, 110
  interpreting normal OCT images of, 22-27
  irregularities of in Vogt-Koyanagi-Harada disease, 388
  layers of, 32
  microstructure of, 24
  morphology of, 25, 32-37
  OCT instrumentation for, 15-17
  pathology of
    general features associated with, 38
    interpreting optical coherence tomography images of, 37-46
  reflectivity of, 103
  thickening of with papillitis, 642
  thickness measurement of, 33, 38, 67
  thickness of, 694
    analysis of, 695
  topographic mapping and analysis of, 33-35
  traction on, 58
retinal angiomatous proliferation (RAP)
  in age-related macular degeneration, 244-245, 312-315, 318-319
  follow-up in, 320-329
  with minimally classic choroidal neovascularization, 271-272
  progression of, 316-318
retinal artery
  macroaneurysms of, 105, 148-154
  occlusion of
    branch (BRAO), 103, 106-109
    central (CRAO), 103-104, 110
retinal detachment
  repair of, 457
    persistent subfoveal fluid after, 467-468
  tractional, with proliferative diabetic retinopathy, 209-213
retinal dystrophy
  clinical evaluation of, 416-454
  diagnosis of, 413
  disorders associated with, 413-414
retinal ganglion cells, 484
retinal lesion anastomoses, 244-245
retinal map analysis, 694, 696
  for acute sympathetic ophthalmia, 391-392
  for birdshot chorioretinopathy, 396
  for central retinal vein occlusion, 131-132
  of cystoid macular edema, 373-374
  for nonproliferative diabetic retinopathy, 166-167, 168
  for proliferative diabetic retinopathy, 186-187, 191-193
  for retinitis pigmentosa, 416-417
  for rod-cone dystrophy, 430-432
  for Stargardt's disease, 440-441, 444-445
  for syphilitic uveitis, 407-408
  for toxoplasmic chorioretinitis, 397-398, 399-400
  in Vogt-Koyanagi-Harada disease, 386-387
retinal nerve fiber layer
  thickness analysis of, 35-37
  thickness protocol for, 692
  visualization of, 3
retinal nerve fiber layer (RNFL)
  map protocol, 692
  thickness analysis of, 692, 696
  thickness analysis protocol of, 694
  thickness average analysis protocol of, 694, 697
  thickness change protocol of, 697
  thickness map analysis of, 697
  thickness serial analysis protocol of, 697
retinal pigment epithelium/Bruch's/choriocapillaris complex, 244, 245
  in age-related macular degeneration, 249, 251, 252, 254
  with geographic atrophy, 257, 259
retinal pigment epithelium/choriocapillaris complex, 103-104, 413
    reflections from, 105
retinal pigment epithelium (RPE), 25. *See also* pigment epithelial detachment (PED)
  abnormalities of, 345
  atrophic patches of, 416
  atrophy of

with choroidal neovascularization, 305
in rod-cone dystrophy, 428, 430
in Stargardt's disease, 436, 438, 442
detached, 38
detachment of, 228, 236
in age-related macular degeneration, 245
in central serous chorioretinopathy, 229
drusenoid, 250
with posterior segment trauma, 458
serous, 221
focal leaks at, 215
identifying, 23
imaging of, 24
loss of, 422-423
loss of retinal tissue in, 58
optical coherence tomography of, 44-46
signal irregularities of, 222
tears in
in age-related macular degeneration, 244, 330-335
formation of, 334-335
occult choroidal neovascularization with, 332-333
window defects in, 160
retinal pigment hyperplasia plaques, 104
retinal probability map, 694
retinal schisis, 96
retinal serous detachment, 658
retinal thickness image-processing techniques, 35
retinal thickness map, 694
for postoperative cystoid macular edema, 461-462
retinal thickness/volume analysis, 694
retinal thickness/volume tabular output, 694, 695
retinal vascular diseases. *See also* specific diseases
in central visual loss, 103
optical coherence tomograms of, 106-154
types of, 103-105
retinal vasculitis, idiopathic, 376-378
retinal vein
occlusion of
branch (BRVO), 104, 111-124
central (CRVO), 104, 125-139
retinal dystrophies and, 413
sclerotic, 123
retinal vessels, 26-27
retinitis pigmentosa, 46, 48, 413
clinical studies of, 416-423
retinitis punctata albescens, 424-427
retinopathy, cancer-associated, 478-479
retinoschisis, 457
rhegmatogenous retinal detachment, 457, 465-466
rod-cone dystrophy, 428-435

sarcoidosis, with choroidal granulomas, 383-385
scan pattern, 14-15
scanning laser biomicroscopy (SLB), 483-484
scanning laser polarimetry (SLP), 483
scanning reference mirror, 681-682
Scheimpflug photography, 668-669
sclera, 28
sclerotic retinal vessels, 207
scotoma, central, 215
segmentation, 32, 33
sensitivity, 681-682
serial radial tomogram, 30-32
serial raster scans, 30
short-pulse laser light sources, 686
signal beam, 679-680
signal-to-noise performance, 684
signal-to-noise ratio (SNR), 682
single circle protocol, 692
slit-lamp biomicroscope, 17, 686
slit-lamp biomicroscopy, 686
for bilateral idiopathic juxtafoveal retinal telangiectasis, 140
for branch retinal vein occlusion, 111
for idiopathic epiretinal membrane, 57
for retinal arterial macroaneurysm, 153
slit-lamp-mounted high-speed OCT system, 668, 671
slit-lamp-mounted scanner, 667
slit-scanning topography, 665
sound scales, 8
spatial resolution, 682-683
spectroscopic OCT, 686
Stargardt's disease, 414
clinical studies of, 436-445
Stargardt's dystrophy, 46, 48
subfoveal fluid, persistent, 467-468
subhyaloid hemorrhage, 470
submacular hemorrhage, 469
subretinal fibrosis
in age-related macular degeneration, 244
multifocal choroiditis with, 381-382
in subretinal hemorrhage with choroidal neovascularization, 361
subretinal neovascularization
in Best's disease, 446, 447
toxoplasmosis with, 401-402
photodynamic therapy for, 403-404
sulfadiazine, 397-399
surgical anatomy, 670-671
Swedish interactive thresholding algorithm (SITA), 500
syphilitic uveitis, 405-406
treatment of, 407-408

telangiectatic retinal veins, 127
telangiectatic vessels, juxtafoveal, 365-366
three-dimensional imaging, 663
time-efficient scan, 692
timolol, 510, 551, 553, 562, 572

timolol gel, 504
timolol maleate, 465
TISA-750, 668-669
tissue
  index of refraction of, 10
  optical properties of, 21-22
  optical reflection and scattering properties of, 13
tomogram
  circular, in peripapillary region, 26-27
  serial horizontal of normal macula, 31
topographic mapping
  for age-related macular degeneration, 245
  of retinal thickness, 35-37
toxic optic neuropathy, 611, 617-620
toxoplasmic chorioretinitis, 371, 397-398
  treatment of, 399-400
toxoplasmosis
  with subretinal neovascularization, 401-402
    photodynamic therapy for, 403-404
trabeculectomy
  for advanced open-angle glaucoma, 587
  cataract extraction and, 602-604
  with mitomycin C, 541
  for open-angle glaucoma, 575, 592, 596
  for pseudoexfoliation glaucoma, 579
  surgical anatomy for, 670-671
trabeculo-iris space area (TISA), 668
tractional retinal detachment, 209-213
transverse pixel density, 685
transverse resolution, 13-14, 682, 683
trauma, posterior segment, 458
travoprost, 559
triamcinolone acetonide injection
  for branch retinal vein occlusion, 111, 113, 115, 119
  for central retinal vein occlusion, 129, 131, 133, 136
  intravitreal
    follow-up after, 322-329
    for pathologic myopia, 355
  for nonproliferative diabetic retinopathy, 175, 178, 183
  in nonproliferative diabetic retinopathy, 168
  with photodynamic therapy, 326-329
  for postoperative cystoid macular edema, 461-462
  for proliferative diabetic retinopathy, 188, 194, 199
  for retinal vein occlusion, 104
tumor, optic nerve, 613
type A personality, 215

UBM photography, 668-669, 671
ultrahigh-resolution OCT imaging, 686-687
ultrasound, 3, 677
  gray-scale display in, 11-13
  high-frequency imaging of, 6-7
  versus optical tomography, 6-8
uveitis
  classification of, 371
  complications of, 371
  with cystoid macular edema, 373-375
  syphilitic, 405-408

valsalva retinopathy, 470
vascular disease, retinal, 103-154
ventriculoperitoneal shunt, 627
vignetting, 46-47, 49
vision loss
  acute, 307-308, 309
  central, 413
  peripheral, 413
visual acuity
  best-corrected (BCVA), 217, 218, 233
    in cystoid macular edema, 373
  central, decreased and distorted, 215-216
  in epiretinal membrane with pseudohole, 63
  poor central, 222
visual field
  abnormalities of
    in advanced glaucoma, 508-509
    early, in glaucoma, 517-520
    nerve fiber layer thinning and, 579
    structural imaging suggesting in glaucoma, 541-544
  in advanced glaucoma, 504-507
  central island remaining, in advanced glaucoma, 510-513
visual field defects
  as artifact, 535-538
  early
    nerve fiber layer and neuroretinal rim loss in, 529-530
    superior, 523-526, 527-528
  fluctuating, in absence of glaucoma, 600-601
  inferior, structural measures of in glaucoma, 545-546
  nerve fiber layer loss prior to, 602-604
visual field loss
  central, 611
  in compressive optic neuropathy, 614
  in glaucoma, 484, 514
  inferior
    as artifact, 539-540
    superior structural abnormalities presaging, 596-597
  with mild optic disc drusen, 649
  nerve fiber layer, macular, and optic nerve head scanning corresponding with, 531-534
  nerve fiber layer and macular thinning with, 557-558
  nerve fiber layer loss paralleling, 608-609
  nerve fiber layer thinning and, 583-586
  nerve fiber layer thinning in advanced glaucoma corresponding with, 587-588
  on one side of horizontal meridian, 521-522
  progressive nerve fiber layer loss with, 605-607

retinal nerve fiber layer, macular, and optic nerve head abnormalities corresponding with, 562-565
with severe optic disc drusen, 651
structural damage as sign of, 592-595
visual field testing
in advanced pseudoexfoliation glaucoma, 551-552
in anterior ischemic optic neuropathy, 639
corresponding with optical coherence tomography and Heidelberg retina tomography, 559-561
corresponding with visual field defects in glaucoma, 535-538
in glaucoma, 483, 517-520
Humphrey, 488, 496, 510, 521
in juvenile diabetic papillopathy, 640-641
nerve fiber layer and macular findings and, 575-578
nerve fiber layer assessment and, 566-567
nerve fiber layer loss in, 602-604
in open-angle glaucoma, 492
in open angle without glaucoma, 598-599
vitelliform lesion, 450
vitelliform macular lesion, 252-255
vitrectomy surgery
closing full-thickness macular hole, 94-95
improved macular edema after, 71-72
for stage 1B macular hole, 84-85
for vitreomacular traction and epiretinal membrane, 75-77
vitreomacular traction, 37
detection of, 371
diabetic, 157
with macular edema, 74
spontaneous resolution of, 81
vitrectomy surgery for, 75-77
vitreomacular traction syndrome, 58
retinal dystrophies and, 413
vitreopapillary traction, 644
vitreoretinal adhesions, 157
vitreoretinal attachments, perifoveal, 256
vitreoretinal interface, 41
abnormalities of, 40
disorders of, 57-101
identification of, 23-24
vitreous abnormalities, 40
vitreous detachment, 41
posterior, 91
Vogt-Koyanagi-Harada disease, 386-388
response to corticosteroid treatment for, 389-390
retinal pattern in, 391-392

x-line protocol, 692
X-linked juvenile retinoschisis, 414, 454
X-ray study, 30